PRIMER
ON
KIDNEY
DISEASES

PRIMER ON KIDNEY DISEASES

FOURTH EDITION

EDITOR

Arthur Greenberg, MD

Division of Nephrology
Department of Medicine
Duke University Medical Center
Durham, North Carolina

ASSOCIATE EDITORS

Alfred K. Cheung, MD

Division of Nephrology and Hypertension
University of Utah
Veterans Affairs Salt Lake City Healthcare System
Salt Lake City, Utah

Thomas M. Coffman, MD

Division of Nephrology
Department of Medicine
Duke University Medical Center
Durham, North Carolina

Ronald J. Falk, MD

Division of Nephrology and Hypertension
Department of Medicine
University of North Carolina
Chapel Hill, North Carolina

J. Charles Jennette, MD

Department of Pathology and Laboratory Medicine
University of North Carolina
Chapel Hill, North Carolina

National Kidney Foundation™

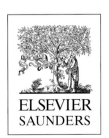

ELSEVIER
SAUNDERS

SAUNDERS
An Imprint of Elsevier

The Curtis Center
170 S Independence Mail W 300E
Philadelphia, Pennsylvania 19106

PRIMER ON KIDNEY DISEASES
Copyright © 2005, by National Kidney Foundation. All rights reserved.

NOTICE

Knowledge and best practice in this field are constantly changing. As new research and experience broaden our knowledge, changes in practice, treatment, and drug therapy may become necessary or appropriate. Readers are advised to check the most current information provided (i) on procedures featured or (ii) by the manufacturer of each product to be administered, to verify the recommended dose or formula, the method and duration of administration, and contraindications. It is the responsibility of the practitioner, relying on their own experience and knowledge of the patient, to make diagnoses, to determine dosages and the best treatment for each individual patient, and to take all appropriate safety precautions. To the fullest extent of the law, neither the Publisher, the National Kidney Foundation, nor the Editors assume any liability for any injury and/or damage to persons or property arising out or related to any use of the material contained in this book.

Previous editions copyrighted 2001, 1998, 1994

ISBN-13: 978–1–4160–2312–8
ISBN-10: 0–1–4160–2312–7

Publishing Director: Susan Pioli
Developmental Editor: Cathy Carroll

Printed in China

Last digit is the print number: 9   8   7   6   5   4   3   2

Contributors

Sharon Adler, MD
Associate Chief; Director, Outpatient Dialysis, Division of Nephrology and Hypertension, Harbor–UCLA Medical Center; Harbor–UCLA Research and Education Institute, Torrance, CA

Michael Allon, MD
Professor of Medicine, University of Alabama–Birmingham, Birmingham, AL

Sharon Anderson, MD
Professor of Medicine, Division of Nephrology and Hypertension, Oregon Health and Science University, Portland, OR

Gerald B. Appel, MD
Professor of Clinical Medicine, College of Physicians and Surgeons, Columbia University; Director of Clinical Nephrology, Columbia University Medical Center, New York, NY

Billy S. Arant, Jr., MD
Professor of Pediatrics, University of Tennessee College of Medicine; Medical Director, Hypertension Management Center, Erlanger Health System, Chattanooga, TN

Vicente Arroyo, MD
Professor of Medicine and Director of Institute of Digestive and Metabolic Diseases, Hospital Clinic, University of Barcelona, Barcelona, SPAIN

Arshad Asghar, MD
Staff Physician, Department of General Medicine, St. Anthony Memorial Hospital, Michigan City, IN

Phyllis August, MD
Professor, Department of Medicine, Weill Medical College of Cornell University, New York, NY

George L. Bakris, MD
Professor, Preventive and Internal Medicine, Rush University Medical Center, Chicago, IL

Jeffrey S. Berns, MD
Associate Professor, Renal Electrolyte and Hypertension Division, University of Pennsylvania, Philadelphia, PA

Gregory L. Braden, MD
Associate Professor, Department of Medicine, Tufts University School of Medicine, Boston; Chief, Renal Division, Baystate Medical Center, Springfield, MA

Josephine P. Briggs, MD
Director, KUH Division, NIDDK, National Institutes of Health, Bethesda, MD

David A. Bushinsky, MD
Professor of Medicine and Pharmacology and Physiology, University of Rochester School of Medicine and Dentistry; Chief, Nephrology Unit, Strong Memorial Hospital, Rochester, NY

M. Luiza Caramori, MD, PhD
Associate Professor, Endocrine Division, Universidade Federal do Rio Grande do Sul, Porto Alegre, RS, BRAZIL

Daniel C. Cattran, MD
Professor of Medicine, Division of Nephrology, University of Toronto; Nephrologist, Toronto General Hospital, Toronto, Ontario, CANADA

Arlene B. Chapman, MD
Professor of Medicine, Renal Division, Emory University School of Medicine, Atlanta, GA

Glenn M. Chertow, MD
Associate Professor, Department of Medicine, Division of Nephrology, University of California–San Francisco, San Francisco, CA

Alfred K. Cheung, MD
Professor of Medicine, Division of Nephrology and Hypertension, University of Utah; Staff Physician, Veterans Affairs Salt Lake City Healthcare System, Salt Lake City, UT

Kerry C. Cho, MD
Clinical Instructor, Department of Medicine, Division of Nephrology, University of California–San Francisco, San Francisco, CA

Thomas M. Coffman, MD
Professor of Medicine, Program Director, Nephrology Training Program, Division of Nephrology, Duke University Medical Center; VA Medical Center, Durham, NC

Peter J. Conlon, MBBS
Department of Nephrology and Renal Transplant Medicine, Beaumont Hospital, Dublin, IRELAND

R. John Crew, MD
Clinical Instructor, Division of Nephrology, College of Physicians and Surgeons, Columbia University, New York, NY

Gary Curhan, MD, ScD
Associate Professor of Medicine, Harvard Medical School; Associate Professor of Epidemiology, Harvard School of Public Health; Assistant Physician, Renal Unit and General Medicine Unit, Massachusetts General Hospital, Boston, MA

Giuseppe D'Amico, MD
Professor, Head Emeritus, Division of Nephrology, San Carlo Borromeo Hospital, Milan, ITALY

Mary Anne Dooley, MD
Associate Professor of Medicine, University of North Carolina–Chapel Hill, Chapel Hill, NC

Thomas D. DuBose, Jr., MD
Professor and Chair, Department of Internal Medicine, Professor, Physiology and Pharmacology; Chief of Internal Medicine Service, North Carolina Baptist Hospital, Winston-Salem, NC

Garabed Eknoyan, MD
Professor of Medicine, Renal Section, Department of Medicine, Baylor College of Medicine, Houston, TX

David H. Ellison, MD
Head, Division of Nephrology and Hypertension, Oregon Health and Science University, Portland, OR

Jonathan T. Fairbank, MD
Professor, University of Vermont, Department of Radiology, Fletcher Allen Health Care, Burlington, VT

Ronald J. Falk, MD
Chief, Division of Nephrology and Hypertension, University of North Carolina–Chapel Hill, Chapel Hill, NC

Robert N. Foley, MD
Chronic Disease Research Group and United States Renal Data System; Associate Professor of Medicine, University of Minnesota, Minneapolis, MN

Richard N. Formica, Jr., MD
Assistant Professor, Department of Medicine, Director of Transplantation Nephrology, Yale University School of Medicine, New Haven, CT

Alessandro Fornasieri, MD
Medical Consultant, Division on Nephrology, San Carlo Borromeo Hospital, Milan, ITALY

Ali Gharavi, MD
Assistant Professor of Medicine, College of Physicians and Surgeons, Columbia University, New York, NY

Richard J. Glassock, MD
Professor Emeritus, The David Geffen School of Medicine, Los Angeles, CA

Ram Gokal, MD
Consultant Nephrologist, Manchester Royal Infirmary; Professor of Medicine, University of Manchester, Manchester, UNITED KINGDOM

Martin Goldberg, MD
Professor Emeritus, Department of Medicine (Nephrology), Temple University School of Medicine, Philadelphia, PA

R. Ariel Gomez, MD
Vice President for Research and Graduate Studies, Office of Research and Graduate Studies, Professor of Biology and Pediatrics, University of Virginia, Charlottesville, VA

Arthur Greenberg, MD
Clinical Professor of Medicine, Division of Nephrology, Department of Medicine, Duke University Medical Center, Durham, NC

Martin C. Gregory, BM, BCh, D.Phil
Professor of Medicine, University of Utah/HSC, Salt Lake City, UT

Antonio Guasch, MD
Associate Professor of Medicine, Renal Division, Emory University, Atlanta, GA

Christlieb Haller, Dr. med
Chief, Department of Cardiology, Hegau Klinik, Singen/Hohentwiel, GERMANY

William L. Henrich, MD
Professor and Chair, Department of Medicine, University of Maryland School of Medicine; Physician-in-Chief, University of Maryland Medical Center, Baltimore, MD

Timothy J. Higgins, MD
Radiology Resident, Department of Radiology, Fletcher Allen Health Care, Burlington, VT

Friedhelm Hildebrandt, MD
Professor of Pediatrics and Human Genetics, Frederick
G. L. Huetwell Professor for the Cure and Prevention of
Birth Defects, Department of Pediatrics, University of
Michigan, Ann Arbor, MI

Jonathan Himmelfarb, MD
Director, Division of Nephrology and Transplantation,
Maine Medical Center, Portland, ME

Jean L. Holley, MD
Professor of Medicine, Division of Nephrology,
Department of Medicine, University of Virginia Health
Systems, Charlottesville, VA

Chi-yuan Hsu, MD, MSc
Assistant Professor in Residence, Division of
Nephrology, University of California–San Francisco, San
Francisco, CA

Alastair J. Hutchison, MD, FRCP
Clinical Director of Renal Medicine, Manchester
Institute of Nephrology and Transplantation, The Royal
Infirmary, Manchester, UNITED KINGDOM

T. Alp Ikizler, MD
Associate Professor of Medicine, Vanderbilt University
Medical Center, Nashville, TN

J. Charles Jennette, MD
Brinkhous Distinguished Professor and Chair,
Department of Pathology and Laboratory Medicine,
University of North Carolina, Chapel Hill, NC

Wladimiro Jiménez, PhD
Laboratorio de Hormonas, Centre de Diagnostic
Biomedic, Barcelona, SPAIN

Bruce A. Julian, MD
Professor, Division of Nephrology, Department of
Medicine, University of Alabama–Birmingham,
Birmingham, AL

Bertram L. Kasiske, MD, FACP
Director of Nephrology, Hennepin County
Medical Center; Professor of Medicine, University
of Minnesota College of Medicine,
Minneapolis, MN

Paul E. Klotman, MD
Murray Rosenberg Professor of Medicine; Chair, Samuel
F. Bronfman Department of Medicine, The Mount Sinai
Medical Center, New York, NY

Stephen M. Korbet, MD
Professor of Medicine, Rush University Medical
Center; Rush Presbyterian–St. Luke's Medical Center,
Chicago, IL

Eugene C. Kovalik, MD, CM, FRCP(C), FACP
Associate Professor of Medicine, Division of Nephrology,
Department of Medicine, Duke University Medical
Center, Durham, NC

Wilhelm Kriz, MD
Institute of Anatomy and Cell Biology, University of
Heidelberg, Heidelberg, GERMANY

Fadi G. Lakkis, MD
Associate Professor of Medicine and Immunobiology,
Director of Transplant Medicine, Department of
Medicine, Section of Nephrology, Yale University School
of Medicine, New Haven, CT

Brent Lee Lechner, DO
Major, Medical Corps, US Army; Postdoctoral Fellow,
Department of Pediatrics, Yale University School of
Medicine, New Haven, CT

Andrew S. Levey, MD
Gerald J. and Dorothy R. Friedman Professor of
Medicine, Tufts University School of Medicine; Chief,
William B. Schwartz, MD Division of Nephrology,
Tufts–New England Medical Center, Boston, MA

Nicolaos E. Madias, MD
Professor of Medicine, Tufts University School of
Medicine; Chair, Department of Medicine, Caritas St.
Elizabeth's Medical Center, Boston, MA

Colin Mason, MB, MRCPI
Department of Nephrology and Transplantation,
Beaumont Hospital, Dublin, IRELAND

Gary R. Matzke, Pharm.D, FCP, FCCP
Professor, Pharmacy and Therapeutics, University of
Pittsburgh School of Pharmacy, Pittsburgh, PA

Michael Mauer, MD
Professor and Co-Director, Department of Pediatric
Nephrology, University of Minnesota, Minneapolis, MN

Tracy A. McGowan, MD
Assistant Professor of Medicine, Division of Nephrology,
Thomas Jefferson University Hospital, Philadelphia, PA

Catherine M. Meyers, MD
Director, Inflammatory Renal Disease Program, Kidney,
Urologic, and Hematologic Diseases Division, National
Institute of Diabetes, Digestive, and Kidney Diseases,
National Institutes of Health; Medical Staff
Nephrologist, NIDDK/Warren G. Magnuson Clinical
Center, Bethesda, MD

Alain Meyrier, MD
Professor of Medicine, Hospital Broussais-Georges
Pompidou, University of Paris, Paris, FRANCE

Howard J. Mindell, MD (deceased)
Department of Radiology, Fletcher Allen Health Care,
Burlington, VT

Marianne Monahan, MD
Instructor, Mt. Sinai School of Medicine, Division of
Nephrology, New York, NY

Narayana S. Murali, MD
Fellow in Nephrology, Mayo Clinic, Rochester, MN

Patrick H. Nachman, MD
Associate Professor of Medicine, Division of Nephrology
and Hypertension, University of North Carolina–Chapel
Hill, Chapel Hill, NC

Cynthia C. Nast, MD
Professor of Pathology, David Geffen School of Medicine
at UCLA; Attending Pathologist, Cedars-Sinai Medical
Center, Los Angeles, CA

Karl A. Nath, MD
Professor of Medicine, Department of Internal Medicine,
Mayo Clinic College of Medicine, Rochester, MN

Lindsay E. Nicolle, MD, FRCPC
Professor of Internal Medicine and Medical
Mircrobiology, University of Manitoba, Winnipeg,
Manitoba, CANADA

Victoria F. Norwood, MD
Associate Professor, Department of Pediatrics; Chief,
Pediatric Nephrology, University of Virginia Children's
Hospital, Charlottesville, VA

Akinlolu O. Ojo, MB, BS, MPH, PhD
Associate Professor of Internal Medicine, University of
Michigan, Ann Arbor, MI

John F. O'Toole, MD
Lecturer, Division of Nephrology, Department of
Internal Medicine, University of Michigan,
Ann Arbor, MI

Paul M. Palevsky, MD
Professor of Medicine, Renal–Electrolyte Division,
University of Pittsburgh; Chief, Renal Section, VA
Pittsburgh Healthcare System, Pittsburgh, PA

Biff F. Palmer, MD
Professor, Department of Internal Medicine, Division of
Nephrology, University of Texas Southwestern Medical
Center, Dallas, TX

Patrick S. Parfrey, MD
University Research Professor, Division of
Nephrology, The Health Sciences Center, University
of Newfoundland, St. John's, Newfoundland,
CANADA

Roberto Pisoni, MD
Clinical Research Center for Rare Diseases, Aldo e Cele
Dacco, Ranica, Bergamo, ITALY

Charles D. Pusey, MSc, FRCP, FRCPath
Professor of Medicine, Renal Section, Division of
Medicine, Imperial College, London, UNITED
KINGDOM

L. Darryl Quarles, MD
Summerfield Endowed Professor of Nephrology, Vice
Chair of Internal Medicine, Director, The Kidney
Institute and Division of Nephrology, University of
Kansas Medical Center, Kansas City, KS

Giuseppe Remuzzi, MD
Negri Bergamo Laboratories, Bergamo, ITALY

Eberhard Ritz, MD
Department of Internal Medicine, Nierenzentrum
Ruperto-Carola-University Heidelberg, Heidelberg,
GERMANY

Dana Rizk, MD
Clinical Instructor, Atlanta Veterans Affairs Medical
Center, Emory University School of Medicine,
Atlanta, GA

Robert L. Safirstein, MD
Professor and Executive Vice Chair, Internal Medicine,
University of Arkansas for Medical Sciences; Chief,
Medicine Science, Central Arkansas Veterans Healthcare
System, Little Rock, AR

Paul W. Sanders, MD
Professor of Medicine, Departments of Medicine and
Physiology and Biophysics, Division of Nephrology,
University of Alabama–Birmingham; Chief, Renal
Section, Department of Veterans Affairs Medical
Center, Veterans Affairs Medical Center
Birmingham, AL

Steven J. Scheinman, MD
Professor of Medicine and Pharmacology; Dean, College
of Medicine; Executive Vice President, SUNY Upstate
Medical University, Syracuse, NY

Arrigo Schieppati, MD
Division of Nephrology and Dialysis, Azienda
Ospedaliera Ospedali Riuniti di Bergamo; Clinical
Research Center for Rare Diseases, Aldo e Cele Dacco,
Ranica, Bergamo, ITALY

Jurgen B. Schnermann, MD
Senior Investigator, Branch Chief, Kidney Diseases
Branch, National Institute of Diabetes, Digestive, and
Kidney Diseases, National Institutes of Health,
Bethesda, MD

Norman J. Siegel, MD
Professor of Pediatrics and Medicine, Director, Section of
Pediatric Nephrology, Yale University School of
Medicine; Attending, Department of Pediatrics, Yale
New Haven's Children's Hospital, New Haven, CT

F. Bruder Stapleton, MD
Pediatrician-in-Chief, Children's Hospital and Regional
Medical Center, Seattle, WA

Lesley A. Stevens, MD, FRCPC
Assistant Professor of Medicine, Division of Nephrology,
Tufts–New England Medical Center, Boston, MA

Harold M. Szerlip, MD
Professor and Vice Chair, Department of Medicine,
Medical College of Georgia, Augusta, GA

Nadine DeLove Tanenbaum, MD
Fellow in Nephrology, Division of Nephrology,
Department of Medicine, Duke University Medical
Center, Durham, NC

Carlos Terra, MD
Research Fellow, Liver Unit, Department of
Medicine, University of Barcelona Medical School;
Institute of Digestive Diseases Hospital, Barcelona,
SPAIN

Joseph G. Verbalis, MD
Professor of Medicine and Physiology, Interim Chair,
Department of Medicine; Director, General Clinical
Research Center, Georgetown University Medical Center;
Physician-in-Chief, Georgetown University Hospital,
Washington, DC

William L. Whittier, MD
Assistant Professor of Medicine, Department of
Medicine, Division of Nephrology, Rush University
Medical Center, Chicago, IL

Christopher S. Wilcox, MD, PhD
Chief, Division of Nephrology, Georgetown University
Medical Center, Washington, DC

Franklin E. Yuan, MD
Resident, Department of Internal Medicine, Oregon
Health and Sciences University, Portland, OR

Martin Zeier, MD
Department of Internal Medicine, Nierenzentrum
Ruperto-Carola-University, of Heidelberg, Heidelberg,
GERMANY

Fuad N. Ziyadeh, MD
Professor of Medicine, Renal–Electrolyte Division,
University of Pennsylvania, Philadelphia, PA

Foreword

I am pleased to introduce the fourth edition of the National Kidney Foundation's *Primer on Kidney Diseases*. By all accounts, the *Primer* serves a very useful role. It provides a succinct yet comprehensive text for practicing physicians, house staff, and students. It is fair to say as well that consulting nephrologists will find some pearls of wisdom in its pages! House staff and students have enthusiastically embraced the *Primer* as an efficient and relatively easy way to understand many of the complex issues of nephrology, including acid base and fluid disorders and hypertension.

This fourth edition is noteworthy as the first to contain the new staging system and terminology established by the K/DOQI Chronic Kidney Disease Guidelines, published in 2002. The book continues to maintain its freshness, in part because nearly one third of the chapters are written by new authors. In dealing with the global nature of nephrology advances and expertise, many of the authors are from outside the United States.

Arthur Greenberg, as editor, continues to provide the vision and guiding spirit for the *Primer*. It is he, more than any other individual, who is responsible for the comprehensiveness, accuracy, and usefulness of this text. Dr. Greenberg has utilized a rigorous review process wherein each chapter was read by himself and an associate or consulting editor.

The ongoing contributions of the healthcare industry should also be acknowledged. The fact that several corporations have purchased large numbers of the *Primer* for distribution to house staff and students has played no small role in making the *Primer* readily available and in increasing its impact on the nephrologic skills of future medical practitioners and the medical care of patients everywhere with kidney disease.

DAVID G. WARNOCK, MD
President
National Kidney Foundation

Preface

The goal of this fourth edition of the *Primer* is the same as that of its predecessors: to be a comprehensive but accessible source of information on the pathophysiology and treatment of kidney diseases and electrolyte disorders. As in past editions, each chapter was written by a nationally or internationally recognized expert who was asked to present the essential features of the topic with clarity and cogency. New and returning authors alike have critically reviewed current developments to put them in perspective for the general audience of students, house officers, nephrology fellows, and practicing physicians who comprise the book's main readership.

A number of chapters have been consolidated and several new ones added. Reflecting the extraordinary growth in understanding of the heritable kidney disorders, a new chapter on the genetic basis of glomerular and structural kidney diseases now complements the one on genetically determined transport disorders introduced in the third edition. The section on hypertension has been reorganized with a new chapter devoted to diagnosis and management of secondary hypertension.

The most striking change in the *Primer* is its adoption of the NKF K/DOQI Clinical Practice Guidelines. This is most apparent in the section on Chronic Kidney Disease, which was renamed to reflect the new terminology and approach adopted by the 2002 K/DOQI Clinical Practice Guidelines for Evaluation, Classification, and Stratification of Chronic Kidney Disease. One chapter is devoted to these guidelines specifically. Throughout the book,

familiar but imprecise terms used in past editions, such as renal insufficiency and chronic renal failure, have been replaced by references to chronic kidney disease and its stages. Although DOQI guidelines originated in 1997, the first guidelines applied only to dialysis care and thus received limited attention in previous editions of the *Primer*. Guidelines introduced since the third edition address management issues of prime concern to generalists and are therefore an important part of this fourth edition. The full set of guidelines is available online (www.kdoqi.org), and in print in the *American Journal of Kidney Diseases* (see the Appendix for references and additional information about the NKF websites).

The other change apparent in this edition is its appearance: Color has been added to text headings and tables, and all of the line drawings have been redrawn in a uniform and harmonious style. This is a welcome upgrade. Cathy Carroll and Susan Pioli have done a superb job with production and with the transition to our new imprint of Saunders at Elsevier.

Throughout the production of this edition, the editors have tried to remember that the essence of a *Primer* is brevity. We are grateful to the authors for their efforts to distill the key facts into as small a package as possible. Once more, I am indebted to Alfred Cheung, Tom Coffman, Ron Falk, and Charles Jennette for their insights, hard work, and unstinting devotion to this project.

Contents

Structure and Function of the Kidneys and Their Clinical Assessment

CHAPTER 1

Overview of Kidney Function and Structure*

Josephine P. Briggs   Wilhelm Kriz   Jurgen B. Schnermann

BASIC CONCEPTS

Functions of the Kidney

The main functions of the kidneys can be categorized as follows:

1. Maintenance of body composition. The kidney regulates the volume of fluid in the body; its osmolarity, electrolyte content, and concentration; and its acidity. It achieves this regulation by variation in the amounts of water and ions excreted in the urine. Electrolytes regulated by changes in urinary excretion include sodium, potassium, chloride, calcium, magnesium, and phosphate.
2. Excretion of metabolic end products and foreign substances. The kidney excretes a number of products of metabolism, most notably urea, and a number of toxins and drugs.
3. Production and secretion of enzymes and hormones.
   a. Renin is an enzyme produced by the granular cells of the juxtaglomerular apparatus that catalyzes the formation of angiotensin from a plasma globulin, angiotensinogen. Angiotensin is a potent vasoconstrictor peptide and contributes importantly to salt balance and blood pressure regulation.
   b. Erythropoietin, a glycosylated, 165–amino acid protein produced by renal cortical interstitial cells, stimulates the maturation of erythrocytes in the bone marrow.
   c. 1,25-Dihydroxyvitamin D_3, the most active form of vitamin D_3, is formed by proximal tubule cells. This steroid hormone plays an important role in the regulation of body calcium and phosphate balance.

In later chapters of this *Primer*, the pathophysiologic mechanisms and consequences of derangements in kidney function are discussed in detail. This chapter reviews the basic anatomy of the kidney and the normal mechanisms for urine formation/glomerular filtration and tubular transport.

The Kidney and Homeostasis

Numerous functions of the body proceed optimally only when body fluid composition and volume are maintained within an appropriate range. For example,

- Cardiac output and blood pressure are dependent on optimum plasma volume.
- Most enzymes function best over rather narrow ranges of pH and ionic concentrations.
- Cell membrane potential depends on K^+ concentration.
- Membrane excitability depends on Ca^{2+} concentration.

The principal job of the kidneys is the correction of perturbations in the composition and volume of body fluids that occur as a consequence of food intake, metabolism, environmental factors, and exercise. Typically, in healthy people, such perturbations are corrected within a matter of hours so that, in the long term, body fluid volume and the concentration of most ions do not deviate much from normal set points. In many disease states, however, these regulatory processes are disturbed, resulting in persistent deviations in body fluid volumes or ionic concentrations. Understanding these disorders requires an understanding of the normal regulatory processes.

The Balance Concept

A central theme of physiology of the kidneys is understanding the mechanisms by which urine composition is altered to maintain the body in balance. The maintenance of stable body fluid composition requires that appearance and disappearance rates of any substance in the body balance each other. Balance is achieved when

$$\text{Ingested amount} + \text{produced amount}$$
$$= \text{excreted amount} + \text{consumed amount.}$$

For a large number of organic compounds, balance is the result of metabolic production and consumption. However, electrolytes are not produced or consumed by the body, balance is achieved by adjusting excretion to match intake. Therefore, when a person is in balance for sodium, potassium, and other ions, the amount excreted must equal the amount ingested. Because the kidneys are the principal organs where regulated excretion takes place, urinary excretion of such solutes closely follows the dietary intake.

---

*This chapter is in the public domain.

TABLE 1-1 Bedside Estimates of Body Fluid Compartment Volumes

Remember	Example for 60-kg Patient
Total body water = 60% × body weight	60% × 60 kg = 36 L
Intracellular water = 2/3 total body water	2/3 × 36 L = 24 L
Extracellular water = 1/3 total body water	1/3 × 36 L = 12 L
Plasma water = 1/4 extracellular water	1/4 × 12 L = 3 L
Plasma water	
Blood volume = $\dfrac{\text{Plasma water}}{1-\text{Hct}}$	3 L ÷ (1 − 0.40) = 6.6 L

Body Fluid Composition

To a large extent, humans are composed of water. Adipose tissue is low in water content; thus, in obese people, the fraction of body weight that is water is lower than that in lean individuals. As a consequence of slightly greater fat content, women contain less water on average than men, about 55% instead of 60%. Useful round numbers to remember for bedside estimates of body fluid volumes are given in Table 1-1. Typical values for the ionic composition of the intracellular and extracellular fluid compartments are given in Table 1-2.

KIDNEY STRUCTURE

The kidneys are two bean-shaped organs lying in the retroperitoneal space, each weighing about 150 g. The kidney is an anatomically complex organ, consisting of many different types of highly specialized cells, arranged in a highly organized three-dimensional pattern. The functional unit of the kidney is called a nephron (there are approximately 1 million nephrons in one human kidney); each nephron consists of a glomerulus and a long tubule, which is composed of a single layer of epithelial cells (the nephron is depicted schematically in Fig. 1-1). The nephron is segmented into distinct parts—proximal tubule, loop of Henle, distal tubule, collecting duct—each with a typical cellular appearance and special functional characteristics.

The nephrons are packed together tightly to make up the kidney parenchyma, which can be divided into

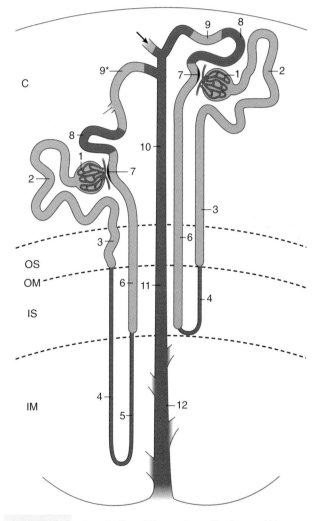

FIGURE 1-1 Organization of the nephron. The human kidney is made up of a million nephrons, two of which are shown schematically here. Each nephron consists of the following parts: glomerulus (1), proximal convoluted tubule (2), proximal straight tubule (3), thin descending limb of the loop of Henle (4), thin ascending limb (5), thick ascending limb (6), macula densa (7), distal convoluted tubule (8), and connecting tubule (9). Several nephrons coalesce to empty into a collecting duct, which has three distinct regions: the cortical collecting duct (10), the outer medullary collecting duct (11), and the inner medullary collecting duct (12). As shown, the deeper glomeruli give rise to nephrons with loops of Henle, which descend all the way to the papillary tips, while the more superficial glomeruli have loops of Henle that bend at the junction between the inner and outer medulla.

TABLE 1-2 Typical Ionic Composition of Plasma and Intracellular Fluid

	Plasma (mEq/L)	Intracellular Fluid (mEq/L)
Cations		
K⁺	4	150
Na⁺	143	12
Ca²⁺ (ionized)	2	0.001
Mg²⁺	1	28
Total cations	150 mEq/L	190 mEq/L
Anions		
Cl⁻	104	4
HCO₃⁻	24	10
Phosphates	2	40
Protein	14	50
Other	6	86
Total anions	150 mEq/L	190 mEq/L

regions. The outer layer of the kidney is called the cortex: it contains all the glomeruli, much of the proximal tubule, and some of the more distal portions as well. The inner section, called the medulla, consists largely of the parallel arrays of the loops of Henle and collecting ducts. The medulla is formed into cone-shaped regions, called pyramids (the human kidney typically has seven to nine), which extend into the renal pelvis. The tips of the medullary pyramids are called papillae. The medulla is important for concentration of the urine; the extracellular fluid in this region of the kidney has much higher solute concentration than plasma—as much as four times higher—with highest solute concentrations reached at the papillary tips.

The process of urine formation begins in the glomerular capillary tuft, where an ultrafiltrate of plasma is formed. The filtered fluid is collected in Bowman's capsule and enters the renal tubule to be carried over a circuitous course, successively modified by exposure to the sequence of specialized tubular epithelial segments with different transport functions. The proximal convoluted tubule, which is located entirely in the renal cortex, absorbs approximately two thirds of the glomerular filtrate. Fluid remaining at the end of the proximal convoluted tubule enters the loop of Henle, which dips down in a hairpin configuration into the medulla. Returning to the cortex, the tubular fluid passes close by its parent glomerulus at the juxtaglomerular apparatus, then enters

the distal convoluted tubule and finally the collecting duct, which courses back through the medulla, to empty into the renal pelvis at the tip of the renal papilla. Along the tubule, most of the glomerular filtrate is absorbed, but some additional substances are secreted. The final product, the urine, enters the renal pelvis and then the ureter, collects in the bladder, and is finally excreted from the body.

RENAL CIRCULATION

Anatomy of the Circulation

The renal artery, which enters the kidney at the renal hilum, carries about one fifth of the cardiac output; this represents the highest tissue-specific blood flow of all larger organs in the body (about 350 mL/min per 100 g tissue). As a consequence of this generous perfusion, the renal arteriovenous O_2 difference is much lower than that of most other tissues (and blood in the renal vein is noticeably redder in color than that in other veins). The renal artery bifurcates several times after it enters the kidney and then breaks into the arcuate arteries, which run, in an archlike fashion, along the border between the cortex and the outer medulla. As shown in Figure 1-2, the arcuate vessels give rise, typically at right angles, to interlobular arteries, which run to the surface of the kidney.

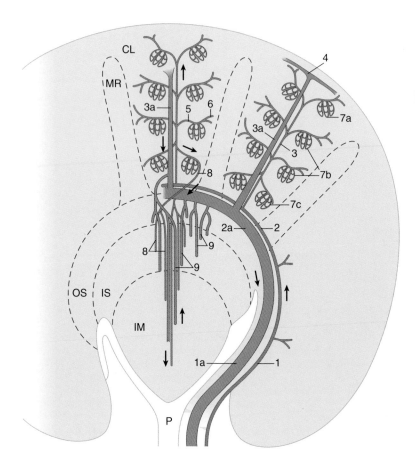

FIGURE 1-2 Organization of the renal vascular system. The renal artery bifurcates soon after entering the kidney parenchyma and gives rise to a system of arching vessels that run along the border between the cortex and the medulla. In this diagram, the vascular elements surrounding a single renal pyramid are shown. The human kidney typically has seven to nine renal pyramids. Here the arterial supply and glomeruli are shown in black, and the venous system is shown in gray. The peritubular capillary network that arises from the efferent arterioles is omitted for the sake of simplicity. The vascular elements are named as follows: interlobar artery and vein (1 and 1a), arcuate artery and vein (2 and 2a), interlobular artery and vein (3 and 3a), stellate vein (4), afferent arteriole (5), efferent arteriole (6), glomerular capillaries (7) (from superficial, 7a; midcortex, 7b; and juxtamedullary, 7c regions), juxtamedullary efferent arteriole, supplying descending vasa recti (8), and ascending vasa recti (9).

The afferent arterioles supplying the glomeruli come off the interlobular vessels.

Two Capillary Beds in Series

The renal circulation is unusual in that it breaks into two separate capillary beds: the glomerular bed and the peritubular capillary bed. These two capillary networks are arranged in series so that all the renal blood flow passes through both. As blood leaves the glomerulus, the capillaries coalesce into the efferent arteriole, but almost immediately the vessels bifurcate again to form the peritubular capillary network. This second network of capillaries is the site where the fluid reabsorbed by the tubules is returned to the circulation. Pressure in the first capillary bed, that of the glomerulus, is rather high (about 40 to 50 mm Hg), whereas pressure in the peritubular capillaries is similar to that in capillary beds elsewhere in the body (about 5 to 10 mm Hg).

About one fourth of the plasma that enters the glomerulus passes through the filtration barrier to become the glomerular filtrate. Blood cells, most of the proteins, and about 75% of the fluid and small solutes stay in the capillary and leave the glomerulus via the efferent arteriole. This postglomerular blood, which has a relatively high concentration of protein and red cells, enters the peritubular capillaries, where the high osmotic pressure from the high protein concentration facilitates the reabsorption of fluid. The peritubular capillaries coalesce to form venules and eventually the renal vein.

Medullary Blood Supply

The blood supplying the medulla is also postglomerular: specialized peritubular vessels, called vasa recta, arise from the efferent arterioles of the glomeruli nearest the medulla (the juxtamedullary glomeruli). Like medullary renal tubules, these vasa recta form hairpin loops dipping into the medulla.

GLOMERULUS

Structure

The structure of the glomerulus is shown schematically in Figure 1-3 and in a photomicrograph in Figure 1-4. The glomerulus is a ball consisting of capillaries, lined by endothelial cells, with the outside of the capillaries covered with specialized epithelial cells, called podocytes. These are large, highly differentiated cells that form an array of lacelike foot processes over the outer layer of these capillaries. An outer epithelial capsule, called Bowman's capsule, acts as a pouch to capture the filtrate and direct it into the beginning of the proximal tubule. As shown in Figures 1-3 and 1-4, the capillaries are held together by a stalk of cells, called the glomerular mesangium.

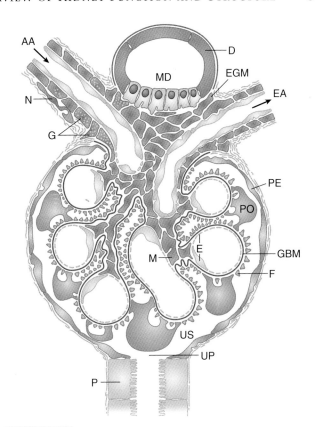

FIGURE 1-3 Schematic diagram of a section of a glomerulus and its juxtaglomerular apparatus. Structures shown are as follows: afferent arteriole (AA), distal tubule (D), endothelial cell (E), efferent arteriole (EA), extraglomerular mesangial cell (EGM), foot process (F), juxtaglomerular granular cell (G), glomerular basement membrane (GBM), mesangial cell (M), macula densa (MD), sympathetic nerve endings (N), proximal tubule (P), parietal epithelial cell (PE), epithelial podocyte (PO), urinary pole (UP), and urinary space (US).

Glomerular Filtration Barrier

Urine formation begins at the glomerular filtration barrier. The glomerular filter through which the ultrafiltrate has to pass consists of three layers: the fenestrated endothelium, the intervening glomerular basement membrane, and the podocyte layer (Fig. 1-5). This complex "membrane" is freely permeable to water and small dissolved solutes, but retains most of the proteins and other larger molecules, as well as all blood particles. The main determinant of passage through the glomerular filter is molecular size. A molecule such as inulin (5 kD) passes freely through the filter, and even a small protein such as myoglobin (16.9 kD) is filtered to a large extent. Substances of increasing size are retained with increasing efficiency until at a size about 60 to 70 kD the amount filtered becomes very small. Filtration also depends on ionic charge, and negatively charged proteins, such as albumin, are retained to a greater extent than would be predicted by size alone. In certain glomerular diseases, proteinuria develops because of loss of this charge selectivity.

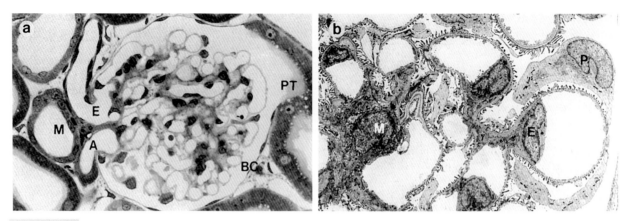

FIGURE 1-4 Structure of the glomerulus. *A,* Light micrograph of a glomerulus, showing the afferent arteriole (A), efferent arteriole (E), macula densa (M), Bowman's capsule (BC), and beginning of the proximal tubule (PT). The typical diameter of a glomerulus is about 100 to 150 μm, which is just barely visible to the naked eye. *B,* Higher-power view of glomerular capillary loops, showing the epithelial podocyte (P), endothelial cells (E), and mesangial cells (M).

Filtration by the Glomerulus

Filtrate formation in the glomerulus is governed by Starling forces, the same forces that determine fluid transport across other blood capillaries. The glomerular filtration rate (GFR) is equal to the product of the net filtration pressure, the hydraulic permeability, and the filtration area,

$$GFR = L_p \times Area \times P_{net},$$

where L_p is the hydraulic permeability, and P_{net} is the net ultrafiltration pressure. Net ultrafiltration pressure or

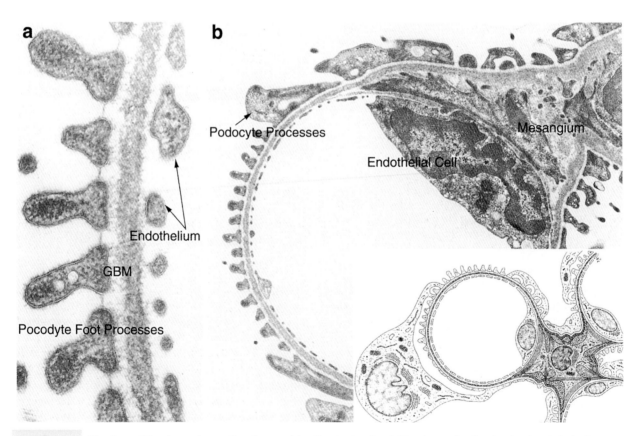

FIGURE 1-5 Structure of the glomerular capillary loop and the filtration barrier. *A,* The glomerular filtration barrier. *B,* A single capillary loop showing the endothelial and foot process layers and the attachments of the basement membrane to the mesangium. Pressure in the glomerular capillary bed is substantially higher than in other capillaries. As shown in the diagrammatic insert, the mesangium provides the structural supports that permit these cells to withstand these high pressures.

effective filtration pressure is the difference between the hydrostatic and osmotic pressure difference across the capillary loop,

$$P_{net} = \Delta P - \Delta \Pi = (P_{GC} - P_B) - (\Pi_{GC} - \Pi_B),$$

where P is hydrostatic pressure, Π is osmotic pressure, and the subscripts GC and B refer to the glomerular capillaries and Bowman's space.

Changes in GFR can result from changes in the permeability/surface area product ($L_p \times$ Area) or from changes in net ultrafiltration pressure. One factor influencing P_{net} is the resistance in the afferent and efferent arterioles. An increase in resistance in the afferent arteriole (before blood gets to the glomerulus) decreases P_{GC} and GFR. However, an increase in resistance as blood exits through the efferent arteriole tends to increase P_{GC} and GFR. Changes in P_{net} can also occur as a result of an increase in renal arterial pressure, which tend to increase P_{GC} and GFR. Obstruction of the tubule increases P_B and decreases GFR, and a decrease in plasma protein concentration tends to increase GFR.

Determination of GFR

Glomerular filtration rate is measured by determining the plasma concentration and excretion of a marker substance that meets the following requirements:

1. The substance must be neither absorbed nor secreted by the renal tubules.
2. The substance should be freely filterable across the glomerular membranes.
3. The substance is not metabolized or produced by the kidneys.

When these conditions are met, the amount excreted equals the amount filtered, and the formula for GFR, as shown in Table 1-3, follows from this relationship. In

---

TABLE 1-3 Derivation of the Formula for GFR

Step 1. Filtered amount of inulin = excreted amount of inulin

$$GFR \times GF_{in} = U_{in} \times V.$$

where GFR is the glomerular filtration rate, GF_{in} is the concentrations of inulin in the filtrate, U_{in} is the concentration of inulin in urine, and V is the urine flow rate.

Step 2. Inulin is freely filterable, so its concentrations in plasma and filtrate are identical. Hence,

$$\text{Filtered amount of inulin} = GFR \times P_{in},$$

where P_{in} is the concentration of inulin in plasma.

Step 3. Substituting produces

$$GFR \times P_{in} = U_{in} \times V$$

and hence

$$GFR = \frac{U_{in} \times V}{P_{in}}$$

GFR, glomerular filtration rate.

classic studies, inulin, a large sugar molecule with a molecular weight of about 5000, was infused to measure GFR. Other molecules with similar properties have been developed, including iothalamate and iohexol, and these compounds can be administered to patients to measure GFR. Creatinine is an endogenous substance that, although not a perfect GFR marker, is handled by the kidney in a similar way so that its plasma concentration can be used to estimate GFR. The clearance of creatinine is slightly greater than GFR (15% to 20%) because the excreted amount exceeds the amount filtered as a result of some tubular secretion of creatinine. Cystatin is another endogenous substance that is cleared by the kidney in rough proportion to the level of GFR; plasma levels of cystatin can also be used to estimate GFR. Filtration markers are discussed in more detail in Chapter 2.

GFR depends on body size, age, and physiologic state. Normal values for GFR for adults are typically given as 100 mL/min for women and 120 mL/min for men. Values in children are given in Chapter 55. High protein diet and high salt intake increase GFR, and GFR increases markedly with pregnancy (see Chapter 56). GFR decreases with a low-protein diet, and declines steadily with aging (see Chapter 57).

Juxtaglomerular Apparatus

Tightly adherent to every glomerulus, in between the entry and the exit of the arterioles, is a plaque of distal tubular cells called the macula densa, which is part of the juxtaglomerular apparatus. This cell plaque is in the distal tubule, at the very terminal end of the thick ascending limb of the loop of Henle, right before the transition to the distal convoluted tubule. This is a special position along the nephron, because at this site NaCl concentration is quite variable. Low rates of flow result in a very low salt concentration at this site, 15 mEq/L or less, while at higher flow rates salt concentration increases to 40 to 60 mEq/L. NaCl concentration at this site regulates glomerular blood flow through a mechanism called tubuloglomerular feedback; increases in salt concentration cause a decrease in glomerular blood flow.

The other unique cells that make up the juxtaglomerular apparatus are the renin-containing juxtaglomerular granular cells. Renin secretion is also regulated locally by salt concentration in the tubule at the macula densa. In addition, the granular cells have extensive sympathetic innervation, and renin secretion is controlled by the sympathetic nervous system.

TUBULAR FUNCTION: BASIC PRINCIPLES

Absorption and Secretion in the Renal Tubules

The glomerular filtrate undergoes a series of modifications before becoming the final urine. These changes

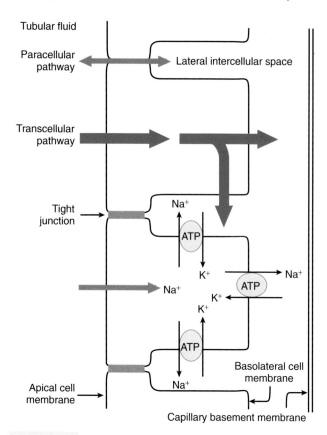

FIGURE 1-6 General scheme for epithelial transport. The driving force for solute movement is primarily generated by the action of the Na⁺ K⁺-ATPase in the basolateral membrane. Solute and water can move through either a paracellular pathway between cells or a transcellular transport pathway, which requires movement across both luminal and basolateral membranes. (From BM Koeppen, BA Stanton: Renal Physiology. St. Louis, CV Mosby, 1992, with permission.)

consist of removal or absorption and addition or secretion of solutes and fluid. Absorption and secretion indicate directions of transport, not mechanisms.

1. Absorption, the movement of solute or water from tubular lumen to blood, is the predominant process in the renal handling of Na⁺, Cl⁻, H₂O, HCO₃⁻, glucose, amino acids, protein, phosphates, Ca²⁺, Mg²⁺, urea, uric acid, and others.
2. Secretion, the movement of solute from blood or cell interior to tubular lumen, is important in the renal

handling of H⁺, K⁺, NH₄⁺, and a number of organic acids and bases.

Substances can move into or out of the tubule either by the transcellular pathway, which requires traversing the luminal and the basolateral cell membranes, or by the paracellular pathway between cells (Fig. 1-6). Many specialized membrane proteins participate in the movement of substances across cell membranes along the renal tubule. Some of the important membrane transport mechanisms, together with examples of substances that use these mechanisms, and proteins that are important for these processes are listed in Table 1-4.

Segmentation of the Nephron

One of the more striking characteristics of the renal tubule is its dramatic cellular heterogeneity. Early renal anatomists recognized that there are marked differences in the appearance of the cells of the proximal tubule, loops of Henle, and distal tubule. These nephron segments also differ markedly in function, distribution of important transport proteins, and responsiveness to drugs such as diuretics that inhibit transport.

Proximal Tubule

The proximal tubules absorb the bulk of filtered small solutes. These solutes are present at the same concentration in proximal tubular fluid as they are in plasma. Approximately 60% of the filtered Na⁺, Cl, K⁺, Ca²⁺, and H₂O and more than 90% of the filtered HCO₃⁻ are absorbed along the proximal tubule. This is also the segment that normally reabsorbs virtually all the filtered glucose and amino acids by Na⁺-dependent cotransport. An additional function of the proximal tubule is phosphate transport, which is regulated by parathyroid hormone. In addition to these reabsorption functions, secretion of solutes also occurs along the proximal tubule. The terminal portion of the proximal tubule, the S3 or pars recta, is the site of secretion of numerous organic anions and cations, a mechanism used by the body for eliminating a number of drugs and toxins. The proximal tubule, as shown in Figure 1-7, has a prominent brush border, extensive interdigitated basolateral infoldings, and large prominent mitochondria, which supply the energy for Na⁺ K⁺-ATPase.

TABLE 1-4 Types of Membrane Transport Mechanisms Used in the Kidney

Mechanism	Examples of Substances	Examples of Transport Protein
Facilitated or carrier mediated	Glucose, urea	GLUT1 carrier, urea carrier
Active transport (pumps)	Na⁺, K⁺, H⁺, Ca²⁺	Na⁺ K⁺-ATPase, H⁺ ATPase, Ca²⁺-ATPase
Coupled transport		
Cotransport	Cl⁻, glucose, amino acids, formate, phosphates	NKCC2 cotransporter
Countertransport	Bicarbonate, H⁺	Cl⁻/HCO₃⁻ exchanger (AE1), Na⁺/H⁺ antiporter (NHE3)
Osmosis	H₂O	Water channels (aquaporins)

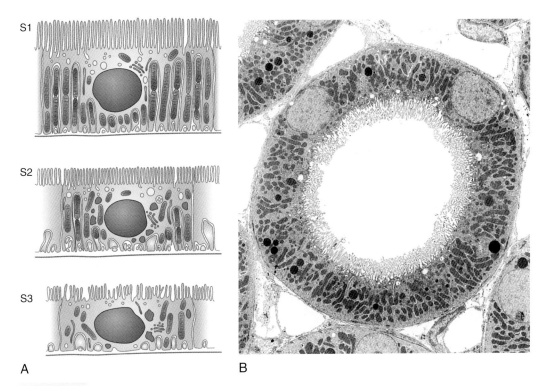

FIGURE 1-7   Proximal tubule. The proximal tubule consists of three segments: S1, S2, and S3. *A,* Schematic diagrams of the typical cells from these three segments. *B,* A cross section of the S1 segment. The S1 begins at the glomerulus, and extends several millimeters, before the transition to the S2 segment. The S3 segment, which is also called the proximal straight tubule, descends into the renal medulla to the inner medulla. The proximal tubule is characterized by a prominent brush border, which increases the membrane surface area by a factor of about 40-fold. The basolateral infoldings, which are lined with mitochondria, are interdigitated with the basolateral infoldings of adjacent cells (in these diagrams, processes that come from adjacent cells are shaded). These adaptations are most prominent in the first parts of the proximal tubule, and are less well developed later along the proximal tubule.

Loop of Henle

The loop of Henle consists of the terminal or straight portion of the proximal tubule, thin descending and ascending limbs, and the thick ascending limb and is important for generation of a concentrated medulla and for dilution of the urine. The thick ascending limb is often called the diluting segment, since transport along this water-impermeable segment results in development of a dilute tubular fluid. The thick ascending limb is also a major site of Mg^{2+} reabsorption along the nephron. The principal luminal transporter expressed in this segment is the Na^+-K^+-$2Cl^-$ cotransporter (NKCC2), which is the target of diuretics such as furosemide. The morphology of the loop of Henle epithelia is illustrated in Figure 1-8.

Distal Nephron

The distal nephron, which includes the distal convoluted tubule, the connecting tubule, and the cortical and medullary collecting duct, is the portion of the nephron where final adjustments in urine composition, tonicity, and volume are made. Distal segments are the sites where the most critical regulatory hormones, such as aldosterone and vasopressin, regulate acid and potassium excretion and determine final urinary concentrations of potassium, sodium, and chloride.

Both the distal convoluted tubule and connecting tubule have well-developed basolateral infoldings with abundant mitochondria, like the proximal tubule, although they are easily distinguished from the proximal tubule by the lack of brush border (Fig. 1-9). The distal convoluted tubule is the principal site of action of thiazide diuretics.

The collecting duct cells are cuboidal, and their basolateral folds do not interdigitate extensively. When there is a sizable osmotic gradient, and water moves across this epithelium, the spaces between cells become wide. The collecting duct changes in its appearance as it travels from the cortex to the papillary tip (Fig. 1-10). In the cortex there are two different cell types in the collecting duct: principal cells and intercalated cells. Principal cells are the main site of salt and water transport, and intercalated cells are the key sites for acid-base regulation. The

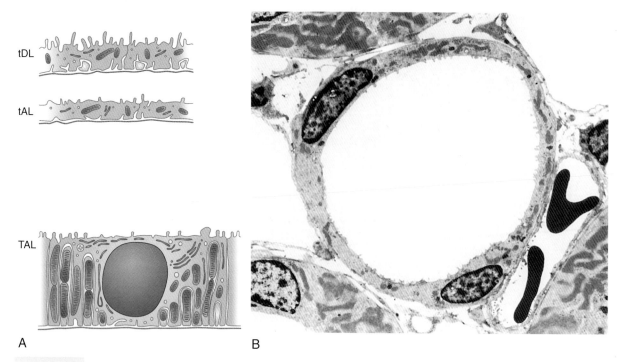

FIGURE 1-8   Loop of Henle. The loop of Henle makes a hairpin loop into the medulla. Segments included in the loop are the terminal portion of the proximal tubule, the thin descending (tDL) and ascending limbs (tAL), as well as the thick ascending limb (TAL). *A,* Schematic drawings of cell morphology. *B,* A cross-section through the thin descending limb in the outer medulla. The thin limbs, as their names suggest, are shallow epithelia without the prominent mitochondria of more proximal segments. The thick limb, in contrast, is a taller epithelium with basolateral infoldings and well-developed mitochondria. This segment is water impermeable, and transport along this segment is important for generation of interstitial solute gradients and a low salt concentration and to dilute fluid in the tubular lumen.

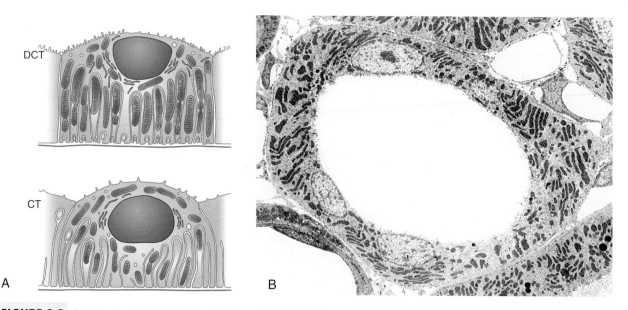

FIGURE 1-9   Distal convoluted tubule. The distal convoluted tubule is customarily divided into two parts: the true distal convoluted tubule and the connecting tubule, where cell morphology is somewhat more similar to the collecting duct. *A,* Schematic diagrams of the true distal convoluted tubule (DCT) and connecting tubule (CT). *B,* Cross-section of DCT.

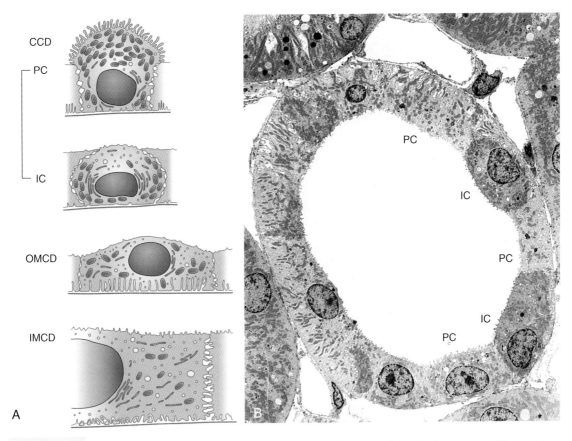

FIGURE 1-10   Collecting duct. The collecting duct changes its morphology as it travels from cortex (CCD, cortial collecting duct) to medulla (OMCD, outer medullary collecting duct; IMCD, inner medullary collecting duct). In the cortex there are two cell types: principal cells (PC) and intercalated cells (IC). *A,* Schematic appearance. *B,* Cross-section.

medullary collecting duct in its most terminal portions comes increasingly to resemble the tall cells typical of transitional epithelium.

SALT AND VOLUME REGULATION

Absorption of Sodium

Because of its high extracellular concentration, large amounts of Na^+ and its accompanying anions are present in the glomerular filtrate, and the absorption of this filtered Na^+ is in a quantitative sense the dominant work performed by the renal tubules. The amount of Na^+ absorbed by the tubules is the difference between the amount of Na^+ filtered and the amount of Na^+ excreted:

$$Na^+ \text{ absorption} = \text{filtered } Na^+ - Na^+ \text{ excretion}$$

or

$$Na^+ \text{ absorption} = (GFR \times P_{Na}) - (V \times U_{Na}),$$

where U_{Na} is the urinary Na^+ concentration and P_{Na} is the plasma Na^+ concentration. With a GFR of 120 mL/min and a plasma Na^+ concentration of 145 mEq/L, 17.4 mEq of Na^+ is filtered every minute, or about 25,000 mEq or 575 g of Na^+ per day. Because only about 100 to 250 mEq

of Na^+ is excreted per day (this reflects the average intake provided by a typical Western diet), one can estimate that the tubule reabsorbs somewhat more than 99% of the filtered Na^+. The fractional excretion of Na^+ (FE_{Na}) is defined as the fraction of filtered Na^+ excreted in the urine. Using creatinine as a GFR estimate, FE_{Na} is calculated from

$$FE_{Na} = \frac{\text{excreted}_{Na}}{\text{filtered}_{Na}} = \frac{U_{Na} \times V}{P_{Na} \times GFR}$$

$$= \frac{U_{Na} \times V}{P_{Na} \times \left(\dfrac{U_{Cr}}{P_{Cr}}\right) \times V} = \frac{U_{Na}/P_{Na}}{U_{Cr}/P_{Cr}}$$

FE_{Na} is usually less than 1%. However, this value depends on Na^+ intake and can vary physiologically from nearly 0% at extremely low intakes to about 2% at extremely high intakes. FE_{Na} can also exceed 1% in disease states where tubular transport of Na^+ is impaired (e.g., in most cases of acute renal failure).

Mechanisms of Na^+ Absorption

Tubular Na^+ absorption is a primary active transport process driven by the enzyme Na^+ K^+-ATPase. In renal epithelial cells, as in most cells of the body, this pump translocates Na^+ out of cells (and K^+ into cells) and thereby lowers intracellular Na^+ concentration (and elevates intracellular K^+ concentration). A key for the generation of net Na^+ movement from tubular lumen to blood is the asymmetrical distribution of this enzyme: it is present exclusively in the basolateral membrane (the blood side) of all nephron segments, but not in their luminal membranes. Delivery of Na^+ to the pump sites is maintained by Na^+ entry into the luminal side of the cells along a favorable electrochemical gradient. Because Na^+ permeability of the luminal membrane is much higher than that of the basolateral membrane, Na^+ entry is fed from the luminal Na^+ pool. The asymmetrical permeability is due to the presence of a variety of different transport proteins or channels exclusively in the luminal membrane.

A number of these luminal transporters are the target molecules for diuretic action. Principal entry mechanisms for Na^+ and Cl^- in the different nephron segments (and effective diuretics) are

1. Early proximal: Na^+-dependent cotransporter, Na/H exchanger (NHE3)
2. Late proximal: Na/H exchanger, Cl-anion exchanger
3. Thick ascending limb of the loop of Henle: NKCC2 cotransporter (furosemide-sensitive carrier)
4. Distal convoluted tubule: Na^+/Cl^- (NCCT) cotransporter (thiazide-sensitive carrier)
5. Collecting duct: Na^+ channel (ENaC, amiloride-sensitive channel)

Regulation of NaCl Excretion

Because Na^+ salts are the most abundant extracellular solutes, the amount of sodium in the body (the total body sodium) determines extracellular fluid volume. Therefore, excretion or retention of Na^+ salts by the kidneys is critical for the regulation of extracellular fluid volume.* Disturbance in volume regulation, particularly enhanced salt retention, is common in disease states. The sympathetic nervous system, renin-angiotensin-aldosterone system, atrial natriuretic peptide, and vasopressin represent the four main regulatory systems that change their activity in response to changes in body fluid volume. These changes in activity mediate the effects of body fluid volume on urinary Na^+ excretion.

Sympathetic Nervous System

A change in extracellular fluid volume is sensed by stretch receptors on blood vessels, principally those located on the low pressure side of the circulation in the

thorax, for example, in the vena cava, cardiac atria, and pulmonary vessels. A decreased firing rate in the afferent nerves from these volume receptors enhances sympathetic outflow from cardiovascular medullary centers. Increased renal sympathetic tone enhances renal salt reabsorption and can decrease renal blood flow at higher frequencies. In addition to its direct effects on kidney function, increased sympathetic outflow promotes the activation of another salt retaining system: the renin-angiotensin system.

Renin-Angiotensin System

Renin is an enzyme that is formed by and released from granular cells in the wall of renal afferent arterioles near the entrance to the glomerulus. These granular cells are part of the juxtaglomerular apparatus (see Fig. 1-3). Renin is an enzyme that cleaves angiotensin I from angiotensinogen, a large circulating protein made principally in the liver. Angiotensin I, a decapeptide, is converted by angiotensin-converting enzyme to the biologically active angiotensin II. Renin catalyzes the rate-limiting step in the production of angiotensin II, and it is therefore the plasma level of renin that determines plasma angiotensin II. The three principal mechanisms in control of renin release are as follows:

1. **Macula densa mechanism.** Macula densa refers to a group of distinct epithelial cells in the wall of the thick ascending limb of the loop of Henle, where it makes contact with its own glomerulus. At this location, NaCl concentration is between 30 and 40 mEq/L, and it varies as a direct function of tubular fluid flow rate; that is, it increases when flow rate is high and decreases when flow rate is low. A decrease in NaCl concentration at the macula densa strongly stimulates renin secretion, whereas an increase inhibits it. The connection to the regulation of body fluid volume is the dependence of the flow rate past the macula densa cells on body Na^+ content. The flow rate is high in states of Na^+ excess and low in Na^+ depletion.
2. **Baroreceptor mechanism.** Renin secretion is stimulated by a decrease in arterial pressure, an effect believed to be mediated by a "baroreceptor" in the wall of the afferent arteriole responding to pressure, stretch, or shear stress.
3. **β-Adrenergic stimulation.** An increase in renal sympathetic activity or in circulating catecholamines stimulates renin release through β-adrenergic receptors on the juxtaglomerular granular cells.

Angiotensin II has direct and indirect effects to promote salt retention. It enhances Na^+ reabsorption in the proximal tubule (stimulation of Na^+/H^+ exchange), and, because it is a potent renal vasoconstrictor, it may reduce GFR by reducing glomerular capillary pressure or plasma flow. Angiotensin II affects salt balance indirectly by stimulating the production and release of the steroid

*Plasma Na^+ concentration does not correlate at all with total body sodium or the extracellular fluid volume. In fact, a low serum Na^+ may be found in sodium excess and sodium deficiency states. However, plasma Na^+ concentration is the principal determinant of extracellular fluid osmolarity. In general, abnormalities in Na^+ concentration arise from defects in tonicity regulation, not volume regulation.

hormone aldosterone from the zona glomerulosa of the adrenal gland. Aldosterone acts on the collecting duct to augment salt reabsorption (and K$^+$ secretion).

Atrial Natriuretic Factor

Atrial natriuretic factor (ANF) is a peptide hormone that is synthesized by atrial myocytes and released in response to increased atrial distention. Thus, ANF secretion is increased in volume expansion and inhibited in volume depletion. The main cause of the ANF-induced natriuresis is an inhibition of Na$^+$ reabsorption along the collecting duct, but an increase in GFR may sometimes play a contributory role.

Vasopressin or Antidiuretic Hormone

Vasopressin or antidiuretic hormone (ADH) is regulated primarily by body fluid osmolarity. However, in states in which intravascular volume is depleted, the set point for vasopressin release is shifted, so that for any given plasma osmolarity, vasopressin levels are higher than they would be normally. This shift promotes water retention to aid in restoration of body fluid volumes.

WATER AND OSMOREGULATION

Regulation of Body Fluid Osmolarity

When water intake is low or water is lost from the body (e.g., in hypotonic fluids such as sweat), the kidneys conserve water by producing a small volume of concentrated urine. In dehydration, urine production is less than a liter per day (less than 0.5 mL/min) and the osmotic concentration may reach 1200 mOsm/kg H$_2$O. When water intake is high, urine flow may increase to as much as 14 L/day (10 mL/min) with an osmolality substantially lower than that of plasma (75 to 100 mOsm/kg). These wide variations in urine volume and osmotic concentration do not obligatorily affect the excretion of the daily solute load. Thus, the daily solute excess of about 1200 mOsm/ day may be excreted in 12 L of urine (with a U$_{osm}$ of 100 mOsm/L) or in 1 L (with a U$_{osm}$ of 1200 mOsm/L). The hormone responsible for the regulatory changes in urine volume and tonicity is ADH (vasopressin).

Role of ADH in Osmolarity Regulation

Antidiuretic hormone is a nonapeptide produced by neurons located in the supraoptic and paraventricular nuclei of the hypothalamus. It is stored in and released from granules in nerve terminals that are located in the posterior pituitary (neurohypophysis). The release of ADH is exquisitely sensitive to changes in plasma osmo-

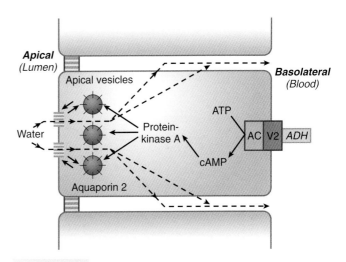

FIGURE 1-11 Mechanism of action of antidiuretic hormone (ADH) on the collecting duct. ADH combines with a basolateral receptor (V2) which is coupled with adenylate cyclase (AC). Generation of cyclic adenosine monophosphate (cAMP) leads to activation of protein kinase A, which in turn phosphorylates the water channel, aquaporin 2. The vesicles containing aquaporin are then inserted into the luminal membrane, increasing water permeability 10-fold.

lality, with increases in P$_{osm}$ above a threshold of about 285 mOsm/kg leading to increases in ADH secretion and plasma ADH concentrations. As has been pointed out, the actual set point for release depends on body fluid volume as well.

The most important function of ADH is the regulation of water permeability of the distal portions of the nephron, particularly the collecting duct. As shown schematically in Figure 1-11, ADH binds to receptors (R) in the basolateral membrane of collecting duct cells. This activates adenylate cyclase (AC) to form cyclic adenosine monophosphate. The latter activates a protein kinase, which leads to the phosphorylation of undefined proteins. This phosphorylation causes membrane fusion of vesicles that contain preformed water channels. The result is an increase of up to 20-fold in water permeability of the apical (luminal) membrane of collecting duct cells. On removal of ADH, water channels are rapidly removed from the apical membrane by endocytosis.

Tubular Water Absorption

At each point along the nephron, the osmotic pressure of the tubular fluid is lower than that in the interstitial space. This transtubular osmotic pressure difference provides the driving force for tubular water reabsorption. The rate of fluid absorption in a given nephron segment is determined by the magnitude of this gradient and the osmotic water permeability of the segment. Even though the osmotic pressure difference across the proximal tubule epithelium is small (3 to 4 mOsm/L), the rate of fluid absorption is high because this segment has a very high water permeability. In contrast, osmotic gradients across the thick ascending limb may be as high as 250 mOsm/L, and yet virtually no water flows across this segment because it is highly water impermeable. This segment dilutes the urine because it absorbs Na⁺ and Cl⁻ without water.

In contrast to the invariability of water conductivity in the proximal tubule and the thick ascending limb, water permeability in the collecting duct can be altered under the influence of ADH. If ADH is absent, water permeability and water absorption are low, and the hypotonicity generated in the thick ascending limb persists along the collecting duct. As a consequence, a dilute urine is excreted. If ADH is present, the collecting duct becomes quite water permeable, and water is reabsorbed until the tubular fluid in the collecting duct equilibrates with the hypertonic interstitium. The final urine in this case is osmotically concentrated and has a low volume.

Medullary Hypertonicity

To allow osmotically driven water absorption, the osmotic concentration in the medullary interstitium must be slightly higher than that in the collecting duct lumen. Thus, when a final urine with an osmolality of 1200 mOsm/kg is excreted, the medullary interstitium at the tips of the papillae must be a little higher than 1200 mOsm/kg. The generation of such a unique extracellular environment is achieved by a countercurrent multiplication system that exists in the renal medulla in the form of the countercurrent arrangement of descending and ascending limbs of the loops of Henle.

Countercurrent Multiplication

In two adjacent tubes with flow in opposite directions, the fluid can attain an osmotic concentration difference in the longitudinal axis of the system that can by far exceed that seen at each level along it. This principle of countercurrent multiplication requires energy expenditure and the presence of unique differences in membrane characteristics between the two limbs of the system.

The countercurrent multiplier represented by the loops of Henle is believed to generate an osmotic gradient for the following reasons:

1. Active NaCl transport across the ascending limb (the so-called single effect of the countercurrent system) generates an osmotic difference between tubular fluid and surrounding local interstitium.
2. A low water permeability of the ascending limb prevents dissipation of this gradient.
3. A high water permeability of the descending limb permits equilibration of descending limb contents with the surrounding local interstitium.

How such a system can result in progressive increases in osmotic concentration along the corticopapillary axis is shown in Figure 1-12. In step 1 (time zero), the fluid in the descending and ascending limbs and the interstitium is isoosmotic to plasma. In step 2, NaCl is absorbed from the ascending limb into the interstitium until a gradient of 200 mOsm/kg is reached. In step 3, the fluid in the descending limb equilibrates osmotically with the interstitium by water movement out of the tubule. In step 4,

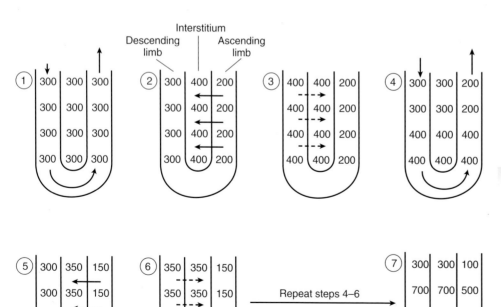

FIGURE 1-12 The process of countercurrent multiplication. (From BM Koeppen, BA Stanton: Renal Physiology. St. Louis, CV Mosby, 1992, with permission.)

the hypertonic fluid is presented to the thick ascending limb (TAL) with an increased solute concentration in the region near the tip of the system. Active NaCl transport along the ascending limb establishes a 200 mOsm/kg gradient, increasing interstitial concentrations and (by water abstraction) descending limb concentration. Note that concentrations near the tip begin to be higher than those near the base. Continued operation of such a mechanism gradually results in generation of a gradient of hypertonicity, with the highest osmolarities at the papillary tip.

The tubular fluid leaving the ascending limb of the loop of Henle countercurrent multiplier is hypotonic. However, the medullary interstitium has been osmotically "charged." Because the collecting ducts on their way to the papillary tip return to the hypertonic medullary environment, their content can be concentrated by water flow along an osmotic gradient.

Role of Urea in the Countercurrent Mechanism

In addition to Na^+ and Cl^-, urea is the other major solute present in the renal medulla in an osmotically concentrated form. Urea enters the medulla by reabsorption across the collecting duct. Marked differences in the permeability to urea allow reabsorption to proceed only across the terminal portions of the medullary collecting duct. In the early portions of the collecting duct, urea permeability is low and reabsorption of urea cannot occur. Because water leaves the tubule under the influence of ADH, the urea staying behind is progressively concentrated. As a consequence, a substantial urea gradient develops, providing the driving force for urea reabsorption when the permeability to urea permits it. The contribution of urea accumulation to osmotic water absorption along the inner medullary collecting duct must be sizable because urea accounts for about half of inner medullary tonicity. Therefore, a reduction in urea synthesis by reducing protein intake markedly impairs the concentrating ability of the kidneys.

Comparison Between Volume Regulation and Osmoregulation

Osmoregulation is under the control of a single hormonal system, ADH, whereas volume regulation is under the control of a set of redundant and overlapping control mechanisms. Lack or excess of ADH results in defined and rather dramatic clinical syndromes of excess water loss or water retention. In contrast, a defect in a single volume regulatory mechanism generally results in more subtle abnormalities, because of the redundant regulatory capacity from the other mechanisms. Thus, excess aldosterone results in a mild volume retention followed by

"escape" and return to normal Na^+ excretion, due to the action of the other mechanisms. Similarly, excess ANF probably produces only a modest decrement in volume, with no persistent abnormality in Na^+ excretion. Severe salt-retaining states, such as liver cirrhosis and congestive heart failure, are characterized by activation of all the volume regulatory mechanisms. Finally, the symptoms characteristic of disorders of osmoregulation and of volume regulation are different, with hypo- and hypernatremia being the hallmarks of deranged osmoregulation, and edema or hypovolemia resulting from deranged volume regulation.

REGULATION OF BODY FLUID POTASSIUM AND ACIDITY

Both potassium and hydrogen ions are present in body fluids at low concentrations, about 4 to 4.5 mEq/L for K^+ and about 40 nEq/L for H^+. Both ions show a number of features:

1. Relatively small deviations in either K^+ or H^+ concentrations can be life threatening, and therefore the regulation of K^+ and H^+ concentration requires control systems with high sensitivity and precision.
2. Constancy of both K^+ and H^+ concentration over the long term is achieved by regulated excretion of these ions in the urine. However, in both cases, other mechanisms exist that provide immediate protection against excessive deviations of plasma concentrations from normal.
3. Regulation in the renal excretion of both K^+ and H^+ is caused to a large extent by variation in the secretion of these ions by collecting ducts. The principal cell of the collecting duct is the cell type responsible for regulated K^+ secretion; the intercalated cell is the cell type responsible for H^+ secretion (see Fig. 1-10).
4. The rate of both K^+ and H^+ secretion is increased by aldosterone.
5. A primary derangement of K^+ balance can cause an acidity disturbance, and a primary acidity disturbance can derange K^+ homeostasis.

Regulation of Body Fluid Potassium

Distribution of Body K^+

Owing to the presence of Na^+ K^+-ATPase in virtually all cell membranes, K^+ is mostly in the intracellular space. Of the 3500 mEq of body potassium, only about 1% to 2% is present in the extracellular space, where it has a concentration of 4 to 5 mEq/L. The remainder (about 98%) is stored in cells.

The distribution poses a potential risk in that the release of even a small amount of K^+ from intracellular stores can elevate plasma K^+ concentration substantially (e.g., in insulin deficiency, cell lysis, severe exercise). On the other hand, the distribution of K^+ between the extracellular and intracellular space is utilized as a means to buffer acute changes in plasma K^+ concentrations. For example, the administration of an acute oral K^+ load induces much smaller changes in plasma K^+ concentration than would occur if all absorbed K^+ were to remain in the extracellular space. Potassium ions are shifted into cells under the stimulatory influence of insulin and epinephrine. The effect of both hormones reflects mainly an activation of the Na^+ K^+-ATPase. Another important factor determining K^+ distribution is plasma H^+ concentration. An increase in H^+ ions causes uptake of H^+ into cells and intracellular buffering and this uptake to some extent occurs in exchange for K^+. Thus, acidosis tends to increase plasma K^+, and alkalosis tends to decrease it.

Renal Handling of K^+

Potassium ion homeostasis in the long term requires the excretion of an amount equivalent to the daily K^+ intake (50 to 150 mEq). This represents a fractional K^+ excretion (FE_{K+}) of about 10%, much higher than FE_{Na+}. About 60% to 70% of filtered K^+ is absorbed along the proximal tubule, and further reabsorption of K^+ takes place in the thick ascending limb of the loop of Henle; only about 10% of filtered K^+ enters the distal tubule. Along the collecting duct, K^+ is both secreted and absorbed. Collecting duct K^+ secretion increases when dietary K^+ intake is elevated. On the other hand, when intake is low, collecting duct K^+ secretion virtually ceases and absorption is dominant. Thus, although K^+ absorption along the proximal tubule and the loop of Henle does not change very much depending on intake, collecting duct K^+ secretion is variable, and this variability accounts almost completely for the variation in urinary K^+ excretion.

Mechanisms of K^+ Secretion

K^+ secretion across the collecting duct epithelium utilizes the transcellular route. K^+ uptake across the basolateral membrane is driven by Na^+ K^+-ATPase, which elevates intracellular K^+ concentration to a level above electrochemical equilibrium. K^+ can then move along a favorable gradient from cell interior to tubule lumen utilizing potassium channels in the luminal membrane.

Three major variables determine the rate at which K^+ is secreted by collecting duct cells:

1. Changes in the activity of Na^+ K^+-ATPase affect uptake and thereby intracellular K^+ concentration. An increase in pump activity increases intracellular K^+ levels and tends to stimulate K^+ secretion.
2. Changes in the electrochemical gradient affect the driving force for K^+ movement across the luminal membrane. Both an increase in intracellular K^+ concentration and in the lumen negative transepithelial potential difference increase the driving force and tend to increase K^+ secretion.
3. Changes in the permeability of the luminal membrane determine the amount of K^+ that can be secreted for a given driving force. Thus, an increase in luminal K^+ conductance increases K^+ secretion.

Regulation of K^+ Excretion

1. **Plasma K^+ concentration.** One important determinant of K^+ excretion is plasma K^+ concentration. For example, the change in K^+ excretion following a change in dietary K^+ intake is mediated by an increase in plasma K^+. The effect of plasma K^+ on secretion is induced partly by a direct effect on intracellular K^+ concentration.
2. **Aldosterone.** At any level of plasma K^+, K^+ secretion also depends on plasma aldosterone levels. Aldosterone enhances K^+ secretion by activation of Na^+ K^+-ATPase and by an increase in K^+ permeability of the luminal membrane. Aldosterone is partly responsible for the diet-induced increase in K^+ excretion because its production and secretion are directly stimulated by plasma K^+ concentration. This effect is independent of angiotensin.
3. **Tubular flow rate.** An increase in tubular flow rate past the K^+-secreting cells stimulates, and a decrease reduces, K^+ secretion. This effect is the consequence of flow-dependent changes in the K^+ gradient across the apical membrane. K^+ secretion causes an increase in K^+ concentration in the tubular fluid, which eventually decreases the K^+ gradient and the rate of K^+ secretion. An increase in flow diminishes the rate of rise of luminal K^+ concentration so that a more favorable K^+ gradient for K^+ secretion is maintained.
4. **Distal sodium delivery.** When more Na^+ is delivered to the distal nephron, if reabsorption increases, the net electrical charge in the lumen becomes more negative. This favorable electrochemical gradient tends to increase urinary K^+ secretion.
5. **Hydrogen ions.** A decrease in H^+ concentration in alkalotic states causes a stimulation of K^+ secretion. This effect is mediated by the increase in intracellular K^+ concentration that occurs in alkalosis.

Diuretics and K^+ Excretion

Diuretics increase tubular flow rate. Agents such as loop diuretics and thiazides that inhibit NaCl and water absorption in segments prior to the collecting duct (in the loop of Henle and in the distal tubule, respectively) increase the flow of fluid past the collecting duct cells, which causes increased K^+ secretion. In addition, the diuretics cause volume depletion, which stimulates aldosterone secretion.

Regulation of Body Fluid Acidity

Basic Considerations

Maintenance of the extracellular pH around 7.4 depends on the operation of buffer systems that accept H^+ when it is produced and liberate H^+ when it is consumed. The state of the demand on total body buffering can be determined by assessing the behavior of the HCO_3^-/CO_2 system, which is the major extracellular buffer. The law of mass action for this buffer system states that

$$pH = 6.1 + \log\frac{[HCO_3]}{CO_2}$$

Because $[CO_2]$ equals the solubility coefficient multiplied by P_{CO_2}, this can be rewritten as

$$pH = 6.1 + \log\frac{[HCO_3]}{0.03 \times P_{CO_2}}$$

This, the familiar Henderson-Hasselbach equation, tells us that pH constancy depends on a constant ratio in the concentration between the two buffer components. If this ratio increases because either HCO_3^- increases or CO_2 decreases, pH increases (alkalosis). If the ratio decreases, because either HCO_3^- decreases or CO_2 increases, pH decreases (acidosis). Regulation of HCO_3^- is mainly a function of the kidneys, and regulation of CO_2 is a respiratory function.

The regulation of HCO_3^- concentration by the kidneys consists of two main components:

1. **Absorption of HCO_3^-.** Because of the high GFR and because plasma HCO_3^- concentrations are also relatively high (24 mEq/L), large amounts of HCO_3^- are filtered. Retrieval of this filtered HCO_3^- is absolutely essential for acid-base balance. It is important to note that this process of renal HCO_3^- absorption does not add new HCO_3^- to the blood, but merely prevents a loss of filtered HCO_3^- into the urine. Therefore, renal HCO_3^- absorption cannot correct an existing metabolic acidosis.
2. **Excretion of H^+.** Under normal dietary conditions, approximately 40 to 80 mmol H^+ is generated daily (mostly sulfuric acid from the metabolism of sulfur-containing amino acids). This H^+ is buffered and therefore consumes HCO_3^-. The kidneys must excrete this H^+ to regenerate the HCO_3^- pool (this second task can therefore also be labeled as generation of "new" HCO_3^-).

Mechanisms of Bicarbonate Absorption

Filtered HCO_3^- (about 4300 mEq/day) is efficiently absorbed by renal tubules, predominantly the proximal tubules, so that under normal acid-base conditions very little HCO_3^- is found in the urine. As a rule, all tubular HCO_3^- absorption is the consequence of H^+ secretion, and not of direct absorption of HCO_3^- ions. H^+ is continuously generated inside the cells from the dissociation of H_2O (or by CO_2 reacting with H_2O) and transported into the lumen. In the lumen, secreted H^+ combines with filtered HCO_3^- to form carbonic acid, which is broken down to CO_2 and H_2O in a reaction that is catalyzed by a carbonic anhydrase located in the apical brush border membrane. CO_2 and H_2O are then absorbed passively. The OH^- generated in the cell during this process combines with CO_2 to form HCO_3^-, a reaction catalyzed by a cytosolic carbonic anhydrase. HCO_3^- exits across the basolateral side of the cell and returns to the blood in association with Na^+. The net balance of this process can be expressed as

$$H_2O + CO_2 \leftarrow H_2CO_3 \leftarrow HCO_3^- + \overset{|}{H}{}^+ \leftarrow H_2O \rightarrow OH^- + CO_2 \rightarrow \overset{|}{H}CO_3^- + Na^+$$

$$\text{tubular lumen} \qquad \text{cell interior} \qquad \text{blood}$$

Specific transport proteins in renal epithelial cells cause the H^+ and HCO_3^- to move in the right directions. Two different mechanisms, both located in the apical membrane, are responsible for the movement of protons into the tubular fluid:

1. The first is an Na^+/H^+ exchanger (NHE3) that is driven by the Na^+ gradient and is found in the proximal tubule. In terms of mEq transported, it contributes most to HCO_3^- absorption.
2. The second is a primary active transport of H^+. An H^+-ATPase has been found in the luminal membrane of one class of intercalated collecting duct cells. There is also some evidence for the presence of an H^+ K^+-ATPase similar to that found in parietal cells of the gastric mucosa. Active H^+ transport is responsible for the secretion of smaller amounts of H^+ than Na^+/H^+ exchange, but it can proceed against a steeper gradient.

There are also at least two mechanisms for the transport of HCO_3^- across the basolateral membrane. The movement of HCO_3^- can be coupled to the movement of Na^+, and this is the major exit mechanism in the proximal tubule. In the collecting duct, HCO_3^- exit occurs predominantly through a basolateral Cl^-/HCO_3^- exchanger (equivalent to the band 3 protein of red cells, AE1).

Bicarbonate Secretion

Although net HCO_3^- transport for the whole kidney is always in the reabsorptive direction, certain intercalated cells in the cortical portion of the collecting duct can actually secrete HCO_3^-. The HCO_3-secreting cells have a polarity that is the reverse of the H^+-secreting cells; that is, they possess a basolateral H^+-ATPase and probably a luminal Cl^-/HCO_3^- exchanger. HCO_3^- secretion may be important during consumption of a diet providing base equivalents and for the correction of metabolic alkalosis.

Excretion of H$^+$ Ions (Formation of New HCO$_3^-$)

Urinary acid excretion cannot to any significant extent occur as free H^+. The absolute minimum urinary pH in humans is about 4.5, corresponding to an H^+ concentration of only 0.03 mEq/L. Because about 40 to 80 mEq of H^+ must be excreted per day, it is clear that most H^+ ions must be excreted in a bound or buffered form. Excretion of bound H^+ is achieved (1) by the titration of luminal nonbicarbonate buffers and (2) by the renal synthesis and excretion of ammonium ions.

Titratable Acidity

Binding of secreted H^+ to filtered nonbicarbonate buffer anions leads to the formation and excretion of urinary titratable acidity (titratable acidity is defined as the number of moles of NaOH that has to be added to bring urine back to pH 7.4). The ability to buffer H^+ depends on its dissociation constant (pK) and the quantity of buffer. Under normal conditions only the $HPO_4^{2-}/H_2PO_4^-$ buffer is present in amounts sufficient to act as an intratubular H^+ acceptor. This buffer pair has a pH of 6.8 and is excreted at a daily rate of about 50 mmol. Applying the Henderson-Hasselbach equation for the phosphate buffer ($pH = 6.8 + \log[HPO_4^{2-}]/[H_2PO_4^-]$), the following relationships can be calculated (considering only that fraction of total phosphate that is actually excreted, about 25% to 30% of the filtered phosphate load):

	pH	HPO_4^{2-} (mmol/day)	$H_2PO_4^-$ (mmol/day)	H^+ Buffered (mmol/day)
Filtrate	7.4	40	10	0
End proximal	6.8	25	25	15
Urine	4.8	0.5	49.5	39.5

This tabulation shows that the buffer capacity of HPO_4^{2-} can be fully utilized if the intratubular pH is lowered sufficiently. In some situations, other urinary buffers become important. In diabetic ketoacidosis, large amounts of β-hydroxybutyrate are excreted (e.g., 300 mmol/L). Even though this buffer component has a pK of 4.8, it carries up to 150 mmol H^+ per liter.

Ammonium Excretion

The second form of bound H^+ in the urine is ammonium. The excretion of NH_4^+ is equivalent to the generation of HCO_3^- or excretion of H^+. Glutamine, formed in the liver from glutamate and extracted from the blood by uptake mechanisms in the luminal and basolateral membranes of renal proximal tubule cells, is the major source of urinary ammonium. Ammonium is generated in the proximal tubule by a metabolic pathway that degrades glutamine to glutamate and further to α-ketoglutarate; this yields $2NH_4^+$ and $2HCO_3^-$ (rather than NH_3, CO_2, and H_2O). While the NH_4^+ ions are secreted through distinct transport pathways into the lumen of the proximal tubule, the new HCO_3^- ions are added to the blood HCO_3^- pool.

It is essential that the NH_4^+ that is formed by renal proximal tubules is preferentially secreted into the tubular lumen and then excreted in the urine. If the generated NH_4^+ was absorbed by the renal tubular epithelium (or secreted preferentially into the blood), it would be used to form urea (H_2NCONH_2). Ureagenesis forms H^+ that would consume the produced HCO_3^- and thereby negate net base production. This is shown in the following reactions:

$$2NH_4^+ + CO_2 \rightarrow urea + H_2O + 2H^+$$

or

$$2NH_4^+ + 2HCO_3^- \rightarrow urea + CO_2 + 3H_2O.$$

Urinary H^+ excretion in the form of NH_4^+ is on the order of 40 to 50 mmol/day. Renal NH_4^+ formation and excretion are greatly enhanced in metabolic acidosis. Failure of proximal tubules to generate NH_4^+ is the main reason that metabolic acidosis occurs in chronic kidney disease.

Regulation of H$^+$ Secretion

1. **Intracellular pH.** Systemic pH changes, whether caused by changes in plasma HCO_3^- (metabolic) or by changes in P_{CO_2} (respiratory), alter H^+ secretion (and therefore HCO_3^- absorption). Intracellular acidification, as occurs in acidosis, stimulates H^+ secretion and intracellular alkalinization (alkalosis) inhibits it.
2. **Aldosterone.** In addition to affecting Na^+ absorption and K^+ secretion, aldosterone stimulates H^+ secretion by collecting ducts.
3. **Potassium.** Changes in plasma K^+ concentration can affect H^+ secretion, in part by changing intracellular pH. Thus, hypokalemia increases intracellular acidity and stimulates H^+ ion secretion. Although the effect of hypokalemia alone is relatively small, a marked stimulation of H^+ secretion results when hypokalemia occurs with high plasma aldosterone levels. In this situation, which can occur in primary hyperaldosteronism or with administration of diuretics, metabolic alkalosis may be generated by the kidneys.

RENAL HANDLING OF GLUCOSE AND AMINO ACIDS

An important function of the renal tubule is retrieval of the glucose and amino acids that are present in glomerular filtrate and which would be lost to the body if they were not reabsorbed. To a large extent, this is a proximal tubule function, and disordered glucose and amino acid transport is characteristic of diseases that disturb proximal tubular function.

Glucose transport by the proximal tubule occurs via a transport protein present in the luminal membrane that carries a glucose molecule together with a sodium ion, the glucose-sodium cotransporter. This transporter uses the sodium concentration gradient (sodium concentration is higher outside the cell than inside the cell) to drive the movement of glucose into the cell. Glucose then diffuses out of the cell across the basolateral membrane, a process facilitated by a second carrier protein. The resulting reabsorption process is highly efficient, and in normal circumstances practically all the filtered glucose is removed from the proximal tubule fluid and glucose is virtually absent from urine.

When plasma glucose concentration rises, increasing amounts of glucose are filtered, and at a certain point the filtered load of glucose exceeds the capacity of the proximal transport mechanisms. This maximum reabsorption rate is called the tubular transport maximum for glucose (T_{mG}; Fig. 1-13). When glucose delivery exceeds the T_{mG}, the excess glucose is excreted in the urine.

Many of the same principles apply to the reabsorption of amino acids. A function of the proximal tubule, amino acid absorption is also highly effective. For most amino acids, less than 1% of the amount filtered escapes into the urine. A number of different luminal and basolateral

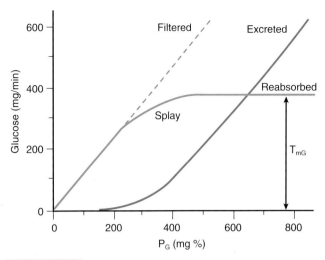

FIGURE 1-13 Glucose reabsorption. Shown is a typical filtration curve for renal glucose reabsorption. At plasma glucose concentrations less than approximately 200 mg/dL, the filtered glucose is completely reabsorbed, and no glucose is excreted in the urine. When plasma glucose exceeds this level, the filtered load of glucose exceeds the transport capacity of the tubule, and glucose appears in the urine.

transport proteins are needed to remove the amino acids from the glomerular filtrate. A specific transporter carries the dibasic amino acids, L-arginine and L-lysine, and another carrier is responsible for removal of the acidic amino acids from the tubular fluid. There also are luminal transporters that, like the sodium-glucose cotransporter, exploit the sodium concentration gradient for cotransport of certain amino acids together with sodium. Other carrier molecules in the basement membrane facilitate the exit of the amino acids from the cell.

BIBLIOGRAPHY

For a more thorough introduction to normal kidney function:

Giebisch G, Windhager E: The urinary system. In Boron WF, Emile L, Boulpaep EL (eds): Medical Physiology. A Cellular and Molecular Approach. Section VI. Philadelphia, WB Saunders, 2003, pp 735–875.
Guyton AC: Textbook of Medical Physiology, 8th ed. Chapters 25–31. Philadelphia, WB Saunders, 1991.
Koeppen B, Stanton B: Renal Physiology. St. Louis, Mosby-Year Book, 1992.
Rose BD: Clinical Physiology of Acid-Base and Electrolyte Disorders, 5th ed. New York, McGraw-Hill, 2001.
Shayman JA: Renal Physiology, Philadelphia, JB Lippincott, 1995.
Stanton BA, Koeppen BM: The kidney. In Berne RM, Levy MN, Koeppen BM, Stanton BA (eds): Physiology, 5th ed. Section VII. St. Louis, CV Mosby, 2004, pp 621–716.

For more detail on topics covered in this chapter:

Adrogue HJ, Madias NE: Management of life threatening acid-base disorders, first of two parts. N Engl J Med 338:26–34, 1998.

Adrogue HJ, Madias NE: Management of life threatening acid-base disorders, second of two parts. N Engl J Med 338: 107–111, 1998.
Baylis C: Glomerular filtration dynamics. In Lote CJ (ed): Advances in Renal Physiology. London, Grune & Stratton, 1986, pp 33–83.
Brater DC: Diuretic therapy. N Engl J Med 339:1505–1511, 2002.
Levey AS: Clinical practice. Nondiabetic kidney disease. N Engl J Med 347:1505–1511, 2002.
Levey AS: Measurement of renal function in chronic renal disease. Kidney Int 38:167–184, 1990.
Lifton RP: Genetic determinants of human hypertension. Proc Natl Acad Sci USA 92:8545–8551, 1995.
Ritz E, Orth SR: Nephropathy in patients with type 2 diabetes mellitus. N Engl J Med 341:1127–1133, 1999.
Scheinman SJ, Guay-Woodford LM, Thakker RV, Warnock DG: Genetic disorders of renal electrolyte transport. N Engl J Med 340:1177–1187, 1999.

CHAPTER 2

Clinical Evaluation of Kidney Function

Chi-yuan Hsu

This chapter discusses the evaluation of kidney function in everyday clinical practice. The approach taken is heavily influenced by the recently promulgated National Kidney Foundation Kidney Disease Outcomes Quality Initiative (K/DOQI) Chronic Kidney Disease (CKD) Clinical Practice Guidelines.

The National Kidney Foundation criteria for diagnosis of CKD are:

1. Kidney damage for greater than or equal to 3 months, as defined by structural or functional abnormalities of the kidney, with or without decreased glomerular filtration rate, manifest by either:
   a. Pathological abnormalities or
   b. Markers of kidney damage, including abnormalities in the composition of the blood or urine, or abnormalities in imaging tests.
2. Glomerular filtration rate less than $60 \, mL/min/1.73 \, m^2$ for greater than or equal to 3 months, with or without kidney damage.

Chronic kidney disease is further divided into stages 1 to 5 as shown in Table 2-1. For further details regarding the rationale behind the definition and staging of CKD, see Chapter 59.

GLOMERULAR FILTRATION RATE: THE KEY PARAMETER

The most important parameter in the clinical evaluation of kidney function is the glomerular filtration rate (GFR), which is generally accepted as the best overall index of kidney function. The level of GFR correlates well (albeit not perfectly) with the likelihood of developing complications of kidney disease, such as anemia, hyperphosphatemia, and uremic symptoms. A chronically low GFR by itself (less than $60 \, mL/min/1.73 \, m^2$) is sufficient to make the diagnosis of CKD, regardless of the presence or absence of other markers of kidney damage.

Measured GFR is the sum of all the single nephron glomerular filtration rates in both kidneys. It is possible for a disease to reduce the number of nephrons without GFR decreasing if a compensatory increase in single nephron glomerular filtration rate occurs. However, because it is not feasible to measure nephron number or single nephron glomerular filtration rate in humans, overall GFR remains the cornerstone of the clinical evaluation of kidney function.

Since its introduction by Homer Smith, the gold standard for measurement of GFR has been the clearance of the small carbohydrate moiety inulin—an ideal filtration marker because it is freely filtered in the glomeruli and is neither reabsorbed nor secreted by the tubules. Because clearance is defined as the volume of plasma cleared entirely of a substance in a unit of time, clearance of inulin equals GFR. Direct measure of GFR using inulin clearance is cumbersome, requiring intravenous infusion and timed urine collection. In research studies, GFR has been measured by clearance of iothalamate (a small polyiodinated radiographic contrast molecule that can be radiolabeled), but that is also not clinically practical.

WHY NOT USE SERUM CREATININE ALONE TO EVALUATE KIDNEY FUNCTION?

In daily clinical practice, serum creatinine concentration (SCr) has been the most commonly used parameter to evaluate kidney function. The small molecule creatinine (molecular weight 113 daltons) is endogenously produced by muscle and excreted by the kidneys. Therefore, reduction in GFR leads to an increase in SCr. Serum creatinine is easy and cheap to measure, and no urine collection is needed. Many laboratories report a normal reference range for SCr of around 0.7 to 1.4 mg/dL.

However, the National Kidney Foundation CKD Guidelines explicitly recommend that clinicians "should not use serum creatinine concentration as the sole means to assess the level of kidney function." This departure from current clinical practice needs an explanation. One known problem is that renal creatinine clearance is not the same as GFR because creatinine is not an ideal filtration marker. It is not only filtered in the glomeruli but also actively secreted by renal tubules. Therefore, creatinine clearance tends to overestimate GFR. More importantly, serum creatinine often does not reflect underlying GFR because SCr is a function not only of creatinine clearance (which reflects kidney function) but also creatinine production (which largely reflects muscle mass). Therefore, the same SCr can represent very different underlying glomerular filtration rates in individuals because of muscle mass differences.

A clinically practical solution to this problem is to use SCr to estimate kidney function via equations that take

TABLE 2-1   The Five Stages of CKD as Defined by the National Kidney Foundation*

Stage	Description	GFR (mL/min/1.73 m²)
1	Kidney damage with normal or ↑ GFR	≥90
2	Kidney damage with mild or ↓ GFR	60–89
3	Moderate ↓ GFR	30–59
4	Severe ↓ GFR	15–29
5	Kidney failure	<15 or dialysis

CKD, chronic kidney disease; GFR, glomerular filtration rate.
*CKD is defined as either kidney damage or GFR <60 mL/min/1.73 m² for ≥3 months. Kidney damage is defined as pathologic abnormalities or markers of damage, including abnormalities in blood or urine test results or imaging studies.
From National Kidney Foundation: K/DOQI Clinical Practice Guidelines for Chronic Kidney Disease: Evaluation, classification, and stratification. Am J Kidney Dis 39(suppl 1):1–266, 2002. With permission.

into account variables such as age, sex, race, and body size (which are all important predictors of muscle mass and hence creatinine production). Numerous such equations have been proposed, but the two endorsed by the National Kidney Foundation as being most valid are the Cockcroft-Gault equation and the Modification of Diet in Renal Disease study (MDRD) equation.

The Cockcroft-Gault equation estimates creatinine clearance (mL/min) as

$$\text{Creatinine Clearance} = [(140 - \text{age}) \times \text{weight} (\times 0.85 \text{ if female})/72]/\text{SCr}$$

There are several versions of the MDRD equation. The abbreviated version estimates GFR (mL/min/1.73 m²) as

$$\text{GFR} = 186 \times [\text{SCr}]^{-1.154} \times [\text{age}]^{-0.203} \times [0.742 \text{ if female}] \times [1.210 \text{ if black}]$$

Online and PDA (personal digital assistant) versions of either of these equations are widely available.

The following example using the MDRD equation is illustrative. A 40-year-old black man with an SCr of 1.1 mg/dL for 3 or more months is estimated to have a normal GFR of 96 mL/min/1.73 m². However, the same chronic stable SCr of 1.1 mg/dL in a 70-year-old white woman corresponds to an underlying GFR of only 52 mL/min/1.73 m². The latter would be classified as having stage 3 CKD but the former would not. In other words, using serum creatinine alone to assess kidney function may result in considerable misclassification of GFR.

Particularly among elderly patients, who are at higher risk for kidney disease, the absolute SCr may be misleadingly low despite substantial reductions in GFR due to decreased muscle mass and hence creatinine production. In these patients, SCr can increase from, say, 0.5 mg/dL to 1.1 mg/dL over 5 years because of kidney disease, but this increase may be missed by clinicians because SCr remains in the normal reference range. Because of the hyperbolic relationship between clearance and serum creatinine, this doubling of SCr in actuality reflects roughly halving of GFR. Other clinical scenarios in which increments in SCr that remain within the normal reference range belie major disease events include young women with progression of lupus nephritis and cachectic cancer patients receiving nephrotoxic medications. It is clear from this discussion that for SCr, the laboratory normal reference range for creatinine has the potential to be misleading.

THE ROLE OF 24-HOUR URINE COLLECTIONS

Timed urine collections such as 24-hour urine collections have long been used clinically to measure creatinine clearance and hence GFR. However, the National Kidney Foundation CKD Guidelines also recommend against this common practice. This is because studies have shown that a single 24-hour urine collection often does not provide a better estimate of GFR than the estimation equations.

Figure 2-1 shows the results of one such study. This pilot investigation for the African American Study of Kidney Disease and Hypertension (AASK) measured SCr, 24-hour urine creatinine clearance, and radioactive-iothalamate clearance GFR in 118 men and women. Compared with the reference standard ¹²⁵I-iothalamate clearance GFR, the creatinine clearance measured from the 24-hour urine collection was not more precise than the Cockcroft-Gault equation estimated clearance.

The notorious difficulties in getting reliable 24-hour urine specimens likely account for the imprecision of this test. In other words, random errors due to under- or over-collection of urine introduce significant mistakes in the calculated creatinine clearance. Because it is difficult even in the research setting to obtain reliable 24-hour urine collections, reliable collections in clinical practice are even less likely.

CAVEATS FOR GLOMERULAR FILTRATION RATE ESTIMATION FORMULAS

Several caveats must be kept in mind when applying SCr-based equations to estimate GFR in clinical practice. First, the patient must be in the steady state. When the SCr is changing rapidly, such as during acute renal failure, it is wrong to estimate GFR using the Cockcroft-Gault or the MDRD equation. It may be possible under those circumstances to model the underlying kidney function from the rate and pattern of change in SCr using complex mathematical models beyond the scope of usual clinical

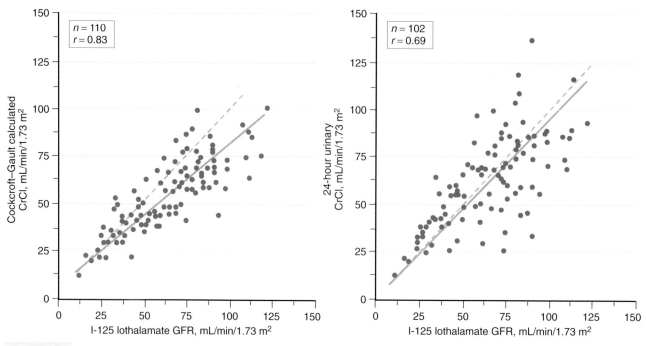

FIGURE 2-1 The single 24-hour urine collection method is not more precise than the equation in estimating glomerular filtration rate. There is less variability in the scatter plot of the Cockcroft-Gault equation creatinine clearance versus gold standard ^{125}I- iothalamate clearance GFR (*left*) compared with the scatter plot of 24-hour urine creatinine clearance versus gold standard ^{125}I- iothalamate clearance GFR (*right*). (From Coresh J, Toto RD, Kirk KA, et al: Creatinine clearance as a measure of GFR in screenees for the African-American Study of Kidney Disease and Hypertension pilot study. Am J Kidney Dis 32:32–42, 1998. With permission.)

practice. An extreme case illustration of this is a patient who has just undergone bilateral nephrectomy; the SCr may be 1.5 mg/dL immediately after the operation but the GFR is zero. Second, a variety of conditions have been known to artifactually increase or decrease SCr without affecting GFR. Some substances (e.g., some cephalosporins) interfere with the measurement of serum creatinine. Others reduce renal tubular creatinine secretion, and hence creatinine clearance, without affecting GFR (one well known example is cimetidine). Of course, these are relevant not only for GFR estimation equations but also when SCr alone is used to assess kidney function. Finally, for patients with unusual body compositions or extremes of body sizes, SCr-based equations will likely give invalid estimates of GFR because of alterations in the usual relationship between muscle mass and parameters such as age, sex, and weight. Examples include patients with hepatic cirrhosis, limb amputation, spinal cord injury, or morbid obesity. For these patients, multiple 24-hour urine collections (to reduce inaccuracies in collection) may be the best practical way to evaluate GFR. Ancillary markers of kidney function, such as blood urea nitrogen (BUN), may also provide clinically useful hints regarding degree of azotemia.

EVALUATION OF PROTEINURIA

Proteinuria is the second most important parameter in the clinical evaluation of kidney function. There are several reasons for this.

One, for many patients with early kidney disease, the GFR may be normal and there is no upward increase in serum creatinine. In these subjects, proteinuria may be the only sign of kidney damage. The best-known example of this is classic diabetic nephropathy where development of albuminuria precedes reduction in GFR. Persistent proteinuria is diagnostic of CKD regardless of GFR level. Recent epidemiologic studies show that there are over 10 million adults in the United States with persistent albuminuria (stages 1 and 2 CKD). This is a larger number than those with decreased GFR below 60 mL/min/1.73 m² (stages 3 to 5 CKD).

Two, proteinuria is the single most important risk factor for future loss of kidney function. Numerous studies have shown that patients with increased proteinuria are the ones at highest risk for further loss of GFR. One popular hypothesis postulates that this is because proteinuria in and of itself perpetuates kidney damage. Another holds that proteinuria is mostly a marker for severity of underlying kidney disease and glomerular hyperfiltration (see Chapter 58). Importantly, interventions that reduce proteinuria (such as blood pressure control) also retard the progression of kidney disease. Therefore, it is important to be able to easily and accurately quantify proteinuria over time among patients being treated.

Three, among patients with CKD, proteinuria is an important and independent risk factor for cardiovascular disease and mortality. This may be because leakage of protein into the urine reflects generalized endothelial damage and capillary injury (see Chapter 65).

SPOT URINE SAMPLES VERSUS 24-HOUR URINE COLLECTIONS TO QUANTIFY PROTEINURIA

The methods most familiar to clinicians for proteinuria assessment are dipstick urinalysis and 24-hour urine collection. The former, however, only provides relatively crude quantification of the concentration of protein and thus is affected by urinary dilution. The latter is susceptible to the same overcollection and undercollection errors that plague 24-hour urine quantification of creatinine clearance. The hassle and inconvenience to patients of collecting 24-hour urine specimens (frequently with instructions to store in a home refrigerator) is also a disadvantage.

The National Kidney Foundation CKD Guidelines recommend that under most circumstances, untimed ("spot") urine samples should be used to detect and monitor proteinuria. The Guideline authors' review of the literature concluded that it is usually not necessary to obtain a timed urine collection (overnight or 24-hour).

This recommendation is supported by data such as those shown in Figure 2-2. This is a study of 101 ambulatory, hospitalized, and bed-bound patients encompassing a wide range of age, SCr, amount of proteinuria, and underlying cause of kidney disease. A random urine specimen and a 24-hour urine collection were obtained on the same day for each patient. A strong correlation was found between the unitless urine protein-to-creatinine ratio and the 24-hour proteinuria as measured in grams. In this study, all patients who excreted more than 3.0 g of protein in 24 hours had protein-to-creatinine ratios that exceeded 3.0. All patients who excreted less than 0.2 g of protein had protein-to-creatinine ratios of less than 0.2.

The underlying physiologic and mathematical reason that the unitless urine protein-to-creatinine ratio is numerically similar to the 24-hour proteinuria measured in grams is because most people produce and excrete on the order of 1 g of creatinine every day. So when both urine protein and urine creatinine are reported in similar units (say, mg/dL), the urine protein-to-creatinine ratio can be thought of as the excretion rate of urinary protein in grams relative to the excretion rate of 1 g of creatinine.

CAVEATS FOR PROTEINURIA ESTIMATES

Several caveats must be kept in mind when applying the spot urine protein-to-creatinine ratio to evaluate proteinuria in clinical practice. Again, patients must be in a steady state and not be in acute renal failure. For patients who generate much less than 1 g of creatinine a day (e.g., a severely malnourished elderly patient) the urine protein-to-creatinine ratio would imply that daily protein excretion is greater than it really is. Conversely, for individuals who generate much more than 1 g of creatinine a day (e.g., a young male body builder), the urine protein-to-creatinine ratio would imply that daily protein excretion is less than what a complete 24-hour urine collection would reveal. Before interpreting proteinuria as a marker of parenchymal kidney disease, numerous causes of transient proteinuria must be kept in mind. These include vigorous exercise, fever, and poor glycemic control among diabetic patients. If possible, proteinuria should be measured in the absence of these conditions. More mundane reasons for false-positive proteinuria include urinary tract infections and contamination with semen, menses, or vaginal discharge. Persistence of proteinuria in several measurements is a more robust indicator of CKD, and a 3-month period is recommended by the National Kidney Foundation CKD Guidelines. Proteinuria is discussed in more detail in Chapter 4.

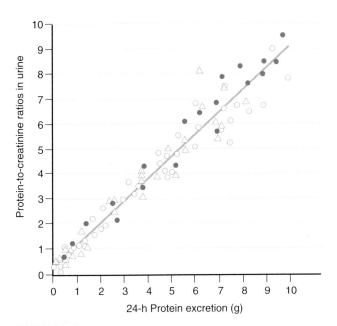

FIGURE 2-2 A tight correlation is seen between the random urine sample protein-to-creatinine ratio and 24-hour urine protein excretion. Linear regression parameters: y = 0.87x + 0.33; r = 0.96, n = 101. Solid circles represent ambulatory outpatients, open circles ambulatory inpatients, and open triangles bed-bound inpatients. (From Schwab SJ, Christensen RL, Dougherty K, Klahr S: Quantitation of proteinuria by the use of protein-to-creatinine ratios in single urine samples. Arch Intern Med 147:943–944, 1987. With permission.)

OTHER SIGNS OF CHRONIC KIDNEY DISEASE

In addition to chronically reduced GFR and persistent proteinuria, other diagnostic criteria for CKD include renal hematuria, pyuria, glycosuria, and other kidney abnormalities defined by radiologic or pathologic studies.

For more information the reader is referred to Chapters 3, 4, and 5.

ON EVALUATING KIDNEY FUNCTION IN ACUTE RENAL FAILURE

As alluded to previously, SCr-based equations cannot be used to estimate GFR in acute renal failure. Historically, acute renal failure has been defined as an acute increase in SCr. Some patients also show other signs of kidney dysfunction such as low urine output, hyperkalemia, or metabolic acidosis. Unfortunately, there is no agreement on how much the serum creatinine has to increase over what time period for it to constitute acute renal failure. Examples of definitions that have been used include "increase in serum creatinine of 0.5 mg/dL within 48 hours" or "50% increase in serum creatinine concentration to at least 2.0 mg/dL." Many of the same limitations of using SCr alone to assess kidney function in CKD also apply in acute renal failure. For example, for any acute GFR decrement, individuals who have more muscle mass and generate more creatinine (e.g., young men) are more likely to reach the threshold value of an increase in SCr of 0.5 mg/dL than those who generate less creatinine (e.g., women and the elderly). This may be one reason why some studies have found that hospitalized men have a higher incidence of acute renal failure than women. The nonlinearity of SCr changes bears emphasis in acute renal failure as it does in CKD. Even though the absolute increment in SCr is the same (0.5 mg/dL), whether the serum creatinine changes from 1.0 to 1.5 mg/dL or from 4.0 to 4.5 mg/dL, the percentage change (50% vs. 12.5%) and the absolute GFR reduction are much greater in the first instance. Restated another way, this example illustrates how the higher the starting value, the more sensitive the SCr is as an indicator of reduced GFR.

In acute renal failure, BUN level is sometimes useful diagnostically. The K/DOQI CKD Guidelines placed relatively little emphasis on BUN as an index of kidney function. This is because BUN is influenced by numerous extrarenal factors, even more so than serum creatinine. For example, independent of GFR, reduced protein intake will lower urea generation and BUN. Increased catabolism (from sepsis or corticosteroid use) as well as protein loading (from high-protein feeds or parenteral nutrition) will elevate BUN. In acute renal failure, the ratio of BUN to creatinine has been used as a diagnostic guide. A BUN:creatinine ratio greater than 20:1 (when both are measured in mg/dL) suggests reduced renal perfusion as the cause of acute renal failure. This is because urea (molecular weight 60 daltons) is not only filtered in the glomeruli but also reabsorbed in the renal tubules, and this reabsorption increases with decreased renal perfusion and urine flow rate, even without a change in GFR.

HOW FUTURE RESEARCH WILL LIKELY IMPACT THE CLINICAL EVALUATION OF KIDNEY FUNCTION

Several areas of research will likely impact the clinical evaluation of kidney function in the future. An important effort is underway to reduce the between-laboratory systematic differences in measured SCr. Currently, because of lack of standardization, calibration differences up to 0.3 mg/dL can occur. In other words, the same patient's SCr may be measured at 0.8 mg/dL in one laboratory and 1.1 mg/dL in another. Although both 0.8 mg/dL and 1.1 mg/dL fall within the normal reference range and may be considered unremarkable by many clinicians, a difference of 0.3 mg/dL may represent very different underlying GFR. Recall our example of the 70-year-old white woman with an SCr of 1.1 mg/dL and MDRD equation estimated GFR of 52 mL/min/1.73 m^2 (stage 3 CKD). If her SCr is measured at 0.8 mg/dL in another laboratory, then her estimated GFR would be 75 mL/min/1.73 m^2 and she would not be considered to have CKD (in the absence of other evidence of kidney damage). It should be noted that this same systematic error exists when timed urine collections are used to evaluate kidney function. In order to apply the National Kidney Foundation CKD Guidelines sensibly, standardization of serum creatinine measures across laboratories is essential. This is analogous to prior successful efforts to standardize measurements of serum cholesterol and hemoglobin A1c.

Some have questioned the classification of elderly patients with reduced GFR as having CKD, arguing that this is merely natural aging. This remains controversial. Not all elderly patients undergo the same age-associated decline in GFR, and elderly patients with decreased GFR are at higher risk for acute renal failure and toxicity from drugs excreted by the kidney such as digoxin. Low GFR at any age, therefore, may indeed represent disease. Further research is needed for clarification (see Chapter 57).

Finally, novel serum markers of kidney function, such as cystatin C, may eventually be adopted in clinical practice if investigations show that they provide clear-cut advantages over current methodologies.

For abrupt declines in kidney function, efforts to standardize the definition of acute renal failure would represent an important advance. One proposed strategy is to consider other dimensions of acute renal failure besides changes in serum creatinine and urine output. These include stage of CKD at baseline, nature of insult precipitating acute renal failure, and whether or not other organs are failing simultaneously. The validity and usefulness of these newer approaches will need to be studied.

BIBLIOGRAPHY

Cockcroft DW, Gault MH: Prediction of creatinine clearance from serum creatinine. Nephron 16:31–41, 1976.

Coresh J, Toto RD, Kirk KA, et al: Creatinine clearance as a measure of GFR in screenees for the African-American Study of Kidney Disease and Hypertension pilot study. Am J Kidney Dis 32:32–42, 1998.

GISEN Group: Randomised placebo-controlled trial of effect of ramipril on decline in glomerular filtration rate and risk of terminal renal failure in proteinuric, non-diabetic nephropathy. Lancet 349:1857–1863, 1997.

Hsu CY, Chertow GM, Curhan GC: Methodological issues in studying the epidemiology of mild to moderate chronic renal insufficiency. Kidney Int 61:1567–1576, 2002.

Levey AS, Bosch JP, Lewis JB, et al: A more accurate method to estimate glomerular filtration rate from serum creatinine: A new prediction equation. Ann Intern Med 130:461–470, 1999.

Levey AS, Coresh J, Balk E, et al: National Kidney Foundation practice guidelines for chronic kidney disease: Evaluation, classification, and stratification. Ann Intern Med 139:137–147, 2003.

Levey AS, Greene T, Kusek JW, Beck GJ: A simplified equation to predict glomerular filtration rate from serum creatinine [abstract]. J Am Soc Nephrol 11:155, 2000.

Mehta RL, Chertow GM: Acute renal failure definitions and classification: Time for change? J Am Soc Nephrol 14:2178–2187, 2003.

Moran SM, Myers BD: Course of acute renal failure studied by a model of creatinine kinetics. Kidney Int 27:928–937, 1985.

National Kidney Foundation: K/DOQI Clinical Practice Guidelines for Chronic Kidney Disease: Evaluation, classification, and stratification. Am J Kidney Dis 39(suppl 1):1–266, 2002.

Schwab SJ, Christensen RL, Dougherty K, Klahr S: Quantitation of proteinuria by the use of protein-to-creatinine ratios in single urine samples. Arch Intern Med 147:943–944, 1987.

CHAPTER 3

Urinalysis

Arthur Greenberg

The microscopic examination of the urine sediment is an indispensable part of the evaluation of patients with impaired kidney function, proteinuria, hematuria, urinary tract infection, or nephrolithiasis. The relatively simple chemical tests performed in the routine urinalysis rapidly provide important information about a number of primary kidney and systemic disorders. Examination of the urine sediment provides valuable clues about the renal parenchyma. The dipstick tests can be performed via machine and optical devices, and flow cytometry can be used to identify some cells in the urine. However, automated tests cannot detect unusual cells or distinguish among casts. There is no substitute for careful examination of the urine under the microscope. This task must not be delegated; it should be performed personally. The features of a complete urinalysis are listed in Table 3-1.

SPECIMEN COLLECTION AND HANDLING

Urine should be collected with a minimum of contamination. A clean-catch midstream collection is preferred. If this is not feasible, bladder catheterization is appropriate in adults; the risk for contracting a urinary tract infection following a single catheterization is negligible. Suprapubic aspiration is used in infants. In the uncooperative male patient, a clean, freshly applied condom catheter and urinary collection bag may be used. Urine in the collection bag of a patient with an indwelling bladder catheter is subject to stasis, but a sample suitable for examination may be collected by withdrawing urine from above a clamp placed on the drainage tube.

The chemical composition of the urine changes with standing, and the formed elements degenerate over time. The urine is best examined when fresh, but a brief period of refrigeration is acceptable. Because bacteria multiply at room temperature, bacterial counts from unrefrigerated urine are unreliable. High urine osmolality and low pH favor cellular preservation. These two characteristics of the first voided morning urine give it particular value in suspected glomerulonephritis.

PHYSICAL AND CHEMICAL PROPERTIES OF THE URINE

Appearance

Normal urine is clear, with a faint yellow tinge due to the presence of urochromes. As the urine becomes more concentrated, its color deepens. Bilirubin, other pathologic metabolites, and a variety of drugs may discolor the urine or change its smell. Suspended erythrocytes, leukocytes, or crystals may render the urine turbid. Conditions associated with a change in the appearance of the urine are listed in Table 3-2.

Specific Gravity

The specific gravity of a fluid is the ratio of its weight to the weight of an equal volume of distilled water. The urine specific gravity is a conveniently determined but inaccurate surrogate for osmolality. Specific gravities of 1.001 to 1.035 correspond to an osmolality range of 50 to 1000 mOsm/kg. A specific gravity near 1.010 connotes isosthenuria, with a urine osmolality matching that of plasma. Relative to osmolality, the specific gravity is elevated when dense solutes such as protein, glucose, or radiographic contrast are present.

Three methods are available for specific gravity measurement. The hydrometer is the reference standard, but it requires a sufficient volume of urine to float the hydrometer as well as equilibration of the specimen to the hydrometer calibration temperature. The second method is based on the well-characterized relationship between urine specific gravity and refractive index. Refractometers calibrated in specific gravity units are commercially available; they require only a drop of urine. Finally, the specific gravity may also be estimated by dipstick.

The specific gravity is used to determine whether the urine is or can be concentrated. During a solute diuresis accompanying hyperglycemia, diuretic therapy, or relief of obstruction, the urine is isosthenuric. In contrast, with a water diuresis due to overhydration or diabetes insipidus, the specific gravity is typically 1.004 or lower.

TABLE 3-1 Routine Urinalysis

Appearance

Specific gravity

Chemical tests (dipstick)
  pH
  Protein
  Glucose
  Ketones
  Blood
  Urobilinogen
  Bilirubin
  Nitrites
  Leukocyte esterase

Microscopic examination (formed elements)
  Crystals: urate; calcium phosphate, oxalate, or carbonate, triple phosphate; cystine; drugs
  Cells: leukocytes, erythrocytes, renal tubular cells, oval fat bodies, transitional epithelium, squamous cells
  Casts: hyaline, granular, red blood cells, white blood cells, tubular cell, degenerating cellular, broad, waxy, lipid-laden
  Infecting organisms: bacteria, yeast, *Trichomonas*, nematodes
  Miscellaneous: spermatozoa, mucous threads, fibers, starch, hair, and other contaminants

In the absence of proteinuria, glycosuria, or iodinated contrast administration, a specific gravity of more than 1.018 implies preserved concentrating ability. Measurement of specific gravity is useful in differentiating between prerenal azotemia and acute tubular necrosis (ATN) and in assessing the import of proteinuria observed in a randomly voided urine. Because the protein indicator strip responds to concentration of protein, the significance of a borderline reading depends on the overall urine concentration.

Chemical Composition of the Urine

Routine Dipstick Methodology

The urine dipstick is a plastic strip to which paper tabs impregnated with chemical reagents have been affixed. The reagents in each tab are chromogenic. After timed development, the color on the paper segment is compared with a chart. Some reactions are highly specific. Others are sensitive to the presence of interfering substances or extremes of pH. Discoloration of the urine with bilirubin or blood may obscure the color changes.

pH

The pH test pads use indicator dyes that change color with pH. The physiologic urine pH ranges from 4.5 to 8. The determination is most accurate if done promptly, because growth of urea-splitting bacteria and loss of CO_2 raise the pH. In addition, bacterial metabolism of glucose may produce organic acids and lower pH. These strips are not sufficiently accurate to be used for the diagnosis of renal tubular acidosis.

Protein

Protein measurement uses the protein-error-of-indicators principle. The pH at which some indicators change color varies with the protein concentration of the bathing solution. Protein indicator strips are buffered at an acid pH near their color change point. Wetting them with a protein-containing specimen induces a color change. The protein reaction may be scored from trace to 4+ or by concentration. Their equivalence is as follows: trace, 5 to 20 mg/dL; 1+, 30 mg/dL; 2+, 100 mg/dL; 3+, 300 mg/dL; 4+, greater than 2000 mg/dL. Highly alkaline urine, especially after contamination with quaternary ammonium

TABLE 3-2 Selected Substances That May Alter the Physical Appearance or Odor of the Urine

Color Change	Substances
White	Chyle, pus, phosphate crystals
Pink/red/brown	Erythrocytes, hemoglobin, myoglobin, porphyrins, beets, senna, cascara, levodopa, methyldopa, deferoxamine, phenolphthalein and congeners, food colorings, metronidazole, phenacetin
Yellow/orange/brown	Bilirubin, urobilin, phenazopyridine urinary analgesics, senna, cascara, mepacrine, iron compounds, nitrofurantoin, riboflavin, rhubarb, sulfasalazine, rifampin, fluorescein, phenytoin
Brown/black	Methemoglobin, homogentisic acid (alcaptonuria), melanin (melanoma), levodopa, methyldopa
Blue or green, green/brown	Biliverdin, *Pseudomonas* infection, dyes (methylene blue and indigo carmine), triamterene, vitamin B complex, methocarbamol, indican, phenol, chlorophyll

Odor	Substance or Condition
Sweet or fruity	Ketones
Ammoniacal	Urea-splitting bacterial infection
Maple syrup	Maple syrup urine disease
Musty or mousy	Phenylketonuria
Sweaty feet	Isovaleric or glutaric acidemia or excess butyric or hexanoic acid
Rancid	Hypermethioninemia, tyrosinemia

skin cleansers, may produce false-positive reactions. Protein strips are highly sensitive to albumin but less so to globulins, hemoglobin, or light chains. When light chain proteinuria is suspected, more sensitive assays should be used. With acid precipitation tests, an acid that denatures protein is added to the urine specimen and the density of precipitate related to the protein concentration. Urine negative by dipstick but positive with sulfosalicylic acid is highly suspicious for light chains. Tolbutamide, high-dose penicillin, sulfonamides, and radiographic contrast may yield false-positive turbimetric reactions. More sensitive and specific tests for light chains, including immunoelectrophoresis or immuno-precipitation, are preferred. If the urine is very concentrated, the presence of a modest protein reaction is less likely to correspond to significant proteinuria in a 24-hour collection. The protein indicator used for routine dipstick analysis is not sensitive enough to detect microalbuminuria.

Blood

Reagent strips for blood rely on the peroxidase activity of hemoglobin to catalyze an organic peroxide with subsequent oxidation of an indicator dye. Free hemoglobin produces a homogeneous color. Intact red cells cause punctate staining. False-positive reactions occur if the urine is contaminated with other oxidants such as povidone-iodine, hypochlorite, or bacterial peroxidase. Ascorbate yields false-negative results. Myoglobin is also detected, because it has intrinsic peroxidase activity. A urine sample that is positive for blood by dipstick analysis but shows no red cells on microscopic examination is suspect for myoglobinuria or hemoglobinuria. Pink discoloration of serum may occur with hemolysis, but free myoglobin is seldom present in a concentration sufficient to change the color of plasma. A specific assay for urine myoglobin will confirm the diagnosis (see Chapter 38).

Specific Gravity

Specific gravity reagent strips actually measure ionic strength using indicator dyes with ionic strength–dependent dissociation constants (pK_a). They do not detect glucose or nonionic radiographic contrast.

Glucose

Modern dipstick reagent strips are specific for glucose. They rely on glucose oxidase to catalyze the formation of hydrogen peroxide, which reacts with peroxidase and a chromogen to produce a color change. High concentrations of ascorbate or ketoacids reduce test sensitivity. However, the degree of glycosuria occurring in diabetic ketoacidosis is sufficient to prevent false-negative results despite ketonuria.

Ketones

Ketone reagent strips depend on the development of a purple color after acetoacetate reacts with nitroprusside. Some strips can also detect acetone, but none react with β-hydroxybutyrate. False-positive results may occur in patients taking levodopa or drugs like captopril or mesna that contain free sulfhydryl groups.

Urobilinogen

Urobilinogen is a colorless pigment produced in the gut from metabolism of bilirubin. Some is excreted in feces and the rest is reabsorbed and excreted in the urine. In obstructive jaundice, bilirubin does not reach the bowel and urinary excretion of urobilinogen is diminished. In other forms of jaundice, urobilinogen is increased. The urobilinogen test is based on the Ehrlich reaction, in which diethylaminobenzaldehyde reacts with urobilinogen in acid medium to produce a pink color. Sulfonamides may produce false-positive results, and degradation of urobilinogen to urobilin may yield false-negative results.

Bilirubin

Bilirubin reagent strips rely on the chromogenic reaction of bilirubin with diazonium salts. Conjugated bilirubin is not normally present in the urine. False-positive results may be observed in patients receiving chlorpromazine or phenazopyridine. False-negative results occur in the presence of ascorbate.

Nitrite

This screening test for bacteriuria relies on the ability of gram-negative bacteria to convert urinary nitrate to nitrite, which activates a chromogen. False-negative results occur owing to infection with enterococcus or other organisms that do not produce nitrite, when ascorbate is present, or when urine has not been retained in the bladder long enough (approximately 4 hours) to permit sufficient production of nitrite from nitrate.

Leukocytes

Granulocyte esterases can cleave pyrrole amino acid esters, producing free pyrrole that subsequently reacts with a chromogen. The test threshold is 5 to 15 white blood cells per high-power field (WBCs/HPF). False-negative results occur with glycosuria, high specific gravity, cephalexin or tetracycline therapy, or excessive oxalate excretion. Contamination with vaginal debris may yield a positive test result without true urinary tract infection.

Microalbumin Dipsticks

Albumin-selective dipsticks are available for screening for microalbuminuria in incipient diabetic nephropathy. The most accurate screening occurs when first morning specimens are examined, because exercise can increase albumin excretion. One type of dipstick uses colorimetric detection of albumin bound to gold-conjugated antibody. Normally the urine albumin concentration is below the 20 µg/L detection threshold for these strips. Unless the urine is very dilute, a patient with no detectable albumin by this method is unlikely to have microalbuminuria. Because urine concentration varies widely, however, this assay has the same limitations as any test that only measures concentration. This strip is useful only as a screening test, and more formal testing is required if albuminuria is found. A second type of dipstick has tabs for measurement of both albumin and creatinine concentration and permits calculation of the albumin:creatinine ratio. In contrast to the other dipstick tests described in this chapter, these strips cannot be read by simple visual comparison with a color chart. An instrument is required, but this system is suitable for point-of-care testing. When present on more than one determination, an albumin:creatinine ratio of 30 to 300 µg/mg signifies microalbuminuria. Details on interpretation of microalbuminuria are discussed further in Chapters 4, 28, and 29.

MICROSCOPIC EXAMINATION OF THE SPUN URINARY SEDIMENT

Specimen Preparation and Viewing

The contents of the urine are reported as the number of cells or casts per high-power (400×) field after resuspension of the centrifuged pellet in a small volume of urine. The accuracy and reproducibility of this semiquantitative method depends on using the correct volume of urine. Twelve milliliters of urine should be spun in a conical centrifuge tube for 5 minutes at 1500 to 2000 rpm (450 g). After centrifugation, the tube is inverted and drained. The pellet is resuspended in the few drops of urine that remain in the tube after inversion by flicking the base of the tube gently with a finger or with the use of a pipette. Care should be taken to fully suspend the pellet without excessive agitation. A drop of urine is poured onto a microscope slide or transferred with the pipette. The drop should be sufficient in size that a standard 22 × 22 mm coverslip just floats on the urine. If too little is used, the specimen rapidly dries out. If an excess of urine is applied, it will spill onto the microscope objective or stream distractingly under the coverslip. Rapid commercial urine stains or the Papanicolaou stain may be used to enhance detail. Most nephrologists prefer the convenience of viewing unstained urine. Subdued light is necessary. The condenser and diaphragm are adjusted to maximize contrast and definition. When the urine is dilute and few formed elements are present, detection of

motion of objects suspended in the urine ensures that the focal plane is correct. One should scan the urine at low power (100×) to get a general impression of its contents before moving to high power (400×) to look at individual fields. It is useful to scan large areas at low power and move to high power when a structure of interest is identified. Cellular elements should be quantitated by counting or estimating the number in at least 10 representative HPFs. Casts may be quantitated by counting the number per low-power field, although most observers use less specific terms such as rare, occasional, few, frequent, and numerous.

Cellular Elements

The principal formed elements of the urine are listed in Table 3-1. The figures constitute an atlas of selected formed elements.

Erythrocytes

Red blood cells (RBCs; Fig. 3-1A and B) may find their way into the urine from any source between the glomerulus and the urethral meatus. The presence of more than two to three erythrocytes per HPF is usually pathologic. Erythrocytes are biconcave disks 7 µm in diameter. They become crenated in hypertonic urine. In hypotonic urine, they swell or burst, leaving ghosts. Erythrocytes originating in the renal parenchyma are dysmorphic, with spicules, blebs, submembrane cytoplasmic precipitation, membrane folding, and vesicles. Those originating in the collecting system retain their uniform shape. Some experienced observers report success differentiating renal parenchymal from collecting system bleeding by systematic examination of erythrocytes using phase contrast microscopy.

Leukocytes

Polymorphonuclear leukocytes (PMNs; Fig. 3-1C) are approximately 12 µm in diameter and are most readily recognized in a fresh urine sample before their multilobed nuclei or granules have degenerated. Swollen PMNs with prominent granules displaying brownian motion are termed "glitter" cells. PMNs indicate urinary tract inflammation. They may occur with intraparenchymal diseases such as glomerulonephritis or interstitial nephritis. They are a prominent feature of upper or lower urinary tract infection. They also may appear with periureteral inflammation, as in regional ileitis or acute appendicitis.

Renal Tubular Epithelial Cells

Tubular cells (Fig. 3-1D) are larger than PMNs, ranging from 12 to 20 µm in diameter. Proximal tubular cells are oval or egg shaped and tend to be larger than the

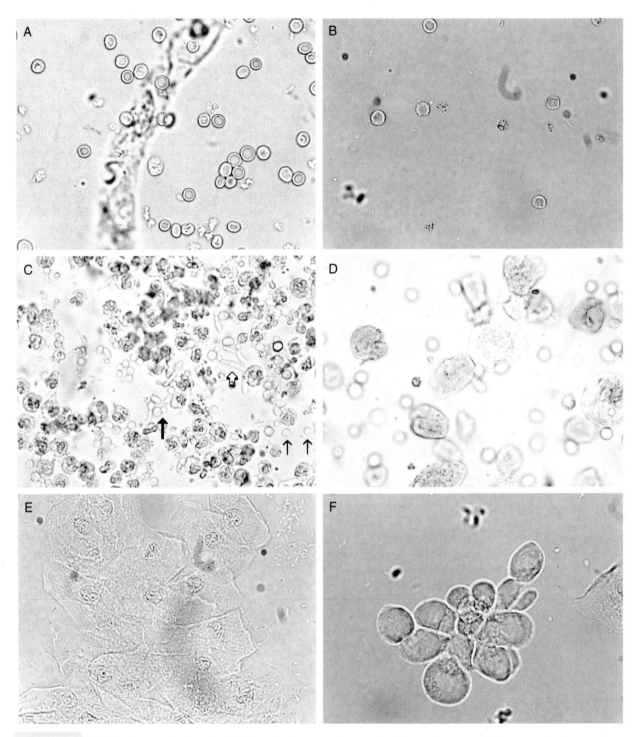

FIGURE 3-1   Cellular elements in the urine. In this and subsequent figures, all photographs were made from unstained sediments and, except as specified, photographed at 400× original magnification. *A,* Nondysmorphic red blood cells. Note that they appear as uniform, biconcave disks. *B,* Dysmorphic red blood cells from a patient with immunoglobulin A nephropathy. Their shape is irregular, with membrane blebs and spicules. *C,* Urine obtained from a patient with an indwelling bladder catheter. Innumerable white blood cells as well as individual (*small arrows*), budding (*single thick arrow*), and hyphal forms (*open arrow*) are present. *D,* Renal tubular epithelial cells. Note the variability of shape. The erythrocytes in the background are much smaller. *E,* Squamous epithelial cells. *F,* Transitional epithelial cells in a characteristic clump.

cuboidal distal tubular cells, but because their size varies with urine osmolality, they cannot be reliably differentiated. In hypotonic urine, it may be difficult to distinguish tubular cells from swollen PMNs. A few tubular cells may be seen in a normal urine sample. More commonly, they indicate tubular damage or inflammation from ATN or interstitial nephritis.

Other Cells

Squamous cells (Fig. 3-1E) of urethral, vaginal, or cutaneous origin are large, flat cells with small nuclei. Transitional epithelial cells (Fig. 3-1F) line the renal pelvis, ureter, bladder, and proximal urethra. They are rounded cells several times the size of leukocytes and often occur in clumps. In hypotonic urine, they may be confused with swollen tubular epithelial cells.

Casts and Other Formed Elements

Based on their shape and origin, casts are appropriately named. Immunofluorescence studies demonstrate that they consist of a matrix of Tamm-Horsfall urinary glycoprotein (uromodulin) in the shape of the distal tubular or collecting duct segment in which they were formed. The matrix has a straight margin helpful in differentiating casts from clumps of cells or debris.

Hyaline Casts

Hyaline casts consist of the protein alone. Because their refractive index is close to that of urine, they may be difficult to see, requiring subdued light and careful manipulation of the iris diaphragm. Hyaline casts are nonspecific. They occur in concentrated normal urine as well as numerous pathologic conditions (Fig. 3-2A).

Granular Casts

Granular casts consist of finely or coarsely granular material. Immunofluorescence studies show that fine granules derive from altered serum proteins. Coarse granules may result from degeneration of embedded cells. Granular casts are nonspecific but usually pathologic. They may be seen after exercise or with simple volume depletion and as a finding in ATN, glomerulonephritis, or tubulointerstitial disease (Fig. 3-2B).

Waxy Casts

Waxy casts or broad casts are made of hyaline material with a much greater refractive index than hyaline casts, hence their waxy appearance. They behave as if they were more brittle than hyaline casts and frequently have fissures along their edge. Broad casts form in tubules that have become dilated and atrophic due to chronic parenchymal disease (Fig. 3-2C).

Red Blood Cell Casts

Red blood cell casts indicate intraparenchymal bleeding. The hallmark of glomerulonephritis, they are seen less frequently with tubulointerstitial disease. RBC casts have been described along with hematuria in normal individuals after exercise. Fresh RBC casts retain their brown pigment and consist of readily discernable erythrocytes in a tubular cast matrix (Fig. 3-2E). Over time, the heme color is lost along with the distinct cellular outline. With further degeneration, RBC casts are hard to distinguish from coarsely granular casts. RBC casts may be diagnosed by the company they keep. They appear in a background of hematuria with dysmorphic red cells, granular casts, and proteinuria. Occasionally the evidence for intraparenchymal bleeding is a hyaline cast with embedded red cells. These have the same pathophysiologic implication as RBC casts.

White Blood Cell Casts

White blood cell casts consist of WBCs in a protein matrix. They are characteristic of pyelonephritis and useful in distinguishing this disorder from lower tract infection. They may also be seen with interstitial nephritis and other tubulointerstitial disorders.

Tubular Cell Casts

These casts consist of a dense agglomeration of sloughed tubular cells or just a few tubular cells in a hyaline matrix. They occur in concentrated urine, but are more characteristically seen with the sloughing of tubular cells that occurs with ATN (Fig. 3-2D).

Bacteria, Yeast, and Other Infectious Agents

Bacillary or coccal forms of bacteria may be discerned even on an unstained urine sample. Examination of a Gram's stain preparation of unspun urine allows estimation of the bacterial count. One organism per HPF of unspun urine corresponds to 20,000 organisms/mm^3. Individual and budding yeasts and hyphal forms occur with *Candida* infection or colonization. *Candida* organisms are similar in size to erythrocytes, but they are greenish spheres, not biconcave disks. When budding forms or hyphae are present, yeast cells are obvious (see Fig. 3-1C). *Trichomonas* organisms are identified by their teardrop shape and motile flagellum.

Lipiduria

In the nephrotic syndrome with lipiduria, tubular cells reabsorb luminal fat. Sloughed tubular cells containing fat droplets are called oval fat bodies. Fatty casts contain lipid-laden tubular cells or free lipid droplets. By light microscopy, lipid droplets appear round and clear with a green tinge. Cholesterol esters are anisotropic;

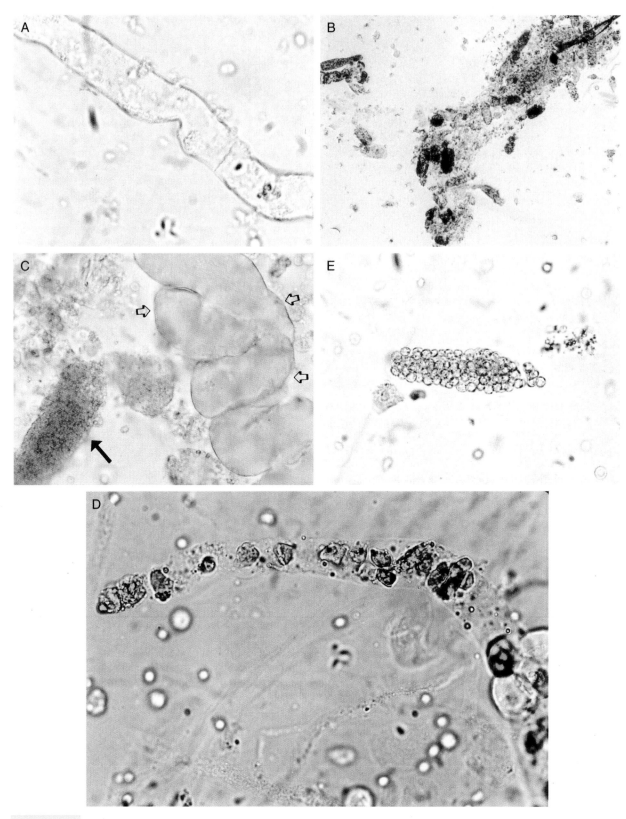

FIGURE 3-2   Casts. *A,* Hyaline cast. *B,* Muddy brown granular casts and amorphous debris from a patient with acute tubular necrosis (original magnification, 100×). *C,* Waxy cast (*open arrows*) and granular cast (*solid arrow*) from a patient with lupus nephritis and a telescoped sediment. Note background hematuria. *D,* Tubular cell cast. Note the hyaline cast matrix. *E,* Red blood cell cast. Background hematuria is also present.

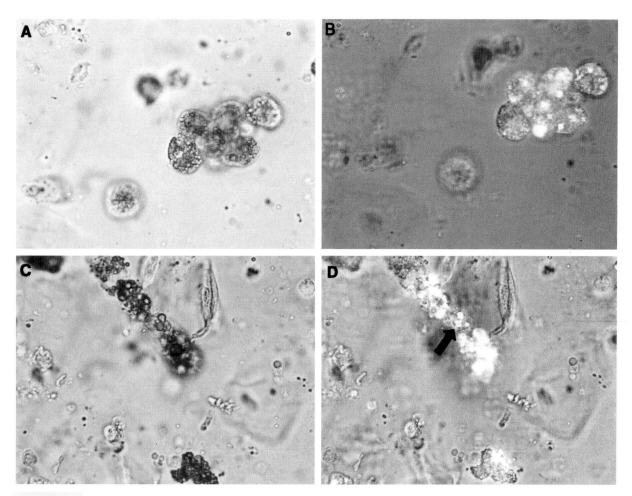

FIGURE 3-3   Lipid. *A,* Oval fat bodies, bright field illumination. *B,* Same field under polarized light. *C,* Lipid-laden cast, bright-field illumination. *D,* Same field under polarized light. Characteristic Maltese cross shown at arrow.

cholesterol-containing droplets rotate polarized light, producing a Maltese cross appearance under polarized light. Triglycerides appear similar by light microscopy, but they are isotropic. Crystals, starch granules, mineral oil, and other urinary contaminants are also anisotropic. Before concluding that anisotropic structures are lipid, the observer must compare polarized and bright-field views of the same object (Fig. 3-3).

Crystals

Crystals may be present spontaneously or precipitate with refrigeration of a specimen. They may be difficult to identify because of similar shapes; the common urinary crystals are described in Table 3-3. The pH is an important clue to identity, because solubility of a number of urinary constituents is pH dependent. The three most distinctive crystal forms are cystine, calcium oxalate, and magnesium ammonium (triple) phosphate. Cystine crystals are hexagonal plates resembling benzene rings. Calcium oxalate crystals are classically described as envelope shaped, but when viewed as they rotate in the urine under the microscope, they appear bipyramidal (Fig.

3-4A). Coffin lid–shaped triple phosphates are rectangular with beveled ends (Fig. 3-4B). Oxalate may also occur in dumbell-shaped crystals (Fig. 3-4C). Urate may have several forms, including rhomboids (Fig. 3-4D) or needles (Fig. 3-4E).

Characteristic Urine Sediments

The urine sediment is a rich source of diagnostic information. Occasionally a single finding (e.g., cystine crystals) is pathognomonic. More often, the sediment must be considered as a whole and interpreted in conjunction with clinical and other laboratory findings. Several patterns bear emphasis.

In the acute nephritic syndrome, the urine may be pink or pale brown and turbid. Blood and moderate proteinuria are detected by dipstick analysis. The microscopic examination shows RBCs and RBC casts as well as granular and hyaline casts. WBC casts are rare. In the nephrotic syndrome, the urine is clear or yellow. Increased foaming may be noted because of the elevated protein content. In comparison with the sediment of

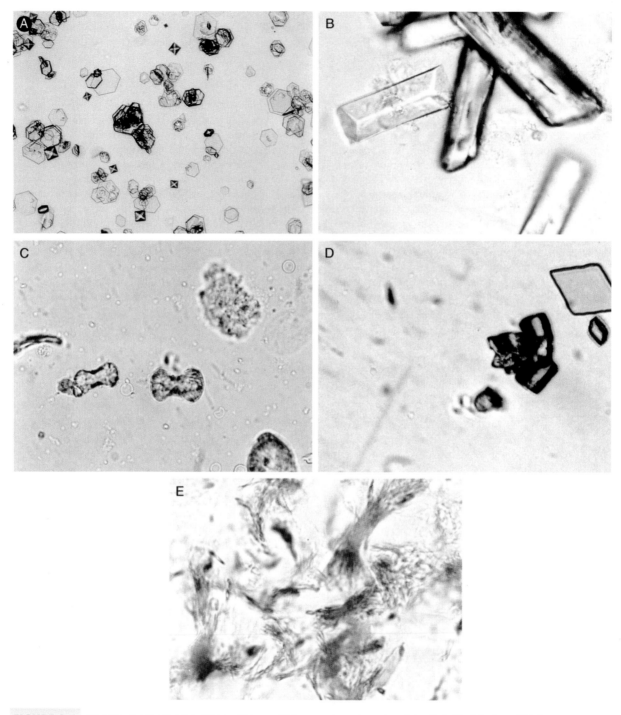

FIGURE 3-4 Crystals. *A,* Hexagonal cystine and bipyramidal or envelope-shaped oxalate. *B,* Coffin lid–shaped triple phosphate. *C,* Dumbell-shaped oxalate. *D,* Rhomboid urate. *E,* Needle-shaped urate. (*A,* Courtesy of Dr. Thomas O. Pitts.)

nephritic patients, the nephrotic sediment is bland. Hyaline casts and lipiduria with oval fat bodies or lipid-laden casts predominate. Granular casts and a few tubular cells may also be present along with a few RBCs. With some forms of chronic glomerulonephritis, a telescoped sediment is observed. This term refers to the presence of the elements of a nephritic sediment together with broad or waxy casts, indicative of tubular atrophy and dipstick

findings of heavy proteinuria (see Fig. 3-2C). In pyelonephritis, WBC casts and innumerable WBCs are present along with bacteria. In lower tract infection, WBC casts are absent. The sediment in ATN shows tubular cells, tubular cell casts, and muddy brown granular casts (see Fig. 3-2B). The typical urinary findings in individual kidney disorders are discussed in their respective chapters.

TABLE 3-3 Common Urinary Crystals

Description	Composition	Comment
Crystals found in acid urine		
Amorphous	Uric acid	Cannot be distinguished from amorphous phosphates except
	Sodium urate	by urine pH, may be orange tinted by urochromes.
Rhomboid prisms	Uric acid	
Rosettes	Uric acid	
Bipyramidal	Calcium oxalate	Also termed "envelope-shaped."
Dumbbell-shaped	Calcium oxalate	
Needles	Uric acid	Clinical history provides useful confirmation.
	Sulfa drugs	Sulfa may resemble sheaves of wheat; urate and contrast crystals
	Radiographic contrast	are thicker.
Hexagonal plates	Cystine	Presence may be confirmed with nitroprusside test.
Crystals found in alkaline urine		
Amorphous	Phosphates	Indistinguishable from urates except by pH.
Coffin lid (beveled rectangular prisms)	Triple (magnesium ammonium) phosphate	Seen with urea-splitting infection and bacteriuria.
Granular masses or dumbbells	Calcium carbonate	Larger than amorphous phosphates.
Yellow brown masses with or without spicules	Ammonium biurate	
Platelike rectangles, fan-shaped, starburst	Indinavir	Causes nephrolithiasis or renal colic. In vitro solubility increased at very low pH. The lowest urine pH achievable in vivo may not actually be acid enough to lessen crystalluria.

BIBLIOGRAPHY

Birch DF, Fairley KF, Becker GJ, Kincaid-Smith P: A Color Atlas of Urine Microscopy. New York, Chapman & Hall, 1994.

Braden GL, Sanchez PG, Fitzgibbons JP, et al: Urinary doubly refractile lipid bodies in nonglomerular renal disease. Am J Kidney Dis 16:332–337, 1988.

Canaris CJ, Flach SD, Tape TG, et al: Can internal medicine residents master microscopic urinalysis? Results of an evaluation and teaching intervention. Acad Med 78:525–529, 2003.

Fairley KF, Birch DF: Hematuria: a simple method for identifying glomerular bleeding. Kidney Int 21:105–108, 1982.

Fassett RG, Owen JE, Fairley J, et al: Urinary red-cell morphology during exercise. Br Med J 285:1455–1457, 1982.

Fogazzi GB, Cameron JS: Urinary microscopy from the seventeenth century to the present day. Kidney Int 50:1058–1068, 1996.

Fogazzi GB, Ponticelli C, Ritz E: The Urinary Sediment. An Integrated View, 2nd ed. Oxford, UK, Oxford University Press, 1999.

Graff L: A Handbook of Routine Urinalysis. Philadelphia, JB Lippincott, 1983.

Henry JB, Fuller CE, Threatte GA: Basic examination of the urine. In Henry JB (ed): Clinical Diagnosis and Management by Laboratory Methods, 20th ed. Philadelphia, WB Saunders, 2001, pp 367–402.

Kincaid-Smith P: Haematuria and exercise-related haematuria. Br Med J 285:1595–1597, 1982.

Kopp JB, Miller KD, Mican JM, et al: Crystalluria and urinary tract abnormalities associated with indinavir. Ann Intern Med 127:119–125, 1997.

Raymond JR, Yarger WE: Abnormal urine color: differential diagnosis. South Med J 81:837–841, 1988.

Rutecki GJ, Goldsmith C, Schreiner GE: Characterization of proteins in urinary casts. Fluorescent-antibody identification of Tamm-Horsfall mucoprotein in matrix and serum proteins in granules. N Engl J Med 284:1049–1052, 1971.

Schumann GB, Harris S, Henry JB: An improved technic for examining urinary casts and a review of their significance. Am J Clin Pathol 69:18–23, 1978.

Stamey TA, Kindrachuk RW: Urinary Sediment and Urinalysis. A Practical Guide for the Health Professional. Philadelphia, WB Saunders, 1985.

Voswinckel P: A marvel of colors and ingredients. The story of urine test strips. Kidney Int 46(suppl):3–7, 1994.

CHAPTER 4

Hematuria and Proteinuria

Richard J. Glassock

Hematuria and proteinuria are two cardinal manifestations of kidney disease. Because of their simplicity and ready availability, tests used to detect these abnormalities serve as cornerstones of nephrologic diagnosis. All physicians should be cognizant of the analytical methods, be aware of the interpretation of results and their pitfalls, and be prepared to conduct a logical follow-up study of abnormal findings. Although hematuria or proteinuria does not always signify an abnormality arising from within the kidneys or urinary tract, the thorough investigation of both abnormalities requires a systematic approach leading toward a definitive diagnosis.

HEMATURIA

Definition and Abnormal Values

Hematuria is defined as the excretion of abnormal numbers of erythrocytes (either intact or damaged) in the urine. It must be distinguished from pigmenturia (e.g., hemoglobinuria or myoglobinuria), in which protein or other substances impart an abnormal coloration to urine that resembles hematuria. Many of these substances are delivered to the kidneys from the circulation and are filtered into the urine. Proteinaceous pigment material also is detected as proteinuria; nonproteinaceous pigment is not.

Normal individuals excrete small numbers of erythrocytes in the urine, and the number may increase following vigorous exercise (e.g., a marathon race). The number of erythrocytes in normal urine (collected at rest or in association with usual activities) is approximately 8000/mL in centrifuged urine and up to 13,000/mL in uncentrifuged urine (some erythrocytes remain in the supernatant of centrifuged urine). In normal individuals, there are usually two or fewer erythrocytes per field when the resuspended sediment from freshly voided urine produced by light centrifugation is examined under the high-power objective of a light microscope (400× magnification). Menstruation or urethral trauma (e.g., urethral catheterization) may increase these values substantially.

Estimation of the degree of hematuria is most commonly performed by counting the number of erythrocytes per high-power field from the resuspended sediment or by direct counting of erythrocytes in a hemocytometer chamber using uncentrifuged urine. Hematuria can be visible to the naked eye (gross or macroscopic hematuria) or visible only by microscopic examination of the urine (covert or microscopic hematuria). Hematuria can occur in several patterns, namely, persistent, transient, intermittent, and recurrent. The coexistence or absence of symptoms referable to the urinary tract confers the designations of "symptomatic" or "asymptomatic" hematuria, respectively. The term *isolated hematuria* refers to the presence of abnormal numbers of erythrocytes in the urine without any other abnormality in the urine (i.e., absence of proteinuria). These patterns of hematuria may have diagnostic significance.

Detection and Quantification

Hematuria is detected in one or both of two ways. The first method is by direct microscopic examination of the urine. Microscopic examination of the urine is always the preferred method because information about the shape and size of the erythrocytes may be obtained, as may information regarding the presence of other cellular elements (e.g., leukocytes) or formed elements (e.g., casts), which may have diagnostic significance. The assessment of erythrocyte dysmorphism is a critical and vital step in the microscopic examination of the urine. Small, poorly hemoglobinized, and distorted erythrocytes (dysmorphic erythocyturia) are a sign of the glomerular origin of the hematuria (see Chapter 3, Fig. 3-1B). Normal-sized and -shaped, well-hemoglobinized erythrocytes (normo- or isomorphic erythrocyturia) (see Chapter 3, Fig. 3-1A) commonly originate in the urinary tract outside of the renal glomeruli. The shape, size, and hemoglobin content of erythrocytes in the urine can be best evaluated by phase-contrast microscopy. Unfortunately, this superior method of detecting dysmorphism in erythrocytes is not widely available and thus not generally used. Supravital staining with Eosin-Y or the Sternheimer-Malbin stain is a reasonable alternative. When these modalities are unavailable, erythrocyte dysmorphism can be assessed, albeit with less accuracy, when unstained specimens of the urine are examined by light microscopy under reduced illumination with the condenser adjusted to increase diffraction. Not all distorted erythrocytes in the urine are suggestive of a glomerular source. Acanthocytes, small erythrocytes with multiple spine-like or bubble-like projections, are most specific for glomerular bleeding. Crenated erythrocytes, seen in very hypertonic urine not freshly examined can be confused for dysmorphic erythrocytes. Very hypotonic urine may cause the erythrocytes to lyse and release hemoglobin, leaving behind the hemoglobin free "ghosts" of intact erythrocytes. *Candida* spherules, oxalate crystals, air bubbles, lipid globules, and starch granules can also be mistaken for erythrocytes by the untrained eye (see Chapter 3). When cellular (especially erythrocyte) casts are also present, dysmorphic erythrocytes are almost always indicative of a glomerular source for the hematuria. Automated cell sorters may allow for the determination of the mean corpuscular volume (MCV) of the erythrocytes in urine. A value for the MCV of less than 70 fL is usually indicative of a glomerular source. Occasionally patients with glomerular disease (especially immunoglobulin A nephropathy, acute glomerulonephritis, and crescentic glomerulonephritis) may initially excrete a combination of dysmorphic and normomorphic cells, but the absolute quantity of dysmorphic cells excreted per milliliter of urine or per minute is always abnormal.

The second method of detecting hematuria, very useful for screening for abnormalities, is via orthotolidine-impregnated paper strips (Hemastix, Clinistix-Ames). These tests are highly sensitive and can detect as few as one to two erythrocytes per high-power field in centrifuged urine. A trace positive result may therefore indicate a normal red blood cell excretion value. The strip will also indicate a positive result in myoglobinuria and hemoglobinuria. Thus, all positive test results (including trace positive results) must be accompanied by a careful and thorough microscopic examination of the urine in order to differentiate hematuria from pigmenturia and to evaluate the possibility of a false-positive qualitative test result. False-negative results may occasionally occur in patients taking large doses of vitamin C.

Although any value for erythrocyte excretion above the upper limit of normal is by definition a sign of potential disease, abnormal findings should usually be confirmed by a repeat test after a short interval. Additional useful information can also be obtained by quantitation of erythrocyte excretion rates. In gross (macroscopic) hematuria, the "urocrit" may be obtained in the same way a hematocrit is obtained. A urocrit greater than 1% often signifies lower urinary tract bleeding. When microscopic hematuria is present, timed overnight or random morning urine specimens (centrifuged or noncentrifuged) may be carefully examined in a hemocytometer chamber, and the number of erythrocytes excreted per hour (or per 12 hours) or the number of erythrocytes excreted per milliliter of urine may be readily calculated. The excretion of large numbers of dysmorphic erythrocytes (e.g., greater than 10^6/mL) may be an indication of an underlying crescentic glomerulonephritis.

Pathophysiology

Abnormal numbers of erythrocytes in the urine may arise from anywhere between the glomerular capillaries and the tip of the distal urethra. Glomerular hematuria presumably arises from small breaks or discontinuities in the integrity of the glomerular capillary wall, such as occur in glomerulonephritis (especially with crescent formation), thin basement membrane nephropathy, and diabetic nephropathy (likely due to ruptured microaneurysms in the glomerular capillaries). It is believed that these erythrocytes acquire their dysmorphic shape during their passage across the glomerular capillary. Other circulating elements, including plasma proteins (high and low molecular weight) also escape via the capillary disruptions into Bowman's space and the urine. Disruption of tubular architecture may also lead to the passage of erythrocytes from peritubular capillaries into tubular lumina, leading to hematuria. In this circumstance, proteinuria is less conspicuous and is usually of tubular origin. Urinary tract abnormalities at any location from the renal pelvis down to the distal urethra lead to microscopic or macroscopic but normomorphic hematuria. Because plasma proteins are excreted only in proportion to the degree of bleeding, lower urinary tract hematuria seldom leads to marked proteinuria. For example, urinary tract bleeding sufficient to result in gross hematuria with a 0.5% urocrit would give rise only to proteinuria of 2+ or less (less than 100 mg/dL) as estimated by the semiquantitative dipstick method. Hemolysis of erythrocytes in dilute urine (when urine is not freshly examined) will increase the protein concentration further, but the urine will have a pinkish hue in the supernatant after centrifugation. The presence of and concentration of hemoglobin in urine can be assessed by urinary electrophoresis. Hemoglobin migrates as a beta globulin. Myoglobinuria can be assessed in a similar fashion or by immunochemical tests. Macroscopic hematuria accompanied by proteinuria of 3+ or greater, in the absence of erythrocyte hemolysis, should always be regarded as being due to glomerular disease. The causes of glomerular, tubulointerstitial, and urinary tract bleeding are quite diverse (Table 4-1).

Approach to the Evaluation of Hematuria

All patients with hematuria should have a complete and thorough history and physical examination, with particular attention directed to weight changes, fever, symptoms referable to the kidneys or urinary tract (flank pain, dysuria, urgency, nocturia, hesitancy, incontinence), drug ingestion or exposure, bleeding tendency, corneal or hearing abnormalities, skin lesions, family history, or abdominal or flank masses or tenderness. One of the first steps in the evaluation of a patient who has been found to have hematuria (assuming that

TABLE 4-1   Causes of Hematuria

Renal Parenchymal Diseases	Urinary Tract Diseases

Glomerular disease
  Primary
    Mesangial IgA nephropathy (Berger's disease)
    Thin basement membrane nephropathy
    Mesangial proliferative glomerulonephritis with IgM and/or
      C3 deposits
    Membranoproliferative glomerulonephritis
    Crescentic glomerulonephritis
    Focal glomerulosclerosis
    Membranous glomerulopathy (<20%)
    Minimal change disease (<20%)
    Fibrillary glomerulonephritis
  Multisystem
    Systemic lupus erythematosus nephritis
    Microscopic polyangiitis
    Wegener's granulomatosis
    Henoch-Schönlein purpura
    Goodpasture's disease
    Thrombotic microangiopathies (e.g., hemolytic-uremic
      syndrome)
  Infection
    Poststreptococcal glomerulonephritis
    Infective endocarditis
    Shunt nephritis
    Other postinfectious glomerulonephritis
  Hereditary disease
    Alport's syndrome
    Nail-patella syndrome
    Fabry's disease
  Other
    Primary idiopathic renal hematuria with or without
      hypercalciuria
 	
Vascular and tubulointerstitial diseases
  Hypersensitivity
    Acute hypersensitivity interstitial nephritis
    Tubulointerstitial nephritis with uveitis
  Neoplastic
    Tumors (renal cell carcinoma, Wilms' tumor, leukemic
      infiltrates, angiomyolipoma)
    Metastatic tumors (uncommon)
  Hereditary
    Polycystic kidney disease (autosomal-dominant variety)
    Medullary sponge kidney
  Vascular
    Malignant hypertension
    Renal arterial emboli or thrombosis
    Loin pain–hematuria syndrome
    Arteriovenous malformations
  Papillary necrosis
    Analgesic abuse nephropathy
    Sickle cell trait
    Diabetes mellitus
    Alcoholism
    Ankylosing spondylitis
    Obstructive uropathy
  Trauma
    Acute bacterial pyelonephritis
    Acquired cystic disease of renal failure and dialysis
	Renal pelvis
	  Transitional cell carcinoma
	  Varices
	  Calculi
	  Trauma
	  Severe hydronephrosis
	  Nevi
	
	Ureter
	  Calculi (uric acid, calcium oxalate, calcium phosphate,
	    struvite, cystine, adenine, xanthine, drugs)
	  Transitional cell carcinoma
	  Periureteritis (appendicitis, ileocolitis, abscess)
	  Retroperitoneal fibrosis
	  Ureterocele
	  Varices
	  Endometriosis
	  Tuberculosis
	
	Bladder
	  Carcinoma of the bladder
	  Cystitis (bacterial, viral, parasitic, fungal)
	  Chronic interstitial cystitis (Hunner's ulcers)
	  Schistosoma haematobium
	  Radiation cystitis
	  Nitrogen mustard or cyclophosphamide cystitis
	  Hypersensitivity (allergic) cystitis
	  Bladder calculi
	  Sudden decompression of severe overdistention
	  Foreign bodies
	  Vascular anomalies
	  Amyloidosis
	  Trauma
	  Jogger's or marathon runner's hematuria (?)
	  Tuberculosis
	
	Prostate
	  Benign prostatic hypertrophy
	  Carcinoma of the prostate
	  Acute or chronic prostatitis
	
	Urethra
	  Meatal ulcers
	  Urethral prolapse
	  Urethral caruncle
	  Acute or chronic urethritis
	  Carcinoma of the urethra or penis
	  Vascular anomalies
	  Trauma
	  Foreign body
	  Condyloma acuminatum
	  Other (endometrosis)
	
	In association with a systemic coagulation disturbance
	(with or without diseases previously listed)
	
	Platelet defect
	  Idiopathic or drug-induced
	  Thrombocytopenic purpura
	  Thrombasthenia
	  Bone marrow diseases
	
	Coagulation protein deficiency
	  Hemophilia A or B
	  Heparin therapy
	  Warfarin therapy
	  Other congenital and acquired defect in coagulation
	
	Other
	  Scurvy
	  Hereditary telangiectasia
	  Surreptitious (malingering)

From Glassock R: Hematuria and pigmenturia. In Massry SG, Glassock RJ (eds): Textbook of Nephrology, 3rd ed. Baltimore, Williams & Wilkins, 1995.

pigmenturia has been excluded) is to assign the patient to one of three categories of probable diagnoses (Table 4-2): glomerular hematuria, indeterminant hematuria, or urinary tract hematuria.

Patients with glomerular hematuria should be further evaluated to detect and diagnose the cause of the glomerular disease (see Table 4-1). In many patients the cause will be evident, whereas in others a systematic clinical and laboratory evaluation will be required. A history of systemic features, such as fever or weight loss, may suggest a multisystem disease such as vasculitis. A family history of hematuria may suggest Alport's syndrome, Fabry's disease, or thin basement membrane nephropathy. The further laboratory evaluation of patients with suspected glomerular hematuria will depend largely on the nature of the findings in the history and physical examination, but most patients will require a hemogram, tests of kidney function (serum creatinine) with estimation of GFR using a prediction equation such as the Modification of Diet in Renal Disease study (MDRD) or Cockroft-Gault equation, and a renal-metabolic panel (electrolytes, calcium, phosphorous, total protein, albumin, globulin, cholesterol, alkaline phosphatase, alanine aminotransferase, aspartic aminotranferase, lactic dehydrogenase, uric acid, and glucose; Table 4-3). Urinary excretion of protein should be quantitated by 24-hour collection or by a protein (or albumin)-to-creatinine ratio in a random untimed first morning voided urine sample. Kidney size, echogenicity, and contour should be evaluated by renal ultrasonography. Small or echogenic kidneys usually indicate a chronic disease process with substantial interstitial fibrosis. Which other tests are required depends greatly on the circumstances and associated findings. In an older patient with associated weight loss and abdominal or pulmonary symptoms, a chest radiograph (or chest computed tomogram [CT]) and analysis of a stool for occult blood looking for evidence of a neoplastic disease or vasculitis would be prudent. A search for an underlying malignancy is especially

TABLE 4-3 Glomerular Hematuria: Laboratory Testing Based on Suspected Disease Causation

Suspected Cause	Laboratory Tests
Vasculitis	ANCA, Cryo-Ig, CRP, blood cultures, Anti-GBM, FANA
Systemic lupus erythematosus	FANA, anti-DNA, C3, C4
Goodpasture's disease	Anti-GBM, ANCA, Cryo-Ig
Crescentic glomerulonephritis	ANCA, anti-GBM, C3, C4, Cryo-Ig
Henoch–Schönlein purpura	IgA-fibronectin, serum IgA
Poststreptococcal glomerulonephritis	ASLOT, anti-DNAse, C3, C4
Membranoproliferative glomerulonephritis	C3, C4, Cryo-Ig, anti–hepatitis C, C3 NeF
Alport syndrome	Audiogram, slit-lamp examination
Infective endocarditis	Blood cultures, rheumatoid factor, C3, C4
Acute interstitial nephritis	Hansel's stain for urine eosinophils, CRP
Fibrillary glomerulonephritis	Serum and urinary electrophoreses, C3, C4

ANCA, antineutrophil cytoplasmic antibody; anti-DNA, anti-double-stranded (native) DNA antibody; anti-DNAse, anti-deoxyribonuclease; anti-GBM, anti-glomerular basement membrane antibody; ASLOT, antistreptolysin O titer; C3 NeF, C3 nephritic factor; CRP, C-reactive protein; Cryo-Ig, cryo-immunoglobulins; FANA, fluorescent antinuclear antibody.

TABLE 4-2 Clinical Categories of Hematuria

Glomerular hematuria
Microscopic or gross hematuria
>70% of erythrocytes are dysmorphic and/or
Proteinuria >1000 mg/day or ≥2+ present
Cellular casts (including erythrocyte casts) present

Indeterminate hematuria
Microscopic or gross hematuria
>30 and <70% of erythrocytes are dysmorphic and/or
Proteinuria <1000 mg/day or ≥2+ present
Cellular casts (except erythrocyte casts) are variably present

Nonglomerular (urinary tract) hematuria
Microscopic or gross hematuria
>70% of erythrocytes are normomorphic and/or
Protein excretion rate normal or slightly increased (≤2+)
Cellular or erythrocyte casts absent

appropriate in high-risk patients such as heavy smokers or those with a strong family history of neoplasia. In contrast, a chest radiograph would be of very low yield in a child with a history suggestive of Henoch-Schönlein purpura or a young adult with known systemic lupus erythematosus. Serologic studies, again critically dependent on the clinical findings in history and physical examination, might include C3, C4, C'H50, antineutrophil cytoplasmic autoantibody (antimyeloperoxidase and anti-PR3 autoantibodies), anti–glomerular basement membrane autoantibody, fluorescent antinuclear antibody, anti-double-stranded DNA antibody, antistreptolysin/anti-DNAse antibody, or cryoimmunoglobulins. Audiograms should be performed when Alport's syndrome is suspected, and a slit-lamp examination of the cornea might be performed in Fabry's disease. As emphasized, the selection of noninvasive diagnostic tests will be greatly influenced by the a priori probability of the presence of specific diseases. In many, but not all, patients, a kidney biopsy will be needed to establish a definitive diagnosis, assess prognosis, and guide therapy. Whether to perform this invasive procedure will be greatly influenced by how likely it is to add information of diagnostic or prognostic value. The kidney biopsy has a low probability of yielding information critical to determination of prognosis or therapeutic decision making when performed in a patient with isolated microscopic hematuria, normal blood pressure, and normal kidney function, since most such patients carry a good prognosis without treatment. Nevertheless, some patients, particularly those with a family history of hematuria or those suspected of having a genetically determined disease, may benefit from the knowledge acquired by kidney biopsy, even when the clinical finding is so mild as to indicate a favorable outcome.

Patients with indeterminant hematuria can have either glomerular or urinary tract bleeding, and further evaluation will depend heavily on clues obtained in the history and physical examination. The greater the absolute degree of erythrocyte dysmorphism in the urine, the greater the likelihood of a glomerular disease. At a minimum, these patients should undergo testing of kidney function (serum creatinine), quantification of urinary protein excretion (by a protein or albumin-to-creatinine excretion ratio, renal-metabolic panel, or hemogram), and renal ultrasonography. Many patients require further imaging studies, including spiral CT, intravenous urograms, and urinary cytology. Invasive procedures, such as cystoscopy, can usually be deferred unless the clinical features strongly suggest malignancy (e.g., weight loss, heavy smoking history, bladder irritation symptoms, older males, positive urinary cytology). Further evaluation, according to the glomerular or urinary tract hematuria approach, may be necessary based on the findings in the initial evaluative steps.

Patients with suspected urinary tract hematuria, in addition to the routine tests of renal function, hemogram, renal metabolic panel, and renal ultrasonography, will nearly always require a thorough and meticulous imaging of the urinary tract (Table 4-4; see Chapter 5). Urinary cytology should also be performed in smokers, those with a history of heavy analgesic consumption, or those who have been exposed to carcinogens (such as cyclophosphamide, ionizing radiation to

TABLE 4-4 Nonglomerular (Urinary Tract) Hematuria: Evaluation Based on Suspected Cause

Suspected Cause	Test
Parenchymal renal mass, cystic or solid	Abdominal CT, IVU, puncture for cytology (if cystic)
Bilateral enlarged kidneys, cystic	Abdominal CT
Pelvic mass or filling defect	IVU, cystoscopy, urine cytology
Papillary necrosis	Urine cytology, cystoscopy, hemoglobin electrophoresis, review analgesic exposure
Medullary sponge kidney	Urine calcium, urine culture
Ureteral stricture	Urine for *M. tuberculosis*, ANCA
Urinary calculus	Urine calcium, oxalate, cystine, urine culture, serum calcium, phosphorus, PTH
Retroperitoneal mass	Abdominal CT
Bladder/prostatic neoplasm	Cystoscopy, IVU, urine cytology

ANCA, antineutrophil cytoplasmic antibody; CT, computed tomography; IVU, intravenous urogram; PTH, parathyroid hormone.

the bladder or abdomen, aniline dyes, or plant or fungal toxins). Cystoscopy often is performed if noninvasive tests are not diagnostic and must always be performed if the urinary cytology result is positive. Intravenous urograms are useful for the detection of lesions in the upper urinary tract (ureter and pelvis), such as stones or uroepithelial tumors.

Although the sequence of investigative studies may vary according to the clinical presentation and the diagnostic suspicion raised by preliminary laboratory findings, at present, spiral (helical) CT followed by urinary cytology and cystoscopy is a frequently recommended sequence of studies when the clinical findings are not definitive in localizing the source of nonglomerular hematuria. CT examinations to evaluate renal masses are usually performed with the administration of contrast. Magnetic resonance imaging (MRI) can be used as an alternative. If gross hematuria is present, cystoscopy should be performed on a semiurgent basis to attempt to ascertain the source of bleeding. If all results are negative, an iodinated contrast angiogram or an MRI angiogram with gadolinium contrast may be necessary to detect an occult arteriovenous malformation or a small tumor.

Coagulation tests (prothrombin time, partial thromboplastin time, bleeding time, and platelet count) will be required if there is a bleeding diathesis in the patient or family history or if anticoagulants have been administered. Bleeding in patients who are anticoagulated should still be regarded as pathologic and investigated per the preceding discussion. Sickle cell hemoglobin should be evaluated in African Americans, since patients with the sickle trait are at risk for painless macroscopic hematuria, perhaps related to papillary necrosis. A tuberculin skin test is indicated when patients are suspected of having *Mycobacterium tuberculosis* infection. Urine cultures for *M. tuberculosis* should also be obtained. Urine should be tested for ova and parasites in patients who have traveled or lived in areas endemic for *Schistosoma haematobium*.

The pattern of urinary bleeding in patients with macroscopic hematuria can be helpful in estimating the site of bleeding. Urinary tract bleeding confined to the first 10 to 15 mL of urine voided suggests a urethral site, bleeding in the final 10 to 30 mL of urine voided suggests bladder bleeding, and bleeding throughout all phases of urination suggests bladder or upper tract bleeding. Significant bleeding at the very end of voiding suggests schistosomal infection or a urinary bladder (trigonal area) source. Significant irritative symptoms (dysuria, frequency) can accompany bladder bleeding even in the absence of infection (e.g., bladder carcinoma). A 24-hour urine calcium or uric acid measurement may detect hypercalciuria or hyperuricosuria in patients with unexplained urinary tract hematuria, particularly in children.

Using the preceding approach, about 85% or more of patients with hematuria can be correctly diagnosed. In the remaining patients with "idiopathic" hematuria, the correct diagnosis may become evident on follow-up with the emergence of new symptoms or signs. Follow-up of patients with "idiopathic" hematuria is encouraged. Although many will undergo a spontaneous remission of hematuria, a small proportion will also develop features of a treatable disease, such as a bladder cancer (missed in the initial cystoscopy), vascular malformations, or low-grade infections with fastidious organisms. Malingering is a rare cause of hematuria but can be very frustrating to detect and manage.

PROTEINURIA

Definition and Abnormal Values

The normal rate of excretion of total protein in the urine is 80 ± 24 mg/day in healthy individuals. Thus, over 95% of normal adults excrete less than 130 mg of total protein in the urine on a daily basis. Protein excretion rates are somewhat higher in children, adolescents, and pregnant women, and the value for the upper limit of normal may be approximately 200 mg/day in these individuals. Over 75% of the total 24-hour urine protein excretion occurs during quiet, upright ambulation. Fever, strenuous exercise, and the acute infusion of pressor agents (e.g., angiotensin, norepinephrine) may cause a transient increase in protein excretion rates in otherwise healthy individuals.

Abnormal proteinuria can be intermittent or constant and can occur predominantly in the upright position (orthostatic proteinuria). It may be isolated (without any other accompanying abnormalities in the urine). On quantification, abnormal proteinuria can be nephrotic if it exceeds 3.5 g/24 hours in adults or 40 mg/hr/m^2 in children. Subnephrotic proteinuria ranges between 0.2 g/day and 3.5 g/day. Overt proteinuria is usually defined as that level that is easily detectable using routine screening methods (usually greater than 300 to 500 mg/day). The excretion of small amounts of protein, principally albumin (30 to 300 mg/day), often below the usual detection limits for routing screening methods, is frequently called microalbuminuria.

Detection and Quantification

Abnormal proteinuria may be detected in several ways. The simplest and least expensive method is the use of a dye-impregnated paper strip (Albustix, Multistix, Ames), which depends on a color change of a pH sensitive dye (tetrabromophenol blue) buffered to pH 3. These tests detect protein, principally albumin, in concentrations from approximately 20 mg/dL to 300 mg/dL and thereby provide a semiquantitiative estimate of protein concentration in the urine. The strips are relatively insensitive to globulin (including Bence Jones proteins) and may underestimate total protein excretion compared with assays that measure both albumin and globulins to an equal extent. False-positive results may occur when highly alkaline urine overwhelms the dye's buffer and in the presence of certain drugs (e.g., tolbutamine, cephalosporins, and radiocontrast agents). These semi-quantitative estimates of proteinuria are concentration values, and their significance is greatly influenced by urinary concentration. The latter can be assessed by measuring urine osmolality or specific gravity. Highly concentrated urine (e.g., osmolality = 1200 mOsm/kg, urine specific gravity of 1.030) may show abnormal results (e.g., 1+, 30 mg/dL) even when the absolute daily excretion is normal. Similarly, highly dilute urine (osmolality 50 mOsm/kg, specific gravity 1.004) may show normal or only modestly elevated results for protein concentration (trace positive) when abnormal amounts of protein (e.g., 1000 mg/day) are excreted in a urine volume of 5000 mL/day. Dye-impregnated strips and special immunoassays are available that can detect albumin excretion below the usual detection limits. These are useful in detecting so-called microalbuminuria, between 15 and 200 μg/min or 30 to 300 mg/day, which is a key finding in incipient diabetic nephropathy (see Chapter 28). Commercial (e.g., biuret) or turbidometric (heat and acetic acid or 3% sulfosalicylic acid) methods can detect lower amounts of total proteinuria (down to about 5 to 10 mg/dL). These tests also detect albumin and globulins to an equal extent. Thus, a negative or borderline positive test result for proteinuria on the dipstick method and a strongly positive test result by a colorimetric or turbidometric assay usually indicate the presence of globulins (e.g., immunoglobulin or light chains) in the urine. False-positive turbidometric assays may also occur with the administration of certain agents (tolmetin, radiocontrast agents, or cephalosporins).

Quantitation of urine protein excretion rates can be determined by subjecting timed urine samples (e.g., 12 to 24 hours) to chemical or immunochemical assay. Alternatively, quantitation of protein excretion can be approximated by a comparison of the total urine protein (or albumin) concentration to a reference substance (also in mg/dL) excreted primarily by glomerular filtration and whose concentration in the final urine is mostly dependent by the extraction of water from urine. Creatinine is conventionally chosen as the reference substance, even though in certain circumstances it may undergo substantial tubular secretion. The protein (or albumin)-to-creatinine ratio (Up or Ualb:Ucr) can be expressed as milligrams of protein (or albumin) per milligram or per gram of creatinine. Because total creatinine excretion differs in male and female subjects, differing ratios may define values for males and females. The Up:Ucr ratio correlates well with 24-hour urine protein excretion rates. When suspected, the presence of orthostatic proteinuria may be confirmed by comparing Up:UCr ratios in a specimen collected upon awakening to one collected during the day after ambulation or by collecting split 24-hour urine samples, with separate containers for urine produced while the patient is recumbent at night and ambulatory during the day. Other tests may be useful in evaluating proteinuria, including cellulose acetate electrophoresis, immunoelectrophoresis, immunofixation, and spectrophotometry. These are well suited for examining the chemical nature of the excreted protein (e.g., hemoglobin, myoglobin, globulins, monoclonal light chains).

Composition of Urine Proteins

The intact proteins found in normal and abnormal urine are derived from three sources: (1) plasma proteins normally or abnormally filtered at the glomerular capillaries and escaping reabsorption or degradation by the proximal tubules; (2) proteins normally secreted by renal tubules (e.g., Tamm-Horsfall mucoprotein) or leaking into tubular lumina as a result of cellular injury; and (3) proteins derived from the lower urinary tract secreted by lining cells or associated glands, or leaking into urine as a result of tissue injury or inflammation. Additional protein fragments, arising from glomerular filtration and partial tubular degradation, are also excreted into the urine. These may not be detected by many of the routine assays for intact proteins (e.g., immunoreactive albumin) in the urine.

The composition of normal urine is shown in Table 4-5. It is noteworthy that albumin comprises 15% of the total urinary protein excreted, with normal values for excretion ranging from 4 to 15 µg/min (5.8 to 21.6 mg/day). Values above the upper limit of normal for albumin excretion rate (e.g., greater than 20 to 30 µg/min) to values which are usually detected by semiquantitative screening methods (about 200 to 300 mg/day) are commonly referred to as microalbuminuria. This corresponds to a Ualb:Ucr ratio of 17 to 250 mg/g in men and 25 to 355 mg/g in women. Approximately half of the protein in normal urine is derived from the kidney, and about half represents filtered plasma protein escaping reabsorption by the tubules or arising in the lower urinary tract (e.g., secretory immunoglobulin A [IgA]).

Pathophysiology of Abnormal Proteinuria

Four pathophysiologic varieties of abnormal proteinuria are recognized: (1) glomerular proteinuria, (2) tubular proteinuria, (3) overflow proteinuria, and (4) tissue proteinuria. Each has diagnostic significance and requires a different approach to evaluation (Table 4-6).

Glomerular proteinuria is the result of a disturbance in the permselectivity properties of the glomerular capillary wall leading to the filtration of plasma proteins in abnormally high amounts, which quickly saturate maximal tubular reabsorptive capacity and are thus excreted into the urine. Some of the filtered proteins are reabsorbed and delivered back into the circulation intact, whereas some are degraded and excreted as peptides or small polypeptides. Two subvarieties of glomerular proteinuria are described. Selective proteinuria, in which albumin and other relatively low-molecular-weight proteins

TABLE 4-5   **Protein Composition of Normal Urine**

		Urinary Protein	
		Excretion Rate	Percentage of Total
	µg/min	mg/day	%
Plasma proteins			
Albumin	8	12	15
	(4–5)	(5–25)	
IgG	2	3	
	(1–3)	(2–7)	
IgA (secretory)	0.7	1	5.4
	(0.2–2.0)	(0.4–3.0)	
IgM	0.2	0.3	
Light chains	2.6	3.7	4.6
κ		2.3	
λ		1.4	
β_2-Microglobulin	0.8	0.12	<0.2
Other plasma proteins and enzymes (total)	13.8	≈20	25
Subtotal of all plasma proteins	27.5 µg/min	40 mg/day	50%
Nonplasma proteins			
Tamm-Horsfall protein	28	40	50
Other renal-derived proteins	<0.7	<1	<1
Subtotal of nonplasma proteins	28 µg/min	40 mg/day	50%
Total protein	55 ± 17 µg/min	80 ± 24 mg/day	100%
	(1 SD)	(1 SD)	

From Glassock R: Proteinuria. In Massry SG, Glassock RJ (eds): Textbook of Nephrology, 3rd ed. Baltimore, Williams & Wilkins, 1995.

TABLE 4-6 Differential Diagnosis of Proteinuria Based on Pathophysiologic Mechanism

Glomerular proteinuria
Primary glomerular disease
 Minimal change lesion
 Mesangial proliferative glomerulonephritis (including IgA and IgM nephropathy)
 Focal and segmental glomerulosclerosis
 Membranous glomerulonephritis
 Mesangiocapillary glomerulonephritis
 Fibrillary glomerulonephritis
 Crescentic glomerulonephritis
Secondary glomerular disease
 Medications (mercurials, gold compounds, heroin, penicillamine, probenecid, captopril, lithium, NSAID)
 Allergens (bee sting, pollen, milk)
 Infectious (bacterial, viral, protozoal, fungal, helminthic)
 Neoplastic (solid tumors, leukemia)
 Multisystem (SLE, Henoch-Schönlein purpura, amyloidosis)
 Heredofamilial (diabetes mellitus, congenital nephrotic syndrome, Fabry's disease, Alport's syndrome)
 Other (transplant rejection, reflux nephropathy, toxemia of pregnancy)
 Other glomerular proteinuria
  Postexercise proteinuria
  Benign orthostatic proteinuria
  Febrile proteinuria

Tubular proteinuria
Toxins and drugs
 Endogenous
  Light chain damage to proximal tubule
  Lysozyme (myelomonocytic leukemia)
 Exogenous
  Mercury
  Lead
  Cadmium
  Outdated tetracycline
  Arginine or lysine infusions
Tubulointerstitial disease (chiefly and predominantly involving proximal nephron)
 Lupus erythematosus
 Acute hypersensitivity interstitial nephritis
 Acute bacterial pyelonephritis
 Obstructive uropathy
 Chronic interstitial nephritis (e.g., Sjögren's syndrome, Balkan endemic nephropathy, tubulointerstitial nephritis with uveitis)
 Fanconi's syndrome

Overflow proteinuria
Multiple myeloma
Light chain disease
Amyloidosis (see also glomerular proteinuria)
Hemoglobinuria
Myoglobinuria
Certain pancreatic or colon carcinomas (rare)

Tissue proteinuria
Acute inflammation of urinary tract
Uroepithelial tumors

IgA, immunoglobulin A; IgM, Immunoglobulin M; NSAID, nonsteroidal antiinflammatory drugs; SLE, systemic lupus erythematosus.
From Glassock RJ: Proteinuria. In Massry SG, Glassock RJ (eds): Textbook of Nephrology, 3rd ed. Baltimore, Williams & Wilkins, 1995.

(e.g., transferrin) are excreted, results from a disturbance in the permselectivity barrier and is principally seen in minimal change disease (a steroid-responsive form of nephrotic syndrome). Nonselective proteinuria, in which globulins (e.g., gamma globulin) and other higher-molecular-weight proteins are excreted in addition to albumin, is another subvariety. This is a reflection of the disturbance in the size-selective barrier of the glomerular capillary wall and is seen particularly in association with diseases that produce significant structural abnormalities in the glomerulus (e.g., focal and segmental glomerulosclerosis). The quantification of the globulin constituents of abnormal urine (e.g., immunoglobulin G [IgG], α_1-microglobulin, β_2-microglobulin, α_1-macroglobulin) have great utility in estimating prognosis and responsiveness to therapy in some glomerular diseases associated with the nephrotic syndrome (e.g., membranous nephropathy, focal and segmental glomerulosclerosis). One should not rely exclusively on the quantity of protein (or albumin) excretion to estimate the likelihood of future progression of kidney disease. The composition of the urine, especially the content of IgG and β_2-microglobulin has important predictive power as well. The total quantity of protein excreted in these various pathophysiologic states varies from slightly above normal (200 mg/day) to over 20 g/day.

Nephrotic range proteinuria is diagnosed when the protein excretion rate exceeds 3.5 gm/day in the adult (corresponding to a Up:Ucr ratio of 3.0 mg/mg). Nephrotic range proteinuria is frequently, but not exclusively, associated with underlying glomerular disease. When nephrotic range proteinuria is accompanied by hypoalbuminemia, edema, and hyperlipidemia, an underlying glomerular disease is almost invariably present. This constellation of findings is termed nephrotic syndrome.

Tubular proteinuria results from inadequate reabsorption or reclamation of normal or abnormally filtered proteins. Glomerular and tubular proteinuria can coexist, especially when tubulointerstitial injury complicates the picture of a primary glomerular disease. Isolated tubular proteinuria is usually the result of a hereditary or acquired defect in proximal tubule function (e.g., Dent's disease, Fanconi's syndrome). The proteinuria chiefly consists of alpha and beta migrating proteins on electrophoresis. Albumin is also almost invariably present. An increase in β_2-microglobulin excretion relative to albumin excretion is characteristic of tubular proteinuria. The total amount of protein excreted is usually modest, generally in the range of 200 to 2000 mg/day, corresponding to a Up:Ucr ratio below 3.0 mg/mg. The detection of tubular proteinuria requires analytic methods involving separation of proteins based on size or charge (electrophoresis, gel filtration) or immunochemical characteristics (immunofixation, immunoelectrophoresis).

Overflow proteinuria is due to the filtration of low-molecular-weight proteins across a normal glomerular capillary bed accompanied by incomplete proximal tubule reabsorption or degradation. The abnormal filtration is due to an increase in the plasma concentration of a protein in a form (size, shape, charge) that can be readily filtered. Examples include free hemoglobin (not bound to haptoglobin), myoglobin, and fragments of monoclonal immunoglobulins (light chains). The amount of protein excreted in overflow proteinuria varies widely, from trace amounts to massive quantities, even exceeding the "nephrotic" range. Detection and identification of the molecular species of overflow proteinuria depends on electrophoretic, immunochemical, or spectrophotometric analysis of urine protein composition. Monoclonal light chains are best detected by immunochemical methods (immunofixation).

Tissue proteinuria is generally associated with an inflammatory or neoplastic process within the urinary tract. It seldom exceeds 500 mg/day and is best detected by electrophoretic or immunochemical assays (e.g., secretory IgA)

These four pathophysiologic categories of abnormal proteinuria can be caused by a wide array of underlying disorders outlined in Table 4-6. The approach to diagnosing these conditions in a patient with abnormal proteinuria depends on appropriate initial classification.

Microalbuminuria is a special case of abnormal proteinuria. It escapes detection if conventional screening methods alone (e.g., dipstick) are used, but it can be detected with albumin-specific test strips and further evaluated by use of sensitive immunochemical assays for intact albumin. Quantification of albumin excretion in the microalbuminuric range (30 to 300 mg/day) is an important step in the follow-up of patients with diabetes mellitus because the development of microalbuminuria is highly correlated with the subsequent development of overt diabetic nephropathy. Microalbuminuria is also an important risk factor for cardiovascular disease.

Approach to the Evaluation of Proteinuria

The approach to the evaluation of a patient with abnormal proteinuria that has been detected on a random urine sample by semiquantitiative screening methods involves three phases: (1) initial confirmation of abnormal proteinuria by repeat measurement under more "controlled" conditions (e.g., a first morning sample of freshly voided urine); (2) preliminary investigation designed to determine the pattern and pathophysiologic type; and (3) definitive evaluation leading to a precise diagnosis.

Initial Confirmation

One should first assess whether the initial abnormal test results using dye-impregnated strips are likely to be false positives (e.g., highly buffered alkaline urine, drugs). The clinical significance of the abnormal result is diminished if the specimen was collected during a high fever, following vigorous exercise, or during the infusion of vasopressor agents. A confirmatory test using a colorimetric or turbidometric assay for total protein (e.g., heat and acetic acid or sulfosalicylic acid or a Up or Ualb:Ucr ratio on a first morning voided urine (after overnight recumbancy) is quite useful and often indicated, especially when the initial test shows only modest proteinuria (trace to 2+). Normal findings in the follow-up examination suggest a laboratory error in the initial sample or possible orthostatic proteinuria. If the Ualb:Ucr is normal, it remains possible that an overflow or tubular proteinuria is present. A wide disparity between the results of the dipstick test (weakly positive) and the turbidometric assays (strongly positive) suggest globulinuria (such as excessive monoclonal light chain excretion). Abnormal findings in the initial and follow-up studies confirm pathologic proteinuria. A freshly voided urine sediment should be examined microscopically. If hematuria or other formed elements, especially erythrocyte casts, are present, glomerular or tubulointerstitial parenchymal disease should be suspected and additional testing should be undertaken as outlined in the following sections. The confirmatory steps mentioned previously can often be omitted if the initial tests demonstrated heavy proteinuria (3+ to 4+) and if the urinary sediment displays dysmorphic hematuria.

Preliminary Investigation

In patients confirmed to have persistent abnormal proteinuria by semiquantitative testing, the urinary protein excretion rate should be quantitated by a 24-hour collection or by a Up or Ualb:Ucr ratio in a random urine specimen; the latter is the preferred method due to inaccuracies in a 24-hour collection. One can also measure the Up or Ualb:Ucr ratio in an aliquot of a 24-hour collection. If the protein excretion is over 3.5 g/day or the Up:Ucr ratio is over 3.0 mg/mg, one should suspect a glomerular or overflow cause. A test of kidney function (serum creatinine with estimation of glomerular filtration rate by use of a formula such as the Cockcroft-Gault or MDRD equations) along with a hemogram and biochemical studies of the serum should be undertaken. This should include albumin, globulin, cholesterol, calcium, phosphorus, uric acid, alkaline phosphatase, bilirubin, alanine aminotransferase, and aspartate transaminase. Ultrasonography of the kidneys should also be performed to assess size, contour, echogenicity, and urinary obstruction or vesicoureteric reflux. The history and physical examination should be thoroughly reevaluated for the possible signs and symptoms of the diseases listed in Table 4-6, with particular attention to systemic diseases and concomitant use of therapeutic agents. Clues present in the history and physical examination and the initial confirmatory tests should be used to direct further preliminary investigations and definitive evaluation. For example, as previously mentioned, a disparity between the results of the dipstick and the quantitative measures of total protein excretion in a patient with anemia, reduced kidney function, reduced anion gap, and elevated serum globulins would raise suspicion for overflow proteinuria due to the excretion of monoclonal light chains secreted by neoplastic plasma cells (multiple myeloma). This would lead to detection of the monoclonal light chain in the urine by immunochemical means and to a bone marrow biopsy to detect the abnormal plasma cell clones. Heavy proteinuria and dysmorphic hematuria associated with abnormal kidney function would lead to a preliminary investigation for glomerular disease (e.g., serologies, serum complement assay) and later to a kidney biopsy for definitive diagnosis. Modest proteinuria (less than 2.0 gm/day, or a Up:Ucr ratio less than 2.0 mg/mg) associated with signs of tubular dysfunction including renal tubular acidosis, hypophosphatemia, hypouricemia, or renal glycosuria would lead to an evaluation of tubular proteinuria (including a urinary β_2-microglobulin:albumin excretion ratio). Patients with features consistent with a systemic disease, drug-related disorder, chronic infectious disease (e.g., hepatitis B or C), or heredofamilial disorder will require additional studies directed at confirming the specific diagnosis.

In the absence of urinary sediment abnormalities, including hematuria, an evaluation for tubular or overflow proteinuria, such as cellulose acetate electrophoresis, acrylamide gel electrophoresis, immunoelectrophoresis, or β_2-microglobulin:albumin excretion ratio might be in order.

Finally, an evaluation of the anatomy of the urinary tract is usually not needed unless there is a history of recurrent urinary tract infections or unless renal masses, hydronephrosis, or multiple renal cysts are noted in the preliminary ultrasound examination. A voiding cystourethrogram may be indicated if vesicoureteric reflux nephropathy is suspected.

Definitive Evaluation

Precise diagnosis of the cause of proteinuria will be guided by the results of the initial and preliminary investigations (Table 4-7). Nephrotic range proteinuria accompanied by hypoalbuminemia, regardless of the findings in the urinary sediment, will often lead to a kidney biopsy, unless a systemic, heredofamilial, infectious, or drug-related cause is obvious. In some circumstances, even when the likely diagnosis is evident, a kidney biopsy may be performed for prognostic purposes or for therapeutic decision making. In patients with the nephrotic syndrome and no apparent underlying disease (i.e., idiopathic nephrotic syndrome), serologic investigations (C3, C4, C'H50, antineutrophil cytoplasm antibodies, anti–glomerular basement membrane antibodies, cryoglobulins, or streptococcal-related antibodies

or enzymes) may be indicated. Older patients (over 60 years of age) with the nephrotic syndrome should be suspected of having covert primary amyloidosis or a malignancy (colon, stomach, lung, breast, other) with associated membranous or membranoproliferative glomerulonephritis and should undergo a thorough physical examination looking for signs of amyloidosis or malignancy as well as urine and serum electrophoresis (or immunofixation), CT scan of the chest, stool occult blood determination, mammography (females), and prostate-specific antigen (males) as appropriate.

Subnephrotic glomerular proteinuria, especially if accompanied by abnormal urinary sediment, may be another indication for a kidney biopsy. Patients with modest proteinuria (less than 1.0 g/day or a Up:Ucr ratio of less than 1.0 mg/mg) without changes in the urinary sediment and with normal kidney function and blood pressure can often be followed without a kidney biopsy, providing overflow and tubular proteinuria have been excluded by the appropriate tests. Patients with overflow proteinuria due to abnormal light chain excretion will require an aggressive diagnostic approach, including bone marrow biopsy and skeletal radiologic survey. Patients with myoglobinuria require an evaluation for muscle damage, including an inherited muscle enzyme deficiency and drug toxicity. Patients with hemoglobinuria should be evaluated for causes of intravascular hemolysis, including erythrocyte enzyme or membrane abnormalities.

Patients with tubular proteinuria, confirmed by electrophoretic studies or an elevated β_2-microglobulin:albumin excretion ratio should undergo evaluation for heavy metal intoxication (cadmium, lead), systemic diseases such as Sjögren's syndrome, leukemia, and exposure to biologic toxins (mycotoxins). Patients

TABLE 4-7 Proteinuria: Initial Evaluation Based on Pathophysiologic Category

Pathophysiologic Category	Test
Glomerular	24-hr protein or Up:Ucr ratio Urine sediment C3, C4 Serum albumin Serum cholesterol Serum and urine immunoelectrophoresis (if amyloid suspected) Renal biopsy
Tubular	β_2-Microglobulin/albumin excretion ratio Heavy metal screen Urinary electrophoresis
Overflow	Urinary electrophoresis Serum electrophoresis Urinary light chains Urinary spectrophotometry

Ucr, urinary creatinine; Up, urinary protein.

with fixed and reproducible orthostatic proteinuria, normal kidney function and blood pressure, and a normal urine sediment examination result do not need further evaluation but should be followed at yearly intervals to be sure that evolution to constant proteinuria has not occurred. Most of the individuals with fixed and reproducible orthostatic proteinuria will eventually enter into a lasting spontaneous remission.

BIBLIOGRAPHY

Cohen RA, Brown RS: Microscopic hematuria. N Engl J Med 348: 2330–2338, 2003.

Fairley K, Birch DF: A simple method for identifying glomerular bleeding. Kidney Int 21:105–108, 1982.

Fogazzi GB, Ponticelli C, Ritz E: The Urinary Sediment: An Integrated View, 2nd ed. Oxford, UK, Oxford University Press, 1999.

Glassock R: Hematuria and pigmenturia. In Massry SG, Glassock RJ (eds): Textbook of Nephrology, 4th ed. Philadelphia, Lippincott Williams & Wilkins, 2001, pp 502–512.

Glassock R: Proteinuria. In Massry SG, Glassock RJ (eds): Textbook of Nephrology, 4th ed. Philadelphia: Lippincott Williams & Wilkins, 2001, pp 545–549.

Mallick N, Short CP: The clinical approach to hematuria and proteinuria. In Davison A, Cameron JS, Grunfeld J-P, et al (eds): Oxford Textbook of Clinical Nephrology, 2nd ed. Oxford, UK, Oxford Medical, 1998, pp 227–236.

National Kidney Foundation: Clinical practice guidelines for chronic kidney disease: Evaluation, classification and stratification. Part 4. Definition and classification of stages of chronic kidney disease. Am J Kidney Dis 39(suppl 1):46–75, 2002.

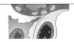

CHAPTER 5

Kidney Imaging Techniques

Timothy J. Higgins   Howard J. Mindell   Jonathan T. Fairbank

GENERAL CONSIDERATIONS

Investigation of patients with kidney disorders often requires obtaining images of the kidneys and urinary tract. Although more helpful in evaluating renal masses or disorders of the urinary outflow tract than intrinsic renal parenchymal disease, imaging studies can either establish the general pathway for further investigation or lead to a specific diagnosis. As in most organ system evaluations in general, the choice of studies proceeds from less to more invasive or expensive studies, unless the expensive or invasive study is much more likely to be definitive.

ULTRASONOGRAPHY

Ultrasonography (US) is safe, independent of kidney function, capable of multiplanar display, and does not require contrast agents or prior patient preparation. However, it lacks specificity in many instances, and it is not especially successful in differentiating among renal parenchymal diseases. Isoechoic kidney masses are often not identified. Technical problems may arise, leading to inadequate imaging. For example, in large patients tissue degrades the interrogating sound waves. In addition, intestinal gas reflects sound and may prevent delineation of the underlying structures. Although US can exquisitely demonstrate vascular occlusive disease, in many patients it is not applicable because of the technical reasons previously cited. Doppler US, even with the use of color to show flow direction, has not enjoyed wide or universal success in screening for renovascular hypertension, although newer techniques and equipment are making inroads. In addition to the limitations noted, multiple renal arteries, present in 14% to 30% of the population, may be impossible to sort out by US alone. Nevertheless, US is a mainstay of kidney imaging and is frequently the first study chosen. US can easily differentiate hydronephrosis (Fig. 5-1) from intrinsic renal parenchymal disease and renal cysts from solid tumors. Color Doppler US has unique potential, such as easily showing the presence of moving blood in a renal artery aneurysm (Fig. 5-2). US is also a useful method for delineating perinephric collections, pyelonephritic scars, and nephrocalcinosis. US can assist in evaluating kidney transplants and guide a variety of interventional approaches to the kidney. Investigations into the use of ultrasound contrast agents in kidney imaging are in progress, and early results show promise in evaluating complex cystic masses of the kidneys and improving the success of renal vascular studies.

EXCRETORY (INTRAVENOUS) UROGRAPHY

The role of the intravenous urography (IVU) is evolving with advances in other imaging techniques. Although other imaging modalities, such as US, magnetic resonance imaging (MRI), and computed tomography (CT), may provide more detail regarding the kidney parenchyma, IVU remains an inexpensive, widely available test that gives excellent detail of the urothelium. Lesions such as transitional cell carcinoma of the renal pelvis, ureters, and bladder may in some cases be seen only with the detail provided by conventional radiography. Indications for IVU include hematuria, tuberculosis, evaluation for scarring in chronic pyelonephritis, papillary necrosis, and a variety of congenital anomalies. However, IVU can no longer be recommended as the sole imaging study to evaluate for a kidney mass. In most institutions, CT sections have been added to IVU, the result being a hybrid, "CTU." CTU offers increased parenchymal resolution over the linear tomographic sections ordinarily available with IVU. CTU may consist of an initial nonenhanced scan for the detection of urinary tract stones, followed by enhanced scans to detect kidney, ureteral, or bladder masses. To completely evaluate the collecting system, delayed conventional plain film urograms are obtained following CT, or a three-dimensional computer work station is used to reconstruct coronal plane images to replicate IVU. Unenhanced helical CT has replaced IVU for the diagnosis of renal colic (see later section on Urolithiasis). Radiation exposure is significantly increased with the CTU technique, which is of concern for pregnant or younger patients. When the collecting systems must be examined, but CTU/IVU is inadequate because chronic kidney disease limits excretion of radiographic contrast and urinary tract visualization, retrograde urography or percutaneous antegrade urography may be needed. Another option in the setting of chronic kidney disease or pregnancy is magnetic resonance urography (MRU), which, although not as well developed as CTU, is

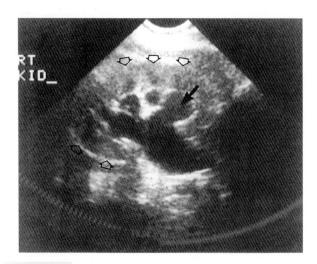

FIGURE 5-1 Ultrasound image showing a sagittal section through the right kidney. The single black arrow indicates a dilated calyx in the lower pole. Note how the calyx connects to the dilated renal pelvis (black, fluid-filled). Multiple open arrows indicate the margin of the renal cortex.

emerging as an alternative in some institutions. MRU is not nearly as sensitive as CT for urinary tract stones. In addition, spatial resolution is poor in comparison with CT and IVU with regard to evaluating calyces, infundibulae, or ureters.

The contrast media used for IVU and other studies may result in acute reactions as an untoward side effect, so-called "idiosyncratic" reactions, or, alternatively, may cause contrast media–induced nephropathy (i.e., acute renal failure). Idiosyncratic reactions involve some 0.1% to 0.2% of patients, and such events may result in allergic-like symptoms of urticaria, wheezing, and dyspnea; hypotension or chest pain less frequently; and in rare instances anaphylaxis and cardiovascular collapse. The fatality rate, difficult to estimate because of its rarity, may approach 1 in 100,000. Pretreatment with steroids or the use of newer nonionic or low osmolality contrast reduces the frequency of mild or severe reactions, but there is no conclusive evidence of a lower fatality rate with the nonionic contrast agents. Low osmolar contrast has become the standard of use in most institutions. The use of isosmolar contrast in the form of iodixanol has been shown in one study to significantly reduce the risk for contrast-induced nephropathy in patients with mild chronic kidney disease and diabetes, and some institutions routinely use this agent for patients at high risk for acute renal failure.

The risk for contrast nephropathy is highest in patients with diabetic nephropathy, intermediate in patients with chronic kidney disease due to other causes, and low or normal for diabetics without kidney disease. There are no absolute contraindications to the use of intravenous contrast, but it should be used with circumspection in such settings as advanced age, debility, congestive heart failure, and multiple myeloma. Patients with volume depletion are at much higher risk. Intravascular volume should be restored by fluid administration before contrast is given. Overnight expansion with 0.5% saline affords protection in patients who are not volume depleted (see Chapter 35). The prophylactic administration of acetylcysteine has also been shown in some studies to reduce the risk of contrast nephropathy in patients with chronic kidney disease.

These comments about side effects of administration of radiographic contrast apply no matter what the procedure for which the contrast material is used. They are not specific to IVU, and concern about contrast

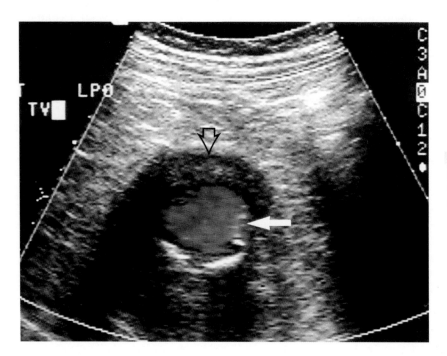

FIGURE 5-2 Color Doppler ultrasound image of renal artery aneurysm. Arrow to the aneurysm "lit up" in red by turbulent arterial flow.

administration must be taken into account when CT with contrast or angiography is requested. Finally, the visualization of the urinary tract is diminished when the serum creatinine exceeds 2 to 3 mg/dL; IVU is unlikely to successfully visualize the collecting system when the serum creatinine exceeds 4 mg/dL. Therefore, the risk for increased contrast administration should be weighed against its diminished potential benefit in these patients. In patients with endstage renal disease who are maintained on dialysis, the issue of contrast-induced nephropathy is not relevant. The sole risks of contrast administration are the idiosyncratic reactions previously described and volume overload due to the small amount of intravascular expansion produced by administration of approximately 100 mL of contrast agent. It is not necessary to follow contrast administration with dialysis unless clinical evidence of volume overload develops after the radiographic procedure.

PLAIN ABDOMINAL RADIOGRAPHY

The plain abdominal (kidney, ureter, and bladder [KUB]) radiograph, while a standard prelude (scout film) for IVU, may be requested alone or in conjunction with US. Renal or ureteric calculi usually contain calcium and are visible on the KUB image, although the former may require oblique views to confirm an intrarenal location (as opposed to the more anterior gallbladder, etc.), and the latter may require IVU to differentiate from pelvic phleboliths. Urinary tract calculi may, when large enough, be followed by plain films after identification by renal colic CT, instead of serial CT scans to reduce radiation exposure.

COMPUTED TOMOGRAPHY

Computed tomography offers far greater contrast resolution than conventional radiography, with detailed anatomic cross-sectional anatomic imaging unaffected by overlying structures such as bone or gas. Virtually the entire urinary system and retroperitoneum are well visualized on CT. This modality has the definitive role in staging kidney neoplasms and in imaging the kidneys in trauma. CT is useful in the diagnosis of pyelonephritis and its complications and of renal cystic disorders. With arterial occlusive disease, CT can show perfusion defects, where contrast fails to opacify segments of the kidney parenchyma, and recent work has shown that three-dimensional reconstruction with helical CT shows the renal arteries directly and can be used to accurately diagnose renal artery stenosis. With venous occlusive disease, CT can show flow abnormalities and stasis in the affected kidney and can directly show thrombus in the renal vein. Unenhanced helical CT has essentially replaced IVU in renal colic because it may show tiny calculi precisely, even urate stones that were invisible on conventional radiography. It also demonstrates hydronephrosis, hydroureter, and other pertinent findings (Fig. 5-3); frequently nonrenal pathologies such as appendicitis or diverticulitis are revealed on a renal colic study. Surgical planning is greatly assisted by three-dimensional reconstruction in the setting of kidney neoplasm. CTU is invaluable in the workup of patients with hematuria, as described earlier. The sensitivity of CTU for upper tract uroepithelial neoplasia has been reported to be 95%. A caveat for CT evaluation of hematuria is the lack of sensitivity for flat transitional cell carcinomas of the bladder.

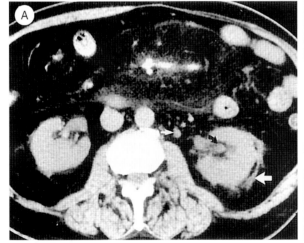 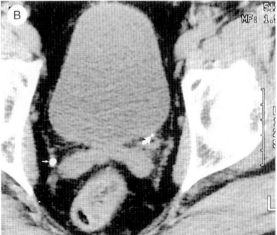

FIGURE 5-3 *A,* Unenhanced CT at the level of the kidneys. Patient with obstruction secondary to calculus at left ureterovesical junction. Black arrow to dilated renal pelvis; small white arrow to proximal hydroureter. Large white arrow to extravasation of urine secondary to ruptured calyx due to acute obstruction. *B,* Same patient, unenhanced CT at the level of the bladder. Curved arrow to 3-mm calculus in the left ureterovesical junction. Note flattening of the ipsilateral bladder wall, left ureter coursing to the calculus. Straight arrow to an incidental phlebolith; note the pelvic vein containing the phlebolith.

MAGNETIC RESONANCE IMAGING

Magnetic resonance imaging depends on first aligning the spins of the hydrogen nuclei (protons) of body tissues with a powerful magnetic field and then applying radiofrequency (RF) pulses to deflect these spins. Energy released in these circumstances can be measured and used to create anatomic images dependent on characteristics of the tissues and the introduced magnetic and RF energy sources. MRI offers superb tissue contrast with multiplanar imaging capabilities, although calcification is not well visualized. MRI is safe and uses no ionizing radiation, although MRI contrast agents such as gadolinium may rarely cause side effects or reactions such as urticaria or bronchospasm. MRI may not be suitable for use in claustrophobic patients or those with implanted ferromagnetic devices, such as pacemakers. MRI has a limited role in defining specific parenchymal lesions at present, although its sensitivity to iron in hemoglobin permits its use to image the kidneys in patients with paroxysmal nocturnal hemoglobinuria, myoglobinuria, and epidemic Korean fever. MRI can effectively show the renal vasculature, and magnetic resonance angiography (MRA) has replaced conventional angiography or is a rival to computed tomographic angiography (CTA) at many centers in assessing various arterial lesions such as renal artery stenosis. MRI has the following roles in kidney imaging:

1. Delineating complex masses, where CT is not definitive.
2. Staging kidney neoplasms, particularly in evaluating for renal vein or inferior vena caval extension of tumor, usually after CT is not definitive or where the patient is reactive to iodinated contrast agents.
3. Diagnosing renovascular lesions.
4. Where reduced kidney function or contrast media reactivity preclude the use of other modalities. MRU, the MR equivalent of KUB radiography, after the use of intravenous gadolinium, offers imaging roughly comparable with IVU. This technique is used at some centers, mainly to show hydronephrosis or hydroureter.
5. Evaluation of potential living kidney donors and transplanted kidneys.

RADIONUCLIDE IMAGING

For nuclear medicine studies, radiopharmaceutical agents with specific renal handling characteristics are used (Table 5-1). These agents are administered, and then the patient is imaged with a gamma camera that can record the number of counts emitted and the location of their source. This permits quantification of function in a specific region as well as anatomic delineation. Nuclear medicine techniques are particularly useful in assessing the adequacy of renal perfusion and in determining

TABLE 5-1 Most Commonly Used Radiopharmaceuticals in Kidney Imaging

Radionuclide	Mechanism of Renal Action	Major Clinical Usefulness
^{99m}Tc DTPA	Glomerular filtration	Perfusion Parenchymal imaging Estimate GFR Excretion
^{99m}Tc DMSA	Tubular binding and tubular secretion	Pyelonephritis Estimation of tubular mass (i.e., cortical scar)
^{99m}Tc GHP	Glomerular filtration, tubular secretion, tubular binding	Perfusion Excretion Estimation of tubular mass
^{99m}Tc MAG3	Tubular secretion and glomerular filtration	High renal extraction and useful images even with moderate kidney dysfunction Estimate ERPF
^{67}Ga citrate	N/A	Pyelonephritis Interstitial nephritis Renal abscess
^{99m}Tc-labeled, ^{111}In-labeled WBCs	N/A	Renal abscess

DMSA, 2,3-dimercaptosuccinic acid; DTPA, diethylenetriamine-penta-acetic acid; ERPF, effective renal plasma flow; GFR, glomerular filtration rate; MAG3, mercaptoacetyltriglycine; N/A, not applicable; WBC, white blood cell.

whether the outflow tract is intact. Kidney parenchymal integrity may also be assessed.

The scanning method is varied according to the nature of the information sought. When anatomic information is desired, the scanning interval for each image typically encompasses several minutes. Late views may be obtained after a delay of hours. In contrast, when flow is being studied, images are typically of only a few seconds in duration. Although the spatial resolution of nuclear medicine studies cannot match the other imaging modalities, it is superior in assessing renal physiology. Modern gamma cameras are equipped with single-photon emission computed tomography, which renders three-dimensional images that greatly enhance anatomic detail. The following are some of the most common uses of nuclear medicine studies:

1. *Measurement of renal function.* Radionuclide studies permit calculation of glomerular filtration rate (GFR) and effective renal plasma flow (ERPF), even in cases of impaired kidney function. Appropriate radionuclides are injected intravenously and images obtained. The most accurate calculations of GFR and ERPF are obtained by withdrawing blood samples at predetermined intervals and using standard clearance calculations, but strictly count-based computer imaging

methods now closely rival this method, without requiring blood samples. These studies may also be performed in patients unsuitable for contrast media injections. Allergic reactions to radiotracers are extremely rare. To determine whether nephrectomy is warranted or safe, it is often important for the surgeon to know the relative contribution to total renal function of each kidney. Computer-enhanced scan techniques can determine the contribution of each kidney to ERPF or GFR. Split renal function measurements are also helpful in follow-up of surgical procedures that relieve unilateral obstruction.

3. *Renovascular hypertension.* Differential renal blood flow studies using technetium 99m mercaptoacetyl-triglycine (MAG3) before and after administration of an angiotensin-converting enzyme inhibitor such as captopril in an appropriately screened hypertensive patient with intact renal function will detect renovascular disease with a sensitivity and specificity exceeding 90%.

4. *Evaluation of kidney transplants.* Radionuclide imaging may detect impaired blood flow at the renal arterial anastomotic site, urinary tract obstruction, and extravasation of urine due to disruption at the ureteric anastomosis (Fig. 5-4A, B). This modality complements US for these purposes.

5. *Obstructive uropathy.* The diuretic renogram is helpful, particularly in children who demonstrate an enlarged renal pelvis by US or IVU. This test distinguishes between true obstruction at the ureteropelvic junction and nonobstructive hydronephrosis. Furosemide is injected before or after administration of ^{99m}Tc diethylenetriamine-penta-acetic acid or MAG3, renal images are obtained, and a renogram curve of activity in each kidney is constructed. Dilation without significant obstruction is suggested when radionuclide accumulation in the dilated area is reduced at high urine flow rates.

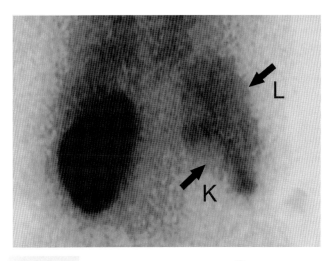

FIGURE 5-5 Posterior image after injection of ^{99m}Tc 2,3-dimercaptosuccinic acid (DMSA). The left kidney is normal. On the right there is evidence of hydronephrosis and marked cortical atrophy (*K arrow*) as a result of chronic obstruction and scarring. The liver is indicated by an L arrow.

6. *Renal infection or scar.* The IVU may appear normal in patients with pyelonephritis, and the differentiation between this and cystitis may be difficult. 99m-Dimercaptosuccinic acid and glucoheptonate are renal cortical scanning agents. Areas of inflammation or scar demonstrate no uptake (Fig. 5-5). The agents are also helpful in determining the amount of remaining renal cortex in children with chronic urinary tract infections and vesicoureteric reflux. ^{99m}Tc- or indium 111–labeled white blood cells (WBCs) may be used to identify kidney abscesses. In patients with low WBC counts, gallium 67 may be used.

Positron emission tomography (PET) is a functional imaging technique using a glucose molecule tagged to a short-lived radioisotope. This compound, fluorodeoxyglucose (FDG), is an indicator of tumor glucose metabolism and is being studied for the detection of renal cell carcinoma and its spread. Because FDG is normally excreted by the kidneys, small primary tumors may be difficult to distinguish, but PET can play an essential role in monitoring progression of disease, metastasis, or local recurrence.

ANGIOGRAPHY

Renal angiography can be used for diagnostic or for therapeutic purposes.

Diagnostic Angiography

1. *Suspected artery lesions.* Renal angiography is the definitive imaging procedure when renovascular hypertension is suspected, although catheter angiography is increasingly challenged at many centers, as previously

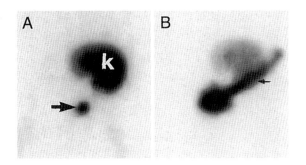

FIGURE 5-4 *A,* Kidney transplant scan (5 minutes after injection) with ^{99m}Tc MAG3 showing tracer in kidney and bladder. K, kidney; arrow to urinary bladder. *B,* Scan at 30 minutes showing leak of tracer due to ureteric necrosis at anastomosis site. Arrow to extravasation of radioactive urine. Note fading activity in kidney, increased size of bladder overlapping inferior margin of extravasation.

indicated, by CTA (Fig. 5-6A, B) and MRA. Such angiography is indicated if medical therapy for hypertension is ineffective, or in young patients with significant hypertension in whom medication may be needed for many decades. The patient also should be a suitable candidate for surgical or angioplastic therapy. Renal vein sampling for renin levels may help in selecting patients for treatment. Patients with acute occlusion or thrombosis of the renal arteries, embolic processes, or post-traumatic renal vascular injury may be candidates for renal angiography. In patients with polyarteritis nodosa, renal angiography is the only method with sufficient resolution to detect the characteristic tiny peripheral aneurysms.

2. *Unexplained hematuria.* Because of the availability of helical CT, angiography is now less likely to be required to investigate the cause of unexplained hematuria, but occasionally angiography is still indispensable. Vascular malformations may be suspected on US or CT but generally require angiography for definitive delineation, especially if the use of catheter injected coils, gelfoam, or other therapeutic agents is contemplated.

3. *Kidney transplantation.* Angiography may be required to map the arterial system in prospective kidney donors, where multiple renal arteries or vascular anomalies may complicate transplant surgery; however, MRA may prove more suitable for this task with its multiprojection capabilities. Angiography may be required to diagnose posttransplantation renal artery stenoses or occlusions. US, CTA, and MRA are increasingly assuming this role, depending on local circumstances and preferences.

4. *Renal vein disorders.* Although renal vein thrombosis or occlusion may be shown by US, CT, or MRI, rarely direct angiographic renal venography may be required when there are problems or uncertainties with the other methods.

5. *Miscellaneous.* Complex or highly unusual renal masses, complications of polycystic disease such as superimposed neoplasm, or trauma may require angiography.

Interventional Angiography

Angiography has become increasingly important as a therapeutic maneuver rather than a diagnostic test alone, and in many angio-interventional radiology sections, therapy far overshadows straight diagnostic imaging in terms of daily workload. Balloon angioplasty treatment is now widely accepted and may be used to dilate renal artery stenosis in both native and transplanted kidneys (see Fig. 5-6B). Ostial lesions previously thought to be refractory to this method may be amenable to endovascular stenting. Angiography may also be used to embolize bleeding sites within the kidney that may have resulted from trauma or as a complication of interventional procedures such as percutaneous biopsy. Angiography may also be used for selective infusion of thrombolytic agents for treatment of renal artery or vein thrombosis.

Voiding Cystourethrography

This study is useful in demonstrating vesicoureteric reflux. Voiding cystourethrography is most commonly performed with fluoroscopic techniques, but radionuclide methods have similar sensitivities in the detection of vesicoureteric reflux.

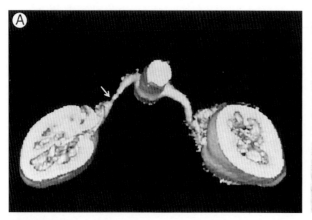 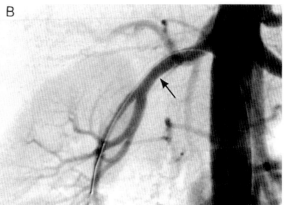

FIGURE 5-6   *A,* Computed tomographic angiography (CTA) showing the computer-generated three-dimensional reconstruction of the aorta and the main renal arteries, possible after a simple intravenous injection of contrast media. The arrow indicates a significant stenosis in the main right renal artery. *B,* Selective right renal angiogram after successful angioplasty, in the same patient as in Figure 5-4A, with an arrow showing the now patent right main renal artery. (Courtesy of Dr. Ken Najarian, FAHC, Burlington, Vermont.)

CHOICE OF IMAGING PROCEDURE FOR SPECIFIC CLINICAL SITUATIONS

Arterial Disease

Ultrasonography can readily diagnose aortic aneurysm, but CT is more accurate where aneurysmal bleeding is suspected, and CT or CTA is better for surgical planning, especially to show the exact levels of the renal arteries. CT can diagnose acute renal infarction by showing parenchymal perfusion defects with a peripheral "rim sign" of collateral flow.

The imaging choices for the diagnosis of renovascular hypertension are now many. Angiotensin-converting enzyme inhibition scintigraphy is useful for evaluating the functional significance of renal artery stenosis, with a sensitivity of 90% and specificity of almost 100% being reported. In the realm of anatomic imaging, strides have been made in the improvement of Doppler US as a screening tool, which can provide significant cost savings in comparison with other methods. Although technical and operator factors have to be considered as described earlier, high sensitivity and specificity can be achieved in experienced hands. MRA of the renal arteries has reported sensitivity and specificity for renal artery stenosis of 97% and 92%, while those of CT angiography are 94% and 99%, respectively. The gold standard, catheter angiography, should be reserved for those patients at highest risk for renal artery stenosis. MRA should be considered the initial screening test of choice for renal artery stenosis secondary to its sensitivity and safety.

Congenital Disorders

The most common congenital renal anomalies for which imaging is used are the various forms of renal ectopia, fusion anomalies such as horseshoe kidney, and obstructive processes of the ureteropelvic junction (UPJ) or distal ureter. US and IVU or CTU are the primary imaging tools in evaluating these lesions, although occasionally horseshoe kidney (Fig. 5-7) or another anomaly presents as an incidental finding on MRI or nuclear medicine study such as a bone scan, where the radiopharmaceutical is excreted by the kidneys. UPJ obstruction may be further evaluated by diuretic urography or radionuclide renography.

Inflammatory Diseases

Computed tomography can be used to diagnose acute pyelonephritis by showing peripheral perfusion defects in the renal parenchyma, frequently with edema in the perinephric fat. When urinary tract infections follow an atypical or protracted course, US (or with better specificity, CT) can delineate infected renal cysts, abscesses,

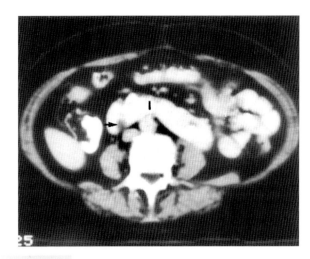

FIGURE 5-7   CT through the isthmus of a horseshoe kidney. *I* is on the isthmus, and the arrow points to an incidental cyst in the attached lower pole of the right kidney.

or infected perirenal collections. Either US or CT can guide interventional procedures for diagnosis and treatment. Tuberculosis causes strictures of the renal collecting systems or ureters, and the diagnosis may be suggested by IVU/CTU findings. Chronic pyelonephritis, frequently associated with reflux nephropathy, produces scarred kidneys readily shown on IVU or cross-sectional imaging.

Neoplasia

The main grouping of kidney tumors divides renal parenchymal masses from urothelial lesions. Although cystic or solid renal parenchymal masses may be first detected by IVU, they require US, CT, or MRI for further differentiation and staging (Fig. 5-8). Urothelial tumors, nearly always transitional cell carcinoma (TCC), are sometimes best shown on IVU or retrograde pyelography, the latter serving as a guide for brush biopsy. The detection of small TCCs of the ureter or bladder is one reason CT has not totally supplanted IVU as a screening tool in hematuria, although in selected patients cross-sectional imaging may be required to confirm or further delineate such lesions. Multiplanar reconstruction with three-dimensional CT or even three-dimensional MRI of renal tumors is used to stage renal neoplasm, especially when partial nephrectomy is considered.

Cystic Disorders

Benign renal cysts occur in up to 30% of normal adults and can nearly always be readily differentiated from solid neoplasms by US. Complex cysts may require CT for definitive evaluation. Both infantile autosomal-recessive and adult autosomal-dominant polycystic renal disease is

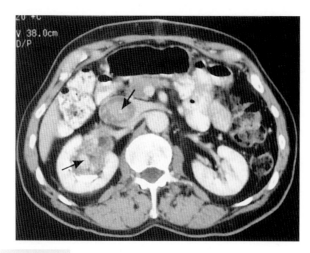

FIGURE 5-8   Computed tomogram showing renal carcinoma. This cross-section through the level of the kidneys was obtained using oral and intravenous contrast media. The lower black arrow points to the irregularly radiolucent, necrotic tumor mass. The second black arrow, higher in position as the reader views the illustration, points to a filling defect in the interior vena cava, representing tumor thrombus. A normal cava would be homogeneously bright with enhancing blood, like the aorta.

readily diagnosed by US. Medullary sponge kidney is diagnosed by IVU or CTU.

Trauma

Helical CT is used in evaluating kidney trauma because of its speed, its accuracy, and its multiorgan sweep. CT also may assess the renal vascular supply, although conventional angiography is required in selected cases or major renovascular trauma, where diagnosis or therapy is required. For suspected bladder rupture, CT cystography is the method of choice. For suspected urethral rupture in men, retrograde urethrography remains the procedure of choice.

Parenchymal Disorders

Renal parenchymal disease consists of a broad range of processes, from inflammatory or immunologic disorders to toxic or ischemic lesions. Imaging can show small kidneys, and US may demonstrate echogenic abnormal parenchyma, but rarely pinpoints the diagnosis, which may require kidney biopsy. The main goal of imaging is to rule out obstruction, polycystic kidney disease, renal papillary necrosis, vascular disease, or reflux nephropathy. For patients presenting with impaired kidney function, US is an excellent noninvasive method to differentiate intrinsic parenchymal disease from obstructive uropathy.

Urolithiasis

Most urinary calculi are calcified and therefore are readily detectable by KUB radiography. Radiolucent stones on plain radiography, primarily composed of uric acid, appear as filling defects within the opacified urinary tract on IVU. IVU also shows obstruction by virtue of demonstrating hydronephrosis or hydroureter related to the obstructing calculus. Retrograde pyelography may be required to plan therapy where stent placement is needed, and KUB images may assist in follow-up of calculus material treated by extracorporeal shock wave therapy. US has a limited role in patients with urinary calculi: it can show nephrocalcinosis or nephrolithiasis and occasionally urinary bladder calculi, but is insensitive for ureteric stones. The major innovation in the diagnosis of renal colic has been the conversion from the use of IVU to unenhanced helical abdominal CT, the so-called renal colic CT protocol. Helical CT (see Fig. 5-3A, B) has completely replaced IVU in many centers when renal colic is suspected. CT is quick, requires no patient preparation, is without any side effects since no intravenous contrast is used, is highly accurate and sensitive, and can precisely locate and measure the size of ureteric stones. CT shows calculi not visible on KUB images; virtually all calculi, regardless of their chemical composition, are visible. CT can show obstruction and extravasation of urine and help in planning therapy.

Kidney Transplantation

Kidney transplantation donors need US preoperatively and, as previously indicated, depending on institutional preferences, angiography, CTA, or MRA, to assess vascular anatomy. In recipients posttransplantation, color flow Doppler US documents the status of vascular perfusion to the transplanted kidney, and US can document hydronephrosis, renal volumes, and extrarenal collections such as lymphocele, but cannot reliably differentiate rejection from acute tubular necrosis. Radionuclide studies can also assess perfusion or obstruction, and rarely retrograde or even percutaneous antegrade pyelography is required to assess ureteral patency. Angiography may be needed to show renal artery stenoses to the transplant. MRI is increasingly being used for both pretransplantation evaluation of donors and posttransplantation evaluation of the transplanted kidney.

Ureteral Obstruction

Bilateral ureteric obstruction causing kidney function to decline is rare in adults in the absence of malignancy. Although specific lesions such as retroperitoneal fibrosis must be considered, US can show hydronephrosis and is generally used as the first imaging procedure in patients with acute renal failure. US can readily differentiate obstructive hydronephrosis with ureterectasis from other causes of renal failure where the calyces may be normal but the kidney parenchyma may be diminished or scarred, such as in chronic pyelonephritis. Acute unilateral ureteric obstruction, commonly due to renal colic with passage of a ureteric calculus, is readily diagnosed by IVU or helical CT.

Renal Vein Lesions

Diagnostic imaging of the renal vein is now nearly always done during the course of cross-sectional imaging (US, CT, or MRI). In difficult presentations, MR or CT venography is the study of choice.

BIBLIOGRAPHY

Aspelin P, Aubry P, Fransson S, et al: Nephrotoxic effects in high risk patients undergoing angiography. N Engl J Med 348:491–499, 2003.

Birck R, Krzossok S, Markowetz F: Acetylcysteine for prevention of contrast nephropathy: Meta-analysis. Lancet 362:598–603, 2003.

Dodd GD, Tublin ME, Shah A, Zajko AB: Imaging of vascular complications associated with renal transplants [Review]. AJR 157:449–459, 1991.

Fielding JR, Silverman SG, Rubin GD: Helical CT of the urinary tract [Review]. AJR 172:1199–1206, 1999.

Hartman RP, Kawashima A, King BF: Evaluation of renal causes of hypertension. Radiol Clin North Am 41:909–929, 2003.

Hussain SM, Kock MC, Ijzermans JN, et al: MR imaging: A "one stop shop" modality for preoperative evaluation of living kidney donors. Radiographics 23:505–520, 2003.

Lanoue MZ, Mindell HJ: Pictorial essay. The use of unenhanced helical CT to evaluate suspected renal colic. AJR 169:1579–1584, 1997.

Kawashima A, Glockner JF, King BF: CT urography and MR urography. Radiol Clin North Am 41:945–961, 2003.

Mindell HJ, Cochran ST: Current perspectives in the diagnosis and treatment of urinary stone disease [Commentary]. AJR 163:1314–1315, 1994.

Robbin ML, Lockhart ME, Barr RG: Renal imaging with ultrasound contrast: Current status. Radiol Clin North Am 41:963–978, 2003.

Shvarts O, Han K, Seltzer M, et al: Positron emission tomography in urologic oncology. Cancer Control 9:335–342, 2002.

Solomon R, Warner C, Mann D, et al: Effects of saline, mannitol and furosemide on acute decreases in renal function produced by radiocontrast agents. N Engl J Med 331:1416–1420. 1994.

Taylor A: Radionuclide renography: A personal approach. Semin Nucl Med 29(2):102–127, 1999.

Tublin ME, Murphy ME, Tessler FN: Current concepts in contrast media-induced nephropathy [Review]. AJR 171:933–939, 1998.

Zagoria RJ, Berchtold RE, Dyer RB: Staging of renal adenocarcinoma: Role of various imaging procedures. AJR 164:363–370, 1995.

Acid-Base, Fluid, and Electrolyte Disorders

CHAPTER 6

Hyponatremia and Hypo-osmolar Disorders

Joseph G. Verbalis

The incidence of hyponatremia depends on the patient population and the criteria used to define hyponatremia. Hospital incidences of 15% to 22% are common if hyponatremia is defined as any serum [Na$^+$] less than 135 mEq/L, but in most studies only 1% to 4% of patients have a serum [Na$^+$] under 130 mEq/L, and fewer than 1% have levels under 120 mEq/L. Recent studies have confirmed prevalences from 7% in ambulatory populations to 28% in acutely hospitalized patients. The elderly are particularly susceptible to hyponatremia, with reported incidences as high as 53% in institutionalized geriatric patients. Although most cases are mild, hyponatremia is important clinically because (1) acute severe hyponatremia can cause substantial morbidity and mortality; (2) mild hyponatremia can progress to more dangerous levels during management of other disorders; (3) general mortality is higher in hyponatremic patients with a wide range of underlying diseases; and (4) overly rapid correction of chronic hyponatremia can produce severe neurologic deficits and death.

DEFINITIONS

Hyponatremia is of clinical significance only when it reflects corresponding hypo-osmolality of the plasma. Plasma osmolality (P$_{osm}$) can be measured directly by osmometry or calculated as follows:

$$P_{osm} \text{ (mOsm/kg H}_2\text{O)} = 2 \times \text{serum [Na}^+\text{] (mEq/L)} +$$
$$\text{glucose (mg/dL)}/18 + \text{blood urea nitrogen (mg/dL)}/2.8$$

Both methods produce comparable results under most conditions, as does simply doubling the serum [Na$^+$]. However, total osmolality is not always equivalent to effective osmolality, sometimes referred to as the tonicity of the plasma. Solutes predominantly compartmentalized to the extracellular fluid (ECF) are effective solutes because they create osmotic gradients across cell membranes, leading to osmotic movement of water from the intracellular fluid (ICF) to ECF compartments. In contrast, solutes that freely permeate cell membranes (urea, ethanol, methanol) are not effective solutes because they do not create osmotic gradients across cell membranes and therefore are not associated with secondary water shifts. Only the concentration of effective solutes in plasma should be used to determine whether clinically significant hypo-osmolality is present.

Hyponatremia and hypo-osmolality are usually synonymous, but with two important exceptions. First, pseudohyponatremia can be produced by marked elevation of serum lipids or proteins. In such cases the concentration of Na$^+$ per liter of serum water is unchanged, but the concentration of Na$^+$ per liter of serum is artifactually decreased because of the increased relative proportion occupied by lipid or protein. Although measurement of serum or plasma [Na$^+$] by ion-specific electrodes currently used by most clinical laboratories is less influenced by high concentrations of lipids or proteins than is measurement of serum [Na$^+$] by flame photometry, such errors nonetheless still occur. However, because direct measurement of P$_{osm}$ is based on the colligative properties of only the solute particles in solution, the measured P$_{osm}$ will not be affected by increased lipids or proteins. Second, high concentrations of effective solutes other than Na$^+$ can cause relative decreases in serum [Na$^+$] despite an unchanged P$_{osm}$; this commonly occurs with hyperglycemia. Misdiagnosis can be avoided again by direct measurement of P$_{osm}$, or by correcting the serum [Na$^+$] by 1.6 mEq/L for each 100 mg/dL increase in blood glucose concentration above 100 mg/dL (although recent studies have suggested that a more accurate correction factor may be closer to 2.4 mEq/L).

PATHOGENESIS

The presence of significant hypo-osmolality indicates excess water relative to solute in the ECF. Because water moves freely between the ICF and ECF, this also therefore indicates an excess of total body water relative to total body solute. Imbalances between water and solute can be generated initially either by depletion of body solute more than body water, or by dilution of body solute from increases in body water more than body solute (Table 6-1). It should be recognized, however, that this distinction represents an oversimplification, because most hypo-osmolar states include variable components of both solute depletion and water retention (e.g., isotonic solute losses, as occurs during an acute hemorrhage, do not produce hypo-osmolality until the subsequent retention

TABLE 6-1 Pathogenesis of Hypo-osmolar Disorders

Depletion (primary decreases in total body solute + secondary water retention)*:
- Renal solute loss
  - Diuretic use
  - Solute diuresis (glucose, mannitol)
  - Salt-wasting nephropathy
  - Mineralocorticoid deficiency
- Nonrenal solute loss
  - Gastrointestinal (diarrhea, vomiting, pancreatitis, bowel obstruction)
  - Cutaneous (sweating, burns)
  - Blood loss

Dilution (primary increases in total body water ± secondary solute depletion)†:
- Impaired renal free water excretion
  - Increased proximal reabsorption
    - Hypothyroidism
  - Impaired distal dilution
    - Syndrome of inappropriate antidiuretic hormone secretion (SIADH)
    - Glucocorticoid deficiency
  - Combined increased proximal reabsorption and impaired distal dilution
    - Congestive heart failure
    - Cirrhosis
    - Nephrotic syndrome
  - Decreased urinary solute excretion
    - Beer potomania
- Excess water intake
  - Primary polydipsia
  - Dilute infant formula

*Virtually all disorders of solute depletion are accompanied by some degree of secondary retention of water by the kidneys in response to the resulting intravascular hypovolemia; this mechanism can lead to hypo-osmolality even when the solute depletion occurs via hypotonic or isotonic body fluid losses.

†Disorders of water retention primarily cause hypo-osmolality in the absence of any solute losses, but in some cases of SIADH secondary solute losses occur in response to the resulting intravascular hypervolemia and this can then further aggravate the hypo-osmolality (however, this pathophysiology does not likely contribute to the hyponatremia of edema-forming states such as congestive heart failure and cirrhosis, since in these cases multiple factors favoring sodium retention will result in an increased total body sodium).

Modified from Verbalis JG: The syndrome of inappropriate antidiuretic hormone secretion and other hypoosmolar disorders. In Schrier RW (ed): Diseases of the Kidney. Philadelphia, Lippincott Williams & Wilkins, 2001, pp 2511–2548.

of water from ingested or infused hypotonic fluids causes a secondary dilution of the remaining ECF solute). Nonetheless, this concept has proven to be useful because it provides a framework for understanding the diagnosis and therapy of hypo-osmolar disorders.

DIFFERENTIAL DIAGNOSIS

The diagnostic approach to hypo-osmolar patients should include a careful history (especially concerning medications); physical examination with emphasis on clinical assessment of the ECF volume status and a thorough neurologic evaluation; serum or plasma electrolytes, glucose, blood urea nitrogen (BUN), creatinine, and uric acid; calculated or directly measured P_{osm}; and simultaneous urine sodium and osmolality. Although prevalences vary according to the population being studied, a sequential analysis of hyponatremic patients admitted to a large university teaching hospital revealed that approximately 20% were hypovolemic, 20% had edema-forming states, 33% were euvolemic, 15% had hyperglycemia-induced hyponatremia, and 10% had impaired kidney function. Consequently, euvolemic hyponatremia generally constitutes the largest single group of hyponatremic patients found in this setting. A definitive diagnosis is not always possible at the time of presentation, but an initial categorization according to the patient's clinical ECF volume status will allow a determination of the appropriate initial therapy in most cases (Fig. 6-1).

Decreased Extracellular Fluid Volume (Hypovolemia)

Clinically detectable hypovolemia, generally determined most sensitively by careful measurement of orthostatic changes in blood pressure and pulse rate, usually indicates some degree of solute depletion. Elevation of BUN and uric acid are useful laboratory correlates of decreased ECF volume. Even isotonic or hypotonic volume losses can lead to hypo-osmolality if water or hypotonic fluids are ingested or infused as replacement. A low urine Na^+ concentration (U_{Na}) in such cases suggests a nonrenal cause of the solute depletion, whereas a high U_{Na} suggests renal causes of solute depletion (see Table 6-1). Diuretic use is the most common cause of hypovolemic hypo-osmolality, and thiazides are more commonly associated with severe hyponatremia than are loop diuretics such as furosemide. Although this represents a prime example of solute depletion, the pathophysiologic mechanisms underlying the hypo-osmolality are complex and are composed of multiple potential components, including free water retention. Many such patients do not manifest clinical evidence of marked hypovolemia, in part because ingested water has been retained in response to nonosmotically stimulated arginine vasopressin (AVP) secretion, as is generally true for all disorders of solute depletion. To further complicate diagnosis, the U_{Na} may be high or low depending on when the last diuretic dose was taken. Consequently, any suspicion of diuretic use mandates careful consideration of this diagnosis. A low serum $[K^+]$ is an important clue to diuretic use, because few other disorders that cause hyponatremia and hypo-osmolality also produce appreciable hypokalemia. Whenever the possibility of diuretic use is suspected in the absence of a positive history, a urine screen for diuretics should be performed. Most other causes of renal or nonrenal solute losses causing hypovolemic hypo-osmolality will be clinically apparent, although some cases of

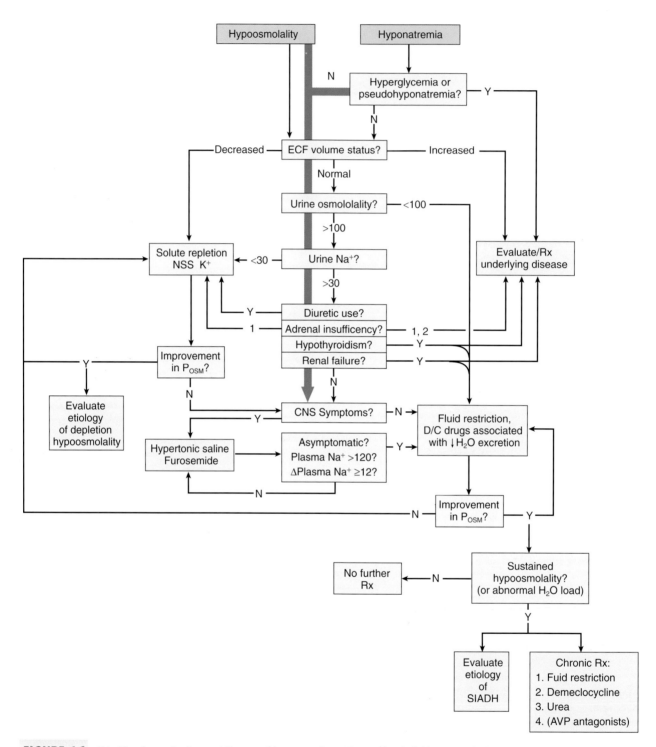

FIGURE 6-1 Algorithm for evaluation and therapy of hypo-osmolar patients. The dark blue arrow in the center emphasizes that the presence of central nervous system dysfunction due to hyponatremia should always be assessed immediately, so that appropriate therapy can be started as soon as possible in symptomatic patients, even while the outlined diagnostic evaluation is proceeding. Values referring to osmolality are in mOsm/kg H_2O; values referring to serum Na^+ concentration are in mEq/L. 1°, primary; 2°, secondary; d/c, discontinue; ECF, extracellular fluid volume; N, no; NSS, normal (isotonic) saline; P_{osm}, plasma osmolality; Rx, treat; SIADH, syndrome of inappropriate antidiuretic hormone secretion; Y, yes;. (Modified from Verbalis JG: Inappropriate antidiuresis and other hypoosmolar states. In Becker KG [ed]: Principles and Practice of Endocrinology and Metabolism. Philadelphia, JB Lippincott, 1995, pp 265–276. With permission.)

salt-wasting nephropathies (e.g., chronic interstitial nephropathy, polycystic kidney disease, obstructive uropathy, or Bartter's syndrome) or mineralocorticoid deficiency (e.g., Addison's disease) can be challenging to diagnose during the early phases of these diseases.

Normal Extracellular Fluid Volume (Euvolemia)

Virtually any disorder associated with hypo-osmolality can present with a hydration status that appears normal by standard methods of clinical evaluation. Because clinical assessment of ECF volume status is not very sensitive, the presence of normal or low levels of serum BUN and uric acid are helpful laboratory correlates of relatively normal ECF volume. Conversely, a low U_{Na} suggests a depletional hypo-osmolality secondary to ECF losses with subsequent volume replacement by water or other hypotonic fluids; as discussed earlier, such patients may appear euvolemic by all the usual clinical parameters used to assess hydration status. Primary dilutional disorders are less likely in the presence of a low U_{Na} (less than 30 mEq/L), although this pattern can occur in hypothyroidism. A high U_{Na} (greater than 30 mEq/L) generally indicates a dilutional hypo-osmolality such as the syndrome of inappropriate antidiuretic hormone secretion (SIADH) (see Table 6-1). SIADH is the most common cause of euvolemic hypo-osmolality in clinical medicine. The criteria necessary for a diagnosis of SIADH remain essentially as defined by Bartter and Schwartz in 1967 (Table 6-2), but several points deserve emphasis. First, true ECF hypo-osmolality must be present and hyponatremia secondary to pseudohyponatremia or hyperglycemia excluded. Second, urinary osmolality (U_{osm}) must be inappropriate for plasma hypo-osmolality. This does not mandate that the U_{osm} be greater than the P_{osm}, but simply that the U_{osm} be greater than maximally dilute (i.e., U_{osm} greater than 100 mOsm/kg H_2O in adults). Furthermore, U_{osm} need not be inappropriately elevated at all levels of P_{osm} but simply at some level under 275 mOsm/kg H_2O, because in patients with a reset osmostat, AVP secretion can be suppressed at some level of osmolality, resulting in maximal urinary dilution and free water excretion at plasma osmolalities below this level. Although some consider a reset osmostat to be a separate disorder rather than a variant of SIADH, such cases nonetheless illustrate that some hypo-osmolar patients can exhibit an appropriately dilute urine at some, but not all, plasma osmolalities. Third, clinical euvolemia must be present to diagnose SIADH, and this diagnosis cannot be made in a hypovolemic or edematous patient. Importantly, this does not mean that patients with SIADH cannot become hypovolemic for other reasons, but in such cases it is impossible to diagnose the underlying SIADH until the patient is rendered euvolemic. The fourth criterion, renal salt wasting, has probably caused

---

TABLE 6-2 Criteria for the Diagnosis of SIADH

Essential
1. Decreased effective osmolality of the extracellular fluid (P_{osm} < 275 mOsm/kg H_2O).
2. Inappropriate urinary concentration (U_{osm} > 100 mOsm/kg H_2O with normal kidney function) at some level of hypo-osmolality.
3. Clinical euvolemia, as defined by the absence of signs of hypovolemia (orthostasis, tachycardia, decreased skin turgor, dry mucous membranes) or hypervolemia (subcutaneous edema, ascites).
4. Elevated urinary sodium excretion while on a normal salt and water intake.
5. Normal thyroid, adrenal, and kidney function.

Supplemental
6. Abnormal water load test (inability to excrete at least 80% of a 20-mL/kg water load in 4 hours and/or failure to dilute U_{osm} to < 100 mOsm/kg H_2O).
7. Plasma AVP level inappropriately elevated relative to plasma osmolality.
8. No significant correction of serum [Na^+] with volume expansion but improvement after fluid restriction.

AVP, arginine vasopressin; P_{osm}, plama osmolality; SIADH, syndrome of inappropriate antidiuretic hormone; U_{osm}, urine osmolality.
Modified from Verbalis JG: The syndrome of inappropriate antidiuretic hormone secretion and other hypoosmolar disorders. In Schrier RW (ed): Diseases of the Kidney. Philadelphia, Lippincott Williams & Wilkins, 2001, pp 2511–2548.

---

the most confusion regarding SIADH. The importance of this criterion lies in its usefulness in differentiating hypo-osmolality caused by a decreased effective intravascular volume, in which case renal Na^+ conservation occurs, from dilutional disorders in which urinary Na^+ excretion is normal or increased due to ECF volume expansion. However, U_{Na} can also be high in renal causes of solute depletion such as diuretic use or Addison's disease, and conversely patients with SIADH can have a low urinary Na^+ excretion if they subsequently become hypovolemic or solute depleted, conditions sometimes induced by imposed salt and water restriction. Consequently, although high urinary Na^+ excretion is generally the rule in most patients with SIADH, its presence does not necessarily confirm this diagnosis, nor does its absence rule out the diagnosis. The final criterion emphasizes that SIADH remains a diagnosis of exclusion, and the absence of other potential causes of hypo-osmolality must always be verified. Glucocorticoid deficiency and SIADH can be especially difficult to differentiate, because either primary or secondary hypocortisolism can cause elevated plasma AVP levels and has direct renal effects to prevent maximal urinary dilution. Therefore, no patient with chronic hyponatremia should be diagnosed as having SIADH without a thorough evaluation of adrenal function, preferably via a rapid adrenocorticotropic hormone (ACTH) stimulation test (acute hyponatremia of obvious etiology, such as postoperatively or in association with pneumonitis, may be treated without adrenal testing as long as there are no other clinical signs or symptoms suggestive of adrenal dysfunction). Many different disorders have been associated with SIADH, and these can be divided into several major etiologic groups (Table 6-3).

Some cases of euvolemic hyponatremia do not fit particularly well into either a dilutional or depletional category. Chief among these is the hyponatremia that sometimes occurs in patients who ingest large volumes of beer with little food intake for prolonged periods, called beer potomania. Even though the volume of fluid ingested may not seem sufficiently excessive to overwhelm renal diluting mechanisms, in these cases free water excretion is limited by very low urinary solute excretion, thereby causing water retention and dilutional hyponatremia. However, because such patients also have very low sodium intakes, it is likely that relative depletion of body Na^+ stores is a contributory factor to the hypo-osmolality in some cases.

Increased Extracellular Fluid Volume (Hypervolemia)

The presence of hypervolemia, as detected clinically by the presence of edema or ascites, indicates whole-body sodium excess, and hypo-osmolality in these patients suggests a relatively decreased effective intravascular volume or pressure leading to water retention as a result of both elevated plasma AVP levels and decreased distal delivery of glomerular filtrate. Such patients usually have a low U_{Na} because of secondary hyperaldosteronism, but under certain conditions the U_{Na} may be elevated (e.g., glucosuria in diabetics, diuretic therapy). Hyponatremia generally does not occur until fairly advanced stages of diseases such as congestive heart failure, cirrhosis, and nephrotic syndrome, so diagnosis is usually not difficult. Retention of both sodium and water may occur due to impaired kidney function, but in this case the factor limiting excretion of excess body fluid is not decreased effective circulating volume but rather decreased glomerular filtration. It should be remembered that even though many edema-forming states have secondary increases in plasma AVP levels as a result of decreased effective arterial blood volume, nonetheless they are not classified as cases of SIADH because they fail to meet the criterion of clinical euvolemia (see Table 6-2, point 3). Although it can be argued that this represents a semantic distinction, it is nonetheless important because it allows segregation of identifiable etiologies of hyponatremia that are associated with different methods of evaluation and therapy.

Several situations can cause hyponatremia because of acute water loading in excess of renal excretory capacity. Primary polydipsia can cause hypo-osmolality in a small subset of patients with some degree of underlying SIADH, particularly psychiatric patients with long-standing schizophrenia on neuroleptic drugs, or even more rarely in patients with normal kidney function if the volumes ingested exceed the maximum renal free water excretory rate of approximately 500 to 1000 mL/hour. Recently, endurance exercising such as marathon and ultramarathon racing has been associated with sometimes fatal hyponatremia, primarily as a result of ingestion of excessive amounts of hypotonic fluids during the exercise that exceeds the water excretory capacity of the kidney. However, these types of patients rarely manifest overt signs of volume excess because water retention alone without sodium excess generally does not cause clinically apparent hypervolemia.

TABLE 6-3   Common Etiologies of SIADH

Tumors
  Pulmonary/mediastinal (bronchogenic carcinoma, mesothelioma, thymoma)
  Nonchest (duodenal carcinoma, pancreatic carcinoma, ureteral/prostate carcinoma, uterine carcinoma, nasopharyngeal carcinoma, leukemia)

Central nervous system disorders
  Mass lesions (tumors, brain abscesses, subdural hematoma)
  Inflammatory diseases (encephalitis, meningitis, systemic lupus, acute intermittent porphyria, multiple sclerosis)
  Degenerative/demyelinative diseases (Guillain-Barré syndrome, spinal cord lesions)
  Miscellaneous (subarachnoid hemorrhage, head trauma, acute psychosis, delirium tremens, pituitary stalk section, transsphenoidal adenomectomy, hydrocephalus)

Drug induced
  Stimulated AVP release (nicotine, phenothiazines, tricyclic antidepressants)
  Direct renal effects and/or potentiation of AVP antidiuretic effects (desmopressin, oxytocin, prostaglandin synthesis inhibitors)
  Mixed or uncertain actions (angiotensin-converting enzyme inhibitors, carbamazepine and oxcarbazepine, chlorpropamide, clofibrate, clozapine, cyclophosphamide, 3,4methylenedioxymethamphetamine ["Ecstasy"], omeprazole, serotonin reuptake inhibitors, vincristine)

Pulmonary diseases
  Infections (tuberculosis, acute bacterial and viral pneumonia, aspergillosis, empyema)
  Mechanical/ventilatory (acute respiratory failure, COPD, positive pressure ventilation)

Other
  AIDS and AIDS-related complex
  Prolonged strenuous exercise (marathon, triathlon, ultramarathon, hot weather hiking)
  Senile atrophy
  Idiopathic

AIDS, acquired immunodeficiency syndrome; AVP, arginine vasopressin; COPD, chronic obstructive pulmonary disease; SIADH, syndrome of inappropriate antidiuretic hormone.

Modified from Verbalis JG: The syndrome of inappropriate antidiuretic hormone secretion and other hypoosmolar disorders. In Schrier RW (ed): Diseases of the Kidney. Philadelphia, Lippincott Williams & Wilkins, 2001, pp 2511–2548.

CLINICAL MANIFESTATIONS OF HYPONATREMIA

Hypo-osmolality is associated with a broad spectrum of neurologic manifestations, ranging from mild non-specific symptoms (e.g., headache, nausea) to more significant deficits (e.g., disorientation, confusion, obtundation, focal neurologic deficits, and seizures). In the most severe cases, death can result from respiratory arrest after tentorial herniation with subsequent brain stem compression. This neurologic symptom complex has been termed hyponatremic encephalopathy and primarily reflects brain edema resulting from osmotic water shifts into the brain caused by the decreased effective P_{osm}. Significant symptoms generally do not occur until the serum [Na^+] falls below 125 mEq/L, and the severity of symptoms can be roughly correlated with the degree of hypo-osmolality. However, individual variability is marked, and for any patient the level of serum [Na^+] at which symptoms will appear cannot be accurately predicted. Furthermore, several factors other than the severity of the hypo-osmolality also affect the degree of neurologic dysfunction. Most important is the period over which hypo-osmolality develops. Rapid development of severe hypo-osmolality is frequently associated with marked neurologic symptoms, whereas gradual development over several days or weeks is often associated with relatively mild symptomatology despite achievement of equivalent degrees of hypo-osmolality. This is because the brain can counteract osmotic swelling by secreting intracellular solutes, both electrolytes and organic osmolytes, via a process called volume regulation. Because this is a time-dependent process, rapid development of hypo-osmolality can result in brain edema before this adaptation can occur, but with slower development of hypo-osmolality brain cells can lose solute sufficiently rapidly to prevent the development of brain edema and subsequent neurologic dysfunction.

Underlying neurologic disease also can significantly affect the level of hypo-osmolality at which central nervous system (CNS) symptoms appear (e.g., moderate hypo-osmolality is generally not of major concern in an otherwise healthy patient, but can cause substantial morbidity in a patient with an underlying seizure disorder). Non-neurologic metabolic disorders (hypoxia, hypercapnia, acidosis, hypercalcemia, etc.) similarly can affect the level of P_{osm} at which CNS symptoms occur. Recent studies have suggested that some patients may be susceptible to a vicious cycle in which hypo-osmolality-induced brain edema causes noncardiogenic pulmonary edema, and the resulting hypoxia and hypercapnia then further impair the ability of the brain to volume regulate, leading to more brain edema, and resulting in neurologic deterioration and death in some cases. Other clinical studies have suggested that young children and menstruating women may be particularly susceptible to the development of neurologic morbidity and mortality during hyponatremia, especially in the acute postoperative setting. The true clinical incidence as well as the underlying pathophysiologic mechanisms responsible for these sometimes catastrophic cases remains to be determined. Finally, the issue of whether mild to moderate hyponatremia is truly "asymptomatic" has been challenged by preliminary studies showing subtle defects in cognition and gait stability in hyponatremic patients that appear to be reversed by correction of the hyponatremia. Confirmation of these findings would have significant import for therapy of chronically hyponatremic patients.

TREATMENT

Despite some continuing controversy regarding the optimal speed of correction of osmolality in hyponatremic patients, there is now a relatively uniform consensus about appropriate therapy in most cases (see Fig. 6-1). If any degree of clinical hypovolemia is present, the patient should be considered to have a solute depletion-induced hypo-osmolality and treated with isotonic (0.9%) NaCl at a rate appropriate for the estimated volume depletion. If diuretic use is known or suspected, this should be supplemented with potassium (30 to 40 mEq/L) even if the serum [K^+] is not low because of the propensity of such patients to have total body potassium depletion. Most often the hypo-osmolar patient is clinically euvolemic, but some circumstances dictate a reconsideration of potential solute depletion even in the patient without clinically apparent hypovolemia: a decreased U_{Na} (less than 30 mEq/L), any history of recent diuretic use, and any suggestion of primary adrenal insufficiency. Whenever a reasonable likelihood of depletion rather than dilution hypo-osmolality exists, it is appropriate to treat initially with a trial of isotonic NaCl. If the patient has SIADH, no harm will have been done with a limited (1 to 2 L) saline infusion, because such patients will simply excrete excess NaCl without significantly changing their P_{osm}. However, this therapy should be abandoned if the serum [Na^+] does not improve, because longer periods of continued isotonic NaCl infusion can worsen the hyponatremia by virtue of gradual water retention.

Treatment of euvolemic hypo-osmolar patients will vary depending on their presentation. A patient meeting all criteria for SIADH except that U_{osm} is low should simply be observed, since this may represent spontaneous reversal of a transient form of SIADH. If there is any suspicion of either primary or secondary adrenal insufficiency, glucocorticoid replacement should be started immediately after completion of a rapid ACTH stimulation test. Prompt water diuresis following initiation of glucocorticoid treatment strongly supports glucocorticoid deficiency, but the absence of a quick response does not negate this diagnosis because several days of glucocorticoids are sometimes required for normalization of P_{osm}. Hypervolemic hypo-osmolar patients are generally treated initially by diuresis and other measures directed at their underlying disorder. Such patients rarely require any therapy to increase P_{osm} acutely, but often benefit from varying degrees of sodium and water restriction to reduce body fluid retention.

In any significantly hyponatremic patient one is faced with the question of how quickly the P_{osm} should be corrected. Although hyponatremia is associated with a broad spectrum of neurologic symptoms, sometimes leading to death in severe cases, too rapid correction of severe hyponatremia can produce pontine and extrapontine myelinolysis, a brain demyelinating disease that also can cause substantial neurologic morbidity and mortality. Recent clinical and experimental results suggest that optimal treatment of hyponatremic patients must entail balancing the risks of hyponatremia against the risks of correction for each patient. Several factors should therefore be considered when making a treatment decision in hyponatremic patients: the severity of the hyponatremia, the duration of the hyponatremia, and the patient's symptomatology. Neither sequelae from hyponatremia itself nor myelinolysis after therapy are likely in patients whose serum [Na$^+$] is equal to 120 mEq/L, although significant symptoms can develop even at higher serum [Na$^+$] levels if the rate of decline of P_{osm} has been rapid. The importance of duration and symptomatology relate to how well the brain has volume regulated to the hyponatremia, and consequently to its degree of risk for subsequent demyelination with rapid correction. Cases of acute hyponatremia (arbitrarily defined as 48 hours in duration) are usually symptomatic if the hyponatremia is severe (i.e., 120 mEq/L). These patients are at greatest risk from neurologic complications from the hyponatremia itself and should be corrected to higher serum [Na$^+$] levels promptly. Conversely, patients with more chronic hyponatremia (greater than 48 hours in duration) who have minimal neurologic symptomatology are at little risk from complications of hyponatremia itself, but can develop demyelination following rapid correction. There is no indication to correct these patients rapidly, and they should be treated using slower-acting therapies such as fluid restriction.

Although the preceding extremes have clear treatment indications, most hyponatremic patients will have hyponatremia of indeterminate duration and will have varying degrees of milder neurologic symptomatology. This group presents the most challenging treatment decision, since the hyponatremia will have been present sufficiently long to allow some degree of brain volume regulation, but not enough to prevent some brain edema and neurologic symptomatology. Most recommend prompt treatment of such patients because of their symptoms, but using methods that allow a controlled and limited correction of their hyponatremia. Reasonable correction parameters consist of a maximal rate of correction of serum [Na$^+$] in the range of 1 to 2 mEq/L/hour as long as the total magnitude of correction does not exceed 25 mEq/L over the first 48 hours. Some argue that these parameters should be even more conservative, with magnitudes of correction that do not exceed 12 mEq/L over the first 24 hours and 18 mEq/L over the first 48 hours of correction. Treatments for individual patients should be chosen within these limits depending on their symptomatology. In patients who are only moderately symptomatic, one should proceed at the lower recommended limits of 0.5 mEq/L/hour, while in those who manifest more severe neurologic symptoms, an initial correction at a rate of 1 to 2 mEq/L/hour would be more appropriate. Controlled corrections are generally best accomplished with hypertonic (3%) NaCl solution given via continuous infusion, because patients with euvolemic hypo-osmolality, such as SIADH, generally do not respond to isotonic NaCl. An initial infusion rate can be estimated by multiplying the patient's body weight (in kilograms) by the desired rate of increase in serum [Na$^+$] (in mEq/L/hour; e.g., in a 70-kg patient an infusion of 3% NaCl at 70 mL/hour will increase serum [Na$^+$] by approximately 1 mEq/L/hour, whereas infusing 35 mL/hour will increase serum [Na$^+$] by approximately 0.5 mEq/L/hour). Furosemide (20 to 40 mg intravenously) should be used to treat volume overload, in some cases anticipatorily in patients with known cardiovascular disease. Patients with diuretic-induced hyponatremia usually respond well to isotonic NaCl and do not require 3% NaCl. However, such patients frequently have a free water diuresis once their ECF volume deficit has been corrected, since this removes the hypovolemic stimulus to vasopressin secretion, resulting in a more rapid correction of the serum [Na$^+$] than predicted from the rate of saline infusion. Regardless of the initial rate of correction chosen, acute treatment should be interrupted once any of three end points is reached: (1) the patient's symptoms are abolished, (2) a safe serum [Na$^+$] (generally equal to 120 mEq/L) is achieved, or (3) a total magnitude of correction of 20 mEq/L is achieved. It follows from these recommendations that serum [Na$^+$] levels must be carefully monitored at frequent intervals (at least every 4 hours) during the active phases of treatment in order to adjust therapy so that the correction stays within these guidelines. Regardless of the therapy or rate initially chosen, it cannot be emphasized too strongly that it is necessary only to correct the P_{osm} acutely to a safe range rather than completely to normal levels. In some situations patients may spontaneously correct their hyponatremia via a water diuresis. If the hyponatremia is acute (e.g., psychogenic polydipsia with water intoxication), such patients do not appear to be at risk for subsequent demyelination; however, in cases where the hyponatremia has been chronic (e.g., hypocortisolism or diuretic therapy), intervention should be considered to limit the rate and magnitude of correction of serum [Na$^+$] (e.g., administration of 1 to 2 μg desmopressin intravenously or infusion of hypotonic fluids to match urine output) using the same end points as for active corrections.

Treatment of chronic hyponatremia entails choosing among several suboptimal therapies. One important exception is those patients with the reset osmostat syndrome; because the hyponatremia of such patients is not progressive but rather fluctuates around their reset level of serum [Na+], no therapy is generally required. For most other cases of mild to moderate SIADH, fluid restriction represents the least toxic therapy and is the treatment of choice. This should always be tried as the initial therapy, with pharmacologic intervention reserved for refractory cases where the degree of fluid restriction required to avoid hypo-osmolality is so severe that the patient is unable, or unwilling, to maintain it. In general, the higher the U_{osm}, indicating higher plasma vasopressin levels, the less likely that fluid restriction will be successful. If pharmacologic treatment is necessary, the preferred drug at present is the tetracycline derivative demeclocycline, which causes nephrogenic diabetes insipidus, thereby decreasing urine concentration. The effective dose of demeclocycline ranges from 600 to 1200 mg/day; several days of therapy are necessary to achieve maximum effects, so one should wait 3 to 4 days before increasing the dose. Demeclocycline can cause reversible nephrotoxicity, especially in patients with cirrhosis; kidney function should be monitored and the medica-tion stopped if increasing azotemia occurs. Several other drugs can decrease AVP hypersecretion in selected cases (diphenylhydantoin, opiates, ethanol), but responses are unpredictable.

Despite current unavailability of an ideal therapeutic agent for chronic dilutional hyponatremias, this will likely change in the near future with development of vasopressin receptor antagonists. Several nonpeptide molecules that antagonize the vasopressin V2 receptor are currently in clinical trials and have proven to be effective at correcting hyponatremia by increasing free water excretion in patients with SIADH, congestive heart failure, and cirrhosis. Because these compounds increase water excretion without stimulating the natriuresis and kaliuresis that are characteristic of standard diuretic agents, they have been termed aquaretic agents. Such drugs will likely become the treatments of choice for dilutional hyponatremias in the future, although their efficacy in some case may be limited by associated increases in AVP concentrations and thirst that counteract the induced free water diuresis. In addition, the use of aquaretic agents to correct established chronic hyponatremia will require judicious adherence to the same guidelines already established for other therapies to prevent complications from brain demyelination. Despite these caveats, the eventual approval of aquaretic agents for clinical use will undoubtedly usher in a new era in the treatment of hyponatremic disorders.

BIBLIOGRAPHY

Anderson RJ, Chung H-M, Kluge R, et al: Hyponatremia: A prospective analysis of its epidemiology and the pathogenetic role of vasopressin. Ann Intern Med 102:164–168, 1985.

Ayus JC, Arieff AI: Pulmonary complications of hyponatremic encephalopathy. Noncardiogenic pulmonary edema and hypercapnic respiratory failure. Chest 107:517–521, 1995.

Ayus JC, Arieff AI: Chronic hyponatremic encephalopathy in postmenopausal women: Association of therapies with morbidity and mortality. JAMA 281:2299–2304, 1999.

Ayus JC, Varon J, Arieff AI: Hyponatremia, cerebral edema, and noncardiogenic pulmonary edema in marathon runners. Ann Intern Med 132:711–714, 2000.

Bartter FC, Schwartz WB: The syndrome of inappropriate secretion of antidiuretic hormone. Am J Med 42:790–806, 1967.

Fraser CL, Arieff AI: Epidemiology, pathophysiology, and management of hyponatremic encephalopathy. Am J Med 102:67–77, 1997.

Gerbes AL, Gulberg V, Gines P, et al: Therapy of hyponatremia in cirrhosis with a vasopressin receptor antagonist: A randomized double-blind multicenter trial. Gastroenterology 124:933–939, 2003.

Hawkins RC: Age and gender as risk factors for hyponatremia and hypernatremia. Clin Chim Acta 337:169–172, 2003.

Miller M, Morley JE, Rubenstein LZ: Hyponatremia in a nursing home population. J Am Geriatr Soc 43:1410–1413, 1995.

Saito T, Ishikawa S, Abe K, et al: Acute aquaresis by the non-peptide arginine vasopressin (AVP) antagonist OPC-31260 improves hyponatremia in patients with syndrome of inappropriate secretion of antidiuretic hormone (SIADH). J Clin Endocrinol Metab 82:1054–1057, 1997.

Schrier RW: Pathogenesis of sodium and water retention in high-output and low-output cardiac failure, nephrotic syndrome, cirrhosis and pregnancy. N Engl J Med 319:1065–1072 and 1127–1134, 1988.

Sterns RH. Severe symptomatic hyponatremia: Treatment and outcome. A study of 64 cases. Ann Intern Med 107:656–664, 1987.

Sterns RH, Cappuccio JD, Silver SM, Cohen EP: Neurologic sequelae after treatment of severe hyponatremia: A multicenter perspective. J Am Soc Nephrol 4:1522–1530, 1994.

Verbalis JG. Inappropriate antidiuresis and other hypoosmolar states. In: Becker KL (ed). Principles and Practice of Endocrinology and Metabolism. Philadelphia, Lippincott Williams & Wilkins, 2001, pp. 293–305.

Verbalis JG: The syndrome of inappropriate antidiuretic hormone secretion and other hypoosmolar disorders. In Schrier RW (ed): Diseases of the Kidney. Philadelphia, Lippincott Williams & Wilkins, 2001, pp 2511–2548.

Verbalis JG: Vasopressin V2 receptor antagonists. J Mol Endocrinol 29:1–9, 2002.

Wong F, Blei AT, Blendis LM, Thuluvath PJ: A vasopressin receptor antagonist (VPA-985) improves serum sodium concentration in patients with hyponatremia: A multicenter, randomized, placebo-controlled trial. Hepatology 37:182–191, 2003.

Zerbe R, Stropes L, Robertson G: Vasopressin function in the syndrome of inappropriate antidiuresis. Annu Rev Med 31:315–327, 1980.

CHAPTER 7

Hypernatremia

Paul M. Palevsky

Hypernatremia is one of the two cardinal disturbances of water homeostasis. Decreases in total body water relative to electrolyte content are characterized by an increase in the electrolyte concentration in all body fluids. In the intracellular compartment this is manifested by a decrease in cell volume and an increase in the intracellular potassium concentration. In the extracellular space, the primary manifestation is an increase in the sodium concentration, resulting in the laboratory finding of hypernatremia.

The development of hypernatremia does not imply an abnormality in sodium homeostasis. Total body sodium content is the primary determinant of extracellular volume. In the setting of intact water homeostasis, alterations in sodium balance result in isotonic volume expansion or volume depletion but do not alter the extracellular fluid sodium concentration. However, hypernatremia may be accompanied by either volume depletion or volume overload if impaired water homeostasis is accompanied by disturbances in sodium balance.

Hypernatremia is a common clinical problem. Its prevalence in hospitalized patients ranges between 0.5% and 2%. In adults, two distinct groups of hypernatremic patients may be identified. Patients developing hypernatremia outside of the hospital setting are generally elderly and debilitated, and often present with an intercurrent acute infection. In contrast, patients developing hypernatremia during the course of hospitalization have an age distribution similar to that of the general hospital population. In these patients, hypernatremia is an iatrogenic complication that develops when impaired thirst or restricted access to water is combined with an inadequate prescription for water administration.

REGULATION OF WATER HOMEOSTASIS

The physiologic response to hypertonicity includes both renal water conservation and stimulation of thirst. Hypertonicity is sensed by osmoreceptors located adjacent to the anterior wall of the third ventricle in the hypothalamus. Activation of these osmoreceptors stimulates the secretion of arginine vasopressin by neurons whose cell bodies are in the supraoptic and paraventricular nuclei in the hypothalamus and whose axons terminate in the posterior pituitary gland. In the kidney, arginine vasopressin modulates the hydraulic permeability of the collecting duct. In the absence of vasopressin, the collecting duct is relatively impermeable to water. Vasopressin exerts its effect on the collecting duct through the activation of V_2-vasopressin receptors located on the basolateral aspect of the tubular epithelium. The V_2-receptor is coupled to adenylate cyclase by guanosine triphosphate–binding proteins; receptor binding activates adenylate cyclase, which catalyzes the conversion of adenosine triphosphate to the second messenger, cyclic adenosine monophosphate (cAMP). cAMP initiates a cascade of intracellular events, ultimately resulting in the fusion of subapical vesicles containing aquaporin 2 water channels with the apical cell membrane. The insertion of these water channels into the apical cell membrane increases its hydraulic permeability and permits the passive reabsorption of water from the collecting duct into the isotonic cortical and hypertonic medullary interstitium. Urinary concentration is therefore dependent on the generation and maintenance of the interstitial corticomedullary osmotic gradient as well as the utilization of the gradient through a normal tubular response to secreted vasopressin.

The osmotic regulation of vasopressin secretion is extremely sensitive. Below a body fluid osmolality of 280 to 285 mmol/kg, vasopressin secretion is inhibited and plasma vasopressin levels are virtually undetectable. As body fluid osmolality increases above this threshold, vasopressin secretion increases linearly. Increases in body fluid osmolality of as little as 1% to 2% result in detectable increases in plasma vasopressin levels. The renal response to changes in vasopressin secretion is also extremely sensitive. Urine is maximally dilute when vasopressin secretion is suppressed; urinary concentration increases linearly as plasma vasopressin levels increase in response to rising plasma tonicity, with maximal urinary concentration achieved at vasopressin levels that correspond to a plasma osmolality of approximately 295 mmol/kg.

Although renal water conservation is important in preventing further renal losses, water conservation is not sufficient for either the prevention of progressive hypertonicity or the restoration of normal plasma tonicity. The ultimate defense against the development of hypertonicity and hypernatremia is the osmotic stimulation of thirst and its resultant increase in water ingestion. Thirst is also mediated by hypothalamic osmoreceptors located in the anterior wall of the third ventricle. Although in proximity to the osmoreceptors modulating vasopressin secretion, the thirst osmoreceptors are anatomically distinct. Impulses from these osmoreceptors are projected to higher levels in the cerebral cortex, where they trigger the perception of thirst and stimulate water-seeking behavior. The osmotic threshold for thirst is approximately 5 mmol/kg higher than the osmotic threshold for vasopressin secretion; once this threshold is exceeded, thirst increases in proportion to increases in body fluid osmolality.

PATHOPHYSIOLOGY

Hypernatremia results when there is net water loss or hypertonic sodium gain. In the normal individual, thirst is stimulated by any increase in body fluid tonicity. Water ingestion increases and the hypernatremic state is rapidly corrected. Therefore, sustained hypernatremia can occur only when the thirst mechanism is impaired and water intake does not increase in response to hypertonicity, or water ingestion is restricted. Although increased water losses or hypertonic sodium gain usually contribute to the development of hypernatremia, impaired osmoregulation or perception of thirst or the inability to gain access to water is required for sustained hypernatremia.

The importance of thirst in the pathogenesis of hypernatremia is illustrated by patients with severe diabetes insipidus. These patients are unable to concentrate their urine and excrete large volumes of dilute urine, occasionally in excess of 10 to 15 L/day. Under normal circumstances they do not develop hypernatremia. In response to their renal water losses, thirst is stimulated and they maintain body fluid tonicity at the expense of profound secondary polydipsia. If, however, they are unable to drink in response to thirst, as may occur during intercurrent illness, hypernatremia rapidly develops.

Isolated defects in thirst (primary hypodipsia) are uncommon but may result from any process involving the hypothalamus in proximity to the anterior wall of the third ventricle (Table 7-1). Lesions may include a wide range of intracranial pathology, including primary and metastatic tumors, granulomatous diseases, vascular abnormalities (most commonly involving the anterior communicating artery), trauma, and hydrocephalus. Hypodipsia has also been described in elderly patients (geriatric hypodipsia) in whom overt hypothalamic pathology is absent. Essential hypernatremia is a rare disorder in which there is an upward resetting of the thresholds for both thirst and vasopressin secretion. Patients with this condition are able to concentrate and dilute their urine, albeit around an elevated body fluid osmolality, and have an elevated set point for thirst perception. More commonly, impaired thirst results from diffuse neurologic disease that interferes with the less well-defined

TABLE 7-1 Defects in Thirst

Primary hypodipsia
  Hypothalamic lesions affecting the osmostat
    Trauma
    Craniopharyngioma or other primary suprasellar tumor
    Metastatic tumor
    Granulomatous disease
    Vascular lesions
  Essential hypernatremia
  Geriatric hypodipsia
Secondary hypodipsia
  Cerebrovascular disease
  Dementia
  Delirium
  Mental status changes

cerebral cortical pathways subserving thirst perception and water ingestion (secondary hypodipsia). Thus, defects in thirst are commonly associated with cerebrovascular disease, dementia, and acute illnesses that result in delirium or obtundation.

CLINICAL CLASSIFICATION

Although impaired thirst and restricted water intake underlie the development of sustained hypernatremia, the hypernatremic states are most commonly classified on the basis of the associated water loss or electrolyte gain and corresponding changes in extracellular fluid volume (Table 7-2). Pure water deficits are associated with minimal change in total body sodium and relative preservation of extracellular fluid volume. When hypotonic fluid deficits are present, hypernatremia coexists with total body sodium depletion and extracellular fluid volume contraction. Hypertonic sodium gain results in hypernatremia and extracellular fluid volume expansion.

Pure Water Deficits

Isolated water deficits are generally not associated with clinical evidence of intravascular volume depletion. Only one third of a pure water deficit is derived from the extracellular compartment, and only one twelfth from the intravascular compartment. In a 70-kg individual, a 5% decrease in total body water, which would result in an increase in the plasma sodium concentration by approximately 7 mmol/L, results in a reduction in extracellular fluid volume by less than 700 mL and intravascular volume by less than 200 mL. This modest degree of volume depletion is generally not detectable on physical examination and may be manifested only by mild prerenal azotemia. With more severe water deficits, hemodynamically significant intravascular volume depletion may develop.

Pure water deficits may occur when thirst is impaired, even in the absence of increased water losses. In patients

TABLE 7-2 Classification of Hypernatremia on the Basis of Associated Changes in Extracellular Volume

Pure water deficit (normal extracellular volume)
Diabetes insipidus
  Hypothalamic
  Nephrogenic
Increased insensible losses

Hypotonic fluid deficit (decreased extracellular volume)
Renal losses
  Diuretic administration
  Osmotic diuresis
  Postobstructive diuresis
  Polyuric phase of ATN
Gastrointestinal losses
  Vomiting
  Nasogastric drainage
  Enterocutaneous fistulae
  Diarrhea
Cutaneous losses
  Burn injuries
  Excessive perspiration

Hypertonic sodium gain (increased extracellular volume)
Salt ingestion
Hypertonic NaCl
Hypertonic NaHCO$_3$
Total parenteral nutrition

ATN, acute tubular necrosis.

with significant hypodipsia, voluntary water ingestion may not be sufficient to replace obligate gastrointestinal and insensible water losses. Despite maximal renal water conservation, progressive hypernatremia will result if supplemental water intake is not provided. Lactation failure resulting in impaired fluid intake is one of the most important causes of hypernatremia in infants.

More commonly, pure water deficits develop when impaired intake is combined with increased insensible or renal water losses. Insensible water losses total approximately 0.6 mL/kg/hour, or about 1 L per day in the average adult. These losses are not subject to osmotic regulation and may be increased by a wide variety of factors, including fever, exercise, increased ambient temperature, and hyperventilation. Increased renal electrolyte-free water losses are the hallmark of diabetes insipidus. Patients with increased insensible losses manifest oliguria with a maximally concentrated urine (urine osmolality greater than 700 mmol/kg). In contrast, patients with diabetes insipidus have polyuria and a less than maximally concentrated urine.

Diabetes Insipidus

Diabetes insipidus results either from failure of the hypothalamic-pituitary axis to synthesize or release adequate amounts of vasopressin (hypothalamic diabetes insipidus) or from impaired collecting duct responsiveness to circulating vasopressin (nephrogenic diabetes insipidus). In both forms, the inability of the kidney to

concentrate the urine leads to polyuria and secondary polydipsia. If water intake is adequate to replace urinary electrolyte-free water losses, hypertonicity and hypernatremia will not develop. Thus, hypernatremia is not a hallmark of diabetes insipidus.

Diabetes insipidus may occur in either complete or partial forms. In complete hypothalamic diabetes insipidus, vasopressin secretion is absent, resulting in the production of large volumes of dilute urine (urine osmolality less than 150 mmol/L). In partial hypothalamic diabetes insipidus, vasopressin secretion is detectable but subnormal, and a less severe defect in renal water conservation is present. Similarly, in complete nephrogenic diabetes insipidus, renal responsiveness to the hydro-osmotic effect of vasopressin is absent, whereas an impaired response occurs in partial nephrogenic diabetes insipidus.

Any pathologic process involving the hypothalamic-pituitary axis may lead to vasopressin deficiency and hypothalamic diabetes insipidus (Table 7-3). Common causes include pituitary surgery, head trauma, primary and metastatic tumors, leukemia, hemorrhage, thrombosis, and granulomatous diseases. Diabetes insipidus following head trauma or surgery may be transient or permanent, or may follow a triphasic course. The transient course is most common, with an abrupt onset followed by resolution over a period of days to weeks. In the triphasic pattern, there is an initial period of vasopressin deficiency lasting 2 to 4 days as the result of axonal injury, a 5- to 7-day period of inappropriate vasopressin release, thought to result from release of hormone by degenerating neurons, and finally permanent diabetes

TABLE 7-3 Hypothalamic Diabetes Insipidus

Pituitary surgery

Head trauma

Neoplasia
Primary: dysgerminoma, craniopharyngioma, suprasellar pituitary tumors
Metastatic: carcinoma of the breast, carcinoma of the lung, lymphoma
Leukemia

Vascular lesions
Aneurysms
Cerebrovascular accidents
Sheehan's syndrome (postpartum pituitary hemorrhage)

Infections
Encephalitis
Meningitis
Tuberculosis
Syphilis

Granulomatous disease
Sarcoidosis
Histiocytosis

Autoimmune

Vasopressin-neurophysin gene mutations

TABLE 7-4 Nephrogenic Diabetes Insipidus

Drug induced
  Lithium
  Demeclocycline
  Methoxyflurane
  Amphotericin B

Electrolyte disorders
  Hypercalcemia
  Hypokalemia

Obstructive uropathy

Congenital
  Vasopressin V_2-receptor mutations
  Aquaporin 2 mutations

insipidus following neuronal death. In 30% of patients, hypothalamic diabetes insipidus is idiopathic, most probably occurring on an autoimmune basis. A rare, hereditary form is due to mutations in the vasopressin-neurophysin gene, which result in an abnormal structure and processing of the vasopressin prohormone and ultimately cell death of the vasopressin-secreting neurons.

The term *nephrogenic diabetes insipidus* should be restricted to those situations in which there is an intrinsic abnormality of the collecting duct that leads to vasopressin insensitivity or hyporesponsiveness. Patients with chronic tubulointerstitial kidney disease may be unable to generate or maintain a normal corticomedullary osmotic gradient and are therefore unable to concentrate their urine normally. However, they rarely have significant polyuria and should not be considered to have nephrogenic diabetes insipidus.

Nephrogenic diabetes insipidus may be either acquired or congenital (Table 7-4). The acquired form is far more common and is most often associated with pharmacologic therapy with lithium or demeclocycline. Both agents have been demonstrated to inhibit intracellular generation of cAMP. In addition, demeclocycline also inhibits its intracellular action. Acquired nephrogenic diabetes insipidus may also result from obstructive uropathy, hypercalcemia, or severe hypokalemia.

A congenital form of nephrogenic diabetes insipidus has been identified in multiple kindreds and is usually inherited in a sex-linked pattern with variable penetrance in hemizygous females. In the majority of kindreds the genetic defect is in the vasopressin V_2-receptor gene. Mutations in the aquaporin 2 gene have been identified in rare patients with an autosomal-recessive form.

The polyuria of diabetes insipidus needs to be differentiated from other forms of polyuria, including primary polydipsia, solute diuresis secondary to glycosuria, mannitol, urea or diuretics, or resolving acute renal failure. Polyuria due to solute diuresis can usually be excluded by demonstrating that the urine osmolality is less than 150 mmol/kg. In a water diuresis (e.g., diabetes insipidus or primary polydipsia), the urine is generally maximally dilute (urine osmolality less than 150 mmol/kg), although a less than maximally dilute urine may be produced by patients with partial forms of diabetes insipidus. Dehydration testing may help differentiate between different forms of polyuria. In patients with severe polyuria formal dehydration testing is usually unnecessary and may result in severe hypernatremia and hypotension. During a dehydration test, patients are placed on a strict fast with special care taken to ensure that they consume no fluids. During the test, urine osmolality is measured hourly and plasma osmolality every 4 to 6 hours. Water deprivation is continued until body weight has declined by 3%, plasma osmolality has reached 295 mmol/kg, or urine osmolality has reached a plateau (variation of less than 5% over 3 hours). In patients with severe diabetes insipidus, urine osmolality will remain lower than plasma osmolality. In partial diabetes insipidus urine osmolality will exceed plasma osmolality, but will remain submaximally concentrated (Table 7-5). The urinary response to exogenous vasopressin (5 units of aqueous vasopressin or 1 μg of desamino-8-D-arginine vasopressin, dDAVP) usually differentiates between the hypothalamic and nephrogenic forms. Measurement of plasma vasopressin levels at maximal dehydration (prior to exogenous vasopressin), although not routinely available, may be extremely useful in equivocal cases.

TABLE 7-5 Diagnosis of DI

	Urine Osmolality		
Diagnosis	**After Dehydration**	**After Exogenous Vasopressin**	**Plasma Vasopressin Level**
Normal individuals	>700 mmol/kg	<10% increase	>2.0 pg/mL
Hypothalamic DI			
Complete	<300 mmol/kg	>50% increase	<1.0 pg/mL
Partial	>300 mmol/kg	>10% increase	<1.5 pg/mL
Nephrogenic DI			
Complete	<300 mmol/kg	<50% increase	>5.0 pg/mL
Partial	>300 mmol/kg	<10% increase	>2.0 pg/mL

DI, diabetes insipidus.

Hypotonic Fluid Deficits

Patients with inadequately replaced hypotonic fluid losses will develop both hypernatremia and extracellular fluid volume depletion. Unlike patients with pure water losses, these individuals manifest the classic findings of intravascular volume depletion: tachycardia, hypotension, and decreased central venous pressure. Hypotonic fluid may be lost from the skin, gastrointestinal tract, or kidney. Cutaneous losses of electrolyte-containing hypotonic fluids are seen in patients with severe burn injuries and with increased sensible perspiration (as opposed to insensible transpirational skin loss). The majority of gastrointestinal fluids, with the exception of pancreatic and biliary secretions, are also hypotonic. Protracted vomiting, nasogastric drainage, and diarrhea commonly contribute to the development of hypovolemic hypernatremia. Diuretic therapy is the most common reason for excessive hypotonic losses from the kidney. Osmotic diureses accompanying hyperglycemia or the administration of mannitol are another common cause of hypotonic renal losses. Postobstructive diuresis, the polyuric phase of acute tubular necrosis, adrenal insufficiency, and a variety of chronic kidney diseases, especially medullary cystic disease and renal tubular acidosis (types I and II) are also associated with renal salt wasting and hypotonic urinary losses. Hypovolemic hypernatremia may also develop in patients with "third space" fluid losses (e.g., bowel obstruction, pancreatitis, or peritonitis) if the sequestration of isotonic fluid is combined with inadequate replacement of ongoing electrolyte-free water losses.

Urinary indices are helpful in ascertaining the source of hypotonic fluid losses. When the losses have a renal origin, the urine sodium concentration is usually elevated (greater than 20 mmol/L) and the urine is less than maximally concentrated. In contrast, nonrenal losses are associated with high renal sodium avidity (urine sodium less than 10 mmol/L) and a maximally concentrated urine (urine osmolality greater than 700 mmol/kg).

Hypertonic Sodium Gain

Hypertonic sodium gain produces hypernatremia and extracellular volume overload. When both thirst and renal function are intact, the volume and tonicity disturbances are transient. The increase in tonicity stimulates thirst, and the resultant increase in water intake ameliorates the hypertonicity. In addition, the associated volume expansion stimulates a natriuresis. Persistent hypernatremia implies impaired thirst or restricted water intake. Hypertonic sodium gain may result from the accidental ingestion of large quantities of sodium salts, but is more commonly iatrogenic, resulting from the administration of hypertonic sodium chloride or sodium bicarbonate solutions, inappropriate electrolyte prescription for parenteral hyperalimentation solutions, or inappropriate sodium supplementation of enteral nutrition. Errors in formula preparation may result in hypernatremia in infants.

Hypertonicity Due to Nonelectrolyte Solutes

Although all hypernatremic patients are hypertonic, hypertonicity can also occur in the absence of hypernatremia. When osmotically active nonelectrolyte solutes accumulate in the extracellular compartment, hypertonicity may be accompanied by a normal, or even depressed, serum sodium concentration. The accumulation of a nonelectrolyte solute increases the osmolality of the extracellular fluids. If the solute is impermeant to cell membranes, water will exit the intracellular compartment to maintain osmotic equilibrium. The net result is intracellular dehydration, cell shrinkage, expansion of the extracellular compartment, and dilution of the extracellular fluid sodium concentration. It is important to recognize nonhypernatremic hypertonicity so as to avoid institution of inappropriate therapy for the resultant dilutional hyponatremia.

Glucose is the most common nonelectrolyte solute associated with hypertonicity. In patients with hyperglycemia, the serum sodium concentration usually declines by 1.6 to 2.0 mmol/L for each 100 mg/dL increase in plasma glucose. Isonatremic and hyponatremic hypertonicity have also been described following administration of mannitol, maltose, sorbitol, glycerol, and radiocontrast agents. The presence of an unmeasured solute may be identified by comparison of the measured plasma osmolality with the estimated plasma osmolality (P_{osm}) derived from measurement of serum sodium, glucose, and urea nitrogen concentrations:

$$P_{osm} = 2 \times [Na^+] + glucose\ (mg/dL)/18 + blood\ urea\ nitrogen\ (mg/dL)/2.8.$$

The presence of an osmolal gap between the measured and calculated plasma osmolality suggests the presence of an unmeasured solute. The specific solute responsible is usually ascertainable from a review of medications administered and may be confirmed by specific biochemical testing.

DIAGNOSTIC APPROACH

The algorithm in Figure 7-1 provides a diagnostic approach to the patient with hypernatremia. The initial step is evaluation of intravascular volume. If intravascular volume is preserved, the hypernatremia is most likely due to pure water losses. Measurement of urine osmolality permits differentiation between nonrenal causes (isolated hypodipsia, increased insensible losses) and renal water loss (diabetes insipidus). Intravascular volume contraction implies combined water and sodium deficits due

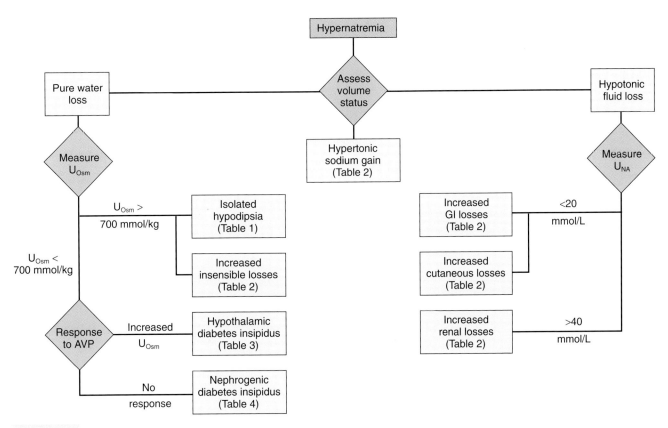

FIGURE 7-1 Algorithm for the evaluation of hypernatremia.

to gastrointestinal, cutaneous, or renal losses, whereas intravascular volume expansion suggests hypertonic sodium gain, but may also be seen when hypernatremia is superimposed on a preexisting edematous disorder.

CLINICAL MANIFESTATIONS

The major clinical manifestations of hypernatremia result from alterations in brain water content. In response to hypertonicity, fluid shifts from the intracellular compartment into the extracellular compartment, maintaining osmotic equilibrium at the expense of a decrease in intracellular volume. In the central nervous system, acute hypernatremia is associated with a rapid decrease in intracellular water content and brain volume (Fig. 7-2). Within 24 hours, adaptive processes are activated, stimulating electrolyte uptake into the intracellular compartment and resulting in partial restoration of brain volume. This acute adaptive response is followed by a second phase of adaptation characterized by an increase in intracellular organic solute content, primarily through the accumulation of amino acids, polyols, and methylamines. This slower chronic adaptive response restores brain volume to normal. The accumulation of these intracellular solutes ("idiogenic osmoles") has important therapeutic implications. Although minimizing cerebral dehydration during hypertonicity, the accumulation of

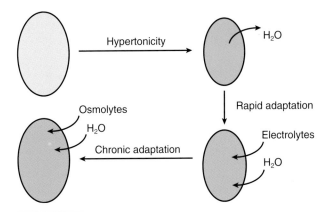

FIGURE 7-2 Brain adaptation to hypernatremia. Brain cell volume is indicated by the size of the oval, intracellular osmolality by the density of shading. Following the acute onset of hypernatremia, there is a rapid loss of water from the intracellular compartment, resulting in a decrease in brain cell volume and an increase in brain cell osmolality. Adaptive processes that restore brain cell volume to normal are then activated. In the initial phase of rapid adaptation, occurring over the first 24 hours, electrolyte uptake into brain cells is stimulated, allowing partial restoration of brain volume. This is followed by chronic adaptation, which is complete by day 7, characterized by accumulation of organic solutes within brain cells and leading to restoration of normal brain volume despite persistent elevation in intracellular osmolality.

intracellular solute increases the risk for cerebral edema during rehydration.

The clinical manifestations of hypernatremia reflect the rapidity of its onset, its duration, and its magnitude. In severe acute hypernatremia, brain shrinkage may be substantial, placing traction on venous sinuses and intracerebral veins and causing their rupture. The resulting intracerebral and subarachnoid hemorrhage may produce irreversible neurologic defects or death. The manifestations of less profound hypernatremia are nonspecific and include nausea, muscle weakness and fasciculations, and alterations in mental status ranging from lethargy to coma. Seizures, although uncommon in chronic hypernatremia, may develop after initiation of therapy in as many as 40% of patients.

The mortality rate associated with hypernatremia ranges from 40% to greater than 70%, depending on its magnitude and the rapidity of its onset. The majority of deaths, however, are not a direct consequence of the hypernatremia per se but result from underlying illnesses. In a study of hypernatremia in hospitalized patients, the overall in-hospital mortality rate was 41%; however, in only 16% of patients did the hypernatremia contribute to the cause of death. When mortality was analyzed on the basis of adequacy of therapy, hypernatremia contributed to mortality in 25% of patients in whom it persisted for more than 72 hours as compared with only 8% of patients in whom the hypernatremia was promptly treated and resolved within 72 hours.

TREATMENT

The treatment of hypernatremia is water. Existing water deficits need to be repleted and any ongoing electrolyte-free water losses replaced. The water deficit may be estimated based on the current serum sodium concentration ($[Na^+]$) and a normal serum sodium concentration of 140 mmol/L. Assuming that the hypernatremia is due to pure water loss and that total body solute has remained constant,

$$[Na^+] \times TBW_{current} = 140 \times TBW_{usual}$$

where TBW_{usual} and $TBW_{current}$ are the patient's normal and current body water content, respectively. Because the water deficit is the difference between the usual and current total body water ($TBW_{usual} - TBW_{current}$), the equation can be arranged as follows:

$$water\ deficit = TBW_{current} \times [([Na^+]/140) - 1]$$

If we assume that total body water is approximately 60% of body weight,

$$water\ deficit = 0.6 \times [body\ weight\ (kg)] \times [([Na^+]/140) - 1]$$

Despite inaccuracies inherent in this formula, this calculation provides a useful first approximation for initiating water replacement.

In acute hypernatremia, repletion of water deficits may be rapid. The electrolytes that accumulate in the brain during acute hypernatremia are rapidly extruded into the extracellular compartment during treatment, minimizing the risk for cerebral edema. In contrast, overly rapid therapy of chronic hypernatremia may produce cerebral edema if the water replacement occurs more rapidly than the brain can dissipate the accumulated organic solutes. This process of deadaptation may take 24 to 48 hours, or longer. Well-controlled clinical studies to ascertain the optimal treatment of chronic hypernatremia have not been performed. However, based on studies of brain deadaptation in animals following chronic hypernatremia, an approach of prompt but gradual correction is most prudent. In symptomatic patients, initial rapid water replacement should be provided; however, the serum sodium concentration should be reduced by no more than 1 to 2 mmol/L/hour. Once symptoms have resolved, replacement of the remainder of the water deficit should occur over 24 to 48 hours. Throughout treatment, the neurologic status of the patient should be closely monitored; deterioration after an initial improvement in neurologic symptoms suggests the development of cerebral edema and mandates temporary discontinuation of water replacement.

No individual regimen of water replacement is of documented superiority. Water may be administered enterally, either orally or by nasogastric tube, or intravenously. Intravenous repletion can consist of either hypotonic saline or 5% dextrose in water; pure water cannot be administered intravenously because the local hypotonicity at the site of administration can produce severe intravascular hemolysis. When using glucose-containing solutions, the blood glucose concentration should be monitored carefully and insulin therapy initiated, as necessary, to forestall hyperglycemia.

In addition to replacing the calculated water deficit, ongoing fluid losses must also be replaced. Urinary, gastrointestinal, and other losses should be quantified and should be replaced on the basis of their volume and electrolyte content. Insensible losses must also be replaced, recognizing that they increase by approximately 20% for each 1°C increase in body temperature.

Prompt attention to reducing excessive water losses is also important. Insensible losses may be reduced by normalizing body temperature with cooling blankets and antipyretics. Hyperglycemia should be controlled and protein loading decreased in order to limit osmotic diuresis. Nasogastric drainage can be reduced by therapy with H_2-receptor antagonists or proton pump inhibitors. Altering enteral feeding, treating infectious causes, discontinuing cathartic agents, or administering antidiarrheal agents can reduce diarrheal losses. Specific therapy for diabetes insipidus should be initiated, when appropriate.

Hypothalamic diabetes insipidus is readily treated with hormone replacement. Although the native hormone, aqueous arginine vasopressin, is available, a synthetic analogue with a longer half-life and less vasoconstrictive effects, dDAVP, is more commonly used for chronic management. Both arginine vasopressin and dDAVP have an onset of action of 30 to 60 minutes, but the duration of action of arginine vasopressin is usually 2 to 8 hours, as compared with 6 to 24 hours for dDAVP. Because of its shorter duration of action and parenteral route of administration, arginine vasopressin (5 to 10 IU subcutaneously) is usually reserved for use in acute situations, such as postoperative diabetes insipidus. dDAVP may be administered either subcutaneously (1 to 2 µg intravenously or subcutaneously every 8 to 24 hours) or by intranasal insufflation (5 to 20 µg every 12 to 24 hours).

Hormone replacement therapy is generally ineffective in nephrogenic diabetes insipidus. Restriction of dietary protein and sodium intake may attenuate the polyuria by reducing obligate urinary solute excretion. Thiazide diuretics may also mitigate renal water losses. Thiazides directly inhibit urinary diluting capacity, reducing free water generation. In addition, they decrease distal tubular fluid delivery by inducing mild intravascular volume contraction. The net effect is decreased delivery of free water to the collecting duct and enhanced vasopressin-independent water reabsorption, thereby moderating the polyuria. Nonsteroidal anti-inflammatory drugs are also useful as adjunctive therapy. Amiloride is beneficial in the treatment of lithium-induced nephrogenic diabetes insipidus. It is postulated that amiloride reduces cellular toxicity by blocking lithium entry into collecting duct cells.

Initial treatment of the patient with coexistent hypernatremia and extracellular volume depletion should be directed at restoring intravascular volume. Frank circulatory compromise should be promptly treated with isotonic saline or colloid solutions. Once adequate volume resuscitation has been achieved, treatment should then be directed toward replacing the water deficit.

The treatment of hypernatremia in patients with volume overload generally requires both water repletion and solute removal. Because hypernatremia often develops rapidly in these patients, the compensatory mechanisms defending brain volume are ineffective and neurologic symptoms may be accentuated. In addition, the concomitant intravascular volume expansion may result in pulmonary edema and exacerbate respiratory failure. Treatment must therefore be promptly instituted in order to prevent neurologic and cardiopulmonary complications. Because water repletion will further exacerbate intravascular volume overload, a loop diuretic should be administered to facilitate solute excretion. In patients with massive volume overload or renal failure, initiation of hemodialysis or hemofiltration may be necessary.

BIBLIOGRAPHY

Adrogue HJ, Madias NE: Hypernatremia. N Engl J Med 342:1493–1499, 2000.

Ayus JC, Armstrong DL, Arieff AI: Effects of hypernatremia in the central nervous system and its therapy in rats and rabbits. J Physiol 492:243–255, 1996.

DeRubertis FR, Michelis MF, Beck N, et al: "Essential" hypernatremia due to ineffective osmotic and intact volume regulation of vasopressin secretion. J Clin Invest 50:97–110, 1971.

Fitzsimons JT: Physiology and pathophysiology of thirst and sodium appetite. In Seldin DW, Giebisch G (eds): The Kidney: Physiology and Pathophysiology, 2nd ed. New York, Raven, 1992, pp 1615–1648.

Gullans SR, Verbalis JG: Control of brain volume during hyperosmolar and hypoosmolar conditions. Ann Rev Med 44:289–301, 1993.

Holtzman EJ, Ausiello DA: Nephrogenic diabetes insipidus: Causes revealed. Hosp Practice 29:67–82, 1994.

LieNYH, Shapiro JI, Chan L: Effects of hypernatremia on organic brain osmoles. J Clin Invest 85:1427–1435, 1990.

Miller M, Dalakos T, Moses AM, et al: Recognition of partial defects in antidiuretic hormone secretion. Ann Intern Med 73:721–729, 1970.

Palevsky PM: Hypernatremia. Semin Nephrol 18:20–30, 1998.

Palevsky PM, Bhagrath R, Greenberg A: Hypernatremia in hospitalized patients. Ann Intern Med 124:197–203, 1996.

Phillips PA, Rolls BJ, Ledingham JGG, et al: Reduced thirst after water deprivation in healthy elderly men. N Engl J Med 311:753–759, 1984.

Robertson GL: Regulation of vasopressin secretion. In Seldin DW, Giebisch G (eds): The Kidney: Physiology and Pathophysiology, 2nd ed. New York, Raven, 1992, pp 1595–1613.

Ross EJ, Christie SBM: Hypernatremia. Medicine 48:441–473, 1969.

Seckl JR, Dunger DB: Diabetes insipidus: Current treatment recommendations. Drugs 44:216–224, 1992.

Snyder NA, Feigal DW, Arieff AI: Hypernatremia in elderly patients. Ann Intern Med 107:309–319, 1987.

Zerbe RL, Robertson GL: A comparison of plasma vasopressin measurements with a standard indirect test in the differential diagnosis of polyuria. N Engl J Med 305:1539–1546, 1981.

CHAPTER 8

Metabolic Acidosis

Harold M. Szerlip

Metabolic acidosis describes a process in which non-volatile acids accumulate in the body. For practical purposes this can result from either the addition of protons or the loss of base. The consequence of this process is a decline in the major extracellular buffer, bicarbonate, and, if unopposed, a decrease in extracellular pH. Depending on the existence and the magnitude of other acid-base disturbances, however, the extracellular pH may be low, normal, or even high. Normal blood pH is between 7.38 and 7.42, corresponding to a hydrogen ion concentration of 42 to 38 nmol/L.

Metabolic acidosis results in a compensatory increase in minute ventilation; respiratory compensation begins promptly. A decrease in pH sensitizes the peripheral chemoreceptors, which triggers an increase in minute ventilation. Because increased ventilation is a compensatory mechanism stimulated by the acidemia, it never returns the pH to normal. The expected partial pressure of carbon dioxide (P_{CO_2}) for any given degree of metabolic acidosis can be predicted using Winters's formula: $P_{CO_2} = (1.5 \times [HCO_3^-]) + 8 \pm 2$.

OVERVIEW OF ACID-BASE BALANCE

In order to maintain extracellular pH within the normal range, the daily production of acid must be excreted from the body (Fig. 8-1). The vast majority of acid production results from the metabolism of dietary carbohydrates and fats. Complete oxidation of these metabolic substrates produces CO_2 and water. The 15,000 mmoles of CO_2 produced daily are efficiently exhaled by the lungs and are therefore known as volatile acid. As long as ventilatory function remains normal, this volatile acid does not contribute to changes in acid-base balance. Nonvolatile or fixed acids are produced by the metabolism of sulfate- and phosphate-containing amino acids. In addition, incomplete oxidation of fats and carbohydrates results in the production of small quantities of lactate and other organic anions, which when excreted in the urine represent loss of base. Individuals consuming a typical meat-based diet produce approximately 1 mmol/kg/day of hydrogen ions. Fecal excretion of a small amount of base also contributes to total daily acid production.

The kidney is responsible not only for the excretion of the daily production of fixed acid but also for the reclamation of the filtered bicarbonate. Bicarbonate reclamation occurs predominantly in the proximal tubule, mainly through the Na^+-H^+ exchanger. Active transporters in the distal tubule secrete hydrogen ion against a concentration gradient. Although urinary pH can fall to as low as 4.5, this, by itself, would account for little acid excretion. Fortunately, urinary phosphate and creatinine help buffer these protons, allowing the kidney to excrete approximately 40% of the daily fixed acid load as titratable acid (TA), so called because they are quantitated by titrating the urine pH back to that of plasma, 7.4. In addition to TA, renal excretion of acid is supported by ammoniagenesis. NH_3 is generated in the proximal tubule by the deamidation of glutamine to glutamate, which is subsequently deaminated to yield NH_3 and α-ketoglutarate. The enzymes responsible for these reactions are up-regulated by acidosis and hypokalemia. Hyperkalemia, on the other hand, reduces ammoniagenesis. NH_3 builds up in the renal interstitium and passively diffuses into the tubule lumen along the length of the collecting duct where it is trapped by H^+.

Under conditions of increased acid production, the normal kidney can increase acid excretion primarily by augmenting NH_3 production. Renal acid excretion varies directly with the rate of acid production. Net renal acid excretion (NAE) is equal to the sum of TA and NH_4^+ minus any secreted HCO_3^- [NAE = (TA + NH_4^+) − HCO_3^-]. Thus, the etiology of a metabolic acidosis can be divided into four broad categories: (1) overproduction of fixed acids, (2) increased extrarenal loss of base, (3) decrease in the kidney's ability to secrete hydrogen ions, and (4) inability of the kidney to reclaim the filtered bicarbonate (Fig. 8-2).

EVALUATION OF URINARY ACIDIFICATION

The cause of metabolic acidosis often is evident from the clinical situation. However, because the kidney is responsible for the reclamation of filtered HCO_3^- and excretion of the daily production of fixed acid, to evaluate a metabolic acidosis it may be necessary to assess whether the kidney is appropriately able to reabsorb HCO_3^-, secrete H^+ against a gradient, and excrete NH_4^+ (Table 8-1). The simplest test is to measure urine pH. Under conditions of

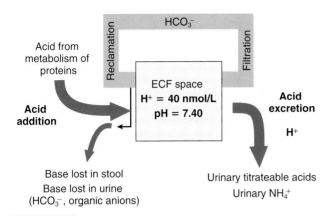

FIGURE 8-1 Maintenance of acid-base homeostasis requires that the addition of acid to the body is balanced by excretion of acid. Production of fixed nonvolatile acid occurs mainly through the metabolism of proteins. A small quantity of base also is lost in the stool and urine. Acid excretion occurs in the kidney through the secretion of H^+ buffered by titratable acids and NH_3. Bicarbonate filtration and reclamation by the kidney is normally a neutral process.

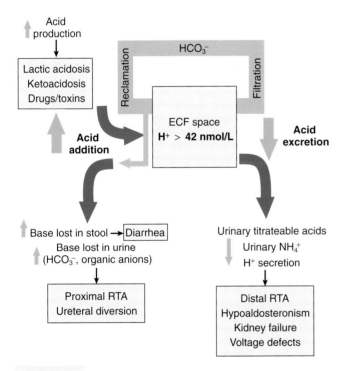

FIGURE 8-2 Metabolic acidosis can result from increased acid production, increased loss of base in stool or urine, or decreased H^+ secretion in the distal tubule. The causes of these processes are shown.

TABLE 8-1   Tests of Renal Acid Excretion

Urine pH (enhanced by furosemide)
NH_4^+ excretion
  Urine NH_4^+
  Urine anion gap
  Urine osmol gap
Urine Pco_2 with bicarbonate loading
Fractional excretion of HCO_3^-

acid loading, urine pH should be below 5.5. A pH of higher than 5.5 usually reflects impaired distal hydrogen ion secretion. Measuring the pH after challenging the patient with the loop diuretic furosemide will increase the sensitivity of this test by providing Na^+ to the distal tubule for reabsorption. The reabsorption of Na^+ creates a negative electrical potential in the lumen and enhances H^+ secretion. It is important, however, to rule out urinary infections with urea-splitting organisms, which will increase pH. An elevated urine pH may also be misleading in conditions associated with volume depletion and hypokalemia, as can occur in diarrhea. In contradistinction to furosemide, volume depletion with decreased sodium delivery to the distal tubule impairs distal H^+ secretion. Furthermore, hypokalemia, by enhancing ammoniagenesis, raises the urine pH.

Because renal excretion of NH_4^+ accounts for the majority of acid excretion, measurement of urine NH_4^+ provides important information. Urinary NH_4^+ excretion can be decreased by a variety of mechanisms, including a primary decrease in ammoniagenesis by the proximal tubule as seen in chronic kidney disease (CKD), or decreased trapping in the distal tubule either secondary to decreased H^+ secretion or an increased delivery of HCO_3^-, which will preferentially buffer H^+, making it unavailable to form NH_4^+. Unfortunately, direct measurement of NH_4^+ is not usually readily available in clinical laboratories. An estimate of NH_4^+ excretion, however, is easily obtained by calculating the urine anion gap (UAG) or urine osmole gap. If, as is usual, the anion balancing the charge of the NH_4^+ is Cl^-, the UAG [$(Na^+ + K^+) - Cl^-$], should be negative because the chloride is greater than the sum of Na^+ and K^+ (Fig. 8-3). Although the measurement of the UAG in conditions of acid loading is often reflective of NH_4^+ excretion, the presence of anions other than Cl^- (such as keto anions or hippurate) makes it a less reliable assessment of NH_4^+ than the urine osmole gap (see Fig. 8-3). The urine osmole gap is calculated as follows: measured urine osmolality − [$2(Na^+ + K^+)$ + urea nitrogen/2.8 + glucose/18]. The osmole gap is made up primarily of NH_4 salts. Thus, half of the gap represents NH_4^+. An osmole gap of greater than 100 mmol/L signifies normal NH_4^+ excretion.

Another test of distal H^+ ion secretory ability is measurement of urine Pco_2 during bicarbonate loading. Distal delivery of HCO_3^- in the presence of normal H^+ secretory capacity results in elevated Pco_2 in the urine. When there is a secretory defect, urine Pco_2 does not increase. Accurate measurement of urine Pco_2 requires that the urine be collected under oil to prevent the loss of CO_2 into the air.

COMPLICATIONS OF ACIDOSIS

Although it has been accepted that a decrease in extracellular pH has detrimental effects on numerous physiologic parameters and should be aggressively treated, this

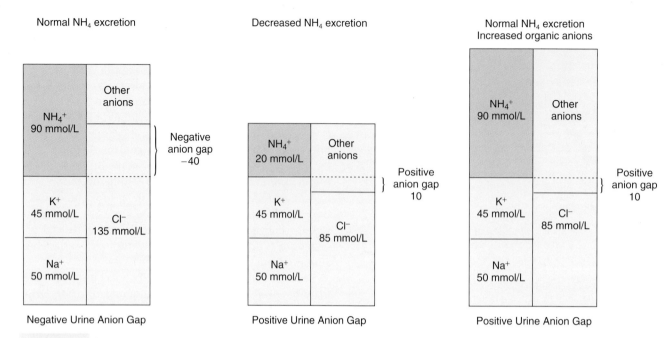

FIGURE 8-3 In the presence of acidemia, the kidney increases NH_4^+ excretion. The urine anion gap (AG) is an indirect method for estimating urine NH_4^+. If the accompanying anion is chloride, the UAG (Na + K − Cl) will be negative, reflecting the large quantity of NH_4^+ in the urine. A decrease in NH_4^+ secretion occurs when ammoniagenesis is diminished, H^+ secretion is impaired, or there is delivery of HCO_3^- to the distal tubule. In these cases the UAG will be inappropriately positive. If anions other than Cl^- are excreted (e.g., ketones, hippurate), the UAG will be positive despite increased NH_4^+ excretion, because these anions are not used in calculation of the gap.

dogma has recently been challenged. The proponents of treatment argue that acidemia depresses cardiac contractility, blocks activation of adrenergic receptors, and inhibits the action of key enzymes. Uncontrolled clinical studies are not easy to interpret because of the difficulties in separating the effects of the acidosis from the effects of the underlying illness. Most controlled studies investigating the role of acidosis on cellular processes have been done in isolated cells or organs; therefore, the effects of acidemia on whole-body physiology and their applicability to humans are unclear.

The effect of pH on cardiac function has been strongly debated. Cardiac output is determined by multiple components, and it is the sum of the effects on these individual components that determines the net effect of acidemia on cardiac function. Myocardial contractile strength and changes in vascular tone determine cardiovascular performance, and the relative contributions of each in the context of acidemia remain to be clarified. Because of differing effects of acidemia on contractile force, vascular tone, and sympathetic discharge, it is difficult to predict what happens to cardiac output from studies using isolated myocytes or perfused hearts.

During continuous infusion of lactic acid, it has been shown that cardiac output and the rate of development of left ventricular force increase. In addition, fractional shortening of the left ventricle as assessed by transthoracic echocardiography appears to be normal even in cases of severe acidemia. At what pH cardiac output and blood pressure falls remains unclear.

APPROACH TO ACID-BASE DISORDERS

Complete evaluation of acid-base status requires a routine electrolyte panel, measurement of serum albumin, and arterial blood gas analysis. The traditional approach to the diagnosis of metabolic acidosis relies on the calculation of the anion gap (AG) and subsequent separation of metabolic acidosis into those with an elevated AG and those in which the AG is normal, or so-called hyperchloremic metabolic acidosis (HCMA; Fig. 8-4). The AG is defined as the difference between the concentration of sodium, the major cation, and the sum of the concentrations of chloride and bicarbonate, the major anions {[Na^+] − ([Cl^-] + [HCO_3^-])}. Because the concentration of potassium changes minimally, its contribution is ignored for convenience. Obviously, electrical neutrality must exist and the sum of the anions must equal the sum of the cations. The gap results because anions such as sulfate, phosphate, organic anions, and especially the weak acid proteins are present but not measured on the routine chemistry panel. There are fewer unmeasured cations. Thus, it would seem upon examination of a chemistry panel that cations exceed anions, creating an AG. The normal AG is $8 \pm 4\,mEq/L$. Any increase in the AG even in the face of a normal or frankly alkalemic pH represents the accumulation of acids and the presence of an acidosis. In many cases the anions that make up the gap are often not easily identifiable.

The one caveat in using the AG is to recognize that the normal gap is predominantly composed of the negative

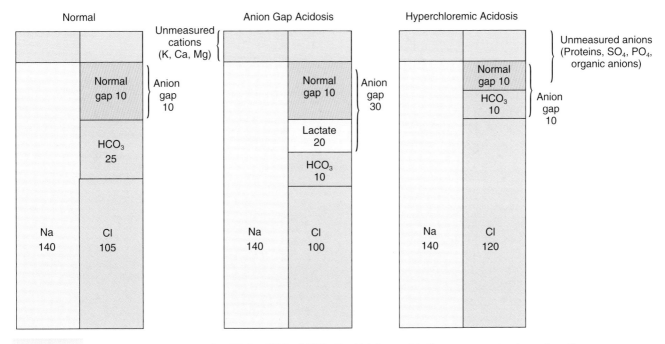

FIGURE 8-4 The anion gap (AG) is equal to $[Na^+] - ([Cl^-] + [HCO_3^-])$, which is equal to the unmeasured anions minus the unmeasured cations. In an AG acidosis there is a decrease in $[HCO_3^-]$ and an increase in organic anions (e.g., lactate), which results in an elevated anion gap. In a hyperchloremic acidosis there is a decrease in $[HCO_3^-]$ and an increase in $[Cl^-]$ with no change in anion gap.

charge on albumin. When hypoalbuminemia is present, the AG must be corrected for the serum albumin. For each 1 g/dL decrease in the serum albumin, the calculated AG should be increased by 2.5 mEq/L. Thus, the corrected AG: $AG_c = AG + 2.5(4 - \text{serum albumin})$. If the AG is not corrected, the presence of a metabolic acidosis may be masked. This is especially true in critically ill patients, who typically have decreased serum albumin.

ANION GAP ACIDOSIS

As previously described, an increased AG represents the accumulation of nonchloride acids. AG acidosis can be divided into four major categories (Table 8-2): (1) lactic

TABLE 8-2 Causes of Anion Gap Acidosis

Lactic acidosis
Type A
Type B
D-Lactic acidosis

Ketoacidosis
Diabetic ketoacidosis
Alcoholic ketoacidosis
Starvation ketosis

Toxins/drugs
Methanol
Ethylene glycol
Salicylate

Kidney failure (with severe reductions in glomerular filtration rate)

acidosis, (2) ketoacidosis, (3) toxin/drugs, and (4) severe kidney failure. In all but kidney failure, the accumulation of acids is caused by their overproduction. These acids dissociate into protons, which are quickly buffered by HCO_3^- and their respective conjugate bases, the unmeasured anions. As long as these anions are retained in the body and not excreted, they contribute to the elevation in the AG.

Lactic Acidosis

Lactic acidosis is a common AG acidosis, and by far the most serious of all AG acidoses. Anaerobic metabolism of glucose (glycolysis) occurs in the extramitochondrial cytoplasm and produces pyruvate as an intermediary. If this were the end of the glycolytic process, there would be a net production of two protons and a metabolically unsatisfactory reduction of NAD to NADH. Fortunately, pyruvate rapidly undergoes one of two metabolic fates: (1) under anaerobic conditions, because of the high NADH/NAD ratio, pyruvate is quickly reduced by lactate dehydrogenase to lactate—releasing energy, consuming a proton, and decreasing the NADH/NAD ratio, thus allowing for continued glycolysis; or (2) in the presence of oxygen, pyruvate diffuses into the mitochondria, and, after oxidation by the pyruvate dehydrogenase (PDH) complex, enters the tricarboxylic acid cycle, where it is completely oxidized to CO_2 and water. Neither of these pathways results in the production of H^+. During glycolysis, glucose metabolism produces two molecules of lactate and two molecules of adenosine triphosphate (ATP). It is the hydrolysis of ATP (ATP → ADP + H$^+$ + P$_i$) that releases protons. Therefore, the acidosis does not occur because of the production of lactate, but because under hypoxic conditions the hydrolysis of ATP is greater than ATP production. Thus, the buildup of lactate is a surrogate marker for ATP consumption during hypoxic states.

Although lactate production averages about 1300 mmol/day, serum lactate levels are normally less than 1 mmol/L because lactate is either reoxidized to pyruvate and enters the tricarboxylic acid cycle or is utilized by the liver and kidney via the Cori cycle for gluconeogenesis. Increased concentration of lactate can therefore result from decreased oxidative phosphorylation, increased glycolysis, or decreased gluconeogenesis. Lactate levels between 2 and 3 mmol/L are frequently found in hospitalized patients. Some of these patients will go on to develop frank acidosis, but others will have no adverse events. Lactic acidosis is defined as the presence of a lactate level of greater than 5 mmol/L.

There is a poor correlation among arterial pH, calculated AG, and serum lactate levels, even in those patients with a serum lactic acid level of greater than 5 mmol/L. Approximately 25% of patients with serum lactate levels between 5 and 9.9 mmol/L have a pH greater than 7.35, and as many as half have AGs of less than 12.

Lactic acidosis has been traditionally divided into types A and B (Table 8-3). Type A, or hypoxic lactic acidosis, results from an imbalance between oxygen supply and oxygen demand. In type B lactic acidosis, oxygen delivery is normal but oxidative phosphorylation is impaired. This is seen in patients who have inborn errors of metabolism or who have ingested drugs or toxins. It has become increasingly clear, however, that lactic acidosis is often caused by the simultaneous existence of both hypoxic and nonhypoxic factors, and in many cases it is difficult to separate one from the other. For example, hereditary partial defects in mitochondrial metabolism as well as age-related declines in cytochrome IV complex activity may result in lactic acidosis with a lesser degree of hypoxia than in patients without such defects. Even in cases of shock in which tissue oxygen delivery is obviously inadequate, decreased portal blood flow and reduced hepatic clearance of lactate contribute to the acidosis. Similarly, in sepsis there is a decrease in both tissue perfusion and in the ability to utilize oxygen. Therefore, this division based solely on cause is largely of historical and conceptual interest.

The presence of lactate acidosis is considered a poor prognostic sign. Studies have found that as lactate levels increase above 2.0 to 2.5 mmol/L the probability of survival decreases precipitously. It remains unclear, however, whether the blood lactate level is an independent contributor to mortality or whether it represents an epiphenomenon confounded by the severity of the patient's illness. Just as important to prognosis is the body's ability to metabolize lactate after restoration of

TABLE 8-3 Lactic Acidosis
Type A
Generalized seizure
Extreme exercise
Shock
Cardiac arrest
Low cardiac output
Severe anemia
Severe hypoxemia
Carbon monoxide poisoning
Type B
Sepsis
Thiamine deficiency
Uncontrolled diabetes mellitus
Malignancy
Hypoglycemia
Drugs/toxins
Ethanol
Metformin
Zidovudine
Didanosine
Stavudine
Lamivudine
Zalcitabine
Salicylate
Propofol
Niacin
Isoniazid
Nitroprusside
Cyanide
Catecholamines
Cocaine
Acetaminophen
Streptozotocin
Pheochromocytoma
Sorbitol/fructose
Malaria
Inborn errors of metabolism
Other
Hepatic failure
Respiratory or metabolic alkalosis
Propylene glycol
D-Lactic acidosis

tissue perfusion. Patients able to reduce their lactate by half within 18 hours of resuscitation have a significantly greater chance of survival. In all likelihood the inability to metabolize lactate is a surrogate marker for organ dysfunction.

Type A Lactic Acidosis

Lactic acidosis is commonly observed in conditions in which oxygen delivery is inadequate, such as low cardiac output, hypotension, severe anemia, and carbon monoxide poisoning. States of hypoperfusion are more prone to the accumulation of lactate than hypoxemic states. In the latter, tissue oxygenation is often preserved due to compensatory mechanisms such as increased cardiac output, augmented red blood cell production, and a reduced affinity of hemoglobin for oxygen. In all cases of type A lactic acidosis, oxygen is unavailable to the mitochondria, and pyruvate, unable to enter the tricarboxylic acid cycle, is reduced to lactate.

Type B Lactic Acidosis

Sepsis

Although sepsis is frequently associated with hypotension and thus type A lactic acidosis, lactic acidosis also may develop during sepsis, even when oxygen delivery and tissue perfusion appear to be unimpeded. It has been postulated that in sepsis there is both an overproduction of pyruvate and an inhibition of PDH activity (the rate-limiting state in oxidative phosphorylation). Because of the increased NADH/NAD ratio, pyruvate is rapidly reduced to lactate. Dichloroacetate, an activator of the PDH complex, lowers lactate levels significantly, suggesting that tissue oxygenation is adequate enough to support oxidative phosphorylation.

Drugs

Numerous drugs and toxins can cause lactic acidosis. The biguanide derivatives phenformin and metformin are recognized causes of lactic acidosis. Phenformin was withdrawn from the United States market in 1976 because of the common occurrence of lactic acidosis. Both of these agents bind to complex 1 of the mitochondrial respiratory chain, inhibiting its activity. Metformin, a newer biguanide, has a markedly lower incidence of lactic acidosis than phenformin, possibly because it is less lipid soluble and thus has limited ability to cross the mitochondrial membrane and bind to the mitochondrial complex. Almost all reported cases of metformin-associated lactic acidosis have occurred in patients with underlying CKD. It has been suggested that the present incidence of lactic acidosis in diabetics is no greater than the incidence of lactic acidosis prior to the introduction of metformin, and thus the association of metformin with lactic acidosis is more "guilt by association." A causative role, however, is suggested by the observations that in isolated mitochondria, metformin inhibits the respiratory chain, and that the incidence of lactic acidosis approaches zero when the drug is prescribed according to recommendations.

Lactic acidosis is being increasingly recognized in patients with human immunodeficiency virus infection who are taking nucleoside reverse-transcriptase inhibitors. These agents, particularly stavudine, but also zidovudine, didanosine, and lamivudine, have been associated with severe lactic acidosis, often with concomitant hepatic steatosis. Nucleoside analogues inhibit mitochondrial DNA polymerase-γ. This causes mitochondrial toxicity and a decrease in oxidative phosphorylation, resulting in both lipid accumulation within the liver and decreased oxidation of pyruvate. Of note, hyperlactatemia without frank lactic acidosis is often present in patients on these medications. What converts these mild elevations in lactate levels into frank lactic acidosis is not known.

Salicylate intoxication often produces lactic acidosis. This occurs both because the salicylate-induced respiratory alkalosis stimulates lactate production and because of the inhibitory effects of salicylates on oxidative metabolism. Ethanol ingestion may cause mild elevations in lactate levels secondary to impaired hepatic conversion of lactate to glucose. In addition, the metabolism of ethanol increases the NADH/NAD ratio, favoring the conversion of pyruvate to lactate. Concomitant thiamine deficiency, as is often seen in alcohol abusers, may exacerbate the acidosis.

Vitamin Deficiency

Deficiency of thiamine, a cofactor for PDH, also can result in lactic acidosis. Patients requiring total parental nutrition may develop thiamine deficiency if not supplemented with this vitamin. During a national shortage of parenteral vitamin preparations, numerous cases of lactic acidosis were reported from inadequate thiamine supplementation.

Systemic Disease

Diabetes is often associated with lactic acidosis. Even under basal conditions, patients with diabetes have mildly elevated lactate levels. This is thought to be secondary to decreased PDH activity caused by free fatty acid oxidation by liver and muscle. Lactate increases even more during diabetic ketoacidosis, possibly secondary to decreased hepatic clearance. This accumulation of lactate contributes to the elevated AG present in ketoacidosis.

Malignancy

Lactic acidosis has been detected in patients with acute rapidly progressive hematologic malignancies such as leukemia or lymphoma. Lactate levels usually parallel disease activity. The increased blood viscosity and microvascular aggregates that are frequently found in acute leukemia cause regional hypoperfusion. Overproduction of lactate may also result from a large tumor burden and rapid cell lysis.

Alternate Sugars

The use of sorbitol or fructose intravenously, as irrigants during prostate surgery or in tube feedings, can cause lactic acidosis. The metabolism of these sugars consumes ATP, inhibiting gluconeogenesis and stimulating glycolysis, leading to the accumulation of excess lactate.

Propylene Glycol

Propylene glycol is a common vehicle for many drugs, including topical silver sulfadiazine and intravenous preparations of nitroglycerin, diazepam, lorazepam, phenytoin, etomidate, and trimethoprim-sulfamethoxazole, among others. Although it is considered relatively safe, many case reports have appeared demonstrating toxicity. Approximately 40% to 50% of administered propylene glycol is oxidized by alcohol dehydrogenase to lactic acid. Toxic patients commonly develop an unexplained AG acidosis with increased serum osmolality. Considering that patients receiving many of the medications solubilized with propylene glycol frequently have other possible causes for their acidosis, it is important to be aware of this iatrogenic cause for the acidosis. Correction of the metabolic abnormalities quickly occurs following discontinuation of the medication

D-*Lactic Acidosis*

This unusual form of AG acidosis is the result of the accumulation of the D-isomer of lactate. Unlike lactate produced by glycolysis in animals, which is the L-isomer, colonic bacteria produce the D-isomer. Overproduction of D-lactate occurs in patients with short-bowel syndrome and is usually precipitated by a high carbohydrate intake. Increased delivery of carbohydrates due to the shortened bowel and an overgrowth of bacteria are responsible for this overproduction. Because D-lactate is not detected on the routine assay, which measures only L-lactate, diagnosis requires a high clinical suspicion. Patients typically present with mental status changes, ataxia, and nystagmus. Treatment consists of an oral fast with intravenous nutrition and restoration of gut flora to normal through the administration of oral antibiotics. In severe cases, hemodialysis can decrease the concentration of D-lactate.

Treatment of Lactic Acidosis

The treatment of lactic acidosis is fraught with controversy. The most important step is treatment of the underlying cause. In sepsis, restoring oxygenation via mechanical ventilation and perfusion via pressors or inotropes are of paramount importance, although these interventions do not always improve the lactic acidosis. In some patients with medication-induced lactic acidosis, withdrawal of the offending agent may be sufficient. There are anecdotal case reports of successful treatment of lactic acidosis associated with nucleoside analogues in patients with acquired immunodeficiency syndrome with riboflavin or L-carnitine.

Often these measures fail and the clinician is faced with the decision of whether to give sodium bicarbonate in an effort to increase serum pH. There are several potential problems with this approach. First, as previously discussed, it is not clear to what extent acidosis is deleterious and therefore whether normalizing pH is of any benefit. Also, increasing pH may actually increase lactic acid production. Sodium bicarbonate is often given as a hypertonic solution, which can lead to hypernatremia and cellular dehydration. Perhaps most important is the possibility that the administration of HCO_3^- can cause a paradoxic decrease in intracellular pH despite an increase

in extracellular pH. Bicarbonate combines with hydrogen, forming carbonic acid, which is then converted to CO_2 and water. Thus, P_{CO_2} increases with the titration of acid by bicarbonate and rapidly diffuses into cells, causing acidification, while bicarbonate remains extracellular. Thus, it is difficult to recommend the use of bicarbonate for the treatment of a low serum pH alone. If the serum bicarbonate is less than 7.1, however, many clinicians, despite the lack of supporting data, opt for treatment because a further small decline in serum bicarbonate can have a profound effect on serum pH.

Other buffers may be better tolerated insofar as they buffer hydrogen ions without increasing CO_2. One such buffer is tris-hydroxymethyl aminomethane (THAM), a biologically inert amino acid that can buffer both CO_2 and protons. It does not cause production of CO_2 and thus works well in a closed system. The protonated molecule is excreted by the kidney and should be used cautiously in patients with kidney failure. Potential side effects include hyperkalemia, hypoglycemia, ventilatory depression, and hepatic necrosis in neonates. Despite its having been available for many years, there are no studies demonstrating improved outcomes with the use of THAM. The acute dose in milliliters of 0.3 mol/L solution can be derived using the following formula: dose in milliliters = 0.3 × body weight (kg) × decrease in HCO_3^- from normal (mmol/L). The first 25% to 50% of the dose is given over 5 minutes, and the rest over 1 hour. Alternatively, a steady infusion of no more than 3.5 L/day can be given for several days.

Dichloroacetate has also been used in the treatment of lactic acidosis. This agent stimulates the activity of PDH, increasing the rate of pyruvate oxidation and thereby decreasing lactate levels. A large multicenter trial in humans showed a reduction in serum lactate, an increase in pH, and an increase in the number of patients able to resolve their hyperlactatemia. Despite these favorable changes, no improvement in either hemodynamic parameters or mortality was found.

Various modes of renal replacement therapy have been used in the treatment of lactic acidosis. Standard bicarbonate hemodialysis treats acidosis primarily by diffusion of bicarbonate from the bath into the blood and is thus another form of bicarbonate administration, albeit with several advantages. Hypernatremia and volume overload are not a concern with hemodialysis as they are with intravenous administration. Also, hemodialysis in addition to adding bicarbonate removes lactate. Although the removal of lactate does not increase serum pH, there is some evidence that the lactate ion itself is harmful. Unfortunately, there are no randomized, prospective trials demonstrating benefit of dialysis in lactic acidosis, and its use in the absence of other indications cannot be routinely recommended.

Several studies have shown that high-volume hemofiltration using either lactate or bicarbonate buffered replacement fluid can rapidly correct metabolic acidosis.

These studies have been small, and the degree and type of acidosis have been poorly characterized. In addition, other treatment measures have usually been instituted, making it difficult to draw conclusions about the effectiveness of this treatment. Nevertheless, hemofiltration remains a viable therapeutic option.

Peritoneal dialysis has also been used in the treatment of metabolic acidosis. Although there are case reports of success using this modality, a randomized study comparing lactate-buffered peritoneal dialysis to continuous hemofiltration showed that hemofiltration corrected acidosis more quickly and more effectively than peritoneal dialysis. Whether newer bicarbonate buffered peritoneal dialysis solution would be more efficacious remains to be determined.

Diabetic Ketoacidosis

Diabetic ketoacidosis (DKA) is another common cause of an AG acidosis. Although, DKA may be the initial presentation of diabetes mellitus, more commonly patients have a known diagnosis of diabetes and either have been noncompliant with their insulin regimen or have some other precipitating factor such as infection. Patients are generally polyuric and polydipsic, but if volume depletion becomes severe enough, polyuria may not be seen. Although DKA is classically seen in type 1 diabetes, it can also occur in patients with type 2 diabetes. DKA results from insulin deficiency and concomitant increase in counter-regulatory hormones such as glucagon, epinephrine, and cortisol. This hormonal milieu leads to an inability of cells to utilize glucose, causing them to oxidize fatty acids as fuel, producing large amounts of ketoacids. A diagnosis of DKA requires a pH less than 7.35, elevated AG, positive serum ketones of at least 1:2 dilutions, and decreased serum bicarbonate. However, not all patients with DKA meet these criteria. If renal perfusion and GFR are well maintained, ketones (anions) are rapidly excreted by the kidney in place of chloride. With the loss of these anions in the urine, the AG acidosis may be replaced by a mixed AG/hyperchloremic acidosis or even a pure hyperchloremic acidosis. Furthermore, an increase in the NADH/NAD ratio, which frequently occurs during DKA, causes ketones to shift from acetoacetate to β-hydroxybutyrate, which is not detected on the standard nitroprusside test used to identify serum and urinary ketones. If this occurs, serum ketones may appear to be negative or only trace positive. Finally, vomiting may result in a metabolic alkalosis, which would raise the serum bicarbonate toward the normal range. In this case, the serum AG would almost certainly be elevated and the astute clinician will not be fooled.

Treatment

The treatment of DKA consists of three parts: fluid resuscitation, insulin administration, and correction of potassium deficits. Patients with DKA often have profound deficits of both sodium and free water. Hypovolemia as demonstrated by hemodynamic compromise should always be treated first. Patients should rapidly receive 1 to 2 L of 0.9% saline until their blood pressure is stabilized. Thereafter, hypotonic fluids in the form of 0.45% saline should be administered to correct free water deficits while continuing to provide volume. Insulin should be administered only after fluid resuscitation is well under way. If insulin is given precipitously, the rapid uptake of glucose by the cells will cause water to osmotically follow, resulting in cardiovascular collapse. A regular insulin bolus of 0.1 unit/kg intravenously is given followed by a continuous infusion of 0.1 unit/kg/hour. If the glucose does not decline by 50 to 100 mg/dL/hour, the infusion should be increased by 50%. The insulin infusion should be continued until the ketosis is resolved, as demonstrated by negative serum ketones, closure of the AG, and near normalization of the serum.

As tissue perfusion improves, β-hydroxybutyrate is converted to acetoacetate, and serum ketones paradoxically increase, but then should decrease. The closure of the AG, by itself, is unreliable because, as discussed previously, with volume resuscitation the ketones are rapidly excreted and the AG acidosis is replaced by a hyperchloremic acidosis. Serum glucose usually approaches normal before ketosis is resolved. When glucose is less than 250 mg/dL, intravenous fluids should be changed to 5% dextrose to avoid hypoglycemia while awaiting resolution of ketosis. The insulin infusion can be discontinued when the ketosis is resolved and the patient is taking food and fluid by mouth. A subcutaneous insulin dose should be given at least 1 hour prior to stopping the drip to avoid rebound ketosis.

Most patients with DKA have total-body potassium depletion. Nevertheless, their serum potassium may be normal to high due to a shift from out of the cells caused by the profound insulinopenia. When insulin is restored, extracellular potassium is rapidly taken up by cells, and severe hypokalemia may ensue. Therefore, addition of potassium to the intravenous fluids is recommended at a concentration of 10 to 20 mEq/L as soon as serum potassium falls below 4.5 mEq/L. Needless to say, this management algorithm requires frequent laboratory tests.

Although bicarbonate therapy has been used in severe DKA, this use is not supported by the literature. In fact, bicarbonate administration even in patients with pH less than 7.0 has not been shown to be advantageous. In almost all cases, the acidosis rapidly improves with appropriate management without the use of bicarbonate. Thus, the administration of sodium bicarbonate to patients with diabetic ketoacidosis cannot be routinely recommended. It is important, however, that these patients be monitored in a setting where they can be closely observed and where frequent analyses of their arterial blood gases and electrolytes can be obtained.

Alcoholic Ketoacidosis

Alcoholic ketoacidosis (AKA) usually presents with an AG acidosis and ketonemia but without significant hyperglycemia. The classic presentation is that of a patient who has been on an alcohol binge, develops nausea and vomiting, and stops eating. The patient typically presents 24 to 48 hours after the cessation of oral intake and may also complain of abdominal pain and shortness of breath. Alcohol levels are low or even unmeasurable by the time AKA develops. AKA is similar to DKA in that it is a state of insulinopenia and increased counter-regulatory hormones; in fact, the levels of these hormones are similar in both disorders. In AKA, normo- to hypoglycemia is usually observed despite a hormonal milieu favoring hyperglycemia because decreased NAD curtails hepatic gluconeogenesis and starvation depletes glycogen stores. Patients with AKA, however, can occasionally present with hyperglycemia, and in those cases distinguishing it from DKA can be difficult. AKA almost always presents with an AG, but acidemia is less universal. Patients often have concurrent metabolic alkalosis from vomiting or respiratory alkalosis from liver disease. Thus, patients with AKA may not be acidemic and rarely do they have a simple metabolic acidosis. Because of the increased NADH/NAD ratio, the primary ketoacid present is β-hydroxybutyrate, and, thus, serum ketones may be reported as negative. This ratio also favors the formation of lactic acid. Finally, electrolyte disorders, including hypokalemia, hypophosphatemia, and hypomagnesemia, are common.

Treatment

Therapy of AKA is straightforward and consists of volume repletion, provision of glucose (except in those patients with hyperglycemia), and correction of any electrolyte abnormalities. Patients are often volume depleted from vomiting combined with poor oral intake. Thiamine must be provided prior to or concurrently with glucose to avoid precipitating Wernicke's encephalopathy. Acidosis resolves as insulin increases and counter-regulatory hormones are turned off in response to glucose infusion. The clinician must maintain a high degree of suspicion for this disorder because the acid-base disturbance may be subtle on routine laboratory analyses, with patients often demonstrating an elevated AG as the only abnormality. Chronic alcoholics often have hypoalbuminemia, which can further obscure the interpretation of the AG. Any patient with nausea and vomiting with a recent history of alcohol abuse should probably be treated for presumptive AKA until the diagnosis is clearly ruled out.

Starvation Ketosis

During prolonged fasting, insulin levels are suppressed, whereas glucagon, epinephrine, growth hormone, and cortisol levels are increased. This hormonal milieu results in increased lipolysis with release of free fatty acids into the blood and stimulation of hepatic ketogenesis. The concentrations of both β-hydroxybutyrate and acetoacetate increase over the course of several weeks, resulting in a mild AG metabolic acidosis.

Toxins and Drugs

Ethylene Glycol

Ingestion of various toxins can cause severe metabolic acidosis with an increased AG and should always be suspected in these cases. Ethylene glycol is a sweet liquid that is found in antifreeze. Ingestion of 100 mL or more can be fatal. Ethylene glycol is metabolized by alcohol dehydrogenase into glycolic acid and subsequently oxalic acid. This generates NADH, which encourages the formation of lactic acid. The AG acidosis results from the accumulation of the various acid metabolites of ethylene glycol as well as lactic acidosis. Diagnosis can be difficult because ethylene glycol is not detected on routine toxicology assays. It should be suspected in anyone who presents with intoxication, a low blood alcohol, and a markedly increased AG metabolic acidosis without ketonemia. The serum osmolar gap may help detect ethylene glycol. Serum osmolar gap is the difference between the calculated serum osmolarity $[([Na^+] \times 2) + (glucose/18) + (BUN/2.8)]$ and the actual serum osmolality as measured by the laboratory. A difference greater than about 10 to 15 mOsm/L suggests the presence of an unmeasured, osmotically active substance, which in the right clinical setting could be a toxin. However, it is important to understand the limitations of this approach. Some laboratories measure serum osmolality using vapor pressure methodology rather than freezing point depression, and volatile substances such as alcohols may not be detected. As the osmotically active alcohol is metabolized into the various acids, the osmolar gap disappears. Thus, early after ingestion, the osmolar gap is elevated without a significant increase in the AG. As the alcohol is metabolized, the osmolar gap decreases while the AG increases. Examination of the urine may reveal calcium oxalate crystals, a finding that can be considered pathognomonic. However, the absence of these crystals does not rule out the ingestion of ethylene glycol. Precipitation of calcium oxalate may occasionally cause hypocalcemia. Because fluorescein is added as a colorant to antifreeze, the urine of a patient with antifreeze ingestion may fluoresce under a Wood's lamp.

Methanol

Methanol is an alcohol often found in solvents or as an adulterant in alcoholic beverages. Toxicity is usually caused by ingestion of as little as 30 mL and has also been reported after inhalation. Methanol is metabolized by alcohol dehydrogenase to formaldehyde and then to formic acid, resulting in an elevated AG acidosis. Similar to ingestions of other alcohols, NAD depletion favors the production of lactate. Methanol is less intoxicating than either ethanol or ethylene glycol. The most characteristic symptom of methanol toxicity is blurry vision. Blindness may occur due to optic nerve involvement, and pancreatitis may be seen in up to two thirds of patients. As described previously, early after ingestion an osmolar gap may be found. The diagnosis of both ethylene glycol and methanol poisoning can be confirmed by specific toxicologic assays, but treatment should never be delayed while awaiting these results.

Treatment of Toxic Alcohol Ingestions

Treatment of both ethylene glycol and methanol toxicity is based on the fact that it is the metabolites of these alcohols that are actually harmful. Both substances are metabolized by alcohol dehydrogenase. Blocking the activity of this enzyme will prevent the metabolic acidosis and allow the alcohol to be excreted by the kidneys or be removed by dialysis. Because alcohol dehydrogenase has a much higher affinity for ethanol than for either ethylene glycol or methanol, use of ethanol as a competitive inhibitor is the traditional treatment. Ethanol is supplied as a 10% solution in 5% dextrose in water (D5W). A loading dose of 0.8 to 1.0 g/kg body weight followed by an infusion of 100 mg/kg/hour should be sufficient to maintain a blood alcohol level of 100 to 150 mg/dL. However, in some patients with marked ethanol tolerance this rate will need to be doubled. More recently 4-methylpyrazole (fomepizole), a competitive inhibitor of alcohol dehydrogenase, has replaced ethanol as the treatment of choice. Fomepizole is a more potent inhibitor of alcohol dehydrogenase than ethanol and does not lead to central nervous system (CNS) depression. An initial loading dose of 15 mg/kg body weight is followed 12 hours later by 10 mg/kg every 12 hours for four doses, then 15 mg/kg every 12 hours for four more doses. Although fomepizole, because of its potency, has begun to call into question the need for dialysis, until more studies are available it is recommended that dialysis be instituted in all patients with suspected ingestions of ethylene glycol or methanol who have end organ damage (kidney failure or visual impairment) and whose pH is less than 7.2. Both compounds can be rapidly removed by hemodialysis. Hemodialysis can also help improve the acidosis by providing a source of bicarbonate. It is important to double the rate of any ethanol infusion or increase the dose of fomepizole while the patient is on hemodialysis. For either ingestion, gastric lavage with charcoal should be performed when ingestion has occurred within the preceding 2 to 3 hours.

Salicylate Toxicity

The ingestion of salicylates is an important cause of mixed acid-base disturbances, producing both a respiratory alkalosis and a metabolic acidosis. Salicylate is a direct respiratory stimulant. Metabolic acidosis results from the accumulation of both lactic and keto-acids. Salicylic acid, by itself, accounts for only a small quantity of the acid load. The common presenting sign of salicylate toxicity is tachypnea. The patient may also complain of tinnitus with serum concentrations of salicylic acid of 20 to 45 mg/dL or higher. Other CNS manifestations are agitation, seizures, and even coma. Both noncardiogenic pulmonary edema and upper gastrointestinal bleeding may occur. Hypoglycemia occurs in children, but is rare in adults. Other symptoms include nausea, vomiting, and hyperpyrexia.

In the setting of salicylate overdose, peak serum concentrations are achieved 4 to 6 hours after ingestion. The severity of the ingestion can be predicted by the Done nomogram, which plots the toxic salicylate level at varying time points following ingestion. This nomogram cannot be used with chronic ingestions or with the ingestion of enteric-coated aspirin. The treatment of salicylate toxicity consists of supportive care, removal of unabsorbed compounds using charcoal lavage, administration of bicarbonate, and, if necessary, hemodialysis. Because the dissociation constant (pK) of salicylic acid is 3.0, alkalinization keeps the drug in its polar dissociated form, preventing diffusion into the CNS. In addition, because tissue salicylic acid is in equilibrium with the nondissociated compound in the plasma, alkalinization also decreases tissue levels. Concurrent alkalinization of the urine traps salicylate in the tubule, promoting its excretion. Hemodialysis is indicated in all patients with altered mental status, kidney failure that causes a decrease in renal excretion, volume overload that prevents the administration of bicarbonate, or when salicylate levels are greater than 100 mg/dL.

Kidney Failure

Kidney failure is also a well-recognized cause of metabolic acidosis. With the reduction in nephron mass that occurs in CKD, there is decreased ammoniagenesis in the proximal tubule. Many patients with diminished kidney function may also have specific acidification defects in the form of a renal tubular acidosis. As the glomerular filtration rate (GFR) declines, the kidney is unable to secrete the daily production of fixed acid. Serum bicarbonate begins to decline when the GFR falls below 40 mL/min/1.73 m^2.

The acidosis of kidney failure can be associated with either an elevated AG or a normal AG. With mild to moderate reductions in glomerular filtration rate, the anions that comprise the gap are excreted normally and the acidosis reflects decreased ammoniagenesis and is therefore hyperchloremic. As kidney failure worsens, the kidney loses its ability to excrete various anions, and the accumulation of sulfate, phosphate, and other anions produce an elevated AG. Because of better control of phosphorus, more intensive dietary modifications and earlier initiation of dialysis provided today, even patients who are beginning renal replacement therapy will often not manifest an AG.

Despite daily net positive acid balance, it is unusual for HCO_3^- to fall below 15 mmol/L. Why the acidosis of CKD is rarely severe is unclear. Whether this lack of severity is secondary to buffering of the retained protons in bone or retention of organic anions, usually lost in the urine, that are instead subsequently converted to HCO_3^- is controversial. The buffering of protons by bone results in the loss of calcium and negative calcium balance. In addition, chronic acidosis causes protein breakdown, muscle wasting, and negative nitrogen balance. Maintaining acid-base balance close to normal can prevent these consequences.

The metabolic acidosis commonly found in patients with CKD can easily be corrected by prescribing oral bicarbonate. Usually two 650-mg (7.8 mEq) tablets three times a day will keep the serum bicarbonate in the normal range. It is rare that hemodialysis has to be initiated solely for the purpose of correcting the acidosis.

HYPERCHLOREMIC ACIDOSIS

Acidosis associated with a normal AG, HCMA, has a limited number of causes (Fig. 8-5). HCMA can occur in CKD when reduced ammoniagenesis impairs the kidney's ability to excrete the daily acid load. In individuals with normal or near normal kidney function, it can be divided into cases caused by the kidney's failure to reabsorb HCO_3^- or secrete the daily fixed load of H^+, commonly known as renal tubular acidosis (RTA), and those in which renal acid-base handling is normal. In contrast to AG acidosis, most cases of HCMA are easily treated with supplemental base.

Renal Causes of Hyperchloremic Metabolic Acidosis

Renal tubular acidoses represent a heterogeneous cause of HCMA in which the kidney is unable to maintain acid-base balance despite preservation of normal or near-normal overall kidney function (normal GFR). There is often confusion regarding the RTAs because no standard nomenclature exists, numerous diverse transport defects have been identified, and the literature often presents contradictory information. A grasp of the underlying pathophysiology makes the approach to these disorders more comprehensible. The RTAs can be divided into four major categories: (1) primary defects in ammoniagenesis, (2) hypoaldosteronism, (3) disorders of the proximal tubule, and (4) disorders of the distal tubule. The distal tubule defects can be further divided into those with hypokalemia and those with hyperkalemia (Fig. 8-6).

Defective Ammoniagenesis

One of the most common causes of an HCMA is the inability of the kidney to generate ammonia because of CKD. By definition, RTA refers to a specific acid excretory defect occurring despite the presence of normal or near-normal kidney function. Thus, it bears emphasis that the HCMA of CKD is not classified as RTA. As the number of nephrons decreases with CKD, there is a proportional decrease in the production of ammonia. As mentioned in the section on AG acidosis, when GFR falls below 40 mL/min/1.73 m², the kidney is unable to excrete the daily acid load and $[HCO_3^-]$ begins to decline with a concomitant increase in the serum $[Cl^-]$, producing HCMA. Only when the GFR falls below 15 to 20 mL/min/1.73 m² does the kidney lose the ability to secrete anions, thus converting this HCMA into an AG acidosis. It needs to be

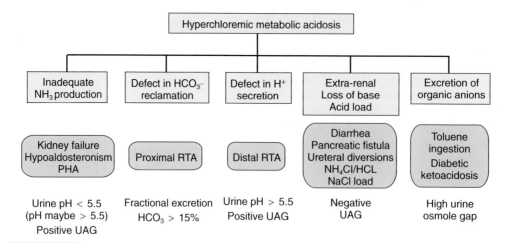

FIGURE 8-5 The etiology of hyperchloremic metabolic acidosis. Shown at the bottom are useful diagnostic tools. AG, anion gap; PHA, pseudohypoaldosteronism; RTA, renal tubular acidosis; UAG, urine anion gap.

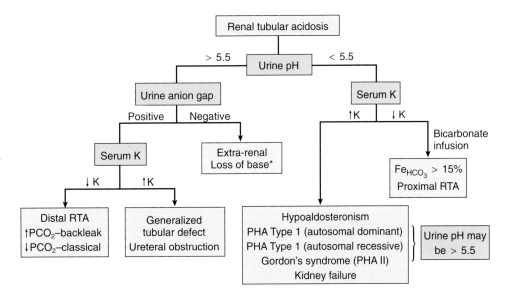

FIGURE 8-6 Evaluation of renal tubular acidosis. FE$_{HCO3}$, fractional excretion of bicarbonate; PHA, pseudo-hypoaldosteronism; RTA, renal tubular acidosis. *Extrarenal loss of base is not a form of renal tubular acidosis. Findings shown since use of this algorithm may lead to its discovery.

stressed that the acidosis in kidney failure, whether manifested by hyperchloremia or an AG, is primarily caused by defective ammoniagenesis. As such, the UAG will be positive because of the decrease in ammonia excretion, whereas urine pH will be less than 5.5.

Hypoaldosteronism

Primary or secondary hypoaldosteronism are common disorders causing hyperkalemia and metabolic acidosis (Table 8-4). Hyporeninemic hypoaldosteronism (type IV RTA) is the most frequently encountered variety of this disorder. This disorder is usually seen in patients with diabetes and mild CKD. The precise cause of hyprorerinemia has not been clearly defined. The finding that hypertension is frequently present and that the disorder may be partly reversed with chronic furosemide use suggests that renin suppression may be secondary to chronic volume overload. Neither has the cause of the hypoaldosteronism been fully explained. Renin lack alone should not cause hypoaldosteronism, because hyperkalemia is a potent stimulus of aldosterone secretion and anephric individuals still secrete aldosterone. The acidosis is primarily caused by decreased ammoniagenesis as a result of the associated hyperkalemia induced by the

TABLE 8-4 Hypoaldosteronism

Primary
    Addison's disease
    Congenital enzyme defects
    Drugs
        Heparin
        Angiotensin converting enzyme inhibitors
        Angiotensin receptor blockers

Hyporeninemic hypoaldosteronism (type IV RTA)

Pseudohypoaldosteronism I (autosomal dominant)—mineralocorticoid resistance

aldosterone deficiency. Hypoadosteronism, by diminishing distal sodium reabsorption, also results in a less negative lumen potential, thus decreasing the rate of H$^+$ secretion but not the electromotive force of the pump. Because the hydrogen pump is not defective, urine pH is usually less than 5.5.

Patients with type IV RTA are usually asymptomatic, with only minor laboratory abnormalities (mild hyperkalemia and decreased HCO$_3^-$). However, when renal potassium handling is further perturbed by various stressors—including sodium depletion, which decreases delivery of sodium to the distal tubule; high potassium diet; and potassium-sparing diuretics or medications that further decrease renin and aldosterone levels, such as angiotensin-converting enzyme inhibitors, angiotensin receptor blockers, nonsteroidal anti-inflammatory drugs, or heparin—marked hyperkalemia ensues with a decline in ammoniagenesis. Most patients can be treated by removing the insult to potassium homeostasis, restricting potassium intake, and providing supplemental bicarbonate. Although the diagnosis of type IV RTA is made by demonstrating low renin and aldosterone levels after sodium depletion, for practical purposes these tests are rarely ordered today.

Autosomal-dominant pseudohypoaldosteronism (PHA) type I is an uncommon disorder caused by a mutation in the renal mineralocorticoid receptor, which results in decreased affinity for aldosterone. This genetic disorder presents in childhood with hyperaldosteronism, hyperkalemia, metabolic acidosis, salt wasting, and hypotension. Autosomal-dominant PHA type I becomes less severe with age. Carbenoxolone and glycyrrhizic acid (found in true licorice) both inhibit 11-β-hydroxysteroid dehydrogenase, the enzyme in the kidney that converts cortisol, which binds the mineralocorticoid receptor to cortisone, which does not bind. They can be used to treat this disorder by increasing the intrarenal supply of mineralocorticoid.

TABLE 8-5 Causes of Proximal Renal Tubular Acidosis

Isolated defects in HCO$_3^-$ reabsorption
Carbonic anhydrase inhibitors
Acetazolamide
Topiramate
Sulfamylon
Carbonic anhydrase deficiency

Generalized defects in proximal tubular transport
Cystinosis
Wilson's disease
Lowe's syndrome
Galactosemia
Multiple myeloma
Light chain disease
Amyloidosis
Vitamin D deficiency
Ifosfamide
Cidofovir
Lead
Aminoglycosides

Proximal Renal Tubular Acidosis

Proximal RTA, often called type II RTA (because it was the second type described) is a defect in the ability of the proximal tubule to reclaim filtered HCO$_3^-$ (Table 8-5). In type II RTA, the proximal tubule has a diminished threshold (approximately 15 mmol/L instead of the normal 24 mmol/L) for HCO$_3^-$ reabsorption. When plasma [HCO$_3^-$] falls below this threshold, complete reabsorption occurs. Proximal RTA can be congenital or acquired and may exist as an isolated defect in HCO$_3^-$ reabsorption or as part of a more generalized transport defect known as Fanconi's syndrome, in which there is diminished reabsorption of most solutes across the proximal tubule. Patients with proximal RTA and Fanconi's syndrome, in addition to the loss of HCO$_3^-$, inappropriately excrete amino acids, glucose, phosphorous, uric acid, and other solutes in their urine.

As would be expected, mutations in the Na$^+$-H$^+$ exchanger on the luminal membrane, the Na$^+$-HCO$_3^-$ cotransporter on the basolateral membrane, and cytosolic carbonic anhydrase have all been implicated in the isolated hereditary and sporadic forms of proximal RTA. Several drugs that block carbonic anhydrase, including the diuretic acetazolamide and the anticonvulsant topiramate, also cause isolated HCO$_3^-$ wasting. Proximal RTA with Fanconi's syndrome is frequently found in patients with cystinosis, Wilson's disease, Lowe's syndrome, multiple myeloma, and light chain disease, among others. A decrease in ATP production, which reduces basolateral Na$^+$ K$^+$-ATPase activity, is the presumed etiology of this global transport defect. Drugs, particularly the cyclophosphamide analogue ifosfamide, and cidofovir, used in the treatment of cytomegalovirus retinitis, have also been associated with a generalized proximal tubulopathy.

Because distal H$^+$ excretion is normal, urine pH during steady state, when the [HCO$_3^-$] is below the lowered threshold and bicarbonaturia is absent, will be less than 5.5. At this time the serum [HCO$_3^-$] will be between 15 and 18 mEq/L. It is important to recognize that whenever the HCO$_3^-$ increases above the reabsorptive threshold, HCO$_3^-$ will appear in the urine and the pH will be greater than 6.5. Although ammoniagenesis is preserved in proximal RTA, direct or indirect measurement of urine NH$_4^+$ may reveal an inappropriately low excretion. This can occur because HCO$_3^-$, which escapes proximal reabsorption, serves as a buffer sink for secreted H$^+$, thus reducing the trapping of NH$_3^+$. The diagnosis of proximal RTA is established by increasing the serum bicarbonate to normal and demonstrating a fractional excretion of HCO$_3^-$ of greater than 15%.

Treatment of proximal RTA is difficult because administered base is rapidly excreted in the urine. Extremely large amounts of base (10 to 15 mmol/kg/day) are frequently needed, and therefore compliance is limited. The increased delivery of HCO$_3^-$ to the distal nephron induces or exacerbates hypokalemia. It is recommended that frequent doses of a mixture of Na and K salts of bicarbonate and citrate be used.

Distal Renal Tubular Acidosis

Classical Distal Renal Tubular Acidosis with Hypokalemia

Distal RTA, also known as type I RTA, represents the inability of the distal tubule to acidify the urine (Table 8-6). As with proximal RTA, the distal variety can be congenital or acquired. Abnormalities have been identified in both the luminal H$^+$-ATPase and the basolateral Cl-HCO$_3^-$ exchanger (AE1). The acquired form is associated with

TABLE 8-6 Causes of Distal Renal Tubular Acidosis with Hypokalemia

Familial
Defective HCO$_3^-$-Cl$^-$ exchanger (AE1) (autosomal dominant)
Defective H$^+$-ATPase (autosomal recessive)

Endemic
Thai endemic distal renal tubular acidosis

Drugs
Amphotericin
Toluene
Lithium
Ifosfamide
Foscarnet
Vanadium
Systemic disorder
Sjögren's syndrome
Cryoglobulinemia
Systemic lupus erythematosus
Kidney transplant rejection

autoimmune diseases, especially systemic lupus and Sjögren's syndrome; dysproteinemia; and kidney transplant rejection. Immunocytochemical studies have revealed decreased staining of the H^+-ATPase and Cl-HCO_3^- exchanger in patients with the acquired form of distal RTA. Ifosfamide, which is also associated with a proximal RTA, can also cause a distal defect. Amphotericin, which literally punches holes in membranes forming ion channels, causes a distal RTA by allowing the back-leak of protons across the luminal membrane. The classic finding in type I RTA is an inappropriately high urine pH (greater than 5.5).

Because H^+ secretion is defective in distal RTA, less NH_4^+ can be trapped in the lumen of the tubule and the UAG will be positive, reflecting this decrease in NH_4^+ excretion. Besides having an inappropriately high urine pH and a positive UAG, distal RTA can be further characterized by measuring urine PCO_2 during an HCO_3^- infusion. Distal delivery of HCO_3^- in the presence of a normal H^+ secretory capacity results in elevated PCO_2 in the urine. When there is a H^+ secretory defect, urine PCO_2 will not increase. As would be expected, in amphotericin-induced RTA, in which H^+ ion secretion is unaffected, urine pCO_2 increases normally. Occasionally it may be difficult to distinguish HCMA induced by diarrhea from a distal RTA. Diarrhea results in HCMA and hypokalemia. Because the hypokalemia increases renal ammoniagenesis, urine pH may be inappropriately elevated. Thus, on the surface, both forms of acidosis appear similar. Measurement of the UAG will easily distinguish the markedly elevated urine NH_4^+ with its negative AG found in diarrheal illness from the low NH_4^+ excretion and positive AG found with distal RTA. The one caveat is that sodium must be delivered to the distal tubule as shown by a urine Na^+ of greater than 20 mmol/L.

Classical distal RTA is associated with hypokalemia (due to augmented distal K^+ secretion in lieu of H^+ secretion in exchange for Na^+ reabsorption), hypocitraturia (from proximal tubule cell reabsorption), hypercalciuria (from the buffering of H^+ in bone and loss of calcium), and nephrocalcinosis. The treatment of distal RTA is simply to supply enough base (2 to 3 mmol/kg/day) to counter the daily fixed production of acid. This can be administered as a mixture of sodium and potassium salts of either bicarbonate or citrate.

Distal Renal Tubular Acidosis with Hyperkalemia

Distal RTA with hyperkalemia can be further divided into two broad general categories: (1) a generalized defect of both distal tubular H^+ and K^+ secretion or (2) a primary defect in Na^+ transport often called a "voltage defect" (Table 8-7).

Generalized Distal Tubule Defect

Unlike classical distal RTA, a more generalized defect of the distal tubule can occur in which both H^+ and K^+ secre-

TABLE 8-7 Causes of Distal Renal Tubular Acidosis with Hyperkalemia

Lupus nephritis

Obstructive nephropathy

Sickle cell anemia

Voltage defects

Familial
  Pseudohypoaldosteronism type I (autosomal recessive)
  Pseudohypoaldosteronism type II (autosomal recessive)—
    Gordon's syndrome

Drugs
  Amiloride
  Triamterene
  Trimethoprim
  Pentamidine

tion is impaired. This has been best identified in cases of ureteral obstruction and in patients with interstitial kidney disease resulting from sickle cell anemia or systemic lupus erythematosus. In animals with ureteral obstruction, immunocytochemical staining has revealed loss of the apical H^+-ATPase. Why hyperkalemia occurs is less clear. Because K^+ excretion cannot be augmented by diuretics, a primary defect in K^+ transport is likely. Similar to classical distal RTA, urine pH is greater than 5.5.

Distal Sodium Transport Defects

Several disorders have been characterized by defective sodium transport in the distal tubule. The reabsorption of Na^+ by the distal tubule generates a lumen-negative potential. This electrical negativity helps promote the secretion of K^+ and H^+. Any drug or disorder that interferes with this lumen-negative potential will diminish both K^+ and H^+ secretion. These are commonly classified as voltage defects. Autosomal-recessive PHA type I is a syndrome in which there is loss of function of the epithelial sodium channel (ENaC) in the distal tubule. Numerous mutations have been described in various subunits of this channel. This disease manifests in childhood with marked hyperkalemia, metabolic acidosis, hyperaldosteronism, and salt wasting. Because the ENaC also exists in other tissue, including lung, colon, and sweat glands, patients with this disorder often have symptoms related to these organs. Treatment consists of providing a high salt intake. Drugs that block ENaC produce a similar metabolic picture. These include the potassium-sparing diuretics amiloride and triamterene, as well as trimethoprim and pentamidine.

Another well-recognized disorder of distal transport is PHA type II, also known as Gordon's syndrome. Individuals with this condition have mild volume overload with suppressed renin and aldosterone, hypertension, hyperkalemia, and metabolic acidosis. Recently, mutations in two members of a family of serine-threonine kinases,

WNK1 and WNK4 (*With No K* [K = lysine]) have been shown to be the cause of this syndrome. These kinases appear to have an important role in the regulation of Cl^- transport in numerous different tissues. It appears that defects in these kinases result in an increase in the number of neutral NaCl transporters (NCCT) and thus increase NaCl transport across the distal convoluted tubule. Less sodium is delivered to the more distal tubule segments for reabsorption, which curtails the generation of the lumen-negative potential. This results in decreased H^+ and K^+ secretion. Supporting this hypothesis is the fact that Gordon's syndrome can be treated with thiazide-type diuretics, which block the NCCT.

The acidosis in all of these sodium transport disorders is secondary to decreased H^+ secretion caused by an unfavorable electrical gradient in the distal tubule and the decreased ammoniagenesis caused by the hyperkalemia. Whether the urine pH is less than 5.5 depends on how severely H^+ secretion is affected.

Combined Proximal and Distal Renal Tubular Acidosis

This is an extremely uncommon disorder, which has been called type 3 RTA. As would be expected, both proximal HCO_3^- reabsorption and distal H^+ secretion is impaired. Mutations in the gene for cytosolic carbonic anhydrase can cause such a defect. As already discussed, ifosfamide can also cause a combined defect.

Incomplete Distal Renal Tubular Acidosis

Patients with incomplete distal RTA will come to medical attention because of calcium stone disease and nephrocalcinosis. Serum $[HCO_3^-]$ is normal, but urine pH never falls below 5.5, even after acid loading with NH_4Cl or $CaCl_2$. This disorder likely represents a milder form of distal RTA. Frank metabolic acidosis may become evident when patients are stressed by diarrhea or other conditions that require compensation by augmented renal proton secretion.

Extrarenal Causes of Hyperchloremic Metabolic Acidosis

Extrarenal Bicarbonate Loss

Loss of base during episodes of diarrhea or with overzealous use of laxatives is associated with HCMA. Loss of HCO_3^- can also occur with pancreatic fistulae or with pancreas transplants if drainage of the pancreatic duct is into the bladder. Ureteral diversions using an isolated sigmoid loop were frequently associated with bicarbonate loss because of $Cl\text{-}HCO_3^-$ exchange in the bowel loop. These ureteral-sigmoidostomies have largely been replaced with ureteral diversions using ileal conduits, which have less surface area and contact time for loss of HCO_3^- to occur. If these become obstructed, however, HCMA can still develop.

Acid Load

An obvious cause of an HCMA is ingestion or infusion of a chloride salt of an acid. Both NH_4Cl and $CaCl_2$ can result in a metabolic acidosis and can be used as a provocative test to assess urinary acidification. In addition, total parenteral nutrition using hydrochloric acid salts of various amino acids can produce a metabolic acidosis if an insufficient quantity of base (usually acetate) is added to the infusion mixture. Another form of acid load is NaCl. Volume resuscitation with 0.9% NaCl will often produce an HCMA. This occurs because of "dilution" of the plasma HCO_3^- by the more acidic saline solution (pH 7.0) and because volume expansion diminishes proximal HCO_3^- reabsorption.

Urinary Loss of Anions

As previously discussed, if organic anions are excreted in the urine, they represent a source of base lost from the body. Although involving the kidney, this cannot be viewed as being caused by an intrinsic kidney defect. Because of the low renal threshold for the excretion of keto-acids, patients with DKA, if they are able to maintain their intravascular volume or are volume resuscitated, will excrete these anions in place of Cl^-. This results in HCMA. A similar metabolic disturbance exists after toluene exposure. Toluene is a common solvent found in paint products and glues. Exposure is generally by inhalation, either accidental or intentional. Toluene is rapidly absorbed through the skin and mucous membranes and metabolized to hippuric acid. Hippurate is quickly excreted by the kidney, leaving behind an HCMA. Although hippurate is not a base, its rapid excretion into the urine conceals the AG origins of this disturbance. Both of these disorders are usually easily discovered on taking an adequate history.

BIBLIOGRAPHY

Alper SL: Genetic diseases of acid-base transporters. Annu Rev Physiol 64:899–923, 2002.

Adrogue HJ, Madias NE: Management of life-threatening acid-base disorders. N Engl J Med 338:26–34 and 107–111, 1998.

Bonny O, Rossier B: Disturbances of Na/K balance: Pseudohypoaldosteronism revisited. J Am Soc Nephrol 13:2399–2414, 2002.

Brent J, McMartin K, Phillips S, et al: Fomepizole for the treatment of methanol poisoning. N Engl J Med 344:424–429, 2001.

Carlisle EJ, Donnelly SM, Vasuvattakul S, et al: Glue-sniffing and distal renal tubular acidosis: sticking to the facts. J Am Soc Nephrol 1:1019–1027, 1991.

Chang CT, Chen YC, Fang JT, Huang CC: Metformin-associated

lactic acidosis: Case reports and literature review. J Nephrol 15:398–394, 2002.

Claessens YE, Cariou A, Monchi M, et al: Detecting life-threatening lactic acidosis related to nucleoside-analog treatment of human immunodeficiency virus-infected patients, and treatment with L-carnitine. Crit Care Med 31:1042–1047, 2003.

Dargan PI, Wallace CI, Jones AL: An evidence based flowchart to guide the management of acute salicylate (aspirin) overdose. Emerg Med J 19:206–209, 2002.

DuBose TD Jr, Mcdonald GA: Renal tubular acidosis. In Dubose TD, Hamm LL Jr (eds): Acid-Base and Electrolyte Disorders: A Companion to Brenners and Rector's The Kidney, Philadelphia, WB Saunders, 2002, pp 189–206.

Figge J, Jabor A, Kazda A: Anion gap and hypoalbuminemia. Crit Care Med 26:1807–1810, 1998.

Fraser AD: Clinical toxicologic implications of ethylene glycol and glycolic acid poisoning. Ther Drug Monit 24:232–238, 2002.

Han J, Kim G-H, Kim J, et al: Secretory-defect distal renal tubular acidosis is associated with transporter defect in H+-ATPase and anion exchanger-1. J Am Soc Nephrol 13:1425–1432, 2002.

Hood VL, Tannen RL: Protection of acid-base balance by pH regulation of acid production. N Engl J Med 339:819–826, 1998.

Igarashi T, Sekine T, Inatomi J, Seki G. Unraveling the molecular pathogenesis of isolated proximal renal tubular acidosis. J Am Soc Nephrol 13:2171–2177, 2002.

Ishihara K, Szerlip HM: Anion gap acidosis. Semin Nephrol 18:83–89, 1998.

Izzedine H, Launay-Vacher V, Isnard-Bagnis C, Derray G: Drug-induced Fanconi's syndrome. Am J Kid Dis 41:292–309, 2003.

Karet FE: Inherited distal renal tubular acidosis. J Am Soc Nephrol 13:2178–2184, 2002.

Kirschbaum B, Sica D, Anderson F: Urine electrolytes and the urine anion and osmolar gaps. J Lab Clin Med 133:597–604, 1999.

Lemann J Jr, Bushinsky DA, Hamm LL: Bone buffering of acid and base in humans. Am J Physiol Renal Physiol 285: F811–F832, 2003.

Levraut J, Grimaud D: Treatment of metabolic acidosis. Curr Opin Crit Care 9:260–265, 2003.

Llushine KA, Harris CR, Holger JS: Methanol ingestion: Prevention of toxic sequelae after massive ingestion. J Emerg Med 24:433–436, 2003.

Mycyk MB, Aks SE: A visual schematic for clarifying the temporal relationship between the anion and osmol gap in toxic alcohol poisoning. Am J Emerg Med 21:333–335, 2003.

Ogedegbe AE, Thomas DL, Diehl AM: Hyperlactataemia syndromes associated with HIV therapy. Lancet Infect Dis 3: 329–337, 2003.

Oh M, Carrrol H: Value and determinants of the urine anion gap. Nephron 90:252–255, 2002.

Reynolds HN, Teiken P, Regan ME, et al: Hyperlactatemia, increased osmolar gap, and renal dysfunction during continuous lorazepam infusion. Crit Care Med 28(5):1631–1634, 2000.

Salpeter SR, Greyber E, Pasternak GA, Salpeter EE: Risk of fatal and nonfatal lactic acidosis with metformin use in type 2 diabetes mellitus: Systematic review and meta-analysis. Arch Intern Med 163:2594–2602, 2003.

Soriano J. Renal tubular acidosis: the clinical entity. J Am Soc Nephrol 13:2160–2170, 2002.

Stacpoole PW: Lactic acidosis and other mitochondrial disorders. Metabolism 46:306–321, 1997.

Uribarri J, Oh MS, Carroll HJ: D-lactic acidosis: A review of clinical presentation, biochemical features, and pathophysiologic mechanisms. Medicine 77:73–82, 1998.

CHAPTER 9

Metabolic Alkalosis

Thomas D. DuBose, Jr.

PATHOGENESIS

Metabolic alkalosis occurs as a result of net gain of [HCO_3^-] or loss of nonvolatile acid (usually HCl by vomiting) from the extracellular fluid. Because it is unusual for alkali to be added to the body, the disorder involves a generative stage, in which the loss of acid usually causes alkalosis, and a maintenance stage, in which the kidneys fail to compensate by excreting HCO_3^- because of volume contraction, a low glomerular filtration rate (GFR), or depletion of Cl^- or K^+.

Under normal circumstances, the kidneys have an impressive capacity to excrete HCO_3^-. Continuation of metabolic alkalosis represents a failure of the kidneys to eliminate HCO_3^- in the usual manner. The kidneys will retain, rather than excrete, excess alkali and maintain the alkalosis if (1) volume deficiency, chloride deficiency, and K^+ deficiency exist in combination with a reduced GFR, which augments distal tubule H^+ secretion; or (2) hypokalemia exists because of autonomous hyperaldosteronism. In the first example, alkalosis is corrected by administration of NaCl and KCl, whereas in the latter example it is necessary to repair the alkalosis by pharmacologic or surgical intervention, not with saline administration.

PATHOPHYSIOLOGY

In assessing a patient with metabolic alkalosis, two questions should be considered: (1) What is the source of alkali gain (or acid loss) that generated the alkalosis? (2) What renal mechanisms are operating to prevent excretion of excess HCO_3^-, thereby maintaining, rather than correcting, the alkalosis?

For HCO_3^- to be added to the extracellular fluid, HCO_3^- must be administered exogenously or retained in some manner. Thus, the development of metabolic alkalosis represents a failure of the kidneys to eliminate HCO_3^- at the normal capacity. The kidneys retain excess alkali and maintain alkalosis if one of two mechanisms is operative:

1. Cl^- deficiency (extracellular fluid volume contraction) exists concurrently with K^+ deficiency to decrease GFR and/or enhance proximal fractional HCO_3^- reabsorption. This combination of disorders evokes secondary hyperreninemic hyperaldosteronism and stimulates H^+ secretion in the collecting duct. Repair of the alkalosis may be accomplished by saline and K^+ administration.

2. Excessive elaboration of mineralocorticoid and hypokalemia are induced by autonomous factors unresponsive to increased extracellular fluid volume. The stimulation of distal H^+ secretion is then sufficient to reabsorb the increased filtered HCO_3^- load of metabolic alkalosis and to overcome the decreased proximal HCO_3^- reabsorption caused by extracellular fluid volume expansion. Repair of the alkalosis in this case rests with removal of the excess autonomous mineralocorticoid; saline is ineffective.

DIFFERENTIAL DIAGNOSIS

To establish the cause of metabolic alkalosis (Table 9-1), it is necessary to assess the status of the extracellular fluid volume, the recumbent and upright blood pressure, the serum [K^+], and the renin-aldosterone system. For example, the presence of chronic hypertension and chronic hypokalemia in an alkalotic patient suggests either mineralocorticoid excess or a hypertensive patient receiving diuretics. Low plasma renin activity and a urine [Na^+] and [Cl^-] above 20 mEq/L in a patient who is not taking diuretics indicate a primary mineralocorticoid excess syndrome. The combination of hypokalemia and alkalosis in a normotensive, nonedematous patient can pose a difficult problem. Possible causes to be considered are Bartter's or Gitelman's syndrome, magnesium deficiency, vomiting, exogenous alkali, or diuretic ingestion. Determination of urine electrolytes (especially the urine [Cl^-]) and screening of the urine for diuretics may be helpful. It is often useful to measure the urine chloride concentration (Table 9-2) and to place this value in context with assessment of the extracellular fluid volume status of the patient. A low urine [Cl^-] (i.e., less than 10 mEq/L) indicates avid Cl^- retention by the kidney and denotes extracellular fluid volume depletion even when urine Na^+ excretion and the urine [Na^+] are high (i.e., greater than 15 mEq/L). A high urine [Cl^-], in the absence of concurrent diuretic use, suggests inappropriate chloruresis due to a tubular defect or mineralocorticoid excess. If the urine is alkaline, with an elevated [Na^+] and [K^+] but a urine [Cl^-] below 10 mEq/L, the diagnosis is usually either vomiting (overt or surreptitious) or alkali ingestion. If the urine is relatively acid and has low concentrations of Na^+, K^+, and Cl^-, the most likely possibilities are prior vomiting, the posthypercapnic state, or prior diuretic ingestion. If, on the other hand, neither the urine sodium, potassium, nor chloride concentrations are

TABLE 9-1   Causes of Metabolic Alkalosis

Exogenous HCO₃⁻ loads
  Acute alkali administration
  Milk-alkali syndrome

Effective ECV contraction, normotension, K⁺ deficiency, and secondary hyper-reninemic hyperaldosteronism
  Gastrointestinal origin
    Vomiting
    Gastric aspiration
    Congenital chloridorrhea
    Villous adenoma
    Combined administration of sodium polystyrene sulfonate (kayexalate and aluminum hydroxide)
  Renal origin
    Diuretics (especially thiazides and loop diuretics)
      Acute
      Chronic
    Edematous states
    Posthypercapnic state
    Hypercalcemia–hypoparathyroidism
    Recovery from lactic acidosis or ketoacidosis
    Nonreabsorbable anions such as penicillin, carbenicillin
    Mg²⁺ deficiency
    K⁺ depletion
    Bartter's syndrome (loss of function mutation of Cl⁻ transport in TALH)
    Gitelman's syndrome (loss of function mutation in Na⁺-Cl⁻ cotransporter)
    Carbohydrate refeeding after starvation

ECV expansion, hypertension, K⁺ deficiency, and hypermineralocorticoidism
  Associated with high renin
    Renal artery stenosis
    Accelerated hypertension
    Renin-secreting tumor
    Estrogen therapy
  Associated with low renin
    Primary aldosteronism
      Adenoma
      Hyperplasia
      Carcinoma
      Glucocorticoid suppressible
    Adrenal enzymatic defects
      11-β-Hydroxylase deficiency
      17-α-Hydroxylase deficiency
    Cushing's syndrome or disease
      Ectopic corticotropin
      Adrenal carcinoma
      Adrenal adenoma
      Primary pituitary
    Other
      Licorice
      Carbenoxolone
      Chewing tobacco
      Lydia Pinkham tablets

Gain of function mutation of ENaC with extracellular fluid volume expansion, hypertension, K⁺ deficiency, and hyporeninemic-hypoaldosteronism
  Liddle's syndrome

ECV, extracellular fluid volume; ENaC, epithelial Na⁺ channel; TALH, thick ascending limb of the loop of Henle.

TABLE 9-2   Diagnosis of Metabolic Alkalosis

Low Urinary [Cl⁻] (<10 mEq/L)	High or Normal Urinary [Cl⁻] (>15–20 mEq/L)
Normotensive	Hypertensive
Vomiting, nasogastric aspiration	Primary aldosteronism
Diuretics	Cushing syndrome
Posthypercapnia	Renal artery stenosis
Bicarbonate therapy of organic acidosis	Renal failure plus alkali therapy
K⁺ deficiency	Normotensive
Hypertensive	Mg²⁺ deficiency
Liddle's syndrome	Severe K⁺ deficiency
	Bartter's syndrome
	Gitelman's syndrome
	Diuretics

depressed, magnesium deficiency, Bartter's or Gitelman's syndrome, or current diuretic ingestion should be considered. Bartter's syndrome is distinguished from Gitelman's syndrome because of hypocalciuria and hypomagnesemia in the latter disorder. The genetic and molecular bases of these two disorders have been elucidated recently.

METABOLIC ALKALOSIS DUE TO EXOGENOUS BICARBONATE LOADS

Alkali Administration

Administration of base to individuals with normal kidney function rarely causes alkalosis because the kidney has a high capacity for bicarbonate excretion. However, in patients with coexistent hemodynamic disturbances, alkalosis can develop because the normal capacity to excrete HCO₃⁻ may be exceeded or there may be enhanced reabsorption of HCO₃⁻. Examples include those who receive oral or intravenous HCO₃⁻, acetate loads (parenteral hyperalimentation solutions), citrate loads (transfusions, continuous renal replacement therapy, or infant formula), or antacids plus cation-exchange resins (aluminum hydroxide and sodium polystyrene sulfonate).

Chronic administration of alkali to individuals with normal kidney function results in minimal, if any, alkalosis. In patients with chronic kidney disease, overt alkalosis can develop after alkali administration, because the capacity to excrete HCO₃⁻ is exceeded or because coexistent hemodynamic disturbances have caused enhanced fractional HCO₃⁻ reabsorption.

Milk-Alkali Syndrome

A long-standing history of excessive ingestion of milk and antacids is an unusual cause of metabolic alkalosis. Both hypercalcemia and vitamin D excess have been suggested to increase renal HCO₃⁻ reabsorption. Patients with this disorder are prone to develop nephrocalcinosis, renal function impairment, and metabolic alkalosis. Discontinuation of alkali ingestion is usually sufficient to repair the alkalosis, but the kidney disease may be irreversible when nephrocalcinosis is advanced.

METABOLIC ALKALOSIS ASSOCIATED WITH EXTRACELLULAR FLUID VOLUME CONTRACTION, K⁺ DEPLETION, AND SECONDARY HYPERRENINEMIC HYPERALDOSTERONISM

Gastrointestinal Origin

Gastrointestinal loss of H⁺ from vomitus or gastric aspiration results in retention of HCO_3^-. The loss of fluid and NaCl results in contraction of the extracellular fluid volume and an increase in the secretion of renin and aldosterone. Volume contraction causes a reduction in GFR and an enhanced capacity of the renal tubule to reabsorb HCO_3^-. During active vomiting, there is continued addition of HCO_3^- to plasma in exchange for Cl^-, and the plasma $[HCO_3^-]$ exceeds the reabsorptive capacity of the proximal tubule. The excess $NaHCO_3$ reaches the distal tubule, where potassium secretion is enhanced by aldosterone and the delivery of the poorly reabsorbed anion HCO_3^-. Thus, the predominant cause of the hypokalemia is renal, rather than gastrointestinal potassium wasting. Hypokalemia has selective effects on renal bicarbonate absorption and ammonium production, which are counterproductive. Hypokalemia dramatically increases the activity of the $H^+ K^+$-ATPase in the cortical collecting tubule to reabsorb K^+, but at the expense of enhanced net acid excretion and bicarbonate absorption. Hypokalemia also increases ammonium production independently of acid-base status, which in the face of enhanced H⁺ secretion results in increased ammonium excretion and the addition of new bicarbonate to the systemic circulation. Therefore, the hypokalemia plays an important role in the seemingly maladaptive response of the kidney to maintain the acidosis. Because of contraction of the extracellular fluid volume and hypochloremia, Cl^- is avidly conserved by the kidney as recognized by a low urinary chloride concentration (see Table 9-2). Correction of the contracted extracellular fluid volume with NaCl and repair of K^+ deficits corrects the acid-base disorder.

Congenital Chloridorrhea

This rare autosomal-recessive disorder is associated with severe diarrhea, fecal acid loss, and HCO_3^- retention. The disease is due to loss of the normal ileal HCO_3^-/Cl^- anion exchange mechanism so that Cl^- cannot be reabsorbed. The parallel Na^+-H^+ ion exchanger remains functional,

allowing Na^+ to be reabsorbed and H^+ to be secreted. Therefore, H⁺ and Cl⁻ exit in the stool, causing Na^+ and HCO_3^- retention in the extracellular fluid. The alkalosis is sustained by concomitant extracellular fluid volume contraction, hyperaldosteronism, and K^+ deficiency. Therapy consists of oral supplements of sodium and potassium chloride. Recently, the use of proton-pump inhibitors has been advanced as a means of reducing chloride secretion by the parietal cells and thus reducing the diarrhea.

Villous Adenoma

Metabolic alkalosis has been described in cases of villous adenoma. K^+ depletion probably causes the alkalosis, because colonic secretion is alkaline.

Renal Origin

Diuretics

Drugs that induce chloruresis, such as thiazides and loop diuretics (furosemide, bumetanide, torsemide, and ethacrynic acid), diminish extracellular fluid volume without altering total body bicarbonate content. Consequently, the serum $[HCO_3^-]$ increases. The chronic administration of diuretics tends to generate metabolic alkalosis by increasing distal salt delivery, so that K^+ and H⁺ secretion are stimulated. The alkalosis is maintained by persistence of the contraction of the extracellular fluid volume, secondary hyperaldosteronism, K^+ deficiency, and activation of the $H^+ K^+$-ATPase, as long as diuretic administration continues. Repair of the alkalosis is achieved by providing isotonic saline to correct the extracellular fluid volume deficit and by repairing the potassium deficit.

Bartter's Syndrome

Both classic Bartter's syndrome and the antenatal type are inherited as autosomal-recessive disorders and involve impaired thick ascending limb of the loop of Henle (TALH) salt absorption, which results in salt wasting, volume depletion, and activation of the renin-angiotensin system. These manifestations are the result of loss of function mutations of one of the genes that encode three transporters involved in vectorial NaCl absorption in the thick ascending limb of Henle's loop. The most prevalent disorder is a mutation of the gene *NKCC2*, which encodes the bumetanide-sensitive Na^+ $2Cl^-$ K^+cotransporter on the apical membrane. A second mutation has been discovered in the gene *KCNJ1*, which encodes the adenosine triphosphate–sensitive apical K^+ conductance channel (ROMK) that operates in parallel with the Na^+ $2Cl^-$ K^+ transporter to recycle K^+. Both defects can be associated with antenatal Bartter's syndrome or classic Bartter's syndrome. A mutation of the *CLCNKb* gene encoding the voltage-gated basolateral chloride channel (ClC-Kb) is associated only with classic

Bartter's syndrome, and is milder and rarely associated with nephrocalcinosis. All three defects have the same net effect, loss of Cl⁻ transport in the TALH.

Antenatal Bartter's syndrome has been observed in consanguineous families in association with sensorineural deafness, a syndrome linked to chromosome 1p31. The responsible gene, *BSND*, encodes a subunit, barttin, that colocalizes with the CLC-Kb channel in the TALH and K-secreting epithelial cells in the inner ear. Barttin appears to be necessary for function of the voltage-gated chloride channel. Expression of ClC-Kb is lost when coexpressed with mutant barttins. Thus, mutations in *BSND* represent a fourth category of patients with Bartter's syndrome.

Such defects would predictably lead to extracellular fluid volume contraction, hyperreninemic hyperaldosteronism, and increased delivery of Na^+ to the distal nephron and thus alkalosis and renal K^+ wasting and hypokalemia. Secondary overproduction of prostaglandins, juxtaglomerular apparatus hypertrophy, and vascular pressor unresponsiveness would then ensue. Most patients have hypercalciuria and normal serum magnesium levels that distinguish this disorder from Gitelman's syndrome.

Bartter's syndrome is inherited as an autosomal-recessive defect, and most patients studied with mutations in these genes have been homozygotes or compound heterozygotes for different mutations in one of these genes. A few patients with the clinical syndrome have no discernible mutation in any of these four genes. Plausible explanations include unrecognized mutations in other genes, a dominant-negative effect of a heterozygous mutation, or other mechanisms. Recently, two groups of investigators have reported features of Bartter's syndrome in patients with autosomal-dominant hypocalcemia and activating mutations in CaSR. Activation of the calcium-sensing receptor CaSR on the basolateral cell surface of the TALH inhibits function of ROMK. Thus, mutations in CaSR may represent a fifth gene associated with Bartter's syndrome.

Distinction from surreptitious vomiting, diuretic administration, and laxative abuse is necessary to make the diagnosis of Bartter's syndrome. The finding of a low urinary Cl⁻ concentration is helpful in identifying the vomiting patient (see Table 9-2). The urinary Cl⁻ concentration in Bartter's syndrome would be expected to be normal or increased, rather than depressed.

The therapy of Bartter's syndrome is generally focused on repair of the hypokalemia by inhibition of the renin-angiotensin-aldosterone system or the prostaglandin-kinin system using K^+ supplementation, Mg^{2+} repletion, propranolol, spironolactone, prostaglandin inhibitors, and angiotensin-converting enzyme inhibitors.

Gitelman's Syndrome

Patients with Gitelman's syndrome resemble the Bartter's syndrome phenotype in that an autosomal-recessive chloride-resistant metabolic alkalosis is associated with hypokalemia, a normal to low blood pressure, volume depletion with secondary hyperreninemic hyperaldosteronism, and juxtaglomerular hyperplasia. However, hypocalciuria and symptomatic hypomagnesemia are consistently useful in distinguishing Gitelman's syndrome from Bartter's syndrome on clinical grounds. These unique features mimic the effect of chronic thiazide diuretic administration. A large number of missense mutations in the gene *SLC12A3*, which encodes the thiazide-sensitive sodium chloride cotransporter in the distal convoluted tubule (NCCT), have been described and account for the clinical features, including the classic finding of hypocalciuria. However, it is not clear why these patients have pronounced hypomagnesemia. A recent study has demonstrated that peripheral blood mononuclear cells from patients with Gitelman's syndrome express mutated NCCT messenger RNA (mRNA). In a large consanguineous Bedouin family, missense mutations were noted in *CLCNKb*, but the clinical features overlapped between Gitelman's and Bartter's syndromes.

Gitelman's syndrome becomes symptomatic later in life and is associated with milder salt wasting than is Bartter's syndrome. A large study of adults with proven Gitelman's syndrome and NCCT mutations showed that salt craving, nocturia, cramps, and fatigue were more common than in sex- and age-matched controls. Women experienced exacerbation of symptoms during menses, and many had complicated pregnancies.

Treatment of Gitelman's syndrome, as with Bartter's syndrome, consists of liberal dietary sodium and potassium salts, but with the addition of magnesium supplementation in most patients. Angiotensin-converting enzyme inhibitors have been suggested to be helpful in selected patients but can cause frank hypotension.

Nonreabsorbable Anions and Magnesium Deficiency

Administration of large quantities of nonreabsorbable anions, such as penicillin or carbenicillin, can enhance distal acidification and K^+ secretion by increasing the transepithelial potential difference (lumen negative). Mg^{2+} deficiency may cause hypokalemic alkalosis by enhancing distal acidification through stimulation of renin and hence aldosterone secretion.

Potassium Depletion

Pure K^+ depletion causes metabolic alkalosis, although generally of only modest severity. Hypokalemia independently enhances renal ammonium production, which increases net acid excretion, and thereby the return of "new" bicarbonate to the systemic circulation. Another explanation for the mild alkalosis is that K^+ depletion also causes positive sodium chloride balance with or without mineralocorticoid administration. The salt retention, in turn, antagonizes the degree of alkalemia. When access to salt and K^+ is restricted, more severe alkalosis develops. Activation of the renal H^+ K^+-ATPase in the collecting duct by chronic hypokalemia likely plays a major role in maintenance of the alkalosis. Specifically, chronic hypokalemia has been shown to markedly increase the abundance of the colonic H^+ K^+-ATPase mRNA and protein in the outer medullary collecting duct. Alkalosis associated with severe K^+ depletion, however, is resistant to salt administration. Repair of the K^+ deficiency is necessary to correct the alkalosis.

After Treatment of Lactic Acidosis or Ketoacidosis

When an underlying stimulus for the generation of lactic acid or ketoacid is removed rapidly, as with repair of circulatory insufficiency or with insulin therapy, the lactate or ketones are metabolized to yield an equivalent amount of HCO_3^-. Other sources of new HCO_3^- are additive to the original amount generated by organic anion metabolism to create a surfeit of HCO_3^-. Such sources include new HCO_3^- added to the blood by the kidneys as a result of enhanced acid excretion during the preexisting period of acidosis, and alkali therapy during the treatment phase of the acidosis. Acidosis-induced contraction of the extracellular fluid volume and K^+ deficiency act to sustain the alkalosis.

Posthypercapnia

Prolonged CO_2 retention with chronic respiratory acidosis enhances renal HCO_3^- absorption and the generation of new HCO_3^- (increased net acid excretion). If the partial pressure of carbon dioxide in arterial blood ($PaCO_2$) is returned to normal by mechanical ventilation or other means, metabolic alkalosis results from the persistently elevated $[HCO_3^-]$. Associated extracellular fluid volume contraction does not allow complete repair of the alkalosis by correction of the $PaCO_2$ alone, and alkalosis persists until isotonic saline is infused.

METABOLIC ALKALOSIS ASSOCIATED WITH EXTRACELLULAR FLUID VOLUME EXPANSION, HYPERTENSION, AND HYPERALDOSTERONISM

Mineralocorticoid administration or excess production [primary aldosteronism of Cushing's syndrome and adrenal cortical enzyme defects] increases net acid excretion and may result in metabolic alkalosis, which may be worsened by associated K^+ deficiency. Extracellular fluid volume expansion from salt retention causes hypertension and antagonizes the reduction in GFR or increases tubule acidification induced by aldosterone and by K^+ deficiency. The kaliuresis persists and causes continued K^+ depletion with polydipsia, inability to concentrate the urine, and polyuria. Increased aldosterone levels may be the result of autonomous primary adrenal overproduction or of secondary aldosterone release due to renal overproduction of renin. In both situations, the normal feedback of extracellular fluid volume on net aldosterone production is disrupted, and hypertension from volume retention can result (see Table 9-2).

Liddle's Syndrome

Liddle's syndrome is associated with severe hypertension presenting in childhood, accompanied by hypokalemic metabolic alkalosis. These features resemble primary hyperaldosteronism, but the renin and aldosterone levels are suppressed (pseudohyperaldosteronism). Liddle originally described patients with low renin and low aldosterone levels that did not respond to spironolactone. The defect is inherited as an autosomal-dominant form of monogenic hypertension and has been localized to chromosome 16q. Subsequently, this disorder was attributed to an inherited abnormality in the gene that encodes the β or the γ subunit of the renal epithelial Na^+ channel (ENaC) at the apical membrane of principal cells in the cortical collecting duct and leads to constitutive activation of this channel. Either mutation results in deletion of the cytoplasmic tails of the β or γ subunits, respectively. The C-termini contain a PY amino acid motif that is highly conserved, and essentially all mutations in Liddle's syndrome patients involve disruption or deletion of this motif. Such PY motifs are important in regulating the number of sodium channels in the luminal membrane by binding to the WW domains of the Nedd4-like family of ubiquitin protein ligases. Disruption of the PY motif dramatically increases the surface localization of the ENaC complex, because these channels are not internalized or degraded (Nedd4 pathway), but remain activated on the cell surface. Persistent Na^+ absorption eventuates in volume expansion, hypertension, hypokalemia, and metabolic alkalosis.

Glucocorticoid-Remediable Hyperaldosteronism

This is an autosomal-dominant form of hypertension, the features of which resemble those of primary aldosteronism (hypokalemic metabolic alkalosis and volume-dependent hypertension). In this disorder, however, glucocorticoid administration corrects the hypertension as well as the excessive excretion of 18-hydroxysteroid in the urine. This disorder results from unequal crossing over between the two genes located in close proximity on chromosome 8, which is the glucocorticoid-responsive promoter region of the gene encoding the 11-β-hydroxylase (*CYP11B1*), where it is joined to the structural portion of the *CYP11B2* gene encoding aldosterone synthase. The chimeric gene produces excess amounts of aldosterone synthase, unresponsive to serum potassium or renin levels, but it is suppressed by glucocorticoid administration. Although a rare cause of primary aldosteronism, the syndrome is important to distinguish because treatment differs and it can be associated with severe hypertension, stroke, and accelerated hypertension during pregnancy.

Cushing's Disease or Syndrome

Abnormally high glucocorticoid production due to adrenal adenoma or carcinoma or to ectopic corticotropin production causes metabolic alkalosis. The alkalosis may be ascribed to coexisting mineralocorticoid (deoxycorticosterone and corticosterone) hypersecretion. Alternatively, glucocorticoids may have the capability of enhancing net acid secretion and NH_4^+ production, which may be due to occupancy of cellular mineralocorticoid receptors.

Miscellaneous Conditions

Ingestion of licorice or licorice-containing chewing tobacco can cause a typical pattern of mineralocorticoid excess. The glycyrrhizinic acid in licorice inhibits 11 β-hydroxysteroid dehydrogenase. This enzyme is responsible for converting cortisol to cortisone, an essential step in protecting the mineralocorticoid receptor from cortisol. When the enzyme is inactivated, cortisol is allowed to occupy type I renal mineralocorticoid receptors, mimicking aldosterone. Genetic apparent mineralocorticoid excess (AME) resembles excessive ingestion of licorice: volume expansion, low renin, low aldosterone levels, and a salt-sensitive form of hypertension, which may include metabolic alkalosis and hypokalemia. The hypertension responds to thiazides and spironolactone but without abnormal steroid products in the urine. In genetic AME, 11 β-hydroxysteroid dehydrogenase is defective, and monogenic hypertension develops.

SYMPTOMS OF METABOLIC ALKALOSIS

With metabolic alkalosis, changes in central and peripheral nervous system function are similar to those of hypocalcemia; symptoms include mental confusion, obtundation, and a predisposition to seizures, paresthesia, muscular cramping, tetany, aggravation of arrhythmias, and hypoxemia in chronic obstructive pulmonary disease. Related electrolyte abnormalities include hypokalemia and hypophosphatemia.

TREATMENT OF METABOLIC ALKALOSIS

The maintenance of metabolic alkalosis represents a failure of the kidney to excrete bicarbonate efficiently because of chloride or potassium deficiency, or continuous mineralocorticoid elaboration or both. Treatment is primarily directed at correcting the underlying stimulus for HCO_3^- generation and restoring the ability of the kidney to excrete the excess bicarbonate. Assistance is gained in the diagnosis and treatment of metabolic alkalosis by directing attention to the urinary chloride, arterial blood pressure, and volume status of the patient (particularly the presence or absence of orthostasis; see Table 9-1). Helpful in the history is the presence or absence of vomiting, diuretic use, or alkali therapy. A high urine chloride level and hypertension suggest that mineralocorticoid excess is present. If primary aldosteronism is present, correction of the underlying cause will reverse the alkalosis (adenoma, bilateral hyperplasia, Cushing's syndrome). Patients with bilateral adrenal hyperplasia may respond to spironolactone. Normotensive patients with a high urine chloride may have Bartter's or Gitelman's syndrome if diuretic use or vomiting can be excluded. A low urine chloride level and relative hypotension suggests a chloride-responsive metabolic alkalosis such as vomiting or nasogastric suction. [H^+] loss by the stomach or kidneys can be mitigated by the use of proton pump inhibitors or the discontinuation of diuretics. The second aspect of treatment is to remove the factors that sustain HCO_3^- reabsorption, such as extracellular fluid volume contraction or K^+ deficiency. Although K^+ deficits should be repaired, NaCl therapy is usually sufficient to reverse the alkalosis if extracellular fluid volume contraction is present, as indicated by a low urine [Cl^-].

Patients with congestive heart failure (CHF) or unexplained volume overexpansion represent special challenges in the critical care setting. Patients with a low urine chloride concentration, usually indicative of a "chloride-responsive" form of metabolic alkalosis, may not tolerate normal saline infusion. Renal HCO_3^- loss can be accelerated by administration of acetazolamide (250 mg intravenously), a carbonic anhydrase inhibitor, if associated conditions preclude infusion of saline (elevated pulmonary capillary wedge pressure, or evidence of CHF). Acetazolamide is usually effective in patients with adequate kidney function, but can exacerbate urinary K^+ losses and exacerbate hypokalemia. Dilute hydrochloric acid (0.1 N HCl) is also effective but can cause hemolysis and may be difficult to titrate. If used, the goal should not be to restore the pH to normal, but to a level of approximately 7.50. Alternatively, acidification can also be achieved with oral NH_4Cl, which should be avoided in the presence of liver disease. Hemodialysis against a dialysate low in [HCO_3^-] and high in [Cl^-] can be effective when kidney function is impaired. Patients receiving continuous renal replacement therapy in the ICU typically develop metabolic alkalosis with high bicarbonate dialysate or when citrate regional anticoagulation is used. Therapy should include reduction of alkali loads via di-alysis by reducing the bicarbonate concentration in the dialysate, or if citrate is being used, by infusion of 0.1 N HCl postfiltration.

BIBLIOGRAPHY

Birkenhager R, Otto E, Schurmann MJ, et al: Mutation of BSND causes Bartter syndrome with sensorineural deafness and kidney failure. Nat Genet 29:310–314, 2001.

Conn JW, Rovner DR, Cohen EL: Licorice-induced pseudoaldos-teronism: Hypertension, hypokalemia, aldosteronopenia, and suppressed plasma renin activity. JAMA 205:492, 1968.

Cruz DN, Shaer AJ, Bia MJ, et al: Gitelman's syndrome revisited: An evaluation of symptoms and health-related quality of life. Kidney Int 59:719–717, 2001.

DuBose TD Jr: Acid-base disorders. In Brenner BM (ed): Brenner and Rector's The Kidney, 7th ed. Philadelphia, WB Saunders, 2003, pp 925–997.

Herbert SC, Gullans SR: The molecular basis of inherited hypokalemic alkalosis: Bartter's and Gitelman's syndromes. Am J Physiol 271:F957–F959, 1996.

Hernandez R, Schambelan M, Cogan MG, et al: Dietary NaCl determines severity of potassium depletion-induced meta-bolic alkalosis. Kidney Int 31:1356, 1987.

Jamison RL, Ross JC, Kempson RL, et al: Surreptitious diuretic ingestion and pseudo-Bartter's syndrome. Am J Med 73:142, 1982.

Kamynina E, Staub O: Concerted action of ENaC, Nedd4-2, and Sgkl in transepithelial Na$^+$ transport. Am J Physiol Renal Physiol 283:F377, 2002.

Lifton RP, Dluhy RG, Powers M, et al: Hereditary hypertension caused by chimaeric gene duplications and ectopic expres-sion of aldosterone synthase. Nat Genet 2:66–74, 1992.

Orwoll ES: The milk-alkali syndrome: Current concepts. Ann Intern Med 97:242, 1982.

Schroeder ET: Alkalosis resulting from combined administration of a "nonsystemic" antacid and a cation-exchange resin. Gas-troenterology 56:868, 1969.

Schwartz WB, Relman AS: Metabolic and renal studies in chronic potassium depletion resulting from overuse of laxatives. J Clin Invest 32:258, 1953.

Seldin DW, Rector FC Jr: The generation and maintenance of metabolic alkalosis. Kidney Int 1:306, 1972.

Shimkets RA, Warnock DG, Bositis CM, et al: Liddle's syndrome: Heritable human hypertension caused by mutations in the beta subunit of the epithelial sodium channel. Cell 79:407, 1994.

Wesson DE, et al: Clinical syndromes of metabolic alkalosis. In Seldin DW, Giebisch G (eds): The Kidney: Physiology and Pathophysiology, 3rd ed. Philadelphia, Lippincott Williams & Wilkins, 2000.

Zelikovic I, Szargel R, Hawash A, et al: A novel mutation in the chloride channel gene, CLCNKB, as a cause of Gitelman and Bartter syndromes. Kidney Int 63:24–32, 2003.

CHAPTER 10

Respiratory Acidosis and Alkalosis

Nicolaos E. Madias

RESPIRATORY ACIDOSIS

Respiratory acidosis, or primary hypercapnia, is the acid-base disturbance initiated by an increase in CO_2 tension of body fluids. Hypercapnia acidifies body fluids and elicits an adaptive increment in plasma bicarbonate that should be viewed as an integral part of the respiratory acidosis. Arterial carbon dioxide tension (pCO_2) measured at rest and at sea level is greater than 45 mm Hg in simple respiratory acidosis. Lower values of pCO_2 might still signify the presence of primary hypercapnia in the setting of mixed acid-base disorders (e.g., eucapnia, rather than the expected hypocapnia, in the presence of metabolic acidosis).

Pathophysiology

Hypercapnia develops whenever CO_2 excretion by the lungs is insufficient to match CO_2 production, thus leading to positive CO_2 balance. Hypercapnia could result from increased CO_2 production, decreased alveolar ventilation, or both. Overproduction of CO_2 is usually matched by increased excretion such that hypercapnia is prevented. However, patients with marked limitation in pulmonary reserve and those receiving constant mechanical ventilation might experience respiratory acidosis due to increased CO_2 production. Established clinical circumstances include increased physical activity, augmented work of breathing by the respiratory muscles, shivering, seizures, sepsis, burns, fever, and hyperthyroidism. Increments in CO_2 production might also be imposed by the administration of large carbohydrate loads (greater than 2000 kcal per day) and parenteral nutrition to semi-starved, critically ill patients as well as during the decomposition of bicarbonate infused in the course of treating metabolic acidosis. By far, most cases of respiratory acidosis reflect a decrease in alveolar ventilation. Decreased alveolar ventilation can result from decreased minute ventilation, increased dead space ventilation, or a combination of the two.

The major threat to life from CO_2 retention in patients breathing room air is the associated obligatory hypoxemia. Thus, in the absence of supplemental oxygen, patients in respiratory arrest develop critical hypoxemia within a few minutes, long before extreme hypercapnia ensues. Because of the constraints of the alveolar gas equation, it is not possible for pCO_2 to reach values much higher than 80 mm Hg while the level of the partial pressure of oxygen (pO_2) is still compatible with life. Extreme hypercapnia can only be seen during oxygen administration and, in fact, is often the result of uncontrolled oxygen therapy.

Secondary Physiologic Response

An immediate increment in plasma bicarbonate concentration owing to titration of nonbicarbonate body buffers occurs in response to acute hypercapnia. This adaptation is complete within 5 to 10 minutes after the increase in pCO_2. On average, plasma bicarbonate increases by about 0.1 mEq/L for each mm Hg acute increment in pCO_2; as a result, plasma hydrogen ion concentration increases by about 0.75 nEq/L for each mm Hg acute increment in pCO_2. Therefore, the overall limit of adaptation of plasma bicarbonate in acute respiratory acidosis is quite small; even when pCO_2 increases to levels of 80 to 90 mm Hg, the increment in plasma bicarbonate does not exceed 3 to 4 mEq/L. Moderate hypoxemia does not alter the adaptive response to acute respiratory acidosis. On the other hand, preexisting hypobicarbonatemia (whether due to metabolic acidosis or chronic respiratory alkalosis) enhances the magnitude of the bicarbonate response to acute hypercapnia, whereas such a response is diminished in hyperbicarbonatemic states (whether due to metabolic alkalosis or chronic respiratory acidosis). Other electrolyte changes observed in acute respiratory acidosis include a mild increase in plasma sodium (1 to 4 mEq/L), potassium (0.1 mEq/L for each 0.1 unit decrease in pH), and phosphorus, and a small decrease in plasma chloride and lactate concentrations (the latter effect originating from inhibition of the activity of 6-phosphofructokinase, and thus glycolysis, by intracellular acidosis). A small reduction in the plasma anion gap is also observed, reflecting the decline in plasma lactate and the acidic titration of plasma proteins.

The adaptive increase in plasma bicarbonate concentration observed in the acute phase of hypercapnia is amplified markedly during chronic hypercapnia as a result of generation of new bicarbonate by the kidneys. Both proximal and distal acidification mechanisms contribute to this adaptation, which requires 3 to 5 days for completion. The renal response to chronic hypercapnia includes chloruresis and generation of hypochloremia. On average, plasma bicarbonate increases by about 0.3 mEq/L for each mm Hg chronic increment in pCO_2, as a result, plasma hydrogen ion concentration increases by about 0.3 nEq/L for each mm Hg chronic increase in pCO_2. Empirical observations indicate a limit of adaptation of plasma bicarbonate on the order of 45 mEq/L. The renal response to chronic hypercapnia is not altered appreciably by dietary sodium or chloride restriction, moderate potassium depletion, alkali loading, or moderate hypoxemia. It is currently unknown to what extent chronic kidney disease of variable severity limits the renal response to chronic hypercapnia. Obviously, patients with endstage kidney disease cannot mount a renal response to chronic hypercapnia; thus, they are more subject to severe acidemia. The degree of acidemia is more pronounced in patients receiving hemodialysis rather than peritoneal dialysis because the former treatment maintains, on average, a lower plasma bicarbonate concentration. Recovery from chronic hypercapnia is crippled by a chloride-deficient diet. In this circumstance, despite correction of the level of pCO_2, plasma bicarbonate concentration remains elevated as long as the state of chloride deprivation persists, thus creating the entity of "posthypercapnic metabolic alkalosis." Chronic hypercapnia is not associated with appreciable changes in the plasma concentrations of sodium, potassium, phosphorus, or anion gap.

Etiology

Respiratory acidosis can develop in patients with normal or abnormal airways and lungs. Tables 10-1 and 10-2 present causes of acute and chronic respiratory acidosis, respectively. This classification takes into consideration the usual mode of onset and duration of the various causes and emphasizes the biphasic time course that characterizes the secondary physiologic response to hypercapnia. Primary hypercapnia can result from disease or malfunction within any element of the regulatory system controlling respiration, including the central and peripheral nervous system, respiratory muscles, thoracic cage, pleural space, airways, and lung parenchyma. Not infrequently, more than one cause contributes to the development of respiratory acidosis in a given patient. Chronic lower airway obstruction resulting from bronchitis and emphysema is the most common cause of chronic hypercapnia.

Clinical Manifestations

Because hypercapnia almost always occurs with some degree of hypoxemia, it is often difficult to determine whether a specific manifestation is the consequence of the elevated pCO_2 or the reduced pO_2. Nevertheless, one should bear in mind several characteristic manifestations

TABLE 10-1 Causes of Acute Respiratory Acidosis

Normal Airways and Lungs	Abnormal Airways and Lungs

Central nervous system depression
  General anesthesia
  Sedative overdosage
  Head trauma
  Cerebrovascular accident
  Central sleep apnea
  Cerebral edema
  Brain tumor
  Encephalitis
	Upper airway obstruction
	  Coma-induced hypopharyngeal obstruction
	  Aspiration of foreign body or vomitus
	  Laryngospasm or angioedema
	  Obstructive sleep apnea
	  Inadequate laryngeal intubation
	  Laryngeal obstruction postintubation

Neuromuscular impairment
  High spinal cord injury
  Guillain-Barré syndrome
  Status epilepticus
  Botulism, tetanus
  Crisis in myasthenia gravis
  Hypokalemic myopathy
  Familial hypokalemic periodic paralysis
  Drugs or toxic agents (e.g., curare, succinylcholine, aminoglycosides, organophosphorus)
	Lower airway obstruction
	  Generalized bronchospasm
	  Severe asthama (status asthmaticus)
	  Bronchiolitis of infancy and adults
	  Disorders involving pulmonary alveoli
	  Severe bilateral pneumonia
	  Acute respiratory distress syndrome
	  Severe pulmonary edema

Ventilatory restriction
  Rib fractures with flail chest
  Pneumothorax
  Hemothorax
  Impaired diaphragmatic function (e.g., peritoneal dialysis, ascites)
	Pulmonary perfusion defect
	  Cardiac arrest
	  Severe circulatory failure
	  Massive pulmonary thromboembolism
	  Fat or air embolus

Iatrogenic events
  Misplacement or displacement of airway cannula during anesthesia or mechanical ventilation
  Bronchoscopy-associated hypoventilation or respiratory arrest
  Increased CO_2 production with constant mechanical ventilation (e.g., due to high carbohydrate diet or sorbent-regenerative hemodialysis)	

Adapted from Madias NE, Adrogué HJ: Respiratory acidosis and alkalosis. In Adrogué HJ (ed): Contemporary Management in Critical Care: Acid-Base and Electrolyte Disorders. New York, Churchill Livingstone, 1991, pp 37–53.

of organ dysfunction to diagnose the condition accurately and to treat it effectively. Clinical manifestations of respiratory acidosis arising from the central nervous system are collectively known as hypercapnic encephalopathy and include irritability, inability to concentrate, headache, anorexia, mental cloudiness, apathy, confusion, incoherence, combativeness, hallucinations, delirium, and transient psychosis. Progressive narcosis or coma might develop in patients receiving oxygen therapy, especially those with an acute exacerbation of chronic respiratory insufficiency in whom pCO_2 levels of up to 100 mm Hg or even higher can occur. In addition,

TABLE 10-2 Causes of Chronic Respiratory Acidosis

Normal Airways and Lungs	Abnormal Airways and Lungs

Central nervous system depression
  Sedative overdosage
  Methadone/heroin addiction
  Primary alveolar hypoventilation (Ondine's curse)
  Obesity-hypoventilation syndrome (pickwickian syndrome)
  Brain tumor
  Bulbar poliomyelitis
	Upper airway obstruction
	  Tonsillar and peritonsillar hypertrophy
	  Paralysis of vocal cords
	  Tumor of the cords or larynx
	  Airway stenosis after prolonged intubation
	  Thymoma, aortic aneurysm

Neuromuscular impairment
  Poliomyelitis
  Multiple sclerosis
  Muscular dystrophy
  Amyotrophic lateral sclerosis
  Diaphragmatic paralysis
  Myxedema
  Myopathic disease
	Lower airway obstruction
	  Chronic obstructive lung disease (bronchitis, bronchiolitis, bronchiectasis, emphysema)

Ventilatory restriction
  Kyphoscoliosis, spinal arthritis
  Obesity
  Fibrothorax
  Hydrothorax
  Impaired diaphragmatic function
	Disorders involving pulmonary alveoli
	  Severe chronic pneumonitis
	  Diffuse infiltrative disease (e.g., alveolar proteinosis)
	  Interstitial fibrosis

Adapted from Madias NE, Adrogué HJ: Respiratory acidosis and alkalosis. In Adrogué HJ (ed): Contemporary Management in Critical Care: Acid-Base and Electrolyte Disorders. New York, Churchill Livingstone, 1991, pp 37–53.

frank papilledema (pseudotumor cerebri) and motor disturbances, including myoclonic jerks, flapping tremor identical to that observed in liver failure, sustained myoclonus, and seizures, might develop. Focal neurologic signs (e.g., muscle paresis, abnormal reflexes) might be observed. The occurrence of neurologic symptomatology in patients with respiratory acidosis depends on the magnitude of the hypercapnia, the rapidity with which it develops, the severity of the acidemia, and the degree of the accompanying hypoxemia. In view of this range of neurologic manifestations, it is not surprising that severe hypercapnia often is misdiagnosed as a cerebral vascular accident or an intracranial tumor.

The hemodynamic consequences of respiratory acidosis reflect a variety of mechanisms, including a direct depressing effect on myocardial contractility. An associated sympathetic surge, sometimes intense, leads to increases in plasma catecholamines, but during severe acidemia (generally blood pH below 7.20), receptor responsiveness to catecholamines is markedly blunted. Hypercapnia results in systemic vasodilatation by a direct action on vascular smooth muscle; this effect is most obvious in the cerebral circulation, where blood flow increases in direct relation to the level of pCO_2. By contrast, CO_2 retention can produce vasoconstriction in the pulmonary circulation as well as in the kidneys; in the latter case, the hemodynamic response might be mediated via an enhanced sympathetic activity. The composite effect of these inputs is such that mild to moderate hypercapnia is usually associated with an increased cardiac output, normal or increased blood pressure, warm skin, a bounding pulse, and diaphoresis. However, when hypercapnia is severe or considerable hypoxemia is present, decreases in both cardiac output and blood pressure might be observed. Concomitant therapy with vasoactive medications (such as β-adrenergic receptor blockers) or the presence of congestive heart failure might further modify the hemodynamic response. Cardiac arrhythmias, particularly supraventricular tachyarrhythmias not associated with major hemodynamic compromise, are common, especially in patients receiving digitalis as therapy for cor pulmonale. They do not result primarily from the hypercapnia, but rather reflect the associated hypoxemia and sympathetic discharge, concomitant medication, electrolyte abnormalities, and underlying cardiac disease. Salt and water retention is commonly observed in sustained hypercapnia, especially in the presence of cor pulmonale. In addition to the effects of heart failure on the kidney, multiple other factors might be involved, including the prevailing stimulation of the sympathetic nervous system and the renin-angiotensin-aldosterone axis, increased renal vascular resistance, and elevated levels of antidiuretic hormone and cortisol.

Diagnosis

In general, one never should rely on clinical evaluation alone to assess the adequacy of alveolar ventilation. Whenever hypoventilation is suspected, arterial blood gases should be obtained. If the acid-base profile of the patient reveals hypercapnia in association with acidemia, at least an element of respiratory acidosis must be present. However, hypercapnia might be associated with a normal or an alkaline pH because of the simultaneous presence of additional acid-base disorders (see Chapter 11). Information from the patient's history, physical examination, and ancillary laboratory data should be used for an accurate assessment of the acid-base status.

Therapeutic Principles

Treatment of acute respiratory acidosis must be directed at prompt removal of the underlying cause whenever possible. Immediate therapeutic efforts should focus on establishing and securing a patent airway, restoring adequate oxygenation by delivering an oxygen-rich inspired mixture, and providing adequate ventilation in order to repair the abnormal gas composition. As noted, acute respiratory acidosis poses its major threat to survival not because of hypercapnia or acidemia, but because of the associated hypoxemia. Mechanical ventilation must be initiated in the presence of apnea, severe hypoxemia unresponsive to conservative measures, progressive CO_2 retention, severe obtundation, or coma. When the need for ventilatory support arises, it is sometimes possible to avoid or delay laryngeal intubation with sedation by using bilevel continuous positive airway pressure (bilevel CPAP) by nasal or facial mask. This method provides partial ventilatory support by assisting both inspiratory and expiratory effort. Despite its overall merit, noninvasive oximetry should not substitute for arterial blood gas measurements in titrating the fraction of inspired oxygen. Use of a CPAP mask can also be effective in obstructive sleep apnea. The presence of a component of metabolic acidosis is the primary indication for alkali therapy in patients with acute respiratory acidosis. Administration of sodium bicarbonate to patients with simple respiratory acidosis is not only of questionable efficacy, but also involves considerable risk. Concerns include pH-mediated depression of ventilation, enhanced CO_2 production due to bicarbonate decomposition, and volume expansion. Alkali therapy might have a special role in patients with severe bronchospasm by restoring the responsiveness of the bronchial musculature to β-adrenergic agonists. Successful management of intractable asthma in patients with blood pH below 7.00 by administering sufficient sodium bicarbonate to raise blood pH to above 7.20 has been reported.

Considering that large tidal volumes often lead to alveolar overdistention and volutrauma, an alternative strategy for management of disorders requiring mechanical ventilation, such as acute respiratory distress syndrome and severe airway obstruction, has been introduced. The strategy entails prescription of tidal volumes of less than 6 mL/kg body weight (instead of the conventional level of 10 to 15 mL/kg body weight) to achieve plateau airway pressures of less than 30 cm H_2O, while blood oxygenation is secured. Because an increase in pCO_2 develops, this approach is termed permissive hypercapnia or controlled mechanical hypoventilation. If the resultant hypercapnia reduces blood pH below 7.15 to 7.20, many physicians prescribe bicarbonate; however, this strategy is controversial and others intervene only for pH values on the order of 7.00. Several studies indicate that permissive hypercapnia affords improved clinical outcomes. Heavy sedation and neuromuscular blockade are frequently needed with this therapy. Following discontinuation of neuromuscular blockade, some patients develop prolonged weakness or paralysis. Contraindications to permissive hypercapnia include cerebrovascular disease, brain edema, increased intracranial pressure, and convulsions; depressed cardiac function and arrhythmias; and severe pulmonary hypertension. Notably, most of these entities can develop as adverse effects of permissive hypercapnia itself, especially when associated with substantial acidemia.

Patients with chronic respiratory acidosis frequently develop episodes of acute decompensation that can be serious or life threatening. Common culprits include pulmonary infection, use of narcotics, or uncontrolled oxygen therapy. In contrast to acute hypercapnia, injudicious use of oxygen therapy in patients with chronic respiratory acidosis can produce further reductions in alveolar ventilation. Respiratory decompensation superimposes an acute element of CO_2 retention and acidemia on the chronic baseline. Unfortunately, only rarely can one remove the underlying cause of chronic respiratory acidosis. Nonetheless, maximizing alveolar ventilation with relatively simple maneuvers is often rewarding in managing respiratory decompensation. Such maneuvers include treatment with antibiotics, bronchodilators, or diuretics; avoidance of irritant inhalants, tranquilizers, or sedatives; elimination of retained secretions; and gradual reduction of supplemental oxygen aiming at a pO_2 of about 60 mm Hg. Administration of adequate quantities of chloride (usually as the potassium salt) prevents or corrects a complicating element of metabolic alkalosis (commonly diuretic induced) that can further dampen the ventilatory drive. Acetazolamide can be used as an adjunctive measure, but care must be taken to avoid potassium depletion. Potassium and phosphate depletion should be corrected because they can contribute to the development or the maintenance of respiratory failure by impairing the function of skeletal muscles. The use of pharmacologic stimulants of ventilation has been generally disappointing, but a measure of benefit can be derived by some patients with central sleep apnea, obesity-hypoventilation syndrome, or chronic obstructive lung disease. Whereas an aggressive approach that favors the early use of ventilator assistance is most appropriate for acute respiratory acidosis, a more conservative approach is advisable in decompensated chronic hypercapnia because of the great difficulty often encountered in weaning such patients from ventilators. As a general rule, if the patient is alert, able to cough, and can cooperate with the treatment program, mechanical ventilation is usually not necessary. On the other hand, if the patient is obtunded or unable to cough, and if hypercapnia and acidemia are worsening, mechanical ventilation should be instituted. Restoration of the pCO_2 of the patient to near its chronic baseline should proceed gradually over a period of many hours to a few days. Overly rapid reduction in pCO_2 in such patients risks the development of sudden, posthypercapnic alkalemia with potentially serious consequences, including reduction in cardiac output and cerebral blood flow, cardiac arrhythmias (including predisposition to digitalis intoxication), and generalized seizures. Noninvasive mechanical ventilation with a nasal or facial mask is increasingly being used to avoid the potential complications of endotracheal intubation. In the absence of a complicating element of metabolic acidosis and with the possible exception of the severely acidemic patient with intense generalized bronchoconstriction undergoing mechanical ventilation, there is no role for alkali administration in chronic respiratory acidosis.

RESPIRATORY ALKALOSIS

Respiratory alkalosis, or primary hypocapnia, is the acid-base disturbance initiated by a reduction in CO_2 tension of body fluids. Hypocapnia alkalinizes body fluids and elicits an adaptive decrement in plasma bicarbonate that should be viewed as an integral part of the respiratory alkalosis. The level of pCO_2 measured at rest and at sea level is lower than 35 mm Hg in simple respiratory alkalosis. Higher values of pCO_2 might still indicate the presence of an element of primary hypocapnia in the setting of mixed acid-base disorders (e.g., eucapnia, rather than the anticipated hypercapnia, in the presence of metabolic alkalosis).

Pathophysiology

Primary hypocapnia most commonly reflects pulmonary hyperventilation owing to increased ventilatory drive. The latter results from signals arising from the lung, the peripheral chemoreceptors (carotid and aortic), the brain stem chemoreceptors, or influences originating in other centers of the brain. Hypoxemia is a major stimulus of alveolar ventilation, but pO_2 values lower than 60 mm Hg are required to elicit this effect consistently. Additional mechanisms for the generation of primary hypocapnia include maladjusted mechanical ventilators, the extrapulmonary elimination of CO_2 by a dialysis device or extracorporeal circulation (e.g., heart-lung machine), and decreased CO_2 production (e.g., due to sedation, skeletal muscle paralysis, hypothermia, hypothyroidism) in patients receiving constant mechanical ventilation.

A condition termed pseudorespiratory alkalosis occurs in patients with profound depression of cardiac function and pulmonary perfusion but with relative preservation of alveolar ventilation, including patients with advanced circulatory failure and those undergoing cardiopulmonary resuscitation. In these patients, there is venous (and tissue) hypercapnia due to the severely reduced pulmonary blood flow that limits the CO_2 delivered to the lungs for excretion. On the other hand, arterial blood evidences hypocapnia owing to the increased ventilation-to-perfusion ratio that causes a larger than normal removal of CO_2 per unit of blood traversing the pulmonary circulation. Absolute CO_2 excretion is decreased, however, and body CO_2 balance is positive. Therefore, respiratory acidosis, rather than respiratory alkalosis, is present. Such patients may have severe venous acidemia (often owing to mixed respiratory and metabolic acidosis) accompanied by an arterial pH that ranges from the mildly acidic to the frankly alkaline. In addition, arterial blood might reveal normoxia or hyperoxia despite the presence of severe hypoxemia in venous blood. Thus, both arterial and mixed (or central) venous blood sampling is needed to assess the acid-base status and oxygenation of patients with critical hemodynamic compromise.

Secondary Physiologic Response

Adaptation to acute hypocapnia is characterized by an immediate decrement in plasma bicarbonate that is principally due to titration of nonbicarbonate body buffers. This adaptation is completed within 5 to 10 minutes after the onset of hypocapnia. Plasma bicarbonate declines, on average, by approximately 0.2 mEq/L for each mm Hg acute decrement in pCO_2; consequently, plasma hydrogen ion concentration decreases by about 0.75 nEq/L for each mm Hg acute reduction in pCO_2. The limit of this adaptation of plasma bicarbonate is on the order of 17 to 18 mEq/L. Concomitant small increases in plasma chloride, lactate, and other unmeasured anions balance the decline in plasma bicarbonate; each of these components accounts for about one third of the bicarbonate decrement. Small decreases in plasma sodium (1 to 3 mEq/L) and potassium (0.2 mEq/L for each 0.1 unit increase in pH) might be observed. Severe hypophosphatemia can occur in acute hypocapnia due to translocation of phosphorus into the cells.

A larger decrement in plasma bicarbonate occurs in chronic hypocapnia as a result of renal adaptation to the disorder and involves suppression of both proximal and distal acidification mechanisms. Completion of this adaptation requires 2 to 3 days. Plasma bicarbonate decreases, on average, by about 0.4 mEq/L for each mm Hg chronic decrement in pCO_2, as a consequence, plasma hydrogen ion concentration decreases by approximately 0.4 nEq/L for each mm Hg chronic reduction in pCO_2. The limit of this adaptation of plasma bicarbonate is on the order of 12 to 15 mEq/L. About two thirds of the decline in plasma bicarbonate is balanced by an increase in plasma chloride concentration, the remainder reflecting an increase in plasma unmeasured anions; part of the remainder is due to the alkaline titration of plasma proteins, but most remains undefined. Plasma lactate does not increase in chronic hypocapnia, even in the presence of moderate hypoxemia. Similarly, no appreciable change in the plasma concentration of sodium occurs. In sharp contrast with acute hypocapnia, the plasma concentration of phosphorus remains essentially unchanged in chronic hypocapnia. Although plasma potassium is in the normal range in patients with chronic hypocapnia at sea level, hypokalemia and renal potassium wasting have been described in subjects in whom sustained hypocapnia was induced by exposure to high altitude. Patients with endstage kidney disease are obviously at risk for developing severe alkalemia in response to chronic hypocapnia because they cannot mount a renal response. Such a risk is higher in patients receiving peritoneal dialysis rather than hemodialysis because the former treatment maintains, on average, a higher plasma bicarbonate concentration.

Etiology

Primary hypocapnia is the most frequent acid-base disturbance encountered, occurring in normal pregnancy and high-altitude residence. Table 10-3 lists the major causes of respiratory alkalosis. Most are associated with the abrupt appearance of hypocapnia, but in many instances the process might be sufficiently prolonged to permit full chronic adaptation to occur. Consequently, no attempt has been made to separate these conditions into acute and chronic categories. Some of the major causes of respiratory alkalosis are benign, whereas others are life threatening. Primary hypocapnia is particularly common among the critically ill, occurring either as the simple disorder or as a component of mixed disturbances. Its presence constitutes an ominous prognostic sign, mortality increasing in direct proportion to the severity of the hypocapnia.

Clinical Manifestations

Rapid decrements in pCO_2 to half the normal values or lower are typically accompanied by paresthesias of the extremities, chest discomfort, circumoral numbness, light-headedness, confusion, and, infrequently, tetany or generalized seizures. These manifestations are seldom present in the chronic phase. Acute hypocapnia decreases cerebral blood flow, which in severe cases might reach values less than 50% of normal, resulting in cerebral hypoxia. This hypoperfusion has been implicated in the pathogenesis of the neurologic manifestations of acute respiratory alkalosis along with other factors, including hypocapnia per se, alkalemia, pH-induced shift of the oxyhemoglobin dissociation curve, and decrements in the level of ionized calcium and potassium. Some evidence indicates that cerebral blood flow returns to normal in chronic respiratory alkalosis.

Actively hyperventilating patients manifest no appreciable changes in cardiac output or systemic blood pressure. By contrast, acute hypocapnia in the course of passive hyperventilation—typically observed during mechanical ventilation in patients with a depressed central nervous system or those under general anesthesia—frequently results in a major reduction in cardiac output and systemic blood pressure, increased peripheral resistance, and substantial hyperlactatemia (exceeding 2 mEq/L). This discrepant response probably reflects the decline in venous return caused by mechanical ventilation in passive hyperventilation and the reflex tachycardia consistently observed in active hyperventilation. Although acute hypocapnia does not lead to cardiac arrhythmias in normal volunteers, it appears that it contributes to the generation of both atrial and ventricular tachyarrhythmias in patients with ischemic heart disease. Chest pain and ischemic ST-T wave changes have been observed in acutely hyperventilating subjects with or without coronary artery disease. Coronary vasospasm and Prinzmetal's angina can be precipitated by acute hypocapnia in susceptible subjects. The pathogenesis of these manifestations has been attributed to the same factors that have been incriminated in the neurologic manifestations of acute hypocapnia.

Diagnosis

Careful observation can detect abnormal patterns of breathing in some patients, yet marked hypocapnia can be present without a clinically evident increase in respiratory

TABLE 10-3 Causes of Respiratory Alkalosis

Hypoxemia or tissue hypoxia	**Central nervous system stimulation**
Decreased inspired O_2 tension	Voluntary
High altitude	Pain
Bacterial or viral pneumonia	Anxiety
Aspiration of food, foreign body, or vomitus	Psychosis
Laryngospasm	Fever
Drowning	Subarachnoid hemorrhage
Cyanotic heart disease	Cerebrovascular accident
Severe anemia	Meningoencephalitis
Left shift deviation of HbO_2 curve	Tumor
Hypotension*	Trauma
Severe circulatory failure*	**Drugs or hormones**
Pulmonary edema	Nikethamide, ethamivan
Stimulation of chest receptors	Doxapram
Pneumonia	Xanthines
Asthma	Salicylates
Pneumothorax	Catecholamines
Hemothorax	Angiotensin II
Flail chest	Vasopressor agents
Acute respiratory distress syndrome	Progesterone
Cardiac failure	Medroxyprogesterone
Noncardiogenic pulmonary edema	Dinitrophenol
Pulmonary embolism	Nicotine
Interstitial lung disease	**Miscellaneous**
	Pregnancy
	Sepsis
	Hepatic failure
	Mechanical hyperventilation
	Heat exposure
	Recovery from metabolic acidosis

*Might produce "pseudorespiratory alkalosis."
Adapted from Madias NE, Adrogué HJ: Respiratory acidosis and alkalosis. In Adrogué HJ (ed): Contemporary Management in Critical Care: Acid-Base and Electrolyte Disorders. New York, Churchill Livingstone, 1991, pp 37–53.

effort. Thus, arterial blood gases should be obtained whenever hyperventilation is suspected. In fact, the diagnosis of respiratory alkalosis, especially the chronic form, is frequently missed; physicians often misinterpret the electrolyte pattern of hyperchloremic hypobicarbonatemia as indicative of normal anion gap metabolic acidosis. If the acid-base profile of the patient reveals hypocapnia in association with alkalemia, at least an element of respiratory alkalosis must be present. Primary hypocapnia, however, might be associated with a normal or an acidic pH due to the concomitant presence of other acid-base disorders. Notably, mild degrees of chronic hypocapnia commonly leave blood pH within the high-normal range. As always, proper evaluation of the acid-base status of the patient requires careful assessment of the history, physical examination, and ancillary laboratory data. Once the diagnosis of respiratory alkalosis has been made, a search for its cause should be performed. The diagnosis of respiratory alkalosis can have important clinical implications: it often provides a clue to the presence of an unrecognized, serious disorder (e.g., sepsis) or signals the severity of a known underlying disease.

Therapeutic Principles

Management of respiratory alkalosis must be directed toward correcting the underlying cause, whenever possible. Taking measures to treat the respiratory alkalosis itself is not commonly required because the disorder, especially in its chronic form, leads to minimal or no symptoms and poses little risk to health. A notable exception is the patient with the anxiety-hyperventilation syndrome; in addition to reassurance or sedation, rebreathing into a closed system (e.g., a paper bag) might prove helpful by interrupting the vicious cycle that can result from the reinforcing effects of the symptoms of hypocapnia. Administration of acetazolamide can be beneficial in the management of signs and symptoms of high-altitude sickness, a syndrome characterized by hypoxemia and respiratory alkalosis. Considering the risks of severe alkalemia, sedation, or, in rare cases, skeletal muscle paralysis, mechanical ventilation might be required to temporarily correct marked respiratory alkalosis. Management of pseudorespiratory alkalosis must be directed at optimizing systemic hemodynamics.

BIBLIOGRAPHY

Adrogué HJ, Madias NE: Management of life-threatening acid-base disorders. N Engl J Med 338:26–34, 107–111, 1998.

Adrogué HJ, Madias NE: Respiratory acidosis, respiratory alkalosis, and mixed disorders. In Johnson RJ, Feehally J (eds): Comprehensive Clinical Nephrology. London, CV Mosby, 2003, pp 167–182.

Adrogué HJ, Rashad MN, Gorin AB, et al: Assessing acid-base status in circulatory failure. Differences between arterial and central venous blood. N Engl J Med 320:1312–1316, 1989.

Amato MB, Barbas CSV, Medeiros DM, et al: Effect of a protective-ventilation strategy on mortality in the acute respiratory distress syndrome. N Engl J Med 338:347–354, 1998.

Arbus GS, Hebert LA, Levesque PR, et al: Characterization and clinical application of the "significance band" for acute respiratory alkalosis. N Engl J Med 280:117–123. 1969.

Brackett NC Jr, Cohen JJ, Schwartz WB: Carbon dioxide titration curve of normal man. Effect of increasing degrees of acute hypercapnia on acid-base equilibrium. N Engl J Med 272:6–12, 1965.

Brackett NC Jr, Wingo CF, Muren O, Solano JT: Acid-base response to chronic hypercapnia in man. N Engl J Med 280:124–130, 1969.

Dries DJ: Permissive hypercapnia. J Trauma 39:984–989, 1995.

Epstein SK, Singh N: Respiratory acidosis. Respir Care 46:366–383, 2001.

Foster GT, Vaziri ND, Sassoon CSH: Respiratory alkalosis. Respir Care 46:384–391, 2001.

Jardin F, Fellahi J, Beauchet A, et al: Improved prognosis of acute respiratory distress syndrome 15 years on. Intens Care Med 25:936–941, 1999.

Krapf R, Beeler I, Hertner D, Hulter HN: Chronic respiratory alkalosis. The effect of sustained hyperventilation on renal regulation of acid-base equilibrium. N Engl J Med 324:1394–1401, 1991.

Madias NE, Adrogué HJ: Respiratory acidosis and alkalosis. In Adrogué HJ (ed): Contemporary Management in Critical Care: Acid-Base and Electrolyte Disorders. New York, Churchill Livingstone, 1991, pp 37–53.

Madias NE, Adrogué HJ: Respiratory alkalosis and acidosis. In Seldin DW, Giebisch G (eds): The Kidney: Physiology and Pathophysiology. Philadelphia, Lippincott Williams & Wilkins, 2000, pp 2131–2166.

Madias NE, Adrogué HJ: Respiratory alkalosis. In DuBose TD, Hamm LL (eds): Acid-Base and Electrolyte Disorders. Philadelphia, WB Saunders, 2002, pp 147–164.

Madias NE, Wolf CJ, Cohen JJ: Regulation of acid-base equilibrium in chronic hypercapnia. Kidney Int 27:538–543, 1985.

Stewart TE, Meade MO, Cook DJ, et al: Evaluation of a ventilation strategy to prevent barotrauma in patients at high risk for acute respiratory distress syndrome. N Engl J Med 338:355–361, 1998.

Tobin MJ: Advances in mechanical ventilation. N Engl J Med 344:1986–1996, 2001.

CHAPTER 11

Approach to Acid-Base Disorders*

Martin Goldberg

Acid-base disorders occur commonly in medical and surgical patients. They are particularly important in severely ill hospitalized patients. They may be present as single (simple) disorders or as a combination of simple disorders (mixed acid-base disturbances). Systematic diagnostic recognition and correction of these simple or mixed disorders is important because they may not only affect the prognosis of the patient, but also may provide clues to the nature of the underlying primary diseases. Before discussing a systematic approach to the diagnosis of acid-base disorders, several fundamental terms require definition.

ACIDEMIA VERSUS ALKALEMIA

These terms represent abnormal hydrogen ion concentrations of blood: either higher (acidemia) or lower (alkalemia) than the normal range of 35 to 45 nEq/L (pH = 7.35 to 7.45).

$$[H^+] = \text{hydrogen ion concentration}$$

$$pH = \log 1/[H^+] = -\log [H^+]$$

The Henderson-Hasselbalch equation is

$$pH = pK + \log ([HCO_3^-]/0.03 \times pCO_2).$$

Normally,

$$\text{Blood } pH = 6.10 + \log (24/0.03 \times 40)$$
$$= 6.10 + \log (20/1) = 7.40.$$

The Henderson equation (modified) is

$$[H^+] = 24 \times pCO_2/[HCO_3^-].$$

Normally,

$$[H^+] = 24 \times (40/24) = 40 \text{ nEq/L}.$$

ACIDOSIS VERSUS ALKALOSIS

These are pathophysiologic processes or abnormal states that, if unopposed by therapy or disease, would cause deviations of extracellular fluid [H⁺] from normal levels. They are defined independently of the [H⁺] or pH since two or more concomitant processes may be present simultaneously. In this instance they may either produce no net change in [H⁺] and/or may modify the body's adaptive response to a single disorder.

Alkalosis is a primary process (e.g., loss of H⁺ from vomiting) which, if unopposed, would produce alkalemia. Acidosis is a primary process (e.g., retention of [H⁺] due to impaired kidney function), which, if unopposed, would produce acidemia.

RESPIRATORY VERSUS METABOLIC DISTURBANCES

Respiratory disturbances are those caused by abnormal pulmonary elimination of CO_2, producing an excess (acidosis) or deficit (alkalosis) of H_2CO_3 (in equilibrium with pCO_2) in extracellular fluid. These primarily alter the pCO_2 in the denominator of the Henderson-Hasselbalch equation. Compensatory (adaptive) adjustments involve changes in [HCO₃⁻] accumulation in body fluids. Adaptation via the kidneys is slow (3 to 4 days); hence, there are operationally four respiratory disorders: acute and chronic respiratory acidosis, and acute and chronic respiratory alkalosis.

Metabolic disturbances are those caused by excessive intake, metabolic production, or losses of fixed (nonvolatile) acids or bases in the extracellular fluid. These are reflected by changes in [HCO₃⁻] in blood and therefore alter primarily the numerator of the Henderson-Hasselbalch ratio. Adaptation to metabolic disorders is relatively rapid (12 to 36 hours). Hence, there are two metabolic disorders: metabolic acidosis (a process that lowers plasma [HCO₃⁻]) and metabolic alkalosis (a process that raises plasma [HCO₃⁻]).

COMPENSATORY (ADAPTIVE) RESPONSES

Primary changes in the metabolic component ([HCO₃⁻]) stimulate adaptive changes in ventilation, producing changes in pCO_2. Additional adaptive changes occur in extracellular and cellular buffers and in the kidney (adjustments in H⁺ secretion, HCO₃⁻ reabsorption and secretion, and generation of HCO₃⁻).

Primary changes in the respiratory component (pCO_2) stimulate adaptive changes in [HCO₃⁻] via reactions with extra- and intracellular buffers and by slower (renal) adjustments in H⁺ secretion, HCO₃⁻ reabsorption and secretion, and HCO₃⁻ generation. As a rule, compensation

---

*Author retains © copyright on his original figure.

restores [H$^+$] or pH toward normal, but not to complete normality.

SIMPLE (SINGLE) VERSUS MIXED DISORDERS

A simple disorder includes the primary process with the initial changes in [H$^+$], arterial carbon dioxide tension (pCO$_2$), or [HCO$_3^-$] and all compensatory processes in reaction to these initial changes.

A mixed disorder is the simultaneous occurrence of two or more simple disturbances in a patient. Mixed disorders may be additive or counterbalancing regarding their net effect on [H$^+$] or pH; they are frequently difficult to diagnose and reflect serious illness. A mixed disorder in which there are three simultaneous primary acid-base disorders present is commonly termed a triple acid-base disturbance.

ACID-BASE MAPS AND FORMULAS IN DIAGNOSIS OF ACID-BASE DISORDERS

The adaptive responses for the six simple disorders (including the acute and chronic respiratory disorders) have been quantified experimentally. The 95% confidence limits can be defined, and several formulas have been developed to reflect the ranges of compensation. The acid-base map provides the graphic representation of these ranges (Table 11-1 and Fig. 11-1).

In a patient with a clinical condition suggesting a simple acid-base disorder, values of pH, pCO$_2$, and [HCO$_3^-$] lying within the ranges defined by the formulas or map are compatible with the diagnosis of the specified simple disorder. However, this does not rule out the possibility of a mixed disorder due to two or more counterbalancing processes, the net effects of which might produce values lying in the normal range, or in an area of a simple disorder. Furthermore, whereas values lying outside the range of a simple disorder suggest the diagnosis of a mixed disorder, a mixed disorder may sometimes be simulated during a transient state in which the adaptive processes to a simple disorder have not yet been completed.

ANION GAP

The anion gap (AG) is the concentration of unmeasured anions (proteinate, phosphates, sulfates, organic acid anions) that are typically associated with H$^+$ as it is initially generated in body fluids. It is commonly calculated as follows:

$$AG = plasma\ [Na^+] - (plasma\ [Cl^-] + plasma\ [HCO_3^-]).$$

Normal values for AG are 6 to 13 mEq/L. An AG greater than 15 mEq/L generally indicates one type of metabolic acidosis (i.e., due to accumulation of organic acids as occurs in lactic acidosis or diabetic ketoacidosis, or after ingestion of toxins). An exception is the widening of the AG that occurs during infusions of fluids containing salts of organic anions (e.g., lactate, amino acids, high doses of penicillins).

APPROACH TO THE DIAGNOSIS OF ACID-BASE DISORDERS

Appropriate diagnosis of acid-base disorders involves analysis and synthesis of all relevant information based on the patient's history, physical examination, and laboratory data. Use of data from one of these areas alone is insufficient to define the various processes that determine the primary disorder and the adaptational responses of

TABLE 11-1 Patterns of Arterial Blood Changes and Adaptation in Simple Acid-Base Disorders

| Primary Disorder | Blood Acid-Base Pattern* | | | | Adaptive Response† | Limits of Adaptation |
	pH	[H$^+$]	[HCO$_3^-$]	pCO$_2$		
Metabolic acidosis	↓	↑	↓‡	↓§	pCO$_2$ = 1.5 × [HCO$_3^-$] + 8 ± 2	pCO$_2$ not <10 mm Hg
Matabolic alkalosis	↑	↓	↑‡	↑§	ΔpCO$_2$ = 0.5 × Δ[HCO$_3^-$]	pCO$_2$ not >55 mm Hg
Respiratory acidosis						
Acute	↓	↑	↑§	↑‡	Δ[HCO$_3^-$] = 0.1 × ΔpCO$_2$	[HCO$_3^-$] not >30 mEq/L
Chronic	↓	↑	↑↑§	↑‡	Δ[HCO$_3^-$] = 0.4 × ΔpCO$_2$	[HCO$_3^-$] not >45 mEq/L
Respiratory alkalosis						
Acute	↑	↓	↓§	↓‡	Δ[HCO$_3^-$] = 0.2 × ΔpCO$_2$	[HCO$_3^-$] not <17–18 mEq/L
Chronic	↑	↓	↓↓§	↓‡	Δ[HCO$_3^-$] = 0.5 × ΔpCO$_2$	[HCO$_3^-$] not <12–15 mEq/L

*Arrows indicate direction of change from normal. A double arrow indicates that the magnitude of the change is considerably greater in the chronic disorder compared to the acute disorder. Units for pCO$_2$ are mm Hg, and units for [HCO$_3^-$] mEq/L.
†Δ, Change from normal.
‡Initial event.
§Secondary adaptive response.
Modified and updated from Goldberg M, Green SB, Moss ML, et al: Computer-based instruction and diagnosis of acid-base disorders. JAMA 223:249–275, 1973. With permission.

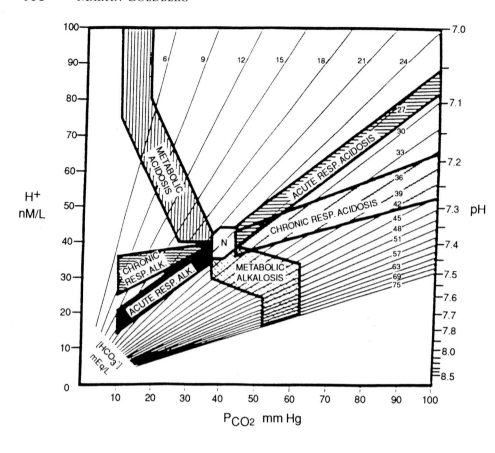

FIGURE 11-1 The acid-base map. Shaded areas represent the 95% confidence limits for zones of adaptation of the simple acid-base disorders. Numbered diagonal lines represent isopleths of plasma bicarbonate concentration. (Modified and updated from Goldberg M, Green SB, Moss ML, et al: Computer-based instruction and diagnosis of acid-base disorders. JAMA 223:269–275, 1973. With permission.)

the body. The important steps in this approach are outlined as follows:

1. Suspect acid-base disturbances from the history.
2. Suspect acid-base disturbances from the physical examination.
3. Evaluate the venous total CO_2 (tCO_2), [Cl⁻], [K⁺], and AG to support suspected diagnoses and to suggest possible additional primary disorders.
4. Obtain arterial pH, pCO_2, and [HCO_3^-] to establish definitive diagnoses using formulas, acid-base map, and limits of compensation.

A careful review of the patient's history may reveal several commonly encountered clinical conditions that are typically associated with one or more acid-base disturbances (Table 11-2). The presence of these conditions should lead one to add the potential disorders to the differential diagnosis. One needs to assess the specific disease states, the various drugs, the presence of mechanical ventilation, and nasogastric suction, all of which may be either causative of primary acid-base disorders or modifiers of the adaptive response to a disorder. Thus, a history of impaired kidney function suggests metabolic acidosis; pneumonia, sepsis, or hepatic failure should raise the suspicion of respiratory alkalosis, and therapy with the common diuretics should alert one to the possibility of metabolic alkalosis. In particular, certain clinical catastrophes such as cardiac arrest, septic shock, various

intoxications, and the hepatorenal syndrome typically involve mixed acid-base disorders (see Table 11-2).

The physical examination may provide additional clues to potential acid-base disorders or may provide evidence in support of those suspected from the history. For example, normocalcemic tetany is compatible with severe alkalemia, and cyanosis may indicate severe hypoxia and the possibility of respiratory acidosis or lactic metabolic acidosis. Rapid or deep respirations in the absence of cardiac or pulmonary failure are compatible with the compensatory hyperventilation associated with severe metabolic acidosis. Metabolic alkalosis is common in patients with signs of extracellular fluid volume contraction, whereas high fever typically stimulates respiratory alkalosis.

Careful analysis of the routine laboratory data, including the venous electrolytes, may provide useful quantitative information enabling the identification of the possible predominant acid-base disturbance and clues to additional disorders. The presence of azotemia strengthens support for the diagnosis of renal metabolic acidosis.

Most useful is examination of the venous plasma tCO_2, [Cl⁻], [K⁺], and the AG. In the clinical laboratory, measurement of venous plasma or serum electrolytes includes an estimation of the tCO_2. This measurement reflects the sum of the numerator and the denominator of the Henderson or Henderson-Hasselbalch equation, that is, [HCO_3^-] + H_2CO_3 + dissolved CO_2 gas. Because normally

TABLE 11-2 Common Clinical Conditions Associated with Acid-Base Disorders

Condition	Metabolic Acidosis	Metabolic Alkalosis	Respiratory Acidosis	Respiratory Alkalosis
Cardiovascular disease				
Cardiopulmonary arrest	+*	+†	+	+†
Pulmonary edema				+
CNS disease			+ or	+
Diabetes mellitus	+*			
Drugs				
Diuretics		+		
Poisonings	+*		+	+
Fever				+
GI disease				
Diarrhea	+			
Vomiting/gastric suction		+		
Hepatic failure	+*			+
Hyperkalemia	+			
Hypokalemia		+		
Pulmonary disease				
Acute asthma			+	
COPD/respiratory failure				+
Emboli				+
Pneumonia			+	
Renal disease				
Renal failure	+*			
Renal tubular acidosis	+			
Sepsis	+*			+

*High anion gap metabolic acidosis.
†During treatment and recovery.
Modified and updated from Goldberg M, Green SB, Moss ML, et al: Computer-based instruction and diagnosis of acid-base disorders. JAMA 223:269–275, 1973. With permission.

and in pathophysiologic states the [HCO_3^-] is greater than 90% of the tCO_2, then the venous tCO_2 is a reasonable approximation of the venous [HCO_3^-]. An abnormal plasma [HCO_3^-] indicates an acid-base disorder (see Table 11-1). An increased [HCO_3^-] indicates either a primary metabolic alkalosis or adaptation to respiratory acidosis. A decreased [HCO_3^-] indicates either primary metabolic acidosis or adaptation to respiratory alkalosis. Applying knowledge of the limits of adaptation (see Table 11-1) may enable the elimination of some diagnostic considerations. For example, if the plasma [HCO_3^-] is less than 12 mEq/L, a value that exceeds the limits of adaptation (see Table 11-1) to respiratory alkalosis, then metabolic acidosis is definitely present. Conversely, if plasma [HCO_3^-] is greater than 45 mEq/L, exceeding the adaptive limit for respiratory acidosis, then metabolic alkalosis may be diagnosed. A plasma [HCO_3^-] in the normal range, on the other hand, does not exclude either a mixture of disorders which have opposing effects on [HCO_3^-] (e.g., metabolic acidosis plus metabolic alkalosis, such as may occur in a patient with impaired kidney function with a high AG metabolic acidosis who is also vomiting due to uremia and is losing hydrochloride), or acute respiratory disorders in which the early adaptive changes in [HCO_3^-] are small (see Table 11-1).

Evaluating changes in plasma [Cl^-] may provide additional insights into possible acid-base disorders. Remember, however, that changes in [Cl^-] are important from the standpoint of acid-base disorders only when they are disproportionate to changes in plasma [Na^+]. When this occurs, the changes in plasma [Cl^-] are typically associated with reciprocal changes in plasma [HCO_3^-]. Thus, in primary metabolic alkalosis and in the adaptation to chronic respiratory acidosis, plasma [Cl^-] decreases as [HCO_3^-] increases, whereas in primary metabolic acidosis (with normal AG) and in the adaptation to chronic respiratory alkalosis, plasma [Cl^-] increases as [HCO_3^-] decreases.

Abnormalities in plasma [K^+] are common in patients with acid-base disorders. There is, however, no consistent quantitative relationship between changes in pH or [HCO_3^-] and changes in [K^+]. This is because [K^+] is influenced by many metabolic and physiologic factors besides acid-base disturbances. Alterations in plasma [K^+] are more pronounced in metabolic than in respiratory disorders. An increase in serum [K^+] is more likely to be associated with an acute metabolic acidosis with normal AG and is least likely to be observed in lactic acidosis. In general, a change in [K^+] is useful only as a qualitative indicator in acid-base disorders; a high K^+ plus a low [HCO_3^-] implies metabolic acidosis, and a low [K^+] with high [HCO_3^-] suggests metabolic alkalosis.

Calculation of the AG is essential in the evaluation of acid-base disorders. An elevated AG commonly signifies the presence of a metabolic acidosis regardless of the change in plasma [HCO_3^-]. One should be aware, however, that uncommonly the AG may be moderately increased (5 to 9 mEq/L) by severe volume contraction, metabolic alkalosis, and infusions of sodium salts of unmeasured anions (e.g., sulfates, lactate, carbenicillin). Nevertheless, the AG is a valuable tool in studying for the presence of metabolic acidosis: an AG greater than 30 mEq/L almost always signifies a metabolic acidosis, and an AG between 20 and 30 mEq/L usually signifies metabolic acidosis.

Examination of the relationship between the changes in AG (Δ AG) and the change in [HCO_3^-] (Δ HCO_3^-) may be useful in diagnosing mixed acid-base disorders. In simple high AG metabolic acidosis, each 1 mEq of H^+ accumulation is associated with 1 mEq of unmeasured anion accumulation: furthermore, each 1 mEq of H^+ has consumed 1 mEq of HCO_3^-. Therefore, increases in the AG are associated with corresponding decreases in plasma [HCO_3^-], and Δ AG approximates Δ HCO_3^-. If Δ AG is greater than Δ HCO_3^-, this suggests the presence of an additional process that generates HCO_3^- (either a metabolic alkalosis or chronic respiratory acidosis), whereas Δ AG less than Δ HCO_3^- suggests the additional presence of a hyperchloremic metabolic acidosis or a chronic respiratory alkalosis.

Arterial blood gases are used to confirm the predominant acid-base disorder and to identify and confirm mixed disturbances. From information derived from the history, physical examination, and routine analyses of venous blood, potential acid-base disturbances can be identified, and in many instances a reasonable acid-base diagnosis can be established without obtaining arterial blood gases. On the other hand, it is extremely difficult to diagnose acute respiratory disturbances and most mixed acid-base disorders without knowledge of arterial pH, pCO_2, and [HCO_3^-]. Thus, if these are distinct possibilities or if the patient is critically ill (a setting in which mixed disorders are common), arterial studies should be obtained.

The data on arterial pH, pCO_2, and [HCO_3^-] should be analyzed and applied to the acid-base formulas, to the acid-base map, and to knowledge of limits of adaptation (see Table 11-1 and Fig. 11-1). The results of these analyses should be coordinated with the differential and potential diagnostic inferences derived from the history, physical examination, and routine laboratory data. Before proceeding further, however, one must ensure the internal consistency of the blood values and their compatibility with the Henderson-Hasselbalch or Henderson equation. This can readily be accomplished using the acid-base map (which also serves as a nomogram for these equations) or by converting pH values to [H^+] and applying the Henderson equation. In the pH range 7.20 to 7.50, each 0.1 unit change in pH from a normal value of 7.40 corresponds to a 10-nEq/L change in [H^+] from a normal value of 40 nEq/L.

If the pH is abnormal, then the major acid-base disturbance may be identified. Acidemia denotes a predominant acidosis, and alkalemia indicates a predominant

alkalosis. Reference should then be made to the patterns for each acid-base disorder summarized in Table 11-1. This will enable confirmation of the major disorder. For example, acidemia, a low [HCO_3^-], and a low pCO_2 support the diagnosis of metabolic acidosis. To rule out an additional primary disorder as a component of a mixed disturbance, the data must be compared with the expected range of adaptation by either plotting the data on the acid-base map (see Fig. 11-1) or using one of the formulas for adaptive response in Table 11-1. When the pCO_2 is above or below the predicted range of compensation for a metabolic disturbance, or when the [HCO_3^-] is above or below the predicted levels for a respiratory disorder, a mixed disturbance is present.

Although many mixed acid-base disorders can be diagnosed using the arterial blood values in conjunction with the map or formulas, the final diagnostic conclusions require a coordinated synthesis of information derived from the clinical and laboratory data in conjunction with the arterial data. Thus, use of the map alone will not identify triple mixed acid-base disorders. Values lying within a specific zone on the map (while suggesting a simple disorder) are also compatible with a mixed disorder with counterbalancing effects on pH, [HCO_3^-], or pCO_2. To dissect out the various components of a mixed disorder, we must apply information on changes in AG, plasma [Cl^-], and plasma [K^+]. In fact, a normal plasma [HCO_3^-], a normal pH, or a normal pCO_2 by themselves do not rule out mixed disorders; nor are normal levels of all three variables simultaneously incompatible with mixed disorders.

Mixed disorders should be suspected in the following circumstances:

1. pH is normal and:
   a. [HCO_3^-] is high (mixed metabolic alkalosis plus respiratory acidosis).
   b. [HCO_3^-] is low (mixed metabolic acidosis plus respiratory alkalosis).
   c. [HCO_3^-] is normal and AG is high (mixed metabolic acidosis plus metabolic alkalosis).
2. [HCO_3^-] is normal and:
   a. pH is in the acidemic range (mixed chronic respiratory acidosis and metabolic acidosis).
   b. pH is in the alkalemic range (mixed metabolic alkalosis and chronic respiratory alkalosis).
3. pCO_2 and [HCO_3^-] are shifted from normal in opposite directions.
4. AG is elevated, and clinical/laboratory data suggest a diagnosis other than a simple metabolic acidosis (metabolic acidosis is a component of a mixed disorder).
5. When AG is high and the Δ AG $\neq$ Δ HCO_3^- (see previous discussion of AG and Δ AG). Remember that a mixed disorder may include two different types or etiologies of a simple disorder (e.g., a high AG plus a

normal AG metabolic acidosis or an acute respiratory disorder superimposed on an underlying chronic respiratory disorder).

In conclusion, a successful approach to resolving the sometimes complex dilemmas associated with the diagnosis of acid-base disorders involves the application of a systematic, orderly, and logical series of steps. Building on knowledge of pathophysiology, these involve a coordinated analysis and resynthesis of information derived from taking a proper history, performing an adequate physical examination, and obtaining relevant laboratory data. Final success is measured not only by the intellectual satisfaction of the physician in making the correct evaluations, but also by the well-being of the patient who has benefited from the appropriate corrective therapy.

BIBLIOGRAPHY

DuBose TD Jr: Acid-base disorders. In Brenner BM (ed): The Kidney, 6th ed. Philadelphia, WB Saunders, 2000, pp 925–997.

Goldberg M, Green SB, Moss ML, et al: Computer-based instruction and diagnosis of acid-base disorders. JAMA 223:269–275, 1973.

Gabow PA: Disorders associated with an altered anion gap. Kidney Int 27:472–483, 1985.

Hamm L: Mixed acid-base disorders. In Kokko JP, Tannen RL (eds): Fluids and Electrolytes. Philadelphia, WB Saunders, 1990, pp 490–495.

Kraut JA, Madias NE: Approach to patients with acid-base disorders. Respir Care 46:392–403, 2001.

Laski ME, Kurtzman NA: Acid-base disorders in medicine. Dis Mon 42:51–125, 1996.

McCurdy DK: Mixed metabolic and respiratory acid-base disturbances: Diagnosis and treatment. Chest 62(suppl):35–44, 1972.

CHAPTER 12

Disorders of Potassium Metabolism

Michael Allon

MECHANISMS OF POTASSIUM HOMEOSTASIS

Total body potassium is about 3500 mmol. Approximately 98% of the total is intracellular, primarily found in skeletal muscle, and to a lesser extent in the liver. The remaining 2% (about 70 mmol) is in the extracellular fluid. Two homeostatic systems help to maintain potassium homeostasis. The first system regulates potassium excretion (kidney and intestine). The second regulates potassium shifts between the extracellular and intracellular fluid compartments.

External Potassium Balance

The average American diet contains about 100 mmol of potassium per day. Dietary potassium intake may vary widely from day to day. To stay in potassium balance, it is necessary to increase potassium excretion when dietary potassium increases, and decrease potassium excretion when dietary potassium decreases. Normally, the kidneys excrete 90% to 95% of dietary potassium, with the remaining 5% to 10% excreted by the gut. Potassium excretion by the kidney is a relatively slow process. It takes 6 to 12 hours to excrete an acute potassium load.

Renal Handling of Potassium

To understand the physiologic factors that determine renal excretion of potassium, it is critical to review the main features of tubular potassium handling. Plasma potassium is freely filtered across the glomerular capillary into the proximal tubule. It is subsequently completely reabsorbed by the proximal tubule and loop of Henle. In the distal tubule and the collecting duct, potassium is secreted into the tubular lumen. For practical purposes, urinary excretion of potassium can be viewed as a reflection of potassium secretion into the lumen of the distal tubule and collecting duct. Thus, any factor that stimulates potassium secretion increases urinary potassium excretion; conversely, any factor that inhibits potassium secretion decreases urinary potassium excretion.

Physiologic Regulation of Renal Potassium Excretion

Five major physiologic factors stimulate distal potassium secretion (increase excretion): aldosterone, high distal sodium delivery, high urine flow rate, high [K$^+$] in tubular cells, and metabolic alkalosis. Aldosterone directly increases the activity of the Na$^+$ K$^+$-ATPase in the collecting duct cells, thereby stimulating secretion of potassium into the tubular lumen. Medical conditions that impair aldosterone production or secretion (e.g., diabetic nephropathy, chronic interstitial nephritis) or drugs that inhibit aldosterone production or action (e.g., nonsteroidal anti-inflammatory drugs [NSAIDs], angiotensin-converting enzyme [ACE] inhibitors, angiotensin receptor blockers [ARBs], heparin, spironolactone) decrease potassium secretion by the kidney. Conversely, medical conditions associated with increased aldosterone levels (primary aldosteronism, secondary aldosteronism due to diuretics or vomiting) increase potassium excretion by the kidney. Although there is profound secondary hyperaldosteronism in congestive heart failure and cirrhosis, each of these conditions may be associated with hyperkalemia due to decreased delivery of sodium. Many diuretics increase renal potassium excretion by a number of mechanisms, including high distal sodium delivery, high urine flow rate, metabolic alkalosis, and hyperaldosteronism due to volume depletion. Poorly controlled diabetes commonly increases urinary potassium excretion due to osmotic diuresis with high urinary flow rate and high distal delivery of sodium.

Reabsorption of sodium in the collecting duct occurs through selective sodium channels. This creates an electronegative charge within the tubular lumen relative to the tubular epithelial cell, which in turn promotes secretion of cations (K$^+$ and H$^+$) into the lumen. Therefore, drugs that block the sodium channel in the collecting duct decrease potassium secretion. Conversely, in Liddle's syndrome, a rare genetic disorder, this sodium channel is constitutively open, resulting in avid sodium reabsorption and excessive potassium secretion.

Adaptation in Kidney Failure

In patients with kidney failure, the kidney compensates by increasing the efficiency of potassium excretion. Clearly, there is a limit to renal compensation, and a significant loss of kidney function impairs the ability to excrete potassium, thereby predisposing to a positive potassium balance and a tendency toward hyperkalemia. In most patients with chronic kidney disease, overt hyperkalemia does not occur until the creatinine clearance (CrCl) falls below 10 mL/min. Serum aldosterone levels are elevated in many patients with chronic kidney disease. Aldosterone stimulates the activity of both Na$^+$ K$^+$-ATPase and H$^+$ K$^+$-ATPase, thereby promoting secretion of potassium in the collecting duct, and defending against hyperkalemia. These adaptive mechanisms are less effective in patients with acute renal failure, as compared with chronic kidney disease. Moreover, patients with acute renal failure are often hypotensive, resulting in tissue hypoperfusion and release of potassium from ischemic limbs. For these reasons, severe hyperkalemia occurs more frequently in patients with acute renal failure, as compared to those with chronic kidney disease.

A subset of patients with chronic kidney disease fail to increase aldosterone levels appreciably; as a result, they develop hyperkalemia impairment of kidney function (CrCl less than 50 mL/min), typically in association with hyperchloremic, normal anion gap metabolic acidosis (type IV renal tubular acidosis [RTA]). This condition is most commonly associated with diabetic nephropathy and chronic interstitial nephritis. Moreover, administration of drugs that inhibit aldosterone production or secretion (e.g., ACE inhibitors, ARBs, NSAIDs, heparin) may provoke hyperkalemia in patients with mild to moderately advanced chronic kidney disease.

Intestinal Potassium Excretion

Like the renal collecting duct, the small intestine and colon secrete potassium. Aldosterone stimulates potassium excretion by the gut. In normal individuals, intestinal potassium excretion plays a minor role in potassium homeostasis. However, in patients with significant kidney failure, intestinal potassium secretion is increased three- to fourfold, thereby contributing significantly to potassium homeostasis. This adaptation is limited and is inadequate to compensate for the loss of excretory function in patients with advanced kidney failure.

Internal Potassium Balance

Overview

Extracellular fluid [K] is approximately 4 mEq/L, whereas the intracellular [K] is approximately 150 mEq/L. Because of the uneven distribution of potassium between the fluid compartments, a relatively small net shift of potassium from the intracellular to the extracellular fluid compartment produces marked increases in plasma potassium. Conversely, a relatively small net shift from the extracellular to the intracellular fluid compartment produces a marked decrease in plasma potassium. Unlike renal excretion of potassium, which requires several hours, potassium shift between the extracellular and intracellular fluid compartment (also referred to as extrarenal potas-

sium disposal) is extremely rapid, occurring within minutes.

In patients with advanced kidney failure, whose capacity to excrete potassium is marginal, extrarenal potassium disposal plays a critical role in the prevention of life-threatening hyperkalemia following potassium-rich meals. The following example will illustrate this important principle. Suppose that a 70-kg dialysis patient with a serum potassium of 4.5 mmol/L eats one cup of pinto beans (approximately 35 mmol potassium). Initially the dietary potassium is absorbed into the extracellular fluid compartment ($0.2 \times 70 = 14$ L). This amount of dietary potassium will increase the serum potassium by 2.5 mmol/L (35 mmol/14 L). In the absence of extrarenal potassium disposal, the patient's serum potassium would increase acutely to 7.0 mmol/L, a level frequently associated with serious ventricular arrhythmias. In practice, the increase in serum potassium is much smaller, due to efficient physiologic mechanisms that promote potassium shifts into the intracellular fluid compartment.

Effects of Insulin and Catecholamines on Extrarenal Potassium Disposal

The two major physiologic factors that stimulate transfer of potassium from the extracellular to the intracellular fluid compartments are insulin and epinephrine. The stimulation of extrarenal potassium disposal by both insulin and β$_2$-adrenergic agonists is mediated by stimulation of the Na$^+$ K$^+$-ATPase activity, primarily in skeletal muscle cells. Interference with these two physiologic mechanisms (insulin deficiency or β$_2$-adrenergic blockade, respectively) predisposes to hyperkalemia. On the other hand, excessive insulin or epinephrine levels predispose to hypokalemia.

The potassium-lowering effect of insulin is dose related within the physiologic range of plasma insulin. The potassium-lowering effect of insulin is independent of its effect on plasma glucose. Even the low physiologic levels of insulin present during fasting promote extrarenal potassium disposal. In nondiabetic individuals, hyperglycemia stimulates endogenous insulin secretion, thereby decreasing the serum potassium. In insulin-dependent diabetics, endogenous insulin production is limited, and significant hyperglycemia may occur. Hyperglycemia results in plasma hypertonicity, which promotes potassium shifts out of the cells, and produces paradoxic hyperkalemia.

The potassium-lowering action of epinephrine is mediated by β$_2$-adrenergic stimulation, and is blocked by nonselective beta blockers, but not by selective β$_1$-adrenergic blockers. Alpha-adrenergic stimulation promotes shifts of potassium out of the cells into the extracellular fluid compartment, tending to increase serum potassium. Epinephrine is a mixed α- and β-adrenergic agonist, such that its net effect on serum potassium reflects the balance between its β-adrenergic (potassium-lowering) and α-adrenergic (potassium-raising) effects. In normal individuals the β-adrenergic effect of epinephrine predominates over the α-adrenergic effect, such that the serum potassium decreases. In contrast, the α-adrenergic effect of epinephrine on potassium shifts is much more prominent in patients with severe kidney failure; as a result, dialysis patients are refractory to the potassium-lowering effect of epinephrine.

Effect of Acid-Base Disorders on Extrarenal Potassium Disposal

Acid-base disorders produce internal potassium shifts in a less predictable manner. As a general rule, metabolic alkalosis shifts potassium into the cells, whereas metabolic acidosis shifts potassium out of the cells. However, the nature of the metabolic acidosis determines its effect on serum potassium. Cells are relatively impermeable to chloride. With inorganic acidosis, entry of protons (but not chloride) into the cell results in a reciprocal extrusion of potassium out of the cell to maintain electric neutrality. In contrast, cells are highly permeable to organic anions. The addition of an organic acid to the extracellular fluid results in parallel shifts of protons and organic anions into the cells, with no net change in the electric balance; as a result, potassium is not extruded out of the cells. Thus, mineral acidosis (i.e., hyperchloremic, normal anion gap metabolic acidosis) typically results in hyperkalemia, whereas organic metabolic acidosis (e.g., lactic acidosis) does not affect the serum potassium. Bicarbonate administration to individuals with normal kidney function decreases serum potassium, but this effect is largely due to enhanced urinary excretion of potassium. In contrast, bicarbonate administration to dialysis patients (in whom the capacity for urinary potassium excretion is negligible) does not lower plasma potassium acutely. Moreover, bicarbonate administration does not potentiate the potassium-lowering effects of insulin or albuterol in dialysis patients.

LABORATORY TESTS FOR DIFFERENTIAL DIAGNOSIS OF POTASSIUM DISORDERS

Differential Diagnosis of Hypokalemia and Hyperkalemia

The clinical history, review of medications, family history, and physical examination are sufficient in the rapid differential diagnosis of the etiology of most potassium disorders. In selected patients the cause of hypokalemia or hyperkalemia is not apparent, and additional specialized laboratory tests may be useful. Measurements of the fractional excretion of potassium (FE_K) and transtubular potassium gradient (TTKG) may be useful in distinguishing between renal and nonrenal

causes of hyperkalemia and hypokalemia. The general principle underlying these tests is that the kidney compensates for hyperkalemia by increasing potassium excretion, and compensates for hypokalemia by decreasing potassium excretion. In contrast, when potassium excretion is inappropriate for the serum potassium, this suggests a renal etiology. The optimal use of FE_K or TTKG in the differential diagnosis requires that these values be obtained before the potassium abnormality (hyperkalemia or hypokalemia) is corrected.

Fractional Excretion of Potassium

The fractional excretion of potassium is the percentage of potassium filtered into the proximal tubule that appears in the urine. It represents potassium clearance corrected for glomerular filtration rate, or Cl_K/Cl_{CR}. Since the clearance of any substance can be calculated from UV/P, this fractional excretion ratio can be algebraically transformed to

$$\frac{(U_K V/P_K)}{(U_{CR}V/P_{CR})} \times 100\%.$$

The V in the numerator and denominator cancel out, giving the simplified formula,

$$\frac{(U_K/S_K)}{(U_{CR}/S_{CR})} \times 100\%,$$

where U_K and U_{CR} are the concentrations of potassium and creatinine in the urine, and S_K and S_{CR} are the corresponding serum concentrations. For an individual with normal kidney function on an average dietary potassium intake, the FE_K is approximately 10%. When hypokalemia is due to extrarenal causes (low potassium diet, gastrointestinal losses, potassium shifts into cells), the kidney conserves potassium, and the FE_K is low. In contrast, hypokalemia due to renal potassium losses is associated with an increased FE_K. Similarly, in the setting of hyperkalemia, a high FE_K suggests an extrarenal etiology, whereas a low FE_K is consistent with a renal etiology. If a urine creatinine measurement is not available, one can often use U_K alone to differentiate between renal and extrarenal causes of hyperkalemia. Specifically, in a hypokalemic patient, U_K that is greater than 20 mEq/L suggests a renal etiology, whereas U_K that is less than 20 mEq/L suggests an extrarenal etiology.

Transtubular Potassium Gradient

The TTKG is a formula that estimates the potassium gradient between the urine and the blood in the distal nephron. It is calculated from $[U_K/(U_{osm}/P_{osm})]/P_K$, where U_{osm} and P_{osm} are the urine and plasma osmolalities. The numerator is an estimate of the luminal potassium concentration. The U_{osm}/P_{osm} term is included to correct for the increase in U_K that is due purely to water abstraction and concentration of urine overall. TTKG values have been derived from empiric measurements in normal individuals under a variety of physiologic conditions. In a normal individual under normal circumstances, the TTKG is about 6 to 8. Hypokalemia with a high TTKG suggests excessive renal potassium losses, whereas hypokalemia with a low TTKG suggests appropriate renal compensation and an extrarenal etiology. Similarly, hyperkalemia with a low TTKG suggests an inadequate renal response and a renal etiology, whereas hyperkalemia with a high TTKG is consistent with an extrarenal etiology.

Several factors limit the utility of the FE_K and TTKG in the differential diagnosis of potassium disorders. The FE_K and TTKG are increased when dietary potassium is increased, and decreased when dietary potassium is decreased. Furthermore, in patients with chronic kidney disease, there is an adaptive increase in potassium excretion per functioning nephron, such that FE_K and TTKG increase. This means that the "normal" value for a given individual can vary substantially, making it difficult to determine the significance of a high or low FE_K or TTKG.

HYPOKALEMIA

Hypokalemia versus Potassium Deficiency

It is important to distinguish between potassium deficiency and hypokalemia. Potassium deficiency is the state resulting from a persistent negative potassium balance (i.e., potassium excretion exceeding potassium intake). Hypokalemia refers to a low plasma potassium concentration. Hypokalemia can be due either to potassium deficiency (inadequate potassium intake or excessive potassium losses) or to net potassium shifts from the extracellular to the intracellular fluid compartment. A patient may have severe potassium depletion without manifesting hypokalemia. An important example is a patient presenting with diabetic ketoacidosis. Such patients have typically had severe hyperglycemia with osmotic diuresis for several days, leading to high levels of renal potassium excretion and potassium deficiency. However, as a result of insulin deficiency, there is a concomitant shift of potassium out of the cells into the extracellular fluid compartment. At presentation to the hospital, such patients are frequently normokalemic or even hyperkalemic. Once they are treated with exogenous insulin, there is a rapid shift of potassium back into the cells, and within a few hours the patients develop significant hypokalemia. Conversely, patients hospitalized with an acute myocardial infarction commonly have hypokalemia due to stress-induced catecholamine release and enhanced extrarenal potassium disposal, even though they have a normal external potassium balance.

TABLE 12-1 Causes of Hypokalemia

Inadequate potassium intake (severe malnutrition)

Extrarenal potassium losses
  Vomiting
  Diarrhea

Hypokalemia due to urinary potassium losses
  Diuretics (loop diuretics, thiazides, acetazolamide)
  Osmotic diuresis (e.g., hyperglycemia)
  Hypokalemia with hypertension
    Primary aldosteronism
    Glucocorticoid-remediable hypertension
    Malignant hypertension
    Renovascular hypertension
    Renin-secreting tumor
    Essential hypertension with excessive diuretics dosing
    Liddle syndrome
    11-β-hydroxysteroid dehydrogenase deficiency
      Genetic
      Drug induced (chewing tobacco, licorice, some French wines)
      Congenital adrenal hyperplasia
  Hypokalemia with a normal blood pressure
    Distal RTA (type I)
    Proximal RTA (type II)
    Bartter's syndrome
    Gitelman's syndrome
    Hypomagnesemia (cis-platinum, alcoholism, diuretics)

Hypokalemia due to potassium shifts
  Insulin administration
  Catecholamine excess (acute stress)
  Familial periodic hypokalemic paralysis
  Thyrotoxic hypokalemic paralysis

RTA, renal tubular acidosis.

Clinical Disorders Associated with Hypokalemia

Table 12-1 provides a list of the most common causes of hypokalemia. The kidney can avidly conserve potassium, such that hypokalemia due to inadequate potassium intake is a rare event requiring prolonged starvation ("tea and toast" diet). Therefore, hypokalemia is usually due to excessive potassium losses from the gut or the urine or from potassium shifts from the extracellular to the intracellular fluid compartments. Prolonged vomiting causes potassium losses, in part due to potassium present in the gastric juice (approximately 10 mEq/L), but primarily due to renal losses because of secondary aldosteronism from volume depletion. Severe diarrhea, due to either disease or laxative abuse, results in significant potassium excretion in the stool.

Excessive renal potassium losses as a cause of hypokalemia are seen with a number of clinical syndromes. Conceptually, it is useful to distinguish between hypokalemia associated with hypertension and hypokalemia associated with a normal blood pressure. When hypokalemia is associated with hypertension, measurements of plasma renin and aldosterone may be helpful in the differential diagnosis. Several physiologic observations are relevant in this regard:

1. Aldosterone, a mineralocorticoid, stimulates sodium reabsorption and potassium secretion in the collecting duct.
2. The physiologic stimulus for aldosterone secretion is activation of the renin-angiotensin axis. Moreover, aldosterone-induced sodium retention suppresses the renin-angiotensin axis by negative feedback.
3. Glucocorticoids at high concentrations bind to mineralocorticoid receptors and mimic their physiologic actions.
4. Glucocorticoids are stimulated by adrenocorticotropic hormone (ACTH) and suppress ACTH production by negative feedback.

Primary aldosteronism is due to autonomous (non-renin-mediated) secretion of aldosterone by the adrenal cortex. This results in avid sodium retention and potassium secretion by the distal nephron. The patients present with volume-dependent hypertension, hypokalemia, and metabolic alkalosis. Biochemical evaluation reveals a high serum aldosterone level and suppressed plasma renin. Abdominal computed tomography scan reveals either a unilateral adrenal adenoma or bilateral adrenal hyperplasia. The former is treated surgically, and the latter with spironolactone. Glucocorticoid-remediable aldosteronism (GRA) is a rare autosomal-dominant condition in which there is fusion of the 11-β-hydroxylase and aldosterone synthase genes. As a result, aldosterone secretion is stimulated by ACTH and can be suppressed by an exogenous glucocorticoid, dexamethasone. Patients with GRA have a clinical presentation similar to those with primary aldosteronism (volume-dependent hypertension, hypokalemia, high serum aldosterone, and low serum renin), except that they are younger and have a family history of hypertension.

Patients with renovascular hypertension, renin-secreting tumors, and severe malignant hypertension may also present with severe hypertension and hypokalemia. In contrast to patients with primary aldosteronism, these patients have secondary aldosteronism (i.e., high serum renin and aldosterone levels). Of course, patients with essential hypertension may also have hypokalemia and high plasma renin and aldosterone levels if they are treated with loop or thiazide diuretics and are volume depleted.

Patients with 11-β-hydroxysteroid dehydrogenase deficiency, a rare genetic disorder, have a defect in the conversion of cortisol to cortisone in the peripheral tissues. This results in high tissue cortisol levels that activate the mineralocorticoid receptors, producing hypokalemia and hypertension. Such patients have low serum renin and aldosterone levels. Chewing tobacco, certain brands of licorice, and some French red wines contain glycyrrhizic acid, which inhibits 11-β-hyroxysteroid dehydrogenase. Ingestion of these foods may produce hypokalemia, volume-dependent hypertension, and low serum renin and aldosterone levels, similar to the clinical presenta-

tion of congenital 11-β-hyroxysteroid dehydrogenase deficiency.

Patients with congenital adrenal hyperplasia have a deficiency of 11-β-hydroxylase, an enzyme required in the common pathways for mineralocorticoids and glucocorticoids. These patients have low serum renin and aldosterone levels, high levels of DOCA (a mineralocorticoid), and high levels of androgen. Males have early puberty, and females exhibit virilization, with hirsutism and clitoromegaly. This condition improves with exogenous corticosteroids to suppress ACTH.

Liddle's syndrome is a rare autosomal-dominant disorder caused by a defect of the epithelial sodium channel, such that there is increased sodium absorption and potassium secretion in the collecting duct. The patients present with hypokalemia, hypertension, and volume overload. Their biochemical profile reveals a low serum renin and aldosterone. The patient's blood pressure and serum potassium improve dramatically with inhibitors of the epithelial sodium channel, such as amiloride.

Hypokalemia due to excessive renal potassium excretion is also seen in a number of clinical conditions in which hypertension is infrequently observed. Both type I (distal) and type II (proximal) RTA are associated with kaliuresis and hypokalemia; both conditions present with a normal anion gap metabolic acidosis. Type I RTA is frequently associated with hypercalciuria and calcium oxalate kidney stones. Type II RTA is rare in adults, and is often associated with a generalized defect in proximal tubular function, manifesting with glycosuria (with a normal serum glucose), hypophosphatemia with phosphaturia, and a low serum uric acid with uricosuria.

Bartter's syndrome is a rare familial disease characterized by hypokalemia, metabolic alkalosis, hypercalciuria, normal blood pressure, and high plasma renin and aldosterone levels. It has been associated with a number of mutations that interfere with sodium reabsorption in the thick ascending limb of Henle, including mutations in the luminal Na-K-2Cl transporter (NKCC2) or potassium secretory channel (ROMK), or the basolateral chloride channel (ClC-Kb) (see Chapter 43). These patients act as if they are chronically ingesting loop diuretics; therefore, they are difficult to distinguish clinically from patients with surreptitious diuretic ingestion. Patients with Gitelman's syndrome, a variant of Bartter's syndrome, differ in that they have hypocalciuria and hypomagnesemia. Gitelman's syndrome has been linked to a mutation in the renal thiazide-sensitive NaCl transporter, or NCCT. These patients act as if they are chronically ingesting thiazide diuretics.

Familial hypokalemic periodic paralysis is a rare autosomal-dominant disorder in which affected individuals develop periodic episodes of severe muscle weakness in association with profound hypokalemia, due to rapid shifts of potassium from the extracellular to the intracellular fluid compartment. Interestingly, even when the patient has complete paralysis, the diaphragm and bulbar muscles are spared, such that the patient is able to breathe, swallow, talk, and blink. The paralysis resolves within hours of potassium ingestion. The patients are asymptomatic, with a normal serum potassium in between the acute episodes. Thyrotoxic hypokalemic paralysis is an unusual manifestation of hyperthyroidism, seen primarily in Asian patients. The clinical presentation is similar to that of hypokalemic periodic paralysis, except that the paralytic episodes cease when the hyperthyroidism is corrected.

Drug-Induced Hypokalemia

A number of drugs have the potential to cause hypokalemia, either by stimulating renal potassium excretion or by blocking extrarenal disposal. Exogenous mineralocorticoids mimic the effects of aldosterone, thereby stimulating distal potassium secretion. High doses of glucocorticoids possess some mineralocorticoid activity and have a similar effect. Most diuretics, including loop diuretics, thiazide diuretics, and acetazolamide, increase renal potassium excretion. A number of drugs, including alcohol, diuretics, and cis-platinum, cause renal magnesium wasting and hypomagnesemia. For reasons that are not well understood, hypomagnesemia impairs renal potassium conservation. Thus, these patients may have associated hypokalemia that is refractory to potassium supplementation until the magnesium deficit is corrected. (Paradoxically, cyclosporine may produce hypomagnesemia in conjunction with hyperkalemia.)

Drugs that promote extrarenal potassium disposal may also result in hypokalemia. This phenomenon can be seen after the administration of an acute dose of insulin. Similarly, β_2-agonists (either intravenous or nebulized), including albuterol and terbutaline, frequently result in acute hypokalemia.

Clinical Manifestations of Hypokalemia

Hypokalemia may produce electrocardiographic (ECG) abnormalities, including a flattened T wave and a U wave (Fig. 12-1). Hypokalemia also appears to increase the risk for ventricular arrhythmias in patients with ischemic heart disease or patients taking digoxin. Severe hypokalemia is associated with variable degrees of skeletal muscle weakness, even to the point of paralysis. On rare occasions diaphragmatic paralysis from hypokalemia can lead to respiratory arrest. There may also be decreased motility of smooth muscle, manifesting with ileus or urinary retention. Rarely, severe hypokalemia may result in rhabdomyolysis.

Severe hypokalemia also interferes with the urinary concentrating mechanism in the distal nephron, resulting in nephrogenic diabetes insipidus. Such patients have

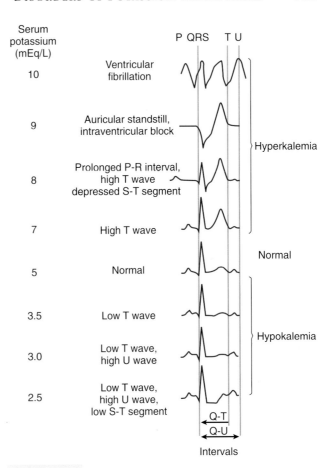

FIGURE 12-1 A schematic representation of electrocardiographic changes and the serum potassium levels at which such changes are typically seen. (From Seldin DW, Giebisch G [eds]: The Regulation of Potassium Balance. New York, Raven, 1989. With permission.)

a low urine osmolality in the face of high serum osmolality, and are refractory to vasopressin.

Treatment of Hypokalemia

The acute treatment of hypokalemia requires potassium supplementation. This can be given either intravenously or orally. The correlation between serum potassium and total potassium deficit in hypokalemia patients is poor. A given patient's serum potassium is a reflection of both external potassium balance and transcellular potassium shifts. The percentage of administered exogenous potassium that remains in the extracellular fluid compartment is variable. Thus, it is difficult to predict how much potassium replacement a given hypokalemic patient will require. Without adequate monitoring, it is possible to give too much potassium and make the patient hyperkalemic. Therefore, one should give multiple small doses of potassium, with frequent checks of serum potassium values.

Oral potassium administration is safer than the intravenous route, and less likely to produce an overshoot in the serum potassium. Each oral dose should not exceed

20 to 40 mEq of potassium. Intravenous KCl should be reserved for severe, symptomatic hypokalemia (less than 3.0 mEq/L) or for patients who cannot ingest oral potassium. Intravenous KCl should not be given any faster than 10 mmol/hour in the absence of continuous electrocardiographic monitoring. The serum potassium should be rechecked every 2 to 3 hours to confirm a clinical response and avoid an overshoot.

Correction of the underlying medical condition may prevent recurrence of hypokalemia after potassium repletion. If the patient has a chronic condition associated with persistent urinary potassium losses, such that hypokalemia is likely to recur, the patient should be encouraged to increase the intake of foods high in potassium (especially fresh fruits, nuts, and legumes). In some patients chronic oral potassium supplementation may be necessary.

HYPERKALEMIA

Pseudohyperkalemia is a factitious elevation of the serum potassium due to in vitro release of potassium from blood cells. It may be seen with in vitro hemolysis, thrombocytosis, or severe leukocytosis. Pseudohyperkalemia due to hemolysis is readily apparent because the serum is pink. Pseudohyperkalemia due to severe thrombocytosis or leukocytosis can be confirmed by drawing simultaneous blood samples in tubes with and without anticoagulant; the serum potassium is higher than plasma potassium in pseudohyperkalemia.

True hyperkalemia is caused by a positive potassium balance (increased potassium intake or decreased potassium excretion) or an increase in net potassium shift from the intracellular to the extracellular fluid compartment. Table 12-2 provides a list of the most common causes of hyperkalemia. In practice, most patients who develop severe hyperkalemia have more than one contributory factor. For example, a patient with moderately advanced chronic kidney disease due to diabetic nephropathy may be medicated with an ACE inhibitor and have mild hyperkalemia. However, when he is started on indomethacin for acute gouty arthritis, the patient rapidly develops severe hyperkalemia.

Drug-Induced Hyperkalemia

A large number of drugs have the potential to cause hyperkalemia, either by inhibiting renal potassium excretion or by blocking extrarenal disposal (Table 12-3). Most individuals taking these drugs will not develop hyperkalemia. Patients at risk are those with kidney failure, especially if they have a high dietary potassium intake or are on an additional medication that predisposes to hyperkalemia. Most diuretics (loop diuretics, thiazide diuretics, acetazolamide) increase urinary potassium excretion and tend to cause hypokalemia. However,

---

TABLE 12-2 Causes of Hyperkalemia

Pseudohyperkalemia
  Hemolysis
  Thrombocytosis
  Severe leukocytosis
  Fist clenching

Decreased renal excretion
  Acute or chronic kidney failure
  Aldosterone deficiency (e.g., type IV renal tubular acidosis)
  Frequently associated with diabetic nephropathy
  Chronic interstitial nephritis or obstructive nephropathy
  Adrenal insufficiency (Addison's disease)
  Drugs that inhibit potassium excretion (see Table 12-3)
  Kidney diseases that impair distal tubule function
    Sickle cell anemia
    Systemic lupus erythematosus

Abnormal potassium distribution
  Insulin deficiency
  Beta blockers
  Metabolic or respiratory acidosis
  Familial hyperkalemic periodic paralysis

Abnormal potassium release from cells
  Rhabdomyolysis
  Tumor lysis syndrome

TABLE 12-3 Mechanisms for Drug-Induced Hyperkalemia

Decrease renal potassium excretion

Block sodium channel in the distal nephron
  Potassium-sparing diuretics: amiloride, triamterene
  Antibiotics: trimethoprim, pentamidine

Block aldosterone production
  ACE inhibitors (e.g., captopril, enalapril, lisinopril, benazepril)
  Angiotensin receptor blockers
  NSAIDs and COX-2 inhibitors
  Heparin
  Tacrolimus

Block aldosterone receptors
  Spironolactone
  Eplerenone

Block Na^+K^+-ATPase activity in the distal nephron
  Cyclosporine

Inhibit extrarenal potassium disposal
  Block β_2-adrenergic mediated extrarenal potassium disposal—nonselective beta blockers (e.g., propranolol, nadolol, timolol)
  Block Na^+K^+-ATPase activity in skeletal muscles: digoxin overdose (not therapeutic doses)
  Inhibit insulin release (e.g., somatostatin)

Potassium release from cells
  Drug-induced rhabdomyolysis (e.g., lovastatin, cocaine)
  Drug-induced tumor lysis syndrome (chemotherapy agents in acute leukemias, high-grade lymphomas)
  Depolarizing paralytic agents (e.g., succinylcholine)

Drug-induced acute renal failure

ACE, angiotensin-converting enzyme; COX-2, cyclo-oxygenase-2; NSAID, nonsteroidal anti-inflammatory drug.

potassium-sparing diuretics inhibit urinary potassium excretion and predispose to hyperkalemia by one of two mechanisms. Spironolactone and eplerenone are competitive inhibitors of aldosterone; they bind to the aldosterone receptors in the collecting duct, thereby inhibiting Na^+ K^+-ATPase activity, and indirectly limiting potassium secretion. Interestingly, the immunosuppressant drug cyclosporine also blocks Na^+ K^+-ATPase activity in the distal nephron. Two other potassium-sparing diuretics, amiloride and triamterene, bind to the epithelial sodium channel in the collecting duct. This inhibits sodium reabsorption in the distal nephron, and thereby limits the establishment of an electrochemical gradient required for potassium secretion. Interestingly, two antibiotics, trimethoprim (one of the components of Bactrim) and pentamidine, have also been shown to block the epithelial sodium channel in the collecting duct, and therefore predispose patients to hyperkalemia. In addition, trimethoprim has been shown to inhibit the collecting tubule H^+ K^+-ATPase.

Because aldosterone plays an important role in enhancing renal potassium excretion in patients with kidney failure, drugs that inhibit aldosterone production (either directly or indirectly) predispose such patients to hyperkalemia. Angiotensin II is a potent stimulator of aldosterone production in the adrenal cortex. ACE inhibitors inhibit the production of angiotensin II, thereby decreasing aldosterone levels. Similarly, angiotensin II receptor blockers also inhibit aldosterone production. Prostaglandins directly stimulate renin production, and prostaglandin inhibitors (NSAIDs) inhibit the production of renin, thereby indirectly decreasing aldosterone production. This effect is seen even with "kidney-sparing" NSAIDs, such as sulindac (a nonselective cyclo-oxygenase-1 [COX-1] and COX-2 inhibitor). Hyperkalemia may also be caused by selective COX-2 inhibitors. Heparin has been shown to directly inhibit the production of aldosterone in the renal cortex, primarily by decreasing the number and affinity of angiotensin II receptors in the zona glomerulosa. This effect occurs even with the low doses of subcutaneous heparin used for prophylaxis of venous thrombosis in hospitalized patients (e.g., 5000 units every 12 hours). Tacrolimus, an immunosuppressant drug, may also cause hyperkalemia by inhibiting aldosterone synthesis.

Given the stimulation of extrarenal potassium disposal by β-adrenergic agonists, it is not surprising that β_2-antagonists can predispose to hyperkalemia. This effect is seen primarily with nonselective beta blockers (e.g., propranolol and nadolol), rather than β_1-selective blockers (e.g., atenolol, metoprolol). There is significant systemic absorption of topical beta blockers, and severe hyperkalemia may rarely be provoked by timolol eyedrops. Drugs inhibiting endogenous insulin release, such as somatostatin, have been implicated rarely as a cause of hyperkalemia in patients with kidney failure. Presumably, long-acting somatostatin analogues, such as octreotide,

would have a similar effect on serum potassium. Digoxin overdose causes inhibition of Na^+ K^+-ATPase activity in skeletal muscle cells, and may manifest with hyperkalemia. This effect is rarely seen at therapeutic doses of the drug. Depolarizing paralytic agents used for general anesthesia, such as succinylcholine, can occasionally produce hyperkalemia by causing potassium to leak out of the cells.

Finally, drugs can also cause hyperkalemia indirectly by causing release of intracellular potassium from injured cells (e.g., rhabdomyolysis with lovastatin and cocaine, or tumor lysis syndrome when chemotherapy is administered in patients with acute leukemia or high-grade lymphoma). Moreover, drug-induced acute renal failure may be associated with secondary hyperkalemia.

Fasting Hyperkalemia in Dialysis Patients

Prolonged fasting decreases plasma insulin concentrations, thereby promoting potassium shifts from the intracellular to the extracellular fluid compartments. In normal individuals the excess potassium is excreted in the urine, such that the plasma potassium remains constant. In dialysis patients the potassium entering the extracellular fluid compartment during fasting cannot be excreted, thereby resulting in progressive hyperkalemia. The phenomenon of fasting hyperkalemia may be clinically significant in dialysis patients who are fasted longer than 8 to 12 hours prior to a surgical or radiologic procedure. Occasionally, such patients develop life-threatening hyperkalemia during a prolonged fast. The hyperkalemia can be prevented by the administration of intravenous dextrose (to stimulate endogenous insulin secretion) for the duration of the fast. If the patient is diabetic, insulin must be added to the dextrose infusion to prevent paradoxic hyperkalemia.

Clinical Manifestations of Hyperkalemia

Hyperkalemia may produce progressive electrocardiographic abnormalities, including peaked T waves, flattening or absence of P waves, widened QRS complexes, and sine waves (see Fig. 12-1). The major risk of severe hyperkalemia is the development of life-threatening ventricular arrhythmias. Severe hyperkalemia with ECG changes is a medical emergency.

Severe hyperkalemia, like severe hypokalemia, can cause skeletal muscle weakness, even to the point of paralysis and respiratory failure. Hyperkalemia impairs urinary acid excretion by decreasing collecting tubule apical H^+ K^+-ATPase and by decreasing ammoniagenesis, which may result in type IV RTA. Hyperkalemia stimulates endogenous aldosterone secretion. Hyperkalemia stimulates insulin secretion in dogs, but not in humans.

Treatment of Hyperkalemia

Severe hyperkalemia associated with ECG changes (see Fig. 12-1) is a life-threatening state requiring emergent intervention. If the patient's ECG is suspicious for hyperkalemia, one should initiate therapy without waiting for the laboratory confirmation. If the patient has kidney failure, urgent dialysis is required for removal of potassium from the body. Because of the inevitable delay in initiating dialysis, the following temporizing measures must be initiated promptly:

1. The first step is to stabilize the myocardium. Acute administration of intravenous calcium gluconate does not change plasma potassium, but does transiently improve the ECG. The effect is almost immediate. Give 10 mL of calcium gluconate over 1 minute. If there is no improvement in the ECG appearance within 3 to 5 minutes, the dose should be repeated.
2. The second step is to shift potassium from the extracellular to the intracellular fluid, so as to rapidly decrease the serum potassium. This involves administration of insulin and a β_2-agonist.
   a. Intravenous insulin is the fastest way to lower the serum potassium. The plasma potassium starts to decrease within 15 minutes. Intravenous glucose is given concurrently to prevent hypoglycemia. One should give 10 units of regular insulin and 50 mL of 50% dextrose (one ampoule of D_{50}) as a bolus, followed by a continuous infusion of 5% dextrose at 100 mL/hour to prevent late hypoglycemia. In diabetic patients the serum glucose should be ascertained with a glucometer; if it is over 300 mg/dL, one can administer the intravenous insulin alone (without concomitant 50% dextrose). One should never give dextrose without insulin for the acute treatment of hyperkalemia; in patients with inadequate endogenous insulin production, the resulting hyperglycemia can produce a paradoxic increase in serum potassium.
   b. Beta-agonists. One should give 20 mg of albuterol (a β_2-agonist) by inhalation over 10 minutes. The onset of action is 30 minutes. Make sure the concentrated form (5 mg/mL) of the drug is used so that the volume that needs to be inhaled is minimized. The dose required to lower plasma potassium is considerably higher than that used to treat asthma, because only a small fraction of nebulized albuterol is absorbed systemically. Thus, 0.5 mg of intravenous albuterol (not available in the United States) produces a comparable change in plasma potassium to that seen after 20 mg of nebulized albuterol. The potassium-lowering effect of albuterol is additive to that of insulin.
   c. Sodium bicarbonate. In patients with chronic kidney disease who are not yet on dialysis, bicarbonate administration can lower serum potassium by enhancing renal potassium excretion. However, bicarbonate administration is of dubious value for treatment of hyperkalemia in patients without residual kidney function. It takes at least 3 to 4 hours for the serum potassium to start to decrease after bicarbonate administration to dialysis patients, so this modality is not useful for the acute management of hyperkalemia. Moreover, bicarbonate administration does not enhance the potassium-lowering effects of insulin or albuterol. Bicarbonate administration is still indicated if the patient has severe metabolic acidosis (serum bicarbonate less than 10 mmol/L).
3. Once the previous temporizing measures have been performed, further interventions are undertaken to remove potassium from the body.
   a. Diuretics only work if the patient has adequate kidney function.
   b. The resin exchanger sodium polystyrene sulfonate (Kayexalate) removes potassium from the blood into the gut, in exchange for an equal amount of sodium. It is relatively slow acting, requiring 1 to 2 hours before plasma potassium decreases. Each gram of resin removes 0.5 to 1.0 mmol of potassium. One should give 50 g in 30 mL sorbitol by mouth, or 50 g in a retention enema. The rectal route is faster and more reliable. A recent study suggested that a single standard oral dose of Kayexalate may not be efficacious in decreasing the serum potassium within 4 hours in normokalemic hemodialysis patients, despite a documented increase in potassium excretion by the gut. Whether this modality is effective in hyperkalemic dialysis patients, or when given in multiple doses, remains to be determined. Given this uncertainty, frequent monitoring of plasma potassium in patients treated with Kayexalate is warranted.
   c. Hemodialysis is the definitive treatment for patients with advanced chronic kidney disease and severe hyperkalemia.

For patients with moderate hyperkalemia, not associated with ECG changes, it is frequently sufficient to discontinue the drugs predisposing to hyperkalemia.

To prevent a recurrence of hyperkalemia once the acute treatment has been provided, the following measures are useful:

1. Counsel the patient on dietary potassium restriction, 40 to 60 mEq per day (Table 12-4).
2. Avoid medications that interfere with renal excretion of potassium (e.g., potassium-sparing diuretics and NSAIDs). ACE inhibitors and ARBs play a major role in slowing the progression of chronic kidney disease. For this reason, when patients on these medications develop hyperkalemia, one should first attempt to

TABLE 12-4 Potassium Content of Selected Foods

Food	Potassium (mg)	Potassium (mEq)
Pinto beans (1 cup)	1370	35
Raisins (1 cup)	1106	28
Honeydew (1/2 melon)	939	24
Nuts (1 cup)	688	18
Black-eyed peas (1 cup)	625	16
Collard greens (1 cup)	498	13
Banana (1 medium)	440	11
Tomato (1 medium)	366	9
Orange (1 large)	333	9
Milk (1 cup)	351	9
Potato chips (10)	226	6

decrease dietary potassium intake, stop other drugs contributing to hyperkalemia, add a diuretic, or reduce the dose of ACE inhibitor or ARB. Only if all other measures fail to control the hyperkalemia should the ACE inhibitor or ARB be discontinued.

3. Avoid drugs that interfere with potassium shifts from the extracellular to the extracellular compartments (e.g., nonselective beta blockers).

4. When hemodialysis patients are fasted in preparation for surgery or a radiologic procedure, administer intravenous 10% dextrose at 50 mL/hour to prevent hyperkalemia. If the patient is diabetic, add 10 units of regular insulin to each liter of 10% dextrose.

5. In selected patients, chronic medication with loop diuretics can be used to stimulate urinary potassium excretion.

6. Specific therapy may be indicated for the underlying etiology, when available. For example, patients with adrenal insufficiency require replacement with exogenous glucocorticoids and mineralocorticoids. In patients with hyperkalemic periodic paralysis (a rare autosomal-dominant disorder in which affected individuals develop periodic episodes of severe muscle weakness in association with profound hyperkalemia), prophylactic aerosolized albuterol can prevent both exercise-induced hyperkalemia and muscle weakness.

BIBLIOGRAPHY

Acker CG, Johnson JP, Palevsky PM, Greenberg A: Hyperkalemia in hospitalized patients: Causes, adequacy of treatment, and results of an attempt to improve physician compliance with published therapy guidelines. Arch Intern Med 158:917–924, 1998.

Allon M: Treatment and prevention of hyperkalemia in endstage renal disease. Kidney Int 43:1197–1209, 1993.

Allon M: Hyperkalemia in endstage renal disease: Mechanisms and management. J Am Soc Nephrol 6:1134–1142, 1995.

Allon M, Takeshian A, Shanklin N: Effect of insulin-plus-glucose infusion with or without epinephrine on fasting hyperkalemia. Kidney Int 43:212–217, 1993.

DuBose TD: Hyperkalemic hyperchloremic metabolic acidosis: Pathophysiologic insights. Kidney Int 51:591–602, 1997.

Ethier JH, Kamel KS, Magner PO, et al: The transtubular potassium concentration in patients with hyperkalemia and hypokalemia. Am J Kidney Dis 15:309–315, 1990.

Farese RV, Biglieri EG, Shackleton CHL, et al: Licorice-induced hypermineralocorticoidism. N Engl J Med 325:1223–1227, 1991.

Gruy-Kapral C, Emmett M, Santa Ana CA, et al: Effect of single dose resin-cathartic therapy on serum potassium concentra-tion in patients with endstage renal disease. J Am Soc Nephrol 9:1924–1930, 1998.

Kamel KS, Halperin ML, Faber MD, et al: Disorders of potassium balance. In Brenner BM (ed): The Kidney. Philadelphia, WB Saunders, 1996, pp 999–1037.

Kamel KS, Wei C: Controversial issues in the treatment of hyperkalemia. Nephrol Dial Transplant 18:2215–2218, 2003.

Krishna GG, Steigerwalt SP, Pikus R, et al: Hypokalemic states. In Narins RG (ed): Clinical Disorders of Fluid and Electrolyte Metabolism. New York, McGraw-Hill, 1994, pp 659–696.

Kurtz I: Molecular pathogenesis of Bartter's and Gitelman's syndromes. Kidney Int 54:1396–1410, 1998.

Lifton RP, Dluhy RG, Powers M, et al: A chimaeric 11 beta-hydroxylase/aldosterone synthase gene causes glucocorticoid-remediable aldosteronism and human hypertension. Nature 355:262–265, 1992.

Salem MM, Rosa RM, Batlle DC: Extrarenal potassium tolerance in chronic renal failure: Implications for the treatment of acute hyperkalemia. Am J Kidney Dis 18:421–440, 1991.

Shimkets RA, Warnock DG, Bositis CM, et al: Liddle's syndrome: Heritable human hypertension caused by mutations in the beta subunit of the epithelial sodium channel. Cell 79:407–414, 1994.

CHAPTER **13**

Disorders of Calcium and Phosphorus Homeostasis

David A. Bushinsky

CALCIUM

Calcium Homeostasis

Distribution

The vast majority (99.5%) of total body calcium is contained within the bone mineral, while only about 0.1% of body calcium is in the extracellular fluid. The mineral phases of bone provide a reservoir of calcium for the far smaller extra and intracellular pools. The concentration of calcium in the cell cytosol is approximately 100 nmol/L or approximately one ten thousandth of the extracellular calcium concentration. Within the cell, the mitochondria and the sarcoplasmic and endoplasmic reticula contain the highest concentrations of calcium.

Serum Concentration

In humans, the concentration of serum calcium is maintained at a constant level between 9.0 and 10.4 mg/dL, or 2.25 to 2.6 mmol/L. Of the total serum calcium, approximately 40% is protein bound, especially to albumin and to a lesser extent to globulins and other proteins. Approximately 10% of the calcium is complexed to phosphate, citrate, carbonate, and other anions, and the remaining 50% exists in the ionized form. The ionized and complexed calcium together constitute that which is filtered by the kidney, the ultrafilterable calcium, which has a concentration of approximately 1.5 mmol/L.

The concentration of ionized calcium is of physiologic importance and remains remarkably constant even with marked variations in the levels of total calcium. Increases in total calcium concentration lead to an increase in calcium binding to albumin, lessening the increase in ionized calcium concentration. While a decrease in serum albumin of 1 g/dL is usually associated with a decrease of 0.8 mg/dL in total calcium concentration, the proportional decline in ionized calcium will be less. The decrease in albumin lessens the fraction of bound calcium and results in only a small decrease in the concentration of ionized calcium. Alterations in systemic pH alter calcium binding by albumin. Because the decrease in ionized calcium is difficult to predict, the best

approach is to measure ionized calcium directly. Most clinical laboratories have this capability.

Intestinal Absorption

The average American diet contains approximately 800 mg (20 mmol) of calcium, of which there is generally a net absorption of approximately 160 mg (4 mmol). Calcium absorption varies widely depending on other dietary components that may bind calcium (oxalate or phosphate) or promote absorption (lactose) and the level of serum $1,25(OH)_2$ vitamin D_3. $1,25(OH)_2$ vitamin D_3 is the principal hormonal regulator of intestinal calcium absorption, and increases in its serum level stimulate absorption. Calcium is absorbed in the duodenum, jejunum, and ileum. Calcium moves across the brush border through calcium channels, down its concentration gradient by a $1,25(OH)_2$ vitamin D_3–facilitated mechanism, through the cell bound to $1,25(OH)_2$ vitamin D_3–induced calcium binding proteins, and then is transported across the basolateral membrane against a steep gradient utilizing a calcium adenosine triphosphatase (ATPase) or through a sodium-for-calcium exchange mechanism.

Renal Excretion

A 70-kg man with a glomerular filtration rate of 180 L/day filters approximately 270 mmol of calcium per day (180 L/day × 1.5 mmol/L). This quantity of calcium, over 10 g, is far more than the calcium content of the entire extracellular fluid. The kidney reabsorbs approximately 98% of the ultrafiltered calcium, leading to a urine calcium excretion of approximately 4 mmol/day.

Approximately 70% of filtered calcium is reabsorbed in the proximal tubule, predominantly through paracellular pathways, with salt and water carrying calcium from the lumen to the interstitium through the transport mechanism of solvent drag. Proximal tubule calcium reabsorption does not appear to be under hormonal control.

Twenty percent of filtered calcium is reabsorbed in the thick ascending limb of the loop of Henle (TALH), via both paracellular and transcellular processes. In this segment, a lumen-positive voltage generated by the Na/K/2Cl transporter (NKCC2/BSC-1) provides the

120

driving force for paracellular transport of calcium. Inhibition of NKCC2 by loop diuretics (bumetanide, furosemide) causes a decrease in the lumen-positive voltage, resulting in decreased paracellular calcium reabsorption that leads to hypercalciuria.

The study of inherited tubulopathies, particularly Bartter's syndrome, has proven valuable for understanding the mechanisms of ion transport in this region of the kidney. The driving force for sodium and chloride uptake in the thick ascending limb is derived from the low intracellular concentrations of these ions maintained by basolateral $Na^+ K^+$-ATPase and chloride channels (CLC-Kb). The activity of NKCC2 is dependent on the presence of luminal potassium. Recycling of potassium ions by the adenosine triphosphate (ATP)-regulated potassium channel ROMK provides the requisite K^+ and generates the lumen-positive potential that drives paracellular calcium transport. In type 1 Bartter's syndrome there is a mutation of NKCC2; in type 2 Bartter's syndrome there is a mutation in the potassium channel ROMK; and in type 3 there is a mutation in the chloride channel CLC-Kb. Each of these mutations leads to a decrease in the lumen-positive voltage and a reduction in calcium reabsorption. Although all of these patients are hypercalciuric, the type 3 patients rarely present with nephrocalcinosis. Mutations in the paracellular channel that result in reduced calcium reabsorption would also be expected to lead to hypercalciuria. Paracellin-1 (PCLN-1) is the principal protein in the tight junctions of the TAL and is a member of the claudin family of tight junction proteins (claudin-16). Primary sequence alterations in PCLN-1 affect calcium and magnesium reabsorption.

The remaining 8% of filtered calcium is reabsorbed in the distal convoluted tubule and connecting tubule; reabsorption in these segments is predominantly active, transcellular transport under hormonal regulation. Similar to transport in the intestine, in the distal convoluted and connecting tubule calcium enters the cell at the apical surface through a calcium channel and binds to the calcium-binding protein calbindin, which serves as a shuttle to transport calcium across the cell. At the basolateral surface, calcium is extruded against an electrochemical gradient. Calcium transport occurs against both electrical and chemical gradients. Distal convoluted tubule calcium reabsorption is stimulated by parathyroid hormone (PTH), phosphorus depletion, and thiazide diuretics and is inhibited by metabolic acidosis and adrenocortical excess. There appears to be some, albeit quite small, calcium reabsorption in the collecting tubule.

In health, daily urine calcium excretion precisely equals intestinal calcium absorption. With impaired kidney function, however, urine calcium excretion declines due not only to the decrease in glomerular filtration rate but also due to enhanced calcium reabsorption secondary to the usual increase in PTH. The increase in PTH is multifactorial; it appears secondary to the decrease in renal $1,25(OH)_2$ vitamin D_3 synthesis, resulting from a decrease in renal mass and from an increase in serum phosphorus due to a decrease in phosphorus excretion. The decline in $1,25(OH)_2$ vitamin D_3 not only decreases calcium absorption, resulting in hypocalcemia and subsequent increased PTH secretion, but $1,25(OH)_2$ vitamin D_3 itself has a significant inhibitory effect on PTH secretion. Increased levels of serum phosphorus increase serum levels of PTH independent of alterations in calcium or $1,25(OH)_2$ vitamin D_3. (These findings and renal osteodystrophy are addressed thoroughly in Chapter 64).

Regulation of Serum Levels

Large amounts of calcium must be transported through the extracellular fluid during periods of rapid skeletal growth and pregnancy, yet the concentration of serum calcium usually varies by less than 10%. This precise regulation of serum calcium concentration is accomplished by a complex interaction of the intestine, bone, and kidney involving the principal calcium-regulating hormones PTH and $1,25(OH)_2$ vitamin D_3.

The calcium-sensing receptor (CaR), present in the TALH as well as in the proximal tubule, distal convoluted tubule, and cortical collecting duct, monitors serum calcium levels and regulates renal tubular calcium reabsorption. Inactivating mutants of the calcium-sensing receptor cause familial hypocalciuric hypercalcemia. A useful model for the regulation of renal calcium reabsorption by the CaR has been proposed. In the presence of elevated basolateral levels of calcium, where reabsorption should be minimized, G_i coupled to the CaR induces a reduction in intracellular cyclic adenosine monophosphate (cAMP) levels, which in turn limits the activation of NKCC2. The CaR can also activate phospholipase A2 to produce arachidonic acid, whose metabolites, including 20-HETE, inhibit NKCC2 and ROMK. CaR is also present in the parathyroid gland. A reduction in ionized calcium leads to secretion of PTH. PTH then stimulates renal calcium reabsorption and bone mineral turnover and increases the serum level of $1,25(OH)_2$ vitamin D_3.

Disorders of Calcium Homeostasis

Hypocalcemia

Hypocalcemia may be defined as a reduction in the ionized component of serum calcium. Patients who have a decrease in total serum calcium concentration may or may not have a reduction in ionized calcium because hypoalbuminemia is prevalent in hospitalized patients and albumin binds the majority of protein-bound calcium. If there is doubt about the diagnosis of hypocalcemia, then ionized calcium should be measured directly.

Clinical Presentation

The clinical presentation of patients with hypocalcemia correlates with the rapidity and magnitude of the decline in serum calcium, but symptoms are observed in many patients with a total serum calcium of 7.0 mg/dL or less. The principal clinical manifestations of hypocalcemia are neurologic. Perioral paresthesias are followed by carpopedal spasm involving the hands and feet. Occasionally patients develop laryngeal stridor. Tetany may be evoked by acute respiratory alkalosis caused by hyperventilation, due to the rapid decrease in ionized calcium concentration. As the pH increases (a decrease in hydrogen ion concentration), hydrogen ions are dissociated from albumin, promoting increased calcium binding at the now vacant negatively charged binding sites.

Two clinical signs may indicate hypocalcemia: Chvostek's and Trousseau's signs. Chvostek's sign is evoked by tapping the facial nerve and observing a grimace and Trousseau's by inflating a blood pressure cuff 3 mm Hg above the systolic pressure for at least 3 minutes and observing spasm of the outstretched hand. Trousseau's sign is more specific because Chvostek's sign is present in approximately 10% of normocalcemic individuals.

Patients with hypocalcemia may also present with generalized seizures, which represent whole-body tetany. The electrocardiogram in hypocalcemic patients has characteristic prolonged corrected QT and ST intervals. There may be peaked T waves, arrhythmias, and heart block.

Causes

Many conditions can lead to hypocalcemia (Table 13-1).

Chronic Kidney Disease

Decreased glomerular filtration decreases renal phosphorus excretion, resulting in hyperphosphatemia. The increased serum phosphorus not only complexes with serum calcium, producing hypocalcemia, but also downregulates the 1-α-hydroxylase responsible for the renal conversion of 25(OH) vitamin D_3 to $1,25(OH)_2$ vitamin D_3. Chronic kidney disease also results in a reduction of functional renal mass and decreased $1,25(OH)_2$ vitamin D_3 production. Serum levels of $1,25(OH)_2$ vitamin D_3 are low, resulting in decreased intestinal calcium absorption and hypocalcemia, and levels of PTH and the osteoblastic enzyme alkaline phosphatase tend to be elevated.

TABLE 13-1 Principal Causes of Hypocalcemia
Chronic kidney disease
Following parathyroidectomy
Hypoparathyroidism
Pseudohypoparathyroidism
Malignant disease
Rhabdomyolysis
Hypomagnesemia
Acute pancreatitis
Septic shock
Vitamin D deficiency

Following Parathyroidectomy

Surgical reduction of the parathyroid mass in patients with chronic kidney disease and secondary or tertiary hyperparathyroidism usually leads to profound hypocalcemia due to rapid bone remineralization. This "hungry bone syndrome" may require prolonged and vigorous calcium replacement. Oral or intravenous $1,25(OH)_2$ vitamin D_3 supplementation promotes intestinal absorption of calcium, providing substrate for bone mineralization.

Hypoparathyroidism

Either idiopathic or postsurgical hypoparathyroidism results in a deficiency of PTH and an increase in renal calcium excretion, a decrease in $1,25(OH)_2$ vitamin D_3 production, and a decrease in bone turnover. Serum levels of PTH are low for the level of serum calcium or may even be undetectable. Isolated hypoparathyroidism may be autosomal dominant (chromosomal location 11p15 in some families) or autosomal recessive (chromosomal location 11p15 or 6p23-24 in some families).

Pseudohypoparathyroidism

In this group of hereditary disorders there is a decrease in the target cell response to PTH. These patients have an elevated PTH level, and in most patients there is a failure of cAMP to respond to PTH. Patients also commonly have shortened metacarpals and metatarsals in addition to short stature, obesity, and heterotopic calcification. A PTH infusion test (300 USP units of bovine parathyroid extract given over 15 minutes) will help to differentiate normal individuals who have a prompt increase in urinary cAMP (50- to 100-fold times basal) from type 1a (reduced levels of guanine nucleotide binding regulatory protein $α_s$) patients and type 1b (normal levels of guanine nucleotide binding regulatory protein $α_s$) patients, in whom there is only a two- to fivefold increase. In type 2 pseudohypoparathyroidism there is a reduced phosphaturic response to PTH despite a normal increase in cAMP. The chromosomal location of the disordered gene is 20q13.2-13.3. Hypomagnesemia must be excluded before the diagnosis can be established.

Malignant Disease

The most frequent cause of a decrease in total calcium concentration in ill patients with malignant disease is a decrease in serum albumin concentration; ionized calcium may be normal. However, certain malignancies, such as of the prostate and breast, may cause enhanced osteoblastic activity and accelerated bone formation, resulting in hypocalcemia. In the tumor lysis syndrome, the rapid cell destruction in response to chemotherapy may result in an increase in serum phosphorus, which then complexes serum calcium, resulting in hypocalcemia. Certain antineoplastic agents such as cis-platinum induce hypocalcemia, due in this case to promotion of hypomagnesemia.

Rhabdomyolysis

Cellular injury, especially due to crush injuries, causes a rapid release of cellular phosphorus, which complexes with extracellular calcium, resulting in hypocalcemia.

Hypomagnesemia

Hypocalcemia and hypomagnesemia frequently coexist and are often due to decreased absorption of dietary divalent cations or poor dietary intake. Hypomagnesemia may both impair PTH secretion and interfere with its peripheral action.

Acute Pancreatitis

Acute pancreatitis leads to the release of pancreatic lipase, which degrades retroperitoneal and omental fat, which then binds calcium in the peritoneum, so-called saponification, removing calcium from the extracellular fluid and resulting in hypocalcemia. Hypomagnesemia and hypoalbuminemia also have been reported to contribute to the hypocalcemia of acute pancreatitis.

Septic Shock

Endotoxic shock is associated with hypocalcemia through mechanisms that are not clear at this time. Because myocardial function and vascular contractility are both correlated directly with ionized calcium concentration, hypocalcemia in this condition may be responsible, in part, for the hypotension.

Vitamin D Deficiency

There are numerous causes of vitamin D deficiency, including chronic kidney disease, as noted previously. Patients with the nephrotic syndrome lose both calcium and vitamin D binding proteins in their urine, resulting in hypocalcemia. Elderly patients, especially during winter when there is a relative lack of sunshine in the northern climates, are frequently vitamin D deficient. This fat-soluble vitamin is subject to malabsorption, and levels may also be low in chronic liver disease and primary biliary cirrhosis. Anticonvulsant therapy with any of several agents increases the turnover of vitamin D into inactive compounds and results in a decrease in serum levels of $1,25(OH)_2$ vitamin D_3.

Treatment

Acute

Patients with symptoms attributable to hypocalcemia must be treated promptly. In addition, asymptomatic patients with a serum calcium of less than approximately 7.0 mg/dL also should generally be treated prophylacti-

cally. Intravenous calcium is the mainstay of treatment. Calcium gluconate may be administered as 10 mL of a 10% solution (94 mg of elemental calcium) over 5 to 10 minutes. Patients on digoxin require electrocardiographic monitoring because administration of calcium may potentiate digitalis toxicity and cause death. Calcium must not be given in the same intravenous line as bicarbonate, or the insoluble salt calcium carbonate will rapidly precipitate. If a patient is acidemic and hypocalcemic, the hypocalcemia generally should be treated first because the acidemia increases the proportion of ionized calcium and thus protects the patient against symptomatic hypocalcemia. If the patient has impaired kidney function, dialysis against a high-calcium, high-bicarbonate bath will correct both the hypocalcemia and acidemia. However, this modality of treatment should be tempered in the presence of significant hyperphosphatemia because the resulting elevated calcium phosphorus product will promote deleterious extraosseous calcification.

More prolonged correction can be accomplished with a constant infusion of calcium gluconate (50 mL of 10% calcium gluconate in 450 mL of D_5W), administered over 4 hours, the rate being titrated by the level of serum calcium. Infusion of 15 mg/kg of elemental calcium over 4 to 6 hours generally increases the total serum calcium by 2 to 3 mg/dL.

Chronic

Treatment of chronic hypocalcemia in patients with normal renal function generally involves administration of oral calcium and $1,25(OH)_2$ vitamin D_3. The former, often given as calcium carbonate, must provide at least 1 g of elemental calcium each day. $1,25(OH)_2$ vitamin D_3 therapy promotes intestinal calcium absorption. In the case of hypoparathyroidism, however, urine calcium excretion is also increased because PTH is not present to promote renal calcium reabsorption. Thus, the goal of therapy in treating patients with hypoparathyroidism and normal renal function is to keep serum calcium concentration at the lower limit of normal, approximately 8.0 mg/dL, and keep urine calcium excretion below 350 mg/day. Thiazide diuretics may be used to help prevent hypercalciuria and promote normocalcemia. $1,25(OH)_2$ vitamin D_3 administered without oral calcium may result in resorption of bone mineral and osteopenia. In patients with chronic kidney disease, the treatment of chronic hypocalcemia often involves lowering the serum phosphorus through a combination of moderate phosphorus restriction, intestinal phosphorus binders, and dialysis. Care should be taken to avoid a calcium phosphorus product of greater than 55 mg^2/dL^2 to prevent extraosseous precipitation of a calcium phosphate solid phase. Patients with chronic kidney disease who are subjected to parathyroidectomy often require prolonged treatment with large doses of oral and intravenous calcium and with $1,25(OH)_2$ vitamin D_3 to prevent hypocalcemia as their bones are being remineralized.

Hypercalcemia

Hypercalcemia is defined as an increase in the concentration of serum ionized calcium.

Clinical Presentation

The clinical signs and symptoms present in patients with hypercalcemia correlate with the rapidity of the increase and the magnitude of the elevation in serum calcium. As with hypocalcemia, neurologic abnormalities predominate in the clinical presentation. Often patients present with drowsiness and lethargy followed by headache and irritability. Confusion may then be observed followed by stupor and coma. Muscle weakness, emotional problems, and depression also may be observed.

Polyuria is frequent in patients with hypercalcemia due to a defect in vasopressin-induced water reabsorption. Hypercalcemia can lead to a decline in kidney function due to a variety of mechanisms. The polyuria may lead to volume depletion and prerenal azotemia. Excess calcium excretion may produce nephrocalcinosis, especially in the presence of alkaline urine, which decreases the solubility of calcium phosphate complexes.

Calcium directly increases cardiac contractility and arterial contraction, and patients with hypercalcemia are thought to have an increased incidence of hypertension. Hypercalcemia shortens the corrected QT interval, may broaden the T waves, and produce first-degree atrioventricular block. Anorexia, nausea, and severe vomiting are associated with hypercalcemia, as is constipation.

Causes

Many conditions can lead to hypercalcemia (Table 13-2).

Primary Hyperparathyroidism

Accounting for more than 50% of patients with hypercalcemia, primary hyperparathyroidism is the leading cause of hypercalcemia. The patients are generally women over 60 years of age, and most have a benign

TABLE 13-2 Principal Causes of Hypercalcemia

Primary hyperparathyroidism
Malignancy
Renal failure
Following kidney transplant
Thiazide diuretics
Lithium
Immobilization
Milk-alkali syndrome
Granulomatous disease
Familial hypocalciuric hypercalcemia
Thyrotoxicosis
Vitamin intoxication

adenoma of a single parathyroid gland; others have hyperplasia of all four glands. Parathyroid carcinoma is extremely rare. The elevated PTH levels increase renal calcium reabsorption and decrease renal phosphorus reabsorption. The excess PTH also increases the serum level of $1,25(OH)_2$ vitamin D_3, increasing enhanced intestinal calcium absorption and bone turnover, with bone resorption predominating over bone formation.

As many as 6% of patients with calcium-containing kidney stones have hyperparathyroidism. In this case, the increased filtered load of calcium exceeds the increased renal calcium reabsorption, leading to hypercalciuria, kidney stone formation, and occasionally nephrocalcinosis. Increased urinary bicarbonate alkalinizes the urine-promoting precipitation of calcium phosphorus complexes. With current routine automated blood chemical analysis, hypercalcemia and the causative hyperparathyroidism are generally detected before stone formation or nephrocalcinosis occurs.

Malignancy

Patients with malignancy are the second largest group presenting with hypercalcemia. The hypercalcemia may be related to direct bone destruction by the growing tumor or to secretion of calcemic factors by malignant cells. Patients with squamous cell lung carcinoma and metastatic carcinoma of the breast develop hypercalcemia most frequently. Patients with myeloma, T-cell tumors, renal cell carcinoma, and other squamous cell tumors are also prone to hypercalcemia. Many tumors produce a PTH-related peptide (PTH-rP) in which the first 13 amino acids are very similar to those in PTH and which binds to PTH receptors in the kidney and bone, yet is not detected on standard PTH assays. Commercial assays are now available for PTH-rP. Other tumors produce factors such as transforming growth factor-α, interleukin-1, cytokines such as lymphotoxin, or hormones such as $1,25(OH)_2$ vitamin D_3.

In general the malignancy is readily evident when patients present with hypercalcemia. The finding of a low level of PTH and an elevated level of PTH-rP supports the diagnosis. Although hypercalcemia due to an occult malignancy is rare, associated symptoms such as weight loss and fatigue should focus the search for tumors that are frequently associated with hypercalcemia such as those in the lung, kidney, and urogenital tract.

Kidney Failure

Hypocalcemia, not hypercalcemia, is generally found in patients with impaired kidney function. In hypercalcemic patients it is important to determine if the hypercalcemia itself was responsible for the kidney failure. Hypercalcemia caused by disorders such as sarcoidosis, myeloma, immobilization, and milk-alkali syndrome not infrequently cause acute renal failure. Hypercalcemia may occur during the recovery phase of rhabdomyolysis-induced acute renal failure because calcium recently deposited in muscle and soft tissues is rapidly mobilized.

Hypercalcemia is frequently observed during excessive vitamin D replacement therapy of patients on dialysis, especially if they are simultaneously being given large amounts of oral calcium as a phosphorus binder. Some patients may develop severe secondary hyperparathyroidism with marked hyperplasia of the parathyroid glands and subsequent hypercalcemia. In addition, patients may have aluminum intoxication, a disorder characterized by low bone turnover, which predisposes them to hypercalcemia. These aluminum-intoxicated patients often have modestly elevated PTH and alkaline phosphatase levels. The calcimimetic agent cinacalcet has recently been approved by the U.S. Food and Drug Administration (FDA). It results in a decrease in PTH secretion through allosteric modification of the calcium receptor, which allows control of PTH with less hypercalcemia than with the combination of vitamin D compounds and calcium-containing phosphate binders. The Kidney Disease Outcome Quality Initiative (K/DOQI) guidelines for control of mineral metabolism in patients with chronic kidney disease are addressed thoroughly in Chapter 64.

Following Kidney Transplantation

Not infrequently patients on long-term dialysis develop parathyroid hyperplasia leading to autonomous secretion of PTH. If these patients then receive a successful kidney graft, the PTH secretion continues and hypercalcemia may develop due to enhanced, PTH-induced, renal calcium reabsorption. The hypercalcemia is generally mild and tends to decrease over the ensuing 6 to 12 months as the hypertrophied parathyroid glands involute; however, patients with prolonged marked hypercalcemia may require surgical parathyroidectomy.

Thiazide Diuretics

Many patients with hypertension or nephrolithiasis are on thiazide diuretic therapy, which is often associated with mild hypercalcemia due to increased renal calcium reabsorption. If the hypercalcemia does not resolve when the thiazides are discontinued, then the patient must be investigated for other causes of hypercalcemia.

Lithium

Approximately 5% of patients treated with lithium carbonate develop hypercalcemia. The hypercalcemia is due to a resetting of the parathyroid gland calcium set point such that PTH secretion is inhibited only by higher-than-normal elevations of serum calcium.

Immobilization

Immobilization leads to a rapid increase in bone resorption and may lead to hypercalcemia, especially if there is any decrement in renal calcium excretion. This disorder is most prevalent in younger patients who sustain a traumatic (especially spinal cord) injury. It is associated with a reduction in levels of both PTH and $1,25(OH)_2$ vitamin D_3.

Milk-Alkali Syndrome

Ingestion of large amounts of calcium-containing nonabsorbable antacids may lead to hypercalcemia, alkalemia, nephrocalcinosis, and chronic kidney disease. With the change in ulcer treatment from antacids to antibiotics and agents that inhibit gastric acid secretion, this disorder has become much less common. However, the increased use of calcium and alkali preparations to prevent and treat osteoporosis may herald an increase in incidence of the milk-alkali syndrome.

Granulomatous Disease

Granulomatous diseases, such as sarcoidosis, tuberculosis, and leprosy, may produce hypercalciuria and hypercalcemia due to the conversion of 25(OH) vitamin D_3 to $1,25(OH)_2$ vitamin D_3 by the granulomatous tissue, as has been observed in anephric patients. Intestinal calcium absorption and bone resorption are increased.

Familial Hypocalciuric Hypercalcemia

This autosomal-dominant disorder causes mild hypercalcemia, hypophosphatemia, and reduced renal calcium excretion (often less than 100 mg/day). These patients have an inactivating mutation in the CaR (chromosomal location 3q21.1), resulting in decreased calcium inhibition of PTH secretion. PTH levels are normal and parathyroidectomy is not indicated.

Thyrotoxicosis

Excess thyroid hormone can stimulate osteoclastic bone resorption, resulting in hypercalcemia. The hypercalcemia is generally mild, and coexistent hyperparathyroidism must be excluded.

Vitamin Intoxication

Vitamin D intoxication, as noted previously, is often observed in patients with endstage renal disease treated with $1,25(OH)_2$ vitamin D_3. Vitamin D intoxication can also occur in food or vitamin faddists, and vitamin A excess can also cause hypercalcemia and may be seen in the same patients.

Treatment

Rational therapy depends on the severity of the hypercalcemia and its cause and should ideally be directed at the underlying disorder. However, if the patient is symptomatic and the serum calcium level is 13.5 mg/dL or higher, acute therapy is indicated. A mainstay of treatment in patients with reasonable kidney and cardiac function is intravenous saline. Rates as high as 200 to 250 mL/hour of normal saline may be used to facilitate renal calcium excretion. Furosemide is calciuric and is often necessary (40 mg intravenously in patients with normal kidney function) during volume repletion with saline to avoid pulmonary congestion. Thiazide diuretics must be avoided because they decrease renal calcium excretion. Patients with impaired kidney function may not be able to excrete the sodium load, and hemodialysis against a low calcium bath may be necessary to acutely lower serum calcium concentration. Patients with cardiac failure or impaired kidney function are at particular risk for volume overload during saline treatment and may require central venous pressure monitoring and a more modest rate of normal saline infusion.

Patients with hypercalcemia mediated by enhanced osteoclastic bone resorption—generally patients with malignancy or immobilization—may benefit from the osteoclastic inhibitor calcitonin (4 to 8 units/kg subcutaneously or intramuscularly every 6 to 12 hours). However, the hypocalcemic effect of calcitonin is often transient. The bisphophonate zoledronic acid (4 mg intravenously) has been shown to reduce serum calcium in a greater number of patients and for a longer period of time than pamidronate (30 to 90 mg/day given as a single 24-hour infusion for 3 days). Most studies have excluded patients with a creatinine greater than 4.5 mg/dL. Bisphosphonates have been reported to cause acute renal failure, which may be reduced by ensuring adequate hydration, reduction of dose amount, and frequency. Gallium nitrate effectively lowers serum calcium, but it is contraindicated in patients with impaired kidney function and in those receiving other nephrotoxic agents.

Patients with hypercalcemia due to enhanced intestinal calcium absorption may benefit from a reduction of dietary calcium intake. Normally Americans consume approximately 800 mg of calcium per day; reducing this by a third is generally effective. However, this should only be a short-term remedy because the provision of a low-calcium diet in a patient with normal renal function and excess $1,25(OH)_2$ vitamin D_3 promotes bone demineralization. Glucocorticoids (initial dose 40 mg of prednisone) inhibit intestinal calcium absorption but may require a week for maximal effect.

Oral phosphorus can be used to treat hypercalcemia, but it should be used only if the serum phosphorus is at or below the lower limit of normal in order to prevent soft tissue calcium deposition. In general, however, this form of outdated therapy should be avoided.

Treatment of hypercalcemia in dialysis patients involves reduction or elimination of both $1,25(OH)_2$ vitamin D_3 and supplemental calcium given for its phosphorus-binding effect. Patients can be treated with the non-calcium-containing phosphorus binder sevelamer hydrochloride. Lanthanum carbonate is a new, recently FDA-approved, non–calcium phosphate binder. Once the

hypercalcemia resolves, $1,25(OH)_2$ vitamin D_3 and oral calcium binders can then be cautiously reinstituted at lower doses while continuing with non-calcium-containing phosphate binders. The recently published K/DOQI guidelines limit the amount of calcium binders in dialysis patients to 1.5 g/day. Analogues of vitamin D such as paricalcitol and doxercalciferol may produce less hypercalcemia than $1,25(OH)_2$ vitamin D_3 itself. As noted previously, the calcimimetic agent cinacalcet appears to allow control of PTH without hypercalcemia.

PHOSPHORUS

Phosphorus Homeostasis

Distribution

Ninety percent of total body phosphorus is contained within the bone mineral, while 10% is contained within the cells and 1% is in the extracellular fluid.

Serum Concentration

The concentration of serum phosphorus in adults ranges from 2.5 to 4.5 mg/dL, or 0.81 to 1.45 mmol/L. Serum phosphorus levels are highest in infants and decrease in childhood, reaching the normal adult levels in late adolescence. Approximately 70% of blood phosphorus is termed organic and contained within phospholipids, and 30% of the blood phosphorus is termed inorganic. Of the inorganic phosphorus, 85% is free and circulates as monohydrogen or dihydrogen phosphate or complexed with sodium, magnesium, or calcium, whereas 15% is protein bound.

Intestinal Absorption

Dietary phosphorus intake varies between 800 and 1850 mg of phosphorus per day (26 to 60 mmol/day) and approximately 25 mmol/day is absorbed. Diets that are adequate in calories and protein generally contain adequate phosphorus. Phosphorus absorption is regulated by $1,25(OH)_2$ vitamin D_3 via a sodium-dependent active transport mechanism principally in the duodenum and by a passive phosphorus concentration–dependent mechanism in the jejunum and ileum. The absorption of phosphorus is hindered by formation of insoluble complexes in the intestine; aluminum, lanthanum, sevelamer, and calcium bind phosphorus and hinder its absorption. During chronic kidney disease, phosphorus absorption continues, and the formation of complexes of intestinal phosphorus by these agents is used to advantage in patients who are unable to excrete absorbed phosphorus. Although aluminum effectively binds phosphorus, its use is discouraged, even transiently, because it is toxic to several organs, including brain and bone.

Renal Excretion

A 70-kg man with a glomerular filtration rate of 180 L/day and a mean serum phosphorus concentration of 1.25 mmol/L filters approximately 200 mmol of phosphorus per day since approximately 85% of serum phosphorus is ultrafilterable (180 liters/day × 1.25 mmol/L × 0.85). Urine phosphorus excretion averages about 25 mmol/day so that approximately 12.5% of the glomerular filtrate is excreted in the urine.

Eighty-five percent of phosphorus reabsorption occurs in the proximal tubule. Proximal phosphorus transport occurs against an electrochemical gradient. Reabsorption appears to be transcellular, absorptive, and dependent on the low concentration of intracellular sodium maintained by the basolateral $Na^+ K^+$-ATPase. The majority of phosphorus absorption occurs in the initial 25% of the proximal tubule. Transport appears more robust in the deeper juxtamedullary nephrons compared with the more cortical nephrons.

Three sodium gradient–dependent phosphate cotransporters (Npt1–Npt3) have been identified. Npt2 is responsible for approximately 85% of proximal tubule renal phosphate transport. It is highly regulated and present on the apical brush border membrane. Npt1 appears responsible for approximately 15% of the proximal phosphate and does not appear to be regulated. Fibroblast growth factor 23 (FGF-23) has been identified as a regulator of Npt2. Because of this action, it has been termed a "phosphatonin." Elevated levels of FGF-23 have been detected in patients with renal phosphate wasting and hypophosphatemia. FGF-23 appears to be metabolized by the *PHEX* gene (phosphate-regulating gene with homologies to the endopeptidases on the X chromosome), and mutations in *PHEX* can also cause hypophosphatemia due to the inability to metabolize FGF-23. Frizzled related protein (FRP4) appears to be another phosphatonin. Infusion of FRP4 into rats and mice reduces fractional reabsorption of phosphate. In longer-term studies, sFRP4 blunts the compensatory increase in 1-α-hydroxylase expression induced by hypophosphatemia.

Parathyroid hormone is another major hormonal regulator of phosphorus excretion, whereas variation in dietary phosphorus intake is the major nonhormonal regulator. PTH is phosphaturic, as is $1,25(OH)_2$ vitamin D_3, extracellular fluid volume expansion, and a high-phosphorus diet, whereas a low-phosphorus diet leads to a decrease in renal excretion. The hypophosphaturia of phosphorus depletion overrides the hyperphosphaturia induced by PTH. With chronic kidney disease, urine phosphorus excretion remains relatively constant until the glomerular filtration rate declines to about 25% of normal. Phosphorus excretion is maintained in the face of a decrease in glomerular filtration rate and the subsequent decline in the filtered load of phosphorus by the phosphaturic effects of elevated PTH levels. Once inside the cell, the absorbed phosphorus equilibrates with cytosolic phosphorus; elimination of luminal phosphorus leads to a marked decline in intracellular phosphorus. Phosphorus transport across the basolateral membrane occurs down a favorable electrochemical gradient using an anion exchanger. It is tightly regulated to prevent depletion of intracellular phosphate.

There appears to be little phosphorus transport in the loop of Henle. A small quantity of phosphorus is reabsorbed in the distal convoluted tubule, especially in the absence of PTH. Whether phosphorus reabsorption occurs more distally is not clear.

The overall tubular maximum for the reabsorption of phosphorus is approximately equal to the normal amount of phosphorus filtered by the glomerulus. Thus, any appreciable increase in the filtered load of phosphorus leads to an increase in urinary phosphorus excretion.

Regulation of Serum Levels

Serum levels of phosphorus are not as tightly regulated as those of calcium, and they may vary by as much as 50% over the course of a day. Although there is diurnal variation in phosphorus levels, alterations in dietary phosphorus intake are principally responsible for the swings in serum levels. In addition, serum levels are controlled by hormones such as PTH and $1,25(OH)_2$ vitamin D_3, and perhaps FGF-23 and FRP, and by the status of extracellular fluid volume and renal function.

Disorders of Phosphorus Homeostasis

Hypophosphatemia

A decrease in the level of serum phosphorus may or may not reflect total body phosphorus content because only 1% of body phosphorus is contained in the extracellular fluid. Moderate hypophosphatemia may be defined as a serum phosphorus level below the lower limit of normal but above 1 mg/dL and severe hypophosphatemia as a serum level below 1 mg/dL. Although moderate hypophosphatemia is generally asymptomatic, severe hypophosphatemia is associated with a variety of clinical disturbances and, occasionally, death. Hypophosphatemia may result from a decrease in intake, an increase in excretion, or a shift of phosphorus from the extracellular environment into the cells.

Clinical Presentation

Patients with severe hypophosphatemia may have neurologic dysfunction characterized by weakness, paresthesias, confusion, seizures, and coma. The weakness may be associated with muscle edema and rhabdomyolysis. Respiratory muscle paralysis may result in death.

Causes

Many conditions can lead to hypophosphatemia (Table 13-3).

Alcohol Related

Many chronic ethanol abusers are hypophosphatemic on hospital admission or become hypophosphatemic with treatment. The cause of their hypophosphatemia is multifactorial but is largely related to poor oral intake.

Refeeding

When patients are fed after prolonged poor intake or starvation, the calories provide a stimulus for tissue growth and utilization of phosphorus in phosphorylated intermediates such as ATP. If the diet does not contain adequate phosphorus, then severe hypophosphatemia may develop. Analogously, if total parenteral nutrition solutions contain inadequate phosphorus, then hypophosphatemia may become evident as the patient regains body mass.

Diabetes Mellitus

In severe diabetic ketoacidosis, especially of prolonged duration, there is excessive urinary phosphorus loss, which, when accompanied by poor oral phosphorus intake, may lead to hypophosphatemia and hypokalemia. The severity of the hypophosphatemia may become apparent only during treatment of the diabetic ketoacidosis.

Alkalosis

Both respiratory and metabolic alkalosis may induce hypophosphatemia; however, hypophosphatemia is far more severe in prolonged respiratory alkalosis. The extracellular alkalosis appears to cause intracellular alkalosis, which results in a shift of phosphorus into the intracellular space and hypophosphatemia.

Following Kidney Transplantation

Hypophosphatemia is commonly observed following kidney transplantation. The cause is multifactorial but is related to a persistent elevation in serum PTH levels and an intrinsic renal tubular defect in phosphorus reabsorption, both resulting in hyperphosphaturia. In addition, glucocorticoids used in immunosuppression inhibit renal phosphorus transport.

Urinary Loss

Renal tubular acidosis, hypokalemia, hypomagnesemia, and other renal tubular disorders are associated with an increased urinary excretion of phosphorus. Hyperparathyroidism results in a marked increase in phosphorus excretion and hypophosphatemia.

Genetic Disorders

X-linked hypophosphatemic rickets and autosomal-dominant hypophosphatemic rickets are associated with a tubular defect in renal phosphorus reabsorption, decreased intestinal phosphate absorption, and rickets or osteomalacia. Serum levels of FGF-23 are elevated in both and are thought to be causal. In vitamin D–dependent rickets there is either a defect in the conversion of 25(OH) vitamin D_3 to 1,25(OH)$_2$ vitamin D_3 (type 1) or a resistance to the actions of vitamin D caused by a defect in the vitamin D receptor (type 2). Type 1 responds to normal doses of 1,25(OH)$_2$ vitamin D_3, whereas type 2 can be treated only with large doses of the hormone.

Tumor Related

Mesenchymal tumors may be associated with hypophosphatemia that is caused by increased urinary phosphate excretion. Some of these tumors have been shown to produce FGF-23 and others FRP4. Resection of the tumors leads to a prompt decrease in circulating levels of the phosphaturic hormone.

Treatment

The treatment of hypophosphatemia is best directed at reversing the underlying disease or nutritional deficiency. Moderate hypophosphatemia can often be treated with oral phosphorus supplementation in the form of milk, an excellent source of phosphorus, containing about 1 g of phosphorus per liter, or Neutra-Phos tablets (250 mg of phosphorus). Oral phosphorus can cause diarrhea, which is usually seen at doses of over 1 g/day. Severe hypophosphatemia usually indicates a significant loss of total body phosphorus. Asymptomatic patients in whom oral replacement is possible should receive approximately 3 g/day for a week. Often the patient is symptomatic and requires intravenous therapy. In this case, treatment may be initiated with 2 mg/kg body weight of phosphorus as the sodium salt is infused over 6 hours. Serum phosphorus levels must be checked frequently during replacement. Intravenous phosphorus may produce hypocalcemia and metastatic calcification, especially if the calcium phosphorus product exceeds 55 mg^2/dL^2. Concurrent electrolyte and mineral disorders, hypokalemia and hypomagnesemia, are often found in patients with hypophosphatemia.

TABLE 13-3 Principal Causes of Hypophosphatemia

Alcohol related
Refeeding
Diabetes mellitus
Alkalosis
After kidney transplantation
Urinary loss
Total parenteral nutrition
Genetic defects
Tumor related

Hyperphosphatemia

In adults, hyperphosphatemia is defined as an increase in the concentration of serum phosphorus to greater than 5.0 mg/dL. Because cells contain abundant phosphorus, hemolysis of the collected sample should be excluded, especially if there is associated hyperkalemia. Hyperphosphatemia may be caused by decreased phosphorus excretion, an increase in phosphorus load, or a shift of phosphorus from the cells into the extracellular fluid.

Clinical Presentation

The clinical presentation of patients with hyperphosphatemia is dominated by the associated decline in serum calcium. As serum phosphorus increases, generally there is a reciprocal decrease in serum calcium. This decrease is multifactorial but includes a decrease in $1,25(OH)_2$ vitamin D_3 synthesis, leading to a decrease in intestinal calcium absorption and formation of calcium phosphorus complexes, resulting in ectopic calcification, especially of previously injured tissues. The symptoms of patients with hyperphosphatemia are those of patients with hypocalcemia: tetany, seizures, and decreased myocardial contractility, along with ectopic calcification, which may occur in virtually any organ in the body, especially when the calcium phosphorus product exceeds $55\,mg^2/dL^2$. Calcification is especially prominent in proton-secreting organs such as the stomach or kidney, in which basolateral bicarbonate secretion results in an increase in pH-promoting calcium hydrogen phosphate (brushite) precipitation. The long-term hyperphosphatemia of chronic kidney disease contributes to development of secondary hyperparathyroidism, chronic kidney disease–associated bone disease, and vascular calcification.

Causes

Many conditions can lead to hyperphosphatemia (Table 13-4).

Chronic Kidney Disease

With a decrease in the glomerular filtration rate below approximately 25 mL/min, renal excretion of phosphorus is less than intestinal absorption, and hyperphosphatemia ensues. Increased levels of phosphorus have been shown to directly increase the level of PTH. The increased levels of phosphorus also suppress renal $1,25(OH)_2$ vitamin D_3 production, resulting in less calcium absorption, and the excess phosphorus may bind

TABLE 13-4 Principal Causes of Hyperphosphatemia

Renal failure
Hypoparathyroidism
Cell injury
Exogenous administration

serum calcium if the calcium phosphorus product exceeds approximately $55\,mg^2/dL^2$. Additionally, levels of serum $1,25(OH)_2$ vitamin D_3 decline due to the reduction in the renal tissue responsible for the conversion of $25(OH)$ vitamin D_3 to $1,25(OH)_2$ vitamin D_3. The resulting hypocalcemia and low levels of $1,25(OH)_2$ vitamin D_3 further increase PTH secretion and urine phosphorus excretion, lowering the level of serum phosphorus at the cost of hyperparathyroidism. Despite the additional phosphorus excretion per nephron, with more advanced chronic kidney disease, serum phosphorus increases because the patient is unable to excrete the absorbed phosphorus. During chronic kidney disease, the hyperphosphatemia is less severe than during the same decrement in glomerular filtration rate in acute renal failure when there has been insufficient time for adaptation (see Chapter 58).

Hypoparathyroidism

Parathyroid hormone promotes renal phosphorus excretion, and hyperphosphatemia is associated with clinical disorders in which there is a lack of PTH or a resistance to its action.

Cell Injury

During effective chemotherapy, especially when there is rapid lysis of a substantial mass of cells, as during treatment of lymphomas, the marked increase in phosphorus release from cells can exceed renal excretory capacity. The hyperphosphatemia is often associated with hyperkalemia and hyperuricemia and leads to hypocalcemia. Phosphorus can also be released from cells during acute rhabdomyolysis, crush injuries, or tissue infarction (see Chapter 38). Hyperphosphatemia is especially severe when the release of cellular phosphorus occurs in the setting of acute renal failure.

Exogenous Administration

Excess phosphorus in total parenteral nutritional solutions or phosphorus in laxatives may result in hyperphosphatemia. Phosphorus-containing enemas can result in hyperphosphatemia and should be avoided in patients with chronic kidney disease. Excess vitamin D not only increases calcium absorption, but phosphorus absorption as well, and can result in hyperphosphatemia.

Treatment

The treatment of hyperphosphatemia must be directed at the underlying cause. If renal function is intact, phosphaturia should be promoted. Extracellular fluid volume expansion with saline lowers renal phosphorus reabsorption, as does increasing urine pH with sodium bicarbonate or acetazolamide. In patients with hyperphosphatemia and acute renal failure, phosphorus is best removed from the extracellular space via dialysis.

The successful treatment of hyperphosphatemia of chronic kidney disease requires a coordinated effort among the patient, dietitian, and physician. A diet devoid of phosphorus is unpalatable and generally contains insufficient protein; however, dietary phosphorus can be reduced substantially with proper dietary supervision. Both hemodialysis and peritoneal dialysis remove phosphorus; however, even with a low-phosphorus diet, dialysis is unable to remove sufficient phosphorus to achieve a neutral phosphorus balance. Agents that bind dietary phosphorus and prevent its absorption are generally necessary in the prevention and treatment of hyperphosphatemia. Calcium salts given with meals are effective in binding dietary phosphorus. Doses are gradually increased until the serum phosphorus is less than approximately 5 mg/dL. If hypercalcemia occurs before the serum phosphorus is controlled or if the intake of calcium from all sources, binders plus diet, exceeds 2.0 g,

then the patient will generally require institution of alternative intestinal phosphorus binders. Aluminum is toxic to the brain, bone, and bone marrow and should be avoided whenever possible. Sevelamer hydrochloride is a calcium-free polymer that binds intestinal phosphate. Lanthanum carbonate is another calcium-free phosphate binder. If patients present with severe hyperphosphatemia (serum phosphorus greater than 6.5 mg/dL), the serum phosphorus should be lowered with a non-calcium-containing phosphate binder or dialysis prior to adding calcium salts to prevent soft tissue calcification. The treatment of hyperphosphatemia in chronic kidney disease is addressed thoroughly in Chapter 64.

ACKNOWLEDGMENTS

This work was supported by Grants AM-39906 and AR-33949 from the National Institutes of Health.

BIBLIOGRAPHY

Brown EM, Pollock AS, Hebert SC: The extracellular calcium-sensing receptor: Its role in health and disease. Annu Rev Med 49:15–29, 1998.

Bushinsky DA, Krieger NS: Integration of calcium metabolism in the adult. In Coe FL, Favus MJ (eds): Disorders of Bone and Mineral Metabolism. New York, Raven, 2002, pp 381–396.

Bushinsky DA: Calcium, magnesium, and phosphorus: Renal handling and urinary excretion. In Favus MJ (ed): Primer on the Metabolic Bone Diseases and Disorders of Mineral Metabolism. Washington, DC, American Society for Bone and Mineral Research, 2003, pp 97–105.

Bushinsky DA, Monk RD: Calcium. Lancet 352:306–311, 1998.

Chertow GM, Burke SK, Raggi P: Sevelamer attenuates the progression of coronary and aortic calcification in hemodialysis patients. Kidney Int 62:245–252, 2002.

Chertow GM, Raggi P, McCarthy JT, et al: The effects of sevelamer and calcium acetate on proxies of atherosclerotic and arteriosclerotic vascular disease in hemodialysis patients. Am J Nephrol 23:307–314, 2003.

Frick KK, Bushinsky DA: Molecular mechanism of hypercalciuria. J Am Soc Nephrol 14:1082–1095, 2003.

Hruska KA, Lederer ED: Hyperphosphatemia and hypophosphatemia. In Favus MJ (ed): Primer on the Metabolic Bone Diseases and Disorders of Mineral Metabolism. Washington, DC, American Society for Bone and Mineral Research, 2003, pp 296–305.

K/DOQI Clinical Practice Guidelines for Bone Metabolism and Disease in Chronic Kidney Disease: *www.kidney.org/professionals/kdoqi/guidelines_bone/index.htm.*

LeBoff MS, Mikulec KH: Hypercalcemia: Clinical manifestations, pathogenesis, diagnosis, and management. In Favus MJ (ed): Primer of the Metabolic Bone Diseases and Disorders of Mineral Metabolism. Washington, DC, American Society for Bone and Mineral Research, 2004, pp 225–230.

Monk RD, Bushinsky D: Treatment of calcium, phosphorus, and magnesium disorders. In Halperin M (ed): Therapy in Nephrology and Hypertension: A Companion to Brenner and Rector's The Kidney. Philadelphia, WB Saunders, 1999, pp 303–315.

Monk RD, Bushinsky DA: Kidney stones. In Larsen PR, Kronenberg HM, Melmed S, Polonsky KS (eds): Williams Textbook of Endocrinology. Philadelphia, WB Saunders, 2003, pp 1411–1425.

Schiavi SC, Kumar R: The phosphatonin pathway: New insights in phosphate homeostasis. Kidney Int 65:1–14, 2004.

Slatopolsky E, Finch J, Denda M, et al: Phosphorus restriction prevents parathyroid gland growth. High phosphorus directly stimulates PTH secretion in vitro. J Clin Invest 97:2534–2540, 1996.

Thakker RV: Hypocalcemia: Pathogenesis, differential diagnosis, and management. In Favus MJ (ed): Primer on the Metabolic Bone Diseases and Disorders of Mineral Metabolism. Washington, DC, The American Society for Bone and Mineral Research, 2003, pp 271–274.

CHAPTER 14

Disorders of Magnesium Homeostasis

Jeffrey S. Berns

MAGNESIUM METABOLISM

The normal adult total body magnesium content is approximately 25 g (approximately 15 mmol/kg); 60% to 65% is in bone, with most of the remainder in the intracellular compartment of muscle and other soft tissues. Much of the intracellular magnesium is bound to various cellular constituents such as adenosine triphosphate, adenosine diphosphate, proteins, and nucleic acids, or within mitochondria, and is only slowly exchangeable with the extracellular fluid (ECF) pool. The free cytosolic concentration is 0.5 to 0.8 mmol/L. Only about 1% of total body magnesium is in the ECF. The normal total plasma magnesium concentration is 1.7 to 2.3 mg/dL (0.71 to 0.96 mmol/L; the molecular weight of magnesium is 24.3 daltons; 1 mmol/L = 2 mEq/L = 2.4 mg/dL). Of the magnesium in the ECF, 30% is protein bound, 60% to 65% is free ionized magnesium, and 5% to 10% is complexed to citrate, phosphate, oxalate, and other anions. Assays to measure ionized, biologically active magnesium have been developed, but are not yet in routine use.

A typical American adult diet contains about 300 to 400 mg/day of elemental magnesium. Cereal, grains, nuts, legumes, green vegetables, some meats and seafoods, and drinking water (especially so-called "hard water") are significant sources of dietary magnesium.

Normally, about 40% to 50% of dietary magnesium is absorbed in the gastrointestinal (GI) tract, primarily in the small intestine. Magnesium is also secreted in the small intestine (approximately 40 mg/day) and reabsorbed in the colon and rectum (approximately 20 mg/day). Absorption of magnesium in the ileum occurs primarily through an active, saturable transcellular pathway; there is also passive absorption in the ileum and remainder of the small intestine. There does not appear to be any important hormonal regulation of GI tract magnesium absorption, although vitamin D may variably increase magnesium absorption.

Renal Handling of Magnesium

Under normal circumstances, 95% to 97% of filtered magnesium is reabsorbed in the kidney, and 3% to 5% appears in the urine. Unlike most other ions, only about 15% to 20% of the filtered load of magnesium is reabsorbed in the proximal tubule. The cortical thick ascending limb of the loop of Henle (TALH) reabsorbs 60% to 70% of the filtered load via a passive, paracellular process, driven largely by the lumen-positive voltage in this segment. A tight junction protein called paracellin-1 (claudin-16) controls paracellular permeability to magnesium in the TALH. The medullary TALH does not appear to reabsorb magnesium in humans. Activation of a basolateral membrane extracellular Ca^{2+}/Mg^{2+}-sensing receptor (CaSR), a member of the G protein–coupled receptor family, by either cation reduces magnesium (and calcium) reabsorption in the TALH. This appears to be due to inhibition of intermediate conductance ROMK apical K^+ channels and Na-2Cl-K cotransport, which reduce the transepithelial voltage and, through modulation of paracellin-1, cause reduced paracellular permeability. Magnesium reabsorption in the distal convoluted tubule (DCT), which accounts for 5% to 10% of the filtered load, is active and transcellular, probably mediated by luminal membrane Mg^{2+}-selective channels and a basolateral membrane Na^+-Mg^{2+} exchanger. Activation of the CaSR in the DCT also inhibits magnesium reabsorption in this segment, but its physiologic role in magnesium handling is not fully established.

The plasma magnesium concentration is the most important determinant of renal magnesium excretion. Magnesium depletion and hypomagnesemia increase magnesium reabsorption, and hypermagnesemia decreases reabsorption in the TALH and DCT. Hypercalcemia also decreases magnesium reabsorption in these segments. These effects of changes in the plasma concentration of magnesium and calcium on urinary magnesium excretion are mediated primarily by the basolateral membrane CaSr. Volume contraction increases and volume expansion decreases magnesium reabsorption in the proximal tubule. Unlike calcium and phosphorous, hormonal control of magnesium handling in the kidney appears to be of relatively minor physiologic importance, although complex direct and indirect hormonal influences on urinary magnesium excretion and renal magnesium transport have been described. Experimentally, parathyroid hormone, calcitonin, $1,25(OH)_2$ vitamin D_3, glucagon, insulin, aldosterone, and vasopressin can be shown to increase magnesium absorption by cells of the TALH or DCT. The effects of aldosterone on renal handling of magnesium are complex. Although aldosterone may increase magnesium absorption in the TALH and DCT, aldosterone-mediated ECF volume expansion reduces magnesium reabsorption in the proximal tubule and can increase urinary magnesium excretion. Loop diuretics decrease magnesium reabsorption in the TALH by reducing the lumen-positive transepithelial voltage that drives paracellular reabsorption in this segment. Acute thiazide diuretic administration and amiloride increase magnesium reabsorption in the DCT by stimulating voltage-sensitive magnesium uptake by DCT cells. Chronic effects of thiazide diuretics on renal magnesium handling are discussed later.

HYPOMAGNESEMIA

The plasma magnesium concentration is not a particularly accurate measure of total body magnesium. It is difficult to predict the extent of magnesium deficiency based on the plasma concentration. Intracellular magnesium depletion can be present with low-normal plasma levels.

Causes of Hypomagnesemia

Impaired GI tract absorption is a common underlying basis for hypomagnesemia, especially when the small bowel is involved due to disorders associated with malabsorption, chronic diarrhea, steatorrhea, or as the result of small intestinal bypass surgery (Table 14-1). Because there is some magnesium absorption in the colon, patients with ileostomies can develop hypomagnesemia. Familial hypomagnesemia with secondary hypocalcemia is a rare autosomal-recessive disorder with impaired intestinal and renal magnesium absorption due to a mutation in the gene for an ion channel, *TRPM6*, which appears to be involved in magnesium transport in the intestine and distal nephron.

Renal causes of hypomagnesemia are listed in Table 14-1. Osmotic and loop diuretics can cause significant urinary magnesium losses and hypomagnesemia. Thiazide diuretics acutely increase magnesium reabsorption in the DCT and do not cause urinary magnesium wasting. With chronic thiazide diuretic use, though, magnesium reabsorption is decreased and magnesium depletion can develop. The mechanisms causing increased urinary magnesium excretion with chronic thiazide use are not fully understood. Experimental studies have shown reduced magnesium uptake by DCT cells in the presence of hypokalemia and cellular K depletion as may occur with chronic thiazide use. Effects of hyperaldosteronism on luminal membrane epithelial sodium channel (ENaC) activity in the DCT leading to an increase in the lumen-negative transepithelial voltage and reduced reabsorption in this segment, as well as possible indirect effects on paracellin-1 function, have also been postulated. Experimental evidence of increased apoptosis of DCT cells with

TABLE 14-1 Causes of Hypomagnesemia

Decreased intake
Chronic alcoholism
Protein calorie malnutrition
Inadequate magnesium content of TPN or intravenous fluids

Gastrointestinal losses
Inflammatory bowel disease
Chronic diarrhea
Laxative abuse
Malabsorption
Surgical resection
Familial hypomagnesemia with secondary hypocalcemia

Renal losses
Osmotic diuretics
Loop diuretics
Thiazide diuretics (chronic use)
Amphotericin B
Aminoglycosides
Cisplatin
Pentamidine
Cyclosporine
Foscarnet
Postobstructive diuresis or diuretic phase of acute tubular necrosis
Inherited disorders with urinary magnesium wasting
  Idiopathic hypermagnesuria
  Familial hypomagnesemia with secondary hypocalcemia
  Isolated hypomagnesemia—autosomal dominant, autosomal recessive
  Familial hypomagnesemia with hypercalciuria and nephrocalcinosis
  Autosomal dominant hypoparathyroidism
  Gitelman's syndrome
  Bartter's syndrome
Alcohol ingestion
Hypercalcemia

Miscellaneous
Acute pancreatitis
Hungry bone syndrome
Diabetic ketoacidosis

thiazide administration has led to the suggestion that this may reduce overall epithelial cell surface area and thus impairs magnesium reabsorption in this segment of the nephron. Several nephrotoxic drugs, such as amphotericin B, the aminoglycosides, cisplatin, and foscarnet, can cause impaired magnesium absorption in the TALH and DCT. The magnesium wasting with these drugs can occur before other evidence of tubular injury develops (i.e., a decline in glomerular filtration rate [GFR]) and persist for months after the drug is stopped. Cisplatin and foscarnet tend to cause the most severe hypomagnesemia.

Urinary magnesium wasting and hypomagnesemia, which may be severe, are seen in most patients with Gitelman's syndrome, which is caused by loss of function mutations in the gene for the DCT NaCl cotransporter (NCCT). The pathophysiologic basis for the urinary magnesium wasting seen in Gitelman's syndrome has not been fully elucidated, but is probably multifactorial. Because thiazide diuretics inhibit the DCT NCCT and thus in some respects create a model of Gitelman's syndrome, the preceding mechanisms proposed for urinary magnesium wasting with chronic thiazide administration may also explain the urinary magnesium wasting of this syndrome. An experimental model of Gitelman's syndrome in which the NCCT gene has been deleted and in which urinary magnesium wasting is present may help in understanding the basis for this disorder. Interestingly, hypokalemia does not develop in these "knock-out" animals, suggesting that in contrast to chronic thiazide administration, hypokalemia and cellular potassium depletion are not responsible for the urinary magnesium wasting in Gitelman's syndrome.

Urinary magnesium wasting and hypomagnesemia are present in only a minority of patients with Bartter's syndrome, and are seen primarily only in those with the classic form, which is mediated by mutations in the gene for the TALH basolateral membrane chloride channel. Urinary magnesium wasting in these patients with Bartter's syndrome is thought to be due to a reduction in the lumen-positive voltage in the TALH, which reduces the driving force for magnesium reabsorption. Why urinary magnesium wasting and hypomagnesemia are not seen in most patients with Bartter's syndrome, but are typical of Gitelman's syndrome, is unclear. Because more magnesium is normally reabsorbed in the loop of Henle than in the DCT, urinary magnesium wasting might be expected more often with the Bartter's syndrome group of disorders than with Gitelman's syndrome, much as urinary magnesium wasting is more common with loop diuretics than with thiazide diuretics. Volume depletion and hyperaldosteronism may attenuate urinary magnesium wasting in patients with Bartter's syndrome, partially explaining why it is less common than otherwise might be expected. Other rare inherited disorders with renal magnesium wasting include mutations in the genes for paracellin-1 (familial hypomagnesemia with hypercalciuria/nephrocalcinosis), the CaSR (autosomal-dominant hypoparathyroidism), and, as mentioned previously, the ion channel *TRPM6* (familial hypomagnesemia with secondary hypocalcemia).

Alcoholics and individuals on magnesium-deficient diets or parenteral nutrition for prolonged periods can become hypomagnesemic without abnormal gastrointestinal or kidney function. Addition of 4 to 12 mmol of magnesium per day to total parenteral nutrition has been recommended to prevent hypomagnesemia. Although urinary magnesium excretion can be reduced to very low levels with magnesium deficiency, hypomagnesemia can still develop due to persistent obligatory losses in urine, stool, and sweat, coupled with the limited and slow exchange of bone and intracellular magnesium with extracellular magnesium. Alcohol ingestion can cause reversible generalized renal tubular dysfunction with urinary magnesium wasting even in the presence of hypomagnesemia. Hypomagnesemia can occur with acute pancreatitis, probably through the same mechanism that contributes to hypocalcemia in this setting,

that is, precipitation of divalent cations in necrotic fat in the pancreatic bed.

Hypomagnesemia is common among patients in intensive care units, particularly in those with sepsis or who are treated with diuretics, and in some studies was associated with higher mortality compared with patients without hypomagnesemia. A beneficial effect of magnesium replacement on outcomes in this setting has not been shown.

In circumstances where the cause of hypomagnesemia is unclear, a 24-hour urinary magnesium excretion of greater than 1 mmol or a calculated fractional excretion of magnesium (FE_{Mg})* of greater than 3% suggests inappropriate renal wasting; the FE_{Mg} can decrease to less than 0.5% with magnesium depletion from nonrenal causes.

Clinical Manifestations of Hypomagnesemia

Hypomagnesemia often coexists with hypokalemia and hypocalcemia, which may be due to the same underlying medical condition (diuretics, diarrhea, etc.). In addition, magnesium depletion enhances renal potassium secretion in the loop of Henle and possibly in the cortical collecting tubules through uncertain mechanisms. The hypocalcemia seen with hypomagnesemia is due to inhibition of parathyroid hormone (PTH) secretion and skeletal resistance to the effects of PTH; inhibition of calcitriol synthesis may also play a role. The hypokalemia and hypocalcemia are often refractory to correction until the hypomagnesemia is corrected.

Neuromuscular manifestations of hypomagnesemia are similar to those of hypocalcemia, including hyper-reflexia, carpopedal spasm, tetany, seizures, and Chvostek's and Trousseau's signs; these can occur in the absence of severe hypocalcemia. Electrocardiographic (ECG) changes include widening of the QRS complex, prolongation of the QT interval, and peaking of T waves; ECG changes related to hypokalemia and hypocalcemia may also be present. Torsade de pointes, premature ventricular contractions (PVCs), ventricular tachycardia, and ventricular fibrillation have also been described with hypomagnesemia, and may respond to intravenous magnesium sulfate. Hypomagnesemia also increases the risk for cardiac toxicity from digitalis glycosides. Magnesium deficiency and reduced dietary magnesium intake have been associated with increased risk for stroke, ischemic coronary artery disease, hypertension, and asthma, albeit through uncertain mechanisms.

Normomagnesemic magnesium depletion should be considered in patients with clinical features consistent

$$*FE_{Mg} = \frac{U_{Mg}/(0.7 \times P_{Mg}) \times 100}{U_{Cr}/P_{Cr}}$$

The plasma magnesium concentration (P_{Mg}) is multiplied by 0.7 because about 70% of total plasma magnesium is not albumin bound and is thus free to be filtered across the glomerulus.

with magnesium depletion, such as unexplained hypokalemia or hypocalcemia, who are at risk for magnesium depletion. The diagnosis may be suggested by a 24-hour urinary magnesium of less than 1 mmol, retention of more than 20% of a standardized dose of magnesium (2.4 mg/kg infused over 4 hours) over 24 hours, or response to empiric treatment with magnesium supplementation.

Treatment of Hypomagnesemia

In patients with asymptomatic or chronic hypomagnesemia that does not respond to increased dietary magnesium, oral replacement therapy is appropriate (Table 14-2). An initial oral dose of 30 to 60 mEq/day in three or four divided doses can be used. Excessive administration of magnesium salts may cause diarrhea. Sustained-release preparations are often recommended. For instance, for Slow-Mag, an enteric-coated preparation of magnesium chloride that contains 64 mg (5.3 mEq) of elemental magnesium per tablet, 6 to 12 tablets in divided doses should be taken daily. Although a single 400-mg tablet of magnesium oxide (with 20 mEq of elemental magnesium) two to three times daily may also be adequate, diarrhea with this preparation tends to be more problematic than with sustained-released magnesium chloride. Repletion of depleted body stores usually takes at least several days. Amiloride and the other K^+-sparing diuretics can reduce renal magnesium wasting due to other diuretics, aminoglycosides, amphotericin B, Gitelman's syndrome, or other similar causes.

Patients with symptomatic or more severe hypomagnesemia should receive intravenous magnesium sulfate. In the presence of normal kidney function, as much as 50% of an administered magnesium dose will be excreted in the urine even when there is substantial magnesium deficiency. An intravenous dose of 1 to 1.5 mEq/kg magnesium can be given over the first 24 hours, with doses of 0.5 to 1.0 mEq/kg daily thereafter until the plasma

magnesium level remains within the normal range, typically requiring several days and magnesium replacement of as much as 3 to 4 mEq/kg. These doses should be reduced commensurate with any reduction in GFR. Intravenous preparations of magnesium sulfate are available in concentrations of 10% to 50%; one commonly used preparation is a 2-mL vial or ampoule of 50% $MgSO_4$ (as $MgSO_4 \cdot 7H_2O$) containing 1 g $MgSO_4$ with 8.1 mEq (98.7 mg) of elemental magnesium. Magnesium sulfate can be painful and sclerosing when administered intravenously, so it should be diluted prior to administration. In emergency situations, 1 to 2 g of $MgSO_4$ (8.1 to 16.2 mEq) can be given intravenously in 50 mL of normal saline or 5% dextrose in water over 5 to 10 minutes. Patients should be monitored during magnesium infusion for hypotension and reduction of deep tendon reflexes. Facial flushing or a feeling of warmth may indicate an overly rapid rate of infusion. Intramuscular injection of magnesium sulfate is painful and should only be used in the absence of intravenous access.

HYPERMAGNESEMIA

Causes of Hypermagnesemia

Because an increase in the plasma magnesium concentration causes decreased reabsorption in the cortical TALH and increased urinary excretion, hypermagnesemia rarely occurs unless there is some degree of kidney impairment (GFR less than 30 mL/min) or a large load of magnesium is delivered by the oral, intravenous, or rectal route. Even among patients on chronic dialysis, symptomatic hypermagnesemia is rare.

Some of the more common causes of hypermagnesemia are shown in Table 14-3. Intentional hypermagnesemia occurs with intravenous magnesium administration for treatment of severe preeclampsia and eclampsia. Severe hypermagnesemia can result from

TABLE 14-2   Preparations for Oral Magnesium Replacement Therapy

Magnesium Salt	Usual Tablet (mg)	Mg Content (mg/tablet)	Mg Content (mEq/tablet)
Oxide			
Mg-Ox 400	400	242	20
UroMag	140	84	7
Gluconate*			
Almora, Magtrate, others	500	27	2.3
Chloride			
Slow-Mag (enteric coated)	535	64	5.3
Mag-SR (sustained release)	535	64	5.3
Lactate			
Mag-Tab SR (sustained release)	840	84	7
L-aspartate HCl			
Maginex (enteric coated)	615	61	5
Maginex DS (enteric coated)	1230	122	10

*Also available in liquid oral formulations.

TABLE 14-3   Principal Causes of Hypermagnesemia

Magnesium infusion
  Therapy for severe preeclampsia and eclampsia
  Total parenteral nutrition
Oral ingestion
  Laxatives
  Antacids
  Epsom salts (magnesium sulfate)
Magnesium-containing enemas
Acute renal failure
Chronic kidney disease

excessive use of magnesium-containing enemas, antacids, laxatives, or nutritional supplements, and accidental ingestion of Epsom salts. Magnesium-containing enemas and laxatives should be avoided in patients with impaired kidney function. Magnesium-containing antacids should be used cautiously in such patients. Uncommon causes of hypermagnesemia include familial hypocalciuric hypercalcemia, which is due to inactivating mutations in the CaSR gene; theophylline intoxication; lithium ingestion; hyperparathyroidism; adrenal insufficiency; hypothyroidism; milk-alkali syndrome; tumor lysis syndrome; and Dead Sea water ingestion.

Clinical Manifestations of Hypermagnesemia

Clinical sequelae of hypermagnesemia are uncommon with plasma concentrations of less than 4.5 to 5 mg/dL. Above this level, cutaneous flushing, nausea, vomiting, and mild hypotension may occur. Hyporeflexia typically occurs at magnesium levels of greater than 5 mg/dL. Loss of deep tendon reflexes, skeletal muscle weakness, and hypotension, which can be severe, develops with levels greater than 7 to 10 mg/dL. Respiratory muscle paralysis typically occurs with levels greater than 12 to 15 mg/dL. ECG manifestations begin to develop with levels greater than 5 mg/dL, including prolonged PR interval, increased QRS duration, and increased QT interval, along with bradycardia that may progress to complete heart block at levels greater than 10 to 15 mg/dL and cardiac arrest when levels exceed 15 to 20 mg/dL.

Symptomatic hypocalcemia due to inhibition of PTH secretion can complicate parenteral magnesium therapy of eclampsia. Although hypermagnesemia decreases the anion gap, this appears not to occur with infusion of magnesium sulfate, because retention of the anionic sulfate moiety counterbalances the unmeasured cation.

Treatment of Hypermagnesemia

Hypermagnesemia usually requires no treatment, provided kidney function is near enough to normal that upon stopping excessive intake, urinary excretion can lower the plasma magnesium concentration. Hemodialysis and, to a much lesser extent, peritoneal dialysis can remove excess magnesium. Intravenous calcium (100 to 200 mg over 5 to 10 minutes) can transiently antagonize effects of hypermagnesemia.

BIBLIOGRAPHY

Agus ZS: Hypomagnesemia. J Am Soc Nephrol 10:1616–1622, 1999.

Al-Ghamdi SMG, Cameron EC, Sutton RAL: Magnesium deficiency: Pathophysiologic and clinical overview. Am J Kidney Dis 24:737–752, 1994.

Blanchard A, Jeunemaitre X, Coudol P, et al: Paracellin-1 is critical for magnesium and calcium reabsorption in the human thick ascending limb of Henle. Kidney Int 59:2206–2215, 2001.

Cholst IN, Steinberg SF, Tropper PJ, et al: The influence of hypermagnesemia on serum calcium and parathyroid hormone levels in human subjects. N Engl J Med 310:1221–1225, 1984.

Cole DEC, Quamme GA: Inherited disorders of renal magnesium handling. J Am Soc Nephrol 11:1937–1947, 2000.

Dai L-J, Friedman PA, Quamme GA: Cellular mechanisms of chlorothiazide and cellular potassium depletion on Mg^{2+} uptake in mouse distal convoluted tubule cells. Kidney Int 51:1008–1017, 1997.

Dai L-J, Ritchie G, Kerstan D, et al: Magnesium transport in the renal distal convoluted tubule. Physiol Rev 81:51–84, 2001.

deRouffignac C, Quamme G: Renal magnesium handling and its hormonal control. Physiol Rev 74:305–322, 1994.

Ellison DH: Divalent cation transport by the distal nephron: Insights from Bartter's and Gitelman's syndromes. Am J Physiol Renal Physiol 279:F616–F625, 2000.

Hebert SC: Extracellular calcium-sensing receptor: Implications for calcium and magnesium handling in the kidney. Kidney Int 50:2129–2139, 1996.

Hebert SC, Brown EM, Harris HW: Role of the Ca^{2+}-sensing receptor in divalent mineral ion homeostasis. J Exp Biol 200:295–302, 1997.

Kelepouris E, Agus ZS: Hypomagnesemia: Renal magnesium handling. Semin Nephrol 18:58–73, 1998.

Kobrin SM, Goldfarb S: Magnesium deficiency. Semin Nephrol 6:525–535, 1990.

Konrad M, Weber S: Recent advances in molecular genetics of hereditary magnesium-losing disorders. J Am Soc Nephrol 14:249–260, 2003.

Mordes JP, Wacker WE: Excess magnesium. Pharmacol Rev 29:273–300, 1977.

Quamme GA: Renal magnesium handling: new insights in understanding old problems. Kidney Int 52:1180–1195, 1997.

Reikes S, Gonzalez EA, Martin KJ: Abnormal calcium and magnesium metabolism. In DuBose TD Jr, Hamm LL (eds): Acid-Base and Electrolyte Disorders. Philadelphia, WB Saunders, 2002, pp 453–487.

Ricci J, Oster JR, Gutierrez R, et al: Influence of magnesium-sulfate-induced hypermagnesemia on the anion gap: Role of hypersulfatemia. Am J Nephrol 10:409–411, 1990.

Simon DB, Lu Y, Choate KA, et al: Paracellin-1, a renal tight junction protein is required for paracellular Mg^{2+} resorption. Science 285:103–106, 1999.

Soliman HM, Mercan D, Lobo SSM, et al: Development of ionized hypomagnesemia is associated with higher mortality rates. Crit Care Med 31:1082–1087, 2003.

Whang R, Whang DD, Ryan MP: Refractory potassium depletion. A consequence of magnesium deficiency. Arch Intern Med 152:40–45, 1992.

CHAPTER 15

Edema and the Clinical Use of Diuretics

David H. Ellison

Edema is usually a manifestation of expanded extracellular fluid (ECF) volume resulting from congestive heart failure, hepatic cirrhosis, nephrotic syndrome, or impaired kidney function, although it can also result from local factors or lymphatic obstruction. Extracellular fluid volume expands when the kidneys retain NaCl in excess of dietary NaCl intake. Renal NaCl retention may reflect an adaptive response to inadequate effective arterial blood volume, as in patients with congestive heart failure, or it may reflect a pathologic response of kidney tubules to damage, as in patients with acute renal failure. Regardless of its cause, the best treatments for edema include restricting dietary NaCl intake and correcting the primary disorder. Despite these interventions, or when they are impossible, ECF volume frequently remains expanded unacceptably and, for this reason, diuretics are prescribed. All of the diuretics used to treat edema increase both Na and water excretion. They are powerful drugs that, if used carefully, play an important role in treating symptomatic edema. The prompt and dramatic symptomatic improvement when intravenous diuretics are administered to a patient suffering from acute pulmonary edema remains one of the most gratifying responses in clinical medicine. For this reason, diuretics remain among the most frequently prescribed drugs.

In addition to their use for edema, diuretic drugs are indicated for a wide variety of nonedematous disorders. Specific details of diuretic treatment of hypertension, acute renal failure, nephrolithiasis, and hyponatremia are discussed in other chapters. This chapter focuses on renal mechanisms of diuretic action and diuretic therapy of edema.

THE PHYSIOLOGIC BASIS OF DIURETIC ACTION

The amount of NaCl excreted by the kidneys is equal to the difference between the filtered amount of Na (plasma Na concentration × glomerular filtration rate) and the quantity reabsorbed by the renal tubules. Assuming a normal glomerular filtration rate (approximately 150 l/day) and a normal plasma Na concentration (approximately 150 mmol/L), approximately 23 moles of Na are filtered each day in normal humans (equivalent to about 3 pounds of table salt). To maintain a normal fractional excretion of Na (FE_{Na}) of under 1%, more than 99% of the filtered Na is reabsorbed. All of the diuretic drugs in clinical use act primarily on the renal tubules to inhibit Na reabsorption and increase fractional Na excretion.

A simple and clinically useful classification of diuretic drugs is based on the sites and mechanisms of their actions along the nephron (Table 15-1). All active NaCl reabsorption by renal epithelial cells is driven by the Na^+ K^+-ATPase pump, which is expressed at the basolateral membrane (the blood side) of epithelial cells along the nephron. This pump uses metabolic energy (derived from hydrolysis of adenosine triphosphate [ATP]) to extrude Na from the cell into the interstitium and blood and to move K into the cell. The action of the Na^+ K^+-ATPase keeps the cellular Na concentration low and the cellular K concentration high. It also contributes to making the cell interior electrically negative with respect to the extracellular fluid (the high intracellular K concentration being the other factor). The low cellular Na concentration and the cell-negative voltage drive positively charged Na ions into the cell across the luminal membrane from tubule fluid. Although Na^+ K^+-ATPase pumps are present at the basolateral cell membranes of nearly every epithelial cell, each nephron segment possesses unique apical mechanisms that permit Na to move across the luminal membrane; these specific transport pathways form the molecular bases of diuretic action. Together, active Na extrusion from the basolateral membrane and passive Na entry across the luminal membrane permit vectorial Na transport in the absorptive direction.

Proximal Tubule Diuretics

Approximately two thirds of filtered water and NaCl are reabsorbed along the proximal tubule. Sodium moves down its electrochemical gradient from tubule lumen into proximal tubule cells coupled to the movement of other solutes against their electrochemical gradients; among these solutes are glucose, amino acids, and phos-

TABLE 15-1   Physiologic Classification of Diuretic Drugs

Proximal Diuretics	Loop Diuretics	DCT Diuretics	CD Diuretics

Carbonic anhydrase inhibitors
   Acetazolamide
	Na-K-2Cl (NKCC2) inhibitors
	   Furosemide
	   Bumetanide
	   Torsemide
	   Ethacrynic acid
		NaCl (NCCT) inhibitors
		   Hydrochlorothiazide
		   Metolazone
		   Chlorthalidone
		   Indapamide*
		   Many others
			Na channel blockers
			  (ENaC Inhibitors)
			   Amiloride
			   Triamterene
			Aldosterone antagonists
			   Spironolactone
			   Eplerenone

CD, collecting duct; DCT, distal convoluted tubule.
*Indapamide may have other actions as well.

phate. The reabsorption of bicarbonate and chloride is indirectly coupled to Na absorption. Because the epithelium is electrically "leaky" (highly permeable to ions), large transepithelial ion gradients do not develop, and solute absorption along this segment is isosmotic.

An important pathway by which Na crosses the luminal membrane of proximal tubule cells involves electroneutral exchange of Na for H (NHE3, gene symbol *SLC9A3*; Fig. 15-1). Protons that are extruded across the luminal membrane of proximal cells titrate bicarbonate (HCO_3), which has been filtered by the glomeruli. This forms carbonic acid (H_2CO_3), which dehydrates to CO_2

and H_2O, a reaction catalyzed by the enzyme carbonic anhydrase in the brush border of proximal tubule cells. Via these events, $NaHCO_3$ is functionally reabsorbed across the luminal membrane into the cell. For transepithelial $NaHCO_3$ reabsorption to continue at steady state, Na and HCO_3 must leave the cell across the basolateral membrane. Sodium leaves via the Na^+ K^+-ATPase pump and also via an $NaHCO_3$ transport pathway. Carbonic anhydrase located within proximal tubule cells generates H^+ ions for extrusion across the apical membrane and bicarbonate ions, which exit across the basolateral membrane.

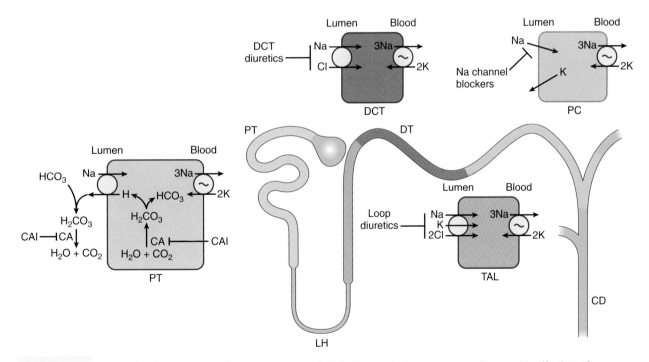

FIGURE 15-1 Predominant sites and mechanisms of action of clinically important diuretic drugs. Patterns identify sites of action along the nephron and corresponding cell types. CA, carbonic anhydrase; CAI, carbonic anhydrase inhibitor; CD, collecting duct; DCT, distal convoluted tubule cell; DT, distal tubule; LH, loop of Henle; PC, principal cell; PT, proximal tubule; TAL, thick ascending limb cell. Both intracellular and luminal actions of carbonic anhydrase inhibitors are important in their ability to reduce Na reabsorption by the renal proximal tubule. Note that Na channel blockers probably act along the connecting tubule as well as the collecting duct. Spironolactone (not shown) is a competitive aldosterone antagonist and acts primarily in the cortical collecting tubule. (From Ellison DH: The physiologic basis of diuretic synergism. Ann Intern Med 114:887, 1991. With permission.)

Carbonic anhydrase inhibitors interfere with enzyme activity both inside the cell and within the brush border. Their action in the brush border inhibits Na^+-H^+ exchange by slowing the rate at which carbonic acid dehydrates. Thus, carbonic acid accumulates in tubule fluid, acidifying it. Their action inside the cell inhibits HCO_3 production, thereby interfering with basolateral base exit. The net result of carbonic anhydrase inhibition is impaired Na, HCO_3, Cl, and water reabsorption by the proximal tubule and increased renal Na, Cl, HCO_3, and water excretion. When administered acutely, these drugs provoke a moderate alkaline diuresis. When administered chronically, their natriuretic potency is relatively weak because compensatory processes develop. First, when $NaHCO_3$ reabsorption along the proximal tubule is inhibited, much of the solute and fluid that escapes reabsorption by the proximal tubule can be reabsorbed by more distal nephron segments. Second, inhibition of solute reabsorption along the proximal tubule increases solute delivery to the macula densa. This activates the tubuloglomerular feedback mechanism, which suppresses glomerular filtration rate and decreases the amount of Na, Cl, and HCO_3 that is filtered. Finally, alkaline diuresis induces metabolic acidosis; when serum HCO_3 concentrations decline, less HCO_3 is filtered and the carbonic anhydrase–dependent component of Na reabsorption declines.

Because carbonic anhydrase inhibitors are relatively weak diuretics in chronic use and because they often result in metabolic acidosis, their use as diuretic drugs is limited. They are commonly used, however, to treat open-angle glaucoma, where they reduce the formation of aqueous humor by as much as 50%. Furthermore, they can be used to prevent acute mountain sickness and to treat metabolic alkalosis at times when Cl cannot be administered because of ECF volume expansion. This is especially useful when respiratory drive is compromised by metabolic alkalosis; careful use of carbonic anhydrase inhibitors may correct alkalosis and improve respiratory drive. Carbonic anhydrase inhibitors may also be used in combination with other classes of diuretics to induce diuresis in otherwise resistant patients (see later section on Diuretic Resistance).

Loop Diuretics

Approximately 25% of the filtered NaCl is reabsorbed along the loop of Henle. Transcellular NaCl reabsorption along the medullary and cortical thick ascending limbs is driven by Na^+ K^+-ATPase at the basolateral membrane. An electroneutral pathway at the luminal membrane (NKCC2, gene symbol *SLC12A1*) carries 1 Na, 1 K, and 2 Cl from tubule fluid into the cell, driven by the electrochemical gradient for Na (see Fig. 15-1). Much of the K that is taken up via this pathway recycles across the luminal membrane through K channels (ROMK, gene

symbol *KCNJ1*). The Na-K-2Cl pathway, therefore, generates net NaCl reabsorption and (because of the K recycling) a voltage across the wall of the tubule that is oriented with the lumen positive relative to blood.

Loop diuretics such as furosemide, bumetanide, and torsemide inhibit the action of the NKCC2 directly. These diuretics are anions that circulate bound to protein; because of the extensive protein binding, very little diuretic reaches tubule fluid by filtration. Instead, loop diuretics are secreted into the lumen of the proximal tubule by the organic anion transport pathway. Once secreted, they travel downstream to the thick ascending limb, where they bind to the transport protein (the Na-K-2Cl transporter) and inhibit its action. Although the mechanism by which ethacrynic acid inhibits NaCl reabsorption is not as clear, its net effect on transport along the thick ascending limb is qualitatively similar. Loop diuretics are potent ("high ceiling") drugs that promote the excretion of Na and Cl, together with K. Although they inhibit K reabsorption along the thick ascending limb, their effects on K excretion predominantly reflect their tendency to increase K secretion along the distal nephron (see later section on Complications of Diuretic Treatment). Loop diuretics increase magnesium and calcium excretion. Bumetanide, furosemide, and torsemide reduce the magnitude of the lumen-positive voltage in the thick ascending limb. This tends to impair Ca and Mg reabsorption because the reabsorption of these cations is driven across the paracellular pathway by the lumen-positive voltage. This accounts for the ability of loop diuretics to increase urinary calcium excretion, a clinically useful phenomenon.

Loop diuretics impair the ability of the kidney to elaborate urine that is either very concentrated or very dilute. The NKCC2 removes Na and Cl from the lumen as fluid courses up the thick ascending limb. Because this segment of the nephron is impermeable to water, solute removal dilutes the tubule fluid. By blocking the predominant solute removal pathway, loop diuretics inhibit free water generation. The action of the NKCC2 also provides the "single effect" that is responsible for countercurrent multiplication (see Chapter 1). Solute removal from the thick ascending limb contributes to generating a high-solute concentration in the medullary interstitium, which drives water reabsorption from the medullary collecting tubule. By blocking the NKCC2, loop diuretics inhibit the kidney's ability to generate a concentrated urine; this is one reason these diuretics can be useful in treating patients with the syndrome of inappropriate antidiuretic hormone secretion.

Loop diuretics have important hemodynamic effects, both within the kidney and systemically. They increase secretion of vasodilatory prostaglandins and often reduce cardiac preload, when administered acutely. In some situations, however, they elicit a vasoconstrictor response that may impair cardiac performance acutely; this anomalous response is probably caused by enhanced renin secretion and may be blocked by angiotensin-converting enzyme inhibitors. Loop diuretics tend to maintain or increase the rate of glomerular filtration, even in the face of ECF volume depletion, because they block the tubuloglomerular feedback mechanism and because diuretic-induced prostaglandin secretion dilates the afferent arteriole.

Distal Convoluted Tubule Diuretics (Thiazides and Others)

The distal tubule, the nephron segment just beyond the loop of Henle, reabsorbs 5% to 10% of the filtered NaCl. The Na concentration in distal convoluted tubule (DCT) cells is maintained low by Na^+ K^+-ATPase. Sodium and Cl enter the cell across the luminal membrane via an electroneutral NaCl cotransport pathway (NCCT or NCC, gene symbol *SLC12A3*; see Fig. 15-1) that is molecularly and functionally distinct from the pathway in the thick ascending limb. Although DCT diuretics are commonly called thiazides, many such drugs (such as chlorthalidone) are not true thiazides; the more general term that defines them by their site of action is preferred. DCT diuretics are anions that, like the loop diuretics, circulate in the bloodstream bound to protein and are secreted into the lumen of the proximal tubule by the organic anion transport pathway. They are carried downstream to the distal tubule, where they bind to the NaCl transport protein and inhibit its action. Because the distal tubule is relatively water impermeable, NaCl reabsorption along the DCT contributes to urinary dilution. DCT diuretics therefore impair urinary diluting capacity, but they have no effect on urinary concentrating ability. Most DCT diuretics, with the possible exception of metolazone, become less effective when the glomerular filtration rate declines below 40 mL/minute.

DCT diuretics increase magnesium excretion but, in contrast to loop diuretics, inhibit urinary calcium excretion. Two mechanisms have been invoked to explain the effects of DCT diuretics on calcium excretion. First, DCT diuretics stimulate calcium reabsorption along the proximal tubule because they contract ECF volume and increase proximal Na reabsorption (Na and Ca transport vary in parallel along the proximal tubule). Second, DCT diuretics stimulate calcium reabsorption along the distal tubule through their action on the NCCT. When this pathway is blocked, intracellular concentrations of Na and Cl decline. Low intracellular Cl concentrations make the cell interior more electrically negative, with respect to interstitium. This is because more chloride, which is negatively charged, tends to diffuse into the cell from the interstitium. This opens voltage-activated epithelial calcium channels in the luminal membrane (the transient receptor potential cation channel, TRPV5). It also stimulates 3Na-Ca exchange at the basolateral cell membrane, which is an electrogenic process. Diuretic-induced reductions in intracellular Na concentrations also stimulate 3Na-Ca exchange because they increase the electrochemical gradient favoring sodium entry. Both processes increase calcium reabsorption. The effects of DCT diuretics on calcium excretion form the basis for the use of these drugs to reduce recurrence of calcium nephrolithiasis.

Collecting Duct Diuretics

Sodium reabsorption by the collecting duct (CD) system, which amounts to only 3% of the filtered NaCl load, is primarily electrogenic (current generating), unlike transport along more proximal segments. An electrical current moves into the cell when Na enters across the luminal membrane through ion channels (ENaC). As in the other tubule segments, the concentration of Na inside CD (also known as principal) cells is maintained below electrochemical equilibrium by the action of the Na^+ K^+-ATPase. As Na moves out of the lumen, it generates a voltage across the tubule wall that is oriented with the lumen negative, relative to blood. This lumen-negative voltage helps to drive K movement in the secretory direction via a separate K channel (ROMK). Although Na and K do not traverse the same channel, transport of one is coupled to transport of the other by the transepithelial voltage.

Two major groups of diuretics act predominantly in the CD. Sodium channel blockers, such as triamterene and amiloride, act from the lumen to inhibit Na movement through Na channels in CD cells. Because these drugs impair Na movement, the transepithelial voltage declines, inhibiting K secretion secondarily. This effect accounts for their K-sparing action. It should be emphasized that, although amiloride inhibits renal Na^+-H^+ exchange in the proximal tubule, the proximal effect probably does not contribute to its diuretic action in humans because the concentrations of amiloride achieved in the lumen of the proximal tubule during oral administration are insufficient to interfere with Na^+-H^+ exchange. The second class of CD diuretics is the aldosterone antagonists, represented by spironolactone and eplerenone. Aldosterone, a mineralocorticoid hormone secreted by the adrenal gland in response to angiotensin II or high serum potassium concentrations, stimulates Na reabsorption and K secretion along the connecting tubule and CD. It also increases the magnitude of the lumen-negative transepithelial voltage. By inhibiting the action of aldosterone, spironolactone and eplerenone cause mild natriuresis and potassium retention. Spironolactone stimulates estrogen receptors, and can lead to troubling estrogenic side effects, especially gynecomastia. Eplerenone binds more specifically to mineralocorticoid receptors than spironolactone and has a lower incidence of estrogenic side effects. Its efficacy appears similar.

Collecting duct diuretics are relatively modest in potency, at least when given acutely, largely because they inhibit distal Na reabsorption incompletely. In the past, their use as sole agents has been limited to situations in which excessive aldosterone secretion plays a central pathogenic role; in patients with cirrhotic ascites, for example, spironolactone has been reported to be more effective than loop diuretics as a single agent. Furthermore, when hypertension is caused by adrenocortical hyperplasia, adequate blood pressure control can often be obtained with oral spironolactone or amiloride. The most common use of the CD diuretics is to prevent excessive potassium wasting when combined with other, more potent, diuretics. Recently, interest in the utility of CD diuretics has been stimulated by suggestions that nonrenal actions of aldosterone may contribute to the pathogenesis of congestive heart failure. Two large trials showed that adding spironolactone, in chronic heart failure, or eplerenone, in post–myocardial infarction heart failure, improves mortality. These findings have led to recommendations to include aldosterone antagonists when treating patients with New York Heart Association class III and IV heart failure.

Osmotic Diuretics

Unlike other classes of diuretics, osmotic diuretics do not interfere directly with specific transport proteins but rather act as osmotic particles in tubule fluid. Water reabsorption throughout the nephron is driven by the osmotic gradients that are generated by solute transport. When an agent such as mannitol is administered, it is filtered but very poorly reabsorbed. Because the mannitol is retained in the tubule lumen, the osmolality of tubule fluid remains higher than normal, inhibiting fluid reabsorption. NaCl reabsorption is also inhibited, in this case because solute reabsorption dilutes tubule fluid, predisposing to NaCl backflux. Thus, these drugs tend to increase the excretion not only of fluid but also of Na, K, Cl, bicarbonate and other solutes. The urinary osmolality during osmotic diuresis tends to approach that of plasma, regardless of the state of hydration. Osmotic diuretics increase renal blood flow and wash out the medullary solute gradient, effects that contribute to the diuretic-induced impairment in urinary concentrating capacity.

Osmotic diuretics have been used in an attempt to prevent acute renal failure following cardiopulmonary bypass, rhabdomyolysis, and radiocontrast exposure. Mannitol is frequently used to reduce cerebral edema, first by osmotic fluid removal from the brain and then by promoting diuresis. Although data in the settings of cardiopulmonary bypass and rhabdomyolysis are inconclusive, a controlled study of patients exposed to radiocontrast agents indicated that hydration with half normal saline was as effective or more effective than mannitol in reducing the incidence of acute renal failure;

thus, mannitol should not be used to reduce the risk for contrast-mediated acute renal failure.

ADAPTATION TO DIURETIC DRUGS

When a loop diuretic drug is administered acutely, Na and fluid excretion increase transiently. This natriuresis is followed by a period of positive NaCl balance, termed postdiuretic NaCl retention (Fig. 15-2). The net effect of the diuretic on ECF volume during a 24-hour period is equal to the sum of NaCl losses during diuretic action (excretion > intake), and NaCl retention during periods when the drug concentration is low (intake > excretion). Factors that influence the relationship between natriuresis and postdiuretic NaCl retention include the dietary NaCl intake, the dose of diuretic, its half-life, and the frequency with which it is administered. When loop diuretics are administered once daily to patients ingesting a high-NaCl diet, postdiuretic NaCl retention often compensates entirely for NaCl losses during the period of drug action; net Na balance remains neutral from the first day (see Fig. 15-2). When NaCl intake is restricted, Na avidity during the postdiuretic period cannot overcome the initial NaCl losses, Na balance is negative, and ECF volume declines. This relationship between dietary NaCl intake and the net effect of diuretics accounts for the central role of dietary NaCl restriction in effective diuretic therapy.

Even when diuretic treatment does induce negative NaCl and fluid balance initially, NaCl balance is restored after several days to weeks because other adaptive mechanisms come into play, limiting the magnitude of the diuretic response (the "braking phenomenon"; see Fig. 15-2). Several mechanisms contribute to adaptation during chronic diuretic treatment. Contraction of the ECF volume, at least relative to pretreatment levels, may stimulate secretion of renin, aldosterone, and antidiuretic hormone, which mediate renal NaCl and fluid retention. Contraction of the ECF volume may increase the activity of renal nerves, which stimulate renal NaCl retention via direct effects on renal tubules. Contraction of the ECF volume may also reduce renal perfusion pressure and the glomerular filtration rate. In addition to adaptations that depend on changes in ECF volume, however, specific intrarenal effects of diuretics may also contribute to adaptation. Loop diuretics inhibit solute reabsorption along the thick ascending limb of Henle's loop, thereby increasing solute delivery to and solute reabsorption from the distal nephron. When solute delivery to the distal tubule is increased chronically (as during long-term diuretic therapy) distal tubule cells undergo substantial hypertrophy and increase the expression of transport proteins. These changes are associated with increases in NaCl transport capacity, which participate in returning the patient to NaCl balance. When these adaptive mechanisms occur prior to the achievement of acceptable levels

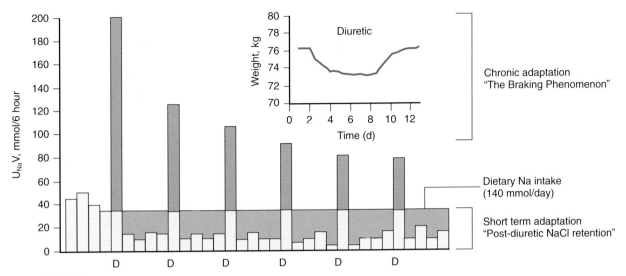

FIGURE 15-2   Effects of a loop diuretic on urinary Na excretion. Bars represent 6 hours. Purple bars indicate periods during which urinary Na excretion exceeds dietary intake. Blue areas indicate postdiuretic NaCl retention, periods during which dietary Na intake exceeds urinary Na excretion. Changes in the magnitude of natriuretic response during several days are indicative of diuretic braking. Black line indicates dietary Na intake per 6-hour period. Inset is effect of diuretics on weight (and extracellular fluid volume) during several days of diuretic administration. (From Ellison DH: Adaptation to diuretic drugs. In Seldin DW, Giebisch G [eds]: Diuretic Agents: Physiology and Pharmacology. San Diego, Academic Press, 1997, pp 209–232. With permission.)

of ECF volume (the desired response to diuretics), they contribute importantly to diuretic resistance, as discussed in the following section. When they occur at acceptable levels of ECF volume, they serve to prevent detrimental ongoing losses of Na, Cl, and water.

It should be emphasized that the goal of diuretic treatment of edema is not simply to increase urinary NaCl or fluid excretion. Instead, the goal is to reduce ECF volume to a clinically acceptable level and to maintain that volume chronically. To achieve this goal, urinary NaCl excretion must increase initially (see Fig. 15-2), but excretion rates of NaCl and fluid always return to pretreatment levels once steady state occurs. Thus, during successful diuretic treatment of edema, when the patient's weight has stabilized, urinary NaCl excretion matches dietary intake; it is not increased above normal values.

COMPLICATIONS OF DIURETIC TREATMENT

The most common complications of diuretic treatment result directly from the effects of these drugs on renal fluid and electrolyte excretion. They include ECF volume depletion, hyponatremia, and hypokalemia. Although both DCT and loop diuretics predispose to hypokalemia, the incidence and the implications of diuretic-induced hypokalemia depend on the indication for treatment, the class of drug, the dose, the dietary Na and K intake, and the duration of treatment. When used to treat essential hypertension, mild hypokalemia occurs more frequently with DCT diuretics, such as hydrochlorothiazide and chlorthalidone, than with loop diuretics, but this side

effect is clearly dose related. Luckily, the antihypertensive efficacy of DCT diuretics depends less on dose than does potassium wasting; for this reason, lower doses of DCT diuretics (12.5 to 25 mg of hydrochlorothiazide or chlorthalidone) than were commonly used in the past are now recommended to treat hypertension. In the recently reported ALLHAT study, serum potassium concentrations of less than 3.5 mEq/L occurred in 12.7% of patients receiving chlorthalidone (12.5 and 25 mg/day) at 2 years and 8.5% at 4 years. Frank hypokalemia during treatment of hypertension with a low dose of a DCT diuretic should alert the clinician that increased renin or aldosterone secretion may be present. This should prompt a search for primary hyperaldosteronism or renovascular disease.

Loop diuretics are prescribed most commonly to treat congestive heart failure. Cardiac dysfunction activates the renin-angiotensin-aldosterone axis, which predisposes to hypokalemia, especially when diuretic drugs are superimposed. Furthermore, many patients with systolic dysfunction or with atrial fibrillation receive digitalis glycosides, which predispose to hypokalemic arrhythmias. Several studies have indicated that the risk of ventricular arrhythmias increases as serum potassium concentrations decline; thus, hypokalemia is often treated more aggressively in this patient population. In one study, serum potassium concentrations of less than 3.5 mEq/L were observed in 25% of patients treated with potassium-losing diuretics, such as loop diuretics. Interestingly, changes in clinical practice during the past 15 years—including the increasing use of angiotensin-converting enzyme inhibitors, aldosterone antagonists, and beta blockers to treat systolic dysfunction—have increased the risk for hyperkalemia in heart failure patients.

Several mechanisms contribute to the tendency of loop and DCT diuretics to cause hypokalemia. First, both classes of diuretics increase fluid flow through the distal nephron, the site at which K secretion determines urinary K excretion rates. High fluid flow rates stimulate K secretion directly. Second, both loop and DCT diuretics stimulate secretion of aldosterone, which further increases K secretion along the distal nephron. Finally, both DCT and loop diuretics predispose to hypomagnesemia, which contributes to the development of hypokalemia through unknown mechanisms. Hypokalemia has several adverse consequences. These include ventricular arrhythmias, especially during the administration of digitalis glycosides or when hypomagnesemia is present. Hypokalemia may also contribute to glucose intolerance, a known complication of DCT diuretic use.

Methods to prevent or treat hypokalemia during diuretic therapy include (1) using the lowest effective diuretic dose (especially for hypertension), (2) supplementing dietary K (best administered as KCl), (3) preventing hypomagnesemia, and (4) using CD (K sparing) diuretics together with loop or DCT diuretics. Serum concentrations of Na and K should be monitored in every patient who is treated with diuretics, and most should be encouraged to consume a diet that is rich in K and low in Na. Many physicians prescribe potassium supplements to patients whose serum K concentration falls below 3.5 mmol/L, although others have suggested that K concentrations between 3.0 and 3.5 mmol/L do not require treatment. Certainly, if a patient is at risk for complications of hypokalemia, such as patients receiving digitalis glycosides or patients with hepatic cirrhosis, K concentrations should be maintained above 3.5 mmol/L. Of note, adding a CD diuretic not only corrects hypokalemia in many patients, but may also prevent hypomagnesemia; hypomagnesemia may act synergistically with hypokalemia to predispose to ventricular arrhythmias.

Hyperkalemia is a complication of CD diuretics. Hyperkalemia occurs most commonly in patients with chronic kidney disease or in patients taking angiotensin-converting enzyme inhibitors, angiotensin receptor blockers, or β-adrenergic-blocking drugs. Unfortunately, recent reports suggest that spironolactone may be contributing to a significant increase in potentially life-threatening hyperkalemia, when it (or presumably eplerenone) is used to treat heart failure patients who have concomitant renal functional impairment. It must be noted that all clinical trials of spironolactone to treat heart failure exclude patients with significant degrees of renal dysfunction. Triamterene metabolism is impaired in patients with cirrhosis, and this drug precipitates hyperkalemia in this group of patients.

Mild metabolic alkalosis occurs frequently during treatment with loop and DCT diuretics. These drugs promote urinary losses of NaCl (leaving HCO_3 behind).

Furthermore, they increase aldosterone secretion, which stimulates H secretion directly. Metabolic alkalosis can exacerbate hepatic encephalopathy and can inhibit the respiratory drive. Severe metabolic alkalosis is often a manifestation of overly aggressive therapy. Loop diuretics or combination diuretic therapy may also lead to excessive ECF volume depletion and vascular collapse.

Hyponatremia may develop during treatment with loop diuretics, but this complication is much more common with DCT diuretics (thiazides and their congeners). Some patients treated with DCT diuretics develop severe and potentially life-threatening hyponatremia, often several days to weeks after initiation of diuretic therapy. This complication is much more common in women and the elderly and can be life-threatening. The mechanisms underlying this response are incompletely understood, but they include the inhibition by DCT diuretics of urinary diluting capacity, the development of potassium deficiency, and central stimulation of thirst. DCT diuretics and, less commonly, loop diuretics also predispose to glucose intolerance, hyperlipidemia, and hyperuricemia, when administered chronically. Although the mechanisms by which these complications develop are not completely clear, hypokalemia and ECF volume contraction may be contributory. Serum concentrations of glucose, lipids, and uric acid should be monitored in patients on chronic diuretic treatment, but the clinical significance of these adverse effects was probably overemphasized in the past.

Some complications of diuretic treatment are drug or group specific and reflect toxic side effects; allergic interstitial nephritis is an idiosyncratic reaction to diuretics that may precipitate skin rash and acute renal failure. Ototoxicity is a toxic effect of loop diuretics that occurs most commonly when high doses are administered rapidly (intravenous furosemide at greater than 15 mg/minute) to patients with impaired kidney function. Triamterene can cause renal stones and may precipitate acute renal failure when administered with indomethacin. Spironolactone causes gynecomastia, especially in patients with cirrhosis of the liver.

DIURETIC TREATMENT OF EDEMA

Edema is a manifestation of disordered NaCl homeostasis. The NaCl retention often reflects a physiologic response to inadequate effective arterial blood volume, as occurs in congestive heart failure. In other situations, NaCl retention may reflect an abnormal renal response, resulting from damage to the kidney, as occurs with impaired kidney function or nephrotic syndrome. In either case, therapeutic maneuvers should be aimed first at correcting the primary disorder. Often, however, such maneuvers are not available or do not contract the ECF volume adequately, and more direct methods of effecting NaCl removal are needed. Before initiating treatment with diuretic drugs, it is important to institute a low NaCl diet. ECF volume varies directly with NaCl intake, both in normal and edematous individuals. For patients with mild ECF volume expansion, a "no added salt" diet may be appropriate (4 g Na per day); for more severe edema, a low-Na diet (2 g Na per day) should be prescribed. Even when dietary restriction alone is unsuccessful and diuretic drugs are administered, the dietary Na intake must be restricted below 4 g/day for diuretics to be effective. A second important consideration before initiating diuretic therapy is to improve the general management of the patient by discontinuing, when possible, drugs that predispose to NaCl retention or interfere with diuretic efficacy. Nonsteroidal anti-inflammatory drugs promote renal NaCl retention directly and interfere with the efficacy of loop and DCT diuretics. Many vasodilators promote edema; minoxidil frequently causes significant ECF volume expansion; nifedipine promotes edema despite intrinsic natriuretic properties, through local vasodilation. Other antihypertensive drugs may also predispose to NaCl retention by reducing renal perfusion.

Once the decision to initiate diuretic therapy has been made, the initial choice of drug and dosage depends on the underlying cause of edema and its severity. Hypertension often responds to very low doses of a DCT diuretic (e.g., 12.5 mg/day of hydrochlorothiazide), doses that tend to cause few side effects. Cirrhotic edema and ascites frequently respond to spironolactone (50 to 300 mg daily); spironolactone appears to be more effective than furosemide in these patients. Moderate edema associated with congestive heart failure may respond to a DCT diuretic such as hydrochlorothiazide, in doses of 25 to 50 mg/day; some studies suggest that a DCT diuretic may reduce extracellular fluid volume more effectively than loop diuretics in patients with mild congestive heart failure. But when edema from congestive heart failure, cirrhosis, or nephrotic syndrome is more than mild, when renal function is impaired, or in the presence of pulmonary congestion or severe symptoms, loop diuretics are the drugs of choice. As mentioned previously, the addition of a small dose of spironolactone (25 to 50 mg/day) or eplerenone to traditional therapy of heart failure was recently shown to reduce morbidity and mortality in patients with left ventricular dysfunction; because this use of mineralocorticoid antagonists is designed primarily to prolong life, rather than to reduce the symptoms of ECF volume overload, it is not discussed at length in this chapter.

Loop diuretics have the highest natriuretic potency, are active at all levels of renal function, and act rapidly, even following oral administration. The drugs have steep dose-response relationships; as the dose is increased, there is little response until a critical threshold is reached, above which diuretic effectiveness increases rapidly to a maximum (Fig. 15-3). When a loop diuretic is administered in a dose that exceeds the threshold, most patients experience an increase in urine output that is noticeable during the several hours after diuretic ingestion. To be effective, each dose of loop diuretic must exceed this threshold. When initiating oral diuretic therapy, a target is set for weight loss and a low dose of loop diuretic (20 mg furosemide or its equivalent) is begun once or twice daily. If urine output increases during the 4 to 6 hours after diuretic ingestion (the patient can usually report a noticeable increase in urine volume), the same dose is continued on a daily basis (unless weight loss exceeds the target value). If urine output does not increase, the patient may double the dose the following day (to 40 mg once daily). If there is no response, the dose can be doubled each day until a response is obtained or until the maximum safe dose is achieved (usually 240 mg furosemide per dose). In normal individuals, 40 mg of furosemide orally produces maximal diuresis, but in patients with edema or abnormal kidney function, larger doses are frequently necessary (see Fig. 15-3). When kidney function is reduced, the loop diuretic dose-response curve shifts to the right. When the fractional Na excretion is plotted, the maximal effectiveness is unchanged. In contrast, when absolute Na excretion is plotted, the maximal effectiveness of loop diuretics can be seen to be reduced dramatically in the setting of chronic kidney disease (see Fig. 15-3). Even with impaired kidney function, however, there is little to be gained by increasing beyond 240 mg furosemide or 8 mg bumetanide per dose, because these doses reach the plateau of the dose-response curve. Some clinicians have reported that much higher doses of loop diuretics can be effective. Figure 15-3C suggests that an increased natriuresis following very high doses of loop diuretics results from more time at which diuretic levels are above the threshold. This prolonged duration, however, comes at the price of potential for toxicity (mostly ototoxicity). Most clinicians believe that more frequent but more moderate doses are just as effective and better tolerated. Adding an afternoon dose of a loop diuretic is often useful or even necessary for therapeutic success; but each dose must exceed the diuretic threshold for it to be useful.

Often the dose that elicits an increase in urine output can be continued indefinitely, because adaptive mechanisms such as those discussed previously bring the patient back into NaCl balance once ECF volume has been reduced. Sometimes, however, patients may be maintained with lower doses than were necessary to elicit diuresis initially, once control of the ECF volume is achieved.

DIURETIC RESISTANCE: CAUSES AND TREATMENT

Control of ECF volume expansion can be attained in most edematous patients using the approach outlined previously. In some circumstances, however, moderate or

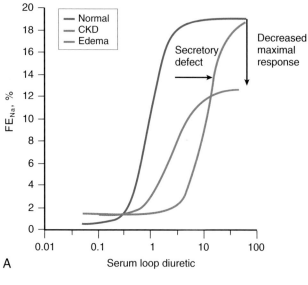

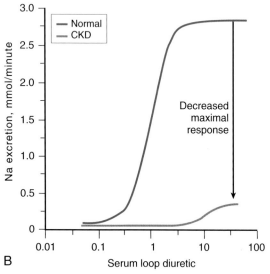

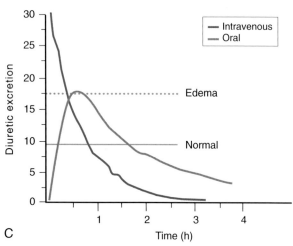

FIGURE 15-3 *A,* Comparison of effects of chronic kidney disease (CKD) and edematous conditions (edema) on the loop diuretic dose response, expressed as the fractional Na excretion (FE_{Na}). *B,* Effect of CKD on the absolute response to a loop diuretic. *C,* Pharmacokinetics of intravenous and oral loop diuretics. The diuretic thresholds (*A*) for normal and edematous individuals are shown as horizontal lines. Whereas a normal individual responds to either intravenous or oral diuretics, some edematous individuals achieve therapeutic levels only following intravenous treatment.

high doses of loop diuretics do not reduce ECF volume to the desired level, even when used appropriately. Such a patient is often deemed resistant to diuretic therapy. Determining what ECF volume is acceptable depends on many factors, including the severity of the underlying disease, patient preference, and comorbid illness. When further reductions in ECF volume are necessary, a systematic approach (Fig. 15-4) to diuretic resistance usually leads to a treatment regimen that is safe and effective. One of the most common causes of apparent resistance to diuretic drugs is dietary indiscretion because, as discussed previously, dietary NaCl excess abrogates the effect of most diuretic regimens; the influence of dietary NaCl intake is most pronounced for the loop diuretics because their half-lives are relatively short. If the patient's weight is stable but edema remains troubling, dietary compliance can be assessed by measuring the amount of Na excreted during 24 hours (always measure creatinine excretion at the same time to validate the collection). A urinary Na excretion rate greater than 100 to 120 mmol/ day (equivalent to 2.3 to 2.8 g Na per day) indicates both that the patient is ingesting too much NaCl and that true diuretic resistance is not present; daily Na excretion rates above 120 mmol should be sufficient to effect weight loss, when patients ingest less than 2 g of Na daily. Of course, dietary compliance cannot always be assured, and more intensive regimens may provide effective diuresis for patients who continue to ingest too much NaCl.

Gastrointestinal absorption of many diuretics is variable. The gastrointestinal absorption of furosemide varies by as much as 60% from day to day in a single individual (this effect is true of both Lasix and unbranded furosemide). It averages only 50% to 60%. Gastrointestinal absorption may be slowed further by edema of the gut, such as occurs in some patients with congestive heart failure. In contrast, the bioavailability of torsemide and bumetanide exceeds 80%, and some studies suggest this may provide more reliable diuresis. Alternatively, intravenous therapy may be necessary until edema is controlled; at this time, diuretic absorption may improve again and oral therapy may again become effective.

Once a loop or DCT diuretic drug has been absorbed into the blood stream, it reaches the lumen of kidney

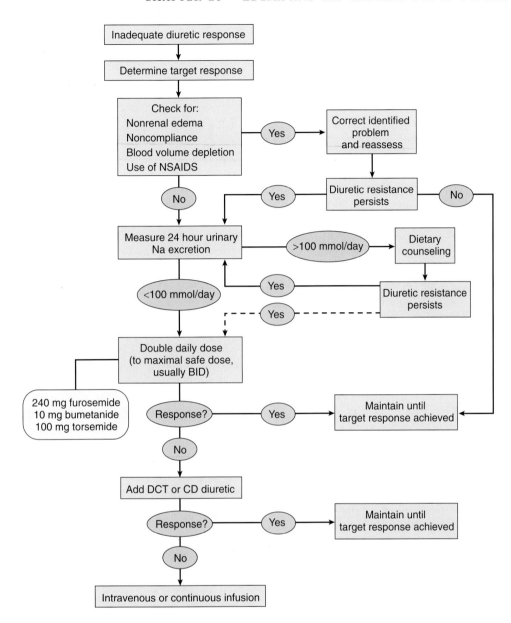

FIGURE 15-4   Algorithm for diuretic-resistant patients. Regimens for combination therapy are given in text. Maximum recommended single doses are provided in the yellow box. Note that higher doses have been used to treat patients with acute renal failure. Higher doses may provide additional natriuresis because of prolonged actions, but at the expense of increases in side effects. NSAIDs, nonsteroidal anti-inflammatory drugs. (Modified from Wilcox CS: Diuretics. In Brenner B [ed]: The Kidney, 5th ed. Philadelphia, WB Saunders, 1996, 2299–2330. With permission.)

tubules via the organic anion secretory pathway located in the proximal tubule. This pathway also interacts with nonsteroidal anti-inflammatory drugs and probenecid, as well as with endogenous anions that accumulate with impaired kidney function. When nonsteroidal anti-inflammatory drugs have been administered and in patients with impaired kidney function, diuretic secretion into the lumen of the proximal tubule is inhibited and less diuretic reaches its active site for any given serum concentration. To overcome the inhibition, higher

serum levels are needed. This is one reason that high doses of diuretic drugs are required to elicit diuresis in patients with impaired kidney function. Of note, although the ratio of equipotent doses of furosemide to bumetanide is 40:1 in patients with normal kidney function, it declines to 20:1 in patients with impaired kidney function because the renal clearance of furosemide is reduced (leading to relatively higher serum levels). In contrast, the clearance of bumetanide is maintained. In general, when switching from intravenous to oral furosemide, the starting oral dose is twice the intravenous dose (because of the limited bioavailability). When switching from intravenous to oral torsemide or bumetanide, the conversion is one to one because bioavailability is higher. In each case, however, it is necessary to confirm that an effective oral dose has been selected.

Diuretic resistance is common in patients with the nephrotic syndrome. Hypoalbuminemia reduces the serum concentration of diuretics because it increases their volume of distribution (diuretics are extensively protein bound), limiting diuretic delivery to the kidney. Furthermore, hypoalbuminemia may predispose to renal vasoconstriction and may inhibit diuretic secretion into kidney tubules directly. In these situations, increasing the diuretic dose, changing from oral to intravenous therapy, or infusing diuretic mixed together with albumin (ratio of 5 mg furosemide per gram of albumin) has been suggested to improve the therapeutic response. The use of albumin with loop diuretics has been extremely controversial. Several recent controlled studies showed modest improvements in natriuresis when albumin was infused with furosemide, compared with furosemide alone in patients with nephrotic syndrome. Yet the effects appear relatively modest. In one study, patients with resistant ascites were effectively treated by adding albumin, thereby increasing natriuresis and reducing hospitalization. The investigators concluded that albumin, in this setting, appeared to be cost effective.

Experiments in animal models suggested that diuretics bind to filtered albumin within kidney tubules of nephrotic patients. In several experimental model systems, this was shown to inhibit diuretic action. A more recent clinical study, however, indicated that urinary protein binding does not contribute significantly to the diuretic resistance of nephrotic patients; several recent studies indicate that changes in diuretic delivery to kidney tubules are also not primary contributors to diuretic resistance. Thus, the main cause of diuretic resistance in nephrosis is the strong primary stimulus to NaCl retention. High doses of loop diuretics, often used in combination with DCT diuretics, may be necessary to achieve diuresis in this patient population.

For patients in whom low cardiac output contributes to diuretic resistance retention, low-dose dopamine (2 to 4 µg/kg/minute) may increase renal plasma flow and increase urine flow (dopamine may also increase urine flow in patients with acute renal failure), but the effects of "renal dose" dopamine are controversial and poorly documented. When edema results from cirrhosis of the liver, removal of ascitic fluid by paracentesis or peritoneovenous shunting may improve renal function and Na excretion. Arterial hypoxemia causes renal vasoconstriction, resulting in antinatriuresis, which reverses promptly when the arterial oxygen tension increases above 60 mm Hg. Renal vasoconstrictors, such as nonsteroidal anti-inflammatory drugs and adrenergic agonists, may also lead to diuretic resistance, in part by reducing

glomerular filtration rate, and should be avoided in the diuretic-resistant patient. The effects of drugs used to reduce cardiac afterload on renal NaCl excretion are complex. When angiotensin-converting enzyme inhibitors or nitroprusside increase cardiac output effectively, they may stimulate natriuresis and reduce edema. On the other hand, when aggressive therapy reduces blood pressure beyond a critical threshold (which may be surprisingly high in patients with severe vascular disease), it may lead to NaCl retention and even acute renal failure. This is especially common during concomitant administration of nonsteroidal anti-inflammatory drugs, when bilateral renal artery stenosis is present, or during very aggressive diuretic therapy.

One new approach to diuretic resistance in patients with systolic dysfunction who are hospitalized is to use intravenous nesiritide (β-type natriuretic peptide). The atrial peptides have many potential benefits for such patients. In addition to increasing urinary Na, Cl, and water excretion, these agents reduce pulmonary capillary wedge pressure and systemic vascular resistance and increase cardiac output. Unlike the loop diuretics, these drugs suppress the renin-angiotensin-aldosterone axis, a potentially beneficial difference. Nevertheless, the role of nesiritide continues to be defined, and outcome studies comparing nesiritide to inotropes and diuretics are limited. Patients who may benefit from nesiritide include those in whom tachycardia or arrhythmias limit the use of positive inotropes, those who appear resistant to loop diuretics, and those in whom impaired kidney function complicates heart failure. Hypotension is a potential complication of this agent.

Not uncommonly, simple approaches to diuretic resistance fail. Several strategies can be used to control ECF volume in such patients (see Fig. 15-4). First, it is often necessary to increase the frequency of loop diuretic administration, especially if postdiuretic Na retention is contributing importantly to NaCl retention. However, each dose must be above the diuretic threshold to be effective (see Fig. 15-3). Patients often can notice a distinct increase in urine output within several hours of each dose of diuretic if the dose is in the appropriate range. Second, another class of diuretic may be added to a regimen that includes a loop diuretic. This strategy produces true synergism; the combination of agents is more effective than the sum of the responses to each agent alone. DCT diuretics are the class of drug most commonly combined with loop diuretics, although diuretic synergism also occurs when loop diuretics are combined with carbonic anhydrase inhibitors. The addition of acetazolamide to a loop diuretic is especially useful for patients in whom metabolic alkalosis is exacerbating hypoventilation, in the setting of volume overload. These drugs may act synergistically for several reasons. Loop diuretics increase NaCl delivery to the distal tubule, a site at which NaCl transport depends on the luminal NaCl concentration. Loop diuretics, there-

TABLE 15-2 Continuous Diuretic Infusion

Diuretic	Loading Dose (mg)	Creatinine Clearance <25 mL/min (mg/hour)	Creatinine Clearance 25–75 mL/min (mg/hour)	Creatinine Clearance >75 mL/min (mg/hour)
Furosemide	40	20–40	10–20	10
Torsemide	20	10–20	5–10	5
Bumetanide	1	1–2	0.5–1	0.5

Data from Brater DC: Diuretic therapy. N Engl J Med 339:387–395, 1998.

fore, stimulate NaCl reabsorption along the nephron segment that is sensitive to DCT diuretics. Adding a DCT diuretic will inhibit NaCl transport along the stimulated segment, thereby eliciting a larger effect than would a DCT diuretic, when given alone. Furthermore, when loop diuretics are administered chronically, cells in the distal tubule become hypertrophic, increasing their ability to reabsorb NaCl. DCT diuretics inhibit the increased NaCl reabsorption that accompanies hypertrophy of the distal nephron and therefore counteract the effects of hypertrophy. Finally, DCT diuretics have longer half-lives than loop diuretics. These drugs therefore prevent or attenuate NaCl retention during the periods when loop diuretic action wanes, thereby increasing their net effect. Thus, at least three mechanisms contribute to the ability of DCT diuretics to act synergistically with loop diuretics.

When two diuretics are combined, the DCT diuretic is generally administered before the loop diuretic (1 hour is reasonable) to ensure that NaCl transport in the distal nephron is blocked when the tubule is flooded with solute. When intravenous therapy is indicated, chlorothiazide (500 to 1000 mg) may be used. Metolazone is the DCT diuretic most frequently combined with loop diuretics because its half-life is relatively long (as formulated in Zaroxolyn) and because it has been reported to be effective even when kidney function is severely impaired. Other thiazide and thiazide-like diuretics, however, are probably equally effective, even with abnormal kidney function. The dramatic effectiveness of combination diuretic therapy is accompanied by complications in a significant number of patients. Massive fluid and electrolyte losses have led to circulatory collapse during combination therapy, and patients must be followed carefully. The lowest effective dose of DCT diuretic should be added to the loop diuretic regimen; patients can frequently be treated with combination therapy for only a few days and then placed back on a single drug regimen; when contin-

uous combination therapy is needed, low doses of DCT diuretic (2.5 mg metolazone or 25 mg hydrochlorothiazide) administered only two or three times per week may be sufficient.

For hospitalized patients who are resistant to diuretic therapy, a different approach is to infuse loop diuretics continuously (Table 15-2 and Fig. 15-4). Continuous diuretic infusions have several advantages over bolus diuretic administration. First, because they avoid peaks and troughs of diuretic concentration, continuous infusions prevent periods of positive NaCl balance (postdiuretic NaCl retention) from occurring. Second, continuous infusions are more efficient than bolus therapy (the amount of NaCl excreted per milligram of drug administered is greater). Third, some patients who are resistant to large doses of diuretics given by bolus have responded to continuous infusion. Fourth, diuretic response can be titrated; in the intensive care unit, where obligate fluid administration must be balanced by fluid excretion, excellent control of NaCl and water excretion can be obtained. Finally, complications associated with high doses of loop diuretics, such as ototoxicity, appear to occur less frequently when large doses are administered as continuous infusion. Total daily furosemide doses exceeding 1 g have been tolerated well when administered over 24 hours, but a more cautious dosing regimen is provided in Table 15-2.

Most patients who are deemed resistant to diuretics respond to these approaches. Increases in serum creatinine and other side effects of diuretic therapy often limit the ability to reduce ECF volume more than does a lack of efficacy. Obtaining effective control of ECF volume without provoking complications requires a thorough understanding of diuretic physiology and a commitment to use diuretics rationally and carefully. When used in this manner, they remain among the most powerful drugs in clinical medicine.

BIBLIOGRAPHY

Agarwal R, Gorski JC, Sundblad K, Brater DC: Urinary protein binding does not affect response to furosemide in patients with nephrotic syndrome. J Am Soc Nephrol 11:1100–1105, 2000.

Brater DC: Diuretic therapy. N Engl J Med 339:387–395, 1998.

Chalasani N, Gorski JC, Horlander JCS, et al: Effects of albumin/furosemide mixtures on responses to furosemide in hypoalbuminemic patients. J Am Soc Nephrol 12:1010–1016, 2001.

Colucci WS, Elkayam U, Horton DP, et al: Intravenous nesiritide, a natriuretic peptide, in the treatment of decompensated congestive heart failure. Nesiritide Study Group. N Engl J Med 343:246–253, 2000.

Ellison DH: Diuretic resistance: Physiology and therapeutics. Semin Nephrol 19:581–597, 1999.

Ellison DH: Diuretic therapy and resistance in congestive heart failure. Cardiology 96:132–143, 2001.

Greenberg A: Diuretic complications. Am J Med Sci 319:10–24, 2000.

Howard PA, Dunn MI: Severe heart failure in the elderly: Potential benefits of high-dose and continuous infusion diuretics. Drugs Aging 19:249–256, 2002.

Okusa MD, Ellison DH: Physiology and pathophysiology of diuretic action. In Seldin DW, Giebisch G (eds): The Kidney: Physiology and Pathophysiology. Philadelphia, Lippincott Williams & Wilkins, 2000, pp 2877–2922.

Pitt B, Williams G, Remme W, Martinez F, et al: The EPHESUS trial: Eplerenone in patients with heart failure due to systolic dysfunction complicating acute myocardial infarction. Eplerenone Post-AMI Heart Failure Efficacy and Survival Study. Cardiovasc Drugs Ther 15:79–87, 2001.

Wilcox CS: New insights into diuretic use in patients with chronic renal disease. J Am Soc Nephrol 13:798–805, 2002.

Glomerular Diseases

CHAPTER 16

Glomerular Clinicopathologic Syndromes

J. Charles Jennette   Ronald J. Falk

Injury to glomeruli results in a multiplicity of signs and symptoms of disease, including proteinuria caused by altered permeability of capillary walls, hematuria caused by rupture of capillary walls, azotemia caused by impaired filtration of nitrogenous wastes, oliguria or anuria caused by reduced urine production, edema caused by salt and water retention, and hypertension caused by fluid retention and disturbed renal homeostasis of blood pressure. The nature and severity of disease in a given patient is dictated by the nature and severity of glomerular injury.

Specific glomerular diseases tend to produce characteristic syndromes of kidney dysfunction, but multiple different glomerular diseases can produce the same syndrome (Tables 16-1 and 16-2). The diagnosis of a glomerular disease requires recognition of one of these syndromes followed by collection of data to determine which specific glomerular disease is present. Alternatively, if reaching a specific diagnosis is not possible or not necessary, the physician should at least narrow the differential diagnosis to a likely candidate disease.

Evaluation of pathologic features identified in a kidney biopsy specimen is often required for a definitive diagnosis. The pathologic features of various glomerular diseases are described in the corresponding chapters of this book. Figure 16-1 depicts some of the clinical and pathologic features used to resolve the differential diagnosis in patients with antibody-mediated glomerulonephritis, Figures 16-2 through 16-5 illustrate the distinctive ultrastructural features of some of the major categories of glomerular disease, and Figure 16-6 illustrates some of the major patterns of immune deposition identified by immunofluorescence microscopy.

ASYMPTOMATIC HEMATURIA AND RECURRENT GROSS HEMATURIA

Hematuria is usually defined as greater than three red blood cells per high-power field observed by microscopic examination of a centrifuged urine sediment (see Chapters 3 and 4 for more details). Hematuria is asymptomatic when a patient is unaware of its presence and it is not accompanied by clinical manifestations of nephritis or nephrotic syndrome, that is, without azotemia, oliguria, edema, or hypertension. Asymptomatic microscopic hematuria occurs in 5% to 10% of the general population. Recurrent gross hematuria may be superimposed on asymptomatic microscopic hematuria, or may occur in isolation. The patient observes urine discoloration, which often is described as tea colored or cola colored.

Most hematuria is not of glomerular origin. Glomerular diseases cause less than 10% of hematuria in patients with no proteinuria, with almost 80% caused by bladder, prostate, or urethral disease. Hypercalciuria and hyperuricosuria also can cause asymptomatic hematuria, especially in children.

Microscopic examination of the urine can help determine whether hematuria is of glomerular or nonglomerular origin. Chemical (e.g., osmotic) and physical damage to red blood cells as they pass through the nephron causes structural changes that are not present in red blood cells that have passed directly into the urine from a gross parenchymal injury in the kidney (e.g., a neoplasm or infection) or from a lesion in the urinary tract (e.g., renal pelvis traumatized by stones or an inflamed bladder). Dysmorphic red blood cells that have transited the urinary tract from the glomeruli usually have lost their biconcave configuration and hemoglobin, and often have multiple membrane blebs, sometimes producing acanthocytes and "Mickey Mouse" cells. The presence of red blood cell casts and substantial proteinuria (more than 2g/24 hours) also supports a glomerular origin for hematuria.

Published kidney biopsy series conducted in patients with asymptomatic hematuria show differences in the frequencies of identified underlying glomerular lesions. Differences in the nature of the population analyzed (e.g., military recruits versus routine physical examination patients), and differences in pathologic analysis (e.g., failure of the earlier studies to recognize thin basement membrane nephropathy) account for the observed disparities. The data presented in Table 16-3 are derived from patients with hematuria who underwent diagnostic kidney biopsy. The data in the first column equate with asymptomatic hematuria and are similar to other

TABLE 16-1   Clinical Manifestations of Glomerular Diseases, and Representative Diseases that Present with These Manifestations*

Asymptomatic proteinuria
  Focal segmental glomerulosclerosis
  Mesangioproliferative GN

Nephrotic syndrome
  Minimal change glomerulopathy
  Membranous glomerulopathy
    Idiopathic (primary)
    Secondary (e.g., lupus)
  Focal segmental glomerulosclerosis
  Mesangioproliferative GN
  Type I membranoproliferative GN
  Type II membranoproliferative GN
  Fibrillary GN
  Diabetic glomerulosclerosis
  Amyloidosis
  Light chain deposition disease

Asymptomatic microscopic hematuria
  Thin basement membrance nephropathy
  IgA nephropathy
  Mesangioproliferative GN
  Alport's syndrome

Recurrent gross hematuria
  Thin basement membrane nephropathy
  IgA nephropathy
  Alport's syndrome

Acute nephritis
  Acute diffuse proliferative GN
    Poststreptococcal GN
    Poststaphylococcal GN

Focal or diffuse proliferative GN
  IgA nephropathy
  Lupus nephritis

Type I membranoproliferative GN

Type II membranoproliferative GN

Fibrillary GN

Rapidly progressive nephritis
  Crescentic GN
    Anti-GBM GN
    Immune complex GN
    ANCA GN

Pulmonary-renal vasculitic syndrome
  Goodpasture's (anti-GBM) syndrome
  Immune complex vasculitis
  Lupus

ANCA vasculitis
  Microscopic polyangiitis
  Wegener's granulomatosis
  Churg-Strauss syndrome

Chronic kidney disease
  Chronic sclerosing GN

ANCA, antineutrophil cytoplasmic antibody; GBM, glomerular basement membrane; GN, glomerulonephritis.
*The same manifestations can be caused by different diseases, and the same disease can manifest in different ways.

TABLE 16-2   Tendencies of Glomerular Diseases to Manifest Nephrotic and Nephritic Features*

	Nephrotic Features	Nephritic Features
Minimal change glomerulopathy	++++	–
Membranous glomerulopathy	++++	+
Diabetic glomerulosclerosis	++++	+
Amyloidosis	++++	+
Focal segmental glomerulosclerosis	+++	++
Fibrillary glomerulonephritis	+++	++
Mesangioproliferative glomerulopathy[†]	++	++
Membranoproliferative glomerulonephritis[‡]	++	+++
Proliferative glomerulonephritis[†]	++	+++
Acute diffuse proliferative glomerulonephritis[§]	+	++++
Crescentic glomerulonephritis[#]	+	++++

*Most diseases can manifest both nephrotic and nephritic features, but there usually is a tendency for one to predominate.
[†]Mesangioproliferative and proliferative glomerulonephritis (focal or diffuse) are structural manifestations of a number of glomerulonephritides, including IgA nephropathy and lupus nephritis.
[‡]Both type I (mesangiocapillary) and type II (dense deposit disease).
[§]Often a structural manifestation of acute poststreptococcal glomerulonephritis.
[#]Can be immune complex mediated, anti–glomerular basement membrane antibody mediated, or associated with antineutrophil cytoplasmic antibodies.
Modified from Jennette JC, Mandal AK: The nephrotic syndrome. In Mandal AK, Jennette JC (eds): Diagnosis and Management of Renal Disease and Hypertension. Durham, NC, Carolina Academic Press, 1994.

TABLE 16-3   Renal Disease in Patients with Hematuria Undergoing Kidney Biopsy*

	Prot <1 Cr <1.5	Prot 1-3	Cr 1.5-3.0	Cr >3
No abnormality	30%	2%	1%	0%
Thin BM nephropathy	26%	4%	3%	0%
IgA nephropathy	28%	24%	14%	8%
GN without crescents[†]	9%	26%	37%	23%
GN with crescents[†]	2%	24%	21%	44%
Other kidney disease[‡]	5%	20%	24%	25%
Total	100% n = 43	100% n = 123	100% n = 179	100% n = 255

BM, basement membrane; Cr, serum creatinine (mg/dL); GN, glomerulonephritis; Prot, proteinuria (g/24 hr).
*An analysis of kidney biopsy specimens evaluated by the University of North Carolina Nephropathology Laboratory. Patients with systemic lupus erythematosus have been excluded from the analysis.
[†]Proliferative or necrotizing GN other than IgA nephropathy or lupus nephritis.
[‡]Includes causes for the nephrotic syndrome, such as membranous glomerulopathy and focal segmental glomerulosclerosis.
Derived from Caldas MLR, Jennette JC, Falk RJ, Wilkman AS: NC Glomerular Disease Collaborative Network: What is found by renal biopsy in patients with hematuria? Lab Invest 62:15A, 1990.

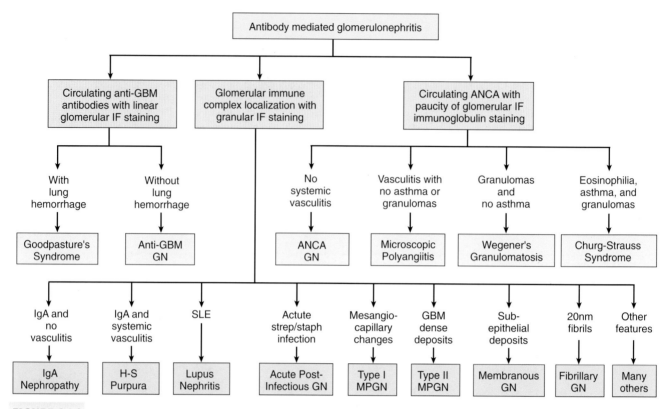

FIGURE 16-1   Features that distinguish among different immunopathologic categories of antibody-mediated glomerulonephritis. ANCA, antineutrophil cytoplasmic antibody; GBM, glomerular basement membrane; GN, glomerulonephritis; H-S, Henoch-Schönlein; IF, immunofluorescence microscopy; MPGN, membranoproliferative glomerulonephritis; SLE, systemic lupus erythematosus.

recent series. In these patients with hematuria, less than 1 g/24 hours proteinuria, and serum creatinine less than 1.5 mg/dL, the three major findings were no pathologic abnormality (30%), thin basement membrane nephropathy (26%), and immunoglobulin A (IgA) nephropathy (28%). Whereas thin basement membrane nephropathy virtually always manifests as asymptomatic hematuria or recurrent gross hematuria, IgA nephropathy can manifest as any of the syndromes listed in Table 16-1.

Alport's syndrome is a hereditary disease caused by a defect in the genes that code for basement membrane type IV collagen (see Chapter 46). Approximately 85% of patients have a mutation in the X-chromosomal α-5 gene and 15% in the autosomal α-3 and α-4 genes. In affected men, Alport's syndrome initially manifests as asymptomatic microscopic hematuria, sometimes with superimposed episodes of gross hematuria. Although relatively similar within a given kindred, the onset of symptoms varies from childhood to adulthood and typically begins with isolated hematuria. Progressively worsening proteinuria and endstage renal disease (ESRD) may eventually develop, although the rate of progression is quite variable. Affected women, who are almost always heterozygous, often have intermittent microscopic hematuria but may have no other manifestations of kidney disease.

Kidney biopsy is not usually performed to evaluate asymptomatic hematuria. Kidney biopsy diagnoses

rarely affect treatment in patients with asymptomatic hematuria, but occasional patients will be found to have disease that might benefit from treatment (e.g., the one patient with early crescentic glomerulonephritis identified in the cohort of patients in the first column of Table 16-3). Kidney biopsy can also be of some prognostic value. For example, thin basement membrane nephropathy has a better prognosis and a much greater propensity for familial occurrence than IgA nephropathy. Many patients with asymptomatic hematuria are subjected to repeated invasive urologic evaluations until a definitive diagnosis can be made. In these patients, additional urologic evaluation can be prevented if kidney biopsy provides a diagnosis.

In kidney biopsy specimens, thin basement membrane nephropathy is suspected if there is thinning of the glomerular basement membrane lamina densa (see Fig. 16-3), whereas Alport's syndrome is suspected if there is marked lamination of the lamina densa. However, it is important to note that in a few patients thin basement membrane lesions rather than laminations may be the ultrastructural manifestation of Alport's syndrome. In Alport's syndrome, the kidney and skin also have diagnostically useful abnormalities in immunohistologic staining for the alpha chains of type IV collagen. The presence of mesangial immune deposits with a dominance or codominance of immunohistologic staining for IgA is diagnostic for IgA nephropathy (see Fig. 16-6).

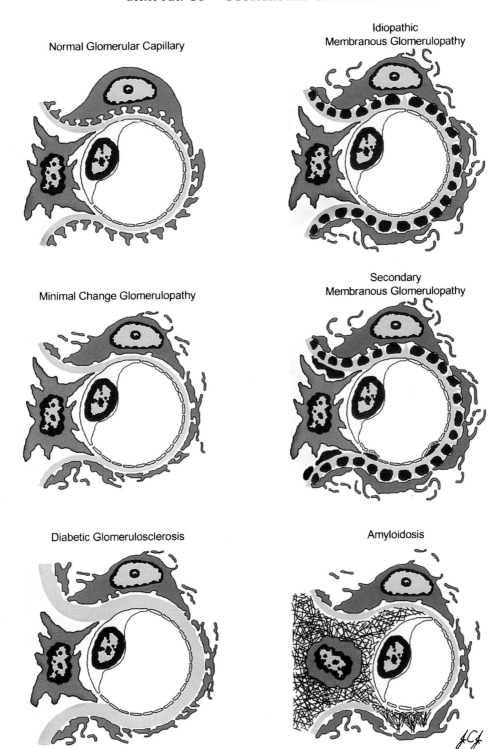

FIGURE 16-2 Ultrastructural changes in glomerular capillaries of glomerular diseases that cause the nephrotic syndrome. Normal glomerular capillary: note the visceral epithelial cell with intact foot processes (*green*), endothelial cell with fenestrations (*yellow*), mesangial cell (*red*) with adjacent mesangial matrix (*light gray*), and basement membrane with lamina densa (*dark gray*) that does not completely surround the capillary lumen but splays out as the paramesangial basement membrane. Minimal change glomerulopathy: note the effacement of foot processes and microvillous transformation. Diabetic glomerulosclerosis: note the thickening of the lamina densa and expansion of mesangial matrix. Idiopathic membranous glomerulopathy: note the subepithelial dense deposits with adjacent projections of basement membrane (see also Fig. 16-5). Secondary membranous glomerulopathy: note the mesangial and small subendothelial deposits in addition to the requisite subepithelial deposits. Amyloidosis: note the fibrils within the mesangium and capillary wall. (From Jennette JC. With permission.)

Thin Basement Membrane
Nephropathy

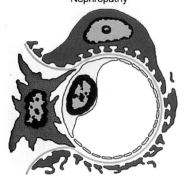

Proliferative Lupus
Glomerulonephritis

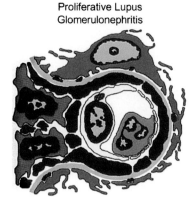

Mesangioproliferative
Glomerulonephritis

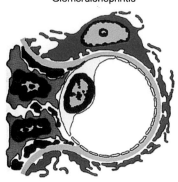

Type I Membranoproliferative
Glomerulonephritis

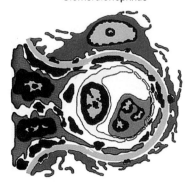

Acute Postinfectious
Glomerulonephritis

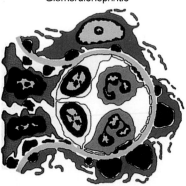

Type II Membranoproliferative
Glomerulonephritis

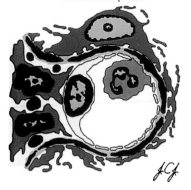

FIGURE 16-3   Ultrastructural changes in glomerular capillaries of glomerular diseases that cause hematuria and the nephritic syndrome. Thin basement membrane nephropathy: note the thin lamina densa of the basement membrane. Mesangioproliferative glomerulonephritis (e.g., mild lupus nephritis or IgA nephropathy): note the mesangial dense deposits and mesangial hypercellularity. Acute diffuse proliferative glomerulonephritis (e.g., poststreptococcal glomerulonephritis): note the endocapillary hypercellularity contributed to by leukocytes, endothelial cells, and mesangial cells, and the dense deposits, including not only conspicuous subepithelial "humps" but also inconspicuous subendothelial and mesangial deposits. Proliferative lupus glomerulonephritis (see also Fig. 16-4): note the extensive subendothelial and mesangial dense deposits. Type I membranoproliferative glomerulonephritis (mesangiocapillary glomerulonephritis): note the subendothelial deposits with associated subendothelial interposition of mesangial cytoplasm and deposition of new matrix material resulting in basement membrane replication. Type II membranoproliferative glomerulonephritis (dense deposit disease): note the intramembranous and mesangial dense deposits. (From Jennette JC. With permission.)

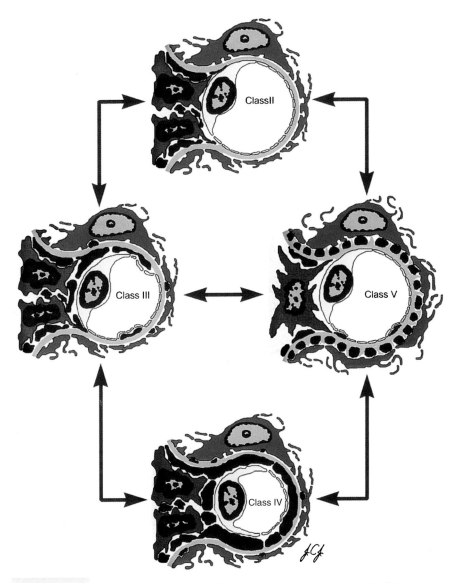

FIGURE 16-4   Ultrastructural features of the major classes of lupus nephritis. The sequestration of immune deposits within the mesangium in class II (mesangioproliferative) lupus glomerulonephritis causes only mesangial hyperplasia and mild renal dysfunction. Substantial amounts of subendothelial immune deposits, which are adjacent to the inflammatory mediator systems of the blood, cause focal (class III) or diffuse (class IV) proliferative lupus glomerulonephritis with overt nephritic signs and symptoms. Localization of immune deposits predominantly in the subepithelial zone causes membranous (class V) lupus glomerulonephritis, which usually manifests predominantly as the nephrotic syndrome. (From Jennette JC. With permission.)

ACUTE GLOMERULONEPHRITIS AND RAPIDLY PROGRESSIVE GLOMERULONEPHRITIS

Acute and rapidly progressive glomerulonephritis often present with acute onset of manifestations of nephritis, such as azotemia, oliguria, edema, hypertension, protein-uria, and hematuria with an "active" urine sediment that often contains red blood cell casts, pigmented casts, and cellular debris. Rapidly progressive glomerulonephritis leads to a 50% or greater loss of kidney function within weeks to months. If kidney dysfunction is severe, manifestations of uremia develop, such as nausea and vomiting, hiccups, dyspnea, lethargy, pericarditis, and encephalopathy. Severe volume overload can cause congestive heart failure and pulmonary edema.

The pathologic processes that most often produce the clinical manifestations of acute or rapidly progressive glomerulonephritis are inflammatory glomerular lesions. The nature and severity of the glomerular inflammation correlate with the clinical features of the glomeru-

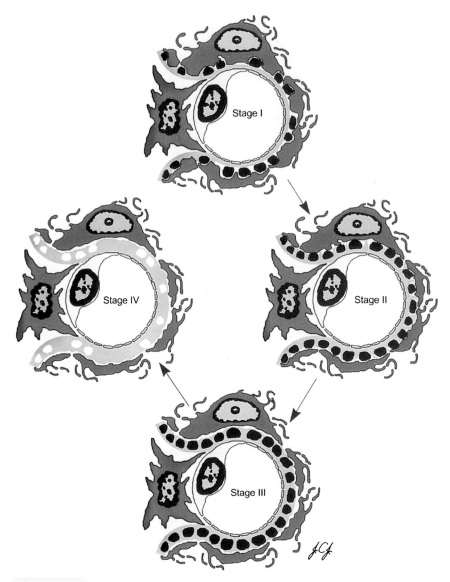

FIGURE 16-5 Ultrastructural stages in the progression of membranous glomerulopathy. Stage I has subepithelial electron dense immune complex deposits without adjacent projections of basement membrane material. Stage II has adjacent glomerular basement membrane (GBM) projections that eventually surround the electron-dense immune deposits in stage III. Stage IV has a markedly thickened GBM with electron lucent zones replacing the electron dense deposits. (From Jennette JC. With permission.)

lonephritis (Fig. 16-7). Note in Figure 16-7 that the structural stages of glomerular inflammation can change over time, and this is reflected by changes in the clinical manifestations of glomerulonephritis.

The least severe structural injury that can be discerned by light microscopy is mesangial hyperplasia alone, which usually is associated with asymptomatic proteinuria or hematuria rather than overt nephritis. Proliferative glomerulonephritis, which may be focal (affecting less than 50% of glomeruli) or diffuse (affecting greater than 50% of glomeruli), is characterized histologically not only by the proliferation of glomerular cells (e.g., mesangial, endothelial, and epithelial cells)

but also by the influx of leukocytes, especially neutrophils and mononuclear phagocytes. Necrosis may be present, especially in disease caused by antineutrophil cytoplasmic antibodies (ANCAs) or anti–glomerular basement membrane (anti-GBM) antibodies. Chronic changes, such as glomerular sclerosis, interstitial fibrosis, and tubular atrophy begin to develop within a week of the onset of destructive glomerular inflammation, and become the dominant features in chronic glomerulonephritis.

Lupus glomerulonephritis (see Chapter 27) provides a paradigm of the interrelationships among pathogenic mechanisms, pathologic consequences, and clinical

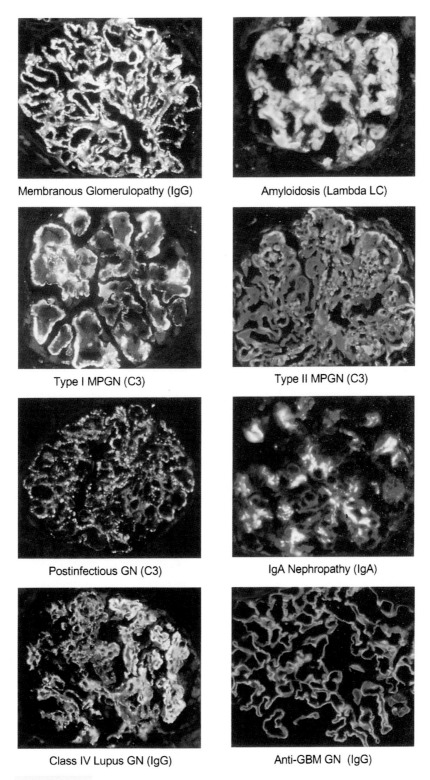

Membranous Glomerulopathy (IgG)   Amyloidosis (Lambda LC)

Type I MPGN (C3)   Type II MPGN (C3)

Postinfectious GN (C3)   IgA Nephropathy (IgA)

Class IV Lupus GN (IgG)   Anti-GBM GN (IgG)

FIGURE 16-6   Immunofluorescence microscopy staining patterns for membranous glomerulopathy: note the global granular capillary wall staining for IgG. AL amyloidosis: note the irregular fluffy staining for light chains. Type I membranoproliferative glomerulonephritis (MPGN): note the peripheral granular to bandlike staining for C3. Type II MPGN: note the bandlike capillary wall and coarsely granular mesangial staining for C3. Acute postinfectious glomerulonephritis: note the coarsely granular capillary wall staining for C3. IgA nephropathy: note the mesangial staining for IgA. Class IV lupus nephritis: note the segmentally variable capillary wall and mesangial staining for IgG. Anti–glomerular basement membrane (anti-GBM) glomerulonephritis: note the linear GBM staining for IgG.

Light Microscopic Morphology

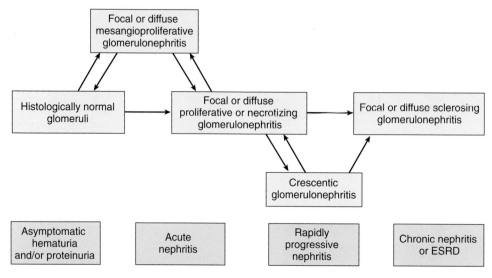

FIGURE 16-7 Morphologic stages of glomerulonephritis (*top*) aligned with the usual clinical manifestations (*bottom*). Certain glomerular diseases, such as anti–glomerular basement membrane (anti-GBM) and ANCA glomerulonephritis, usually have crescentic glomerulonephritis with rapid decline in kidney function if not promptly treated. Others, such as lupus nephritis, have a predilection for causing focal or diffuse proliferative glomerulonephritis with variable rates of progression dependent on the activity of the glomerular lesions. IgA nephropathy tends to begin as mild mesangioproliferative lesions but may progress into more severe proliferative lesions. Poststreptococcal glomerulonephritis typically initially develops an active acute proliferative glomerulonephritis but then resolves through a mesangioproliferative phase to normal. Still others, such as IgM mesangial nephropathy, rarely progress past the mesangioproliferative phase. (Reprinted from Jennette JC, Mandal AK: Syndrome of glomerulonephritis. In Mandal AK, Jennette JC [eds]: Diagnosis and Management of Renal Disease and Hypertension, 2nd ed. Durham, NC, Carolina Academic Press, 1994. With permission.)

manifestations of immune complex glomerular disease (see Fig. 16-4). The mildest expression of lupus nephritis (mesangioproliferative lupus glomerulonephritis, class II lupus nephritis) is induced by exclusively mesangial localization of immune complexes, which usually causes only mild nephritis or asymptomatic hematuria and proteinuria. Localization of substantial amounts of nephritogenic immune complexes in the subendothelial zones of glomerular capillaries where they are adjacent to the inflammatory mediator systems in the blood induces overt glomerular inflammation (focal or diffuse proliferative lupus glomerulonephritis, class III or IV lupus nephritis) and usually causes severe clinical manifestations of nephritis. Qualitative and quantitative characteristics of the pathogenic immune complexes that result in localization predominantly in subepithelial zones where they are not in contact with the inflammatory mediator systems in the blood induces membranous lupus glomerulonephritis (class V lupus nephritis). This variant is usually associated with the nephrotic syndrome rather than nephritis. As the nephritogenic immune response in a given patient changes over time, sometimes modified by treatment, transitions may occur between different lupus nephritis phenotypes.

The structurally most severe form of active glomerulonephritis is crescentic glomerulonephritis, which usually manifests clinically as rapidly progressive glomerulonephritis. In patients with new-onset kidney disease who have a nephritic sediment and a serum creatinine of greater than 3 mg/dL, glomerulonephritis with crescents is the most common finding in kidney biopsy specimens (see Table 16-3). Crescents are proliferations of cells within Bowman's capsule that include both mononuclear phagocytes and glomerular epithelial cells. Crescent formation is a response to glomerular rupture, and therefore is a marker of severe glomerular injury. Crescents do not indicate the cause of glomerular injury, however, because many different pathogenic mechanisms can cause crescent formation. There is no consensus on how many glomeruli should have crescents in order to use the term *crescentic glomerulonephritis* in the diagnosis. Most pathologists use the term when greater than 50% of glomeruli have crescents, but the percentage of glomeruli with crescents should be specified in the diagnosis even if it is less than 50% (e.g., IgA nephropathy with focal proliferative glomerulonephritis and 25% crescents). Within a specific pathogenic category of glomerulonephritis (e.g., anti-GBM disease, ANCA disease, lupus glomerulonephritis, IgA nephropathy, poststreptococcal glomerulonephritis), the higher the fraction of glomeruli with crescents, the worse the prognosis. Among pathogenetically different forms of glomerulonephritis, however, the pathogenic category may be more important in predicting outcome than the presence of crescents. For example, a patient with poststreptococcal glomerulonephritis with 50% crescents has a much better prognosis for kidney survival, even without immunosuppressive treatment, than a patient with anti-GBM glomerulonephritis or ANCA glomerulonephritis with 25% crescents.

This importance of pathogenic category in predicting the natural history of glomerulonephritis indicates that the pathologic diagnosis of glomerulonephritis into the light microscopic morphologic categories in Figure 16-7 is not adequate for optimum patient management. In addition to determining the morphologic severity of glomerular inflammation, the pathogenic or immunopathologic category of disease must be determined. If a kidney biopsy is performed, this is usually done by immunohistology and electron microscopy (see Figs. 16-1 through 16-6). Immunohistology reveals the presence or absence of immunoglobulins and complement components. The distribution (e.g., capillary wall, mesangium), pattern (e.g., granular, linear), and composition (e.g., IgA-dominant, IgG-dominant, IgM-dominant) of immunoglobulin is useful for determining specific types of glomerulonephritis, as will be discussed in detail in later chapters that address specific types of glomerular disease.

Table 16-4 gives the frequencies of the major pathologic categories of glomerulonephritis in patients with crescents who have undergone kidney biopsy. The immune complex category contains a variety of diseases, including lupus nephritis, IgA nephropathy, and poststreptococcal glomerulonephritis. Note that most patients with greater than 50% crescents have little or no immunohistologic evidence for immune complex or anti-GBM antibody localization within glomeruli (i.e., pauci-immune glomerulonephritis). Over 80% of these patients with pauci-immune crescentic glomerulonephritis have circulating ANCAs. Thus, ANCA glomerulonephritis is the most common form of crescentic glomerulonephritis, especially in older adults.

Because both the structural severity (e.g., see morphologic stages in Fig. 16-7) and immunopathologic category of disease (e.g., see the categories given in Figs. 16-1 through 16-6, such as IgA nephropathy, lupus nephritis, and anti-GBM disease) are important in predicting the course of disease in a patient with glomerulonephritis, the most useful diagnostic term should include information about both (e.g., focal proliferative IgA nephropathy, diffuse proliferative lupus glomerulonephritis, crescentic anti-GBM glomerulonephritis).

Because they often are immune-mediated inflammatory diseases, many types of glomerulonephritis are treated with corticosteroids, cytotoxic drugs, or other anti-inflammatory and immunosuppressive agents. The aggressiveness of the treatment, of course, should match the aggressiveness of the disease. For example, active class IV lupus nephritis warrants immunosuppressive treatment, whereas class II lupus nephritis does not.

The two most aggressive forms of glomerulonephritis are anti-GBM crescentic glomerulonephritis and ANCA crescentic glomerulonephritis. The most important factor in improving renal outcome is early diagnosis and treatment. Once extensive sclerosis of glomeruli and advanced chronic tubulointerstitial injury have developed, significant response to treatment is unlikely. Both diseases are treated with immunosuppressive regimens, for example, pulse methylprednisolone and intravenous or oral cyclophosphamide. Plasmapheresis is usually added to the regimen for anti-GBM disease and for ANCA disease with pulmonary hemorrhage. Immunosuppressive treatment generally can be terminated after 4 to 5 months in patients with anti-GBM glomerulonephritis with little risk for recurrence (see Chapter 22). The initial induction of remission for ANCA glomerulonephritis often is performed for 6 to 12 months, and even then there is an approximately 25% risk for recurrence that will require additional immunosuppression (see Chapter 26).

TABLE 16-4   Frequency of Different Type of Crescentic Glomerulonephritis* Relative to Age in Consecutive Native Kidney Biopsy Specimens

	Pauci-Immune	Immune Complex	Anti-GBM	Other[†]
All (n = 632)	60%	24%	15%	1%
Age 1–20 yr (n = 73)	42%	45%	125	0%
Age 21–60 yr (n = 303)	48%	35%	15%	3%
Age 61–100 yr (n = 256)	79%	65%	15%	0%

*Crescentic glomerulonephritis was defined as glomerular disease with 50% or more crescents.
[†]The "other" category includes all other glomerular diseases, such as thrombotic microangiopathy, diabetic glomerulosclerosis, monoclonal immunoglobulin deposition disease, etc.
Modified from Jennette JC: Rapidly progressive and crescentic glomerulonephritis. Kidney Int 63:1164–1172, 2003.

GLOMERULONEPHRITIS ASSOCIATED WITH SYSTEMIC DISEASES

Some patients with acute or rapidly progressive glomerulonephritis have a pathogenetically related systemic disease. Immune complex–mediated glomerulonephritis that is induced by infections may have an antecedent or concurrent infection, such as streptococcal pharyngitis or pyoderma preceding acute poststreptococcal glomerulonephritis or hepatitis C infection concurrent with type I membranoproliferative glomerulonephritis (MPGN). As noted earlier, glomerulonephritis with any of the morphologic expressions shown in Figure 16-7, as well as membranous glomerulopathy, can be caused by systemic lupus erythematosus (see Fig. 16-4).

Because glomeruli are vessels, glomerulonephritis is a frequent manifestation of systemic small vessel vasculitides, such as Henoch-Schönlein purpura, cryoglobulinemic vasculitis, microscopic polyangiitis, Wegener's granulomatosis, or Churg-Strauss syndrome (see Chapter 26). Henoch-Schönlein purpura is caused by vascular localization of IgA-dominant immune complexes, which manifests as IgA nephropathy in the glomeruli. Cryoglobulinemic vasculitis is caused by cryoglobulin deposition in vessels, and often is associated with hepatitis C infection. In glomeruli, cryoglobulinemia usually causes type I MPGN, but other phenotypes of proliferative and even membranous glomerulonephritis may develop. Microscopic polyangiitis, Wegener's granulomatosis, or Churg-Strauss syndrome have a paucity of immune deposits in vessel walls and are associated with circulating ANCAs. Glomerulonephritis caused by ANCAs is characterized pathologically by fibrinoid necrosis and crescent formation, and often manifests as a rapidly progressive decline in kidney function. Patients with vasculitis-associated glomerulonephritis typically have clinical manifestations of vascular inflammation in multiple organs, such as skin purpura caused by dermal venulitis, hemoptysis caused by alveolar capillary hemorrhage, abdominal pain caused by gut vasculitis, and mononeuritis multiplex caused by vasculitis in the small epineural arteries of peripheral nerves.

A distinctive and severe clinical presentation for glomerulonephritis is pulmonary-renal vasculitic syndrome, which has rapidly progressive glomerulonephritis combined with pulmonary hemorrhage. Table 16-1 lists the most common causes for pulmonary-renal vasculitic syndrome. Histologic and immunohistologic examination of involved vessels, including glomeruli in kidney biopsy specimens, is useful in making a definitive diagnosis (see Fig. 16-1). Serologic analysis for anti-GBM antibodies, ANCA, and markers for immune complex disease (e.g., antinuclear antibodies, cryoglobulins, anti–hepatitis C and B antibodies, complement levels) also may indicate the appropriate diagnosis (see Fig. 16-1). ANCA small vessel vasculitis is the most frequent cause for pulmonary-renal vasculitic syndrome.

ASYMPTOMATIC PROTEINURIA AND NEPHROTIC SYNDROME

When proteinuria is severe, it causes the nephrotic syndrome. Less severe proteinuria, or severe proteinuria of short duration, may be asymptomatic. The nephrotic

syndrome is characterized by massive proteinuria (greater than 3 g/24 hours per 1.73 m^2), hypoproteinemia (especially hypoalbuminemia), edema, hyperlipidemia, and lipiduria. The most specific microscopic urinalysis finding is the presence of oval fat bodies. These are sloughed tubular epithelial cells that have reabsorbed some of the excess lipids and lipoproteins in the urine (see Chapter 3).

Severe nephrotic syndrome predisposes to thrombosis secondary to loss of hemostasis control proteins (e.g., antithrombin III, protein S, and protein C), infection secondary to loss of immunoglobulins, and, possibly, accelerated atherosclerosis because of the hyperlipidemia. Volume depletion and inactivity may increase the risk for venous thrombosis in nephrotic patients. In nephrotic patients with frequent bacterial infections, administration of intravenous gamma globulin may be required.

Any type of glomerular disease can cause proteinuria. In fact, proteinuria is a sensitive indicator of glomerular damage. All proteinuria, however, is not of glomerular origin. For example, tubular damage can cause proteinuria, but rarely more than 2 g/24 hours.

As noted in Table 16-2, some glomerular diseases are more likely to manifest as nephrotic syndrome than others, although virtually any form of glomerular disease may be the cause. The two primary kidney diseases that most often manifest as nephrotic syndrome are minimal change glomerulopathy and membranous glomerulopathy, and the two secondary forms of kidney disease that most often manifest as nephrotic syndrome are diabetic glomerulosclerosis and amyloidosis.

As shown in Figure 16-8, age has a major influence on the frequency of causes for the nephrotic syndrome. The data in Figure 16-8 are derived from patients with nephrotic range proteinuria who have undergone kidney biopsy. The frequencies of causes for the nephrotic syndrome that are not always examined by kidney biopsy, especially diabetic glomerulosclerosis, are not accurately represented in Figure 16-8. In children under 10 years of age, about 80% of the nephrotic syndrome is caused by minimal change glomerulopathy. Throughout adulthood, minimal change glomerulopathy accounts for only about 10% to 15% of primary nephrotic syndrome.

Race also influences the predilection for different forms of glomerular disease. Membranous glomerulopathy is the most common cause for primary nephrotic syndrome in white adults, and focal segmental glomerulosclerosis is the most common cause in African-American adults.

Membranous glomerulopathy (see Chapter 20) is most frequent in the fifth and sixth decades of life. It is characterized pathologically by numerous subepithelial immune complex deposits (see Figs. 16-2, 16-5, and 16-6). The glomerular lesion evolves over time, with progressive accumulation of basement membrane material around the capillary wall immune complexes (see Fig. 16-5) and eventual development of chronic tubulointer-

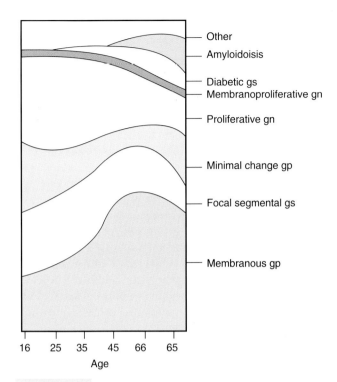

FIGURE 16-8 Diagram demonstrating the approximate frequency of different kidney diseases in patients with the nephrotic range proteinuria who had kidney biopsy samples that were evaluated in the University of North Carolina Nephropathology Laboratory. Note the variation in frequency with age. The proliferative glomerulonephritis category includes all forms of proliferative glomerulonephritis, including lupus nephritis, IgA nephropathy, IgM mesangial nephropathy, and others. gn, glomerulonephritis; gp, glomerulopathy; gs, glomerulosclerosis. (Reprinted from Jennette JC, Mandal AK: The nephrotic syndrome. In Mandal AK, Jennette JC [eds]: Diagnosis and Management of Renal Disease and Hypertension, 2nd ed. Durham, NC, Carolina Academic Press, 1994. With permission.)

stitial injury in those patients with progressive disease. If the Heymann nephritis animal model is analogous to human disease, idiopathic (primary) membranous glomerulopathy may be caused by autoantibodies specific for antigens on visceral epithelial cells, which would allow immune complex formation in the subepithelial zone but not in the subendothelial zone or mesangium of glomeruli. In addition to the numerous subepithelial immune deposits, membranous glomerulopathy secondary to immune complexes composed of antigens and antibodies in the systemic circulation often has immune complex deposits in the mesangium, and may have small subendothelial deposits (see Fig. 16-2). Thus, the ultra-structural identification of mesangial or subendothelial deposits should raise the level of suspicion for secondary membranous glomerulopathy, such as membranous glomerulopathy caused by a systemic autoimmune disease (e.g., lupus, mixed connective tissue disease, autoimmune thyroiditis), infection (e.g., hepatitis B or C,

syphilis), or neoplasm (e.g., lung or gut carcinoma). In very young and very old patients, the likelihood of secondary membranous glomerulopathy is greater, although still uncommon. Membranous glomerulopathy occurring in young patients raises the possibility of systemic lupus erythematosus or hepatitis B infection, and in very old patients raises the possibility of occult carcinoma.

Both type I and type II MPGN (see Chapter 18) typically manifest as mixed nephrotic and nephritic features, sometimes accompanied by hypocomplementemia and C3 nephritic factor, which is an autoantibody against the C3 convertase of the alternative complement activation pathway. Both types often have glomerular capillary wall thickening and hypercellularity by light microscopy. Type I MPGN (mesangiocapillary glomerulonephritis) is characterized ultrastructurally by subendothelial immune complex deposits that stimulate subendothelial mesangial interposition and replication of basement membrane material, whereas type II MPGN (dense deposit disease) has pathognomonic intramembranous dense deposits (see Fig. 16-3). Both types have extensive glomerular staining for C3 (see Fig. 16-6), with type I having more immunoglobulin staining than type II. Type I MPGN may be secondary to cryoglobulinemia, neoplasms, or chronic infections (e.g., hepatitis C and B, and infected prostheses, such as a ventriculoatrial shunt, chronic bacterial endocarditis, or chronic mastoiditis).

When taken as a group, the various forms of proliferative glomerulonephritis account for a substantial proportion of patients who have nephrotic range proteinuria (see Fig. 16-8). Patients with proliferative glomerulonephritis and marked proteinuria usually also have features of nephritis, especially hematuria. Included in this group would be patients with lupus nephritis and IgA nephropathy who have nephrotic range proteinuria.

Amyloidosis as a cause for the nephrotic syndrome is most frequent in older adults. Currently in the United States, amyloid causing the nephrotic syndrome is approximately 75% AL amyloid rather than AA amyloid. Approximately 75% of AL amyloid is composed of λ rather than κ light chain. Patients with κ light chain paraproteins and the nephrotic syndrome are more likely to have light chain deposition disease (i.e., nodular sclerosis without amyloid fibrils) rather than amyloidosis (see Chapter 30). Amyloid composition can be determined by immunofluorescence microscopy (see Fig. 16-6). In less developed areas of the world, where chronic infections are more prevalent, AA amyloidosis is more frequent than AL amyloidosis.

CHRONIC GLOMERULONEPHRITIS AND ENDSTAGE RENAL DISEASE

Most glomerular disease, with possible exceptions being uncomplicated minimal change glomerulopathy and thin basement membrane nephropathy, can progress to chronic glomerular sclerosis with progressively declining kidney function and eventually to ESRD. Chronic glomerular disease is the third leading cause of ESRD in the United States, following hypertensive and diabetic kidney disease in frequency. Clinicopathologic studies of different glomerular diseases have revealed marked differences in their natural histories. Some diseases have a high risk for rapid progression to ESRD unless treated, such as anti-GBM and ANCA crescentic glomerulonephritis. Other diseases have more indolent but persistent courses, with ESRD eventually ensuing in a significant number of patients, such as IgA nephropathy and focal segmental glomerulosclerosis. Some forms of glomerulonephritis, for example, acute poststreptococcal glomerulonephritis, may initially manifest a rather severe nephritis, but usually resolve completely with little risk for progression to ESRD. And some diseases are unpredictable, for example, membranous glomerulopathy, which may remit spontaneously, have persistent nephrosis for decades without a decline in kidney function, or progress over several years to ESRD.

Chronic glomerulonephritis is characterized pathologically by varying degrees of glomerular scarring, which is always accompanied by cortical tubular atrophy, interstitial fibrosis, interstitial infiltration by chronic inflammatory cells, and arteriosclerosis. As the glomerular, interstitial, and vascular sclerosis worsen, they eventually reach a point at which histologic evaluation of the kidney tissue cannot reveal the initial cause for the kidney injury, and a pathologic diagnosis of ESRD is all that can be concluded.

Clinically, chronic glomerulonephritis that is progressing to ESRD eventually results in uremia that must be managed by dialysis or kidney transplantation. As the term implies, patients with uremia have accumulation of nitrogenous wastes (urea, uric acid, creatinine) in the blood. Other clinical manifestations of uremia include nausea and vomiting, hiccups, anorexia, pruritus, lethargy, pericarditis, myopathies, neuropathies, and encephalopathy.

KIDNEY BIOPSY: INDICATIONS AND METHODS

In a patient with kidney disease, a kidney biopsy provides tissue that can be used to determine the diagnosis, indicate the cause, predict the prognosis, direct treatment, and collect data for research, although not all potential applications are accomplished by every kidney biopsy.

Kidney biopsy is indicated in a patient with kidney disease when all three of the following conditions are met: (1) the cause cannot be determined or adequately predicted by less invasive diagnostic procedures, (2) the signs and symptoms suggest parenchymal disease that can be diagnosed by pathologic evaluation, and (3) the

differential diagnosis includes diseases that have different treatments, different prognoses, or both. Situations in which a kidney biopsy serves an important diagnostic function include nephrotic syndrome in adults, steroid-resistant nephrotic syndrome in children, glomerulonephritis in adults other than clear-cut acute poststreptococcal glomerulonephritis or lupus nephritis, and acute renal failure of unknown cause. In some kidney diseases for which the diagnosis is relatively definite from clinical data, a kidney biopsy may be of value not only for confirming the diagnosis but also for assessing the activity, chronicity, and severity of injury; for example, in patients with suspected lupus glomerulonephritis. Although the diagnosis is strongly supported by positive serologic results in patients with anti-GBM and ANCA glomerulonephritis, the extremely toxic treatment that is used for these diseases warrants the additional level of confirmation that a kidney biopsy provides; and a kidney biopsy also provides information about the severity and potential reversibility of the glomerular damage. Table 16-5 demonstrates the types of native kidney disease that have prompted kidney biopsy among the nephrologists who refer specimens to the University of North Carolina Nephropathology Laboratory. Approximately 80% of these biopsies were performed by nephrologists in community practice. Diseases that typically cause nephrotic syndrome were the most frequent impetus for biopsy (e.g., membranous glomerulopathy and focal segmental glomerulosclerosis), followed by diseases that cause nephritis (e.g., lupus nephritis and IgA nephropathy).

Contraindications to percutaneous kidney biopsy include an uncooperative patient, solitary kidney, hemorrhagic diathesis, uncontrolled severe hypertension, severe anemia or dehydration, cystic kidney, hydronephrosis, multiple renal arterial aneurysms, acute pyelonephritis or perinephric abscess, renal neoplasm, and ESRD. Transjugular kidney biopsy and wedge kidney biopsy are advocated by some as safer procedures in patients with these risk factors.

Clinically significant complications of kidney biopsy are relatively infrequent but must be kept in mind when determining the risk/benefit ratio of the procedure. Small perirenal hematomas that can be seen by imaging studies (e.g., ultrasonography) are relatively common if sought carefully. Gross hematuria occurs in less than 10% of patients, arteriovenous fistula in less than 1%, hemorrhage that requires surgery in less than 1%, and death in less than 0.1%.

Current percutaneous needle biopsy procedures usually employ localization of the kidney by real-time ultrasound guidance determination of kidney location and depth by ultrasonography immediately prior to biopsy, or computed tomography (CT)-guided localization of the kidney. Many varieties of biopsy needles have been used over the years, most of which are effective in experienced hands. Currently, most kidney biopsies are performed with spring-loaded disposable gun devices.

TABLE 16-5 Frequency of Various Diagnoses among 7257 Kidney Biopsy Samples Evaluated in the University of North Carolina Nephropathology Laboratory*

Diseases that often cause nephrotic	3067		**Diseases that often cause hematuria and**	2109
idiopathic membranous glomerulopathy	847		**nephritis (29%)**	
(42%)			Lupus nephritis (all classes)	636
Focal segmental glomerulosclerosis (FSGS)	768		IgA nephropathy	538
Minimal change glomerulopathy	398		Other immune complex proliferative GN	375
Diabetic glomerulosclerosis	246		Pauci-immune/ANCA GN	301
Type I membranoproliferative GN	190		Acute diffuse proliferative (postinfectious) GN	86
Mesangioproliferative GN	145		Thin basement membrane nephropathy	82
Amyloidosis	108		Anti-GBM GN	56
Clq nephropathy	99		Alport's syndrome	35
Collapsing variant of FSGS	87			
Glomerular tip lesion variant of FSGS	65		**Diseases that often cause chronic kidney disease**	
Fibrillary GN	59		**(8%)**	583
Light chain deposition disease	26		Arterionephrosclerosis	229
Type II membranoproliferative GN	14		Chronic sclerosing GN	166
Preeclampsia/eclampsia	6		Chronic sclerosing GN	166
Immunotactoid glomerulopathy	6		Endstage renal disease	114
Collagenofibrotic glomerulopathy	3		Chronic tubulointerstitial nephritis	74
			Miscellaneous other diseases (3%)	199
			No pathologic lesion identified (2%)	141
Diseases that often cause acute renal	371			
failure[†] (5%)			**Adequate tissue with nonspecific abnormalities**	370
Thrombotic microangiopathy (all types)	126		**(5%)**	
Acute tubulointerstitial nephritis	101			
Acute tubular necrosis	69		**Inadequate tissue for definitive diagnosis (6%)**	417
Atheroembolization	34			
Light chain cast nephropathy	31			
Cortical necrosis	10			

GN, glomerulonephritis.

*Specimens with nonspecific abnormalities (e.g., interstitial fibrosis, tubular atrophy, glomerular scarring, arteriosclerosis), specimens with no identifiable pathologic abnormality (e.g., in a patient with asymptomatic hematuria), and some specimens with inadequate tissue for definitive diagnosis (e.g., a very small specimen with only a few glomeruli but with negative immunofluorescence microscopy) may nevertheless provide useful clinical information, especially with respect to ruling out diseases that were in the differential diagnosis.

[†]Other than glomerulonephritis.

Light microscopy alone is not adequate for the diagnosis of native kidney diseases, although it may be adequate for assessing the basis for kidney allograft dysfunction during the first few weeks after transplantation. All native kidney biopsy samples should be processed for at least light microscopy and immunofluorescence microscopy. Most renal pathologists advocate performing electron microscopy on all native kidney biopsy specimens, but some fix tissue for electron microscopy but perform the procedure only if the other microscopic findings suggest that it will be useful.

The needle biopsy core sample should be examined with a magnifying glass or a dissecting microscope to confirm that kidney tissue is present and to determine whether it is cortex or medulla. When gently prodded and pulled with forceps, adipose tissue is mushy and strings out, skeletal muscle tissue falls apart into little clumps, and kidney tissue maintains a cylindrical shape. At 15× or higher magnification, adipose tissue looks like clusters of tiny fat droplets (i.e., adipose cells), skeletal muscle is red-brown with irregular bundles of fibers, and kidney tissue is pale pink to tan. Glomeruli in the renal cortex appear as reddish blushes or hemispheres projecting from the surface of the core. Straight red striations produced by the vasa recta are markers for the medulla. When there is extensive glomerular hematuria, the con-

voluted tubules in the cortex appear as red corkscrews. Once the tissue landmarks are identified, portions of tissue should be separated for processing for light, immunofluorescence, and electron microscopy.

In our experience with kidney biopsy specimens sent to us from over 200 different nephrologists per year, most of whom are in community practice, approximately 6% of kidney biopsy specimens are inadequate for a definitive diagnosis (see Table 16-5). The most common inadequacy is kidney tissue with too little or no cortex. This can be remedied by beginning the sampling procedure with the biopsy needle just barely penetrating the outer cortex. Obviously, if the biopsy needle is inserted too deeply into or through the cortex, the specimen will contain only medulla. Even specimens that are considered inadequate for a definitive diagnosis may provide useful information. For example, in a patient with nephrotic syndrome, a kidney biopsy specimen that has no glomeruli for light or electron microscopy, but has one glomerulus that stains negative for immunoglobulins and complement by immunofluorescence microscopy, rules out any form of immune complex glomerulonephritis, such as membranous glomerulopathy, and focuses the differential diagnosis on minimal change glomerulopathy versus focal segmental glomerulosclerosis.

BIBLIOGRAPHY

Appel GB: Renal biopsy: The clinician's viewpoint. In Silva FG, D'Agati VD, Nadasdy T (eds): Renal Biopsy Interpretation. New York, Churchill Livingstone, 1996, pp 21–29.

Bolton WK: Goodpasture's syndrome. Kidney Int 50:1753–1766, 1996.

Cameron JS: Nephrotic syndrome in the elderly. Semin Nephrol 16:319–329, 1996.

Cohen AH, Nast CC, Adler SG, Kopple JD: Clinical utility of kidney biopsies in the diagnosis and management of renal disease. Am J Nephrol 9:309–315, 1989.

D'Agati VD, Fogo AB, Bruijn JA, et al: Pathologic classification of focal segmental glomerulosclerosis: A working proposal. Am J Kidney Dis 43:368–382, 2004.

Dische F, Parsons V, Taube D: Thin-basement-membrane nephropathy. N Engl J Med 320:1752–1753, 1989.

Eddy AA, Symons JM: Nephrotic syndrome in childhood. Lancet 362:629–639; 2003.

Feneberg R, Schaefer F, Zieger B, et al: Percutaneous renal biopsy in children: A 27-year experience. Nephron 79:438–446, 1998.

Galla JH: IgA nephropathy. Kidney Int 47:377–387, 1995.

Glassock RJ: Diagnosis and natural course of membranous nephropathy. Semin Nephrol 23:324–32; 2003.

Glassock RJ, Cohen AH: The primary glomerulopathies. Dis Mon 42:329–383, 1996.

Haas M, Spargo BH, Coventry S: Increasing incidence of focal-segmental glomerulosclerosis among adult nephropathies: A 20-year renal biopsy study. Am J Kidney Dis 26:740–750, 1995.

Jennette JC: Rapidly progressive and crescentic glomerulonephritis. Kidney Int 63:1164–1172, 2003.

Jennette JC, Falk RJ: Diagnosis and management of glomerulonephritis and vasculitis presenting as acute renal failure. Med Clin North Am 74:893–908, 1990.

Jouet P, Meyrier A, Mai F, et al: Transjugular renal biopsy in the treatment of patients with cirrhosis and renal abnormalities. Hepatology 24:1143–1147, 1996.

Mariani AJ, Mariani MC, Macchioni C, et al: The significance of adult hematuria: 1,000 hematuria evaluations including a risk-benefit and cost-effectiveness analysis. J Urol 141:350–355, 1989.

Niles JL, Bottinger EP, Saurina GR, et al: The syndrome of lung hemorrhage and nephritis is usually an ANCA-associated condition. Arch Intern Med 156:440–445, 1996.

Schena FP: Survey of the Italian Registry of Renal Biopsies. Frequency of the renal diseases for 7 consecutive years. The Italian Group of Renal Immunopathology. Nephrology Dial Transplant 12:418–426, 1997.

Tiebosch AT, Frederik PM, van Breda Vriesman PJ, et al: Thin-basement-membrane nephropathy in adults with persistent hematuria. N Engl J Med 320:14–28, 1989.

van der Loop FT, Monnens LA, Schroder CH, et al: Identification of COL4A5 defects in Alport's syndrome by immunohistochemistry of skin. Kidney Int 55(4):1217–1224, 1999.

Weening JJ, D'Agati VD, Schwartz MM, et al: The classification of glomerulonephritis in systemic lupus erythematosus revisited. Kidney Int 65:521–530, 2004.

CHAPTER 17

Minimal Change Disease

Brent Lee Lechner   Norman J. Siegel

TERMINOLOGY AND HISTOPATHOLOGY

Minimal change nephropathy, or minimal change disease (MCD), is a histopathologic lesion that is almost always associated with the nephrotic syndrome at the onset of disease. Other terms such as lipoid nephrosis, nil disease, and idiopathic nephrotic syndrome have been used interchangeably.

Minimal change disease is defined on light microscopy by a lack of definitive alteration in glomerular structure from that seen in normal patients. Although the degree of alterations that may remove a biopsy result from this category has been debated, it is generally agreed that the cellularity of the glomerulus must be minimal and that the tubular and interstitial structures must also be normal. There may be some doubly refractile appearance or lipid droplets in the tubule cells, but there should be no evidence of tubular atrophy or interstitial fibrosis. Immunofluorescent staining also shows no change from normal and an absence of immunoglobulin or complement protein deposition. The most obvious and consistent finding in patients with MCD is a characteristic swelling of epithelial foot processes seen on electron microscopy (Fig. 17-1). Fenestration of the endothelial cells lining the capillary loop is normal. The glomerular basement membrane is uniform in thickness and structure, but the epithelial cells show a continuous layer of contact with the glomerular basement membrane. Because a biopsy is susceptible to sampling error, it must be remembered that lesions which affect only some glomeruli, such as focal and segmental glomerulosclerosis, may be inadvertently misdiagnosed as MCD.

The role of a kidney biopsy in the initial management of patients who present with nephrotic syndrome is controversial. In most cases, children are treated with a course of steroids, and biopsies are reserved for those who are steroid resistant. Because of their lower prevalence of steroid-responsive lesions, biopsy samples are usually taken from adolescents and adults prior to treatment. In patients of any age with a complicated clinical presentation or course of disease, an assessment of histopathologic changes is recommended.

CLINICAL PRESENTATION

The pathogenesis of MCD is poorly understood. As the understanding of podocyte biology has increased, new proteins that are specifically expressed in these cells have been identified, and lesions such as MCD, which are thought to be idiopathic, are becoming better understood. Although generally considered a childhood disease, MCD presents in both children and adults. The insidious onset of nephrotic syndrome, usually manifested by edema formation, is the most common presentation. In children, the onset of disease is after the first year of life, with a peak incidence between 24 and 36 months of age and a strong male predominance. In preadolescent children, 85% to 95% with idiopathic or primary nephrotic syndrome will have MCD. In adolescents and young adults, the prevalence of MCD declines to approximately 50%, and the male predominance begins to disappear. In patients over the age of 40 years with primary nephrotic syndrome, the incidence of MCD is 20% to 25%, and there is a nearly equal distribution between men and women.

In patients presenting with the typical features of MCD, a relatively "pure" nephrotic syndrome is usually observed. Nephritic features such as hypertension, hematuria, and reduced kidney function are relatively uncommon. Any one of these features may occur in 15% to 20% of patients with MCD, but the presence of two or more is decidedly unusual and should make one consider a different diagnosis. The finding of gross hematuria or red cell casts would generally not be considered to be compatible with the diagnosis of MCD. Thus, the predominant clinical features are those of nephrotic syndrome with heavy proteinuria, low serum albumin, edema formation, and elevated serum cholesterol. Other than the findings of oval fat bodies that appear as maltese crosses on examination of the urine under a polarized lens, results of the urinalysis are normal (see Chapter 3, Fig. 3-3). Serum complement levels are normal, and antinuclear antibodies and cryoglobulins are absent. Serum immunoglobulins may be abnormal, with a reduction of serum IgG levels to 20% or less of normal values, a less severe reduction in IgA, and a mild increase in IgM and IgE levels.

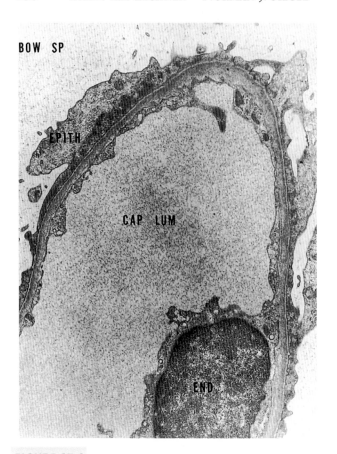

FIGURE 17-1 Electron micrograph of glomerular capillary loop in a patient with minimal change disease. The endothelial cell (end) and basement membrane are normal in content and structure. The epithelial cell (epith) demonstrates diffuse swelling of the pseudopods and foot-process fusion. Note Bowman's space (bow sp). There are no electron-dense deposits.

Although MCD is usually associated with a primary or idiopathic nephrotic syndrome, secondary MCD also occurs (Table 17-1). In 80% to 90% of children, MCD is idiopathic, although cases associated with the ingestion of heavy metals such as mercury or lead as well as acquired immunodeficiency syndrome have been reported. In adult patients, especially the elderly, the association of this MCD with nonsteroidal anti-inflammatory drugs is particularly important because of their frequent use. Hodgkin's disease and lymphoproliferative disorders must be kept in mind when older patients present with MCD. Although most patients with obesity and nephrotic syndrome have focal segmental glomerulosclerosis, some of these patients have responded to steroids or have been documented to have MCD.

RESPONSE TO THERAPY

The benchmark for therapy in MCD is the use of corticosteroids. No other cause of nephrotic syndrome is as exquisitely sensitive to treatment with steroid therapy as MCD. Because of the high prevalence of this lesion in

children, disappearance of proteinuria in response to the oral administration of prednisone is considered diagnostic for MCD. Characteristically, these young children respond to treatment with a diuresis and clearing of proteinuria within about 2 weeks of initiation of prednisone therapy, usually at a dose of 2 mg/kg/day, not to exceed 60 mg daily. Some children may have a slower response to initial therapy and not clear their proteinuria for 6 to 8 weeks. A response to therapy in 80% to 90% of adolescents and adults with MCD has also been documented. However, in these age groups, the response is slower and a prolonged period of therapy, in some cases up to 16 weeks, may be required before complete remission of proteinuria is achieved. In addition, adults more frequently develop a partial remission of proteinuria that is uncommon in children with MCD.

The clinical course of MCD is frequently described in terms of the response of the patient to steroids. Complete remission is defined as complete resolution of proteinuria for at least 3 to 5 consecutive days; a partial remission is a reduction in the degree of proteinuria without complete clearing, and a relapse is a recurrence of proteinuria for at least 3 to 5 consecutive days. The clinical outcome for children with MCD, as related to steroid therapy, is outlined in Figure 17-2. About 10% of children initially treated with steroid therapy do not respond to treatment and will have early steroid resistance. Alternative methods of administration of steroids have been attempted in this group of patients, but have not been particularly successful. These patients may respond to cytotoxic or immunosuppressive therapies.

Adult patients usually undergo kidney biopsy prior to initiation of therapy. A similar, although not identical, pattern of response to initial steroid therapy can be expected in adults. In adult patients, alternative initial therapy should be given in situations in which an underlying condition such as diabetes mellitus, hypertension, or osteoporosis may complicate steroid usage. In those

TABLE 17-1 Secondary Causes of Minimal Change Nephropathy

Drugs
  Nonsteroidal anti-inflammatory agents
  Ampicillin/penicillin
  Trimethadione
Toxins
  Mercury
  Lead
  Bee stings
Infection
  Mononucleosis
  Human immunodeficiency virus
  Immunizations
Tumors
  Hodgkin's lymphoma
  Other lymphoproliferative diseases
  Carcinoma
Obesity

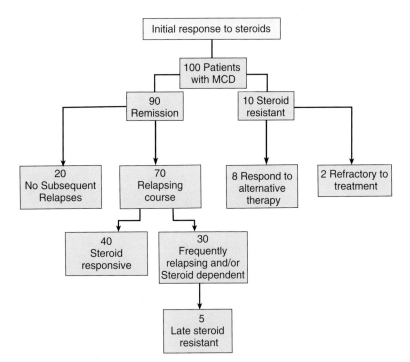

FIGURE 17-2 Clinical outcome for children with minimal change disease.

circumstances, initial therapy with an alkylating agent or mycophenolate mofetil (MMF) may be preferred.

Of the patients who achieve a remission on initial steroid therapy, 75% to 85% experience one or more relapses (see Fig. 17-2). Reports have suggested that prolonged treatment of the initial episode can reduce the incidence of subsequent relapses. In those patients who are destined to follow a relapsing course, the first relapse usually occurs within 6 to 12 months of the onset of their disease, although in some patients the first relapse may be delayed as long as 24 to 30 months. In patients with a relapsing course, 50% to 65% can be expected to have a steroid-responsive clinical profile with frequent relapses occurring over a 3- to 5-year period. However, for 25% to 30% of patients with MCD, a more protracted clinical course occurs, and their disease is described as being frequently relapsing or steroid dependent. A small proportion of these patients may develop late steroid resistance, at which point a repeat kidney biopsy may show evolution to other histopathologic patterns such as focal segmental glomerular sclerosis. Thus, the majority of patients with MCD have a good response to initial steroid therapy, and a disease course characterized by relapses of their nephrotic syndrome but, overall, an excellent long-term prognosis.

Patients with frequently relapsing, steroid-dependent MCD present the greatest therapeutic challenge. In the long run, the relapsing nature of their disease is likely to disappear but, over the short term, deleterious side effects of continued steroid therapy may occur, particularly in adults and geriatric patients. To decrease the frequency of relapses, these patients may be treated with low doses of prednisone on a daily or alternate-day basis without significant side effects. For those patients who require

large doses of medication to remain in remission or who develop significant side effects, alternative therapy must be considered. Adult patients poorly tolerate relapses of edema or recurrent treatment with corticosteroids. Consequently, in this group of patients, compared with children, therapy with cytotoxic agents or other immunosuppressive agents are frequently used earlier in the clinical course.

Cyclophosphamide and chlorambucil have proven to be the most effective alternative therapies for patients with MCD. These drugs have been shown to be effective in both children and adults with frequently relapsing, steroid-dependent nephrotic syndrome. The most pronounced and dramatic effect is the prolonged period of remission of the nephrotic syndrome that is achieved in patients treated with these agents. After cessation of the cytotoxic agent, 30% to 40% of patients have no subsequent relapses. Among relapsers, the average period of remission is 18 to 24 months. Subsequent relapses are usually more steroid responsive than prior to cytotoxic therapy. Thus, steroid-related side effects such as a cushingoid appearance, growth retardation in children, or abnormalities in bone metabolism can be markedly diminished and reversed. Nonetheless, cytotoxic agents have a number of serious side effects, which include cystitis, alopecia, leukopenia, gonadal toxicity, potential for malignancy formation, and seizures; their use requires caution and careful judgment.

Other medications have also been used for the treatment of patients with either steroid-refractory or frequently relapsing, steroid-dependent disease. Cyclosporine has been reported to be effective in some adult and pediatric patients with an initial steroid-resistant course. Its primary utility is to achieve a steroid-sparing effect because the relapse rate is high and prolonged remission is not sustained after cyclosporine is discontinued. Levamisole and MMF have been used to achieve a steroid-sparing effect. In patients, predominantly adults, with frequently relapsing, steroid-dependent MCD, treatment with MMF has been associated with sustained remission after cessation of steroid therapy. The primary side effect of treatment with MMF has been diarrhea.

For patients unresponsive to these therapeutic interventions, symptomatic control of edema with the use of diuretics and a low-salt diet are the mainstays of therapy. If complications of anasarca occur such as pleural or pericardial effusions, severe hyponatremia, or cellulitis, the infusion of albumin can be beneficial to mobilize the extracellular fluid and prevent pulmonary or cardiac decompensation. This therapy, however, should be undertaken with caution because the shifts in intravascular volume associated with albumin infusion can result in severe hypertension or congestive heart failure, particularly in children, and because the beneficial effect is short-term since the albumin is rapidly excreted in a patient with heavy proteinuria. Proteinuria can be reduced with nonsteroidal anti-inflammatory drugs, angiotension-converting enzyme (ACE) inhibitors, and angiotension receptor blockers (ARBs). These therapies may be of benefit in patients who are refractory to treatment of their nephrotic syndrome, have severe proteinuria, and are developing malnutrition because of the quantity of protein lost in the urine. There has been some recent interest in the combined use of ACE inhibitors and ARBs in refractory patients. Although these drugs are generally well tolerated and may be beneficial in a selected subset of patients, the associated complications, including hyperkalemia and acute renal failure, must be carefully monitored.

COMPLICATIONS AND LONG-TERM OUTCOME

The primary complications of MCD are related to persistent nephrotic syndrome or to side effects of therapy. The most common complications of steroid therapy include cushingoid facies, striae, acne, and cataracts. Steroid therapy is also associated with alterations in glucose, lipid and bone metabolism, cosmetic appearance, and emotional lability. In general, these medications are much better tolerated in children than in adults. The induction of a prolonged remission by a cytotoxic agent permits regression of the majority of the steroid-related side effects. Striae and cataracts usually persist; however, catch-up growth in children frequently occurs. The cushingoid appearance disappears, and decreased osteopenia may occur. Complications of cytotoxic agents are substantial but can be minimized with careful dosing of these drugs, short courses, and appropriate precautions such as adequate hydration. Indeed, in the majority of

studies in children and adults, minimal side effects of either chlorambucil or cyclophosphamide have been reported, and the drugs have been well tolerated. One of the most disturbing side effects of cyclophosphamide therapy, gonadal toxicity, appears to be dose related and reversible in the majority of young patients treated with this medication. For adult patients, oligospermia and cessation of menses may occur during a course of treatment but are frequently reversible. Gonadal suppression strategies may be used to lessen the risk for permanent sterility.

Peritonitis is an important complication of the nephrotic syndrome for those patients who are unable to achieve a remission of their proteinuria. Peritonitis occurs during periods of severe edema formation, particularly when ascites is present. The most common infecting agent is *Streptococcus pneumoniae*. However, infections with *Escherichia coli* and *Haemophilus influenzae* have also been reported. Prior to antibiotic therapy, peritonitis was the major cause of death in children and adults with MCD.

Reversible acute renal failure has been reported in patients with MCD. This complication appears to occur much more frequently in adult patients than in children. It usually develops in patients with severe edema formation and those who have been taking nonsteroidal anti-inflammatory drugs or ACE inhibitors. A period of rapid weight accumulation immediately precedes the onset of the renal failure. The pathophysiology of acute renal failure in patients with MCD is poorly understood and cannot be clearly related to intravascular volume depletion, acute tubular necrosis, or vascular obstruction such as renal vein thrombosis. In some cases, the combination of infusions of albumin and diuretics to reduce interstitial edema has been effective.

The development of chronic kidney failure in patients with MCD is rare in children or adults with a steroid-responsive clinical course. Patients at highest risk are those who either do not have an initial response to steroid therapy or those who become late steroid nonresponders (see Fig. 17-2). In both of these situations, the possibility that the histopathologic lesion may be different or may have evolved into a pattern different from MCD must be considered and may be the dominant factor in overall prognosis. For the majority of children, the relapsing nature of their disease begins to dissipate after about 10 years from onset, and the majority will be free of proteinuria after puberty. However, late relapses after long-term remissions of the nephrotic syndrome in patients who had their initial episode at a very young age have been well documented. Patients who have had frequently relapsing, steroid-dependent nephrotic syndrome in childhood do not appear to be at increased risk for cardiovascular disease. Similarly, adult patients with MCD have a very good prognosis, with an 85% to 90% survival rate at 10 years or more after the onset of disease. The major morbidity is related to complications of therapy.

BIBLIOGRAPHY

Berns JS, Gaudio KM, Krassner LS, et al: Steroid-responsive nephrotic syndrome of childhood: A long-term study of clinical course, histopathology, efficacy of cyclophosphamide therapy, and effects on growth. Am J Kidney Dis 9:108–114, 1987.

Habib R, Kleinknecht C: The primary nephrotic syndrome of childhood: Classification and clinicopathologic study of 406 cases. In Sommers SC (ed): Pathology Annual. New York, Appleton-Century-Crofts, 1971, pp 417–474.

International Study of Kidney Disease in Children: Nephrotic syndrome in children: Prediction of histopathology from clinical and laboratory characteristics at time of diagnosis. Kidney Int 13:159–165, 1996.

Nolasco F, Cameron JS, Heywood EF, et al: Adult-onset minimal change nephrotic syndrome: A long-term follow-up. Kidney Int 29:1215–1223,1986.

Mundel P, Shankland S: Podocyte biology and response to injury. J Am Soc Nephrol 13:3005–3015, 2002.

Choi M, Eustace A, Gimenez L, et al: Mycophenolate mofetil treatment for primary glomerular diseases. Kidney Int 61:1008–1114, 2002.

Niaudet P: Steroid-sensitive idiopathic nephrotic syndrome in children. In Avner ED, Harmon WE, Niaudet P (eds): Pediatric Nephrology, 5th ed. Philadelphia, Lippincott Williams & Wilkins, 2004, pp 543–556.

Smith JD, Hayslett JP: Reversible renal failure in the nephrotic syndrome. Am J Kidney Dis 21:201–213, 1992.

Korbet SM: Management of idiopathic nephrosis in adults, including steroid-resistant nephrosis. Curr Opin Nephrol Hypertens 4(2):169–176, 1995.

Bargman JM: Management of minimal lesion glomerulonephritis: Evidence-based recommendations. Kidney Int 55(suppl):3–16, 1996.

Lechner BL, Siegel NJ: The risk of cardiovascular disease in adults who have had childhood nephrotic syndrome. Pediatr Nephrol 19:744–748, 2004.

CHAPTER 18

Membranoproliferative Glomerulonephritis and Cryoglobulinemia

Giuseppe D'Amico   Alessandro Fornasieri

The term *membranoproliferative glomerulonephritis* (MPGN) is used to describe a histopathologic entity characterized by intense glomerular hypercellularity, capillary loop thickening due to subendothelial or intramembranous deposits, and interposition of mesangial cells and matrix into the capillary loops, which produces a double-contour appearance to the basement membrane.

This entity includes both forms of unknown cause (idiopathic MPGN) and forms associated with systemic and infectious disorders (Table 18-1). Its morphologic pattern should be integrated within an etiologic context whenever possible.

IDIOPATHIC MEMBRANOPROLIFERATIVE GLOMERULONEPHRITIS

Epidemiology

In Africa and Asia, "idiopathic" MPGN is a common disease, probably related to uncharacterized infectious or parasitic diseases. In the United States and in Europe, however, it is rare, and its incidence has declined over the past three decades. It occurs equally in males and females, and presents mainly in childhood.

Pathology

Two major and distinct categories of idiopathic MPGN have been identified, termed type I and type II. Type I is characterized by the presence of glomerular subendothelial deposits, associated with proliferation of mesangial cells and mesangial matrix expansion, moderate leukocyte infiltration, and duplication of the peripheral glomerular basement membrane (GBM), with a double-contour appearance due to interposition of mesangial cells (and sometimes also monocytes) in the capillary wall. A more marked mesangial expansion, occluding the capillary lumina of some loops, gives some cases a lobular pattern (Fig. 18-1).

By immunofluorescence, deposition of immunoglobulin M (IgM), IgG, C3, and sometimes also C1q and C4, in a granular capillary wall distribution, is seen (Fig. 18-2).

In type II, homogeneous dense deposits in many renal basement membranes (glomerular, tubular, and arteriolar) are the characterizing feature by electron microscopy (Fig. 18-3), and sometimes also by light microscopy. The immunofluorescence pattern is similar to that seen in type I, but only C3 stains the capillary wall.

A variant of type I MPGN, designated type III MPGN, has also been described. It is characterized by the simultaneous presence of subendothelial and subepithelial deposits associated with lamination and disruption of the lamina densa of GBM.

Pathogenesis

Three interrelated mechanisms contribute to the development of the morphologic features of MPGN: (1) accumulation on the subendothelial side of the GBM (type I) or within the GBM (type II) of electron-dense deposits that are probably immune complexes (ICs) in the first type and deposits of undefined origin in the second; (2) mesangial proliferation involving both cells and matrix, with a tendency of the activated mesangium to expand the peripheral capillary walls and to extend into the subendothelial space, causing the specific splitting (double-contour appearance) of the GBM; and (3) inflow of blood-borne inflammatory cells, mainly monocytes.

The accumulated experience with experimental models of chronic IC-induced GN and with humans, in whom ICs deposit on the internal aspect of the GBM (chronic infectious diseases, systemic lupus erythematosus, or cryoglobulinemia), suggests that deposits come first. The activation of the mesangium, such that it expands to the periphery of capillary walls with cytoplasmic extensions that engulf the deposits, and the inflow of leukocytes are both secondary events. However, these two mechanisms of defense are not necessarily activated to the same extent. When the broad spectrum of lesions associated with protracted deposition of IC and complement is considered, sometimes (in lupus,

TABLE 18-1 Classification of MPGN

Primary
Idiopathic MPGN

Secondary
Infectious diseases
    Hepatitis C with type II mixed cryoglobulinemia
    Subacute endocarditis
    Infected ventriculoatrial shunt
    Malaria
    Schistosomiasis
Systemic connective tissue disorders
    Systemic lupus erythematosus
Neoplasms
    Leukemia and lymphoma

MPGN, membranoproliferative glomerulonephritis.

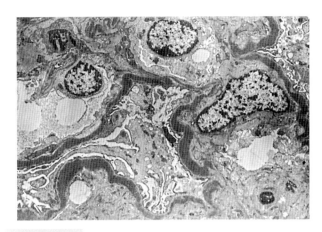

FIGURE 18-3 Diffuse dense intramembranous deposits within glomerular basement membrane. Some portions of glomerular basement membrane are preserved (lead citrate, uranyl acetate, original magnification ×2800).

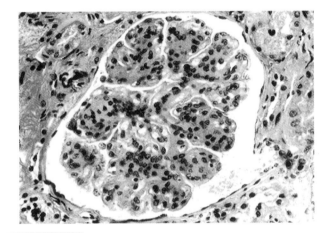

FIGURE 18-1 Type I membranoproliferative glomerulonephritis. Marked mesangial proliferation with mesangial matrix expansion and pronounced lobulation of the glomerular tuft (hematoxylin and eosin, original magnification ×250).

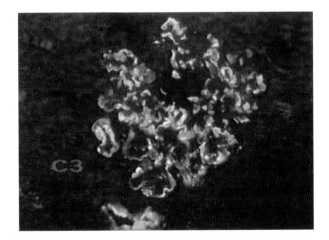

FIGURE 18-2 Type I membranoproliferative glomerulonephritis. Immunofluorescence: diffuse and intense mesangial and capillary loop deposits (C3, original magnification ×250).

cryoglobulinemic GN, and the exudative variant of idiopathic MPGN) the predominant mechanism of defense is the accumulation of monocytes and neutrophils in the subendothelial space. This is also responsible for the thickening and duplication of the GBM, with mesangial interposition being less evident. At the other end of the spectrum, as in the classic type I idiopathic MPGN, little or no cell influx occurs, and mesangial activation with peripheral interposition is the principal mechanism of defense.

It is possible that not only the quantity, but also the nature and composition of the subendothelial deposits account for the endothelial damage and the prevailing cytokine-mediated activation of mesangium or inflammatory cells, mainly monocytes. It is also possible that the recruitment of monocytes and polymorphonuclear cells is the important mechanism when ICs are deposited acutely on the subendothelial aspect of the GBM (see later section on Cryoglobulinemic Glomerulonephritis), whereas mesangial activation and peripheral interposition are later, more chronic phenomena, favored by the cytokine-mediated stimulation of resident glomerular cells induced by the infiltrating monocytes. However, in some circumstances (cryoglobulinemic GN and some cases of idiopathic MPGN), monocyte infiltration can be demonstrated even in less acute stages of the disease, in the absence of evident mesangial interposition.

When ICs are deposited on the internal side of the GBM, it can be postulated that mesangial interposition is a consequence of deposition of complement and immunoglobulins. The regression of the mesangial expansion when exogenous bacterial antigens are eliminated from the body, as in shunt nephritis, confirms this hypothesis. However, it is more difficult to explain mesangial interposition when no deposits are present or when such deposits stain only with complement, without accompanying immunoglobulins. It is possible that other mechanisms of injury of the capillary wall, especially if they induce endothelial cell damage and detachment from the basement membrane, may also eventually stimulate the accumulation of plasma proteins and the ingrowth of the mesangium in the resulting subendothelial space, independent of the presence of deposits.

A characteristic feature, when the sequence of immunopathogenetic events described previously (i.e., long-term accumulation of electron-dense deposits on the internal aspect of the GBM, recruitment of monocytes, and chronic mesangial activation with peripheral interposition) takes place, is the frequent coexistence of persistent hypocomplementemia. In idiopathic MPGN, the association with low complement levels is so frequent that this GN has also been called hypocomplementemic GN.

However, the cause of hypocomplementemia in idiopathic and secondary MPGN, its relationship to the pathogenesis, and its possible role in perpetuating the glomerular disease are still obscure. We also do not yet understand why in some cases (type II idiopathic MPGN) the activation of the alternative pathway predominates, whereas in other cases (type I idiopathic MPGN, lupus nephritis, cryoglobulinemic GN, shunt nephritis), there is activation of the classical pathway. Similarly, it is unknown whether the hypocomplementemia is always a secondary phenomenon, derived from increased consumption triggered by subendothelial or intramembranous deposits, or whether it may precede such deposition and favor it, as proposed many years ago. To make things more complicated, hypocomplementemia per se does not appear to correlate with the clinical course of MPGN. Complement levels are not of value for monitoring the course or predicting the final outcome of MPGN. When persistently depressed, they can only be considered markers of this group of glomerular diseases.

It is now evident that hypocomplementemia can be ascribed to at least two mechanisms: (1) the activation of the classic pathway produced by circulating IC and (2) the presence in the blood of anticomplement autoantibodies, called nephritic factors. At least two nephritic factors have been described: one that acts on the amplification loop of the complement cascade (Nef_a) and another that acts on the terminal pathway (Nef_t). Activation of the classic pathway by circulating IC is probably the major mechanism responsible for hypocomplementemia in idiopathic type I MPGN, lupus nephritis, and shunt nephritis. Nef_a is probably the major mechanism responsible for the hypocomplementemia of type II idiopathic MPGN. However, nephritic factors are sometimes found in sera of patients of the former group, and hypocomplementemia may be multifactorial in origin. The classic pathway is activated in some. In others, the presence of the nephritic factors Nef_t or Nef_a better explains the abnormalities of the serum complement profile. In other words, different nephritic factors can be present in the same morphologic type of MPGN, and the same nephritic factor can coexist in heterogeneous types of MPGN with quite different abnormalities of glomerular ultrastructure.

Clinical Features and Outcome

Idiopathic MPGN presents with nephrotic syndrome in more than 50% of cases, and with non-nephrotic proteinuria with microscopic hematuria in another 20%. Less marked urinary abnormalities occur in the remaining patients. An impairment of kidney function, usually slowly progressive, is present in 20% to 25% of cases at presentation, whereas an acute nephritic syndrome, with rapid deterioration of kidney function, usually associated with the presence of crescents at biopsy, characterizes the onset in less than 10% of patients. Arterial hypertension, sometimes very severe, is present in more than half of the patients. Hypocomplementemia is frequently but not invariably noted at presentation. In type I MPGN, the classic complement pathway is preferentially activated (normal or low C3, low C4, and low CH50). In type II the alternative pathway is activated (low C3, normal C4, and low CH50). With type III, C3 is generally low, in association with a depression of terminal complement components (C3 through C9).

The clinical course of idiopathic MPGN is characterized by spontaneous variations in severity of proteinuria and a variable rate of deterioration of kidney function, with periods of prolonged remission in many patients (total remission being reported in 7% to 10% of patients), or episodes of acute deterioration of kidney function. The few studies on the final outcome of the disease report kidney survivals at 10 years after onset of 60% to 64%. These studies showed that an elevated serum creatinine, severe proteinuria, and arterial hypertension at presentation are the most significant clinical predictors of an unfavorable outcome, whereas the presence of marked tubulointerstitial lesions is the only significant histologic sign of bad prognosis.

Treatment

The role of steroids or cytotoxic drugs in the treatment of idiopathic MPGN, in both children and adults, has remained controversial. In the absence of convincing controlled trials, the use of these drugs is not recommended. Cyclosporine and anticoagulants have been used in some studies, without beneficial results.

Antiplatelet drugs (aspirin and persantine) demonstrated a beneficial effect in a single trial in the United States. They are now commonly used as a long-term therapy, in part because they lack significant adverse effects.

As in all proteinuric diseases, angiotensin-converting enzyme inhibitors should be administered, even in the absence of arterial hypertension, to reduce urinary protein loss. When patients are hypertensive, blood pressure should be treated aggressively.

CRYOGLOBULINEMIC GLOMERULONEPHRITIS

Mixed cryoglobulins are immunoglobulins that precipitate from cooled serum. They are composed of a polyclonal IgG bound to another immunoglobulin with rheumatoid factor (RF) activity (usually IgM). According to the classification of Brouet, two types of mixed cryoglobulins can be identified. In type II, the antiglobulin component is monoclonal (usually an IgM κ); in type III mixed cryoglobulins, it is polyclonal. Type I cryoglobulins are monoclonal IgG or IgM or, less commonly, IgA. The majority of mixed cryoglobulins, defined as secondary mixed cryoglobulinemias, have been detected in patients with connective tissue disorders, lymphoproliferative disorders, noninfectious hepatobiliary diseases, or immunologically mediated glomerular diseases. Until recently, in 30% of all mixed cryoglobulinemias, the etiology was undetermined and cryoglobulinemia was considered essential. With the availability of new serologic markers of hepatitis C virus (HCV) infection, it was recognized that the majority of these patients have antibodies against viral antigens and HCV RNA. This finding may explain why the prevalence of mixed cryoglobulinemia differs according to geographic area and is greater in countries such as in Italy, France, Spain, and Israel, where HCV infection is endemic.

However, in a proportion of cases that amounts to approximately 10% in the previously mentioned countries, but is definitely higher in Northern Europe and probably also in North America, no serologic markers of HCV infection can be found, even after a repetitive search over an extended period. The etiologic agents responsible for essential cryoglobulinemia in this residual group of patients, who have a kidney disease identical, both morphologically and clinically, to that associated with HCV infection, is still unknown.

The clinical syndrome of mixed cryoglobulinemia is characterized by purpura, weakness, arthralgias, and, in some patients, by glomerular involvement. This syndrome can be associated with both type II and type III mixed cryoglobulinemia, whereas kidney involvement has a higher prevalence in type II mixed cryoglobulinemia with monoclonal IgM component (usually IgM κ). Although in the few reported cases of type III mixed cryoglobulinemia with kidney involvement glomerular lesions were variable and nonspecific, in type II mixed cryoglobulinemia a specific and well-characterized pattern of glomerular lesions has been described.

Pathology

In most patients with type II mixed cryoglobulinemia, a peculiar type of exudative membranoproliferative glomerulonephritis (MPGN) is found. Especially in its more acute stage, this cryoglobulinemic glomerulonephritis has distinctive features that differentiate it from idiopathic type I MPGN as well as lupus nephritis.

The glomeruli are markedly hypercellular, due to an evident infiltration of leukocytes, which are mainly monocytes (Fig. 18-4). The average number of infiltrating leukocytes is greater than in diffuse proliferative lupus nephritis. Electron microscopy demonstrates that these leukocytes are in close contact with endocapillary and subendothelial IC deposits, and contain phagolysosomes, indicative of their phagocytic function.

The intraglomerular deposits, which are commonly found in a subendothelial position, as is typical of all glomerulonephritides with the membranoproliferative pattern, may sometimes also fill the capillary lumen, especially in patients with an acute and rapidly progressive deterioration of kidney function. Both these intraluminal deposits and the subendothelial deposits are eosinophilic, periodic acid-Schiff positive, and usually amorphous. They are electron dense and resemble ICs. However, electron microscopic examination sometimes demonstrates a specific fibrillar or cylindrical structure identical to that seen in the in vitro cryoprecipitate of the same patients. These structures are 100 to 1000 µm long and have a hollow axis, appearing in cross-sections like annular bodies (Fig. 18-5).

The peripheral interposition of mesangial matrix and mesangial cells between the GBM and the newly formed basement membrane–like material, which accounts for the double-contour appearance on stains that show basement membrane, is usually less evident than in other primary and secondary type I MPGNs. This milder mesangial involvement may explain both why glomerular segmental and global sclerosis is less severe than in other types of idiopathic or secondary MPGN, even many

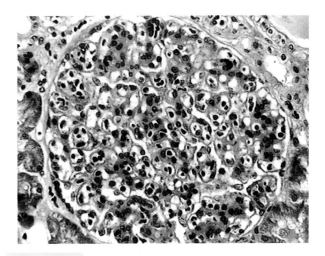

FIGURE 18-4   Glomerulus with prominent endocapillary hypercellularity, mainly due to massive infiltration of inflammatory mononuclear leukocytes. Mesangial cell proliferation and mesangial matrix expansion are mild (Masson trichrome, original magnification ×250).

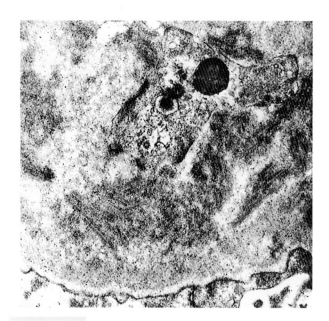

FIGURE 18-5 Electron microscopy: subendothelial deposit showing a specific annular and cylindrical structure (uranyl acetate and lead citrate, original magnification ×22,000). (Courtesy of Dr. E. Schiaffino, Pathology Department, S. Carlo Borromeo Hospital, Milan, Italy.)

years after the onset of the kidney disease and why evolution toward kidney failure with sclerosing nephritis is so rarely observed. In about 20% of cases, these distinctive features may be absent, and the histologic and immunohistologic picture at biopsy can be that of a type I lobular MPGN indistinguishable from that of idiopathic MPGN. Lobular MPGN is more likely to be found in patients with marked proteinuria associated with a moderate reduction in kidney function without a rapidly progressive course. In these patients, when signs of systemic involvement due to mixed cryoglobulinemia, especially purpura, are mild or absent at the time of biopsy, only serologic data, particularly detection of circulating cryoglobulins, make a correct diagnosis possible.

The histologic features of MPGN with subendothelial deposits, including the lobular type, are found in about 80% of patients with HCV-associated type II mixed cryoglobulinemia and glomerular involvement. In the remaining 20% of cases, the biopsy at presentation (the clinical renal syndrome usually being characterized by mild urinary abnormalities) shows the histologic pattern of a mild mesangial proliferative GN, with moderate or no infiltration of leukocytes. A similar pattern may be observed after intensive immunosuppressive therapy.

At least one third of patients with cryoglobulinemic GN have acute vasculitis of the small and medium-sized renal arteries, which is characterized by fibrinoid necrosis of the arteriolar wall and infiltration of monocytes in and around the vessel wall. This renal vasculitis, which is sometimes associated with other signs of systemic vas-

culitis, including purpura and mesenteric vasculitis, can also be found in the absence of obvious glomerular involvement. Even when the fibrinoid necrosis of the renal arterial walls is severe, segmental necrosis of the capillary loops is never observed and crescentic extracapillary proliferation is rare, suggesting that the vasculitic damage is limited to arterial vessels of larger size.

In the case of MPGN with intraluminal deposits, immunofluorescence microscopy reveals intense staining with antisera directed against the immunoglobulins in the mixed cryoglobulins, namely, IgM, IgG, and C3, usually associated with faint irregular segmental subendothelial staining of some peripheral loops. In more chronic stages, when intraluminal deposits are absent, the pattern is that of intense diffuse, granular, subendothelial staining of peripheral loops, similar to that of type I idiopathic MPGN.

Pathogenesis

It appears that HCV directly infects circulating peripheral blood mononuclear cells and bone marrow cells in the majority of patients with types II and III mixed cryoglobulinemia, and even some patients without concomitant cryoglobulinemia, although the occurrence of viral replication within cells is still controversial. It has been hypothesized that HCV infection may stimulate the B lymphocytes to synthesize the cryoprecipitating polyclonal rheumatoid factors responsible for type III mixed cryoglobulinemia. Some additional, as yet uncharacterized, event might induce, in only some of the total population with viral replication in B lymphocytes, abnormal proliferation of the specific clone of B cells producing the monoclonal RF that characterizes type II mixed cryoglobulinemia. The factors that cause this shift are as yet uncharacterized. Factors potentially responsible include duration of the HCV infection as well as superimposed infection with other viruses, such as hepatitis B virus or Epstein-Barr virus. Clonal expansion of IgM-producing cells has been reported, and its reversibility after interferon-α (IFN-α) therapy in some patients has also been documented. This hypothesis, which considers mixed cryoglobulinemia to be a benign lymphoproliferative disorder, may explain why overt B-cell malignancy occurs during its course in a minority of patients. The induction in mice of an MPGN similar to human cryoglobulinemic GN by injecting solubilized type II mixed cryoglobulins from patients with this kidney disease and HCV infection suggests a role of circulating cryoglobulins rather than host-specific factors in the pathogenesis of nephritis. The monoclonal IgM κ RF isolated from such mixed cryoglobulins is devoid of viral antigenic components. Nonetheless when injected separately into these animals, it was able to deposit in the glomerulus, suggesting a specific affinity of the IgM κ RF component of the cryoglobulins for some glomerular structure. Data demonstrate that the same purified IgM κ binds to cellular fibro-nectin, a known constituent of mesangial matrix. In contrast, purified monoclonal IgM from patients with Waldenström's macroglobulinemia, polyclonal IgM from patients with rheumatoid arthritis, or polyclonal IgM from normal subjects lack this affinity.

Host factors may be responsible for initiating disease once cryoglobulins are present; peripheral blood monocytes isolated from patients with cryoglobulinemic MPGN are less effective in removing cryoglobulins in vitro and release excess amounts of cathepsin D precursors in response to cryoglobulins. These cathepsin precursors could then be activated locally to induce tissue injury.

Thus, the prevalent pathogenetic mechanism seems to be the deposition in the glomerulus of a monoclonal IgM RF with particular affinity for the glomerular matrix. This IgM RF is produced by permanent clones of B lymphocytes infected by HCV. We do not yet know whether the IgM RF deposits in the glomerulus (1) alone, with subsequent in situ binding of IgG (perhaps bound already to viral antigens); (2) as a mixed IgG-IgM cryoglobulin, not bound to HCV antigens; or (3) as a complex composed of HCV antigens, IgG anti-HCV antibodies, and IgM κ RF. Demonstration of HCV RNA or virus antigens in glomeruli has remained elusive, and only recently have specific HCV-related proteins been detected in glomerular and tubulointerstitial vascular structures by indirect immunohistochemistry. Evidence that immune complexes containing intact virion are the main component of the glomerular deposits is scanty, and complexes containing HCV capsular antigens cannot be excluded.

Clinical Features and Outcome

Cryoglobulinemic GN is a disease of individuals in the fifth and the sixth decades of life. Extrarenal symptoms include purpura, arthralgias, leg ulcers, systemic vasculitis, Raynaud's phenomenon, and peripheral neuropathy. Renal symptoms are usually a late manifestation of type II MC, and they typically do not appear until a few years after the extrarenal signs. However, the simultaneous appearance of renal and systemic signs of the disease is rather frequent. In some patients, kidney involvement may be the main manifestation of the disease, before the appearance of the more suggestive purpura.

The most frequent renal syndrome is isolated proteinuria with microscopic hematuria, sometimes associated with signs of moderate chronic kidney failure or, less frequently, proteinuria in the nephrotic range. The corresponding histologic picture is that of MPGN, although patients with isolated urinary abnormalities occasionally present with the nonspecific findings of mild segmental mesangial proliferation.

An acute nephritic syndrome, characterized by macroscopic hematuria, severe proteinuria, hypertension, and rapid development of azotemia is present at the onset of kidney disease in 25% of cases, and is complicated by acute oliguric renal failure in 5%. In these individuals, the biopsy shows the typical cryoglobulinemic GN, that is, a severe MPGN characterized by intense monocyte infiltration and massive intraluminal deposits filling many capillary lumina.

Hypertension is frequent (more than 80%) at the time of presentation with kidney disease, even in patients without the nephritic syndrome. Hypertension is often severe and difficult to control.

The kidney disease has a variable course. In nearly one third of patients, a remission of renal symptoms, partial or complete, has been described, even if an acute nephritic syndrome or severe nephrotic syndrome was present. Remission after acute nephritic syndrome may occur before any treatment is started, and is associated with the disappearance of the massive intraluminal deposits that characterize this disorder. In another third of patients, the kidney disease is indolent, taking several years to progress to kidney failure, despite the persistence of urinary abnormalities. In 20% of patients, reversible clinical exacerbations such as nephritic syndrome occur, sometimes associated with flare-ups of systemic signs of the disease. The new episodes of nephritic syndrome can be accompanied by recurrence of massive intraluminal deposits and monocyte infiltration. Repeated exacerbations may occur in a single patient. A moderate degree of kidney failure, if not already present at clinical onset, frequently develops at later stages. Endstage renal disease requiring dialysis is relatively rare, even after many years of cryoglobulinemic GN. In the large series of patients with cryoglobulinemic GN studied in Milan, only 15% required regular dialysis after a mean follow-up of 131 months. Of these 105 patients, 42 patients died during the period of follow-up because of extrarenal complications. Cardiovascular disease (12 patients), infections (9 patients), liver failure (8 patients), and neoplasms, usually of hematologic origin (4 patients) were the most important causes of death. The 10-year probability of being alive without dialysis was 49%. Older patients and patients with recurrent purpura, high serum cryocrit, low serum C3 levels, and high serum creatinine at presentation were more like to die or to reach endstage renal disease.

The quantity of circulating cryoglobulins varies among patients, and may vary in the same patient over time. This laboratory parameter does not correlate with the degree of activity of the disease, but higher cryoglobulin concentrations appear to be associated with a poor prognosis. The serum complement pattern demonstrates characteristic abnormalities in cryoglobulinemic GN. Concentrations of the early complement components (C1q, C4,) and CH50 are usually greatly reduced; C4 can be undetectable. Variably, a moderate decrease in the level of C3 is also observed. Consumption of the early serum complement components, with characteristic sparing of C3, may be attributable to a change in the C4-binding protein that controls activity of classic pathway C3 convertase. Serum complement values do not change much with clinical evolution of the disease. In addition, RF can be detected. Serum protein electrophoresis frequently shows a monoclonal band (IgM κ), and in some cases a monoclonal light chain (usually κ) is evident in the urine.

Treatment

Before the recognition of the etiologic role of HCV infection, when most cryoglobulinemia was considered "essential," acute flare-ups of the kidney disease were treated with glucocorticoids, plasmapheresis, and frequently also with cyclophosphamide. High-dose steroid therapy, including initial treatment with intravenous boluses of methylprednisolone (0.5 to 1.0 g/day), was useful for controlling acute exacerbations of the disease associated with a rapidly progressive deterioration of kidney function, especially when given in combination with plasmapheresis and cyclophosphamide. The former was used to remove circulating cryoglobulins during stages of massive deposition in the glomeruli and vessel walls and the latter to limit vasculitic injury and inhibit production of monoclonal RF by the B lymphocytes. Despite the potential of these modalities to increase viral titers, no consistent evidence of a detrimental effect on hepatic disease accompanied their use. Oral steroids were also used, at lower doses, to control the systemic signs of mixed cryoglobulinemia.

With recognition of the association between cryoglobulinemic GN and HCV infection, the rationale for treatment of the systemic disease and its renal complications has shifted to use of an antiviral therapy. IFN-α has become the most extensively used antiviral agent. Despite its frequent use, the efficacy of IFN-α in cryoglobulinemic GN is still controversial. The three controlled trials that used IFN-α were performed in patients with clinically active mixed cryoglobulinemia associated with HCV infection, but without clearly established kidney involvement.

Based on these trials and a review of the literature on IFN-α treatment of patients with HCV infection (with or without mixed cryoglobulinemia and cryoglobulinemic GN), the following conclusions can be drawn:

- Sustained virologic response (defined as undetectable serum HCV RNA levels 6 months after completion of treatment) is obtained in no more than 15% to 20% of patients after an initial 12-month course of IFN-α at the standard dose of 3 million units three times a week.

- More intensive treatment courses of IFN-α (6 to 10 million units three times a week, or each day for the first 4 to 6 weeks) give only marginally better results.
- Combined treatment of IFN-α at the standard dose and ribavirin (1000 to 1200 mg/day), for at least 6 months, increases the sustained virologic response to 40% to 45% of patients.
- The recent trials with the pegylated forms of interferon (peginterferon-α_{2a} or peginterferon-α_{2b}) indicate an even more frequent sustained virologic response, in comparison with IFN-α. Overall response rates to a 48-week course of combination therapy of peginterferon and ribavirin were around 55%.
- Response to antiviral therapy is poorer in patients with genotype 1. Therefore, for these patients, a 48-week course of combined treatment is the recommended schedule, whereas a 24-week course can give similar beneficial results in patients with genotypes 2 and 3.
- Sustained virologic response interrupts the progression of hepatic damage, and can control the clinical signs of kidney involvement in less severe cases, but it does not prevent progression of kidney damage in the presence of acute exacerbations of cryoglobulinemic GN (characterized by an acute nephritic syndrome with rapidly deteriorating kidney function or nephrotic syndrome with slower deterioration of kidney function), usually associated with recurrence of the systemic signs of mixed cryoglobulinemia. Combination therapy with inflammatory and cytotoxic drugs, used in the past, is still necessary. In this clinical setting, our current policy is to give:
  - Peginterferon-α_{2a} (180 μg) or peginterferon-α_{2b} (1.5 μg/kg) weekly for 24 to 48 weeks, according to virus genotype.
  - Ribavirin (1000 to 1200 mg/day) for 24 to 48 weeks, according to virus genotype.
  - Steroids: Methylprednisolone (0.75 to 1.00 g/day intravenously for 3 consecutive days), followed by oral prednisone for 6 months (0.5 mg/kg body weight per day, tapered over a few weeks until small mainten-ance doses of 10 mg/day or 20 mg/alternate days are achieved).

In the most severe cases, especially if signs of systemic and renal vasculitis are present, we add also:

- Cyclophosphamide: 2 mg/kg body weight per day for 2 to 4 months.
- Plasmapheresis: exchanges of 3 L of plasma three times a week for 2 to 3 weeks.

A controlled trial is needed to verify that the benefits of the addition of steroids and cyclophosphamide outweigh their potential to increase infectious or hepatic complications.

Primary IgA Nephropathy

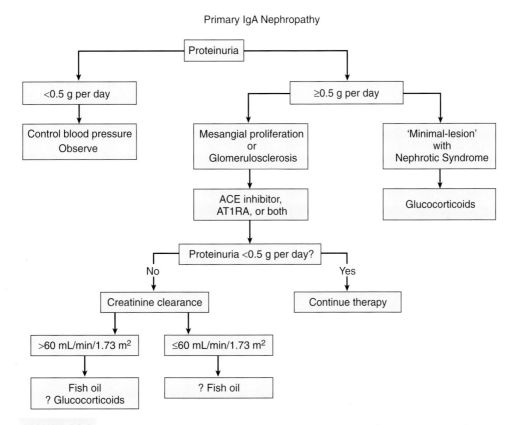

FIGURE 21-3   Treatment of IgA nephropathy in patients with stable kidney function with no or few glomerular crescents and no focal necrotizing lesions on biopsy. It is not yet clear whether glucocorticoids or fish oil offer additional benefit for preservation of kidney function if proteinuria has been reduced to less than 0.5 g/day by using an angiotensin-converting enzyme (ACE) inhibitor, angiotensin II type I receptor antagonist (AT1RA), or both. Fish oil may be beneficial for patients with relatively preserved kidney function, and this effect may be dose dependent. The use of glucocorticoids is more controversial; some studies have shown that treatment reduces proteinuria, preserves kidney function, or both. The sitting systolic blood pressure should be controlled to 120 to 125 mm Hg with additional medications, as needed. Adjunctive therapies to slow the loss of kidney function in proteinuric patients also apply, as reviewed by Wilmer and colleagues.

treatment. Regimens have ranged from intermittent intravenous high-dose methylprednisolone combined with alternate-day oral prednisone over 6 months to a 2-year tapering schedule of oral prednisone. Proteinuria frequently decreases, and one study showed a decrement in mesangial matrix in posttreatment kidney biopsies. However, concomitant use of angiotensin-converting enzyme inhibitors was infrequent, and the benefit of therapy on kidney function was sometimes not statistically significant after including reduction in proteinuria as a covariate in the multivariate analysis. Fish oil rich in omega-3 fatty acids (to provide a daily dose of 1.9 g eicosapentaenoic acid and 1.4 g docosahexaenoic acid) given for 2 years slowed the decline in kidney function in patients with proteinuria at least 1 g/day in a multicenter, placebo-controlled, randomized study, but proteinuria was not reduced. Prior results with fish oil had been controversial; only two of four trials showed a benefit. A recent prospective, placebo-controlled, randomized treatment trial with children and young adults evaluated 2-year treatment with alternate-day prednisone or daily fish oil. Preliminary analysis found that prednisone no more effectively preserved kidney function than placebo, although proteinuria significantly declined. In contrast, patients on fish oil showed improvement in the clinical outcome score (factoring glomerular filtration rate and proteinuria) that correlated with circulating levels of phospholipid and arachidonic acid. Therefore, the benefit from treatment with fish oil may be dose dependent.

Several immunosuppressive or anti-inflammatory agents, alone or in combination, have not consistently shown efficacy: azathioprine, mycophenolate mofetil, cyclosporine, intravenous immunoglobulin, mizoribine, sodium chromoglycate, aspirin, dipyridamole, dapsone, and danazol. Gluten-free and low-antigen diets offer minimal, if any, benefit.

Other general recommendations for treatment of proteinuric patients with chronic kidney disease apply, as recently reviewed by Wilmer and colleagues. Reducing salt intake to 80 to 120 mmol/day optimizes the antiproteinuric effects of angiotensin-converting enzyme inhibitors or angiotensin II type 1 receptor antagonists. Restriction of dietary protein intake to 0.7 to 0.8 g/kg body weight per day may slow loss of kidney function, but patients should be carefully monitored to avoid protein malnutrition. Statin therapy to control hyperlipidemia has been shown to reduce proteinuria. Obese patients should lose weight. Use of tobacco should cease. Correction of metabolic acidosis and elevated homocysteine or uric levels may be beneficial.

A few patients with normal kidney function develop nephrotic syndrome with light microscopic histologic features of minimal change glomerulonephritis. After achieving a glucocorticoid-induced remission of proteinuria, the IgA1 deposits sometimes disappear.

For patients reaching endstage renal failure due to IgA nephropathy, transplantation affords an excellent option. However, disease recurs in about 50% to 60% of patients by 5 years after transplantation, and, unfortunately, loss of the kidney may ensue. Nonetheless, overall survival rates of the patients and allografts are excellent. The frequency of recurrent disease has not been reduced by any of the newer immunosuppressive agents, such as sirolimus or mycophenolate mofetil. Recurrence in some patients with Henoch-Schönlein purpura nephritis is limited to the kidney (with immunohistologic features indistinguishable from Berger's disease), without systemic manifestations of a vasculitis. No consensus has been reached whether a laboratory or clinical parameter confers a greater risk of recurrent disease. Once proteinuria due to recurrent disease occurs, treatment with an angiotensin-converting enzyme inhibitor or angiotensin II type 1 receptor antagonist may not significantly ameliorate the laboratory findings or progressive clinical course. Therefore, instituting therapy with these agents before overt evidence of recurrence seems reasonable. Although a few transplant centers have shown a higher rate of recurrence in kidneys from living-related donors than deceased donors, survival of the allografts did not differ by donor source. Donation from a living donor remains the best choice for kidney transplantation.

BIBLIOGRAPHY

Alexopoulos E: Treatment of primary IgA nephropathy. Kidney Int 65:341–355, 2004.

Appel GB, Glassock RJ: Glomerular, vascular, and tubulointerstitial diseases. Nephrology self-assessment program. Am Soc Nephrol 2:247–251, 2003.

Berger J, Hinglais N: [Intercapillary deposits of IgA-IgG.] Les depots intercapillaires d'IgA-IgG. J Urol Nephrol 74:694–695, 1968.

Davin J-C, ten Berge IJ, Weening JJ: What is the difference between IgA nephropathy and Henoch-Schönlein purpura nephritis? Kidney Int 59:823–834, 2001.

Del Prete D, Gambaro G, Lupo A, et al: Precocious activation of genes of the renin-angiotensin system and the fibrogenic cascade in IgA glomerulonephritis. Kidney Int 64:149–159, 2003.

Donadio JV, Bergstralh EJ, Grande JP, et al: Proteinuria patterns and their association with subsequent endstage renal disease in IgA nephropathy. Nephrol Dial Transplant 17:1997–1203, 2002.

Donadio JV Jr, Grande JP: IgA nephropathy. N Engl J Med 347:738–748, 2002.

Fervenza FC: Henoch-Schönlein purpura nephritis. Int J Dermatol 42:170–177, 2003.

Floege J: Evidence-based recommendations for immunosuppression in IgA nephropathy: Handle with caution. Nephrol Dial Transplant 18:241–245, 2003.

Frimat L, Kessler M: Controversies concerning the importance of genetic polymorphism in IgA nephropathy. Nephrol Dial Transplant 17:542–545, 2002.

Geddes CC, Rauta V, Gronhagen-Riska C, et al: A tricontinental view of IgA nephropathy. Nephrol Dial Transplant 18:1541–1548, 2003.

Itoh A, Iwase H, Takatani T, et al: Tonsillar IgA1 as a possible source of hypoglycosylated IgA1 in the serum of IgA nephropathy patients. Nephrol Dial Transplant 18:1108–1114, 2003.

Julian BA, Novack J: IgA nephropathy: An update. Curr Opin Nephrol Hypertens 13:171–179, 2004.

Liu Y: Epithelial to mesenchymal transition in renal fibrogenesis: Pathologic significance, molecular mechanism, and therapeutic intervention. J Am Soc Nephrol 15:1–12, 2004.

Nakao N, Yoshimura A, Morita H, et al: Combination treatment of angiotensin-II receptor blocker and angiotensin-converting-enzyme inhibitor in non-diabetic renal disease (COOPERATE): A randomized controlled trial. Lancet 361:117–124, 2003.

Pozzi C, Andrulli S, Del Vecchio L, et al: Corticosteroid effectiveness in IgA nephropathy: Long-term results of a randomized, controlled trial. J Am Soc Nephrol 15:157–163, 2004.

Praga M, Gutierrez E, Gonzalez, et al: Treatment of IgA nephropathy with ACE inhibitors: A randomized and controlled trial. J Am Soc Nephrol 14:178–1583, 2003.

Smith AC, Feehally J: New insights into the pathogenesis of IgA nephropathy. Springer Semin Immunopathol 24:477–493, 2003.

Tumlin JA, Lohavichan V, Hennigar R: Crescentic, proliferative IgA nephropathy: Clinical and histological response to methylprednisolone and intravenous cyclophosphamide. Nephrol Dial Transplant 18:1321–1329, 2003.

Urizar RE, Michael A, Sisson S, et al: Anaphylactoid purpura. II. Immunofluorescent and electron microscopy studies of the glomerular lesions. Lab Invest 19:437–440, 1968.

Wilmer WA, Rovin BH, Hebert CJ, et al: Management of glomerular proteinuria: A commentary. J Am Soc Nephrol 14:3217–3232, 2003.

CHAPTER 22

Goodpasture's Syndrome and Other Anti-Glomerular Basement Membrane Disease

Charles D. Pusey

The term *Goodpasture's syndrome* was first used by Stanton and Tange in 1957 in their report of nine patients with pulmonary renal syndrome, which referred back to the original patient described by Goodpasture in 1919. It was not until the 1960s that the development of immunofluorescence techniques led to the detection of immunoglobulin deposited along the glomerular basement membrane (GBM) in this condition. Today Goodpasture's syndrome is often used to describe the combination of rapidly progressive glomerulonephritis (RPGN), pulmonary hemorrhage, and anti-GBM antibodies. However, some researchers use the term *Goodpasture's syndrome* to describe the characteristic clinical features from any cause, and the term *Goodpasture's disease* to describe those who in addition have anti-GBM antibodies. The term *anti-GBM disease* is also widely used to describe any patient with the typical autoantibodies, regardless of clinical features.

CLINICAL FEATURES

There is a bimodal age distribution with peak incidence in the third and sixth decades of life, and a slight preponderance toward males. Most patients present with RPGN and lung hemorrhage, although about a third may present with isolated glomerulonephritis. Rarely, patients present with isolated lung hemorrhage without renal failure, although many of these have hematuria and proteinuria. General malaise, fatigue, and weight loss are the most common systemic features and may relate to anemia.

Pulmonary Disease

Pulmonary hemorrhage occurs in about two thirds of patients and is more common in young men. It may precede the development of kidney disease. Patients often complain of breathlessness and cough, which may be accompanied by minor or massive hemoptysis. Hemoptysis can be triggered by cigarette smoking, inhaled toxins, sepsis, or fluid overload. Clinical signs include tachypnea, respiratory crackles, and eventually cyanosis, but these are often indistinguishable from those of pulmonary edema or infection. Radiographic features are nonspecific, but usually involve patchy or diffuse alveolar shadowing in the central lung fields (Fig. 22-1). The most sensitive test is an elevation in the carbon monoxide diffusion capacity of the lungs due to the presence of hemoglobin in the alveolar spaces. Bronchoscopy may reveal diffuse hemorrhage, but is perhaps of more importance in excluding infection.

Renal Disease

Patients may present with isolated hematuria or mild renal functional impairment, but most commonly present with acute renal failure due to RPGN. The clinical features are not distinguishable from those of any other cause of RPGN. Urine microscopy reveals numerous erythrocytes of glomerular origin, red cell casts, and mild to moderate proteinuria (nephrotic range proteinuria is rare). Hypertension and oliguria are late features. Renal ultrasonography usually reveals normal-sized kidneys and is helpful in excluding other kidney disorders.

PATHOLOGY

Light microscopy of the kidney biopsy usually reveals a diffuse crescentic glomerulonephritis, with most of the crescents at the same stage of evolution (Fig. 22-2). There is often segmental necrosis of glomeruli and some cellular proliferation. Blood vessels are usually normal, but vasculitis has been reported rarely. There is usually a prominent interstitial cellular infiltrate. The immunohistology is characteristic, with linear deposits of immunoglobulin G (IgG; sometimes accompanied by IgA or IgM) and complement C3 along the GBM (Fig. 22-3). Less intense linear staining with IgG may occasionally be seen in diabetes, systemic lupus erythematosus, myeloma, and transplanted kidneys. Lung histology is rarely obtained, since transbronchial biopsy does not provide adequate specimens. Open-lung biopsy can

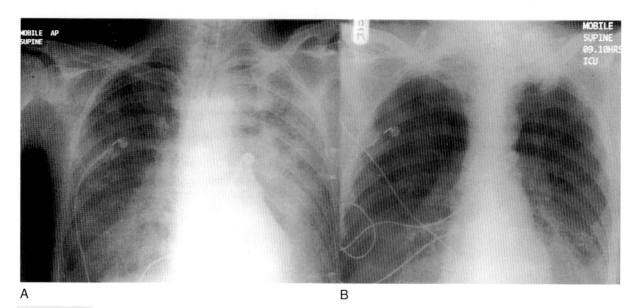

A

B

FIGURE 22-1   Chest radiographs of a patient with Goodpasture's disease. *A,* Alveolar hemorrhage. *B,* Resolution after 4 days of treatment.

reveal alveoli full of red cells, hemosiderin-laden macrophages, and fibrin. Immunofluorescence is technically difficult but may reveal linear deposits of IgG along the alveolar basement membrane.

DIFFERENTIAL DIAGNOSIS

It is important to distinguish anti-GBM disease from other causes of pulmonary renal syndrome and RPGN, because treatment and prognosis are different. Primary systemic vasculitis associated with antineutrophil cytoplasmic antibodies (ANCAs) is the most common cause of Goodpasture's syndrome and is the main differential diagnosis. Occasional patients have both anti-GBM antibodies and ANCAs. Other conditions to consider include systemic lupus erythematosus, cryoglobulinemia,

Henoch-Schönlein purpura, and various causes of pulmonary renal syndrome (Table 22-1). The diagnosis of anti-GBM disease can be made by kidney biopsy and by the detection of circulating anti-GBM antibodies. Various enzyme-linked immunosorbent assays are available for serologic testing, but may vary in their specificity and sensitivity. A screen for other relevant antibodies (e.g., ANCAs and anti-DNA antibodies) is usually performed at the same time.

ASSOCIATED DISEASES

Anti-GBM disease is rarely associated with other autoimmune disorders, except for systemic vasculitis. Up to 30% of patients have been shown to have ANCAs, most commonly perinuclear ANCA (P-ANCA) specific for myeloper-

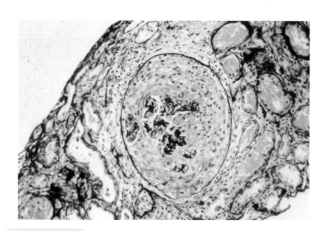

FIGURE 22-2   Renal biopsy from a patient with Goodpasture's disease showing acute crescentic glomerulonephritis (silver stain).

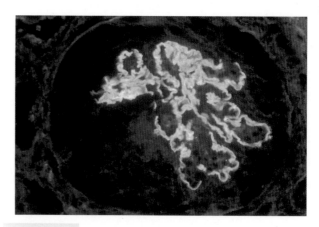

FIGURE 22-3   Renal biopsy from a patient with Goodpasture's disease: immunofluorescence showing linear deposition of IgG along the glomerular basement membrane.

TABLE 22-1 Causes of Pulmonary Renal Syndrome

More common
  Microscopic polyangiitis
  Wegener's granulomatosis
  Goodpasture's disease
  Systemic lupus erythematosus

Less common
  Churg-Strauss syndrome
  Henoch-Schönlein purpura
  Hemolytic uremic syndrome
  Behçet's disease
  Essential mixed cryoglobulinemia
  Rheumatoid vasculitis
  Penicillamine therapy

oxidase. Conversely, relatively few patients with ANCA-associated vasculitis also have anti-GBM antibodies (5% to 10%). There are some reports that these "double-positive" patients behave more like those with systemic vasculitis, but a recent series shows that they are unlikely to recover kidney function once on dialysis. Several patients with membranous nephropathy have been reported to develop anti-GBM disease. It has also been reported following lithotripsy and urinary tract obstruction. Anti-GBM disease may develop in the transplanted kidney in patients with Alport's syndrome. Patients with X-linked Alport's syndrome inherit a defect in the α5 chain of type IV collagen, but also lack the α3 chain, which contains the Goodpasture antigen. Transplantation of a normal kidney therefore exposes the immune system to an antigen to which tolerance has not developed, and an immune response is provoked. The antibodies may be against either the α5 or the α3 chain. Although many patients show antibody deposition along the GBM of the allograft, only a minority develop severe glomerulonephritis.

EPIDEMIOLOGY

Limited epidemiologic studies suggest that anti-GBM disease has an incidence of 0.5 to 1 case per million population per year. It is found in up to 2% of kidney biopsies and may account for up to 7% of patients with endstage renal failure. It is predominantly a disease of whites and is less common in those of African or Asian origin.

Genetic Predisposition

Goodpasture's disease has been reported in siblings and in two sets of identical twins. However, discordant twins have also been documented. As in other autoimmune diseases, there are associations with the major histocompatibility complex. There is a strong association with HLA DR2, which is carried by about 85% of patients with

Goodpasture's disease. Molecular analysis of HLA class II alleles has confirmed the positive association with DRB1*1501 and DRB1*1502, and has shown weaker associations with DRB1*04 and DRB1*03. There are negative associations with DRB1*07 and DRB1*01. Because of linkage disequilibrium, there are also positive associations with the DQ genes DQA1*01 and DQB1*06.

Environmental Factors

There are several case reports documenting exposure to hydrocarbons prior to the onset of clinical disease. There are also case control studies showing a higher incidence of anti-GBM antibodies (usually borderline levels) in those exposed to inhaled industrial hydrocarbons. Cigarette smoking undoubtedly precipitates pulmonary hemorrhage, but is of uncertain relevance to the etiology. Several clusters of cases have been reported, and there are suggestions of associations with viral infection. However, no clear association with any specific infectious agent has been proved.

PATHOGENESIS

There is good evidence that anti-GBM disease is due to the development of autoimmunity to a component of the GBM known as the Goodpasture antigen. The GBM is formed from a network of type IV collagen molecules, of which the α1 and α2 chains are widespread in vascular basement membranes, while the α3, α4, and α5 chains are restricted to the GBM and certain other specialized basement membranes. The Goodpasture antigen is present in the noncollagenous 1 (NC1) domain of the α3 chain of type IV collagen [α3(IV)NC1]. Recent work shows that the main antibody epitope is localized to the amino terminus of the molecule. The antigen is also found in basement membranes of the alveoli, choroid plexus, cochlea, and eye.

Autoimmunity

In Goodpasture's disease, the presence of anti-GBM antibodies is closely linked to the development of clinical features. There is a broad correlation between anti-GBM antibody levels at presentation and severity of disease, and the disease recurs immediately in kidney transplants if the recipient still has circulating antibodies. Importantly, the transfer of anti-GBM antibodies from patients to squirrel monkeys has confirmed that the antibodies are directly pathogenic. However, T cells are also involved in pathogenesis, both by providing help for autoreactive B cells and probably by contributing to cell-mediated glomerular injury. Recent work shows that a population of regulatory T cells can be detected in patients who have recovered from the disease, and this regulatory mechanism may account for the rarity of recurrence.

TABLE 22-2 Initial Treatment of Goodpasture's Disease

Plasma exchange	Daily 4-L exchange for 5% human albumin solution. Use 300–600 mL fresh plasma within 3 days of invasive procedure (e.g., biopsy) or in patients with pulmonary hemorrhage. Continue for 14 days or until antibody levels fully suppressed. Withhold if platelet count <70 × 10^9/mL, or hemoglobin <9 g/dL. Watch for coagulopathy, hypocalcemia, and hypokalemia.
Cyclophosphamide	Daily oral dosing at 2–3 mg/kg/day (round down to nearest 50 mg; use 2 mg/kg/day in patients over 55 years). Stop if white cell count <4 × 10^9/mL, and restart at lower dose when count >4 × 10^9/mL.
Prednisone	Daily oral dosing at 1 mg/kg/day (maximum 60 mg). Reduce dose weekly to 20 mg by week 6, and then more slowly. No evidence of benefit of intravenous methylprednisolone and may increase infection risk (possibly use if plasma exchange not available).
Prophylactic treatments	Oral nystatin and amphotericin (or fluconazole): oropharyngeal fungal infection. H2 blocker or proton-pump inhibitor: steroid promoted gastric ulceration. Low-dose cotrimoxazole: *Pneumocystis carinii* pneumonia.

TREATMENT

Untreated anti-GBM disease is usually rapidly fatal, and kidney function does not recover. However, the introduction in the 1970s of treatment with plasma exchange, cyclophosphamide, and corticosteroids (together with dialysis when required) now allows the great majority of patients to survive. The rationale behind this treatment regimen is that plasma exchange rapidly removes circulating anti-GBM antibodies, while cyclophosphamide prevents further antibody synthesis. There has been only one small trial of plasma exchange compared with drug treatment alone, and this suggested a trend toward improved outcome. However, the widely reported improvement in mortality and in kidney function following introduction of the treatment regimen described previously has led to its widespread use. The protocol we currently use is shown in Table 22-2. Some patients have been treated with intravenous methylprednisolone, but there is no convincing evidence that it confers a benefit, and it may be associated with a greater risk for infection. Cyclosporine has been used in occasional patients unresponsive to other therapy, but its role is not yet clear. In general, long-term treatment is not necessary and patients can stop cyclophosphamide after 3 months. Some authors then change to azathioprine, but there is little evidence that this is necessary. Steroids may be tailed off after about 6 months.

PROGNOSIS

Most patients now survive the acute disease, although pulmonary hemorrhage and infection remain important causes of death. In recent series, 1-year patient survival was 75% to 90%, but only around 40% of survivors recovered independent kidney function. Serum creatinine usually starts to decrease within 1 or 2 weeks of starting treatment and most of those with a creatinine level of less than 6.8 mg/dL at presentation will recover kidney function. However, it has been reported that those with a creatinine level of greater than 6.8 mg/dL, or who are oliguric, rarely recover kidney function. More recently, a single-center study of 71 treated patients showed that almost all of those with a creatinine level of less than 5.7 mg/dL recovered kidney function, as did the majority of those with a creatinine level of greater than 5.7 mg/dL, but not those on dialysis. As in previous studies, very few patients recovered kidney function once on dialysis. Crescent scores of greater than 50% are generally, but not always, associated with a poor renal prognosis. Patients presenting with dialysis-dependent renal failure may therefore not benefit from immunosuppression, unless they also have pulmonary hemorrhage. This is in marked contrast to the outcome in patients with ANCA-associated RPGN, in whom the majority should recover kidney function, even if presenting with a creatinine level of greater than 6.8 mg/dL or on dialysis. Exacerbations of pulmonary hemorrhage and worsening kidney function may occur early in the disease, in the presence of anti-GBM antibodies, and are often triggered by infection. True late recurrence after anti-GBM antibodies have become undetectable is rare. Kidney transplantation may be performed once anti-GBM antibodies are undetectable, but we usually delay this until at least 6 months after disappearance of antibodies.

BIBLIOGRAPHY

Herody M, Bobrie G, Gouarin C, et al: Anti-GBM disease: Predictive value of clinical, histological and serological data. Clin Nephrol 40:249–255, 1993.

Johnson JP, Moore JJ, Austin HJ, et al: Therapy of anti-glomerular basement membrane antibody disease: Analysis of prognostic significance of clinical, pathological and treatment factors. Medicine 64:219–227, 1985.

Lerner RA, Glassock RJ, Dixon FJ: The role of anti-glomerular basement membrane antibodies in the pathogenesis of human glomerulonephritis. J Exp Med 126:989–1004, 1967.

Levy JB, Hammad T, Coulthart A, et al: Clinical features and outcome of patients with both ANCA and anti-GBM antibodies. Kidney Int 66:1535–1540, 2004.

Levy JB, Turner AN, Rees AJ, Pusey CD: Long-term outcome of anti-glomerular basement membrane antibody disease treated with plasma exchange and immunosuppression. Ann Intern Med 134:1033–1942, 2001.

Lockwood CM, Rees AJ, Pearson TA, et al: Immunosuppression and plasma exchange in the treatment of Goodpasture's syndrome. Lancet 1:711–715, 1976.

Merkel F, Pullig O, Marx M, et al: Course and prognosis of anti-basement membrane antibody mediated disease: A report of 35 cases. Nephrol Dial Transplant 9:372–376, 1994.

Phelps RG, Rees AJ: The HLA complex in Goodpasture's disease: A model for analyzing susceptibility to autoimmunity. Kidney Int 56:1638–1653, 1999.

Pusey CD: Anti-glomerular basement membrane (anti-GBM) disease. Kidney Int 64:1535–1550, 2003.

Salama AD, Pusey CD: Immunology of anti-glomerular basement membrane disease. Curr Opin Nephrol Hypertens 11:279–286, 2002.

Saus J, Wieslander J, Langeveld JPM, et al: Identification of the Goodpasture antigen as the α3(IV) chain of collagen IV. J Biol Chem 263:13374–13380, 1988.

Turner N, Mason PJ, Brown R, et al: Molecular cloning of the human Goodpasture antigen demonstrates it to be the alpha 3 chain of type IV collagen. J Clin Invest 89:592–601, 1992.

Wilson CB, Dixon FJ: Anti-glomerular basement membrane antibody-induced glomerulonephritis. Kidney Int 3:74–89, 1973.

The Kidney in Systemic Disease

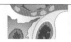

CHAPTER 23

Kidney Function in Congestive Heart Failure

Christlieb Haller   Martin Zeier   Eberhard Ritz

Congestive heart failure (CHF) is the only major cardiovascular disease with an increasing incidence and prevalence in industrialized countries. Despite considerable progress in the clinical management of CHF, its prognosis continues to be worse than in many common cancers. The kidney is the principal organ affected by the decline of cardiac function. At the same time, the kidney contributes to the development of the clinical syndrome of heart failure. Its characteristic hemodynamic and neuroendocrine abnormalities determine the pathophysiology, clinical presentation, and prognosis of this disorder.

EPIDEMIOLOGY

Impaired kidney function is an important determinant of mortality in CHF. It also increases the rate of adverse effects of medications that are commonly used in such patients (e.g., angiotensin-converting enzyme [ACE] inhibitors, angiotensin receptor blockers, or digoxin). Surprisingly, there is little well-documented information on the frequency of impaired kidney function in CHF. In patients with moderate CHF (SOLVD trial), one third had an estimated glomerular filtration rate (GFR) of less than $60\,mL/min/1.73\,m^2$, and in patients with more severe CHF (PRIME trial), one half had that same GFR. Numerous studies documented that estimated GFR is a highly potent predictor of cardiovascular events and mortality, and this is true even for minor degrees of kidney dysfunction. An elevated serum creatinine at discharge is also a significant predictor of hospital readmission. In intervention studies on patients with CHF, estimated GFR emerged as the most powerful predictor of death, followed by New York Heart Association (NYHA) class and use of ACE inhibitors. The mortality rate was higher by a factor of 2.85 in the lowest compared with the highest quartile of estimated GFR.

PATHOPHYSIOLOGY

The Role of Effective Arterial Volume in Congestive Heart Failure

The kidney senses cardiac dysfunction and responds with functional alterations, including salt and volume retention. Initially adaptive, these changes become maladaptive, causing further cardiac compromise by increasing preload and afterload through activation of the sympathetic nervous system and the renin-angiotensin-aldosterone system, which leads to volume expansion and increased vascular tone. The primary lesion, a decrease in cardiac pump function, reduces the filling of the arterial vasculature and tends to lower blood pressure in the aorta. In response, the sympathetic nervous system is activated and the peripheral resistance increases to maintain blood pressure.

Information on filling of the arterial tree and blood pressure is conveyed from vascular baroreceptors to the kidney via the sympathetic nervous system. The impaired cardiac pump function is perceived as a decrease in effective arterial volume irrespective of the actual blood volume, which may be normal, but in CHF it is frequently increased. The perceived decrease in arterial volume stimulates renal mechanisms that are ideally suited to counteract hemorrhage but are less useful to compensate for a chronic reduction of effective arterial volume (Fig. 23-1). The counterregulatory responses include an increase in preload through the renal retention of sodium and an increase in afterload as vascular resistance rises. Although renal plasma flow is reduced, the decrease in GFR is initially not as marked and the filtration fraction is increased. Ultrafiltration of a larger than normal fraction of plasma increases the oncotic pressure in the plasma that reaches the postglomerular

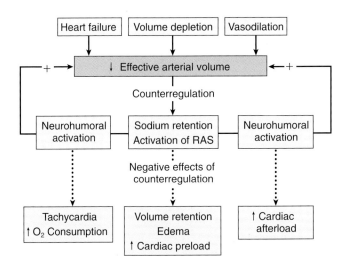

FIGURE 23-1 Cardiorenal volume regulation. Counterregulatory adaptive mechanisms may have negative, maladaptive effects. Heart failure or any other decrease in effective arterial volume activates several counterregulatory cardiorenal mechanisms to increase the effective arterial volume by stimulating renal sodium and volume retention and by increasing vascular resistance. In heart failure, the chronic activation of these counterregulatory mechanisms has a multiplicity of negative effects that characterize the clinical syndrome of congestive heart failure.

renal capillaries and results in increased sodium reabsorption in the proximal tubule. The net effect of the renal responses to a decreased effective arterial volume is sodium and water retention, decreased urine output, and the stimulation of salt and water intake. Many of the clinical signs and symptoms as well as prognostic indicators of CHF are in fact not directly related to the impaired cardiac performance, but rather to the renal counterregulatory mechanisms. Correction of such maladaptive responses of the kidney is therefore an important part of patient management.

Neuroendocrine Activation and Renal Mechanisms

Catecholamines

Arterial underfilling due to cardiac pump failure is sensed by arterial baroreceptors in the large vessels. Their activation results in increased sympathetic tone, which raises cardiac output by stimulating heart rate and cardiac contractility via adrenergic β receptors. Sympathetic activation causes arterial constriction and results in an increased peripheral vascular resistance or afterload, an action mediated by adrenergic α receptors. Sympathetic venoconstriction can increase cardiac filling, or preload. Although these effects are useful for maintaining blood pressure and arterial filling in the short run, they are counterproductive in the failing heart. They increase cardiac work and oxygen consumption and may con-

tribute unfavorably to cardiac remodeling and electrical stability. The primary sympathetic transmitter is norepinephrine, which acts predominantly as a vasoconstrictor. In the kidney, efferent sympathetic nerves induce renal vasoconstriction and stimulate the intrarenal renin-angiotensin system.

Renal vessels also have receptors for dopamine, but the contribution of endogenous dopamine to the physiologic regulation of renal blood flow and function is not clear. The infusion of exogenous dopamine in low doses induces a renal vasodilation and natriuresis, whereas high doses cause renal arterial constriction.

Renin-Angiotensin-Aldosterone System

Sympathetic activation changes intrarenal hemodynamics and stimulates the secretion of renin by the juxtaglomerular apparatus of the kidney. As a consequence, angiotensin II is generated. In concert with the sympathetic nervous system, this hormone induces vasoconstriction in the systemic circulation in an effort to increase or at least maintain blood pressure. At the same time, the intrarenal renin-angiotensin systems are activated. Locally generated angiotensin II has two principal effects: (1) it directly stimulates sodium reabsorption in the proximal tubule, and (2) it preferentially constricts the efferent arteriole, leaving the afferent arteriole relatively unaffected. This differential regulation of afferent and efferent arteriolar resistance increases intraglomerular capillary pressure and filtration fraction and maintains GFR despite decreased overall renal blood flow.

Angiotensin II and aldosterone are the predominant mediators of renal sodium retention in CHF. In addition to its hemodynamic effects, angiotensin II stimulates proximal tubular epithelial cells directly to absorb sodium from the tubular fluid. This effect is linked to secretion of protons generated from CO_2 by the action of carbonic anhydrase. Furthermore, locally synthesized angiotensinogen spills over into tubular fluid, is locally converted to angiotensin II, and further promotes sodium reabsorption in the collecting duct by activating the epithelial sodium channel (ENaC). Angiotensin II in the circulation also induces the synthesis and secretion of aldosterone in the zona glomerulosa of the adrenal cortex. Thus, angiotensin II acts in different ways to reduce salt and water excretion. At the same time, it increases fluid intake, since it is also a potent dipsogen.

Aldosterone acts on the distal nephron. In response to aldosterone, more sodium channels are inserted into the luminal membrane of aldosterone-responsive tubular cells. Because these sodium channels mediate the electrogenic absorption of sodium in this nephron segment, the tubular lumen becomes more negatively charged relative to the peritubular fluid. The negative luminal potential is a strong stimulus for the secretion of K^+ and

H+. The net effect of aldosterone is therefore the reabsorption of sodium and the secretion of protons and potassium ions.

A decrease in effective arterial volume stimulates the secretion of antidiuretic hormone (ADH) from the posterior pituitary. Normally, the secretion of this peptide hormone is regulated by hypothalamic osmoreceptors, and ADH secretion rises with increasing serum osmolality. However, in heart failure ADH secretion occurs despite a normal or even low serum osmolality. The signal for the nonosmotic secretion of ADH arises in the arterial baroreceptors, which override the osmotic control of ADH. ADH stimulates a specific subtype of vasopressin receptors (V2) in renal collecting duct cells. As a consequence, the hydraulic permeability of these cells increases due to the insertion of specific water channels, or aquaporins, into their plasma membrane. Water can thus flow down its concentration gradient from the hypotonic urine into the hypertonic interstitium of the renal medulla. The net result is the retention of osmotically "free" water as a counterregulatory response to the reduction of effective arterial volume. Human ADH is also termed arginine vasopressin, a name that emphasizes its potent vasoconstrictor properties. Furthermore, arginine vasopressin is also an effective dipsogen.

Natriuretic Peptides

Under physiologic conditions of balance, ingestion or administration of salt results in a prompt natriuresis until the excess sodium is excreted. Such fine-tuned control results from tubuloglomerular feedback mechanisms and the action of atrial and brain natriuretic peptides (ANP and BNP) on distal tubular segments. ANP is secreted by the cardiac atrium in response to increased wall stretch as a consequence of volume expansion. These hormones increase the GFR through afferent arteriolar vasodilatation and efferent arteriolar vasoconstriction. In addition, they reduce sodium reabsorption in the renal collecting duct. Together, these effects lead to a natriuresis. The natriuretic peptides are also systemic vasodilators; in total, their effects counter the increase in effective arterial volume.

In CHF, the plasma concentration of natriuretic peptides is usually increased due to cardiac dilatation and increased wall stretch. Natriuretic peptides oppose the action of the renin-angiotensin system, of endothelin 1, and of the sympathetic nerve system, and limit salt and water retention in CHF. However, the other sodium-retentive mechanisms previously mentioned override the effects of the natriuretic peptides and render the kidney relatively resistant to their action. Recently, BNP has emerged as a powerful predictor of cardiac prognosis. The therapeutic effects of pharmacologic doses of exogenous natriuretic peptides are currently under investigation.

Acute Kidney Failure in Congestive Heart Failure

Patients with intrinsically normal kidneys may develop prerenal azotemia, a reversible decline in kidney function due to inadequate perfusion. As CHF begins to develop, the GFR initially remains normal. It is maintained by an increased filtration fraction despite the reduced cardiac output and renal plasma flow. The glomerular afferent arteriole remains dilated despite concurrent efferent arteriolar constriction. These opposite hemodynamic changes result from different vasoactive mediators. Afferent arteriolar dilatation is mediated by renal prostaglandins, whereas the efferent vasoconstriction is an effect of intrarenal angiotensin II. As cardiac output declines further, these compensatory mechanisms are no longer sufficient to maintain GFR, and the latter decreases in parallel with the decline in renal perfusion. These alterations in glomerular hemodynamics also explain why patients with heart failure are at increased risk for acute renal failure after administration of nonsteroidal anti-inflammatory drugs or ACE inhibitors. The former class of agents inhibits prostaglandin synthesis, and the latter reduces generation of angiotensin II. Angiotensin receptor blockers have a similar effect on the glomerulus. Deterioration of kidney function is clinically important, because in the patient with heart failure an increased serum creatinine, and particularly an early increase of serum creatinine after admission, is an independent predictor of mortality.

Hyponatremia in Congestive Heart Failure

In addition to the nonosmotic stimulation of vasopressin release that results from the decrease in effective arterial volume, other factors may reduce water excretion in CHF. Elaboration of a maximal amount of dilute urine occurs only when three conditions are satisfied. ADH must be completely suppressed, solute and fluid delivery to the diluting sites must be unimpaired, and the diluting sites (the loop and distal convoluted tubule) must function normally. With the decrease in effective circulating volume, augmentation of proximal sodium reabsorption results from the increased angiotensin II levels and the increased peritubular capillary oncotic pressure. These effects diminish sodium delivery to the diluting sites. In addition, the use of loop or distal convoluted tubule diuretics to treat CHF interferes with the action of the diluting sites. Development of hyponatremia is associated with a poor outcome. Hyponatremia is a marker for severe CHF, and it is unclear that the increased mortality results from the reduction in serum sodium concentration itself.

MANAGEMENT OF THE PATIENT WITH CONGESTIVE HEART FAILURE

The heart and the kidney are both targets and mediators in CHF. Renal homeostatic mechanisms play a central role in the clinical presentation and the prognosis of CHF. Therapeutic strategies to reverse the renal abnormalities in this condition are not limited to the reduction of volume overload by diuretics, but also include efforts to reverse the neuroendocrine activation.

Management of Edema

Most patients with CHF have edema, that is, sodium and volume overload. A negative sodium balance is therefore a central goal of all CHF treatment strategies (Table 23-1). A moderate decrease in dietary sodium intake is always appropriate. A 4-g daily intake of Na^+ is feasible and can be generally recommended. Some patients can follow tighter restrictions. One potential source of increased sodium intake is sodium-containing intravenous fluid or medications. The fluid prescription and drug list should be reviewed with this in mind. Additional benefits of sodium restriction include the reduction of thirst and the limitation of urinary potassium loss during diuretic treat-

TABLE 23-1   Management of the Edematous Patient with Congestive Heart Failure

Ancillary measures	
Bed rest	Decreased cardiac work
Anticoagulation	Prevention of thromboembolic complications during aggressive diuresis
Sodium restriction	Negative sodium balance, decreased kaliuresis, decreased diuretic requirement, decreased thirst
Diuretic therapy	
Proximal tubule	Angiotensin-converting enzyme inhibition: indirect effect
	Acetazolamide: metabolic acidosis
Henle's loop	Furosemide, bumetanide, torsemide, ethacrynic acid: most effective, but rebound effect (repeated/continuous administration is necessary)
Distal tubule	Thiazides/metolazone: high risk for hypokalemia with relatively small natriuretic effect, not applicable in patients with renal failure
Collecting tubule	Potassium-sparing agents, spironolactone: little diuretic effect, but potassium-sparing effect useful in combination with other diuretics
	Spironolactone: prognostic benefit? (RALES trial)
Collecting duct	Vasopressin (V2) antagonists: aquaresis, rather than natriuresis (these currently investigational agents may be useful for the treatment of hyponatremia in congestive heart failure in the future)

ment. Urinary potassium loss is lower when less sodium is delivered to the sodium/potassium exchange site in the distal renal tubule.

Bed rest has traditionally been an ancillary therapeutic measure, because it reduces the hydrostatic work of the failing heart and thus improves renal perfusion. The aggressive mobilization of edema fluid increases the risk for venous thromboembolic events during this period of bed rest. Patients who are not already anticoagulated because of cardiac dysfunction should receive appropriate prophylactic measures, that is, (low-dose) anticoagulation and compression stockings.

In the majority of patients with CHF, these measures are not sufficient to reduce the markedly increased extracellular volume. Hence, most patients require diuretics. Diuretic therapy is discussed in detail in Chapter 15, but several points bear emphasis here. Although a significant proportion of sodium absorption occurs in the proximal tubule in exchange for protons that derive from CO_2 via the action of carbonic anhydrase, carbonic anhydrase inhibitors such as acetazolamide play only a limited role in the treatment of heart failure, as distal nephron segments compensate for the reduced proximal sodium absorption. Distal tubule diuretics, such as thiazides, are not very effective as monotherapy, since 90% of the filtered sodium load will already have been absorbed proximal to the site of thiazide action. The potassium-sparing agents (amiloride, triamterene, and spironolactone) are weak natriuretic agents at best and act even further downstream than the thiazides. Their principal role is in combination with other diuretics to reduce K^+ and H^+ secretion. In a large-scale randomized trial, spironolactone reduced mortality in patients with CHF, presumably in part through additional direct effects on the heart. Loop diuretics are the most effective agents available for the treatment of volume overload. They inhibit a specific Na^+-K^+-$2Cl^-$ symporter (NKCC2) in the thick ascending limb of Henle's loop, which accounts for the reabsorption of some 20% of the filtered sodium load. However, even their efficacy may be reduced by a compensatory increase in the sodium avidity at distal nephron sites.

In mild heart failure, fluid retention may respond to thiazide diuretics (e.g., hydrochlorothiazide 25 to 50 mg/day), but thiazides can cause severe hypokalemia. Therefore, the use of low doses and their combination with a potassium-sparing diuretic (e.g., triamterene 50 mg/day) are preferred. Most patients with advanced CHF require loop diuretics in doses titrated to the clinical response. Because of a rebound increase in renal sodium retention after the action of the loop diuretic has worn off, repeated administration or the use of a longer-acting compound such as torsemide is necessary. Intravenous administration is preferred in emergency situations or in patients with massive fluid overload. In severe cases, the continuous infusion of a loop diuretic can be helpful. When even high doses of intravenous loop diuretics fail to achieve a negative sodium balance, combination of different classes of diuretics is required. A rational approach is the combination of agents that act on different sites of the nephron, that is, the combination of a loop diuretic with a distally acting compound such as metolazone or chlorothiazide. The addition of a potassium-sparing agent is useful to reduce diuretic-induced hypokalemia. Close clinical and biochemical monitoring of the patient is essential during this intensive diuretic therapy. Potassium-sparing agents are more effective than oral or intravenous potassium supplementation, but one must be aware of the potential risk for life-threatening hyperkalemia, especially during concomitant treatment with high doses of ACE inhibitors and when kidney function is decreased. The risk for hyperkalemia is further increased by a high intake of a high-potassium diet, of potassium supplements, or of potassium-containing salt substitutes. The risk is reduced by the concomitant administration of kaliuretic loop diuretics.

Angiotensin-Converting Enzyme Inhibition and Aldosterone Antagonism

Angiotensin-converting enzyme inhibitors have become the cornerstone of the modern treatment of CHF for a variety of reasons. ACE inhibitors reduce cardiac afterload, thereby improving cardiac function by lowering cardiac energy requirements and allowing the heart to perform on a more favorable point of the Starling curve. The resulting improvement in cardiac function reduces sympathetic drive. This is in contrast to the administration of pure vasodilators or diuretics, which cause a more pronounced reflex activation of the sympathetic nervous system, partially obviating their cardiac benefits. Apart from these systemic effects, ACE inhibitors also inactivate the local renin-angiotensin systems in the cardiovascular system. Inhibition of the renin-angiotensin system in the heart and blood vessels has favorable effects on cardiovascular remodeling in hypertensive heart disease or after myocardial infarction. The inactivation of the renin-angiotensin system by ACE inhibitors (and more recently by angiotensin II antagonists) reduces morbidity and mortality in patients with heart failure. In large trials (e.g., CONSENSUS, SOLVD, and ATLAS), the benefit also extended to the subgroup of CHF patients with moderately impaired kidney function. Potential side effects include a usually transient increase of serum creatinine (aggravated in patients with advanced primary kidney disease or hypovolemia and in individuals receiving nonsteroidal anti-inflammatory agents or cyclosporine). In patients with a persistent major increase of serum creatinine, renovascular disease must be excluded.

Because activation of the sympathetic system and the renin-angiotensin-aldosterone system plays a key role in the development of the renal sodium avidity that charac-terizes CHF, antagonism of this system should reduce renal sodium retention. Consequently, inhibition of the converting enzyme may lower the diuretic requirement in some patients. Usually this effect is obscured, however, by a decrease in blood pressure that stimulates sodium retention. Therefore, most patients with advanced CHF require diuretics despite adequate inhibition of the renin-angiotensin system.

Congestive heart failure is characterized by secondary hyperaldosteronism, which may persist despite treatment with ACE inhibitors because aldosterone secretion by the adrenal cortex may escape control by angiotensin II. In addition, local synthesis of aldosterone has been documented in the hearts of patients with heart failure. The mechanisms for the persistent secretion of aldosterone are still unknown. Blockade of the renin-angiotensin system is insufficient to achieve a lasting reduction of the serum concentration of aldosterone. Persistent secondary hyperaldosteronism explains the propensity of many patients with cardiac failure to develop hypokalemia. The latter increases the risk of life-threatening dysrhythmias and is an adverse prognostic factor in CHF. In addition to its mineralocorticoid effects on the kidney and extrarenal epithelial organs, aldosterone also acts on cardiovascular tissues and causes myocardial and vascular fibrosis.

Because of the adverse effects of aldosterone in heart failure, aldosterone antagonism makes sense, although its combination with ACE inhibition entails the potential risk for inducing life-threatening hyperkalemia in patients with reduced kidney function. However, this risk is small with low doses of the aldosterone antagonist spironolactone; the addition of spironolactone (up to 25 mg/day) to a baseline regimen of ACE inhibitors, digoxin, and diuretics effectively reduces the risk for hypokalemia in patients with moderate heart failure (NYHA classes II to III). The Randomized Aldactone Evaluation Study (RALES) in patients with severe CHF (NYHA classes III and IV) compared low doses of spironolactone with placebo. Patients receiving spironolactone in addition to ACE inhibitors, diuretics, and digoxin had a 30% reduction of mortality and a 35% lower rate of CHF-related hospital admissions. Moreover, there was a significant symptomatic improvement in the spironolactone group. More recently, similar benefit was seen from the administration of the mineralocorticoid receptor antagonist eplerenone, which is devoid of some major side effects of spironolactone (Eplerenone Post-Acute Myocardial Infarction Heart Failure Efficacy and Survival Study [EPHESUS]). Nevertheless, moderate renal dysfunction (serum creatinine concentration of greater than 2.5 mg/dL) was an exclusion criterion in RALES. Thus, the impressive results of RALES cannot necessarily be extrapolated to patients with greater reductions in the GFR, because the higher incidence of hyperkalemia with life-threatening cardiac dysrhythmia may outweigh the benefits of aldosterone antagonism in this group of patients.

Prevention and Treatment of Acute Renal Failure in Congestive Heart Failure

Nonsteroidal anti-inflammatory agents, both cyclooxygenase 1 (COX1) and COX2 inhibitors, should be avoided in patients with decreased effective arterial volume. If they are indispensable for the treatment of comorbid conditions, they should not be used before the intravascular volume is replete.

When used in patients who have undergone aggressive diuresis with a decrease in intravascular volume, ACE inhibitors and angiotensin receptor blockers may be associated with a reversible decrease in GFR. It is often necessary to discontinue these drugs when acute renal failure develops. Cautious reinitiation at a reduced dose after repletion of any intravascular volume depletion may permit their use. In any event, treatment should be started at low doses, preferably initially with a short-acting ACE inhibitor, and with monitoring of serum creatinine concentration. Risk factors for a decline in kidney function include hypertension, diabetes, excessive diuretic use, recent volume loss, and generalized atherosclerosis. Not infrequently, patients with CHF due to coronary artery disease have renal artery stenosis. Patients with bilateral renal artery stenosis are at risk for ACE inhibitor–induced reductions in GFR.

Dopamine infusion in low doses has been advocated in an effort to increase renal blood flow and to induce a natriuresis by stimulating vasodilatory dopamine receptors in the renal arteries and restoring favorable glomerular hemodynamics. However, the clinical benefits of such "renal dose" dopamine therapy are unproven, and the use of this agent in CHF solely to improve kidney function cannot be endorsed.

Management of Anemia

Approximately half of patients with CHF are anemic. Large population-based analyses documented that even after adjustment for confounding, mortality in anemic patient with heart failure was higher by 34%. Interestingly, in CHF high erythropoietin (EPO) concentrations, presumably indicative of renal hypoxia, were found to be independent predictors of mortality. Small studies showed that correction of anemia with EPO and parenteral iron improves functional capacity and reduces hospitalization rates. Studies are underway to establish whether there is also a benefit with respect to hard end points.

Management of Hyponatremia

Except in rare circumstances, hyponatremia indicates an excess of body water rather than a lack of sodium. Administration of high doses of sodium in this setting is thus inappropriate. Because of its complex pathophysiology, the hyponatremia of CHF is notoriously difficult to treat. The mainstay of therapy is the restriction of free water intake. Limitation of fluid intake (including infusions) to 500 mL in addition to the measured daily fluid output is appropriate. Reduction of diuretic therapy allows partial correction of any element of central hypovolemia and permits restoration of function of the diluting mechanism. Rarely, in patients with advanced prerenal azotemia and hyponatremia, it may be necessary to administer loop diuretics and normal saline simultaneously. The loop agent interferes with urinary concentration, resulting in a decrease in the inappropriately elevated urine osmolality and an increase in excretion of electrolyte-free water. Normal saline, which has a higher sodium concentration than the serum of the hyponatremic patient, is administered in an amount matching urinary sodium losses, and intravascular volume is thus maintained. Meticulous monitoring of urinary urine sodium concentration, urine output, and intravascular volume is essential in these patients. Finally, ultrafiltration or even hemodialysis may be required acutely in patients with cardiac insufficiency and severe prerenal failure. Impressive long-term improvement has been seen in CHF patients with therapy resistant volume retention and hyponatremia who were put on peritoneal dialysis or hemodialysis.

Specific V2 vasopressin receptors as well as nonselective V1+V2 vasopressin receptor antagonists were effective in animal models of CHF. They interfere with the effect of vasopressin on the renal collecting tubule, thereby promoting water excretion, and thus eliminating the major cause of hyponatremia. Nonselective antagonists provide additional benefit, relieving V1-mediated vasoconstriction and afterload as well as abrogating the effects of vasopressin locally synthesized in the heart. These agents are undergoing therapeutic trials in humans and may be of benefit for patients with CHF in the future.

BIBLIOGRAPHY

Andreoli TE: Pathogenesis of renal sodium retention in congestive heart failure. Miner Electrolyte Metab 25:11–20, 1999.

Dormans TP, Gerlag PG, Russel FG, Smits P: Combination diuretic therapy in severe congestive heart failure. Drugs 55:165–172, 1998.

Eiskjaer H, Bagger IP, Danielsen H, et al: Mechanisms of sodium retention in heart failure: Relation to the renin-angiotensin-aldosterone system. Am J Physiol 260:F883–F889, 1991.

Ezekowitz JA, McAlister FA, Armstrong PW: Anemia is common in heart failure and is associated with poor outcomes: Insights from a cohort of 12,065 patients with new-onset heart failure. Circulation 107:223–225, 2003.

Forman DE, Butler J, Wang Y, et al: Incidence, predictors at admission, and impact of worsening renal function among patients hospitalized with heart failure. J Am Coll Cardiol 43:61–67, 2004.

Gurm HS, Lincoff AM, Kleiman NS, et al: Double jeopardy of renal insufficiency and anemia in patients undergoing percutaneous coronary interventions. Am J Cardiol 94:30–34, 2004.

Hampton JR, Van Veldhuisen DJ, Cowley AJ, et al: Achieving appropriate endpoints in heart failure trials: The PRIME-II protocol. The second perspective randomized study of ibopamine on mortality and efficacy. Eur J Heart Fail 1:89–93, 1999.

Hillege H, van Gilst W, de Zeeuw D, van Veldhuisen DJ: Renal function as a predictor of prognosis in chronic heart failure. Heart Fail Monit 2:78–84, 2002.

Ichikawa I, Pfeffer JM, Pfeffer MA, et al: Role of angiotensin II in the altered renal function of congestive heart failure. Circ Res 55:669–675, 1984.

McCullogh PA, Kuncheria J, Mathur VS: Diagnostic and therapeutic utility of B-type natriuretic peptide in patients with renal insufficiency and decompensated heart failure. Rev Cardiovasc Med 5:16–25, 2004.

Pitt B, Remme W, Zannad F, et al: Eplerenone Post-Acute Myocardial Infarction Heart Failure Efficacy and Survival Study Investigators (EPHESUS). Eplerenone, a selective aldosterone blocker, in patients with left ventricular dysfunction after myocardial infarction. N Engl J Med 348:1309–1321, 2003.

Pitt B, Zannad F, Remme W, et al: The effect of spironolactone on morbidity and mortality, in patients with severe heart failure. N Engl J Med 341:709–717, 1999.

The RALES Investigators: Effectiveness of spironolactone added to an angiotensin-converting enzyme inhibitor and a loop diuretic for severe chronic congestive heart failure: The randomized aldactone evaluation study (RALES). Am J Cardiol 78:902–907, 1996.

Sarnak MJ, Levey AS, Schoolwerth AC, et al: Kidney disease as a risk factor for development of cardiovascular disease: A statement from the American Heart Associations Councils on Kidney in Cardiovascular Disease, High Blood Pressure Research Council, Clinical Cardiology, and Epidemiology and Prevention. Circulation 108:2154–2169, 2003.

Schepkens H,Vanholder R, Billiouw JM, Lameire N: Life-threatening hyperkalemia during combined therapy with angiotensin-converting enzyme inhibitors and spironolactone: An analysis of 25 cases. Am J Med 110:438–441, 2001.

Schrier RW, Abraham WT: Hormones and hemodynamics in heart failure. N Engl J Med 341:577–585, 1999.

Schrier RW, Martin PY: Recent advances in the understanding of water metabolism in heart failure. Adv Exp Med Biol 449:415–426, 1998.

Shlipak MG: Pharmacotherapy for heart failure in patients with renal insufficiency. Ann Intern Med 138:917–924, 2003.

Silverberg DS, Wexler D, Iaina A. The importance of anemia and its correction in the management of severe congestive heart failure. Eur J Heart Fail 4:681–686, 2002.

Siscovick DS, Raghunathan TE, Psaty BM, et al: Diuretic therapy for hypertension and the risk of primary cardiac arrest. N Engl J Med 330:1852–1857, 1994.

The SOLVD Investigators: Effect of enalapril on survival in patients with reduced left ventricular ejection fractions and congestive heart failure. N Engl J Med 325:293–302, 1991.

Weber KT, Brilla CG: Pathological hypertrophy and cardiac interstitium: Fibrosis and renin-angiotensin-aldosterone system. Circulation 83:1849–1865, 1991.

CHAPTER 24

Kidney Function in Liver Disease

Vicente Arroyo   Carlos Terra   Wladimiro Jiménez

The Peripheral Arterial Vasodilation Hypothesis of Renal Sodium and Water Retention and the Forward Theory of Ascites Formation are the most accepted mechanisms of kidney dysfunction and ascites formation in cirrhosis and constitute the rationale in which modern treatments of these patients are based. The Peripheral Arterial Vasodilation Hypothesis considers that the primary event of renal sodium and water retention in cirrhosis is splanchnic arterial vasodilation due to the massive release of local vasodilators secondary to portal hypertension. At the initial phase of the disease, compensation occurs through the development of a hyperdynamic circulation (high plasma volume, cardiac index, and heart rate). However, as the disease progresses and splanchnic arterial vasodilation increases, these compensatory mechanisms are insufficient to maintain circulatory homeostasis. Arterial pressure decreases, leading to stimulation of baroreceptors, homeostatic activation of the sympathetic nervous and renin-angiotensin systems and antidiuretic hormone, and renal sodium and water retention. This Peripheral Arterial Vasodilation Hypothesis is the basis of a new concept in the pathophysiology of ascites, the Forward Theory of Ascites Formation. According to this theory, the arterial vasodilation in the splanchnic circulation would induce the formation of ascites by simultaneously impairing the systemic circulation, leading to sodium and water retention, and the splanchnic microcirculation, leading to the leakage of fluid into the abdominal cavity.

NATURAL HISTORY OF KIDNEY DYSFUNCTION IN CIRRHOSIS

A reduction of renal ability to excrete sodium and free water and a decrease in renal perfusion and glomerular filtration rate (GFR) are the main kidney function abnormalities in cirrhosis. Their course is usually progressive, except that in alcoholic cirrhotics, kidney function may improve following alcohol withdrawal. The main consequence of the reduced ability to excrete sodium in cirrhosis is the development of sodium retention and ascites, and this occurs when renal sodium excretion decreases below the sodium intake. This represents a marked impairment in renal sodium handling. The kidney's ability to excrete free water is reduced in most patients with cirrhosis and ascites. Dilutional hyponatremia (arbitrarily defined as a serum sodium concentra-

tion of less than 130 mEq/L) develops when electrolyte-free water clearance is severely reduced. Finally, the main consequence of the impaired renal perfusion and GFR is hepatorenal syndrome (HRS), which is defined as a GFR below 40 mL/min (or a serum creatinine of over 1.5 mg/dL) in the absence of any other potential cause of kidney dysfunction. Sodium retention, dilutional hyponatremia, and HRS appear at different times during the evolution of the disease. Therefore, the clinical course of cirrhosis can be divided into phases according to the onset of each of these complications.

Phase 1: Impaired Renal Sodium Metabolism in Compensated Cirrhosis

Chronologically, the first kidney function abnormality occurring in cirrhosis is an impairment in renal sodium metabolism, which can already be detected before the development of ascites, when the disease is still compensated. At this phase of the disease, patients have portal hypertension, increased cardiac output, reduced peripheral vascular resistance, normal or reduced mean arterial pressure, and normal renal perfusion, GFR, and free water clearance. They remain able to excrete the sodium ingested with the diet. However, they present subtle abnormalities in renal sodium excretion. For example, they have a reduced natriuretic response to the acute administration of sodium chloride (i.e., after the infusion of a saline solution) and may not be able to escape from the sodium-retaining effect of mineralocorticoids. Abnormal natriuretic responses to changes in posture are another relevant feature at this phase of the disease. Urinary sodium excretion is reduced in the upright and increased in the supine posture as compared with normal subjects.

Phase 2: Renal Sodium Retention Without Activation of the Renin-Angiotensin-Aldosterone and Sympathetic Nervous Systems

At some point in the progression of the disease, patients become unable to excrete their regular sodium intake. Sodium is then retained together with water, and the fluid accumulates in the abdominal cavity as ascites.

Urinary sodium excretion, although reduced, is usually higher than 10 mEq/day, and in some cases it is over 50 to 90 mEq/day, which means that a negative sodium balance and, therefore, the loss of ascites, may be achieved only by reducing the sodium content in the diet. Renal perfusion, GFR, the ability to excrete free water, plasma renin activity, and the plasma concentrations of antidiuretic hormone are normal. Sodium retention is therefore unrelated to any abnormality of the renin-aldosterone or sympathetic nervous systems, the two most important regulators of renal sodium excretion so far identified. The plasma levels of atrial natriuretic peptide, brain natriuretic peptide, and natriuretic hormone are increased in these patients, indicating that sodium retention is not due to a reduced synthesis of endogenous natriuretic peptides. It has been suggested that circulatory dysfunction at this phase, although greater than in compensated cirrhosis without ascites, is not intense enough to stimulate the sympathetic nervous activity and the renin-angiotensin-aldosterone systems. However, it would activate a still unknown, extremely sensitive, sodium-retaining mechanism (renal or extrarenal).

Phase 3: Stimulation of the Endogenous Vasoconstrictor Systems with Preserved Renal Perfusion and Glomerular Filtration Rate

When sodium retention is intense (urinary sodium excretion below 10 mEq/day), the plasma renin activity and the plasma concentrations of aldosterone and norepinephrine are invariably increased. Aldosterone increases sodium reabsorption in the distal and collecting tubules. In contrast, renal sympathetic nervous activity stimulates sodium reabsorption in the proximal tubule and loop of Henle. Thus, sodium retention in these patients is due to increased sodium reabsorption throughout the nephron.

The plasma volume, cardiac output, and peripheral vascular resistance do not differ from the previous phases. Circulatory dysfunction, however, is more intense because increased activity of the sympathetic nervous system and renin-angiotensin system is needed to maintain circulatory homeostasis. Arterial pressure at this phase of the disease is critically dependent on increased activity of the renin-angiotensin and sympathetic nervous systems and antidiuretic hormone, and the administration of drugs that interfere with these systems (angiotensin receptor blockers, angiotensin-converting enzyme inhibitors, clonidine, V1-vasopressin receptor antagonists) may precipitate arterial hypotension.

Although angiotensin II, norepinephrine, and vasopressin are powerful renal vasoconstrictors, renal perfusion and GFR are normal or only moderately reduced because the effects of these hormones on the renal circulation are antagonized by intrarenal vasodilator mechanisms, particularly prostaglandins and nitric oxide. Cirrhosis is the human condition in which renal perfusion and GFR are most dependent on the renal production of prostaglandins, and severely impaired kidney function may occur at this phase if renal prostaglandins are inhibited with nonsteroidal anti-inflammatory drugs.

The ability to excrete free water is reduced at this phase of the disease owing to the high circulating plasma levels of antidiuretic hormone. However, few patients have significant hyponatremia because the effect of antidiuretic hormone is partially inhibited by an increased renal production of prostaglandin E_2.

Phase 4: Development of Type 2 Hepatorenal Syndrome

Hepatorenal syndrome is functional impairment in kidney function that develops secondary to intense renal hypoperfusion. Type 2 HRS is characterized by a moderate and steady decrease in kidney function (serum creatinine between 1.5 and 2.5 mg/dL) in the absence of other potential causes of renal failure. The International Ascites Club considers that serum creatinine should be higher than 1.5 mg/dL or GFR lower than 40 mL/min for the diagnosis of HRS. However, many patients with a GFR lower than 40 mL/min have normal serum creatinine concentration. Therefore, the frequency of type 2 HRS is underestimated when serum creatinine alone is used in the clinical evaluation.

Type 2 HRS develops in advanced phases of cirrhosis in the setting of a significant deterioration of circulatory function. Patients with type 2 HRS have high plasma levels of renin, norepinephrine, and antidiuretic hormone, as well as significant arterial hypotension. The arterial vascular resistance in these patients is increased not only in the kidneys, but also in the brain, muscle, and skin, indicating a generalized arterial vasoconstriction to compensate for intense splanchnic arterial vasodilation. Type 2 HRS is probably due to the extreme overactivity of the endogenous vasoconstrictor systems that overcome the intrarenal vasodilatory mechanisms. Some studies suggest that in these patients the cardiac output may not be as high as in the previous phase. However, further studies are needed to confirm this feature.

The degree of sodium retention is intense in patients with type 2 HRS. The mechanism is a reduction in filtered sodium and a marked increase in sodium reabsorption in the proximal tubule. The delivery of sodium to the distal nephron, the site of action of diuretics, is very low. Therefore, most of these patients do not respond to diuretics and have refractory ascites. Free water clearance is also markedly reduced and most patients have significant hyponatremia. The prognosis of patients with type 2 HRS is poor, with a mortality rate of 50% 6 months after the onset of impaired kidney function.

Phase 5: Development of Type 1 Hepatorenal Syndrome

Type 1 HRS is characterized by a rapidly progressive decline in kidney function, defined as a doubling of serum creatinine reaching a level greater than 2.5 mg/dL in less than 2 weeks. Although type 1 HRS may arise spontaneously, it frequently occurs in close chronologic relationship with a precipitating factor such as severe bacterial infection, acute hepatitis (ischemic, alcoholic, toxic, viral) superimposed on cirrhosis, a major surgical procedure, or massive gastrointestinal hemorrhage. Severe bacterial infections are the most common precipitating event. Patients with type 2 HRS are predisposed to develop type 1 HRS, although it may also develop in patients with normal serum creatinine concentration. The prognosis of patients with type 1 HRS is extremely poor, with 80% of patients dying less than 2 weeks after the onset of HRS. Patients succumb from progressive circulatory, hepatic, and renal failure, along with encephalopathy.

Type 1 HRS has been closely examined in spontaneous bacterial peritonitis (SBP) since 30% of patients with SBP develop this type of renal failure. The two most important predictors of type 1 HRS in SBP are an increased serum creatinine prior to the infection and an intense intra-abdominal inflammatory response, as suggested by high ascitic fluid concentration of polymorphonuclear leukocytes and cytokines (tumor necrosis factor-α and interleukin-6), at infection diagnosis.

Type 1 HRS after SBP occurs in the setting of a severe deterioration of circulatory function, as indicated by a marked increase in the plasma levels of renin and noradrenalin. A recent study assessed systemic hemodynamics and kidney function in a series of patients at the time of onset of SBP (prior to development of HRS) and after their subsequent development of type 1 HRS. The results of this study suggest that the impairment in circulatory function in patients with HRS is far more complex than initially considered. In addition to an accentuation of the arterial vasodilation, a significant decrease in cardiac output compared with values obtained at infection diagnosis was observed. In some cases cardiac output decreased to values below normal (5 L/min). Whether this decrease in heart function is related to the cirrhotic or septic cardiomyopathy, to a decreased cardiac preload due to central hypovolemia, or to both is currently unknown. The demonstration that using albumin to expand the plasma volume of patients with SBP at infection diagnosis reduces the incidence of type 1 HRS by more than 60% and decreases hospital mortality is consistent with the second hypothesis.

The development of HRS in patients with SBP is not only associated with a deterioration of circulatory and kidney functions, but also with an impairment in hepatic function leading to hepatic encephalopathy. It has been shown that in these patients there is an increase in intrahepatic vascular resistance and portal pressure that correlates closely with an increase in renin and norepinephrine. Circulatory dysfunction in HRS, therefore, also affects the liver.

MANAGEMENT OF KIDNEY DYSFUNCTION AND ASCITES IN CIRRHOSIS

Low-Sodium Diet

Mobilization of ascites occurs when a negative sodium balance is achieved. In 10% of patients, those with normal plasma aldosterone and norepinephrine concentration and relatively high urinary sodium excretion, this can be obtained simply by reducing the sodium intake to 60 to 90 mEq/day. A greater reduction in sodium intake interferes with nutrition and is not advisable. In the majority of cases, however, urinary sodium excretion is very low and a negative sodium balance cannot be achieved without diuretics. Even in these cases, sodium restriction is important because it reduces diuretic requirements. Sodium restriction is essential in patients responding poorly to diuretics. A frequent cause of apparently refractory ascites is inadequate sodium restriction. This should be suspected when ascites does not decrease despite a good natriuretic response to diuretics (see Chapter 15).

Diuretics

Furosemide and spironolactone are the diuretics most commonly used in the treatment of ascites in cirrhosis. In contrast to what occurs in healthy subjects, in whom furosemide is more potent than spironolactone, in cirrhotic patients with ascites, spironolactone is more effective than furosemide. Cirrhotic patients with ascites and marked hyperaldosteronism (50% of the patients with ascites) do not respond to furosemide. In contrast, most cirrhotic patients with ascites respond to spironolactone. Patients with normal or slightly increased plasma aldosterone concentrations respond to low doses of spironolactone (100 to 150 mg/day), but as much as 300 to 400 mg/day may be required in patients with marked hyperaldosteronism. The mechanism of the resistance to furosemide in patients with hyperaldosteronism is pharmacodynamic. With reduced GFR and avid proximal sodium reabsorption, delivery of sodium to the loop of Henle where furosemide acts is reduced. In addition, most of the sodium not reabsorbed in the loop because of the action of furosemide is subsequently reabsorbed in the distal nephron due to stimulation by aldosterone. Therefore, spironolactone is the preferred drug for the management of patients with cirrhosis and ascites. The simultaneous administration of furosemide and spironolactone increases the natriuretic effect of both agents and reduces the incidence of hypo- or hyperkalemia that may be observed when these drugs are given alone. There is general agreement that patients not responding to 400 mg/day of spironolactone and 160 mg/day of furosemide will not respond to higher diuretic dosage.

Diuretic treatment in cirrhosis is not free of complications, particularly in patients requiring high diuretic dosage. Approximately 20% of patients develop significant renal functional impairment (increase in blood urea and serum creatinine concentration), which is usually moderate and always reversible after diuretic withdrawal. Hyponatremia secondary to a decrease in the ability to excrete free water also occurs in approximately 20% of these patients. The most severe complication related to diuretic treatment is hepatic encephalopathy, which occurs in approximately 25% of patients hospitalized with tense ascites requiring a high diuretic dosage.

The term *refractory ascites* is applied when ascites cannot be mobilized, when its early recurrence after therapeutic paracentesis cannot be prevented due to a lack of response to sodium restriction and maximal diuretic treatment (diuretic-resistant ascites), or when diuretic-induced complications preclude the use of an effective diuretic dosage (diuretic-intractable ascites). Refractory ascites is an infrequent condition, occurring in less than 10% of patients hospitalized with tense ascites. Most of these patients have type 2 HRS (serum creatinine concentration greater than 1.5 mg/dL) or less severe but still significant decreases of GFR (serum creatinine between 1.2 and 1.5 mg/dL). It has been estimated that a serum creatinine over 1.2 mg/dL reflects a decrease in GFR of more than 50%. Both an impaired access of diuretics to the renal tubules due to reduced renal perfusion and a reduced delivery of sodium to the loop of Henle and distal nephron secondary to the low GFR and increased sodium reabsorption in the proximal tubule are the mechanisms of diuretic-resistant ascites. Deficient sodium restriction or treatment with nonsteroidal anti-inflammatory drugs should be excluded prior to the diagnosis of diuretic-resistant ascites.

Arterial Vasoconstrictors

It is well known that plasma volume expansion alone (e.g., after the insertion of a LeVeen shunt) does not improve kidney function in patients with HRS despite a significant suppression of plasma renin activity and norepinephrine concentration. Also, the administration of vasoconstrictors alone does not produce clinically significant increases in GFR in these patients. In contrast, simultaneous treatment using intravenous albumin as a plasma expander along with vasoconstrictors over 7 to 14 days in patients with type 1 HRS is associated with an increase in arterial pressure, a suppression of plasma

renin activity and norepinephrine concentration to normal levels, a marked increase in GFR, and a normalization of serum sodium and serum creatinine concentrations in most patients. Interestingly enough, HRS usually does not recur following discontinuation of therapy. These data are consistent with the hypothesis that type 1 HRS is related to both an accentuation of arterial vasodilation, which is corrected by the vasoconstrictor, and decreased cardiac output related to central hypovolemia, which is corrected by the administration of albumin. Very few patients develop side effects related to treatment. The probability of survival after normalization of serum creatinine increases and a significant proportion of patients may reach liver transplantation. Terlipressin (0.5 to 2.0 mg every 4 hours) has been the most frequently used vasoconstrictor for the treatment of type 1 HRS. However, the α-adrenergic agonists noradrenalin and midodrine at doses increasing arterial pressure by more than 10 mm Hg are also effective. An initial dose of albumin of 1 g/kg body weight followed by 20 to 40 g/day over 7 to 14 days is the schedule for volume expansion recommended by some investigators. Although serum creatinine is normalized in many patients with type 1 HRS responding to treatment with vasoconstrictors and albumin, GFR remains very low (it increases from values below 10 mL/min to 30 to 50 mL/min), suggesting that treatment with vasoconstrictors and albumin is effective for correcting the type 1 HRS component of the syndrome but not the reduced GFR present prior to the development of type 1 HRS in most patients. Two features further support this contention. First, and contrary to what occurs with type 1 HRS, type 2 HRS frequently recurs soon after discontinuation of therapy with vasoconstrictors and albumin. Second, sequential treatment with vasoconstrictors and albumin followed by the insertion of a transjugular intrahepatic shunt normalizes serum creatinine and GFR in most patients with type 1 HRS.

Therapeutic Paracentesis

Paracentesis is a rapid, effective, and safe treatment of ascites in cirrhosis. It is considered the treatment of choice of tense ascites. The mobilization of ascites by paracentesis is associated with a deterioration of circulatory function, as manifested by a marked increase in plasma renin activity and aldosterone concentration, in 60% to 70% of the patients. This impairment in circulatory function is due to an accentuation of the arterial vasodilation already present in these patients. The incidence of this complication is reduced to 30% to 40% if paracentesis is accompanied by plasma volume expansion with synthetic plasma volume expanders (dextran 70 or polygeline) and to only 18% if it is accompanied by plasma volume expansion with albumin (8 g per liter of ascitic fluid removed). The prevalence of circulatory dysfunction after paracentesis also depends on the amount of ascitic fluid removed. In patients receiving synthetic plasma expanders it was 18%, 30%, and 54% when the ascitic fluid removed was less than 5 L, between 5 and 9 L, and more than 9 L, respectively. The corresponding values in patients receiving albumin as a plasma expander were 16%, 19%, and 21%, respectively. Paracentesis-induced circulatory dysfunction, therefore, is a frequent event in patients with massive ascites, which is partially prevented by synthetic plasma expanders and almost totally prevented by the administration of intravenous albumin. Paracentesis-induced circulatory dysfunction is asymptomatic. However, it adversely affects the clinical course of the patients and may be associated with a shorter survival.

Transjugular Intrahepatic Portacaval Shunt

Transjugular intrahepatic portacaval shunt (TIPS) is the most recent treatment introduced for the management of portal hypertension. It works as a side-to-side portacaval shunt. TIPS is extremely effective in improving circulatory and kidney function and in the management of ascites in these patients. It induces a marked increase in cardiac output, a decrease in systemic vascular resistance, and an elevation in right atrial pressure and pulmonary wedge pressure. These changes are probably due to an increased venous return secondary to the portacaval fistula. The decrease in systemic vascular resistance is a physiologic response to accommodate the increase in cardiac output and does not represent an impairment in systemic hemodynamics. In fact, TIPS insertion is associated with a significant reduction in the plasma levels of renin, aldosterone, norepinephrine, and antidiuretic hormone, indicating an improvement in effective arterial blood volume. Suppression of the renin-angiotensin system is observed within the first week following TIPS and persists during follow-up. Suppression of norepinephrine and antidiuretic hormone requires a longer period of time. The improvement in circulatory function induces a rapid increase in urinary sodium excretion, which is already observed within the first 1 to 2 weeks and persists during follow-up. A significant increase in serum sodium concentration and GFR is also observed, indicating an improvement in renal perfusion and free water clearance. However, these later changes require 1 to 3 months to occur.

TIPS only partially decompresses the portal venous system, and although the suppression of the renin-aldosterone system is intense, the plasma levels of renin and aldosterone do not decrease to normal levels. The improvement in systemic and splanchnic hemodynamics is associated with complete disappearance of ascites or partial response (no need for paracentesis) in most patients. Only 10% of patients fail to respond to TIPS. Ascites characteristically resolves slowly (1 to 3 months),

but continuous diuretic treatment at lower doses is required in more than 90% of cases, either for the treatment of ascites or to reduce the peripheral edema. The persistence of portal hypertension and hyperaldosteronism may account for this feature.

Hepatic encephalopathy is the most important complication in cirrhotic patients with refractory ascites treated by TIPS. More than 40% of these patients develop hepatic encephalopathy. Although hepatic encephalopathy prior to TIPS is a predictor of post-TIPS encephalopathy, new or worsened hepatic encephalopathy develops in approximately 30% of cases. Shunt dysfunction requiring replacement is also a major problem.

USE OF THESE TREATMENTS AT THE DIFFERENT PHASES OF THE DISEASE

Phase 1: Preascitic Cirrhosis

At present, specific treatment for the prevention of ascites is not recommended in patients with compensated cirrhosis. Therefore, these patients should receive a normal sodium diet and should not be treated with diuretics.

Phases 2 and 3: Moderate and Tense Ascites

Patients with moderate ascites respond easily to sodium restriction and low doses of spironolactone with few complications. Therefore, diuretic treatment (spironolactone 100 to 200 mg/day) is the therapy of choice in these patients. In contrast, most patients with tense ascites require a high diuretic dosage. Several randomized controlled trials show that paracentesis is preferred to diuretic therapy in patients with tense ascites not only because it reduces the duration of hospital stay but also because it is associated with a significantly lower incidence of renal functional impairment and hepatic encephalopathy. Once ascites has been mobilized, phase 3 patients require sodium restriction and diuretics to prevent a recurrence.

Phase 4: Refractory Ascites

Several randomized controlled trials comparing TIPS to therapeutic paracentesis for patients with refractory or recurrent ascites clearly show that TIPS is better for the long-term control of ascites but worse when the development of severe hepatic encephalopathy is considered. The total time in the hospital during follow-up and the probability of survival is similar with either procedure. Based on these results, the International Ascites Club considers paracentesis to be the first-line treatment of refractory ascites. TIPS may be indicated in patients requiring frequent paracentesis (more than 3 times per month) who are without previous episodes of hepatic encephalopathy or cardiac dysfunction, under 70 years of age, and have Child-Pugh scores less than 12.

Phase 5: Type 1 Hepatorenal Syndrome

Patients with type 1 HRS must be treated with intravenous albumin and vasoconstrictors drugs for 1 to 2 weeks. Reversal of HRS is achieved in more than 60% of patients. This is associated with an increase in survival, and a significant proportion of patients may reach liver transplantation. It is well known that early morbidity and mortality after liver transplantation is higher and long-term survival shorter in patients with HRS than in those without HRS. These differences have not been observed if HRS is reversed preoperatively with intravenous albumin and terlipressin. Therefore, pharmacologic treatment of HRS should also be considered in patients with HRS prior to liver transplantation.

BIBLIOGRAPHY

Angeli P, Volpin R, Gerunda G, et al: Reversal of type 1 hepatorenal syndrome with the administration of midodrine and octeotide. Hepatology 29:1690–1697, 1999.

Arroyo V, Bosch J, Mauri M, et al: Renin, aldosterone and renal haemodynamics in cirrhosis with ascites. Eur J Clin Invest 9:69–73, 1979.

Arroyo V, Ginès P, Gerbes AL, et al: Definition and diagnostic criteria of refractory ascites and hepatorenal syndrome in cirrhosis. International Ascites Club. Hepatology 23:164–176, 1996.

Arroyo V, Jimenez W. Complications of cirrhosis. II. Renal and circulatory dysfunction. Lights and shadows in an important clinical problem. J Hepatol 32:157–170, 2000.

Arroyo V, Planas R, Gaya J, et al: Sympathetic nervous activity, renin-angiotensin system and renal excretion of prostaglandin E_2 in cirrhosis. Relationship to functional renal failure and sodium and water excretion. Eur J Clin Invest 13:271–278, 1983.

Caregaro L, Menon F, Angeli P, et al: Limitations of serum creatinine level and creatinine clearance as filtration markers in cirrhosis. Arch Intern Med 154:201–205, 1994.

Duvoux C, Zanditenas D, Hezode C, et al: Effects of noradrenalin and albumin in patients with type I hepatorenal syndrome: a pilot study. Hepatology 36:374–380, 2002.

Epstein M: Renal prostaglandins and the control of renal function in liver disease. Am J Med 80:46–55, 1986.

Follo A, Llovet JM, Navasa M, et al: Renal impairment after spontaneous bacterial peritonitis in cirrhosis: Incidence, clinical course, predictive factors and prognosis. Hepatology 20:1495–1501, 1994.

Ginès A, Fernandez-Esparrach G, Monescillo A, et al: Randomized trial comparing albumin, dextran 70, and polygeline in cirrhotic patients with ascites treated by paracentesis. Gastroenterology 111:1002–1010, 1996.

Ginès P, Tito L, Arroyo V, et al: Randomized comparative study of therapeutic paracentesis with and without intravenous albumin in cirrhosis. Gastroenterology 94:1493–1502, 1988.

Gines P, Uriz J, Calahorra B, et al: Transjugular intrahepatic portosystemic shunting versus paracentesis plus albumin for refractory ascites in cirrhosis. Gastroenterology 123:1839–1847, 2002.

Guevara M, Gines P, Fernandez-Esparrach G, et al: Reversibility of hepatorenal syndrome by prolonged administration of ornipressin and plasma volume expansion. Hepatology 27:35–41, 1998.

Huonker M, Schumacher YO, Ochs A, et al: Cardiac function and haemodynamics in alcoholic cirrhosis and effects of the transjugular intrahepatic portosystemic stent shunt. Gut 44:743–748, 1999.

Maroto A, Ginès P, Arroyo V, et al: Brachial and femoral artery blood flow in cirrhosis: Relationship to kidney dysfunction. Hepatology 17:788–793, 1993.

Martin PY, Ginès P, Schrier RW: Nitric oxide as a mediator of hemodynamic abnormalities and sodium and water retention in cirrhosis. N Engl J Med 339:533–541, 1998.

Moreau R, Durand F, Poynard T, et al: Terlipressin in patients with cirrhosis and type 1 hepatorenal syndrome: A retrospective multicenter study. Gastroenterology 122:923–930, 2002.

Navasa M, Follo A, Filella X, et al: Tumor necrosis factor and interleukin-6 in spontaneous bacterial peritonitis in cirrhosis: Relationship with the development of renal impairment and mortality. Hepatology 27:1227–1232, 1998.

Ortega R, Ginès P, Uriz J, et al: Terlipressin therapy with and without albumin for patients with hepatorenal syndrome: Results of a prospective, nonrandomized study. Hepatology 36:941–948, 2002.

Rimola A, Gines P, Arroyo V, et al: Urinary excretion of 6-keto-prostaglandin F1 alpha, thromboxane B_2 and prostaglandin E_2 in cirrhosis with ascites. Relationship to functional renal failure (hepatorenal syndrome). J Hepatol 3:111–117, 1986.

Ruiz-del-Arbol L, Urman J, Fernandez J, et al: Systemic, renal, and hepatic hemodynamic derangement in cirrhotic patients with spontaneous bacterial peritonitis. Hepatology 38:1210–1218, 2003.

Schrier RW, Arroyo V, Bernardi M, et al: Peripheral arterial vasodilation hypothesis: A proposal for the initiation of renal sodium and water retention in cirrhosis. Hepatology 8:1151–1157, 1988.

Sherman DS, Fish DN, Teitelbaum I: Assessing renal function in cirrhotic patients: Problems and pitfalls. Am J Kidney Dis 41:269–278, 2003.

Sort P, Navasa M, Arroyo V, et al: Effect of intravenous albumin on renal impairment and mortality in patients with cirrhosis and spontaneous bacterial peritonitis. N Engl J Med 341:403–409, 1999.

Wiest R, Groszmann RJ: Nitric oxide and portal hypertension: Its role in the regulation of intrahepatic and splanchnic vascular resistance. Semin Liver Dis 19:411–426, 1999.

CHAPTER 25

Postinfectious Glomerulonephritis

Alain Meyrier

Infection remains a common cause of proliferative glomerulonephritis (GN). Kidney biopsies demonstrate that the same agent may induce more than one histologic type of GN and that a given glomerular lesion may be the consequence of a wide array of pathogens. Thirty years ago, this chapter would have been almost entirely devoted to poststreptococcal acute glomerulonephritis (AGN). However, the epidemiology of postinfectious GN has considerably evolved in the Western world. In fact, what is now true in industrialized countries is not entirely applicable to all parts of the world, and poststreptococcal AGN remains a significant public health problem in Latin America, in Africa, and most probably in eastern Europe. Any proliferative GN whose etiology is unclear should prompt consideration of an infectious origin, even if this etiology is not readily suggested by the clinical context.

CLINICAL APPROACH

The clinical presentation of postinfectious GN spans a large spectrum. A bacterial cause should be considered in any patient with the acute nephritic syndrome, acute or rapidly progressive GN, or nephrotic syndrome with progressively declining kidney function. An infectious cause is readily suggested when any of these glomerular syndromes follows or accompanies evident bacterial infection. However, the infection may be covert, or it may be overlooked in the patient's history. These considerations justify wide indications for kidney biopsy, since it may be the renal pathologist who alerts the clinician to the presence of a possible infectious cause. One such example is a biopsy performed in the course of a febrile episode that discloses glomerular lesions strongly suggestive of infective endocarditis.

Acute Nephritic Syndrome

This is the typical clinical presentation of AGN, irrespective of the offending organism. *Streptococcus* and *Staphylococcus* are the most common agents. However, this syndrome is not pathognomonic of postinfectious GN and can be observed in immunoglobulin A (IgA) nephropathy, Schönlein-Henoch purpura, idiopathic membranoproliferative glomerulonephritis (MPGN), and occasionally crescentic pauci-immune GN, among others.

The illness is characterized by rapid onset of edema, hypertension, and oliguria, with heavy proteinuria, micro- or macroscopic hematuria, and low urinary sodium as well as a concentrated urine. In contrast to nephrotic syndrome, volume expansion involves both the intravascular and the interstitial compartments. Thus, hypertension, cardiac enlargement, and pulmonary edema may be present. The clinical presentation in children can be fulminant, with abdominal pain, acute cerebral edema, and seizures. In the elderly, volume overload may lead to a presentation with acute pulmonary edema. Kidney function ranges from normal to oliguric acute renal failure.

In contrast to IgA nephropathy, where macroscopic hematuria follows soon after upper respiratory tract infection (synpharyngitic hematuria), in postpharyngitic forms of postinfectious GN, the episode of bloody urine is delayed by 10 to 20 days after infection (see Chapter 21).

Acute or Rapidly Progressive Renal Functional Impairment

Postinfectious GN can manifest as rapidly progressive or even acute renal functional impairment that is not necessarily correlated with the type of the glomerular lesions. Some patients with purely proliferative and exudative GN may be oliguric at onset but resolve completely. However, severely impaired kidney function may also indicate the presence of extracapillary proliferation. A kidney biopsy is almost always required in this setting, both to establish the diagnosis and to guide therapy.

Nephrotic Syndrome and Progressive Renal Functional Impairment

Hypertension, usually edema, abundant proteinuria, and microscopic hematuria point to a chronic form of glomerular disease. Except when the initial infectious focus is identified, as in shunt nephritis (discussed later) or following a clearly identified clinical episode, the date of onset is generally not known. The membranoproliferative variant of postinfectious GN usually leads to chronic kidney disease and endstage renal disease (ESRD). Chronic GN with nephrotic proteinuria is an indication for kidney biopsy.

219

PATHOLOGY

The glomerular lesions found in postinfectious GN fall into three patterns: acute endocapillary exudative GN, endo- plus extracapillary (crescentic) GN, and MPGN.

Acute Endocapillary Exudative Glomerulonephritis

This is the classical appearance of acute poststreptococcal GN. However, no routine markers are available for histologic identification of the offending microorganism, and the lesions are the same in AGN due to *Staphylococcus*, other bacteria, and viruses. Many pediatricians would defer a biopsy when the clinical picture is typical. This approach is certainly arguable in adults.

Cell Proliferation

By light microscopy (LM), diffuse hypercellularity involves all glomeruli, so that the diagnosis can be made on a kidney sample comprising just a few or only a single glomerulus. The glomerular tufts are greatly enlarged with minimal urinary space remaining and few open capillaries (Fig. 25-1). Hypercellularity results both from proliferation of resident glomerular cells, mainly mesangial, and the influx of polymorphonuclear leukocytes, monocytes/macrophages, and plasma cells. The term *exudative* refers to the presence of abundant polymorphonuclear cells, some of which may be eosinophils. It is possible, although unusual, to find small focal regions of necrosis with fibrin in some glomeruli. Overall, cell proliferation may range from massive infiltration obstructing virtually all capillary lumina to mild inflammation with a moderate increase in mesangial cellularity and a greater than normal number of polymorphonuclear leukocytes. (Normal is fewer than five per glomerulus.)

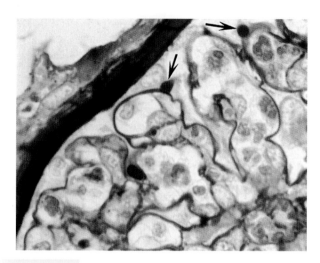

FIGURE 25-2 Acute poststaphylococcal glomerulonephritis. Typical humps on the outer aspect of the glomerular basement membranes (*arrows*) (silver methenamine stain).

Glomerular Basement Membrane Changes

The most characteristic change in acute GN is the postinfectious subepithelial hump. It is usually easily detected on silver stain (Fig. 25-2) and appears as a triangular or oval structure on the outer aspect of the glomerular basement membrane (GBM) overlain by a continuous layer of podocyte cytoplasm. The rest of the GBM is normal. Humps are not absolutely pathognomonic of postinfectious GN, but LM and immunofluorescence (IF) easily eliminate other causes such as Henoch-Schönlein purpura and MPGN. Humps are especially prominent within the first weeks of disease. In most cases, typical silver stain and IF appearance makes electron microscopy unnecessary.

Immunofluorescence

Specific antisera disclose granular IgG and C3 deposits along the capillary wall and within the mesangium (Fig. 25-3). Humps appear brightly fluorescent. Two IF patterns have been described. The "garland" type mainly follows the outline of capillary walls. IF shows numerous humps. This type is often associated with heavy proteinuria. The "starry sky" pattern consists of coarser deposits with mesangial predominance and comprises fewer humps. Proteinuria is less abundant than in the garland type. It should be stressed that absence of complement components on IF preparations casts strong doubt on the infectious origin of a glomerulopathy.

Endo- plus Extracapillary (Crescentic) Glomerulonephritis

The classical picture of GN associated with systemic bacterial infection consists of focal GN with cellular and necrotic lesions in some of the glomerular tuft lobules.

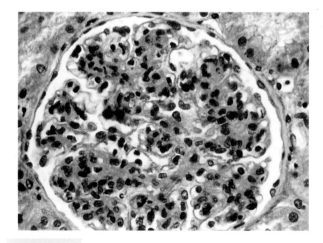

FIGURE 25-1 Acute glomerulonephritis. Marked endocapillary proliferation. Few capillary lumina remain open (Masson's trichrome stain).

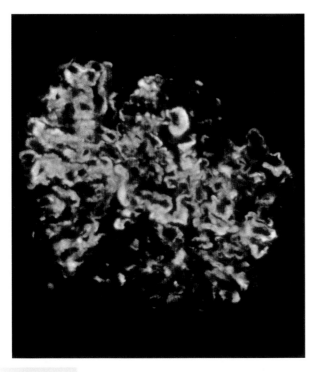

FIGURE 25-3   Acute poststreptococcal glomerulonephritis. Immunofluorescence with an anti-C3 antiserum discloses widespread "garland type" C3 labeling, mostly along the glomerular basement membranes.

This was described a century ago as "embolic" GN in the course of subacute bacterial endocarditis. However, the most common picture complicating endocarditis and other forms of septicemia as well as visceral abscesses with negative blood cultures consists of endo- plus extra-capillary proliferation (Fig. 25-4). Crescent formation is an ominous finding that is often accompanied by inter-stitial edema, inflammation, and tubular atrophy. Crescents appear as layers of inflammatory cells comprising parietal (Bowman's capsule) cells and macrophages.

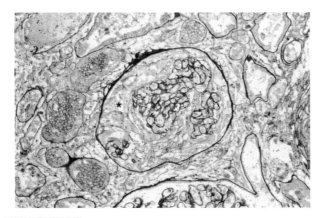

FIGURE 25-4   Crescentic glomerulonephritis complicating a case of infective endocarditis in an elderly patient with urinary tract infection due to *Enterococcus faecalis*. A circumferential crescent (*asterisk*) surrounds the remaining glomerular tuft (silver methenamine stain).

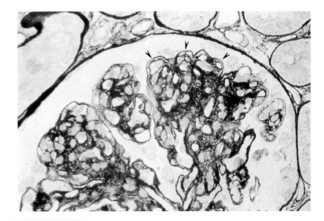

FIGURE 25-5   Membranoproliferative glomerulonephritis in a 50-year-old man with a life-long history of acne. Typical GBM double contours (*arrowheads*) (silver methenamine stain).

Necrosis is characterized by the presence of fibrin. The size and distribution of crescents varies from one glomerulus to another. Circumferential crescents antici-pate glomerular obsolescence. The spared lobules show the same proliferative changes as described previously. IF shows IgG and C3 deposits, as well as fibrin within crescents.

Membranoproliferative Glomerulonephritis

That MPGN may be the consequence of infection has been demonstrated in the case of shunt nephritis. The lesions comprise mesangial proliferation, exudative poly-morphonuclear cell infiltration, and characteristic GBM changes consisting of double contours due to interposi-tion of mesangial cells beneath the basement membrane, elaborating an additional layer of silver-stained mesan-gial matrix (Fig. 25-5). Humps and abundant C3 deposits are strongly suggestive of a postinfectious origin of this type of glomerulopathy, and help to differentiate it from the more common idiopathic variety.

ETIOLOGY AND EPIDEMIOLOGY

Acute Postinfectious Glomerulonephritis

Acute poststreptococcal GN due to nephritogenic strains of *Streptococcus pyogenes* group A remains common in tropical and subtropical regions. It mostly affects children and otherwise healthy adults, including the elderly. The illness can be epidemic. The nephropathy is characterized by the rapid onset of acute nephritic syndrome 10 to 20 days after pharyngeal or cutaneous infection. The offend-ing microorganism is not always identified, but serologic markers usually confirm that the etiologic agent is *Strep-tococcus*. The complement profile is characterized by hypocomplementemia with activation of both the classical and the alternative pathways and depressed C3 and C4 levels, followed by normalization within approximately 6 weeks.

Spontaneous recovery is the rule. Proteinuria wanes over weeks. Microscopic hematuria can last a few months before disappearing. Poststreptococcal AGN is in the majority of cases a benign disease. However, in some cases AGN with an initial histologic appearance of acute exudative GN may progress without remission to crescentic GN. Persistently low complement levels, weeks and months following the initial episode, along with heavy proteinuria and hematuria and rising serum creatinine levels indicate that the disease is not following its usual self-limited course and is progressing to chronic GN. Such progression is an incentive to carry out repeat kidney biopsy.

Regarding long-term prognosis, some publications dating back three decades have indicated that in the long run, after a protracted period of apparent cure, some patients experience hypertension and renal vascular lesions and can progress to ESRD.

However, it is difficult to determine the actual long-term outcome of AGN, because in many early publications, biopsies were not performed. The reported rate of recovery varied from 28% to 100%. The course appears to be more benign in children than in adults. Studies conducted during epidemics have determined that in a substantial number of affected children, the kidney disease is clinically silent, with GN detectable only with screening urinalyses, which demonstrate proteinuria and microscopic hematuria. How many of these clinically silent cases might later eventuate in chronic GN is an unsettled issue. This ascertainment bias may account for the impression that the disease is less severe in children. It has never been clearly established whether cases that are clinically mild and detected only by screening have a better long-term prognosis than the sporadic adult cases that come to attention because kidney involvement is more severe.

AGN can follow infection with a host of microorganisms. AGN complicating staphylococcal infection is virtually indistinguishable from poststreptococcal AGN. This is also true of AGN due to most of the etiologic agents found in Table 25-1. In the Western world, the incidence of classical poststreptococcal AGN has steadily declined in recent decades. It has become rare in children. On the other hand, microorganisms other than *Streptococcus* are increasingly recognized as etiologic agents for AGN. Thus, the overall incidence of postinfectious GN has remained the same but with a different distribution of glomerular lesions. In adults, an immunocompromised background is emerging as a predisposing factor, especially in alcoholic, cirrhotic, and diabetic patients. However, individuals with human immunodeficiency virus (HIV) infection, acquired immunodeficiency syndrome (AIDS), and those receiving immunosuppressive medications do not seem to be at increased risk for AGN.

TABLE 25-1 Infectious Agents Associated with Glomerulonephritis

Bacteria	Viruses
Streptococcus	Hepatitis B
Staphylococcus	Hepatitis C
Pneumococcus	Echovirus
Enterobacteriaceae	Adenovirus
Salmonella typhi	Cytomegalovirus
Meningococcus	Enteroviruses, including coxsackievirus
Treponema pallidum	Epstein-Barr virus
Brucella	Measles
Leptospira	Mumps
Yersinia	Parvovirus
Rickettsia	Rubella
Legionella	SV40
	Varicella

Postinfectious Glomerulonephritis with Rapid or Subacute Development

As noted previously, the typical endocapillary exudative AGN does not always resolve spontaneously. However, an unfavorable course is now mainly, although not exclusively, restricted to patients whose kidney involvement consists of endo- plus extracapillary (crescentic) GN. This variety of postinfectious GN is not new; crescentic GN following septicemia such as infectious endocarditis has been known for nearly a century. Nevertheless, its relative frequency, as indicated previously, at least in industrialized countries, has grown in inverse proportion to that of acute poststreptococcal GN. Its mode of onset and clinical features are more varied. The onset may be heralded by acute nephritic syndrome or rapidly progressive renal functional impairment; alternatively, the disorder may not be detected until chronic kidney disease has developed. The initial focus of infection is not always easy to identify. Most cutaneous, dental, and visceral infections can be complicated by endo- and extracapillary GN. Several candidate foci may be found in a given patient growing both gram-positive and gram-negative organisms. In contrast to acute poststreptococcal GN, extrarenal manifestations, especially purpura, may be present. In a febrile patient with GN and purpura, a search for endocarditis by ultrasonography and repeated blood cultures is mandatory. In our experience, low serum complement levels were found in only 24% of 25 cases with crescentic GN.

Risk factors for this form of postinfectious GN include alcoholism, drug addiction, malnutrition, and low socioeconomic level, because of poor dental and cutaneous hygiene and delayed access to medical care. The prognosis depends on the severity of infection, the immunologic status and age of the host, and the findings on kidney biopsy. The extent of crescentic proliferation on a biopsy comprising a sufficient number of glomeruli is the best predictor of progression to ESRD. Early recognition and eradication of the infectious foci by antibiotic treatment and, if necessary, by visceral or dental surgery are probably the best means of preventing progression of kidney disease.

Postinfectious Membranoproliferative Glomerulonephritis

Membranoproliferative glomerulonephritis was long considered idiopathic in a majority of cases. However, some forms were evidently postinfectious, such as shunt nephritis. Ventriculoatrial shunting was devised three decades ago to relieve hydrocephalus, mostly in children. It consists of a silicon catheter and a valve connecting the cerebral ventricle to the right atrium. This prosthetic material can become colonized with *Staphylococcus epidermidis* or, more rarely, with other organisms. About 160 cases have been published. The disease is characterized by fever, arthralgias, wasting, purpura, and severe anemia. Laboratory findings are suggestive of immune complex disease, with low serum complement levels, complement-driven hemolytic anemia, antinuclear antibodies, rheumatoid factor, and cryoglobulins. Renal signs and symptoms consist of proteinuria, microscopic hematuria, and renal functional impairment that can be rapidly progressive. Kidney biopsy usually discloses type I MPGN, often with numerous endocapillary polymorphonuclear cells and abundant C3 deposits. Endo- and extracapillary GN have also been observed. Removal of the shunt and antibiotic treatment may be followed by stabilization and even regression of the glomerular lesions, a demonstration that type I MPGN is not invariably irreversible. Nevertheless, only half of the patients experience a complete remission.

Several observations are consistent with the theory that some cases of "idiopathic" MPGN also are of infectious origin. These include the presence of C3 by IF and epidemiologic studies demonstrating the striking simultaneous decrease in incidence of both AGN and MPGN in western Europe.

PATHOGENESIS

The Offending Microorganisms

A host of microorganisms, including microbes, viruses, and parasites, can be responsible for postinfectious GN. For historical reasons, the most consistent data deal with streptococci. It has been established that only certain strains of group A streptococci lead to acute GN, especially Lancefield type 12, although not all strains of type 12 are nephritogenic. The main sites of streptococcal infection are the throat, especially in the winter and early spring, and the skin in the late summer and early fall. Tropical or subtropical climate favors skin infection, whereas in temperate climates, a pharyngeal origin is more common. In highly populated areas with low socioeconomic status, poststreptococcal GN is often epidemic. Studies from both the United States and western Europe have documented a decline in poststreptococcal AGN incidence in recent decades in urban areas, contrasting with a stable incidence in rural areas. The same has been observed in the Shanghai area in China. In fact, the sharply declining incidence of poststreptococcal AGN as well as acute rheumatic fever in industrialized countries contrasts with a continuing high incidence in the tropical regions of Africa, Latin America, and the Caribbean. Its prevalence remains high in the countries of Mediterranean Africa, which have a dry climate but a low per capita income.

Is this declining incidence just the consequence of better socioeconomic conditions? A French government–sponsored study that focused on eradication of rheumatic heart disease using the systematic free distribution of oral phenoxymethylpenicillin in the French Caribbean was immediately followed by a dramatic decrease in the annual incidence of both rheumatic fever and acute GN. Thus, the weight of the evidence is that early eradication of *Streptococcus pyogenes* group A infection is effective in preventing AGN. The same is likely true for staphylococcal and other etiologic agents.

The Complex Issue of Postinfectious Glomerular Inflammation

Acute postinfectious GN is an immunologic disease. A good clinical argument for this contention is the latent interval between clinical signs of infection and the onset of GN, at least when the onset of infection can be identified. This interval is usually easy to determine in acute GN, but less readily discerned in endo- and extracapillary forms, and rarely apparent in cases of MPGN. Overall, all forms of proliferative GN appear to follow a triphasic course: (1) induction, depending on an antigen; (2) transduction, characterized by immunoglobulin deposits; and (3) mediation. This last phase involves a host of cytokines that originate from monocytes and macrophages, glomerular mesangial cells, platelets, and endothelial cells, including the C5a and C3a complement fractions, and interferon-γ as well as interleukin-2 (IL-2). Activation of these mediators leads to generation of IL-1, tumor necrosis factor-α, interferon-γ, platelet-derived growth factor, and transforming growth factor-β. The role of C5b-9 in inducing arachidonic acid, free oxygen radicals, and IL-1 release is probably important. The initial event might be deposition of circulating immune complexes, including a bacterial component, or fixation of bacterial antigens with in situ immune complex formation. In human disease, the nephritogenic bacterial antigens are seldom identified within the glomeruli, except in some studies dealing with streptococcal or staphylococcal infections. In this respect, it is noteworthy that hepatitis B viral epitopes have been identified within the glomeruli of carriers of hepatitis B surface antigen having various types of GN. Nephritis-associated plasmin receptor, a group A streptococcal antigen, might have a pathogenic role in patients with acute poststreptococcal GN. However, considering the diversity of microorganisms and viruses capable of inducing postinfectious GN, identification of specific antigens appears to be a formidable task.

Whatever the triggering mechanism, the usual course of poststreptococcal and poststaphylococcal endocapillary exudative AGN is that of a self-limited disease. This is not the case for crescentic GN. Crescent formation in various conditions seems to be related to segmental destruction of the GBM by polymorphonuclear and macrophagic enzymes. Through these gaps, immune cells, plasma, fibrin, and inflammatory mediators gain access to Bowman's space and induce an intense proliferative reaction of Bowman's capsule parietal epithelial cells. The natural history of untreated crescentic GN is evolution to fibrosis and glomerular obsolescence. Why other forms of postinfectious GN produce the chronic form of MPGN is not readily apparent. The fact that the incidence of acute poststreptococcal GN and of MPGN have diminished in parallel suggests that, at least in some cases, the latter might be a mode of progression of an initial occult streptococcal glomerular injury.

PROGNOSTIC INDICATORS AND OUTCOME

Prognostic indicators stem from both the patient's background and the severity of the infectious focus, as well as from features of the glomerulopathy. Patients with poor general health due to malnutrition or cirrhosis are more likely to follow an unfavorable course. Patients with septicemia and those having such sites of infection as visceral abscesses, empyema, meningitis, or endocarditis are more likely to die from the primary disorder than from the consequences of their glomerulopathy. Risk of death is significantly higher in older patients and in those with purpura. Initial presentation with nephrotic syndrome or a serum creatinine above 2.7 mg/dL and the presence of crescents and interstitial fibrosis on kidney biopsy usually herald irreversible kidney damage. Two factors at presentation apparently predict a favorable prognosis: the upper respiratory tract as initial site of infection, and pure endocapillary proliferation with an IF starry sky pattern. Proteinuria below 1.5 g/day is well correlated with recovery in patients with pure endocapillary proliferation, whereas nephrotic syndrome at presentation is often followed by persistent chronic GN.

TREATMENT

In the cases of pure endocapillary GN from three decades ago, the course was considered nearly uniformly favorable. More recent experience indicates that the location of the infectious focus is much more varied than the throat and the skin, and it is often still present at the time of kidney biopsy. When repeat kidney biopsy is performed months and even years after the initial one, it discloses ongoing inflammatory lesions in patients whose infection persists, whereas in those in whom infection had been eradicated, the glomerular lesions are mainly inactive and fibrous. This reinforces the need to eradicate any persistent infection with appropriate antibiotic therapy and if necessary by a surgical or dental procedure.

Definitive treatment recommendations for the crescentic form of postinfectious GN are not available. Anecdotal experience with glomerular complications of endocarditis suggests that corticosteroid therapy, cyclophosphamide, or plasmapheresis have a favorable effect on kidney function. Such observations are uncontrolled. However, they suggest that the prognosis of postinfectious crescentic GN is not necessarily disastrous when an aggressive anti-inflammatory and possibly immunosuppressive regimen is used after achieving eradication of infection.

In addition, postinfectious GN is a public health problem with significant cost implications. In this respect, early, easy access to medical and dental care, control of drug addiction, and the same prophylactic measures that have proven effective in preventing bacterial endocarditis should be implemented to reduce the incidence of the kidney disease.

GLOMERULONEPHRITIS RELATED TO VIRAL INFECTION

Viral infections can be complicated by various types of glomerulopathies, both proliferative and nonproliferative. This confirms that the same agent can induce different histologic types of glomerular diseases.

Hepatitis B Virus–Related Glomerulopathies

The main type of hepatitis B virus (HBV)-related glomerulopathy is membranous glomerulopathy (MGN). It is endemic in Asia and usually affects children infected via maternal-fetal transmission. In the United States, it is essentially found in immigrant children from endemic areas and in adult drug addicts. The second most common form of GN reported with HBV infection is MPGN. The clinical picture consists of nephrotic syndrome. A history of recent acute hepatitis is usually found in adults. The patients carry hepatitis B surface antigen (HBsAg), hepatitis B core antigen (HBcAg), and hepatitis B early antigen (HBeAg). Hypocomplementemia and circulating immune complexes are frequent. Viral antigens can be identified in the glomeruli by immunohistochemistry. Electron microscopy shows viruslike particles incorporated into the GBM. Some forms of HBV infection are accompanied by vasculitis in the form of polyarteritis nodosa. Vasculitic lesions may be found in renal arteries. The natural history of HBV-MGN in children is usually characterized by spontaneous clinical remission with only rare progression to ESRD. Corticosteroid treatment is contraindicated. Specific antiviral therapy is indicated for the liver disease, because it has the potential to eventuate in cirrhosis and hepatocellular carcinoma. The effect of lamivudine to suppress HBV replication in chronic active hepatitis B might lead to new approaches for treatment of the kidney disease.

Hepatitis C Virus–Related Glomerulopathies

That hepatitis C virus (HCV) infection is related to cryoglobulinemia and kidney disease was recognized in 1993. Arthralgias, peripheral neuropathy, and purpura are common and indicate that the cryoglobulinemia induces a generalized vasculitis. The patients may have elevated serum aminotransferase levels, but this laboratory indication of liver involvement waxes and wanes and may be negative at times. The glomerulopathy is characterized by moderate to nephrotic proteinuria and impaired kidney function. In rare cases, the kidney biopsy shows membranous glomerulopathy. Typically, it discloses a particular form of MPGN comprising diffuse thickening of the glomerular capillary walls and double contours, but also massive glomerular infiltration by macrophages and eosinophilic thrombi in some capillary loops that are characteristic of cryoglobulinemia. IF shows glomerular capillary wall and mesangial deposition of large amounts

of IgG, IgM, and C3, especially on the thrombi. Viruslike particles and HCV RNA were identified by electron microscopy in the kidney tissue of half of a series of Egyptian patients with HCV infection and glomerulopathy. Cryoglobulins are present in serum. They contain HCV RNA and IgG anti-HCV antibodies to the nucleocapsid core antigen (c22-3). Circulating IgM rheumatoid factors are usually present. Treatment is based on antiviral therapy. Interferon-γ2b may suppress viremia and simultaneously ameliorate the course of the glomerulopathy. The combination of interferon and ribavirin may be more effective than interferon alone in preventing the frequent relapses that occur after conclusion of a treatment course, but to date the available data are scarce. Regarding the treatment of the glomerulopathy, reports using plasmapheresis, methylprednisolone pulses, and cyclophosphamide provide encouraging results, but large, long-term controlled studies are required before such treatments can be endorsed. Hepatitis C–related cryoglobulinemia is covered in Chapter 18.

Glomerulonephritis Associated with Other Viruses

Numerous publications report anecdotal cases of virus-associated GN. They are listed in Table 25-1. In children, viral glomerulopathies may be accompanied by the hemolytic-uremic syndrome.

Nephrotic focal segmental glomerulosclerosis (FSGS), especially assuming the histologic appearance of collapsing glomerulopathy, is a typical picture of HIV-associated nephropathy. Recent observations indicate that parvovirus B19 and simian virus SV40 may also injure the glomerular podocytes. In this respect, some forms of FSGS can also be listed among glomerulopathies of viral origin (FSGS is covered in Chapter 19).

BIBLIOGRAPHY

Bach JF, Chalons S, Forier E, et al: 10-year educational programme aimed at rheumatic fever in two French Caribbean Islands. Lancet 347:644–648, 1996.
Beaufils M, Gibert C, Morel-Maroger L, et al: Glomerulonephritis in severe bacterial infection with and without endocarditis. In Hamburger J, Crosnier J, Maxwell MH (eds): Advances in Nephrology. Chicago, Yearbook Medical, 1977, pp 217–234.
Daimon S, Mizuno Y, Fujii S, et al: Infective endocarditis-induced crescentic glomerulonephritis dramatically improved by plasmapheresis. Am J Kidney Dis 32:309–313, 1998.
Gallo GR, Neugarten J, Baldwin DS: Glomerulonephritis associated with systemic, bacterial and viral infections. In Tisher CC, Brenner BM (eds): Renal Pathology, 2nd ed. Philadelphia, JB Lippincott, 1994, pp 564–595.
Haffner D, Schindera F, Aschoff A, et al: The clinical spectrum of shunt nephritis. Nephrol Dial Transplant 12:1143–1148, 1997.
Lai KN, Ho RTH, Tam JS, et al: Detection of hepatitis B virus DNA and RNA in kidneys of HBV-related glomerulonephritis. Kidney Int 50:1965–1977, 1996.
Masuda M, Nakanishi K, Yoshizawa N, et al: Group A streptococ-

cal antigen in the glomeruli of children with Henoch-Schönlein nephritis. Am J Kidney Dis 41:366–370, 2003.
Montseny JJ, Meyrier A, Kleinknecht D, et al: The current spectrum of infectious glomerulonephritis. Experience with 76 patients and review of the literature. Medicine 74:63–73, 1995.
Parra G, Rodriguez-Iturbe B, Batsford S, et al: Antibody to streptococcal zymogen in the serum of patients with acute glomerulonephritis: A multicentric study. Kidney Int 54:509–517, 1998.
Roy SI, Stapleton FB: Changing perspectives in children hospitalized with poststreptococcal acute glomerulonephritis. Pediatr Nephrol 4:585–589, 1990.
Sabry AA, Sobh MA, Irving WL, et al: A comprehensive study of the association between hepatitis C virus and glomerulopathy. Nephrol Dial Transplant 17:239–245, 2002.
Silva FG: Acute postinfectious glomerulonephritis and glomerulonephritis complicating persistent bacterial infection. In Jennette JC, Olson JL, Schwartz MM, Silva FG (eds): Heptinstall's Pathology of the Kidney, 5th ed. Philadelphia, Lippincott-Raven, 1998, pp 389–453.

CHAPTER **26**

Kidney Involvement in Systemic Vasculitis

J. Charles Jennette   Ronald J. Falk

The kidneys are affected by many forms of system vasculitis (Fig. 26-1), which cause a wide variety of sometimes confusing clinical manifestations. Large vessel vasculitides, such as giant cell arteritis and Takayasu's arteritis, can narrow the abdominal aorta or renal arteries, resulting in renal ischemia and renovascular hypertension. Medium-sized vessel vasculitides, such as polyarteritis nodosa and Kawasaki's disease, also can reduce flow through the renal artery, and may affect intrarenal arteries, resulting in infarction and hemorrhage. Small vessel vasculitides, such as microscopic polyangiitis, Wegener's granulomatosis, Henoch-Schönlein purpura, and cryoglobulinemic vasculitis, frequently involve the kidneys and especially glomerular capillaries, resulting in glomerulonephritis.

PATHOLOGY

As depicted in Figure 26-1 and described in Table 26-1, different types of systemic vasculitis affect different vessels within the kidney. In addition, each type of vasculitis has different histologic and immunohistologic features.

Giant cell arteritis and Takayasu's arteritis predominantly affect the aorta and its major branches. Takayasu's arteritis is an important cause of renovascular hypertension, especially in young patients. Giant cell arteritis only rarely causes clinically significant kidney disease, although asymptomatic pathologic involvement is common. Giant cell arteritis often involves the extracranial branches of the carotid arteries, including the temporal artery. Some patients, however, do not have temporal artery involvement, and patients with other types of vasculitis (e.g., microscopic polyangiitis and Wegener's granulomatosis) may have temporal artery involvement. Therefore, temporal artery disease is neither a required nor sufficient pathologic feature of giant cell arteritis.

Histologically, both giant cell arteritis and Takayasu's arteritis are characterized by focal chronic granulomatous inflammation, often but not always with multinucleated giant cells. With chronicity, the inflammatory injury evolves into fibrosis and frequently results in vascular narrowing, which is the basis for renovascular hypertension when a renal artery is involved.

Polyarteritis nodosa and Kawasaki's disease affect medium-sized arteries (i.e., main visceral arteries), such as the mesenteric, hepatic, coronary, and main renal arteries. These diseases also may involve small arteries, such as arteries within the parenchyma of skeletal muscle, liver, heart, pancreas, spleen, and kidney (e.g., interlobar and arcuate arteries). By the definitions in Table 26-1, polyarteritis nodosa and Kawasaki's disease affect arteries exclusively and not capillaries or venules. Thus, they do not cause glomerulonephritis. The presence of arteritis with glomerulonephritis indicates some form of small vessel vasculitis rather than a medium-sized vessel vasculitis.

Histologically, the acute arterial injury of Kawasaki's disease and polyarteritis nodosa is characterized by focal artery wall necrosis and infiltration of inflammatory cells. The acute injury of polyarteritis nodosa typically has conspicuous fibrinoid necrosis, which is absent or less apparent in Kawasaki's disease. Fibrinoid necrosis results from plasma coagulation factors spilling into the necrotic areas, where they are activated to form fibrin. Early in the acute injury of polyarteritis nodosa, neutrophils predominate, but within a few days mononuclear leukocytes are most numerous. Thrombosis may occur at the site of inflammation, resulting in infarction. Focal necrotizing injury to vessels erodes into the vessel wall and adjacent tissue, producing an inflammatory aneurysm, which may rupture and cause hemorrhage. Thrombosis of the inflamed arteries causes downstream ischemia and infarction.

Although small vessel vasculitides may affect medium-sized arteries, these disorders favor small vessels such as arterioles, venules (e.g., in the dermis), and capillaries (e.g., in glomeruli and pulmonary alveoli; see Fig. 26-1). As described in Table 26-1, there are a variety of clinically and pathogenetically distinct forms of small vessel vasculitis that have in common focal necrotizing inflammation of small vessels. In the acute phase, this injury is characterized histologically by segmental fibrinoid necrosis and leukocyte infiltration (Fig. 26-2), sometimes

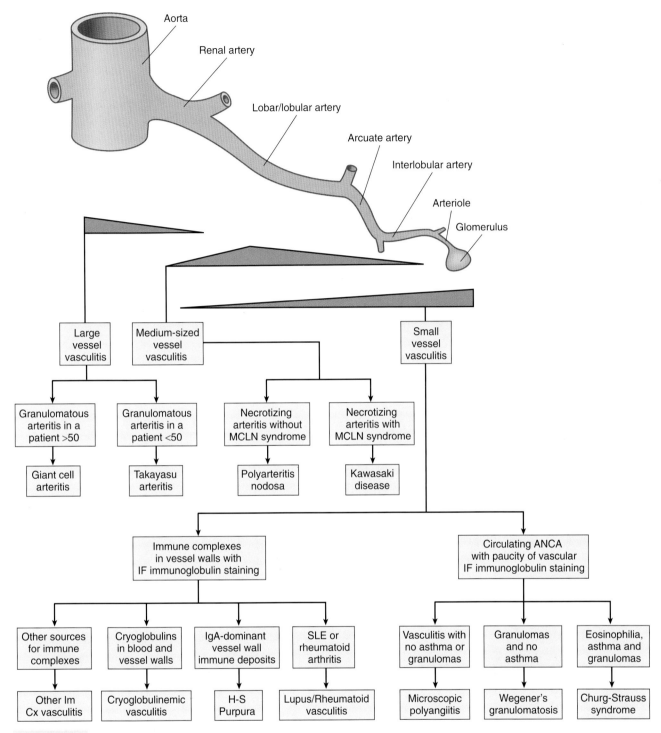

FIGURE 26-1 Predominant distribution of renal vascular involvement by systemic vasculitides, and diagnostic clinical and pathologic features that distinguish among them. The width of the blue triangles indicates the predilection of small, medium-sized, and large vessel vasculitides for various portions of the renal vasculature. Note that medium-sized renal arteries can be affected by large, medium-sized, and small vessel vasculitides, but arterioles and glomeruli are affected by small vessel vasculitides alone, based on the definitions in Table 26-1. H-S, Henoch-Schönlein; IF, immunofluorescence; MCLN, mucocutaneous lymph node syndrome; SLE, systemic lupus erythematosus.

TABLE 26-1   Names and Definitions of Vasculitis Adopted by the Chapel Hill Consensus Conference on the Nomenclature of Systemic Vasculitis

Large vessel vasculitis*	
Giant cell arteritis	Granulomatous arteritis of the aorta and its major branches, with a predilection for the extracranial branches of the carotid artery. Often involves the temporal artery. Usually occurs in patients over 50 and often is associated with polymyalgia rheumatica.
Takayasu arteritis	Granulomatous inflammation of the aorta and its major branches. Usually occurs in patients under 50.
Medium vessel vasculitis*	
Polyarteritis nodosa	Necrotizing inflammation of medium-sized or small arteries without glomerulonephritis or vasculitis in arterioles, capillaries, or venules.
Kawasaki's disease	Arteritis involving large, medium-sized, and small arteries, and associated with mucocutaneous lymph node syndrome. Coronary arteries are often involved. Aorta and veins may be involved. Usually occurs in children.
Small vessel vasculitis*	
Wegener's granulomatosis[†,‡]	Granulomatous inflammation involving the respiratory tract, and necrotizing vasculitis affecting small to medium-sized vessels (e.g., capillaries, venules, arterioles, and arteries). Necrotizing glomerulonephritis is common.
Churg-Strauss syndrome[†,‡]	Eosinophil-rich and granulomatous inflammation involving the respiratory tract and necrotizing vasculitis affecting small to medium-sized vessels, and associated with asthma and blood eosinophilia.
Microscopic polyangiitis[†,‡]	Necrotizing vasculitis with few or no immune deposits affecting small vessels (i.e., capillaries, venules, or arterioles). Necrotizing arteritis involving small and medium-sized arteries may be present. Necrotizing glomerulonephritis is common. Pulmonary capillaritis often occurs.
Henoch-Schönlein purpura[‡]	Vasculitis with IgA-dominant immune deposits affecting small vessels (i.e., capillaries, venules, or arterioles). Typically involves skin, gut, and glomeruli, and is associated with arthralgias or arthritis.
Essential cryoglobulinemic vasculitis[‡]	Vasculitis with cryoglobulin immune deposits affecting small vessels (i.e., capillaries, venules, or arterioles) and associated with cryoglobulins in serum. Skin and glomeruli are often involved
Cutaneous leukocytoclastic angiitis	Isolated cutaneous leukocytoclastic angiitis without systemic vasculitis or glomerulonephritis.

*Large artery refers to the aorta and the largest branches directed toward major body regions (e.g., to the extremities and the head and neck); medium-sized artery refers to the main visceral arteries (e.g., renal, hepatic, coronary, and mesenteric arteries), and small vessel refers to the distal arterial branches that connect with arterioles (e.g., renal arcuate and interlobular arteries), as well as arterioles, capillaries, and venules. Note that some small and large vessel vasculitides may involve medium-sized arteries; but large and medium-sized vessel vasculitides do not involve vessels ther than arteries.
[†]Strongly associated with antineutrophil cytoplasmic antibodies (ANCAs).
[‡]May be accompanied by glomerulonephritis and can manifest as nephritis or pulmonary-renal vasculitic syndrome.
Modified from Jennette JC, Falk RJ, Andrassy K, et al: Nomenclature of systemic vasculitides: The proposal of an international consensus conference. Arthritis Rheum 37:187–192, 1994. Copyright © 1994 John Wiley & Sons, Inc. Reprinted by permission of John Wiley & Sons, Inc.

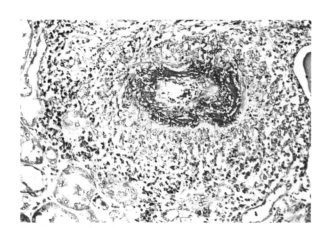

FIGURE 26-2   Renal interlobular artery with fibrinoid necrosis from a patient with microscopic polyangiitis (Masson trichrome stain).

with secondary thrombosis. The neutrophils often undergo karyorrhexis (leukocytoclasia). With chronicity, mononuclear leukocytes become predominant and fibrosis develops.

The various forms of small vessel vasculitis differ from one another with respect to the presence or absence of distinctive features, as summarized in Table 26-1 and Figure 26-1. For example, Wegener's granulomatosis has necrotizing granulomatous inflammation, Churg-Strauss syndrome has blood eosinophilia and asthma, Henoch-Schönlein purpura has immunoglobulin A (IgA)-dominant vascular immune deposits, and cryoglobulinemic vasculitis has circulating cryoglobulins.

The glomerular lesions of microscopic polyangiitis, Wegener's granulomatosis, and Churg-Strauss syndrome are identical pathologically, and are characterized by segmental fibrinoid necrosis, crescent formation (Fig. 26-3), and a paucity of glomerular staining for immunoglobulin (i.e., pauci-immune glomerulonephritis). Leukocytoclastic angiitis of medullary vasa recta (Fig. 26-4) also occurs

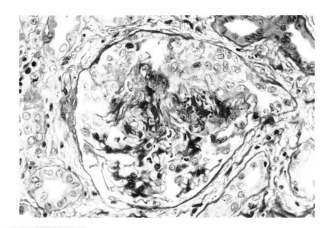

FIGURE 26-3 Glomerulus with segmental fibrinoid necrosis with red (fuchsinophilic) fibrinous material and an adjacent cellular crescent from a patient with antineutrophil cytoplasmic antibody small vessel vasculitis (Masson trichrome stain).

in the antineutrophil cytoplasmic antibody (ANCA) vasculitides, and rarely is severe enough to cause papillary necrosis. Patients with these three vasculitides often have ANCAs.

The glomerulonephritis of Henoch-Schönlein purpura is identical to IgA nephropathy. The glomerulonephritis of cryoglobulinemic vasculitis usually manifests as type I membranoproliferative glomerulonephritis (mesangiocapillary glomerulonephritis), although other patterns of proliferative glomerulonephritis occur less often. Cryoglobulinemic vasculitis frequently is associated with hepatitis C infection.

PATHOGENESIS

Vasculitis is caused by the activation of inflammatory mediator systems in vessel walls. The initiating event (i.e., the cause), however, is unknown for many forms of vasculitis. An immune response to heterologous antigens

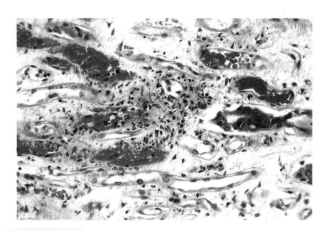

FIGURE 26-4 Medullary vasa recta with leukocytoclastic angiitis from a patient with Wegener's granulomatosis (hematoxylin and eosin stain).

TABLE 26-2 Putative Immunologic Causes of Vasculitis

Immune complex mediated
  Henoch-Schönlein purpura*
  Cryoglobulinemic vasculitis*
  Lupus vasculitis*
  Serum sickness vasculitis*
  Rheumatoid vasculitis
  Polyarteritis nodosa
  Infection-induced immune complex vasculitis*
    Viral (e.g., hepatitis B and C virus)
    Bacterial (e.g., streptococcal)
  Goodpasture's syndrome (anti–glomerular basement
    membrane antibodies)*

Antineutrophil cytoplasmic antibody–mediated
  Wegener's granulomatosis*
  Microscopic polyangiitis*
  Churg-Strauss syndrome*

Cell mediated
  Allograft cellular vascular rejection
  Giant cell arteritis
  Takayasu's arteritis

*May be accompanied by glomerulonephritis and can manifest as nephritis or pulmonary-renal vasculitic syndrome.

(e.g., hepatitis B or C antigens in some forms of immune complex vasculitis) or autoantigens (e.g., proteinase 3 or myeloperoxidase in ANCA vasculitis) is presumed to be the etiologic event in many patients with vasculitis. A number of types of vasculitis are categorized based on putative immunologic mechanisms in Table 26-2.

Primarily because of the pattern of inflammation, T cell–mediated inflammation has been incriminated in the pathogenesis of giant cell arteritis and Takayasu's arteritis. Several mechanisms of antibody-mediated injury are thought to be important in the pathogenesis of necrotizing small vessel vasculitides, but there is evidence that T cells also may play a role.

The vasculitides listed in the immune complex–mediated category in Table 26-2 all have immunohistologic evidence for vessel wall immune complex localization, that is, granular staining for immunoglobulins and complement. Antibodies bound to antigens in vessel walls activate humoral inflammatory mediator systems (e.g., complement, coagulation, plasmin, and kinin systems), which attract and activate neutrophils and monocytes. These activated leukocytes generate toxic oxygen metabolites and release enzymes that cause matrix lysis and cellular apoptosis, resulting in necrotizing inflammatory injury to vessel walls.

This same final pathway of inflammatory injury also can be reached if antibodies bind to antigens that are integral components of vessel walls. The best documented example is anti–glomerular basement membrane (anti-GBM) antibody–mediated glomerulonephritis and Goodpasture's syndrome (see Chapter 22). T cells with specificity for basement membranes or cells also may participate in the mediation or regulation of glomerular injury.

An important group of necrotizing systemic small vessel vasculitides, which frequently involve the kidneys, occurs without immunohistologic evidence for vascular immune complex localization or direct antibody binding. This paucity of immune deposits is the basis for the designation "pauci-immune" for this group of vasculitides, which includes microscopic polyangiitis, Wegener's granulomatosis, and Churg-Strauss syndrome. Approximately 85% of patients with pauci-immune glomerulonephritis and vasculitis have circulating ANCAs. In vitro and in vivo experimental evidence indicate that the vascular inflammation is caused by activation of neutrophils and monocytes by ANCAs.

ANCAs are specific for proteins within the granules of neutrophils and the peroxidase-positive lysosomes of monocytes. They often are detected in patient serum by indirect immunofluorescence microscopy using alcohol-fixed normal human neutrophils as substrate. Using this assay, two patterns of neutrophil staining discriminate between the two major subtypes of ANCAs: cytoplasmic-staining (C-ANCA) and perinuclear staining (P-ANCA). Using specific immunochemical assays such as enzyme-linked immunosorbent assays or radioimmunoassays, most C-ANCAs are specific for a neutrophil and monocyte proteinase called proteinase 3 (PR3-ANCA), and most P-ANCAs are specific for myeloperoxidase (MPO-ANCA).

One hypothesis about the pathogenesis of ANCA-associated vasculitides proposes that ANCAs react with cytoplasmic antigens (e.g., PR3 and MPO) that are released at the surface of cytokine-stimulated leukocytes, causing the leukocytes to adhere to vessel walls, degranulate, and generate toxic oxygen metabolites. The interaction of ANCAs with neutrophils involves Fc receptor engagement, perhaps by immune complexes formed between ANCAs and ANCA antigens in the microenvironment surrounding the leukocyte. ANCA binding to ANCA antigens on the surface of neutrophils also may be involved in neutrophil activation. ANCA antigens also may become planted in vessel walls or even produced by endothelial cells, thus providing a nidus for in situ immune complex formation in vessel walls. If such in situ formation is present, it must be at a level that cannot be detected by immunofluorescence microscopy; ANCA vasculitides are characteristically pauci-immune. The most compelling evidence that ANCAs cause vasculitis is the observation that mouse antibodies specific for MPO cause pauci-immune crescentic glomerulonephritis and small vessel vasculitis when injected intravenously.

CLINICAL FEATURES

The diagnosis and management of systemic vasculitis can be very challenging. The clinical features are extremely varied and are dictated by the category of vasculitis, the type of vessel involved, the organ system distribution of vascular injury, and the stage of disease. Irrespective of the type of vasculitis, most patients have accompanying constitutional features of inflammatory disease, such as fever, arthralgias, myalgias, and weight loss. These probably are caused by increased circulating levels of proinflammatory cytokines.

Giant cell arteritis and Takayasu's arteritis typically present with evidence for ischemia in tissues supplied by involved arteries. Patients with Takayasu's arteritis often develop claudication (especially in the upper extremities), absent pulses, and bruits. Approximately 40% of patients with Takayasu's arteritis develop renovascular hypertension, a feature that only rarely complicates giant cell arteritis. Giant cell arteritis can affect virtually any organ in the body, but signs and symptoms of involvement of arteries in the head and neck are the most common clinical manifestations. Superficial arteries, for example, the temporal artery, may be swollen and tender. Arterial narrowing causes ischemic manifestations in affected tissues, such as headache, jaw claudication, and loss of vision. About half of the patients with giant cell arteritis have polymyalgia rheumatica, which is characterized by aching and stiffness in the neck, shoulder girdle, or pelvic girdle.

Medium-sized vessel vasculitides, such as polyarteritis nodosa and Kawasaki's disease, often present with clinical evidence for infarction in multiple organs, such as abdominal pain with occult blood in the stool, and skeletal muscle pain and cardiac pain with elevated serum muscle enzymes. Laboratory evaluation often demonstrates clinically silent organ damage, such as liver injury with elevated liver function tests and pancreatic injury with elevated serum amylase.

Polyarteritis nodosa frequently causes multiple renal infarcts and aneurysms. Unlike microscopic polyangiitis, polyarteritis nodosa typically does not cause severe impairments in kidney function. Rupture of arterial aneurysms with massive retroperitoneal or intraperitoneal hemorrhage is a life-threatening complication of polyarteritis nodosa.

Kawasaki's disease almost always occurs in children under 6 years of age and has a predilection for coronary, axillary, and iliac arteries. Kawasaki's disease is accompanied by the mucocutaneous lymph node syndrome, which includes fever, nonpurulent lymphadenopathy, and mucosal and cutaneous inflammation. Although the renal arteries frequently are affected pathologically, clinically significant renal involvement is rare in patients with Kawasaki's disease.

The small vessel vasculitides often present with evidence of inflammation in vessels in multiple organs, but may initially manifest with involvement of only one organ, followed later by development of disease in other organs. Hematuria, proteinuria, and impaired kidney function caused by glomerulonephritis are frequent clinical features of all forms of small vessel vasculitis listed in

Table 26-1. Other manifestations include purpura caused by leukocytoclastic angiitis in dermal venules and arterioles, abdominal pain and occult blood in the stool from mucosal and bowel wall infarcts, mononeuritis multiplex from arteritis in peripheral nerves, necrotizing sinusitis from upper respiratory tract mucosal angiitis, and pulmonary hemorrhage from alveolar capillaritis.

In addition to these features, which are shared by patients with any type of small vessel vasculitis, patients with Wegener's granulomatosis and Churg-Strauss syndrome have distinctive clinical features that set them apart. Patients with Wegener's granulomatosis have necrotizing granulomatous inflammation, most often in the upper or lower respiratory tract, and rarely in other tissues (e.g., skin, orbit). In the lungs, this inflammation produces irregular nodular lesions that can be observed by radiography. These lesions may cavitate and hemorrhage. However, massive pulmonary hemorrhage in patients with Wegener's granulomatosis is usually caused by capillaritis rather than granulomatous inflammation. By definition, patients with Churg-Strauss syndrome have blood eosinophilia and a history of asthma. They also develop eosinophil-rich tissue inflammation, especially in the lungs and gut.

DIAGNOSIS

Multisystem disease in a patient with constitutional signs and symptoms of inflammation, such as fever, arthralgias, myalgias, and weight loss, should raise suspicion of systemic vasculitis. Data that will assist in resolving the differential diagnosis include the age of the patient, organ distribution of injury, concurrent syndromes (e.g., mucocutaneous lymph node syndrome, polymyalgia rheumatica, asthma), type of vessel involved (e.g., large artery, visceral artery, small vessel other than an artery), lesion histology (e.g., granulomatous, necrotizing), lesion immunohistology (e.g., immune deposits, pauci-immune), and serologic data (e.g., cryoglobulins, hepatitis C antibodies, hypocomplementemia, antinuclear antibodies, ANCAs; see Fig. 26-1).

Signs and symptoms of tissue ischemia along with angiography demonstrating irregularity, stenosis, occlusion, or, less commonly, aneurysms of large and medium-sized arteries should suggest giant cell arteritis or Takayasu's arteritis. A useful discriminator between giant cell arteritis and Takayasu's arteritis is age. The former is rare in individuals under 50 years of age, and the latter is rare in patients over 50. The presence of polymyalgia rheumatica is a clinical marker for giant cell arteritis.

Polyarteritis nodosa and Kawasaki's disease cause visceral ischemia, particularly in the heart, kidneys, liver, spleen, and gut. Arteritis in skeletal muscle and subcutaneous tissues causes tender erythematous nodules that can be identified on physical examination. Angiographic demonstration of medium-sized artery aneurysms (e.g., in renal arteries) indicates that some type of vasculitis

is present, but it is not disease specific because giant cell arteritis, Takayasu's arteritis, polyarteritis nodosa, Kawasaki's disease, Wegener's granulomatosis, microscopic polyarteritis, and Churg-Strauss syndrome all can produce arterial aneurysms. Kawasaki's disease almost always occurs in children under 6 years of age and is by definition accompanied by the mucocutaneous lymph node syndrome.

A small vessel vasculitis should be suspected when there is evidence for inflammation of vessels smaller than arteries, such as glomerular capillaries (hematuria and proteinuria), dermal venules (palpable purpura), or alveolar capillaries (hemoptysis). To discriminate among the small vessel vasculitides, evaluation of serologic data, vessel immunohistology, or concurrent nonvasculitic disease (e.g., asthma, eosinophilia, lupus) is required (see Fig. 26-1).

Evaluation of vessels in biopsy specimens, such as glomerular capillaries in kidney biopsies or alveolar capillaries in lung biopsies, can be helpful, especially if immunohistology is performed. The pauci-immune vasculitides lack immune deposits, anti-GBM disease has linear immunoglobulin deposits, and immune complex vasculitides have granular immune deposits.

Serology, especially ANCA analysis, is useful in differentiating among the small vessel vasculitides. Wegener's granulomatosis, microscopic polyangiitis, and Churg-Strauss syndrome are strongly associated with ANCAs (Table 26-3). As depicted in Figure 26-5 and listed in Table 26-3, most patients with active untreated Wegener's granulomatosis have C-ANCA (PR3-ANCA). A minority of patients have P-ANCA (MPO-ANCA). Therefore, C-ANCA is not completely specific for Wegener's granulomatosis because some patients with C-ANCA have systemic small vessel vasculitis without granulomatous inflammation (i.e., microscopic polyangiitis), and others have pauci-immune necrotizing and crescentic glomerulonephritis alone. Patients with Churg-Strauss syndrome have the lowest frequency of ANCAs and the lowest frequency of renal involvement by glomerulonephritis. A minority of patients with immunopathologic evidence for immune complex mediated or anti-GBM-mediated vasculitis or glomerulonephritis have concurrent ANCA (see Fig. 26-5). Approximately one fourth to one third of patients

TABLE 26-3 Approximate Frequency of PR3-ANCA or MPO-ANCA in Pauci-Immune Small Vessel Vasculitis

	Microscopic Polyangiitis	Wegener's Granulomatosis	Churg-Strauss Syndrome
PR3-ANCA	40%	75%	10%
MPO-ANCA	50%	20%	60%
ANCA negative	10%	5%	30%

MPO-ANCA, myeloperoxidase antineutrophil cytoplasmic antibody; PR3-ANCA, proteinase 3 antineutrophil cytoplasmic antibody.

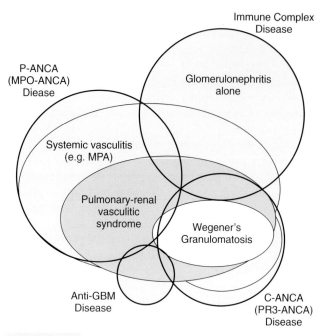

FIGURE 26-5 Relationship of vasculitic clinicopathologic syndromes to immunopathologic categories of vascular injury in patients with crescentic glomerulonephritis. The circles represent the major immunopathologic categories of vascular inflammation that affect the kidneys, and the shaded ovals the clinicopathologic expressions of the vascular inflammation. Note that clinical syndromes can be caused by more than one immunopathologic process; for example, pulmonary-renal vasculitic syndrome can be caused by anti–glomerular basement membrane antibodies (i.e., Goodpasture's syndrome), immune complex localization (e.g., lupus erythematosus), or antineutrophil cytoplasmic antibody–associated disease (e.g., microscopic polyangiitis and Wegener's granulomatosis). (Reproduced from Jennette JC: Anti-neutrophil cytoplasmic autoantibody-associated disease: A pathologist's perspective. Am J Kidney Dis 18:164–170, 1991. With permission.)

with anti-GBM disease are ANCA positive. These patients have kidney disease that is intermediate in severity between ANCA disease and anti-GBM disease (which has the worst prognosis), and they may have persistence or recurrence of ANCA disease after the anti-GBM disease remits.

Diagnostic serologic tests for immune complex–mediated vasculitides include assays for circulating immune complexes (e.g., cryoglobulins in cryoglobulinemic vasculitis), assays for antibodies known to participate in immune complex formation or to mark the presence of a disease that generates immune complexes (e.g., antibodies to hepatitis B or C, streptococci, DNA), and assays for consumption or activation of humoral inflammatory mediator system components (e.g., assays for reduced complement components or for activated membrane attack complex).

THERAPY AND OUTCOME

All of the vasculitides discussed in this chapter respond to anti-inflammatory or immunosuppressive therapy. The aggressiveness of treatment should match the aggressiveness of the disease.

Takayasu's arteritis and giant cell arteritis usually respond well to high-dose corticosteroid treatment (e.g., prednisone, 1 mg/kg body weight per day) during the acute phase of the disease, followed by tapering and low-dose maintenance for several months to a year depending on disease activity. Patients with severe disease or steroid toxicity benefit from other immunosuppressive agents, including methotrexate, cyclophosphamide, or azathioprine. If present, renovascular hypertension should be controlled. After the inflammatory phase is past and the sclerotic phase has developed, reconstructive vascular surgery may be required to improve flow to ischemic tissues, especially in patients with Takayasu's arteritis.

Many patients with polyarteritis nodosa have a persistent viral infection, especially hepatitis B virus infection. These patients are usually ANCA negative. In these cases, antiviral therapy with or without plasma exchange is recommended. Patients with no evidence for infection usually are managed with corticosteroids with or without cytotoxic drugs.

Corticosteroid treatment is not recommended for Kawasaki's disease because it appears to worsen coronary artery disease, which is the most life-threatening aspect of Kawasaki's disease. The preferred treatment is a combination of aspirin and high-dose intravenous gamma globulins. This controls the inflammatory manifestations of the disease (e.g., the mucocutaneous lymph node syndrome), prevents thrombosis of injured arteries, and retards the frequency of coronary artery involvement. With appropriate treatment, over 90% of patients with Kawasaki's disease have complete resolution of the disease.

Most patients with Henoch-Schönlein purpura have mild self-limited disease that requires only supportive care (see Chapter 21). Arthralgias are relieved by non-steroidal anti-inflammatory drugs. Corticosteroid treatment is beneficial in patients who have severe abdominal pain caused by intestinal vasculitis. The treatment of severe glomerulonephritis in patients with Henoch-Schönlein purpura is controversial. There is anecdotal evidence that aggressive crescent glomerulonephritis should be treated with high-dose corticosteroids, cytotoxic agents, or plasmapheresis, but this has not been documented in controlled trials. Data from a large pediatric population suggest that corticosteroid treatment may decrease the risk for developing kidney involvement in those patients with severe abdominal pain and rash.

Cryoglobulinemic vasculitis caused by hepatitis C may respond to α-interferon in combination with antiviral therapy (e.g., ribavirin). The relative response to treatment varies according to the study population. As many as 25% to 50% of patients may have some kind of either partial or complete response.

High-dose corticosteroids (e.g., pulse methylprednisolone) and cytotoxic agents (e.g., cyclophosphamide) are the treatments of choice for necrotizing and crescentic glomerulonephritis associated with microscopic polyangiitis, Wegener's granulomatosis, and the Churg-Strauss syndrome or for renal-limited vascular inflammation. Patients with pulmonary-renal vasculitic syndromes in whom hemoptysis is a major clinical feature require emergent therapy with plasma exchange.

Induction therapy includes pulse methylprednisolone at a dose of 7 mg/kg/day for 3 days followed by daily oral prednisone or plasmapheresis therapy for 7 to 14 days in additional to daily oral prednisone. Prednisone treatment is typically converted to alternate-day treatment during the second month of therapy. Corticosteroid treatment is terminated by the fourth or fifth month after diagnosis. There are a number of cyclophosphamide protocols, including intravenous administration at a starting dose of 0.5 g/m^2 with adjustment upward to 1 g/m^2 based on the leukocyte count. Alternatively, oral cyclophosphamide can be initiated at a dose of 2 mg/kg/day and adjusted on the basis of the leukocyte count. The optimal duration of cyclophosphamide treatment has not been defined. In a recent study, oral cyclophosphamide was terminated at 3 to 6 months of therapy if the patient was in remission, and azathioprine continued for a total treatment of 12 months. This form of therapy was equivalent to 12 months of oral cyclophosphamide. It is possible that some patients may not require any kind of immunosuppressive therapy once they are in remission after 6 to 12 months of overall therapy.

As many as 75% to 85% of ANCA-vasculitic patients enter remission with aggressive immunosuppressive therapy, but approximately 20% to 40% have a relapse within 2 years. Relapses typically occur in the same organ system as the primary disease, although relapses may occur in another organ system as well. Depending on the severity of the relapse, patients may be treated either with another course of corticosteroids and cyclophosphamide or with less toxic therapy, including mycophenolate mofetil, glucocorticoids, or azathioprine.

BIBLIOGRAPHY

Agnello V, Chung RT, Kaplan LM: A role for hepatitis C virus infection in type II cryoglobulinemia. N Engl J Med 327:1490–1495, 1992.

Alric L, Plaisier E, Thebault S, et al: Influence of antiviral therapy in hepatitis C virus–associated cryoglobulinemic MPGN. Am J Kidney Dis 43:617–623, 2004.

Falk RJ, Hogan S, Carey TS, Jennette JC: Clinical course of antineutrophil cytoplasmic autoantibody-associated glomerulonephritis and systemic vasculitis. Ann Intern Med 113:656–663, 1990.

Guillevin L, Durand-Gasselin B, Cevallos R, et al: Microscopic polyangiitis: Clinical and laboratory findings in eighty-five patients. Arthritis Rheum 42:421–430, 1999.

Guillevin L, Lhote F, Gherardi R: The spectrum and treatment of virus-associated vasculitides. Curr Opin Rheumatol 9:31–36, 1997.

Hagen EC, Ballieux Be, van Es LA, Daha MR, van der Woude FJ: Antineutrophil cytoplasmic autoantibodies: A review of the antigens involved, the assays, and the clinical and possible pathogenetic consequences. Blood 81:1996–2002, 1993.

Hoffman GS, Kerr GS, Leavitt RY, et al: Wegener's granulomatosis: An analysis of 158 patients. Ann Intern Med 116:488–498, 1992.

Jennette JC, Falk RJ, Andrassy K, et al: Nomenclature of systemic vasculitides: Proposal of an international consensus conference. Arthritis Rheum 37:187–192, 1994.

Jayne D, Rasmussen N, Andrassy K, et al: A randomized trial of maintenance therapy for vasculitis associated with antineutrophil cytoplasmic autoantibodies. N Engl J Med 349:36–44, 2003.

Jennette JC, Falk RJ: Small vessel vasculitis. N Engl J Med 337:1512–1523, 1997.

Jennette JC, Falk RJ: Pathogenesis of the vascular and glomerular damage in ANCA-positive vasculitis. Nephrol Dial Transplant 13(suppl 1):16–20, 1998.

Jennette JC, Thomas DB, Falk RJ: Microscopic polyangiitis (microscopic polyarteritis). Semin Diagn Pathol 18:3–13, 2001.

Kaku Y, Nohara K, Honda S: Renal involvement in Henoch-Schönlein purpura: A multivariate analysis of prognostic factors. Kidney Int 53:1755–1759, 1998.

Kamesh L, Harper L, Savage CO. ANCA-positive vasculitis. J Am Soc Nephrol 13:1953–1960, 2002.

Klemmer PJ, Chalermskulrat W, Reif MS, et al: Plasmapheresis therapy for diffuse alveolar hemorrhage in patients with small-vessel vasculitis. Am J Kidney Dis 42:1149–1153, 2003.

Langford CA, Balow JE: New insights into the immunopathogenesis and treatment of small vessel vasculitis of the kidney. Curr Opin Nephrol Hypertens 12:267–272, 2003.

Leung DYM, Collins T, Lapierre LA, et al: Immunoglobulin M antibodies present in the acute phase of Kawasaki syndrome lyse cultured vascular endothelial cells stimulated by gamma interferon. J Clin Invest 77:1428–1435, 1986.

Nachman PH, Hogan SL, Jennette JC, Falk RJ: Treatment response and relapse in ANCA-associated microscopic polyangiitis and glomerulonephritis. J Am Soc Nephrol 7: 23–32, 1996.

Niles JL, Pan GL, Collins AB, et al: Antigen-specific radioimmunoassays for antineutrophil cytoplasmic antibodies in the diagnosis of rapidly progressive glomerulonephritis. J Am Soc Nephrol 2:27–36, 1991.

Rieu P, Noel LH: Henoch-Schönlein nephritis in children and adults. Morphological features and clinicopathological correlations. Ann Intern Med 150:151–159, 1999.

Rossi P, Bertani T, Baio P, et al: Hepatitis C virus–related cryoglobulinemic glomerulonephritis: Long-term remission after antiviral therapy. Kidney Int 63:2236–2241, 2003.

Serra A, Cameron JS, Turner DR, et al: Vasculitis affecting the kidney: Presentation, histopathology and long-term outcome. Q J Med 53:181–207, 1984.

Smith DL: Spontaneous rupture of a renal artery aneurysm in polyarteritis nodosa: Critical review of the literature and report of a case. Am J Med 87:464–467, 1989.

CHAPTER 27

Kidney Manifestations of Systemic Lupus Erythematosus and Rheumatoid Arthritis

Mary Anne Dooley   Patrick H. Nachman

SYSTEMIC LUPUS ERYTHEMATOSUS

Systemic lupus erythematosus (SLE) is a severe, multisystem autoimmune disease characterized by the production of several autoantibodies, including antibodies to nuclear antigens (ANAs), double-stranded DNA (anti-dsDNA), histones, ribonucleoproteins (RNPs), and the marker autoantibody anti-Sm. A diagnosis of SLE is a clinical diagnosis, based on combined clinical, pathologic, and laboratory findings enumerated in the criteria established by the American College of Rheumatology (Table 27-1). These criteria are useful in establishing a clinical diagnosis of SLE, although the requirement that a patient exhibit at least 4 of 11 signs or symptoms applies only to clinical research. Kidney disease secondary to SLE affects about 25% of patients and is largely mediated by deposition of immune complexes in the kidneys. The clinical diagnosis of lupus nephritis is usually made following a diagnostic kidney biopsy in the presence of proteinuria and/or hematuria, positive serology, and extrarenal manifestations of SLE. The presence of kidney disease is the most important predictor of morbidity and mortality in patients with SLE.

The clinical course of SLE involves periods of flare-ups and remissions, sometimes requiring the extensive use of corticosteroids and other immunosuppressants. The disease process, in conjunction with the effects of long-term drug therapy, causes significant morbidity, including frequent hospitalizations, increased susceptibility to infections, and increased risk for cardiovascular disease.

Epidemiology of Systemic Lupus Erythematosus and Lupus Nephritis

Systemic lupus erythematosus affects predominantly young women of childbearing age with a peak incidence between the ages of 15 and 40 years. Adult women are affected about 10 times more often than men. In the United States, SLE is estimated to affect 1 in 2000 women. The incidence and prevalence of SLE differ among different ethnic groups. African Americans have a threefold increased incidence of SLE, develop it at a younger age, more frequently develop anti-Sm and RNP antibodies, and have increased mortality when compared with whites. They also develop nephritis earlier in the course of SLE. In an inception cohort of lupus patients in the southeastern United States, the difference in kidney disease in African Americans versus whites within a median of 13 months from diagnosis was significant (31% of black patients vs. 13% of white patients). Hispanics and Asians also have greater frequency and severity of nephritis compared with whites. The proportion of patients receiving dialysis for endstage renal disease (ESRD) due to lupus nephritis is increasing.

Several demographic, serologic, and genetic risk factors are associated with an increased risk for developing kidney disease. Patients with lupus nephritis are more likely than SLE patients without kidney involvement to have a family history of SLE, anemia, high anti-dsDNA antibody titers, and hypocomplementemia. Children with SLE develop nephritis more frequently than adults (approximately 85% vs. 20%) and so do males. The presence of anti-Sm autoantibodies is associated with more severe expressions of SLE, including lupus nephritis, and some studies suggest that anti-dsDNA and antihistone autoantibodies are associated with an increased risk for proliferative lupus nephritis. Expression of the FcγIIIA F151 polymorphism also appears to be associated with an increased risk for developing lupus nephritis, at least in some populations.

Despite investigative attention, racial differences in lupus expression remain poorly understood. Once they have lupus nephritis, African Americans and Hispanics are more likely to progress to ESRD than whites. Factors influencing renal outcomes may include socioeconomic and psychosocial variables. In the LUMINA study, however, the worse outcome for African-American patients with lupus nephritis was independent of healthcare access, compliance with medications, and socioeconomic status. Mortality rates from SLE have been relatively stable among whites but have increased among African Americans since the 1970s. Mortality rates in

TABLE 27-1   The 1982 Revised Criteria for the Classification of Systemic Lupus Erythematosus

Criteria	Definition
Malar rash	Fixed erythema, flat or raised, over the malar eminences, tending to "skip over" the nasolabial folds
Discoid rash	Erythematous raised patches with adherent keratotic scaling and follicular plugging; atrophic scarring may occur in older lesions
Photosensitivity	Skin rash as a result of unusual reaction to sunlight
Oral ulcers	Oral or nasopharyngeal ulceration, usually painless
Arthritis	Nonerosive arthritis involving two or more peripheral joints, characterized by tenderness, swelling, or effusion
Serositis	Pleuritis—convincing history of pleuritic pain, rubbing heard by a clinician, or evidence of pleural effusion *or* Pericarditis—documented by electrocardiography or rub, or evidence of pericardial effusion
Renal disorder	Persistent proteinuria >0.5 g/day or >3+ if quantitation is not performed *or* Cellular casts—may be red cell, hemoglobin, granular, tubular, or mixed
Neurologic disorder	Seizures—in the absence of offending drugs or known metabolic derangements, e.g., uremia, ketoacidosis, or electrolyte imbalance *or* Psychosis—in the absence of offending drugs or known metabolic derangements, e.g., uremia, ketoacidosis, or electrolyte imbalance
Hematologic disorder	Hemolytic anemia with reticulocytosis *or* Leukopenia—<4000/mm^3 total on two or more occasions *or* Lymphopenia—1500/mm^3 on two or more occasions *or* Thrombocytopenia—<100,000/mm^3 in the absence of offending drugs
Immunologic disorder	Positive lupus erythematosus cell preparation *or* Anti-DNA—Antibody to native DNA in abnormal titer *or* Anti-Sm—presence of antibody to Sm nuclear antigen *or* False-positive serologic test for syphilis known to be positive for at least 6 months and confirmed by *Treponema pallidum* immobilization or fluorescent treponemal antibody absorption test
Antinuclear antibody	An abnormal titer of antinuclear antibody by immunofluorescence or an equivalent assay at any point in time and in the absence of drugs known to be associated with drug-induced systemic lupus erythematosus

Reprinted from Tan EM, Cohen AS, Fries JF: The 1982 revised criteria for the classification of systemic lupus erythematosus. Arthritis Rheum 1982; 25:1271. With permission.

lupus patients on dialysis do not differ from the overall dialysis population.

The level of serum creatinine at the time therapy is initiated and the biopsy findings have been suggested as predictors of eventual renal outcome. Histologic evidence of substantial interstitial fibrosis, glomerulosclerosis, and tubular atrophy are likely predictors of subsequent progression to ESRD.

Types of Systemic Lupus Erythematosus Nephritis

Lupus nephritis is an immune complex–mediated glomerulonephritis. Most patients with SLE have deposition of immunoglobulin and complement, even in the absence of clinically significant kidney dysfunction. The location, quantity, and associated host response to the immune reactants result in a spectrum of kidney lesions categorized into different classes of lupus nephritis. A mesangial pattern of injury with mesangial hypercellularity and matrix accumulation results from immune

complex deposition predominantly in the mesangium. Alternatively, immune complex deposition may occur predominantly in a subepithelial distribution, leading to complement activation and cytotoxic injury to the podocytes (epithelial pattern of injury associated with a membranous histopathology). The endothelial pattern of injury is characterized by leukocyte accumulation, endothelial cell injury, and endocapillary proliferation, and is associated with capillary wall destruction, mesangial proliferation, and crescent formation. Immune complex accumulation occurs in the subendothelial space.

Clinical Presentation and the Role of Kidney Biopsy

Clinically, lupus nephritis varies in its expression from mild, asymptomatic proteinuria to an overt nephrotic syndrome or acute nephritis associated with rapidly progressing azotemia. The patterns of injury described previously correlate to some degree with a spectrum of clinical presentations of lupus nephritis. The mesangial pattern is typically associated with subnephrotic proteinuria, microscopic hematuria, and preservation of the glomerular filtration rate (GFR). Similarly to idiopathic membranous nephropathy, a predominantly subepithelial accumulation of immune complexes is associated with nephrotic proteinuria and preservation or gradual reduction in GFR. In contrast, the endothelial pattern of injury is frequently associated with dysmorphic erythrocyturia, red cell casts, sterile pyuria, various degrees of proteinuria, and an acute reduction in GFR. Despite these general correlations, there is substantial overlap in the clinical presentation of patients with the various histopathologic findings, and it is difficult to ascertain the type or severity of kidney disease based on clinical grounds alone. For this reason, a kidney biopsy is useful—if not essential—in the management of patients with suspected lupus nephritis. It provides an invaluable guide to therapy by clarifying the clinicopathologic syndrome and assessing the relative degrees of active inflammation and chronic scarring. It may also identify unsuspected causes for an acute worsening in kidney function such as the development of thrombotic microangiopathy or drug-induced tubulointerstitial nephritis.

The Old and New Classifications of Lupus Nephritis

Because of the recognized spectrum of kidney lesions seen in lupus nephritis, and their diverse outcomes, the classification of lupus nephritis into discrete classes has been essential to facilitate the communication between and among pathologists and clinicians, as well as to define homogeneous groups of patients enrolled in clinical trials.

The initial classification of lupus nephritis was proposed in 1974 (World Health Organization [WHO]) and was modified in 1982 and 1995. The latter was until recently the most commonly, although not universally, used classification. Because of some difficulties associated with the 1995 classification, and in order to take into account recent data pertaining to the clinical outcomes of the various types of lupus nephritis, an international panel of pathologists, rheumatologists, and nephrologists recently proposed a new revision for the classification of lupus nephritis (International Society of Nephrology/Renal Pathology Society [ISN/RPS] classification of lupus nephritis, 2003). Overall, the new proposal bears strong resemblance to the 1974 classification, but introduces several important modifications concerning differences between class III and IV lesions as well as the subclasses of class V lesions. Because this proposal has been published only recently, it is not yet implemented in the design and reporting of clinical studies, and most of the publications refer to the previous versions of the classification of lupus nephritis. For this reason, the following paragraphs describe the 1982/1995 classification. The 2003 ISN/RPS classification of lupus nephritis is described in Table 27-2.

The WHO class I type is the mildest pathologic expression of lupus nephritis and is associated with normal renal histology. Class II is characterized by immune complex deposition confined to the mesangium, with (class IIB) or without (class IIA) varying degrees of focal to diffuse mesangial hypercellularity. Focal proliferative

---

TABLE 27-2 International Society of Nephrology/Renal Pathology Society Classification of Lupus Nephritis 2003*

Class I	**Minimal mesangial lupus nephritis**
	Normal glomeruli by light microscopy, but mesangial immune deposits by immunofluorescence.
Class II	**Mesangial proliferative lupus nephritis**
	Purely mesangial hypercellularity of any degree of mesangial matrix expansion by light microscopy, with mesangial immune deposits.
Class III	**Focal lupus nephritis**[†]
	Active or inactive diffuse, segmental, or global endo- or extracapillary glomerulonephritis involving <50% of all glomeruli, typically with focal subendothelial immune deposits, with or without mesangial alterations.
Class IV	**Diffuse lupus nephritis**[†]
	Active or inactive diffuse, segmental, or global endo- or extracapillary glomerulonephritis involving ≥50% of all glomeruli, typically with diffuse subendothelial immune deposits, with or without mesangial alterations. This class is divided into diffuse segmental (IV-S) lupus nephritis when ≥50% of the involved glomeruli have segmental lesions and diffuse global (IV-G) lupus nephritis when ≥50% of the involved glomeruli have global lesions.
Class V	**Membranous lupus nephritis**
	Global or segmental subepithelial immune deposits or their morphologic sequelae by light microscopy and by immunofluorescence or electron microscopy, with or without mesangial alterations.
	Class V lupus nephritis may occur in combination with class III or IV in which case both will be diagnosed.
Class VI	**Advanced sclerosis lupus nephritis**
	≥90% of glomeruli globally sclerosed without residual activity.

*Classes III and IV are subdivided according to whether the lesions are active (A) or chronic (C) with glomerular scars.
[†]Focal, involving <50% of glomeruli; diffuse, involving >50% of glomeruli; segmental, involving only part of an affected glomerulus; global, involving the entirety of an affected glomerulus.
Modified from Weening JJ, D'Agati VD, Schwartz MM, et al: International Society of Nephrology Working Group on the Classification of Lupus Nephritis; Renal Pathology Society Working Group on the Classification of Lupus Nephritis. The classification of glomerulonephritis in systemic lupus erythematosus revisited. Kidney Int, 65:521–530, 2004; and J Am Soc Nephrol 15:241–250, 2004. With permission.

(class III) and diffuse proliferative (class IV) lupus nephritis are characterized by endocapillary hypercellularity caused not only by mesangial and endothelial proliferation, but also by leukocyte infiltration. The most active lesions are complicated by necrosis and crescent formation (Fig. 27-1). Classes III and IV are the most likely to lead to progressive loss of kidney function or present as a rapidly progressive glomerulonephritis.

Class V lupus nephritis is characterized by the localization of immune complexes predominantly in the subepithelial zone. Similarly to idiopathic membranous nephropathy, class V lupus nephritis usually causes a nephrotic rather than nephritic syndrome, unless substantial proliferative changes are also present. Class V lupus nephritis is further categorized as class Va when membranous changes are found exclusively, class Vb when there is concurrent mesangial hypercellularity, class

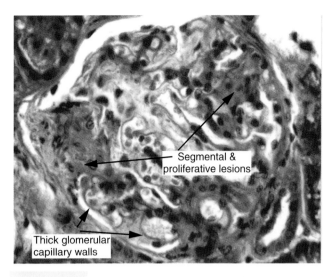

FIGURE 27-2 Membranous lupus glomerulonephritis (evidenced by thickening of the glomerular capillary walls). In addition, focal proliferative changes are present (class V and class III).

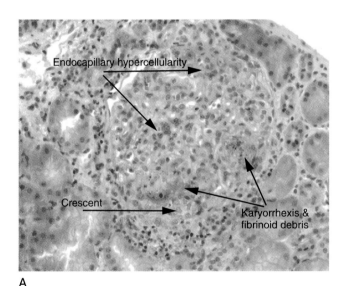

A

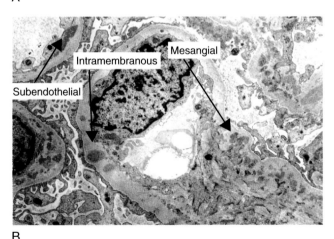

B

FIGURE 27-1 *A,* Single glomerulus from a patient with diffuse proliferative lupus nephritis (class IV). In 60% of glomeruli, cellular crescents were observed. *B,* Electron microscopy of immune complex deposition. In this example, deposits are found in the mesangial, subendothelial, and epithelial compartments.

Vc when there are focal endocapillary proliferative changes, and class Vd in the presence of diffuse proliferative changes. Clinically, patients with class Vc or Vd nephritis follow a clinical course resembling that of focal or diffuse proliferative lupus glomerulonephritis (classes III and IV), whereas patients with class Va or Vb have a predominantly nephrotic course similar to that of idiopathic membranous nephropathy. Therefore, patients with combined membranous and proliferative lesions (classes Vc and Vd) should be treated as if they had class III or IV lupus nephritis. For these reasons, classes Vc and Vd have been abandoned by the 2003 ISN/RPS classification. Patients with features of membranous and proliferative lesions are reported as having class V in addition to class III or IV lesions (Fig. 27-2).

Because of the typically relapsing and remitting nature of SLE, the nephritis eventually results in extensive glomerular sclerosis, adhesions, fibrous crescents, interstitial fibrosis, and arteriosclerosis (class VI). The relative histologic markers of active inflammation and chronic injury can be expressed as activity and chronicity indices. The 2003 ISN/RPS classification explicitly differentiates between predominantly active or scarring lesions, especially for the proliferative lesions.

Some patients with SLE develop a thrombotic microangiopathy that may be associated with antiphospholipid antibodies or with an overlap syndrome with systemic sclerosis. Thrombotic thrombocytopenic purpura is increased in frequency in SLE. This complication is characterized by subendothelial expansion in glomerular capillaries, fibrinoid necrosis of arterioles, and edematous intimal expansion in arteries. The resultant narrowing of lumina, as well as superimposed thrombosis, may cause severe and rapid renal failure and microangiopathic hemolytic anemia.

One difficulty in managing patients with lupus nephritis lies in the fact that the pathologic lesion may change from one form of glomerular injury to another. It is common for a class III lesion to progress to class IV lupus nephritis. Both class III and class IV lesions can transform into membranous (class V) lupus nephritis, either spontaneously or with immunosuppressive therapy. It is less common, but possible, for membranous lesions to transform into more proliferative lesions. Even repetitive clinical evaluations may not be sufficiently insightful in detecting these changes, and repeated kidney biopsies are sometimes needed.

Laboratory Findings

Antinuclear antibodies are more than 90% sensitive but only 70% specific for SLE because they are also found with other rheumatic diseases, infections, and neoplasms, and among older patients. Conversely, up to 10% of patients who meet diagnostic criteria for lupus do not test positive for ANAs. Tests for antibodies to nuclear or cytosolic antigens other than DNA are more specific for SLE. For example, antibodies to the Sm antigen are very specific for lupus, but are found in only 25% of patients. Patients with anti-Sm antibodies have a higher risk for severe lupus, renal disease, central nervous system disease, cutaneous vasculitis, and death. The total hemolytic complement (CH50), C4, and C3 are typically low during active disease. Because some patients with SLE have a genetic decrease in the synthesis of complement components (especially C4), a low complement concentration does not always indicate active disease. Longitudinally repeated measurements of these factors are more helpful in determining the relative state of disease activity of a patient.

Treatment of Systemic Lupus Erythematosus Nephritis

Therapeutic decisions for individual patients with lupus nephritis should be based on consideration of their clinical presentation, laboratory features, and histologic findings on biopsy.

In general, patients with mesangial lupus nephritis (class II) do not require immunosuppressive treatment beyond that for their extrarenal manifestations of disease. In patients with advanced glomerulosclerosis, the risks of immunosuppression outweigh the potential benefits.

Therapy of Proliferative Lupus Nephritis

Patients with mild focal proliferative lupus nephritis (class III lesions without crescents, normal and stable GFR, modest proteinuria, and no demographic risk factors for poor outcome) may be followed closely without the immediate institution of immunosuppressive agents. In contrast, patients with more severe focal proliferative or diffuse proliferative glomerulonephritis (class III and IV, respectively) are at risk for progressive loss of renal function and warrant aggressive immunosuppressive therapy. In patients with proliferative lesions, use of the cytotoxic drug cyclophosphamide or azathioprine in addition to corticosteroids leads to improved kidney survival as compared to treatment with corticosteroids alone. Delay of therapy is associated with an increase in renal scarring, which is poorly responsive to immunosuppressive therapy.

Typically, treatment for class IV or severe class III lupus nephritis is initiated with pulse methylprednisolone (7 mg/kg/day for 3 days) followed by cyclophosphamide and prednisone. Prednisone is started at a dose of 1 mg/kg/day for the first month, followed by a gradual taper over the following 3 to 4 months. Intravenous cyclophosphamide is given once a month for 6 consecutive months, starting at a dose of $0.5\,g/m^2$ body surface area and increasing by $0.25\,g/m^2$ on successive treatments (not to exceed $1\,g/m^2$), provided that the 2-week leukocyte count remains above $3000\,mm^3$. After the first 6 months, pulse cyclophosphamide is given every 3 months for a total of 24 months. Patients with significantly impaired kidney function may need a reduction in the first dose of parenteral cyclophosphamide. The role for intermittent intravenous cyclophosphamide therapy was established by two prospective, controlled clinical trials performed at the National Institutes of Health (NIH). These trials demonstrated greater long-term kidney survival, but not patient survival, with the use of cyclophosphamide as compared with corticosteroids alone. Continuing quarterly pulse cyclophosphamide for at least 1 year after renal remission decreases the frequency of nephritic relapses and the risk of kidney function deterioration.

Azathioprine

The role of azathioprine in the treatment of proliferative lupus nephritis is less well established than that of cyclophosphamide. Early studies suggested improved outcomes with the use of azathioprine in combination with corticosteroids over corticosteroids alone, whereas in the NIH randomized, controlled trial azathioprine was no more effective than prednisone alone in preventing loss of kidney function. However, azathioprine has fewer side effects than cyclophosphamide and may be considered for patients at low risk for ESRD, typically with focal proliferative (WHO class III) nephritis. Recent data suggest a role for azathioprine for maintenance therapy after induction with cyclophosphamide in lieu of the quarterly doses of cyclophosphamide.

Pulse Methylprednisolone

In two controlled trials for the treatment of proliferative lupus nephritis, the combination of cyclophosphamide and pulse methylprednisolone afforded a more rapid response and greater probability of renal remission.

Plasmapheresis

Plasmapheresis has been used in the treatment of lupus nephritis to eliminate pathogenic antibodies and circulating immune complexes. However, a large-scale, prospective controlled clinical trial showed no additional benefit of plasmapheresis compared with corticosteroids and short-course oral cyclophosphamide therapy alone.

Mycophenolate Mofetil

Because of its favorable safety profile when compared with cyclophosphamide, there is great interest in the use of mycophenolate mofetil (MMF) for the treatment of lupus nephritis. Several pilot studies have reported promising results with its use for induction therapy or for maintenance after a course of cyclophosphamide. Three randomized controlled trials of MMF in lupus nephritis have been completed. Two studies compared MMF and corticosteroids to cyclophosphamide and corticosteroids for induction therapy. Although the patient selection of the study by Chan raises questions as to its generalizability, both studies report comparable efficacy of MMF in attaining remission and decreased adverse effects. However, both studies are of relatively short duration and do not provide sufficient data as to the long-term outcomes of patients. Similarly, data in support of the use of MMF after an induction with cyclophosphamide are increasing. In a randomized trial comparing maintenance therapy with MMF, azathioprine, or quarterly doses of intravenous cyclophosphamide, the rate of relapse-free survival was higher in the MMF group than in the cyclophosphamide group and was associated with a lower rate of amenorrhea and infections. Despite these encouraging results, it is currently premature to advocate the use of MMF as a first-line drug in the treatment of class IV lupus nephritis because data on long-term outcomes are still lacking.

Cyclosporine

Cyclosporine has been shown to be effective in reducing clinical and histologic activity in proliferative lupus nephritis. Autoantibody formation and hypocomplementemia do not uniformly improve, and the frequent occurrence of hypertension and nephrotoxicity limit the utility of this therapy.

The last few years have witnessed the advent of a number of "biologic" agents targeting specific inflammatory pathways. Several are currently under investigation for the treatment of SLE and lupus nephritis. These include monoclonal antibodies directed against CD40 ligand, BLYS, BAFF, CTLA-4Ig, C5, and CD20. None has so far been sufficiently evaluated to warrant use outside of controlled clinical trials.

It is unclear whether high-dose prednisone, cyclophosphamide, or azathioprine is necessary in the treatment of patients with mild to moderate focal proliferative glomerulonephritis (class III). However, when there is necrosis or crescent formation in addition to the focal proliferative disease, the long-term outcome is probably similar to that of diffuse proliferative glomerulonephritis (class IV) and should be treated in the same fashion.

Therapy of Membranous Lupus Nephritis

The therapy of membranous lupus nephritis (WHO class Va and Vb; ISN/RPS class V) has not been evaluated in controlled trials. Current treatment recommendations include the use of angiotensin-converting enzyme inhibitors to reduce proteinuria and lipid-lowering agents for cardiovascular protection. In patients with debilitating nephrotic syndrome or with protracted symptomatic severe proteinuria, treatment options include the use of cyclosporine or cyclophosphamide. Cyclosporine reduces the degree of proteinuria, but is associated with the development of hypertension and risk for nephrotoxicity and may not halt progression of glomerular damage when assessed by repeat kidney biopsy. Preliminary results of a randomized controlled trial suggest that the addition of alternate-month pulse cyclophosphamide or low-dose cyclosporine to alternate-day prednisone is more effective in achieving remission than prednisone alone. Patients with WHO class Vc and Vd should be treated similarly to patients with class III and IV lupus nephritis, respectively.

Kidney Transplantation in Patients with Systemic Lupus Erythematosus

Studies addressing the outcome of kidney transplantation in patients with SLE compared with that of non-SLE patients have yielded conflicting results. A case control study of 97 kidney transplant recipients with SLE, matched for age, gender, race, type of allograft, number of previous transplants, and year of transplantation, revealed a relative risk of graft loss of 2 when SLE was the cause of ESRD. Conversely, recent data from the United States Renal Data System compared the outcomes of 772 adults with ESRD from lupus nephritis and 32,644 adults with ESRD due to other causes who received a transplant between 1987 and 1994. After adjusting for potential confounding factors, the risk for graft failure or patient mortality was not increased in patients with SLE after first cadaveric and first living-related kidney transplant. The reported rates of recurrent SLE disease posttransplantation are also widely variable; however, recurrent lupus nephritis appears to account for graft loss in less than or equal to 4% of grafts. The presence of antiphospholipid antibodies may be associated with an elevated risk for thrombotic complications and graft loss, raising the question as to whether patients with a history of antiphospholipid syndrome should receive anticoagulant therapy following transplantation.

Adjunctive and Supportive Care

The institution of attentive supportive care is crucial in maintaining the short- and long-term side effects of therapy to a minimum. Compulsive attention must be focused on the early detection and aggressive treatment of infections because this accounts for about 20% of deaths among patients with SLE. Whenever corticosteroids are used, measures must be taken to minimize the development of osteoporosis. These include calcium and vitamin D supplementation, weight-bearing exercise as tolerated, and potential therapy with pharmacologic agents, including calcitonin if kidney function is reduced, bisphosphonates (unless contraindicated by azotemia or esophagitis), or recombinant parathyroid hormone. Contraception, fertility, and pregnancy are important issues in this predominately female patient population. Advice on the choice of contraceptive method should be given, keeping in mind thrombotic risk factors of hormonal contraceptives such as the presence of antiphospholipid antibodies, hypertension, and nephrotic syndrome. Clinical trials of oral contraceptives in antiphospholipid antibody–negative premenopausal and hormone replacement therapy in postmenopausal women with SLE have recently been completed. In a small uncontrolled study of 25 women with SLE, the use of the gonadotropin-releasing hormone agonist leuprolide during the period of treatment with cyclophosphamide appeared to prevent cyclophosphamide-induced ovarian failure, since these patients resumed normal menstrual cycles within 6 months after discontinuing cyclophosphamide and leuprolide. Similarly, results of a small study suggested that treatment with testosterone during cyclophosphamide therapy may afford a recovery of normal sperm counts in males with nephrotic syndrome. However, this intervention should not replace attempts at storing sperm.

RHEUMATOID ARTHRITIS

The most common renal abnormalities encountered in the setting of rheumatoid arthritis result from the toxicity of the anti-inflammatory drugs used in this disease. Nonsteroidal anti-inflammatory drugs, including cyclo-oxygenase 2 inhibitors, can cause an interstitial nephritis, tubular damage, as well as a nephrotic syndrome associated with a minimal change or membranous histopathology. Similarly, gold salts and D-penicillamine can cause membranous nephropathy. In these cases, the proteinuria usually resolves after discontinuing the offending agent. Rarely, rheumatoid arthritis can lead to an immune complex–mediated nephropathy when rheumatoid factors form circulating immune complexes. Rheumatoid arthritis may also lead to secondary amyloidosis, which is characterized by the extracellular deposition of a fraction of serum amyloid A protein (AA amyloidosis) and results in proteinuria and varying degrees of renal function impairment.

BIBLIOGRAPHY

Balow JE, Austin HA: Therapy of membranous nephropathy in systemic lupus erythematosus. Semin Nephrol 23:386–391, 2003.

Chan TM, Li FK, Tang CS, et al: Efficacy of mycophenolate mofetil in patients with diffuse proliferative lupus nephritis. Hong Kong-Guangzhou Nephrology Study Group. N Engl J Med 343:1156–1162, 2000.

Contreras G, Pardo V, Leclercq B, et al: Sequential therapies for proliferative lupus nephritis. N Engl J Med 350:971–980, 2004.

Reveille JD, Moulds JM, Ahn C, et al: Systemic lupus erythematosus in three ethnic groups: I. The effects of HLA Class II, C4, and CR1 alleles, socioeconomic factors, and ethnicity at disease onset. LUMINA Study Group. Arthritis Rheum 41:1161–1172, 1998.

Stone JH, Amend WJC, Criswell LA: Outcome of renal transplantation in ninety-seven cyclosporine-era patients with systemic lupus erythematosus and matched controls. Arthritis Rheum 41:1438–1445, 1998.

Su W, Madaio MP: Recent advances in the pathogenesis of lupus nephritis: Autoantibodies and B cells. Semin Nephrol 23:564–568, 2003.

Tan EM, Cohen AS, Fries JF: The 1982 revised criteria for the classification of systemic lupus erythematosus. Arthritis Rheum 25:1271, 1982.

Ward MM: Outcomes of renal transplantation among patients with endstage renal disease caused by lupus nephritis. Kidney Int 57:2136–2143, 2000.

Weening JJ, D'Agati VD, Schwartz MM, et al; International Society of Nephrology Working Group on the Classification of Lupus Nephritis; Renal Pathology Society Working Group on the Classification of Lupus Nephritis: The classification of glomerulonephritis in systemic lupus erythematosus revisited. Kidney Int 65:521–530, 2004; and J Am Soc Nephrol 15:241–250, 2004.

CHAPTER 28

Pathogenesis and Pathophysiology of Diabetic Nephropathy

M. Luiza Caramori   Michael Mauer

Diabetic nephropathy is the single most common disorder leading to kidney failure in adults. In the United States, more than 40% of patients entering endstage renal disease (ESRD) programs are diabetic, most of whom (80% or more) have type 2 diabetes. The annual cost of caring for these patients, in the United States alone, exceeds $9 billion. The mortality rate of patients with diabetic nephropathy is high, and a marked increase in cardiovascular risk accounts for more than half of the increased mortality among these patients. Once overt diabetic nephropathy, manifesting as proteinuria, is present, ESRD can be postponed (but in most instances not prevented) by effective antihypertensive treatment and careful glycemic control. Thus, in the past 10 to 15 years, there has been intensive research into early predictors of diabetic nephropathy risk, pathophysiologic mechanisms of diabetic kidney injury, and early intervention strategies.

EPIDEMIOLOGY

About 0.5% of the population in the United States and Central Europe has type 1 diabetes. The prevalence is higher in the northern Scandinavian countries and lower in southern Europe and Japan. Diabetic nephropathy will develop in 25% to 35% of these patients, with a peak in the incidence after 20 years of having diabetes. Type 2 diabetes is about nine times more prevalent than type 1 diabetes, accounting in part for the greater contribution of type 2 diabetic patients to ESRD incidence. Studies in type 2 diabetic patients from western Europe and in Pima Indians from Arizona showed rates of progression to nephropathy similar to those of type 1 diabetic patients. ESRD is much more common in black compared with white type 2 American diabetic patients. Glycemic control, blood pressure levels, and genetic factors seem to be important in determining diabetic nephropathy risk.

NATURAL COURSE OF DIABETIC NEPHROPATHY

For simplicity, the progression of kidney involvement in type 1 diabetes can be divided into five stages. Stage I, present at diagnosis, is that of renal hypertrophy-hyperfunction. At this stage, patients at risk and not at risk for diabetic nephropathy cannot be clearly separated. Although the results of some studies suggest that glomerular filtration rate (GFR) above the normal range (glomerular hyperfiltration) is an important risk factor, this remains controversial. Genetic factors associated with predisposition to or protection from diabetic nephropathy could, in the future, be identified during this period. Stage II is defined by the presence of detectable glomerular lesions in patients with normal albumin excretion rate and normal blood pressure levels (Table 28-1). Normoalbuminuric patients with more severe glomerular lesions might be at increased risk for progression. Twenty-four-hour blood pressure monitoring may reveal a failure of normal nocturnal blood pressure decline (i.e., night/day ratios greater than 0.9) as an early diabetic nephropathy indicator that may often precede the development of persistent microalbuminuria. Microalbuminuria defines stage III, typically occurring after 5 or more years of diabetes, but it may be present earlier, particularly during adolescence, and in patients with poor glycemic control and high normal blood pressure levels. Compared with normoalbuminuric patients, patients with persistent microalbuminuria are at 300% to 400% increased risk for progression to proteinuria and ESRD. Current studies indicate that 20% to 45% of microalbuminuric type 1 diabetic patients progress to proteinuria after about 10 years of follow-up, whereas 20% to 25% return to normoalbuminuric levels, and the rest remain microalbuminuric. At this stage, glomerular lesions are generally more severe than in the previous stages, and blood pressure tends to be increasing, often into the hypertensive range. Other laboratory abnormalities, such as increased levels of cholesterol, triglycerides, fibrinogen, Von Willebrand factor, and prorenin can be detected in some patients. Diabetic retinopathy, lower extremity amputation, coronary heart disease, and stroke are also more frequent in this group. GFR is usually normal and stable or slowly declining. Stage IV occurs after 10 to 20 years of diabetes and is characterized by the presence of dipstick-positive proteinuria. Hypertension is present in about 75% of these patients, and reduced GFR and dyslipidemia are also common. Retinopathy and autonomic neuropathy are present in most patients. In addition, the risk for cardiovascular disorders is extremely

TABLE 28-1   Categories of Urinary Albumin
Excretion

Category	Timed Collection (μg/min)	24 hr Collection (mg/24 hr)	Spot Collection (μg/mg creatinine)
Normoalbuminuria	<20	<30	<30
Microalbuminuria	20–200	30–300	30–300
Macroalbuminuria	>200	>300	>300

high, and asymptomatic myocardial ischemia is frequent. Without therapeutic interventions, GFR declines by about 1.2 mL/min/month in proteinuric type 1 diabetic patients. Progression to ESRD (stage V) will occur 5 to 15 years after the development of proteinuria.

In type 2 diabetic patients, microalbuminuria may reflect a state of generalized endothelial dysfunction in addition to or rather than kidney damage per se, and type 2 diabetic patients can have proteinuria at diagnosis, at least in part because diagnosis is often delayed. In this group of patients, GFR decline is more variable, and patients with a faster GFR decline usually have more advanced diabetic glomerulopathy and worse metabolic control. In these patients, diabetes duration is usually not precisely known, and they can be diabetic for 5 to 10 years before diagnosis. Interestingly, in studies of Pima Indians where type 2 diabetes duration was known, the clinical course of diabetic kidney disease was similar to that of type 1 diabetic patients.

It is important to keep in mind that these categories are general and that progression is highly variable and is often not linear. The expression and natural history of these overlapping stages may be influenced by complex genetic, environmental, and treatment interactions, which may greatly affect outcome. Thus, the scheme presented here can serve as a useful general guide, but not as an accurate predictor of the course of individual patients.

PATHOGENESIS

Although important modulating factors may exist, diabetic nephropathy is secondary to the long-term metabolic aberrations found in diabetes, and exposure to elevated glucose levels is necessary for the expression of this disorder. Studies in type 1 and type 2 diabetes found that improved glycemic control could reduce the risk for the development of diabetic nephropathy. Moreover, the development of the earliest diabetic kidney lesions can be slowed or prevented by strict glycemic control, as was demonstrated in a randomized clinical trial in type 1 diabetic kidney transplant recipients. Also, intensive insulin treatment decreased the progression rates of glomerular lesions in a controlled trial in microalbuminuric type 1 diabetic patients. Finally, regression of established diabetic glomerular lesions has been demonstrated in the

native kidneys of type 1 diabetic patients with prolonged normalization of glycemic levels after successful pancreas transplantation. These studies strongly suggest that hyperglycemia is necessary not only for diabetic nephropathy lesions to develop, but also to sustain established lesions. Removal of hyperglycemia allows reparative mechanisms to be expressed, which ultimately results in healing of the original diabetic glomerular injuries.

Hemodynamic mechanisms also may be involved in the pathogenesis of diabetic nephropathy. Glomerular hyperfiltration could directly promote extracellular matrix (ECM) accumulation by mechanisms such as increased expression of transforming growth factor-β (TGF-β), modeled in vitro by the mechanical stretching of mesangial cells. Glomerular hyperfiltration could also be a marker of other processes, such as increased activity of the renin-angiotensin, TGF-β, and protein kinase C (PKC) systems. However, patients with other causes of hyperfiltration, such as patients with uninephrectomy, do not develop diabetic lesions. Thus, glomerular hyperfiltration alone cannot fully explain the genesis of the early lesions of diabetic nephropathy. Clinical observations suggest that hemodynamic factors may be more important in modulating the rate of progression of already well-established diabetic lesions. It is worth noting that the presence of reduced GFR in normoalbuminuric patients with type 1 diabetes has been associated with the presence of more severe glomerular lesions, and these patients may be at increased risk for progression to diabetic nephropathy. Systemic blood pressure levels are implicated in progression and, as noted previously, blood pressure circadian variation may be implicated in the genesis of diabetic nephropathy. Blood pressure reduction has been associated with decreased rates of progression to micro- and macroalbuminuria in both type 1 and type 2 diabetic patients.

Genetic predisposition to or protection from diabetic nephropathy appears to be the most important determinant of diabetic nephropathy risk in both type 1 and type 2 diabetic patients. Differences in the prevalence of microalbuminuria, proteinuria, and ESRD in different patient populations (e.g., marked excess of diabetic nephropathy among black type 2 diabetic patients) support this view. Moreover, only about half of patients with decades of poor glycemic control will develop diabetic nephropathy, whereas some patients will develop lesions despite relatively good control, findings consistent with genetically modulated susceptibility or resistance factors. Genetic predisposition to diabetic nephropathy has been suggested by studies in type 1 and type 2 siblings concordant for diabetes. These studies show extremely high concordance in diabetic nephropathy risk. Moreover, there is a strong correlation for the severity and patterns of glomerular lesions in type 1 diabetic sibling pairs. Diabetic patients with advanced nephropathy had higher mean arterial blood pressures during adolescence. Prediabetic blood pressure levels predicted albumin excretion rate after diabetes onset in type 2 diabetic Pima Indians. Diabetic patients with a family history of hypertension or cardiovascular disease also have a higher risk for diabetic nephropathy, thus linking the pathogenesis of diabetic nephropathy to factors also favoring the development of atherosclerosis. Recent data also suggest that albumin excretion rate and blood pressure are heritable and linked in white families with type 2 diabetes.

There are ongoing searches for genetic loci related to diabetic nephropathy susceptibility through genome screening and through candidate gene approaches. Neither approach has yet yielded definitive results, but indications are that multiple genes may be involved. Genetic polymorphism affecting background vascular risk in the general population, such as polymorphisms of genes related to the renin-angiotensin system, have been evaluated in many studies in diabetic patients. A polymorphism in the angiotensin-converting enzyme (ACE) gene, consisting of an insertion or deletion of a 287–base pair sequence has been associated with development of diabetic nephropathy. Positive results also have been found for polymorphisms in other genes related to hemodynamic factors, such as angiotensinogen and angiotensin II type 1 receptor genes. The Pittsburgh Epidemiology of Diabetes Complication Study found estimated glucose disposal rate to strongly predict diabetic nephropathy in type 1 diabetic patients, and polymorphisms in genes related to insulin resistance—such as the ecto-nucleotide pyrophosphatase/phosphodiesterase-1 gene (previously known as PC-1), peroxisome proliferator-activated receptor-γ2, glucose transporter-1, and apolipoprotein E—have been associated with diabetic nephropathy risk. The frequency of Q carriers of K121Q polymorphism in the ecto-nucleotide pyrophosphatase/phosphodiesterase-1 gene was higher among proteinuric and ESRD patients than among normoalbuminuric type 1 diabetic patients. Similarly, the ecto-nucleotide pyrophosphatase/phosphodiesterase-1 Q121 variant and the ACE DD genotype were associated with a faster GFR decline in microalbuminuric and proteinuric type 1 diabetic patients. The Ala12 allele type 2 diabetic carriers of the peroxisome proliferator-activated receptor-γ2 had lower albumin excretion rates than noncarriers. Also, the Ala allele was more frequent in normoalbuminuric type 2 diabetic patients than in those with diabetic nephropathy, suggesting that the presence of the Ala allele may confer protection from diabetic nephropathy in patients with type 2 diabetes. Polymorphisms in the glucose transporter-1, apolipoprotein E, and lipoprotein lipase HindIII gene were also associated with diabetic nephropathy risk. There is increasing interest in monocyte/macrophage renal infiltration in diabetic nephropathy. The chemokine receptor 5 promoter 59029 A-positive genotype (G/A or A/A) and the leukocyte-endothelial adhesion molecule-1 P213 genotype were associated with increased diabetic nephropathy risk in Japanese patients.

PATHOPHYSIOLOGY

The kidney lesions of diabetic nephropathy appear to be mainly related to ECM accumulation. ECM accumulation occurs in the glomerular (GBM) and tubular (TBM) basement membranes, is the principal cause of mesangial expansion, and contributes to interstitium expansion late in the disease. The ECM accumulation is secondary to an imbalance between synthesis and degradation of ECM components. Many regulatory mechanisms have been proposed to explain the linkage between a high ambient glucose concentration and ECM accumulation.

Increased levels of growth factors, particularly TGF-β, can be associated with increased production of ECM molecules. TGF-β can also down-regulate the synthesis of ECM degrading enzymes and up-regulate the inhibitors of these enzymes. Angiotensin II can stimulate ECM synthesis through TGF-β activity. High glucose can directly activate PKC, stimulating ECM production through the cyclic adenosine monophosphate pathway. A link between PKC activation and the stimulation of TGF-β action may exist, but TGF-β action is not directly mediated by PKC signaling.

It has been suggested that the accumulation of glycosylation products (generated by nonenzymatic reactions between reducing sugars, such as glucose, with free amino groups, lipids, or nucleic acids) may contribute to the development of diabetic complications. Increased advanced glycation end products (AGE) can stimulate the synthesis of various growth factors, including insulin-like growth factor-I and TGF-β. Binding of AGE proteins to AGE receptors on cell surfaces induces increased intracellular oxidative stress in vitro, characterized by increased nuclear factor κB. These glycosylation products may influence ECM dynamics or may change ECM molecules to render them less degradable. In diabetic patients, oxidative or nonoxidative products of glycated proteins or lipids could accumulate in the vascular wall and induce cytokine and growth factor release, contributing to vascular injury. Further studies of glycation's role in the pathogenesis of diabetic nephropathy are warranted. However, the fact that glycation is a nonenzymatic process dependent on the duration and magnitude of glycemia currently leaves unexplained why only about half of patients with poor glycemic control develop clinical diabetic nephropathy. Hypothetically, genetic variability in cellular responses to AGEs could explain these variabilities in risk.

Aldose reductase, the enzyme that catalyses the reduction of glucose to sorbitol in the polyol pathway, has been associated with diabetic nephropathy and other microvascular complications of diabetes. Increased activity of aldose reductase leads to accumulation of sorbitol, which is further converted to fructose by the sorbitol dehydrogenase enzyme, using NAD$^+$ as substrate. The ratio of NAD$^+$/NADH decreases and the conversion of glyceraldehyde 3-phosphate to 1,3 bisphosphoglycerate is blocked, leaving more substrate (glyceraldehyde 3-phosphate) for the synthesis of α-glycerol phosphate, a diacylglycerol precursor. Diacylglycerol is a PKC activator that could regulate ECM synthesis and removal. Also, increased activity of aldose reductase consumes NADPH, leading to decreased or depleted glutathione. Glutathione is an antioxidant coenzyme used by glutathione peroxidase to reduce peroxide or superoxide, yielding oxidized glutathione. Glutathione can also detoxify carbonyl compounds.

There is rapidly growing evidence that oxidative stress is increased in diabetes and related to diabetic nephropathy. Skin fibroblasts from type 1 diabetic patients with diabetic nephropathy do not show the expected increase in activity and messenger RNA (mRNA) expression for the antioxidant enzymes catalase and glutathione peroxidase when exposed to a high glucose condition in vitro. Siblings concordant for type 1 diabetes and glomerular lesions are concordant for catalase mRNA expression levels. These findings suggest that increased oxidative stress in type 1 diabetic patients with diabetic nephropathy is associated with a decreased response of antioxidant enzymes to high glucose. Recent studies have demonstrated increased oxidative stress in families of type 1 diabetic patients, suggesting that an abnormal redox state could even precede diabetes onset. Interestingly, erythrocyte glutathione content is correlated to Na$^+$-H$^+$ exchanger activity, linking oxidative stress to an ion transport system associated with diabetic nephropathy risk.

There is an association between oxidative stress, altered nitric oxide (NO) production and action, and endothelial dysfunction. Endothelium-derived NO is a potent vasodilator that also has antiatherogenic properties, including decreased platelet and leukocyte adhesion to the endothelium, and inhibition of smooth muscle cell migration. Exposure to high glucose concentrations increases endothelial NO synthase gene expression and NO release, with a concomitant increase in superoxide production. Superoxide inactivates and reacts with NO to form peroxynitrite, a potent oxidant, leading to endothelial dysfunction. Normalization of NO-mediated vasorelaxation in high-glucose conditions by superoxide dismutase, a scavenger that transforms superoxide anion into hydrogen peroxide, further adds to this association. Increased oxidative stress has been linked to alterations in other key downstream pathways, including PKC and nuclear factor κB activation, AGE formation, and increased flux through the aldose reductase and hexosamine pathways.

Glomerular mononuclear cell infiltration may also be associated with diabetic nephropathy. Monocyte chemoattractant protein 1 (MCP-1) recruits monocytes and lymphocytes to the glomerulus. High-glucose leads to increased human mesangial cell MCP-1 mRNA expression and to down-regulation of MCP-1 receptor mRNA expression. Plasma and urinary MCP-1 levels and fluorescent products of lipid peroxidation and malondialdehyde content are higher in micro- and macroalbuminuric than in normoalbuminuric type 1 and type 2 diabetic patients or controls. Plasma levels of intercellular adhesion molecule 1, a glomerular leukocyte recruitment mediator, were also higher in micro- and macroalbuminuric than in normoalbuminuric type 2 diabetic patients or controls.

Insulin resistance, associated with obesity, blood pressure elevation, and disturbed lipid metabolism, may also be a risk factor for diabetic nephropathy. As described previously, insulin sensitivity was the strongest predictor of overt nephropathy in type 1 diabetic patients, and polymorphisms in genes related to insulin resistance have been associated with diabetic nephropathy in type 1 and type 2 diabetes. Other mechanisms possibly associated with diabetic nephropathy include abnormalities of the endothelin and prostaglandin pathways and decreased glycosaminoglycan content in basement membranes.

Thus, the various hypotheses overlap and intersect. Polyol pathway-induced redox changes or hyperglycemia-induced formation of reactive oxygen species could potentially account for most of the other biochemical abnormalities. These mechanisms could also be influenced by genetic determinants of susceptibility or resistance to hyperglycemic damage.

PATHOLOGY

Type 1 Diabetes

Glomerular lesions are absent at onset, but they can be demonstrated after diabetes has been present for a few years. The same is true when a normal kidney is transplanted into a diabetic patient. The changes in kidney structure caused by diabetes are specific, creating a pattern not seen in any other disease. The severity of these diabetic lesions is related to the functional disturbances of the clinical kidney disease and it is also related to diabetes duration, degree of glycemic control, and genetic factors. However, the relationship between duration of type 1 diabetes and extent of glomerular pathology is not precise. This is consonant with the marked variability in susceptibility to this disorder such that some patients may be in kidney failure after having diabetes for 15 years while others escape complications despite having type 1 diabetes for many decades.

Light Microscopy

The earliest renal structural change in type 1 diabetes, renal hypertrophy, is not reflected in any specific light microscopic (LM) changes. In many patients, glomerular structure remains normal or near normal even after decades of diabetes. Others develop progressive diffuse mesangial expansion seen mainly as increased periodic acid-Schiff (PAS)-positive ECM mesangial material (Fig. 28-1). In about 40% to 50% of patients developing proteinuria, there are areas of extreme mesangial expansion called Kimmelstiel-Wilson nodules or nodular mesangial expansion. Mesangial cell nuclei in these nodules are palisaded around masses of mesangial matrix material with compression of surrounding capillary lumina. Nodules are thought to result from earlier glomerular capillary microaneurysm formation. Note that about half of patients with severe diabetic nephropathy do not have these nodular lesions. Thus, although Kimmelstiel-Wilson nodules are diagnostic of diabetic nephropathy, they are not necessary for severe kidney dysfunction to develop. Early changes often include arteriolar hyalinosis lesions involving replacement of the smooth muscle cells of afferent and efferent arterioles with PAS-positive waxy homogeneous material (see Fig. 28-1). The severity of these lesions is directly related to the frequency of global glomerulosclerosis, perhaps as the result of glomerular ischemia. One may also detect GBM and TBM thickening by LM, although this is often more easily seen by electron microscopy (EM). Atubular glomeruli and glomerulo-tubular junction abnormalities are present in proteinuric type 1 diabetic patients and may be important in the progressive loss of GFR in diabetic nephropathy. Finally, usually quite late in the disease, there is tubular atrophy and interstitial fibrosis, common to most forms of chronic kidney disease. Light microscopy changes of nephropathies such as amyloidosis might resemble diabetes but the mesangial expansion is not fibrillar as in diabetic nephropathy, and the vascular hyalinosis is absent. Moreover, clinical and laboratory features and immunofluorescence and electron microscopy studies can easily differentiate these entities.

Immunofluorescence

Diabetes is characterized by linear GBM, TBM, and Bowman's capsule increased staining, especially for immunoglobulin G (IgG; mainly IgG_4) and albumin. This staining is removed only by strong acid conditions, consistent with strong ionic binding. The intensity of staining is not related to the severity of the underlying lesions. The immunofluorescence reader needs to avoid confusing these findings with anti–basement membrane antibody disorders.

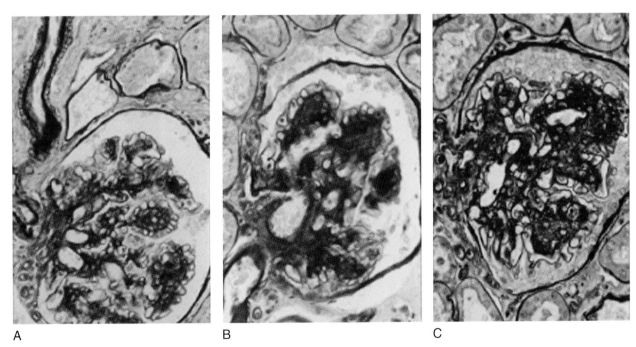

A B C

FIGURE 28-1 Light microscopy photographs of glomeruli in sequential kidney biopsies performed at baseline and after 5 and 10 years of follow-up in a long-standing normoalbuminuric type 1 diabetic patient with progressive mesangial expansion and kidney function deterioration. *A,* Note the diffuse and nodular mesangial expansion and arteriolar hyalinosis in this glomerulus from a patient who was normotensive and normoalbuminuric at the time of this baseline biopsy, 21 years after diabetes onset (periodic acid-Schiff [PAS], original magnification ×400). *B,* Five-year follow-up biopsy showing worsening of the diffuse and nodular mesangial expansion and arteriolar hyalinosis in this now microalbuminuric patient with a declining glomerular filtration rate (PAS, original magnification ×400). *C,* Ten-year follow-up biopsy showing more advanced diabetic glomerulopathy in this now proteinuric patient with further reduced GFR. Note also the multiple small glomerular probably efferent arterioles in the hilar region of this glomerulus (PAS, original magnification ×400), and in the glomerulus in (*A*).

Electron Microscopy

Using morphometric techniques, the first measurable nephropathy change is thickening of the GBM, which can be detected as early as $1^1/_2$ to $2^1/_2$ years after onset of type 1 diabetes. TBM thickening can also be detected, and it is parallel to GBM thickening. Increase in the relative area of the mesangium becomes measurable by 4 to 5 years. The fraction of the volume of the glomerulus that is mesangium increases from about 0.2 in the normal state to about 0.4 when proteinuria begins, and 0.6 to 0.8 in patients with GFRs that are about 40% to 50% of normal. Immunohistochemical studies indicate that these changes in mesangium, GBM, and TBM represent expansion of the intrinsic ECM components at these sites, most likely including types IV and VI collagen, laminin, and fibronectin. Qualitative and quantitative changes in the renal interstitium are observed in patients with various kidney diseases. Interstitial fibrosis is characterized by an increase in ECM proteins and cellularity. Preliminary studies suggest that the pathogenesis of interstitial changes in diabetic nephropathy is different from the mesangial matrix, GBM, and TBM changes. Initial observations indicate that, for all but the later stages of the disease, GBM, TBM, and mesangial matrix changes represent the accumulation of basement membrane ECM material, whereas interstitial expansion, early on, is largely due to cellular alterations. Only later, when GFR is already compromised, is interstitial expansion associated with increased interstitium fibrillar collagen and peritubular capillary loss.

Type 2 Diabetes

Glomerular structure in type 2 diabetic patients is less well studied, but appears to be more heterogeneous than in type 1 patients. One third to one half of type 2 patients with clinical features of diabetic nephropathy have typical changes of diabetic nephropathy, including diffuse and nodular mesangial expansion and arteriolar hyalinosis. Other patients, despite microalbuminuria or even proteinuria, may have no or only mild glomerulopathy. Some patients have disproportionately severe tubular and interstitial and/or vascular lesions, and/or an increased number of globally sclerosed glomeruli. Microalbuminuric type 2 diabetic patients, as a group, more frequently have morphometric glomerular structural measures in the normal range and less severe lesions than microalbuminuric type 1 diabetic patients. Many of these observations have been confirmed in Japanese type 2 diabetic patients. On the other hand, Pima Indian type 2 diabetic patients, who are known to be at high risk for ESRD, appear to have lesions more similar to those seen in type 1 diabetic patients. It is currently unclear why some studies show more structural heterogeneity in type 2 than in type 1 diabetes while others do not. Whether this is due to differences in patient populations or to other as yet unknown variables remains to be determined. However, this is an important question since the rate of progression towards ESRD in type 2 diabetes appears to be at least partially related to the severity of the classical changes of diabetic glomerulopathy. There are reports that type 2 diabetic patients have an increased incidence of nondiabetic lesions, such as proliferative glomerulonephritis and membranous nephropathy, but this is most likely because biopsies were performed in atypical cases. When biopsies are performed for research purposes, the incidence of other definable kidney diseases is very low (less than 5%).

STRUCTURAL-FUNCTIONAL RELATIONSHIPS IN DIABETIC NEPHROPATHY

The progression rates vary greatly between individuals. Type 1 diabetic patients with proteinuria always have advanced glomerular, and usually vascular, tubular, and interstitial lesions. Microalbuminuric patients usually have well-established lesions, but these vary from mild to levels of pathology bordering on those regularly seen in proteinuric patients. There is considerable overlap in glomerular structure between long-standing normo- and microalbuminuric patients because normoalbuminuric patients with long-standing type 1 diabetes can have quite advanced kidney lesions. On the other hand, many long-standing normoalbuminuric diabetic patients have structural measurements within the normal range.

Expansion of the mesangium, mainly due to ECM accumulation, is believed to ultimately reduce or obliterate glomerular capillary luminal space, decreasing glomerular filtration surface and GFR. The fraction of the glomerulus occupied by mesangium is a good predictor of GFR in type 1 diabetic patients, and it is also related to albumin excretion rate and hypertension. The total peripheral GBM filtration surface per glomerulus is directly correlated with GFR and inversely correlated with the degree of mesangial expansion. Thickness of GBM is also directly related to albumin excretion rate, but increasing albuminuria is, in paired biopsy studies, related to increasing mesangial expansion and not to other structural changes. The percentage of global glomerulosclerosis and of interstitial expansion are also correlated with the clinical manifestations of diabetic nephropathy (proteinuria, hypertension, and declining GFR). Progressive tubular atrophy, interstitial fibrosis, glomerular arteriolar hyalinosis, arteriosclerosis, and glomerulosclerosis are also important components of diabetic nephropathy that may contribute to the reduction in GFR. Finally, larger vessel atherosclerosis, perhaps especially in type 2 diabetes, may lead to ischemic kidney tissue damage.

In type 1 diabetic patients, glomerular, tubular, interstitial, and vascular lesions tend to progress more or less in parallel, whereas in type 2 diabetic patients this is often not the case. Preliminary observations suggest that long-standing normoalbuminuric type 1 diabetic patients who progress to diabetic nephropathy have more advanced glomerular lesions than patients who remain normoalbuminuric after long-term follow-up, but these findings are, as yet, unconfirmed. In type 2 diabetes, current evidence suggests that microalbuminuric patients with typical diabetic glomerulopathy have a higher risk of progressive GFR loss than those with fewer glomerular changes.

Recent studies in progressive type 1 diabetic patients found a remarkably high frequency of glomerular tubular junction abnormalities. Most of these abnormalities are associated with tuft adhesions of podocytes and Bowman's capsule at or close to the glomerular tubular junction (tip lesions). The frequency and severity of these lesions and, perhaps their alternate expression, completely atubular glomeruli, greatly increases the understanding of the structural basis of GFR loss in this disease.

NOVEL THERAPEUTIC STRATEGIES

Better understanding of the process involved in diabetic nephropathy pathogenesis may lead to the development of new therapeutic strategies for the prevention, arrest, or reversal of diabetic nephropathy. These novel strategies might include AGE inhibitors and cross-link breakers, PKC inhibitors, and oxidative stress inhibitors. Treatment with an inhibitor of glycated albumin formation reduced albumin excretion, prevented GFR decline, reduced mesangial matrix accumulation, and normalized $\alpha 1(IV)$ collagen cortical mRNA expression in db/db mice. Recently, pimagedine, a second-generation AGE inhibitor, was shown to reduce urinary protein excretion and GFR decline in proteinuric type 1 diabetic patients in a randomized placebo-controlled study. Also, treatment with the cross-link breaker ALT-711 reduced albumin excretion, blood pressure, and kidney lesions in experimental diabetes. Treatment with a PKCβ inhibitor normalized GFR, decreased albumin excretion, and ameliorated glomerular lesions in diabetic rodents. High doses of thiamine and benfotiamine retarded the development of microalbuminuria in experimental diabetic nephropathy. This was associated with decreased activation of PKC and decreased protein glycation and oxidative stress. Sulodexide, a drug that might be capable of repleting glomerular capillary wall charge sites, was associated with albuminuria reduction in microalbuminuric and microalbuminuric type 1 and type 2 diabetic patients. Thus, the effects of a number of novel therapies related to the mechanisms of diabetic nephropathy are currently being evaluated in experimental and human diabetic nephropathy, and will probably be available for clinical use in the near future.

BIBLIOGRAPHY

American Diabetes Association: 2003 United States Renal Data System Annual Report. National Technical Information Service. Nephropathy in diabetes. Diabetes Care 27(suppl): 79–83, 2004.

Babaei-Jadidi R, Karachalias N, Ahmed N, et al: Prevention of incipient diabetic nephropathy by high-dose thiamine and benfotiamine. Diabetes 52:2110–2120, 2003.

Baynes JW, Thorpe SR: Role of oxidative stress in diabetic complications: A new perspective on an old paradigm. Diabetes 48:1–9, 1999.

Bolton WK, Cattran DC, Williams ME, et al: Randomized trial of an inhibitor of formation of advanced glycation end products in diabetic nephropathy. Am J Nephrol 24:32–40, 2004.

Bennet PH, Haffner S, Kasiske BL, et al: Screening and management of microalbuminuria in patients with diabetes mellitus: Recommendations to the Scientific Advisory Board of the National Kidney Foundation from an ad hoc committee of the Council on Diabetes Mellitus of the National Kidney Foundation. Am J Kidney Dis 25:107–112, 1995.

Bilous RW, Mauer SM, Viberti GC: Genetic aspects of diabetic nephropathy. In Morgan SH, Grünfeld J-P (eds): Inherited Disorders of the Kidney, Investigation and Management. Oxford, UK, Oxford University Press, 1998, pp 427–448.

Caramori ML, Canani LH, Costa LA, et al: The human peroxisome proliferator activated receptor γ2 (PPARγ2) Pro12Ala polymorphism is associated with decreased risk of diabetic nephropathy in patients with type 2 diabetes. Diabetes 52:3010–3013, 2003.

Caramori ML, Fioretto P, Mauer M: Low glomerular filtration rate in normoalbuminuric type 1 diabetic patients. An indicator of more advanced glomerular lesions. Diabetes 52:1036–1040, 2003.

Caramori ML, Kim Y, Huang C, et al: Cellular basis of diabetic nephropathy: 1. Study design and structural-functional relationships in patients with long-standing type 1 diabetes. Diabetes 51:506–513, 2002.

The Diabetes Control and Complications Trial Research Group: Effect of intensive therapy on the development and progression of diabetic nephropathy in the Diabetes Control and Complications Trial. Kidney Int 47:1703–1720, 1995.

Fioretto P, Mauer M, Brocco E, et al: Patterns of renal injury in NIDDM patients with microalbuminuria. Diabetologia 39: 1569–1576, 1996.

Fioretto P, Steffes MW, Mauer SM: Glomerular structure in nonproteinuric insulin-dependent diabetic patients with various levels of albuminuria. Diabetes 43:1358–1364, 1994.

Forbes JM, Thallas V, Thomas MC, et al: The breakdown of preexisting advanced glycation end products is associated with reduced renal fibrosis in experimental diabetes. FASEB J 17:1762–1764, 2003.

Hansson L, Zanchetti A, Carruthers SG, et al: Effects of intensive blood-pressure lowering and low-dose aspirin in patients with hypertension: Principal results of the Hypertension Optimal Treatment (HOT) randomised trial. Lancet 351: 1755–1762, 1998.

Huang C, Kim Y, Caramori ML, et al: Cellular basis of diabetic nephropathy: II. The transforming growth factor-beta system and diabetic nephropathy lesions in type 1 diabetes. Diabetes 51:3577–3581, 2002.

Katz A, Caramori ML, Sisson-Ross S, et al: An increase in the cell component of the cortical interstitium antedates interstitial fibrosis in type 1 diabetic patients. Kidney Int 61:2058–2066, 2002.

Kelly DJ, Zhang Y, Hepper C, et al: Protein kinase C beta inhibition attenuates the progression of experimental diabetic nephropathy in the presence of continued hypertension. Diabetes 52:512–518, 2003.

Kiritoshi S, Nishikawa T, Sonoda K, et al: Reactive oxygen species from mitochondria induce cyclooxygenase-2 gene expression in human mesangial cells: Potential role in diabetic nephropathy. Diabetes 52:2570–2577, 2003.

Krolewski AS: Genetics of diabetic nephropathy: Evidence for major and minor gene effects. Kidney Int 55:1582–1596, 1999.

Lewis EJ, Hunsicker LG, Bain RP, et al: The effects of angiotensin-converting-enzyme inhibition on diabetic nephropathy. The Collaborative Study Group. N Engl J Med 329:1456–1462, 1993.

Lurbe E, Redon J, Kesani A, et al: Increase in nocturnal blood pressure and progression to microalbuminuria in type 1 diabetes. N Engl J Med 347:797–805, 2002.

Mauer M, Mogensen CE, Friedman EA: Diabetic nephropathy. In Schrier RW, Gottschalk CW (eds): Diseases of the Kidney. Boston, Little, Brown, 1996, pp 2019–2061.

Mauer SM, Steffes MW, Ellis EN, et al: Structural-functional relationships in diabetic nephropathy. J Clin Invest 74:1143–1155, 1984.

Meltzer S, Leiter L, Daneman D, et al: 1998 Clinical practice guidelines for the management of diabetes in Canada. Canadian Diabetes Association. Can Med Assoc J 159(suppl 8):1–29, 1998.

Mogensen CE: Microalbuminuria, blood pressure and diabetic renal disease: Origin and development of ideas. Diabetologia 42:263–285, 1999.

Nishikawa T, Edelstein D, Brownlee M: The missing link: A single unifying mechanism for diabetic complications. Kidney Int 77(suppl):26–30, 2000.

Orchard TJ, Chang YF, Ferrell RE, et al: Nephropathy in type 1 diabetes: A manifestation of insulin resistance and multiple genetic susceptibilities? Further evidence from the Pittsburgh Epidemiology of Diabetes Complication Study. Kidney Int 62:963–970, 2002.

Østerby R: Glomerular structural changes in type 1 (insulin-dependent) diabetes mellitus: Causes, consequences, and prevention. Diabetologia 35:803–812, 1992.

Tuttle KR, Anderson PW: A novel potential therapy for diabetic nephropathy and vascular complications: Protein kinase C beta inhibition. Am J Kidney Dis 42:456–465, 2003.

United Kingdom Prospective Diabetes Study Group: Intensive blood-glucose control with sulphonylureas or insulin compared with conventional treatment and risk of complications in patients with type 2 diabetes (UKPDS 33). Lancet 352:837–853, 1998.

United Kingdom Prospective Diabetes Study Group: Tight blood pressure control and risk of macrovascular and microvascular complications in type 2 diabetes: UKPDS 38. BMJ 317:703–713, 1998.

CHAPTER 29

Clinical Course and Management of Diabetic Nephropathy

Tracy A. McGowan Fuad N. Ziyadeh

SUMMARY OF CLINICAL FEATURES

Both the incidence and prevalence of endstage renal disease (ESRD) in the United States are projected to increase by 75% from 2000 to 2010. This growth is largely due to the increasing number of people who develop type 2 diabetes mellitus. Thus, diabetic nephropathy is now the leading cause of ESRD in the United States, accounting for approximately 45% of all new cases. Up to 35% of all type 1 or type 2 diabetic patients eventually develop nephropathy after 15 to 20 years of diabetes. Because of the much higher prevalence of type 2 diabetes in the overall diabetic population (90% to 95%), the number of type 2 diabetic patients with ESRD in the United States in 2000 far exceeded that of type 1 (38% and 6% of the total dialysis population, respectively).

Five clinical stages characterize the progression of diabetic nephropathy (Table 29-1). These are best delineated in the setting of type 1 diabetes because the patients are often young and typically do not have other coexisting systemic diseases (e.g., essential hypertension) and because the onset of diabetes is more easily pinpointed. In these patients, proteinuria due to diabetic nephropathy rarely develops before 10 years from diabetes onset. On the other hand, if a patient has diabetes for more than 25 years and has not developed proteinuria, the future risk for developing nephropathy is only about 1% per year. The five clinical stages of diabetic nephropathy are classified on the basis of the values of the glomerular filtration rate (GFR), urinary albumin excretion (UAE), and systemic blood pressure. The natural history for patients with type 2 diabetes is not as easily characterized because 5% to 20% of these patients have some degree of albuminuria at the time of recognition of diabetes. Unlike type 1 diabetic patients, patients with type 2 diabetes commonly have hypertension at presentation. Moreover, due to increased cardiovascular mortality, many type 2 diabetic patients die before they ever progress to ESRD. Nevertheless, longitudinal observations in the Pima Indians, a native American tribe with an alarmingly high incidence of early-onset type 2 diabetes, have revealed that the course of diabetic nephropathy is similar to that of patients with type 1 diabetes.

The patient with diabetes who has proteinuria has a two- to fourfold increased risk for morbidity and mortality from cardiovascular disease. Even with chronic dialysis, the cardiac death rate of diabetic patients is approximately 50% higher than that of nondiabetic patients, reaching 120 deaths per thousand patients after 1 year of dialysis.

The discrete structural lesions in the renal parenchyma and vasculature generally become more severe with advancing stages and roughly track the functional changes in GFR, UAE, and blood pressure, but the diagnosis of diabetic nephropathy is often made on clinical grounds without the need for kidney biopsy except in atypical presentations. The earliest renal manifestations in type 1 diabetes are nephromegaly and glomerular hypertrophy, which are accompanied by afferent arteriolar vasodilation, renal hyperperfusion, and glomerular hyperfiltration (stage 1). Microscopically, there is thickening of the glomerular and tubular basement membranes, which appear even if the patient is not destined to develop established diabetic nephropathy. During stage 2 there is a significant degree of mesangial matrix expansion or diffuse glomerulosclerosis with further thickening of the glomerular and tubular basement membranes. Podocyte loss may also manifest. In stage 3 and beyond, the glomeruli typically demonstrate diffuse glomerulosclerosis or nodular glomerulosclerosis, and there is further podocyte loss and focal areas of foot process effacement. Arteriolar hyalinosis develops in both the afferent and efferent arterioles, and there are variable degrees of tubulointerstitial fibrosis.

SCREENING

The Diabetes Control and Complications Trial (DCCT) and the Stockholm Diabetes Intervention Study (SDIS) in type 1 diabetes, and the United Kingdom Prospective Diabetes Study (UKPDS) and the Kumamoto Study in type 2 diabetes, all show that the onset and progression of nephropathy can be delayed by interventions, provided they are instituted early in the course of disease. For this reason, screening is of paramount importance. It is recommended that a urinalysis be performed annually, starting at approximately 5 years after the onset of type 1 diabetes or at the time of recognition of type 2 diabetes. In the absence of overt proteinuria, a test for microalbu-

249

TABLE 29-1   Clinical Stages of Diabetic Nephropathy

Stage	GFR	UAE	Blood Pressure	Years after Diagnosis
1. Hyperfiltration	Supernormal	<30 mg/day	Normal	0
2. Microalbuminuria	High normal–normal	30–300 mg/day	Rising	5–15
3. Overt proteinuria	Normal–decreasing	>300 mg/day	Elevated	10–20
4. Progressive nephropathy	Decreasing	Increasing	Elevated	15–25
5. ESRD	<15 mL/min	Massive	Elevated	20–30

ESRD, endstage renal disease; GFR, glomerular filtration rate; UAE, urinary albumin excretion.

minuria should be conducted. Conveniently, this is done by measuring the albumin/creatinine ratio on a random urine sample. A 24-hour urine collection is also useful for measuring total protein excretion and creatinine clearance. It is important to note that a transient increase in UAE can be caused by uncontrolled hyperglycemia or hypertension, fever, urinary tract infection, congestive heart failure, or physical exertion. Thus, persistent microalbuminuria should be confirmed by two more urine samples over the following 3 to 6 months.

Once a patient develops proteinuria, it is important to rule out causes other than diabetes. This is particularly important in type 1 patients who have had the diagnosis of diabetes for less than 5 or greater than 30 years or who do not exhibit concomitant signs of diabetic retinopathy. In these cases, the patient should be evaluated for conditions such as viral hepatitis B or C, human immunodeficiency virus infection, lupus nephritis, multiple myeloma, amyloidosis, or use of nonsteroidal antiinflammatory drugs. In many of these cases there may be a nephritic urine sediment with either red blood cells or casts. Some studies have suggested that patients with type 2 diabetes are at increased risk for developing primary glomerulopathies as compared with the general population. The diagnosis of glomerulonephritis may need to be established with a kidney biopsy. Finally, in addition to causing chronic kidney disease (CKD), diabetes can affect the urinary system, causing neurogenic bladder, pyelonephritis, and papillary necrosis. Renal ultrasonography should be performed to rule out obstruction.

MEDICAL MANAGEMENT

Treatment of diabetic nephropathy should be addressed based on the clinical stage of the disease process. Therefore, therapeutic options are discussed for the following categories: prevention of diabetic nephropathy, treatment of established nephropathy, and management options for renal replacement therapy (RRT).

Prevention of Diabetic Nephropathy

Both the DCCT and the SDIS in type 1 diabetes and the UKPDS in type 2 diabetes have shown the benefit of intensive glucose control in the prevention of microvascular complications (i.e., the development of retinopathy or microalbuminuria). Tight glucose control has also been shown to reduce the degree of nephromegaly and glomerular hyperfiltration in type 1 diabetes. In the DCCT, intensive control of blood glucose with multiple daily insulin injections (hemoglobin A1c less than 7%) reduced the occurrence of microalbuminuria (defined in that study as a UAE greater than or equal to 40 mg/day) by 39% in the primary and secondary cohorts combined (with and without baseline retinopathy). Nevertheless, 16% of patients treated to an average blood glucose of 155 mg/dL progressed from normoalbuminuria to microalbuminuria over an average period of 9 years of follow-up. Therefore, there appear to be additional risk factors for the development of microalbuminuria other than chronic hyperglycemia.

Treatment with antihypertensive agents that block the renin-angiotensin system (RAS), such as the angiotensin-converting enzyme (ACE) inhibitors captopril or enalapril, has been demonstrated in small studies to prevent the development of microalbuminuria in normoalbuminuric type 1 or type 2 diabetic patients even in the absence of hypertension. However, there is no current recommendation for initiating therapy with RAS-blocking drugs such as ACE inhibitors or angiotensin receptor blockers (ARBs) in normotensive, normoalbuminuric patients for the primary prevention of diabetic nephropathy. This is because only 20% to 40% of these patients are at risk for ever developing this complication.

It is important to note that RAS-blocking drugs may be prescribed for cardioprotective indications in all diabetic patients irrespective of the presence or absence of kidney disease. The diabetic subgroups of patients who were enrolled in either the Heart Outcomes Prevention Evaluation (HOPE) trial (and received the ACE inhibitor ramipril) or the Losartan Intervention for Endpoint Reduction in Hypertension (LIFE) study (and received the ARB losartan) had significantly fewer cardiovascular events than the patients in the control groups who did not receive RAS-blocking drugs.

Nonpharmacologic interventions and life-style modifications are encouraged to reduce the risk for overt nephropathy; these include regular physical exercise, reduction in body mass index, dietary restriction of salt and saturated fat, and smoking cessation. These interventions can also decrease cardiovascular morbidity and mortality. An important component of therapy for the primary or secondary prevention of cardiovascular events is the use of aspirin (81 to 162 mg/day) in all diabetic patients over 40 years of age.

Therapy of Incipient and Overt Diabetic Nephropathy

Blood Pressure Control

The single most effective measure for delaying the progression of CKD from diabetes in patients with overt proteinuria is the reduction of systemic blood pressure. Treatment of hypertension is vital during any stage of CKD. Clinical trials such as the UKPDS have shown that strict control of blood pressure (as compared with strict glycemic control) provides the greatest favorable impact on patient outcomes, including progression of CKD and cardiovascular end points. Thus, it is of paramount importance to treat hypertension to the recommended target of less than 130/80 mm Hg in all diabetic patients and to 125/75 mm Hg in patients with UAE of greater than 1 g/day. More than one medication is usually required; diabetic patients with overt nephropathy require on average of three different antihypertensive drugs, including a diuretic, to achieve this goal. Any of the different classes of antihypertensive agents can be effectively used in the diabetic population, and the choice is tailored to the needs of the particular patient and to the tolerability of the individual drugs. Increasing doses of loop diuretics rather than low-dose thiazide diuretics become necessary to control the fluid retention and the accompanying hypertension when the nephrotic syndrome develops or there is advanced CKD. Metolazone may be added to loop diuretics to increase fluid removal in some cases. With optimal blood pressure control, it is possible to slow down the progression of chronic kidney disease from a rate of approximately 12 mL/min per year to approximately 5 mL/min per year or lower.

Renoprotection with Renin-Angiotensin System Blockade

Multiple experimental and clinical studies in various chronic kidney diseases including diabetic nephropathy have provided conclusive evidence for the concept of additional renoprotection by RAS-blocking drugs that exceeds the benefit achieved by reduction of systemic blood pressure. Because the changes in blood pressure with either ACE inhibitors or ARB therapy cannot entirely explain the antiproteinuric and nephroprotective responses, it has been suggested that both the intraglomerular hemodynamic and nonhemodynamic renal effects of angiotensin II, which are likely mediated by the fibrotic agent transforming growth factor-β (TGF-β), best explain the observed nephroprotection. The Collaborative Study Group, which published its results in 1993, was the first large trial (approximately 400 patients) to definitively show the benefit of ACE inhibitor therapy compared with traditional antihypertensive agents in the delay of progression of overt nephropathy in patients with type 1 diabetes over a 4-year period of follow-up. The blood pressure in the experimental group treated with captopril was roughly similar to that achieved in the control group who received conventional antihypertensive agents. However, treatment with captopril was associated with nearly 50% reduction in the relative risk of doubling of serum creatinine concentration or the combined end points of death, dialysis, and kidney transplantation. Interestingly, in 1999, the same group performed a prospective randomized, clinical trial on 129 patients with type 1 diabetes with total proteinuria greater than 500 mg/day and serum creatinine less than or equal to 2.5 mg/dL. All patients received an ACE inhibitor (ramipril) at different doses to achieve either a mean arterial pressure (MAP) of less than or equal to 92 mm Hg or a range from 100 to 107 mm Hg. Not surprisingly patients achieving MAP of no more than 92 mm Hg had lower total urinary protein excretion as well as a slower decline in GFR. These studies suggest that both the use of an ACE inhibitor and the absolute reduction in systemic blood pressure are important in preservation of kidney function in type 1 diabetic patients with overt nephropathy. With such an approach, it is possible to reduce the decline in GFR to approximately 3 to 4 mL/min per year. The clinical indications for ACE inhibitors in type 1 diabetic patients have been expanded so that therapy should be initiated as soon as persistent microalbuminuria is documented, even if blood pressure is not elevated; in this setting, treatment with ACE inhibitors has been shown to delay or prevent the development of overt nephropathy.

The benefits of RAS blockade beyond blood pressure control in type 2 diabetic patients with incipient or overt nephropathy have been achieved with the addition of an ARB. Compelling evidence from two recent trials in type 2 diabetic patients with microalbuminuria (Irbesartan in Patients with Type 2 Diabetes and Microalbuminuria [IRMA2] and the Microalbuminuria Reduction with Valsartan [MARVAL]) showed that an ARB-based regimen significantly reduces the number of patients who progress to macroalbuminuria as compared with conventional antihypertensive agents. The benefits of either irbesartan or valsartan were more pronounced with higher doses and were significantly greater when compared with conventional antihypertensive agents in the control groups in which the same degree of blood pressure reduction was achieved. In these trials, normoalbuminuria was restored in more subjects enrolled in the ARB groups compared with the control groups.

Two other large clinical trials in type 2 diabetic patients with overt nephropathy published in 2001 (Reduction of End Points in Type 2 Diabetes with Angiotensin-II Antagonist Losartan [RENAAL] and the Irbesartan Type 2 Diabetic Nephropathy Trial [IDNT]) showed significant reductions in proteinuria and time to doubling of serum creatinine as compared with the control groups who achieved the same degree of blood pressure reduction with antihypertensive agents that do not specifically target the RAS. The RENAAL trial also showed significant reduction in the number of patients progressing to ESRD, and the IDNT established the superiority of irbesartan over the calcium channel blocker amlodipine. Further analysis of data from the RENAAL trial found that the most significant risk factor for progressive nephropathy was the initial amount of UAE. Post-hoc analyses of both the RENAAL trial and IDNT also show that the greatest renoprotection was observed in those subjects with the greatest reduction in systemic blood pressure.

Specific kidney protection by ACE inhibitors compared with various other antihypertensive treatment regimens has not been demonstrated consistently in patients with type 2 diabetes. Several clinical trials on the use of various ACE inhibitors in these patients showed variable degrees of reduction in proteinuria and stabilization of kidney function, and none of them evaluated the effect of therapy on progression of ESRD. Because of one or more major shortcomings in the design of these trials, with regard to assessing the impact on nephropathy progression, there are currently no firm recommendations to select an ACE inhibitor in lieu of other antihypertensive agents in type 2 diabetic patients with overt nephropathy as a means to slow the progression to ESRD. Of course, ACE inhibitors can be prescribed for cardioprotective benefits and as part of a multidrug regimen to effectively lower the blood pressure.

Of note, none of the completed clinical trials included a head-to-head comparison between an ARB and an ACE inhibitor. Therefore, pending trials that are designed for such comparison, no definitive statement can be made regarding the superiority of an ARB over an ACE inhibitor in the diabetic patient with incipient or overt nephropathy (whether in type 1 or type 2 diabetes). The significant occurrence of cough with an ACE inhibitor but not with an ARB (beyond placebo) and the better tolerability of the latter have increased the popularity of an ARB-based antihypertensive regimen despite the increased cost.

Dual Renin-Angiotensin Blockade

In addition to controlling systemic hypertension, a major aim of RAS blockade is to decrease the magnitude of proteinuria to achieve further renoprotection. The degree of reduction in proteinuria by RAS-blocking agents varies from patient to patient, but on average it is approximately 40% from baseline. Many nephrologists advocate an increase in the dosage of either an ACE inhibitor or an ARB (or a combination of both) to achieve further reductions in the UAE even if the target blood pressure has been reached. Fortunately, increased dosage can often be successful in decreasing the UAE without reducing the blood pressure below the normal range. Recently, there has been increased interest in the use of ACE inhibitor and ARB combination therapy in patients with chronic kidney disease including diabetic nephropathy. The clinical trials of dual blockade published thus far show favorable results of combination therapy in terms of better blood pressure control and further reductions in the UAE, but larger studies of longer duration that assess the impact on kidney function are needed to show whether the effects are sustained and lead to long-term renoprotection. The Candesartan and Lisinopril Microalbuminuria (CALM) study, published in 2000, randomized type 2 diabetic patients with hypertension and microalbuminuria to receive monotherapy with either agent (lisinopril 20 mg/day or candesartan 16 mg/day) or combined therapy at the same doses. The combination regimen showed a significant reduction in blood pressure and a greater decrease in the urinary albumin/creatinine ratio compared with either agent alone. Because the doses of lisinopril and candesartan were not maximal, it is possible that more complete blockade of the RAS may be responsible for these beneficial effects. However, a recent study in type 1 diabetic patients with overt nephropathy published in 2003 showed a greater degree of blood pressure reduction and proteinuria when the patients received maximal doses of enalapril 40 mg/day plus irbesartan 300 mg/day as compared with 40 mg/day of enalapril alone. Thus, there is some merit in combining these agents to achieve additional benefits that cannot be obtained from maximal doses of each agent alone.

There is an increased risk for hyperkalemia with either ACE inhibitors or ARBs or a combination of both. Serum potassium and creatinine should be monitored closely within 1 week after the initiation of therapy, and periodically thereafter. Loop diuretics or occasionally the use of cation exchange resins (polystyrene sulfonate or Kayexalate) may be effective in controlling the hyperkalemia during therapy. Patients should be instructed to avoid foods that have high concentrations of potassium (e.g., bananas, oranges, dried fruits, nuts, potatoes, chocolate) and to limit their total daily intake of potassium to less than 2000 mg/day. Interventions other than blood pressure medications used to delay progression of CKD include dietary sodium restriction to less than or equal to 2000 mg/day, limited alcohol consumption (no more than two drinks per day for men and one drink per day for women), control of hyperlipidemia, cessation of smoking, and dietary protein restriction.

Glycemic Control

Attempts at sustained reductions in hyperglycemia continue to be of therapeutic importance in type 1 and type 2 diabetic patients with either incipient or overt nephropathy. In the DCCT, intensive control of blood glucose reduced the occurrence of macroalbuminuria by 54% in the primary and secondary cohorts combined (with and without baseline retinopathy). Also, tight glucose control has been shown to stabilize or even decrease UAE in patients with microalbuminuria, but this effect may take a few years to be clinically evident.

Caution should be exercised in the management of hyperglycemia when the patient has significant CKD. Because insulin is degraded by the kidney, dose reduction may be needed to prevent hypoglycemia. Reduction in the doses of oral hypoglycemic agents may also be necessary, especially some sulfonylurea compounds that are metabolized by the kidney. The insulin-sensitizing agent metformin is contraindicated in the presence of kidney dysfunction, defined as a serum creatinine of greater than 1.5 mg/dL in males or greater than 1.4 mg/dL in females or a creatinine clearance of less than 60 mL/min, because of the risk for life-threatening lactic acidosis. Metformin should also be discontinued before surgery or administration of contrast media. Thiazolidinediones, such as rosiglitazone or pioglitazone, may aggravate edema and congestive heart failure. No data are available on the long-term safety and efficacy of thiazolidiones in patients with CKD.

Dietary Protein Restriction

A meta-analysis of five clinical trials in type 1 diabetic patients with nephropathy concluded that dietary protein restriction (approximately 0.6 g/kg/day of high biologic value protein and adequate calorie intake) has a significant long-term beneficial effect to slow the rate of decline in GFR and to lower the UAE without demonstrable evidence of malnutrition. Currently the American Diabetes Association recommends 0.8 g/kg/day of protein restriction for diabetic patients with increased UAE, which is a manageable and safe recommendation for the majority of patients with challenging dietary prescriptions related to their diabetes and CKD. Dietary counseling by a nutritionist is desirable for patients with advanced CKD in order to avoid protein-calorie malnutrition prior to renal replacement therapy, which has been shown to be a strong predictor for subsequent increased morbidity and mortality during maintenance dialysis. Dietary counselors can also advise on issues of salt, potassium, and phosphate restriction and can counsel patients on the choice of carbohydrates and fats.

Lipid Management

The treatment of hyperlipidemia is known to be important in the prevention of atherosclerosis. There is some circumstantial evidence that the treatment of hyperlipidemia with 3-hydroxy-3-methylglutaryl coenzyme A reductase inhibitors (statins) may protect against the development of glomerulosclerosis, as reflected by decreased UAE and improved serum creatinine. There are a number of proposed mechanisms for this finding, including beneficial effects on nitric oxide and endothelin-1 as well as suppression of glucose-mediated up-regulation of TGF-β. The current American Diabetes Association treatment goals for lipids are low-density lipoprotein cholesterol of less than 100 mg/dL, triglycerides less than 150 mg/dL, and high-density lipoprotein of greater than 40 mg/dL. A multipronged approach of intensive combined therapy, aimed at lowering hemoglobin A1c, blood pressure, serum cholesterol, and body mass index, as well as a program for anemia management, increased physical activity, and smoking cessation, can lead to a significant decrease in cardiovascular events and slowing of progressive nephropathy, not to mention a greater sense of well-being.

Treatment of Endstage Renal Disease in Diabetes

Once a diabetic patient approaches ESRD, various options for RRT should be offered: peritoneal dialysis (PD), hemodialysis (HD), or kidney transplantation. Survival on either modality of dialysis is generally worse for patients with diabetes versus nondiabetic patients. Survival is also inversely related to age, presumably due to less cardiovascular disease in younger patients, because greater than 70% of deaths in this population are attributed to a cardiovascular cause. In the United States about 80% of diabetic patients with ESRD are treated with HD, with more than 80% of these patients doing in-center HD. Choice of dialysis modality in diabetic patients should be similar in consideration to that for any patient with ESRD. However, there are some special considerations in patients with diabetes. Some patients with autonomic neuropathy may have frequent episodes of hypotension associated with large fluid shifts during HD; these may be avoided with the more gradual fluid shifts by PD. On the other hand, patients with diabetes on PD are at risk for absorption of the dextrose present in the dialysate and may have worsened blood glucose control and hypertriglyceridemia and increased insulin requirements. Older diabetic patients may have severe peripheral vascular disease, limiting the success of HD vascular access. Similarly, peripheral vascular disease may also make the peritoneum less than optimal for fluid and electrolyte exchange. Diabetic patients tend to be more prone to infection; however, this would put them more at risk for both peritonitis and vascular access infections. After adjusting for appropriate comorbidities and potential confounders, there is no great body of evidence to suggest that diabetic patients do significantly better with one form of dialysis over the other. In both forms of dialysis, diabetic patients tend to be more sensitive than other ESRD patients to the symptoms of underdialysis.

In diabetic patients eligible for transplantation, survival is much improved compared with dialysis. Two-year survival may be up to four times better for the diabetic patient receiving a kidney transplant compared with staying on dialysis. It could be argued that there is a selection bias for survival after transplantation, because younger and healthier patients are more likely to receive transplants. However, studies looking at the survival of transplant patients compared with matched controls of similar health awaiting a transplant show a survival benefit for the patients who have undergone transplantation. Although statistics vary by center, 5-year patient survival after transplantation is approximately 70%. Although these survival data are worse than for nondiabetic transplant patients, they are better than those for dialysis patients with diabetes, in whom 5-year survival is generally less than 35%. As in patients with other forms of kidney disease, kidney allografts from living-related or -unrelated donors survive significantly longer than those from deceased donors.

Recurrent diabetic nephropathy develops in almost all solitary kidney allografts (i.e., without pancreas or islet cell transplantation). Within 2 years after solitary kidney transplantation, glomerular ultrastructural changes can be seen on biopsy, pointing to the importance of glycemic control in the development of nephropathy. However, graft failure due to recurrent disease is rare because most patients die before their allografts fail.

Pancreas transplantation can be the preferred option for relatively young patients with type 1 diabetes whose blood glucose is especially difficult to control or who have hypoglycemic unawareness but are otherwise in reasonably good health. If the patient also has early nephropathy (microalbuminuria), but well-preserved kidney function, pancreas transplantation alone (PTA) may be considered. Based on the sequential morbidities of the surgery and long-term immunosuppression, the American Diabetes Association recommends that PTA be considered only in patients who exhibit the following: frequent, acute, and severe metabolic complications requiring medical attention (e.g., recurrent hypoglycemia); incapacitating clinical and emotional problems with exogenous insulin therapy; and medical failure of exogenous insulin to prevent acute complications. If the patient has advanced CKD and is approaching dialysis or is already on dialysis, a simultaneous pancreas-kidney (SPK) transplantation is a good alternative. For this procedure, the patient receives the pancreas and the kidney from the same deceased donor (or rarely from different donors) during the same operation. The goal of pancreatic transplantation is to restore euglycemia and thereby attempt to prevent or improve secondary complications of diabetes, including CKD. Sustained euglycemia improves the renal lesions of diabetes in the native kidney (in PTA) and prevents their appearance in the kidney allograft (in SPK transplantation). At the present time, it is not clear whether transplantation of the pancreas as an SPK confers an additive patient survival advantage over kidney transplantation alone. However, benefits of chronic euglycemia after pancreas transplantation may include stabilization of peripheral neuropathy, improved life expectancy in patients with autonomic insufficiency, improved fertility and pregnancy outcomes, and improved quality of life.

Another option is for the patient to receive a kidney allograft, preferably from a living donor, which is followed at a later time by transplantation of a pancreas from a deceased donor (i.e., pancreas-after-kidney [PAK] transplantation). There are no prospective controlled trials to compare outcomes of the different transplantation approaches. Observational surveys show that 1-year pancreas graft survival is about 95% in SPK transplantation and about 75% in PAK transplantation. These differences likely reflect the fact that there is not an easily measured, sensitive marker for early pancreatic rejection, whereas an elevation in the serum creatinine provides an advantage to timely diagnosis and treatment of kidney allograft rejection. In general, minimizing or avoiding the need for dialysis altogether is associated with the best survival rates after transplantation. For this reason and because kidney transplantation alone has a dramatic impact on patient longevity, living kidney donation is recommended for all patients with type 1 diabetes, even if they are potential candidates for pancreatic transplantation. Moreover, kidney graft survival rates are generally superior with live-donor compared with deceased-donor kidney transplants. In this scenario, live-donor recipients may then be eligible for subsequent PAK transplantation.

Recent data with isolated islet cell transplantation using the Edmonton approach have demonstrated promising short-term benefits, but large multicenter trials are awaited to appreciate the full impact of this novel treatment. The greatest hurdle for islet cell transplantation is organ shortage because of the need for two or more donor pancreata per recipient.

BIBLIOGRAPHY

Adler AI, Stratton IM, Neil HA, et al: Association of systolic blood pressure with macrovascular and microvascular complications of type 2 diabetes (UKPDS 36): Prospective observational study. BMJ 321:412–419, 2000.

American Diabetes Association: Standards of medical care in diabetes. Diabetes Care 27(suppl 1):15–35, 2004.

American Diabetes Association; The National Heart, Lung, and Blood Institute; The Juvenile Diabetes Foundation International; The National Institute of Diabetes and Digestive and Kidney Diseases; and The American Heart Association (joint editorial statement): Diabetes mellitus: A major risk factor for cardiovascular disease. Circulation 100:1132–1133, 1999.

Brenner BM, Cooper ME, de Zeeuw D, et al: Effects of losartan on renal and cardiovascular outcomes in patients with type 2 diabetes and nephropathy. N Engl J Med 345:861–869, 2001.

Diabetes Control and Complications (DCCT) Research Group: Effect of intensive therapy on the development and progression of diabetic nephropathy in the Diabetes Control and Complications Trial. Kidney Int 47:1703–1720, 1995.

Fioretto P, Steffes MW, Sutherland DER, et al: Reversal of lesions of diabetic nephropathy after pancreas transplantation. N Engl J Med 339:69–75, 1998.

Hamilton RA: Angiotensin-converting enzyme inhibitors and type 2 diabetic nephropathy: A meta-analysis. Pharmacotherapy 23:909–915, 2003.

Hansen HP, Tauber-Lassen E, Jensen BR, et al: Effect of dietary protein restriction on prognosis in patients with diabetic nephropathy. Kidney Int 62:220–228, 2002.

Hovind P, Rossing P, Tarnow L, et al: Remission and regression in the nephropathy of type 1 diabetes when blood pressure is controlled aggressively. Kidney Int 60:277–283, 2001.

Jacobsen P, Andersen S, Rossing K, et al: Dual blockade of the renin-angiotensin system versus maximal recommended dose of ACE inhibition in diabetic nephropathy. Kidney Int 63:1874–1880, 2003.

Kirpichnikov D, McFarlane SI, Sowers JR: Metformin: An update. Ann Intern Med 137:25–33, 2002.

Lewis EJ, Hunsicker LG, Bain RP, et al: The effect of angiotensin-converting enzyme inhibition on diabetic nephropathy. N Engl J Med 329:1456–1462, 1993.

Lewis EJ, Hunsicker LG, Clarke WR, et al: Renoprotective effect of the angiotensin-receptor antagonist irbesartan in patients with nephropathy due to type 2 diabetes. N Engl J Med 345:851–860, 2001.

McGowan T, McCue P, Sharma K: Diabetic nephropathy. Clin Lab Med. 21:111–146, 2001.

Mogyorosi A, Ziyadeh FN: Diabetic nephropathy. In Massry SG, Glassock RJ (eds): Textbook of Nephrology, 4th ed. Philadelphia, Lippincott, Williams & Wilkins, 2001, pp 874–895.

Nesto RW, Bell D, Bonow RO, et al: Thiazolidinedione use, fluid retention, and congestive heart failure: A consensus statement from the American Heart Association and American Diabetes Association. Diabetes Care 27:256–263, 2004.

Parving HH, Lehnert H, Bröchner-Mortensen J, et al: The effect of irbesartan on the development of diabetic nephropathy in patients with type 2 diabetes. N Engl J Med 345:870–878, 2001.

Pedrini MT, Levey AS, Lau J, et al: The effect of dietary protein restriction on the progression of diabetic and nondiabetic renal diseases: A meta-analysis. Ann Intern Med 124:627–632, 1996.

Tonolo G, Ciccarese M, Brizzi P, et al: Reduction of albumin excretion rate in normotensive microalbuminuric type 2 diabetic patients during long-term simvastatin treatment. Diabetes Care 20:1891–1895, 1997.

Venstrom JM, McBride MA, Rother KI, et al: Survival after pancreas transplantation in patients with diabetes and preserved kidney function. JAMA 290:2817–2823, 2003.

Wolf G, Ritz E: Diabetic nephropathy in type 2 diabetes prevention and patient management. J Am Soc Nephrol 14:1396–1405, 2003.

Wolfe RA, Ashby VB, Milford EL, et al: Comparison of mortality in all patients on dialysis, patients on dialysis awaiting transplantation, and recipients of a first cadaveric transplant. N Engl J Med 341:1725–1730, 1999.

The Writing Team for the Diabetes Control and Complications Trial/Epidemiology of Diabetes Interventions and Complications Research Group: Sustained effect of intensive treatment of type 1 diabetes mellitus on development and progression of diabetic nephropathy. The Epidemiology of Diabetes Interventions and Complications (EDIC) study. JAMA 290:2159–2167, 2003.

Ziyadeh FN, Hoffman BB, Han DC, et al: Long-term prevention of renal insufficiency, excess matrix gene expression, and glomerular mesangial matrix expansion by treatment with monoclonal antitransforming growth factor-beta antibody in db/db diabetic mice. Proc Natl Acad Sci USA 97:8015–8020, 2000.

CHAPTER 30

Dysproteinemias and Amyloidosis*

Paul W. Sanders

LIGHT CHAIN–RELATED KIDNEY DISEASES

Bence Jones proteins, which were originally found by Dr. William Macintyre in the urine of an ill patient, were characterized by Dr. Henry Bence Jones in 1847. Bence Jones proteins are now known to consist of immunoglobulin light chains, and the multiple kidney lesions associated with deposition of these proteins have been studied extensively. Plasma cells synthesize light chains that become part of the immunoglobulin molecule. Each light chain possesses two independent globular regions, termed constant and variable domains. Light chains can be isotyped as kappa or lambda, based on sequences in the constant region of the protein. The variable domain forms part of the antigen-binding site of the immunoglobulin molecule and derives from rearrangement of more than 20 gene segments. Thus, despite similar biochemical properties, no two light chains are identical. Disulfide bonding among light chains with higher-molecular-weight proteins (known as heavy chains) occurs during or shortly after heavy chain synthesis and forms the immunoglobulin molecule that is then secreted by plasma cells. A slight excess production of light, compared to heavy, chains appears to be required for efficient immunoglobulin synthesis, but may result in release of free light chains. Careful analysis of serum or urine from healthy individuals can reveal polyclonal light chains, albeit in very small amounts. Light chains, particularly the lambda isotype, can also form homodimers through disulfide bonding to another light chain before secretion.

Once in the blood stream, light chains are handled similarly to other low-molecular-weight proteins that are removed from the circulation by the kidney. Unlike albumin, monomers (molecular weight approximately 22 kD) and dimers (approximately 44 kD) are readily filtered through the glomerulus and reabsorbed by the proximal tubule. In the proximal tubule, endocytosis of light chains occurs through a single class of receptors with relative selectivity for these proteins. These receptors have now been identified as megalin and cubilin. The isoelectric point of light chains does not influence reabsorption rate. After endocytosis, lysosomal enzymes hydrolyze the proteins, and the amino acid components are returned to the circulation. Reabsorption is

saturable and allows delivery of light chains to the distal nephron and appearance in the urine as Bence Jones proteins.

Urinary Bence Jones proteins possess unusual heat solubility properties. When heated to 60°C, the proteins precipitate, but upon further heating to 100°C, the proteins resolubilize. Although this distinctive thermal property was initially used as a screening test for the presence of urinary Bence Jones proteins, it is insensitive and positive only when significant quantities are excreted in the urine. The qualitative urine dipstick test for protein also has a low sensitivity for detection of light chains. Although some Bence Jones proteins react with the chemical impregnated onto the strip, other light chains cannot be detected; the net charge of the protein may be an important determinant of this interaction. In healthy adults, the urinary concentration of light chain proteins, which are polyclonal because of escape into the circulation of small amounts of free light chain produced during normal immunoglobulin assembly, is about 2.5 μg/mL. Urinary light chain concentration is generally between 20 and 500 μg/mL in patients with monoclonal gammopathy of undetermined significance, and is often much higher (range 0.02 to 11.8 mg/mL) in patients with multiple myeloma or Waldenström's macroglobulinemia. The amount of monoclonal light chain excreted is often insufficient for detection using turbidimetric and heat tests. In addition, because of the insensitivity of routine serum protein electrophoresis and urinary protein electrophoresis, these tests are no longer recommended as screening tools in the diagnostic evaluation of the underlying etiology of kidney disease. Identification therefore rests with antibody detection assays (such as immunofixation electrophoresis or immunoelectrophoresis) using serum and urine. Immunofixation electrophoresis is sensitive and detects monoclonal light chains and immunoglobulins even in very low concentrations, but is basically a qualitative assay and is limited by interobserver variation. A more recent test, known as FREELITE, is now available and quantifies free light chains in the serum. Documenting the presence of monoclonal free light chains is of potential benefit since the vast majority of kidney lesions observed in plasma cell dyscrasias involve deposition of monotypic light chains and not heavy chains or intact immunoglobulins. Causes of monoclonal light chain proteinuria, a hallmark of plasma cell

*This chapter is in the public domain.

TABLE 30-1   Causes of Bence Jones Proteinuria

Multiple myeloma
AL-amyloidosis
Light chain deposition disease
Waldenström's macroglobulinemia
Monoclonal gammopathy of undetermined significance
POEMS syndrome (rare)
Heavy (mu) chain disease (rare)
Lymphoproliferative disease (rare)
Rifampin therapy (very rare)

POEMS, polyneuropathy, organomegaly, endocrinopathy, M protein, and skin changes.

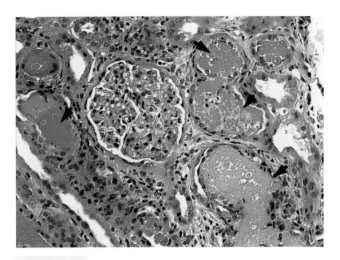

FIGURE 30-1   Renal biopsy tissue from a patient who had cast nephropathy. The findings include tubules filled with cast material (*arrows*) and presence of multinucleated giant cells. Glomeruli are typically normal in appearance (hematoxylin-eosin stain, original magnification ×20).

dyscrasias, are listed in Table 30-1. The most common cause of light chain proteinuria is multiple myeloma.

Virtually every compartment of the kidney can be damaged by monoclonal light chain deposition (Table 30-2). Histologic examination of necropsy specimens from 57 patients demonstrated kidney lesions in approximately 48%. Sixty-five percent of those patients with kidney lesions had cast nephropathy, or "myeloma kidney," whereas 21% had AL-amyloidosis and 11% had monoclonal light chain deposition disease (LCDD). The simultaneous occurrence of two or more of these lesions in the same patient is unusual. Light chains take the center stage in the pathogenesis of these kidney lesions. The type of kidney lesion induced by light chains depends on the physicochemical properties of these proteins.

CAST NEPHROPATHY

Pathology

Cast nephropathy is an inflammatory tubulointerstitial kidney lesion. Characteristically, multiple intraluminal proteinaceous casts are identified mainly in the distal

TABLE 30-2   Light Chain–Related Kidney Lesions

Glomerulopathies
  Light chain deposition disease
  AL-amyloidosis
  Cryoglobulinemia
Tubulointerstitial lesions
  Cast nephropathy ("myeloma kidney")
  Fanconi's syndrome
  Proximal tubule injury (acute tubular necrosis)
  Tubulointerstitial nephritis (rare)
Vascular lesions
Asymptomatic Bence Jones proteinuria
Hyperviscosity syndrome
Neoplastic cell infiltration (rare)

portion of the nephrons (Fig. 30-1). Casts may also be seen in the proximal tubule, or even in glomeruli when they are abundant. The casts are usually acellular, homogeneous, and eosinophilic with multiple fracture lines. Immunofluorescence and immunoelectron microscopy confirm that the casts contain light chains and Tamm-Horsfall glycoprotein. Persistence of the casts produces the giant cell inflammation and tubular atrophy that typify myeloma kidney. Glomeruli are usually normal in appearance.

Clinical Features

Renal failure from this lesion may present acutely or as a chronic progressive disease and may develop at any stage of myeloma. Diagnosis of multiple myeloma is usually evident when chronic bone pain, pathologic fractures, and hypercalcemia are complicated by proteinuria and impaired kidney function. However, many patients present to nephrologists primarily with symptoms of reduced kidney function or undefined proteinuria; further evaluation then confirms a malignant process. Cast nephropathy should therefore be considered when proteinuria (often more than 3 g/day), particularly without concomitant hypoalbuminemia or albuminuria, is found in a patient who is in the fourth decade of life or older. Hypertension is not a common consequence of cast nephropathy. Diagnosis of myeloma may be confirmed by finding monoclonal immunoglobulins or light chains in the serum and urine and by bone marrow examination, although typical intraluminal cast formation on kidney biopsy is virtually pathognomonic. Nearly all patients with cast nephropathy have detectable monoclonal light chains in the urine or blood.

Pathogenesis

Intravenous infusion of nephrotoxic human light chains in rats elevates proximal tubule pressure and simultaneously decreases single-nephron glomerular filtration rate; intraluminal protein casts can be identified in these kidneys. Myeloma casts contain Tamm-Horsfall glycoprotein and occur initially in the distal nephron, which provides an optimum environment for precipitation of light chains. Tamm-Horsfall glycoprotein, which is synthesized exclusively by cells of the thick ascending limb of the loop of Henle, comprises the major fraction of total urinary protein in healthy individuals and is the predominant constituent of urinary casts. Cast-forming light chains bind to a single domain in the peptide backbone of Tamm-Horsfall glycoprotein; binding results in coaggregation of these proteins and subsequent occlusion of the tubule lumen by the precipitated protein complexes, leading to intranephronal obstruction and renal functional impairment. Light chains with binding affinity for Tamm-Horsfall glycoprotein are potentially nephrotoxic.

Coaggregation of Tamm-Horsfall glycoprotein with light chains also depends on the ionic environment and the physicochemical properties of the light chain, because not all patients with myeloma develop cast nephropathy, even when the urinary excretion of light chains is very high. Increasing concentrations of sodium chloride or calcium, but not magnesium, facilitate coaggregation. The loop diuretic furosemide augments coaggregation and accelerates intraluminal obstruction in vivo in the rat. Finally, the lower tubule fluid flow rates of the distal nephron allow more time for light chains to interact with Tamm-Horsfall glycoprotein and subsequently to obstruct the lumen. Conditions that further reduce flow rates, such as volume depletion, can accelerate tubule obstruction or convert nontoxic light chains into cast-forming proteins. Volume depletion and hypercalcemia are recognized factors that promote acute renal failure from cast nephropathy.

Treatment and Prognosis

The principles used to treat cast nephropathy include decreasing the concentration of circulating light chains and preventing coaggregation of light chains with Tamm-Horsfall glycoprotein (Table 30-3). Prompt and effective

TABLE 30-3 Standard Therapy for Cast Nephropathy

Chemotherapy to decrease light chain production
Increase free water intake to 2–3 L per day as tolerated
Treat hypercalcemia aggressively
Avoid exposure to loop diuretics, radiocontrast agents, and nonsteroidal anti-inflammatory agents

chemotherapy should start upon diagnosis of multiple myeloma. Standard treatment includes alkylating agents and steroids. Intermittent treatment with melphalan and prednisone decreases circulating levels of light chains and stabilizes or improves kidney function in two thirds of patients who present with impaired kidney function. Fanconi's syndrome may also resolve with this therapy. Because the primary route of elimination of melphalan is through the kidneys, impaired kidney function complicates dosing. In addition, gastrointestinal absorption of melphalan is unpredictable. An alternative chemotherapeutic regimen that includes vincristine, adriamycin, and either methylprednisolone (VAMP) or dexamethasone (VAD) has been used successfully. VAD can induce a remission more rapidly than melphalan and prednisone and allows faster reduction in the amount of circulating light chains. Often only two courses of treatment are necessary to determine whether a patient will respond to this chemotherapy. Thus, VAD may be particularly beneficial in the setting of impaired kidney function related to deposition of light chains, and the physician can rapidly determine the efficacy of such an approach. Myeloablative therapy with allogeneic bone marrow transplantation is effective in controlling kidney dysfunction in myeloma, but has a significant mortality and is currently limited to the small population who is suitable and has an HLA-compatible relative. Although not curative, high-dose chemotherapy followed by autologous stem cell transplantation is considered by many investigators to be an appropriate choice for the suitable patient with myeloma. Although the morbidity and mortality of this treatment are not inconsequential, there does appear to be a survival advantage of this treatment over other chemotherapeutic approaches.

Plasmapheresis removes light chains from the blood stream effectively over a short time period. Although there is no apparent therapeutic advantage of plasmapheresis in the management of chronic kidney disease associated with multiple myeloma and light chain deposition, this therapy is useful in the setting of acute renal failure or hyperviscosity syndrome. In particular, the patient who has a documented acute decline in kidney function and multiple myeloma with light chain proteinuria may benefit from plasmapheresis.

Prevention of aggregation of light chains with Tamm-Horsfall glycoprotein is a cornerstone of therapy. Volume repletion, normalization of electrolytes, and avoidance of complicating factors such as loop diuretics and nonsteroidal anti-inflammatory agents are helpful in preserving and improving kidney function. Although not all patients with light chain proteinuria develop acute renal failure following exposure to radiocontrast agents, predicting who is at risk for this complication is difficult, suggesting caution in the use of radiocontrast agents in all patients with multiple myeloma. Daily fluid intake of up to 3 L in the form of electrolyte-free fluids should be encouraged, although serum sodium concentration should be monitored periodically. Alkalinization of the urine with oral sodium bicarbonate (or citrate) to keep the urine pH greater than 7 may also be therapeutic, but may be mitigated by the requisite sodium loading, which favors coaggregation of these proteins and also should be avoided in patients who have symptomatic extracellular fluid volume overload. At present, there is little definitive clinical evidence to support the use of oral bicarbonate therapy in myeloma patients, unless there is another indication for treatment, such as acidemia.

Hypercalcemia occurs in more than 25% of patients with multiple myeloma. In addition to being directly nephrotoxic, hypercalcemia enhances the nephrotoxicity of light chains. Treatment of volume contraction with the infusion of saline often corrects mild hypercalcemia. Loop diuretics also increase calcium excretion, but furosemide, because it may facilitate nephrotoxicity from light chains, should not be administered until the patient is clinically euvolemic, and can usually be avoided by using bisphosphonates. Glucocorticoid therapy (such as prednisone, 60 mg/day) is helpful for acute management of the multiple myeloma as well as hypercalcemia. Bisphosphonates, such as pamidronate and zoledronic acid, are used to treat moderate hypercalcemia (serum calcium greater than 3.25 mmol/L, or 13 mg/dL) unresponsive to other measures. Bisphosphonates lower serum calcium by interfering with osteoclast-mediated bone resorption. Although hypercalcemia of myeloma responds to bisphosphonates, these agents can be nephrotoxic and should be administered only to euvolemic patients. Kidney function should be monitored closely during therapy. Treatment with pamidronate or zoledronic acid allows outpatient management of mild hypercalcemia. Besides controlling hypercalcemia, bisphosphonates appear to inhibit growth of plasma cells and have therefore become part of the standard treatment of multiple myeloma, particularly in patients with osseous lesions and bone pain.

Dialysis should be used as indicated. Perhaps 5% to 10% of patients who are dialysis dependent because of cast nephropathy regain sufficient kidney function to stop dialysis, so intensive efforts to reverse this lesion, including plasmapheresis, should be considered, especially in suitable patients who present with acute kidney failure. Kidney transplantation has also been successfully performed in selected patients with multiple myeloma in remission. Because the light chain is the underlying cause of cast nephropathy, tests that ensure absence of circulating free light chains are useful in the evaluation of candidacy for kidney transplantation.

Renal functional impairment decreases survival in multiple myeloma. Median survival for patients with reduced kidney function is 20 months, compared with a median survival of 20 to 40 months for the general population of patients with myeloma. Major predictors of prolonged survival include the stage of the disease, decline in serum creatinine concentration at 1 month into treatment to less than 3.4 mg/dL, and response to chemotherapy. Response to chemotherapy is important: median survival time for responders is 36 months, but only 10 months for nonresponders.

OTHER TUBULOINTERSTITIAL KIDNEY LESIONS

Proximal tubule injury, including Fanconi's syndrome, and tubulointerstitial nephritis can occur. Although there is growing concern that proteinuria alone may be nephrotoxic, elegant studies by Batuman's group demonstrated that endocytosis of monoclonal light chains into proximal tubular cells activates nuclear factor κB. In turn, nuclear factor κB promotes expression of cytokines and chemokines that participate in tubulointerstitial inflammation and scarring. Fanconi's syndrome may precede overt multiple myeloma. Plasma cell dyscrasia should therefore be considered in the differential diagnosis when this syndrome occurs in adults. More severe damage to the proximal tubule epithelium can produce clinical manifestations of acute renal failure. A major mechanism of damage to the proximal epithelium is related to accumulation of toxic light chains in the endolysosomal system. An inflammatory tubulointerstitial nephritis with cellular infiltrates including eosinophils and active tubular damage has also been described. A careful search usually detects subtle light chain deposits along the tubular basement membranes almost exclusively in the areas of interstitial inflammation. This interstitial inflammatory pattern is sometimes associated with glomerular involvement, and cast formation is rare. Without detection of the deposits of light chains along the basement membrane, this lesion may be mistakenly considered to be a hypersensitivity reaction to drugs, most notably nonsteroidal anti-inflammatory agents.

LIGHT CHAIN DEPOSITION DISEASE

Light chain deposition disease is a systemic disease, but typically presents initially with isolated renal injury related to a glomerular lesion associated with nonamyloid electron-dense granular deposits of monoclonal light chains with or without heavy chains. Isolated deposition of heavy chains, termed heavy chain deposition disease, is extremely rare. LCDD may be accompanied by the other clinical features of multiple myeloma or another lymphoproliferative disorder, or may be the sole manifestation of a plasma cell dyscrasia.

Pathology

Nodular glomerulopathy with distortion of the glomerular architecture by deposition of amorphous, eosinophilic material is the most common pathologic finding

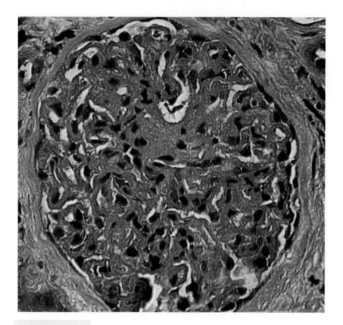

FIGURE 30-2 Glomerulus from a patient with kappa light chain deposition disease showing expansion of the mesangium, related to matrix protein deposition, and associated compression of capillary lumens (hematoxylin-eosin stain, original magnification ×40).

observed with light microscopy (Fig. 30-2). These nodules, which are composed of light chains and extracellular matrix proteins, begin in the mesangium. This appearance is reminiscent of diabetic nephropathy. Less commonly, other glomerular morphologic changes besides nodular glomerulopathy can be seen in LCDD. Immunofluorescence microscopy demonstrates the presence of monotypic light chains in the glomeruli. Under electron microscopy, deposits of light chain proteins are present in a subendothelial position along the glomerular capillary wall, along the outer aspect of tubular basement membranes, and in the mesangium. Tubular cell damage is also notable and obvious even in the early stage of the disease in some patients.

Clinical Features

The typical clinical presentation is reminiscent of a rapidly progressive glomerulonephritis. The major findings in LCDD include proteinuria, sometimes in the nephrotic range, microscopic hematuria, and impaired kidney function. Albumin and monoclonal free light chains are the dominant proteins in the urine. The presence of albuminuria and other findings of nephrotic syndrome are important clues to the presence of glomerular injury and not cast nephropathy. The amount of excreted light chain is usually less than that found in cast nephropathy. Reduced kidney function in untreated patients is common. Because renal manifestations gener-

ally predominate and are often the sole presenting features, it is not uncommon for nephrologists to diagnose the plasma cell dyscrasia. Kidney biopsy is necessary to establish the diagnosis. Other organ dysfunction, especially liver and heart, can develop and is related to deposition of light chains in those organs. Although extrarenal manifestations of overt multiple myeloma can manifest at presentation or over time, a majority (approximately 74%) of patients with LCDD will not develop myeloma or other malignant lymphoproliferative disease.

Pathogenesis

The pathogenesis of LCDD differs from that of cast nephropathy. The response to light chain deposition includes expansion of the mesangium by extracellular matrix proteins to form nodules and eventually glomerular sclerosis. Experimental studies have shown that mesangial cells exposed to light chains obtained from patients with biopsy-proven LCDD produce transforming growth factor-β (TGF-β), which serves as an autacoid to stimulate these same cells to produce matrix proteins, including type IV collagen, laminin, and fibronectin. Thus, TGF-β plays a central role in glomerular sclerosis from LCDD.

Although deposition of light chain is the prominent feature of these glomerular lesions, heavy chains, along with light chains, can occasionally be identified in the deposits, prompting some researchers to suggest the term *monoclonal light and heavy chain deposition disease*. In those specimens, the punctate electron-dense deposits appear larger and more extensive than those deposits that contain only light chains, but it is unclear whether the clinical course of these patients differs from the course of isolated light chain deposition without heavy chain components.

Treatment and Prognosis

The treatment of LCDD is difficult. Randomized controlled trials are unavailable, but patients appear to benefit from the same chemotherapy as that given for multiple myeloma, particularly if the reduction in kidney function is mild at presentation. Five of eight patients with serum creatinine concentrations less than 4.0 mg/dL at the time of diagnosis did not progress with chemotherapy, whereas 9 of 11 patients with higher creatinine concentrations at presentation progressed to endstage renal disease despite therapy. Early diagnosis is therefore important. Caution should be exercised to limit the total dose of the alkylating agent that is used. The role of plasmapheresis in this disease has not been determined and cannot currently be recommended. The 5-year survival rate is approximately 70%, but is reduced by coexistent myeloma.

CHAPTER 31

Thrombotic Microangiopathies

Sharon Adler   Cynthia C. Nast

The thrombotic microangiopathies (TMAs) are a group of diverse disorders that are classified together based on common morphologic features in the kidney. Table 31-1 lists some of the more common underlying causes. This review focuses on four of the most common: thrombotic thrombocytopenic purpura (TTP), hemolytic uremic syndrome (HUS), the antiphospholipid syndrome, and scleroderma renal crisis.

PATHOLOGY

Figure 31-1 demonstrates the characteristic features of the thrombotic microangiopathies. The histopathologic changes are characterized by fibrin accumulation in the lumina and walls of arteries, arterioles, and glomerular capillaries. By light microscopy, fibrin and platelet thrombi are present in many or few capillaries of variable numbers of glomeruli. As the disease progresses, glomeruli may have a lobular appearance with capillary wall double contours, or may be ischemic, characterized by wrinkled and partially collapsed capillaries (see Fig. 31-1A, B). Arterioles and to a lesser extent arteries are thrombosed and contain fibrin in the walls, which also show muscular hypertrophy and mucoid intimal thickening, resulting in luminal narrowing (see Fig. 31-1C, D). Immunofluorescence reveals fibrin in glomerular capillaries and vascular walls, and lumina without immune complexes. Ultrastructurally, glomerular capillary walls have wide subendothelial zones containing flocculent electron-lucent and -dense material representing altered fibrin, which may contain trapped erythrocytes (see Fig. 31-1E, F). There may be a new layer of basement membrane material beneath the widened subendothelial zone, accounting for the double-contour appearance of capillaries. Endothelial cells are swollen, capillary lumina are narrowed, and occasionally capillaries contain tactoids of fibrin. In ischemic glomeruli, capillary basement membranes are wrinkled. There are no electron-dense (immune complex) deposits.

All thrombotic microangiopathic renal lesions are morphologically similar. Subtle differences have been described. Some have suggested that in biopsies from patients with HUS, there may be more fibrin and erythrocytes within the thrombi compared with more platelets in TTP thrombi. Patients with HUS may also be more likely to have cortical necrosis than those with TTP.

However, the pathologic findings are not sufficiently different to allow a specific diagnosis based on histology. The distinction among the thrombotic microangiopathies requires clinical assessment.

THROMBOTIC THROMBOCYTOPENIC PURPURA

Pathogenesis

Thrombotic thrombocytopenic purpura was once thought to be a disorder pathogenetically linked to HUS, but differing somewhat in the involvement of end organs or severity. However, recent information regarding pathogenesis underscores the notion that TTP and HUS are actually pathogenetically distinct entities. TTP is characterized by diminished activity of von Willebrand factor (vWF) cleaving protein, due to either an inherited mutation or to the presence of an immunoglobulin interfering with the function of the vWF cleaving protein, resulting in abnormal amount or size of the circulating vWF multimers. In TTP, unusually large vWF binds to extracellular matrix and platelets, induces platelet aggregation and activation, and leads to intravascular platelet thrombi, organ ischemia, and necrosis. Unusually large vWF is due to defective vWF cleavage. It is found in active TTP but not in remission, and distinguishes TTP from other causes of hemolysis, thrombosis, or thrombocytopenia. The vWF cleaving protein is a member of a recently described family of zinc metalloproteinases named "a disintegrin and metalloprotease with thrombospondin type 1 repeat" (ADAMTS). Mutations of ADAMTS13 are observed in patients with familial and recurrent forms of TTP. Diminished ADAMTS13 activity distinguishes patients with TTP from those with hemolytic uremic syndrome, in that patients with TTP tend to have functional vWF cleaving protein activity that is less than 5% that of healthy controls. Inhibition of a less severe nature may be seen in other disorders, including HUS.

Clinical Presentation and Laboratory Manifestations

The classic pentad of TTP consists of fever, microangiopathic hemolytic anemia, thrombocytopenic purpura, kidney disease, and central nervous system symptoms

TABLE 31-1   Causes of Thrombotic Microangiopathy

Infectious	Medications
Enteric pathogens	Mitomycin C
Escherichia coli 0157:H7	Cyclosporine
Shigella species	Clopidogrel
Salmonella species	Ticlopidine
Campylobacter jejuni	Vinblastine
Yersinia	Cisplatinum
HIV	Bleomycin
Mycoplasma pneumoniae	Cytosine arabinoside
Legionella infection	Daunorubicin
Coxsackie A and B virus	
Systemic Diseases	**Miscellaneous**
Systemic lupus erythematosus	Vaccinations
Malignant hypertension	
Neoplasms	
Thrombotic thrombocytopenic	
purpura	
Hemolytic uremic syndrome	
Antiphospholipid syndrome	
Scleroderma	

ranging from lethargy, somnolence, and confusion to focal neurologic signs, seizures, or coma. The neurologic symptoms often dominate the overall clinical picture. The hemolytic anemia is characterized by the presence of numerous circulating fragmented erythrocytes in the form of schistocytes and helmet cells, which are presumably produced by shear stress injury as blood flows through vessels narrowed by platelet thrombi. Associated high lactate dehydrogenase (LDH) levels correlate with the severity of the disease. Renal signs and symptoms are common but often mild. Some have estimated that kidney involvement is present in as many as 88% of patients. Manifestations include microscopic (rarely gross) hematuria, mild to moderate proteinuria, and azotemia. Acute renal failure occurs in up to 10% of patients, and the need for dialysis is uncommon. The disorder may occur either as an acquired acute disease or in a chronic relapsing form. The acquired forms may be triggered by certain medications, of which quinine, mitomycin-C, calcineurin inhibitors, and ticlopidine are the most common. Antibodies to vWF cleaving protein have been identified in patients with ticlopidine-associated TTP, but a systematic search for antibodies associated with other medication-related TTP has not been reported. TTP rarely has been reported in association with clopidogrel therapy. Acquired TTP may also complicate collagen-vascular disorders such as systemic lupus erythematosus (SLE). Neoplasms and infections (most notably human immunodeficiency virus) have been associated with TTP. For many patients with acquired TTP, no underlying cause is established. ADAMTS13 activity may be modestly low in patients with some of these conditions, including those with neoplasms, liver disease, and chronic inflammatory conditions. However, antibodies to the ADAMTS13 vWF cleaving protein are not always identi-

fied, suggesting other potential mechanisms whereby its function may be disturbed. Most often, TTP in adults does not recur, particularly if an underlying causative factor can be eliminated. However, in 11% to 36% of patients, recurrences are experienced at irregular intervals.

The chronic relapsing form, due to mutations in the gene for ADAMTS13 on chromosome 9q34, is rare. These patients usually present in childhood, although for unknown reasons, some may present later in life. Recurrences at regular intervals are frequent. This disorder is sometimes referred to as Upshaw-Schulman syndrome.

Currently, the measurements of ultralarge vWF, the activity of the vWF cleaving protein, and genetic assessments for mutations in the ADAMTS 13 gene are research tools that are not readily available clinically.

Therapy

Plasma or cryosupernatant (cryoprecipitate-poor plasma) infusion is the mainstay of therapy and provides missing enzyme activity. However, plasma exchange may provide synergism by removing any circulating vWF cleaving protein inhibitor (e.g., in the acquired form) and by facilitating the infusion of large amounts of fresh frozen plasma (FFP) (average course of FFP is approximately 21 L). Steroids may be useful adjunctive therapy. Supportive dialysis therapy may be required in cases with severe kidney involvement. Rituximab has been used with some success in a few refractory patients. Splenectomy and platelet inhibitors are of unproven value but are occasionally used in desperation in patients refractory to standard therapy. Platelet infusions and aspirin are contraindicated. Response to therapy is best monitored by following serial serum LDH levels.

Course and Prognosis

Untreated, the mortality of TTP approaches 90%. With the advent of plasma infusion with or without plasma exchange therapy in the early 1990s, 60% to 90% of patients now survive. Most patients who go into remission have an excellent long-term prognosis. A subset of patients develop chronic TTP or have TTP as a result of an inherited mutation and require long-term treatment, including repetitive infusions of plasma or cryosupernatant for acute exacerbations.

HEMOLYTIC UREMIC SYNDROME

Pathogenesis

As described previously, HUS and TTP were once thought to be different clinical expressions of a single disease

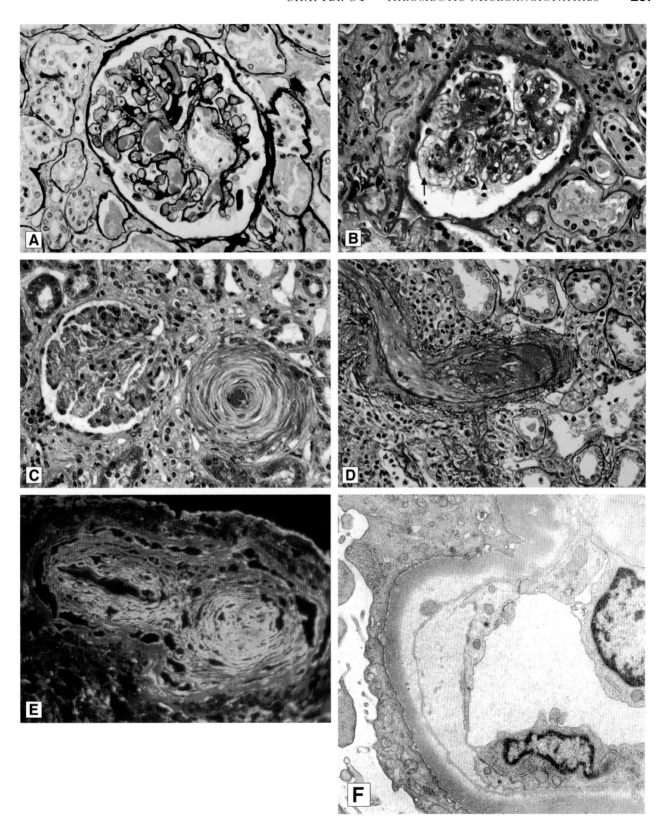

FIGURE 31-1 Kidney biopsy findings in thrombotic microangiopathy. *A,* Glomerulus showing many capillary lumina occluded by fibrin thrombi (periodic acid–methenamine silver, original magnification ×20). *B,* Glomerulus with an membranoproliferative glomerulonephritis type I pattern of injury including capillary wall double contours (*arrowheads*) and a capillary microaneurysm (*arrow*) overlying an area of mesangiolysis (periodic acid–Schiff, original magnification ×20). *C,* Ischemic glomerulus with wrinkled and partially collapsed capillary walls is adjacent to an arteriole. The arteriole has typical "onion skin" thickening of the wall and a fibrin thrombus (Masson's trichrome, original magnification ×10). *D,* An interlobular artery with mucoid intimal thickening, fibrin in the wall and lumen, and swollen endothelial cells (periodic acid–methenamine silver, original magnification ×10). *E,* Immunofluorescence for fibrin showing positive staining in the wall and lumen of an artery, similar to (*D*) (original magnification ×10). *F,* Electron microscopy of a capillary wall from an involved glomerulus. There is a wide subendothelial lucent zone containing flocculent material, the endothelial cell is swollen, and podocyte foot processes are effaced (original magnification ×6,000).

process, with HUS presenting predominantly with features of hemolytic anemia and kidney disease. However, recent biochemical and genetic information regarding defective vWF cleaving protein and ADAMTS13 in TTP but not HUS challenge that assumption, and these disorders are now believed to be distinct.

Hemolytic uremic syndrome has two major clinical presentations: a diarrheal form (D+HUS) and a nondiarrheal form (D-HUS). In D+HUS, it is postulated that a Shiga-like toxin binds to colonic epithelium and induces elaboration of chemokines and cytokines resulting in polymorphonuclear (PMN) influx, and abrogation of barrier function, permitting the Shiga-like toxin to enter the circulation free or bound to PMNs. Circulating toxin then binds to glomerular/renal arteriolar and proximal tubular epithelial cell receptors, resulting in local inflammation, endothelial injury, thrombosis, and acute renal failure.

The pathogenesis of D-HUS is less well understood. In circumstances associated with medication use, neoplasms, infections, pregnancy, or collagen-vascular disease, presumably a change in the coagulation cascade or in the endothelial cell membrane creates a prothrombotic environment. Deficiency in the antithrombotic prostacyclin prostaglandin I_2 has been implicated in some cases of HUS. In addition, D-HUS may rarely present as a familial disease associated with impaired regulation of complement activation. Familial forms of D-HUS have been associated with a genetic deficiency or loss of activity of complement factor H, and with genetic mutations in membrane cofactor protein, a surface-bound complement regulator. In those with reduced levels of factor H there is an autosomal-recessive mode of inheritance associated with low C3 levels and earlier onset of disease. Autosomal-dominant inheritance is related to abnormal function of factor H with normal serum levels, and patients have normal complement levels and later onset. This latter form also is associated more often with a number of underlying factors or events detailed following, which may initiate complement activation. In all forms of D-HUS, the loss of regulatory proteins permits excess complement activation likely through the alternate pathway, resulting in production of complement cleavage products. These products injure endothelial cells and stimulate platelet aggregation, thus initiating or exacerbating HUS.

Clinical Presentation and Laboratory Manifestations

Hemolytic uremic syndrome presents as a classic triad consisting of microangiopathic hemolytic anemia, thrombocytopenia, and kidney disease, with peak incidence in the summer. The signs and symptoms tend to overlap with those of TTP, but in HUS the hematologic and especially the renal features predominate. The

D+HUS is associated with infection with organisms producing a Shiga-like toxin (predominantly *Escherichia coli* O157:H7) or other enteric infections (*Shigella, Salmonella, Campylobacter,* or *Yersinia*). Epidemics associated with ingestion of undercooked hamburger occur sporadically. The nondiarrheal form (D-HUS) is associated with a number of underlying clinical predisposing factors detailed in Table 31-1, which include genetic predisposition, medication use, nongastrointestinal infections, pregnancy, neoplasms, collagen-vascular diseases, systemic vasculitis, and bone marrow transplantation.

In the D+HUS form, diarrhea ranges from watery to hemorrhagic. The other systemic manifestations of the diarrheal and nondiarrheal forms are similar. The classical features are microangiopathic hemolytic anemia and kidney dysfunction, frequently manifesting as acute renal failure in adults, and less commonly in children. Leukocytosis and fever are seen frequently. Other systemic manifestations include fluid and electrolyte disturbances, severe hypertension, cerebral edema and seizures, congestive heart failure, pulmonary edema, and cardiac arrhythmias.

Therapy

Therapy is supportive only. The replacement of factor H by FFP infusion has not been efficacious even in those individuals from families with documented factor H deficiency, but recombinant factor H is being developed as a potential therapy for these individuals. There is no proven value for treatment with antibiotics, anticoagulants, fibrinolytics, intravenous immunoglobulin, plasma infusion, plasmapheresis, prostacyclin infusion, or antiplatelet agents.

Course and Prognosis

A poor outcome has been associated with marked leukocytosis, older age at onset, the presence of D-HUS, pregnancy, *Shigella* or pneumococcal infection, anuria, persistent proteinuria, hypertension, or cortical necrosis.

ANTIPHOSPHOLIPID SYNDROME

Pathogenesis

The antiphospholipid syndrome is induced by the actions of a family of autoantibodies with broad reactivity to phospholipid epitopes or the phospholipid-binding protein β_2-glycoprotein I, resulting in TMA. It now appears that most autoimmune anticardiolipin antibodies are directed against the phospholipid-binding protein rather than the phospholipid and do not actually interact unless the binding protein is present. The syndrome may be present as a primary disorder or as a secondary disorder, the latter usually in association with SLE. Numerous mechanisms have been proposed to account for the hypercoagulable state. Activation of endothelial cells with up-regulation of adhesion molecules, the elaboration of cytokines, and alterations in the balance of prothrombotic thromboxane and anticoagulant prostacyclins have been postulated. Oxidant-mediated endothelial injury may play a role, with autoantibodies to oxidized low-density lipoprotein (LDL) occurring along with anticardiolipin antibodies. In fact, some anticardiolipin antibodies crossreact with oxidized LDL. Finally, antiphospholipid antibodies may interfere with the function of phospholipid-binding proteins involved in the regulation of coagulation. Candidates for such interference include β_2-glycoprotein I, prothrombin, protein C, and tissue factor.

Clinical and Laboratory Manifestations

A diagnostic classification has recently been adopted and requires at least one laboratory and one clinical manifestation.

Diagnostic laboratory studies fall into one of three categories: lupus anticoagulants, anticardiolipin antibodies, and antibodies to phospholipid-binding proteins. Lupus anticoagulants are identified by abnormalities in coagulation assays. These include prolonged prothrombin time or partial thromboplastin time, particularly when the latter is not normalized when mixed with normal serum (i.e., indicating the presence of an antibody-mediated process rather than a factor deficiency); abnormal Russell viper venom test results; or abnormalities in the kaolin cephalin clotting time or the thromboplastin inhibition test. Anticardiolipin antibodies are identified by immunoassays that measure pathologic reactivity to anionic phospholipids, including the anticardiolipin antibody or antiphospholipid antibody, or by a false-positive VDRL test result. Finally, antibodies to the phospholipid-binding protein β_2-glycoprotein I are frequent, but this characteristic is not yet included in the diagnostic classification. The anticardiolipin antibody or lupus anticoagulant must be detected twice at least 6 weeks apart. Approximately 1% to 5% of healthy individuals have circulating anticardiolipin antibodies. It is unclear how many of these results are false positives and how many occur in individuals who will eventually develop a clinical syndrome. The presence of these antibodies and anticoagulants are associated with venous thromboses, premature myocardial infarction, and cerebrovascular accidents. In patients with SLE, it has been estimated that 12% to 30% have anticardiolipin antibodies and 15% to 34% have evidence of a lupus anticoagu-

lant. As many as 50% to 70% of these individuals may have an associated clinical event over the course of 20 years of follow-up.

The clinical diagnostic criteria include a vascular occlusion involving veins, arteries, or capillaries in any organ or pregnancy complications including at least three spontaneous premature abortions before the 10th gestational week, death of a normal fetus after 10 weeks, or prematurity of a normal fetus (earlier than 34 weeks). The antiphospholipid syndrome may involve numerous organs, including the central nervous system, kidney, endocrine, gastrointestinal tract, lungs, skin, and cerebrovascular and cardiovascular systems. Thrombocytopenia is frequent.

Kidney manifestations in the antiphospholipid syndrome were recognized relatively recently, and are usually mild, although there are exceptions. Kidney involvement is noted in fewer than 25% of patients with the anticardiolipin syndrome. The kidney manifestations are protean, and include microscopic hematuria, proteinuria, rarely acute renal failure, mild to malignant hypertension, cortical necrosis, thrombotic microangiopathy, progressive chronic kidney disease sometimes culminating in endstage renal disease, and thrombosis of kidney allografts. Reports of these manifestations include case reports and small series, and the actual frequencies of these manifestations are not known. It is unclear whether the superimposition of the antiphospholipid syndrome on a classical form of lupus nephritis worsens the prognosis.

The syndrome may occur in a "catastrophic" form, defined by involvement of at least three organ systems virtually contemporaneously in time. The kidney is the most frequently affected organ in the crisis form and is involved in 78% of cases. This is accompanied by hypertension, which is often malignant. Dialysis is required in 25% of those with kidney involvement. Other end organ involvement includes pulmonary (66%), central nervous system (56%), cardiac (50%), and dermatologic (50%) types. Disseminated intravascular coagulation is uncommon.

Therapy

The mainstay of therapy is anticoagulation. Therapy with warfarin is recommended for the primary syndrome and for those with SLE. In the past, it was recommended that the international normalized ratio (INR) should be at least 3. A recently published study suggested that there were low rates of recurrent thrombosis in patients in whom the INR was kept in the range of 2 to 3. In addition to anticoagulation, therapy should include avoidance of prothrombotic drugs such as calcineurin inhibitors, oral contraceptives, hydralazine, procainamide, and chlorpromazine. Aspirin should be prescribed for women with prior pregnancy complications. The role of hydroxychloroquine or chloroquine to prevent thrombosis in patients with SLE is controversial. Although not evidence based, glucocorticosteroids, plasmapheresis, and intravenous immunoglobulin have been implemented as salvage therapy in patients with severe or multiple organ involvement.

Course and Prognosis

The antiphospholipid syndrome requires long-term anticoagulation. Mortality for patients with the catastrophic syndrome is high, approximating 50%.

SCLERODERMA RENAL CRISIS

Pathology

The renal parenchymal changes in scleroderma are similar to those in other forms of thrombotic microangiopathy, but there are subtle features more often associated with scleroderma. The involved vessels usually are the arcuate and interlobular arteries, with less common abnormalities of arterioles. Arteries are thickened, with loose edematous and mucinous intimal fibrosis and swollen endothelial cells, without inflammation. There often is a concentric appearance to proliferating intimal cells producing an "onion skin" effect in the artery walls. In more chronic disease, this pattern may be observed due to reduplication of the internal elastic lamina. Muscular hypertrophy is variable, and fibrin is found in the walls or lumina of arteries and arterioles with luminal narrowing. There may be fibrosis of the adventitia of arteries. Glomeruli display varying degrees of ischemia with capillary wall wrinkling and other features of thrombotic microangiopathy, although capillary thrombi are comparatively rare. The juxtaglomerular apparatus often is expanded. Areas of infarcted renal parenchyma are found in patients with cortical necrosis. The immunofluorescence and electron microscopic changes are similar to those of the other thrombotic microangiopathies.

Pathogenesis

The pathogenesis of scleroderma is complex and not fully understood, involving genetic and environmental factors. Exposure to infectious agents, chemicals, and physical agents has been proposed as a predisposing event, but no findings are conclusive. Scleroderma is a lesion of fibrosis and vascular injury, encompassing abnormalities of the microvasculature, cell- and humoral-mediated immune alterations, and aberrant production and accumulation of extracellular matrix. It is possible that this heterogeneous disorder may have different pathogenetic mechanisms operative in different affected individuals.

Vascular dysfunction likely is initiated by endothelial injury, which appears to be the primary process in scleroderma renal crisis. Causes of the damage to endothelium may include effects of antiendothelial antibodies with up-regulation of growth factors and cytokines, decrease in intrinsic complement regulatory proteins, proteolytic activities in serum, and cell-mediated immunity. Endothelial injury results in permeability and vascular intimal edema, myointimal proliferation with increased extracellular matrix production, platelet aggregation and adhesion, and fibrin deposition. The subsequent vascular narrowing and reduced renal perfusion increase renin production, exacerbating hypertension. There is no firm evidence that cold temperatures, cardiac dysfunction, pregnancy, or specific drugs such as nonsteroidal anti-inflammatory drugs (NSAIDs) or calcium channel blockers induce this process, although high steroid doses over time have been linked to renal crisis.

A plethora of autoantibodies is associated with scleroderma, and there appears to be some specificity linked to the pattern of clinical disease presentation. Anti-RNA polymerase III and anti-Th/To ribonucleoprotein are identified frequently in patients who develop scleroderma renal crisis. It is not known whether these phenotype-specific antibodies have a pathogenetic role or are merely markers of disease. Abnormal immune response may influence the onset or progression of scleroderma via several mechanisms. Antibody binding can change the sites of antigen proteolysis or promote the uptake of complexed proteins, which can spread the immune response to different antigenic components (epitope spreading), enhancing the immune reaction. Autoantibodies may be directly pathogenic; 25% to 85% of patients with scleroderma have antiendothelial cell antibodies, which could induce injury, resulting in vascular damage as described previously. Affected tissues often are infiltrated with T cells and macrophages, possibly in response to environmental stimuli, with subsequent cytokine and growth factor release. In addition, altered B cells may up-regulate complement receptor signaling, further inducing target cell injury and augmenting T-cell effector responses.

In patients with scleroderma, fibroblasts overproduce extracellular matrix components, but it is not known whether this is an abnormal response to injury or a dysregulation of the relevant gene expression. Fibroblasts in scleroderma patients express increased levels of TGF-β receptors and become persistently activated by small amounts of TGF-β. When there is immune activation due to one or more inciting events, fibroblasts produce excessive amounts of extracellular matrix material, which accumulates in the target organs. Fibroblast stimulation appears to be a final pathway, regardless of the upstream pathogenetic mechanisms involved.

Clinical and Laboratory Manifestations

Kidney disease was not noted as a major cause of morbidity and mortality in systemic sclerosis until 1952. Classical scleroderma renal crisis, defined by the presence of new-onset often severe hypertension or rapidly progressive acute renal failure occurring in a patient with systemic sclerosis, occurs in approximately 10% of patients. Patients with diffuse systemic sclerosis carry the greatest risk, with up to 25% of patients developing this complication. In contrast, patients with the CREST syndrome (calcinosis, Raynaud's phenomenon, esophagitis, sclerodactyly, and telangiectasias) and limited or localized systemic sclerosis are much less likely to develop renal crisis (approximately 1%). Increased risk for developing renal crisis is associated with the presence of diffuse disease, especially rapid skin thickening on the trunk or proximal limbs; antitopoisomerase III (Scl-70) as opposed to anticentromere antibodies; African-American ethnicity; male gender; onset of scleroderma within the prior 5 years, especially the prior 1 year; fatigue, weight loss and polyarthritis; carpal tunnel syndrome; edema; and tendon friction rubs. Nevertheless, patients with minimal signs of scleroderma have on occasion been reported to develop renal crisis.

The hypertension and increased plasma renin levels characteristic of the disease emerge abruptly, and there are cases in which these were clearly normal within days of an acute presentation. Microscopic hematuria, proteinuria, and diminished GFR frequently accompany accelerated or malignant hypertension at presentation, but they are not helpful in predicting the onset of renal crisis. Striking blood pressure elevation is the most common presenting manifestation, occurring in 90% of patients. The diastolic blood pressure exceeds 120 mm Hg in 30%. In the minority of patients with normal blood pressures, a significant increment for that individual within the normal range is often observed. In the latter setting, microangiopathic hemolytic anemia and thrombocytopenia are clinical clues to the presence of scleroderma renal crisis. The occasional occurrence of scleroderma, acute renal failure, hemolytic anemia, and thrombocytopenia in the absence of severe hypertension suggests that thrombotic microangiopathy may occur in scleroderma via a mechanism independent of or in addition to malignant hypertension.

Extrarenal manifestations occasionally precede the onset of renal crisis, including pericardial effusions, congestive heart failure, ventricular arrhythmias, microangiopathic hemolytic anemia, and thrombocytopenia. Seizures occur rarely with renal crisis.

Plasma renin levels are invariably high in these patients, but whether this is the cause of the hypertension and renal ischemia or a reflection of it has not been resolved. In an era of angiotensin-converting enzyme (ACE) inhibitor therapy, which causes increased renin levels, following this parameter does not have any clinical utility. Other laboratory features on presentation include non-nephrotic proteinuria, dysmorphic (usually microscopic) hematuria, and an elevated serum creatinine. Microscopic angiopathic hemolytic anemia occurs in 43% of patients. Thrombocytopenia occurs, but the platelet count rarely falls below 50,000/mm³.

Mild hypertension, proteinuria, microhematuria, and azotemia may be noted in as many as 50% to 60% of patients with systemic sclerosis who do not have renal crisis, and up to 80% may have kidney disease if abnormalities on kidney biopsy are included in the definition. However, most often, causes of these processes other than systemic sclerosis are identifiable. These include use of D-penicillamine, severe congestive heart failure, prerenal azotemia, and NSAID use. Membranous nephropathy and perinuclear-staining antineutrophil cytoplasmic antibody (P-ANCA)-positive pauci-immune crescentic glomerulonephritis have also occasionally been reported in patients with systemic sclerosis.

Therapy

The use of ACE inhibitors is the mainstay of treatment for patients with renal crisis. Inasmuch as they are effective in patients with hypertension and in the occasional patient without hypertension, their mechanism of action likely reaches beyond blood pressure control. If ACE inhibitors alone cannot adequately control hypertension, other antihypertensives should be prescribed to achieve a goal blood pressure of 125/75 mm Hg. In the treatment of renal crisis, stopping the ACE inhibitor because of concerns that it may be diminishing renal perfusion pressure and exacerbating the decline in kidney function is not recommended. Anecdotal case reports suggest that combining ACE inhibitors with angiotensin receptor blockers may worsen the renal outcome.

Course and Prognosis

Once nearly universally fatal at 1 year, patients with renal crisis treated with ACE inhibitors can anticipate a 5-year survival rate of 65%. Late initiation of ACE inhibitor therapy (e.g., after serum creatinine exceeds 3 mg/dL) worsens prognosis, as does inadequate blood pressure control. For those who progress to require dialysis, continued ACE inhibitor therapy is recommended, because approximately 50% of patients may recover sufficient kidney function over 3 to 18 months to discontinue dialysis. In those on dialysis, graft survival and patient survival were somewhat poorer than in the general dialysis population. Few patients have undergone transplantation, but recurrence in an allograft from an identical twin has been reported.

BIBLIOGRAPHY

Andreoli SP, Trachtman H, Acheson DWK, et al: Hemolytic uremic syndrome: Epidemiology, pathophysiology, and therapy. Pediatr Nephrol 17:293–298, 2002.

Atamas SP, White B: The role of chemokines in the pathogenesis of scleroderma. Curr Opin Rheumatol 15:772–777, 2003.

Crowther MA, Ginsberg JS, Julian J, et al: A comparison of two intensities of warfarin for the prevention of recurrent thrombosis in patients with the antiphospholipid antibody syndrome. N Engl J Med 349:1133–1138, 2003.

Fogo A: Atlas of renal pathology: Thrombotic microangiopathy. Am J Kidney Dis 34:E7, 1999

Harris ML, Rosen A: Autoimmunity in scleroderma: Pathogenetic role and clinical significance of autoantibodies. Curr Opin Rheumatol 15:778–784, 2003.

Hosler GA, Cusumano AM, Hutchins GM: Thrombotic thrombocytopenic purpura and hemolytic uremic syndrome are distinct pathologic entities. Arch Pathol Lab Med 127:834–839, 2003.

Jimenez SA, Derk CT: Following the molecular pathways toward an understanding of the pathogenesis of systemic sclerosis. Ann Intern Med 140:37–50, 2004.

King AJ: Acute inflammation in the pathogenesis of hemolytic-uremic syndrome. Kidney Int 61:1553–1564, 2002.

Levine JS, Branch DW, Rauch J: The antiphospholipid syndrome. N Engl J Med 346:752–763, 2002.

Moake JL: Mechanisms of disease: Thrombotic microangiopathies. N Engl J Med 347:589–600, 2002.

Nochy D, Daugas E, Hill G, Grunfeld JP: Antiphospholipid syndrome nephropathy. J Nephrol 15:446–461, 2002.

Remuzzi G, Galbusera M, Noris M, et al, and the Italian Registry of Recurrent and Familial HUS/TTP: Von Willebrand factor cleaving protease (ADAMTS13) is deficient in recurrent and familial thrombotic thrombocytopenic purpura and hemolytic uremic syndrome. Blood 100:778–785, 2002.

Rock GA, Shumack KH, Buskard NA, et al, and the Canadian Apheresis Group: Comparison of plasma exchange with plasma infusion in the treatment of thrombotic thrombocytopenic purpura. N Engl J Med 325:393–397, 1991.

Ruggenenti P, Noris M, Remuzzi G: Thrombotic microangiopathy, hemolytic uremic syndrome, and thrombotic thrombocytopenic purpura. Kidney Int 60:831–846, 2001.

Steen VD, Medsger TA: Long-term outcomes of scleroderma renal crisis. Ann Intern Med 133:600–603, 2000.

Steen VD: Scleroderma renal crisis. Rheum Dis Clin North Am 29:315–333, 2003.

Takehara K: Pathogenesis of systemic sclerosis. J Rheumatol 30:755–759, 2003.

Tsai H-M, Lian C-Y: Antibodies to von Willebrand factor cleaving protease in acute thrombocytopenic purpura. N Engl J Med 339:1585–1594, 1998.

Tsai H-M: Von Willebrand factor, ADAMTS13, and thrombotic thrombocytopenic purpura. J Mol Med 80:639–647, 2002.

Tsai H-M: Advances in the pathogenesis, diagnosis and treatment of thrombotic thrombocytopenic purpura. J Am Soc Nephrol 14:1072–1081, 2003.

CHAPTER 32

Kidney Disorders Associated with HIV Infection

Marianne Monahan   Paul E. Klotman

Kidney disease occurs frequently in the course of human immunodeficiency virus (HIV) disease and has become the fourth leading condition contributing to death in acquired immunodeficiency virus (AIDS) patients after septicemia, pneumonia, and liver disease. Kidney complications of HIV infection can be subdivided into several categories, including disturbances of fluid and electrolyte metabolism, disturbances in acid-base balance, acute renal failure, chronic kidney disease (particularly HIV-associated nephropathy [HIVAN]), and immune-mediated glomerulopathies (Table 32-1). Many of these disorders are similar to those seen in the HIV-negative population. Others, such as HIVAN, are attributable to HIV infection itself or are the side effects of therapeutic agents used commonly in the treatment of AIDS-related illnesses. Many of these complications are preventable or treatable, making early recognition and intervention essential.

FLUID AND ELECTROLYTES

Sodium

Electrolyte and acid-base abnormalities are common in AIDS patients. Of these, hyponatremia is the most common. Approximately 30% of hospitalized patients with AIDS develop a serum sodium less than 130 mmol/L. Most cases can be attributed to volume depletion from diarrhea, emesis, poor oral intake, or increased insensible losses from fever or pulmonary disease. Other causes of low serum sodium include the syndrome of inappropriate antidiuretic hormone secretion (SIADH; a frequent complication of pulmonary infection and central nervous system lesions), adrenal insufficiency, and renal sodium wasting due to such nephrotoxic medications as amphotericin and pentamidine. Common drug-related toxicities are listed in Table 32-2.

Hypernatremia, though much less common, can also be observed in AIDS patients. This also occurs in the setting of volume depletion from impaired oral intake and may be associated with acquired nephrogenic diabetes insipidus from medications such as amphotericin or foscarnet.

Potassium

Hyperkalemia has been reported in 16% to 21% of hospitalized AIDS patients. Similar to seronegative patients with hyperkalemia, increased serum potassium levels may be due to impaired kidney function, adrenal insufficiency, and acidemia. Medications used commonly in the treatment of opportunistic infections such as *Pneumocystis carinii* pneumonia have been shown to increase potassium blood levels through more direct mechanisms. Trimethoprim's effect on the distal nephron is similar to that of the potassium-sparing diuretics; it inhibits sodium reabsorption and thereby limits potassium secretion. Pentamidine has been shown to act on the distal tubule in a similar manner. Unexplained hyperkalemia has been attributed to hyporeninemic hypoaldosteronism in some AIDS patients. In addition to increased serum potassium, these patients also develop a metabolic acidosis. In these patients, fludrocortisone has been efficacious in the treatment of hyperkalemia.

Hypokalemia, like hyponatremia, occurs most often in the setting of volume depletion. Amphotericin nephrotoxicity can also present with hypokalemia, often associated with magnesium depletion. More recently, hypokalemia has been observed as a complication of the Fanconi syndrome associated with the antiviral nucleotides adefovir and tenofovir.

Calcium

Abnormal serum calcium levels are frequently observed in hospitalized AIDS patients; hypocalcemia occurs in approximately 18% and hypercalcemia in approximately 3%. In many patients, hypocalcemia can be attributed to hypoalbuminemia, a condition highly prevalent in AIDS patients. Medications including foscarnet, pentamidine, and didanosine have also been implicated in hypocalcemia. Severe, symptomatic hypocalcemia manifested by paraesthesias and Trousseau's or Chvostek's signs has been reported in patients treated concurrently with pentamidine and foscarnet. Increased serum calcium levels are seen in patients with granulomatous disease and in patients with disseminated cytomegalovirus.

TABLE 32-1   Renal Disorders in Patients with HIV Infection

Fluid-electrolyte and acid-base disturbances
  Hyponatremia and hypernatremia
  Hypokalemia and hyperkalemia
  Hypocalcemia and hypercalcemia
  Hypomagnesemia
  Hypophosphatemia and hyperphosphatemia
  Syndrome of inappropriate ADH
  Nephrogenic diabetes insipidus
  RTA
  Lactic acidosis
  Fanconi's syndrome

ARF syndromes
  Acute tubular necrosis
  Acute interstitial nephritis
    Allergic
    Infectious
  HUS/TTP
  Crystalluria/obstructive uropathy

Glomerular syndromes
  HIVAN
  Membranoproliferative GN
  Minimal change disease
  Membranous glomerulopathy
  Postinfectious GN

ADH, antidiuretic hormone; ARF, acute renal failure; GN, glomerulonephritis; HIVAN, HIV-associated nephropathy; HUS/TTP, hemolytic uremic syndrome and thrombotic thrombocytopenic purpura; RTA, renal tubular acidosis.

Magnesium

Renal magnesium wasting, resulting in hypomagnesemia, occurs as a complication of treatment with both pentamidine and amphotericin. Drug-induced tubular injury is the proposed mechanism.

ACID-BASE BALANCE

Non–anion gap metabolic acidosis from bicarbonate loss in the stool is not unusual. Many AIDS patients develop acute or chronic diarrheal syndromes given their increased susceptibility to opportunistic enteric pathogens, including *Cyclospora cayetanensis*, *Cryptosporidium parvum*, cytomegalovirus, and disseminated *Mycobacterium avium-intracellulare* (MAI). Lactic acidosis can occur in the setting of sepsis from bacterial or fungal infections or severe hypoxemia due to overwhelming pulmonary infection. Type B lactic acidosis, the lactic acidosis not related to hypoxia or hypoperfusion, is associated with exposure to many of the nucleoside reverse transcriptase inhibitors (NRTIs). The presumed mechanism is inhibition of DNA γ-polymerase resulting in mitochondrial dysfunction in liver and skeletal muscle cells and overproduction of lactic acid. Didanosine and stavudine have been associated with a higher risk as compared with other NRTIs.

Other medications have also been implicated in the generation of acid-base disturbances. Renal tubular aci-

dosis (RTA) complicates treatment with gentamicin, amphotericin B, and adefovir. A series of patients who developed unexplained RTA while receiving high-dose trimethoprim-sulfamethoxazole (Bactrim) has also been reported.

Pulmonary infections can induce a respiratory alkalosis due to hyperventilation or, later in the course of illness, a respiratory acidosis as the ability of the patient to ventilate adequately decreases secondary to fatigue or acute pulmonary decompensation.

Proximal Tubule Injury

Nephrotoxicity is the dose-limiting side effect of cidofovir and adefovir, two nucleotide analogues with potent antiviral activity. The mechanism of toxicity is unclear, but the mechanism of uptake is probably through several organic anion transporters including the human organic acid transporter hOAT1.

TABLE 32-2   Drug-Induced Nephrotoxicity in Patients with HIV-I Infection

Drug	Toxicity
Acyclovir	Acute tubular necrosis Crystalluria Obstructive nephropathy
Adefovir	Fanconi's syndrome
Aminoglycosides	Acute tubular necrosis RTA
Amphotericin	Acute tubular necrosis Hypokalemia Hyperkalemia Hypomagnesemia RTA
Cidofovir	Proximal tubular damage Bicarbonate wasting Proteinuria
Foscarnet	Hypocalcemia Hypercalcemia Hypomagnesemia Hyperphosphatemia Hypophosphatemia Nephrogenic diabetes insipidus
Indinavir	Crystalluria Urinary tract obstruction
NSAIDs	Acute tubular necrosis Allergic interstitial nephritis
Pentamidine	Acute tubular necrosis Hyperkalemia Hypocalcemia
Rifampin	Allergic interstitial nephritis
Sulfadiazine	Crystalluria Urinary tract obstruction Allergic interstitial nephritis

NSAIDs, nonsteroidal anti-inflammatory drugs; RTA, renal tubular acidosis.

Cidofovir is available for the treatment of cytomegalovirus retinitis and has activity against many of the other herpesviruses. In clinical trials, approximately 5% to 7% of patients taking cidofovir develop signs of proximal tubule damage manifested as an elevated creatinine concentration, glycosuria, and bicarbonate wasting. Toxicity can be reduced by coadministration of probenecid, which decreases renal cellular uptake. The related nucleotide analogues adefovir and tenofovir have demonstrated antiretroviral activity against HIV-1 and hepatitis B. Adefovir was found to have activity against HIV isolates that had developed resistance to other antiretrovirals, particularly AZT (azidothymidine). Unfortunately, with the use of adefovir in clinical trials for HIV therapy, Fanconi's syndrome developed in up to 30% of patients on treatment for longer than 6 months at a dose of 30 mg or more. Manifestations included a proximal RTA with bicarbonate wasting, hypophosphatemia, glycosuria, aminoaciduria, and hypokalemia. This resolved with discontinuation of the drug. Recently a dose of 10 mg has been approved for the treatment of hepatitis B infection. At this dose, adefovir has not been associated with significant nephrotoxicity, although occasional cases of Fanconi's syndrome continue to be reported. Tenofovir, a related nucleotide, has been approved for the treatment of HIV-1 infection. Renal tubular dysfunction is rarely associated with tenofovir, but occasional cases of Fanconi's syndrome have been reported with long-term tenofovir use.

ACUTE RENAL FAILURE

The etiologies of acute renal failure (ARF) in AIDS patients are similar to those identified in patients without AIDS and can be subdivided into prerenal, intrarenal, and postrenal causes. Patients with AIDS are at increased risk of developing ARF from many prerenal causes. Volume depletion resulting from vomiting, diarrhea, fever, and poor oral intake is a frequent complication of the underlying illness of hospitalized AIDS patients. In addition, patients with AIDS may have a true salt-wasting syndrome, although the mechanism is unclear. As a result, AIDS patients are particularly sensitive to many potentially nephrotoxic therapeutic and diagnostic agents as well as changes in hemodynamic status. Not surprisingly, ARF is attributed to ischemic renal injury from sepsis in about 50% of cases; to nephrotoxic agents, including aminoglycosides, amphotericin, pentamidine, and intravenous radiocontrast materials in about 25% of cases; and to other causes including acute interstitial nephritis, rhabdomyolysis, massive GI bleeding, cardiac failure, and hepatic failure in the remaining 25%.

Acute interstitial nephritis is not unusual in the HIV-infected patient and can be caused by infection or by a hypersensitivity drug reaction from virtually any medication. Infectious agents associated with interstitial disease in the immunocompromised include cytomegalovirus, candida, tuberculosis, and histoplasmosis. Medications used frequently in the treatment of AIDS-related illness that are associated with acute interstitial nephritis include penicillins, cephalosporins, ciprofloxacin, cotrimoxazole, rifampin, and nonsteroidal anti-inflammatory drugs. Treatment requires discontinuation of the medication.

Vascular causes of ARF, particularly hemolytic uremic syndrome/thrombotic thrombocytopenic purpura (HUS/TTP), are increasingly recognized in the HIV-infected patient. In 25% of seropositive patients with HUS/TTP, the hematologic disturbance is the presenting manifestation of HIV infection. Centers located in areas with a high prevalence of HIV infection have reported that up to one third of patients diagnosed with HUS/TTP are HIV positive. The clinical manifestations and pathologic findings of HIV-related HUS/TTP are similar to the idiopathic forms. Patients present with constitutional symptoms of fever and malaise, signs of a bleeding diathesis including mucosal bleeding and easy bruising, and a variety of neurologic signs and symptoms. Laboratory examination reveals a microangiopathic hemolytic anemia and impaired kidney function. Kidney biopsy reveals platelet and fibrin thrombi in renal and glomerular vessels, interstitial fibrosis, and acute tubular necrosis. Treatment with plasmapheresis and fresh-frozen plasma replacement may be effective.

Postrenal causes of ARF are also common in the seropositive patient. Crystal-induced obstructive nephropathy from various drugs should be considered when evaluating ARF in HIV-positive patients. The drugs most commonly implicated in seropositive patients are sulfadiazine, intravenous acyclovir, and indinavir. Treatment consists of discontinuation of the drug and vigorous hydration. Indinavir therapy is associated with asymptomatic crystalluria in up to 20% of patients. Symptoms of dysuria and renal colic and signs of mildly elevated serum creatinine occur in approximately 8%. Most patients improve with hydration or discontinuation of the drug. Nephrolithiasis associated with the use of nelfinavir has also been reported.

Finally, many seropositive patients are enrolled in clinical trials with investigational drugs whose side effect profiles are poorly characterized. A high index of suspicion for drug toxicity should be maintained and explored whenever evaluating a seropositive patient with ARF.

CHRONIC KIDNEY DISEASE

HIVAN is a disease with unique clinical, pathologic, and epidemiologic features that progresses rapidly to endstage renal disease (ESRD). HIVAN was first described in the early 1980s but was rarely reported as a complication of HIV infection even as late as 1990. Since then, however, HIVAN has increased in incidence and is now the most common cause of chronic kidney disease in HIV-sero-

TABLE 32-3   Clinical Presentation of HIV-Associated Nephropathy

Epidemiology	Third leading cause of ESRD in African Americans ages 20–64
	Incidence increased each year until introduction of HAART
Presentation	Proteinuria
	Azotemia
	Normal or large, echogenic kidneys on sonogram
	CD4⁺ cells usually <200 cells/μL
Pathology	Focal segmental glomerulosclerosis, collapsing variant
	Microcystic dilatation of tubules
Pathogenesis	Direct effect of HIV infection or viral proteins on renal epithelium
	Race cofactor
Treatment	HAART
	ACE inhibition

ACE, angiotensin-converting enzyme; ESRD, endstage renal disease; HAART, highly active antiretroviral therapy.

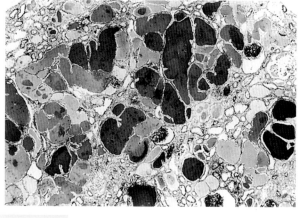

FIGURE 32-1 Kidney biopsy sample of a patient with HIV-associated nephropathy. The classic features of HIVAN are present in this specimen, with microcystic tubular dilatation, proteinaceous casts, modest interstitial infiltrate, and collapsing glomerulosclerosis. (Periodic acid–Schiff stain; magnification ×50.) (Courtesy of Dr. Vivette D'Agati.)

positive patients; moreover, it is the third leading cause of ESRD in African Americans between the ages of 20 and 64. The salient features of HIVAN are indicated in Table 32-3.

Presentation

The morphologic diagnosis of HIVAN is remarkably restricted to black patients; almost 90% of cases occur in African Americans. The remaining 10% of cases are almost exclusively observed in mixed-heritage or Hispanic patients. The disorder is only very rarely seen in seropositive white patients. Patients with HIVAN usually present with azotemia and proteinuria. Most patients are normotensive, and on renal sonogram, kidneys are typically normal or slightly increased in size. By ultrasound, the kidneys are often described as echogenic. HIVAN was initially believed to be a late complication of HIV-1 infection, because it appeared in patients with low CD4 counts and a history of opportunistic infections. In a series of 114 patients with biopsy-proven HIVAN, all but 6 patients had CD4 counts less than 200 cells/μL. However, there have been case reports of HIVAN occurring in the setting of acute HIV-1 seroconversion, indicating that HIVAN may develop at any time in the course of HIV-1 infection.

Pathology

The histopathologic features of HIVAN include focal segmental glomerular sclerosis (FSGS) in combination with microcystic distortion of the tubulointerstitium (Fig. 32-1). Collapsing glomerulosclerosis is a common variant in patients with HIVAN (Fig. 32-2A and B),

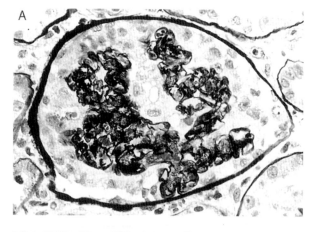

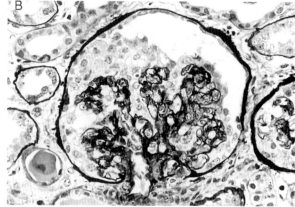

FIGURE 32-2 Focal segmental glomerulosclerosis of the collapsing variant. Both focal (A) and global (B) collapse can be seen in association with HIV infection. (Jones methenamine silver stain; magnification A, ×500, B, ×325.)

although patients who are seronegative have also been reported with this form of FSGS. Microcysts are often filled with proteinaceous casts, and in some patients there is modest interstitial infiltration by lymphocytes, plasma cells, and monocytes. Immunofluorescence is generally nonspecific. Electron microscopic examination may reveal tubuloreticular arrays, but the prevalence of this finding has been decreasing more recently, probably as a result of more effective antiretroviral therapy. Biopsy confirmation of HIVAN is extremely important. Even when HIVAN is suspected, 40% of biopsy samples from patients will be found to have another diagnosis on pathologic examination. The relationship of HIV-1 infection to pathogenesis of other glomerular lesions is not as well understood as it is for the constellation of findings present in HIVAN.

Pathogenesis

Much has been learned about the cellular mechanisms responsible for the development of HIVAN. Increasing evidence from both clinical and animal studies supports a direct role for HIV-1 infection of renal parenchymal cells in the pathogenesis of HIVAN. Transgenic mice expressing a replication-defective HIV-1 construct develop proteinuria, reduced kidney function, and histologic renal disease almost identical to HIVAN. Reciprocal transplantation studies using this mouse model demonstrate that HIVAN develops only in kidneys expressing the transgene. Moreover, HIV-1 RNA and DNA have been detected in podocytes and renal tubular epithelial cells of patients with HIVAN. The mechanism by which HIV-1 enters renal epithelial cells is unknown. Recent studies indicate that the renal epithelial cell is able to support a productive viral life cycle, and the renal epithelium is an important reservoir for HIV-1 infection.

Kidney biopsy samples of patients with HIVAN demonstrate increased epithelial proliferative and apoptotic changes. Proliferation of tubular epithelial cells probably contributes to microcyst formation and may explain why kidneys are normal or large in size. Increased proliferation of podocytes is also present and is an important component of the collapsing glomerulosclerosis found in HIVAN.

The racial predilection of HIVAN for black patients indicates that host factors are important determinants of response to renal epithelial cell infection by HIV-1. Recently, in an effort to determine the influence of genetic background on HIVAN pathogenesis, investigators used the HIV-1 transgenic mouse model of HIVAN to identify genetic loci that are associated with the development of kidney disease. This approach may soon elucidate novel candidate genes that are important for the development of kidney dysfunction in HIVAN.

Treatment

Approaches to the treatment of HIV-related kidney diseases can be divided into three categories: (1) management of the ESRD patient who is seropositive, (2) treatment of HIVAN directed at slowing progression to ESRD, and (3) treatment of the HIV-1 infection.

Management of ESRD

Treatment options for the seropositive patient with ESRD are similar to those when HIV-1 is not the cause of kidney failure. Options include hemodialysis, peritoneal dialysis, and, more recently, kidney transplantation. Studies to evaluate kidney transplantation in patients infected with HIV-1 are now underway. Eligible patients are ESRD patients with undetectable viral burden on a stable HAART (highly active antiretroviral therapy) regimen, who have no evidence of neoplasms or opportunistic infections, and who do not have CD4 counts less than 200 cells/µL. Although the number of HIV-1 patients who have received kidney transplants is small, preliminary data are promising. One-year patient survival rates are similar to unmatched survival data from the United Network for Organ Sharing (UNOS) database. Progression of HIV-1 disease does not appear to be increased by transplantation. In this small group of patients, median CD4 counts have remained stable and HIV-1 viral loads have remained suppressed. The risk of acute rejection, however, appears to be increased in HIV-1 seropositive patients.

Initial reports described a very poor prognosis for HIV-1 seropositive patients with ESRD undergoing chronic hemodialysis. Survival has improved in recent years, probably as a result of improved viral treatment in the form of HAART. Despite improvement, survival remains low compared with age-, race-, and gender-matched HIV-1 negative patients. Transmission of HIV-1 in dialysis units is very unlikely if standard blood precaution practice guidelines are followed. The Centers for Disease Control does not recommend special machines or isolation for HIV-1 seropositive patients undergoing hemodialysis.

Treatment of HIVAN

Studies have suggested that ACE (angiotensin-converting enzyme) inhibitors or immune modulators, including prednisone and cyclosporine, may be efficacious in slowing the progression of HIVAN to ESRD. ACE inhibitors seem to be particularly effective when initiated early in the clinical course, when serum creatinine is still less than 2 mg/dL. The mechanism by which ACE inhibition slows progression of HIVAN is unknown. Studies demonstrating efficacy were not randomized and lacked proper controls, and the findings must be viewed in this context. Therapy with ACE inhibitors is likely to be of little risk to the patient, and as long as serum potassium is carefully monitored, it may be a reasonable approach, in the absence of more definitive evidence. In addition, angiotensin receptor blockers (ARBs) may be beneficial, in light of evidence from studies of other proteinuric glomerular diseases. However, use of ACE inhibitors and ARBs should not detract from an aggressive antiviral strategy.

The use of immunosuppression in the treatment of late-stage HIVAN has also been explored in a small prospective study. Treatment with prednisone at 60 mg/day for up to 11 weeks reduced serum creatinine and lowered proteinuria. Long-term outcome, however, was not substantially different from historical controls, and serious opportunistic infections were observed in 30%. Cyclosporine has been used in a small number of seropositive children with FSGS; in some, the nephrotic syndrome resolved.

Treatment of the HIV-1 Infection

No randomized controlled clinical trials to evaluate HAART in HIVAN have been completed. Case series and retrospective studies suggest that the rate of progression of HIVAN to ESRD has been slowed by the introduction of protease inhibitors and HAART. Data provided by the United States Renal Data System provides further evidence that HAART has improved the natural history of HIVAN. During the first half of the 1990s, the incidence of ESRD due to HIVAN rose rapidly, increasing by more than 550%. Incidence rates dropped slightly from 1995 to 1996 and then reached a plateau. The plateau in incidence of HIVAN coincided with the introduction of HAART. In addition, there are several case reports of patients with biopsy-proven HIVAN who experienced clinical and histologic improvement in their kidney disease after initiating therapy with HAART.

OTHER FORMS OF GLOMERULAR AND KIDNEY DISEASE ASSOCIATED WITH HIV INFECTION

Although FSGS secondary to HIVAN is the most common glomerular lesion seen in HIV-positive patients, biopsy series have revealed a wide spectrum of lesions in seropositive patients, including membranoproliferative glomerulonephritis, minimal change disease, membranous glomerulopathy, IgA nephropathy, amyloidosis, and a variety of parenchymal infections. Coinfection with hepatitis B or C is common in HIV-positive patients, especially in those with a history of intravenous drug use. Because hepatitis B and C are also associated with immune-mediated kidney disease independent of HIV infection, the specific etiology of the kidney disease should be addressed in an individual patient. With the exception of the few cases of IgA nephropathy in HIV-seropositive patients, the importance of immune complex disease in the pathogenesis of HIV-related kidney disease remains unclear.

BIBLIOGRAPHY

Ahuja TS, Grady J, Khan S: Changing trends in the survival of dialysis patients with human immunodeficiency virus in the United States. J Am Soc Nephrol 13:1889–1993, 2002.

Burns GC, Paul SK, Toth IR, Sivak SL: Effect of angiotensin converting enzyme inhibition in HIV-associated nephropathy. J Am Soc Nephrol 8:1140–1146, 1997.

Carbone LG, Bendixen B, Appel GB: Sulfadiazine-associated obstructive nephropathy occurring in a patient with the acquired immunodeficiency syndrome. Am J Kidney Dis 12:72–75, 1988.

Chattha G, Arieff AI, Cummings C, Tierney LM, Jr: Lactic acidosis complicating the acquired immunodeficiency syndrome. Ann Intern Med 118:37–39, 1993.

Cusano AJ, Thies HL, Siegal FP, et al: Hyponatremia in patients with acquired immune deficiency syndrome. J Acquir Immune Defic Syndr 3:949–953, 1990.

D'Agati V, Appel GB: Renal pathology of human immunodeficiency virus infection. Semin Nephrol 18:406–421, 1998.

Dusheiko G: Adefovir dipivoxil for the treatment of HbeAg-positive chronic hepatitis B: A review of the major clinical studies. J Hepatol 39:116–123, 2003.

Gharavi AG, Ahmad T, Wong RD, et al: Mapping a locus for susceptibility to HIV-1–associated nephropathy to mouse chromosome 3. Proc Natl Acad Sci USA 101:2488–2493, 2004.

Herman ES, Klotman PE: HIV-associated nephropathy: Epidemiology, pathogenesis and treatment. Semin Nephrol 23:200–208, 2003.

Kahn J, Lagakos S, Wulfsohn M, et al: Efficacy and safety of adefovir dipivoxil with antiretroviral therapy: A randomized controlled trial. JAMA 282:2305–2312, 1999.

Kimmel PL, Bosch JP, Vassalotti JA: Treatment of human immunodeficiency virus (HIV)–associated nephropathy. Semin Nephrol 18:446–458, 1998.

Klotman PE: HIV-associated nephropathy. Kidney Int 56:1161–1176, 1999.

Kopp JB, Miller KD, Mican JA, et al: Crystalluria and urinary tract abnormalities associated with indinavir. Ann Intern Med 127:119–125, 1997.

Rao TK, Friedman EA: Outcome of severe acute renal failure in patients with acquired immunodeficiency syndrome. Am J Kidney Dis 25:390–398, 1995.

Roland ME, Adey D, Carlson LL, et al: Kidney and liver transplantation in HIV-infected patients: Case presentations and review. AIDS Patient Care and STDs 17:501–507, 2003.

Ross MJ, Klotman PE: Recent progress in HIV-associated nephropathy. J Am Soc Nephrol 13:2997–3004, 2002.

Ross MJ, Klotman PE. HIV-associated nephropathy. AIDS 18:1089–1099, 2004.

Stokes MB, Chawla H, Brody RI, et al: Immune complex glomerulonephritis in patients coinfected with human immunodeficiency virus and hepatitis C virus. Am J Kidney Dis 29:514–525, 1997.

Vrouenraets SM, Treskes M, Regez RM, et al: Hyperlactataemia in HIV-infected patients: The role of NRTI-treatment. Antivir Ther 7:239–244, 2002.

Winston JA, Burns GC, Klotman PE: The human immunodeficiency virus (HIV) epidemic and HIV-associated nephropathy. Semin Nephrol 18:373–377, 1998.

Winston J, Klotman ME, Klotman PE: HIV-associated nephropathy is a late, not early, manifestation of HIV-1 infection. Kidney Int 55:1036–1040, 1999.

SECTION V

Acute Renal Failure

CHAPTER 33

Pathophysiology of Acute Renal Failure

Robert L. Safirstein

The syndrome of acute renal failure (ARF) is defined as a reduction of glomerular filtration rate (GFR) that is often reversible. The syndrome may occur in three clinical settings: (1) as an adaptive response to severe volume depletion and hypotension with structurally and functionally intact nephrons, (2) in response to cytotoxic insults to the kidney when both renal structure and function are abnormal, and (3) when the passage of urine is blocked. Thus ARF may be classified as prerenal, intrinsic, or postrenal. Although this classification is useful in establishing a differential diagnosis (see Chapter 34), it is now evident that many pathophysiologic features are shared among the different categories. The intrinsic form of the syndrome may be accompanied by a well-defined sequence of events: an initiation phase characterized by daily increases in serum creatinine and reduced urinary volume; a maintenance phase, where GFR is relatively stable and urine volume may be increased; and a recovery phase in which serum creatinine falls and tubule function is restored. This sequence of events is not always apparent, and oliguria may not be present at all. The reason for this lack of uniform clinical presentation is most probably a reflection of the variable nature of the injury. It is also useful to classify ARF as oliguric or nonoliguric, with the daily urine excretion as criterion. Oliguria is defined as a daily urine volume of less than 350 to 400 mL/day. Stratification of the renal failure along these lines helps in decision making, such as the timing of dialysis, and seems to be an important criterion for response to therapy (see later). This chapter considers the pathophysiology of the syndrome, focusing especially on the intrinsic form of the disease, and introducing newer concepts of what causes the syndrome based on more recent observations in human and animal forms of the disease. This better understanding of ARF has led to newer approaches to treatment.

MORPHOLOGY OF ACUTE RENAL FAILURE

The changes in renal epithelial morphology that accompany ARF are subtle. At least four cellular fates can be identified in ARF: cells may die either by frank necrosis or by apoptosis; they may replicate and divide; or they may appear indifferent to the stress (Fig. 33-1). Frank necrosis, as is often seen experimentally, is not prominent in the vast majority of human cases. Necrosis is usually patchy, involving individual cells or small clusters of cells, sometimes resulting in small areas of denuded basement membrane. Less obvious injury is more often noted, including loss of brush borders, flattening of the epithelium, detachment of cells, intratubular cast formation, and dilatation of the lumen. Although proximal tubules show many of theses changes, injury to the distal nephron can also be demonstrated when human biopsy material is closely examined. The distal nephron is also the site of obstruction by desquamated cells and cellular debris.

Apoptosis has been noted in ischemic and nephrotoxic forms of ARF. This form of cell death differs from frank necrosis in that it requires the activation of a regulated program that leads to DNA fragmentation, cytoplasmic condensation, and cell loss without precipitating an inflammatory response (Table 33-1). In contradistinction to necrosis, the principal site of apoptotic cell death is the distal nephron.

Disruption of the cell cytoskeleton seems to be an important determinant of many of the early morphologic changes, especially in ischemic injury. Loss of the integrity of the actin cytoskeleton leads to flattening of the epithelium, with loss of the brush border, loss of focal cell contacts, and subsequent disengagement of the cell from the underlying substratum. Membrane proteins, including the integrins and the $Na^+ K^+$-ATPase, redistribute in the plasma membrane as cells lose their polarity. The functional impact of these changes is great, in that cells lose their capacity to achieve vectorial transport, and the redistribution of the adhesion molecules from the basolateral membrane sites provokes intratubular obstruction.

Even more subtle is the injury to the vascular endothelium that takes place in many forms of ARF, especially after cyclosporine administration and in sepsis, where there is little morphologically apparent epithelial cell death. The best evidence that the renal vasculature undergoes permanent injury is the reduction in capillary bed area that occurs after renal ischemia. These and the other changes in cell integrity noted earlier may help to explain the often disproportionate decline in renal function that occurs in certain forms of ARF when compared with the minor morphologic changes observed.

TABLE 33-1   Comparison Between Apoptotic and Necrotic Cell Death

	Apoptosis	Necrosis
Stimuli	Physiologic	Pathologic
Occurrence	Single cells	Groups of cells
Adhesion between cells	Lost (early)	Lost (late)
Nucleus	Convolution of nuclear outline and breakdown (karyorrhexis)	Disappearance (karyolysis)
Nuclear chromatin	Compaction in uniformly dense masses	Clumping not sharply defined
DNA cleavage	Internucleosomal, "laddering" appearance of distinct fragments on agarose gels	Random: "smear" pattern on agarose gels
Phagocytosis by other cells	Present	Absent
Inflammation	Absent	Present

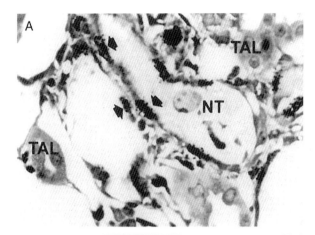

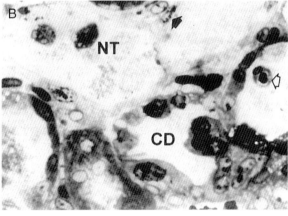

FIGURE 33-1   Representative photomicrographs of outer stripe of outer medulla of rat kidney 5 days after cisplatin injection (5 mg/kg body weight) demonstrating cell fate during ARF. *A,* Necrosis of the S3 segment of the proximal convoluted tubule is apparent (NT). The solid arrows show regenerating tubules, indicated by the uptake of [³H]thymidine. *B,* The open arrow shows an apoptotic body. Thick ascending limbs (TAL) and collecting ducts (CD) are without apparent morphologic damage. (Original magnification ×400.)

Molecular Responses to Renal Injury: Implications for Cell Fate

In sections of the kidney taken from patients with ARF, regeneration and necrosis coexist, so that injury and repair are closely linked. Even in its most severe form, few patients who survive initial dialysis require long-term dialysis, indicating the effectiveness of this repair process. The regeneration process is accompanied by increased DNA synthesis in cells relining the injured epithelium. These regenerating cells are thought to be derived from at least three sources: surviving epithelial cells that dedifferentiate and reacquire the ability to reenter the cell cycle, resident kidney stem cells, and bone marrow–derived stem cells that migrate to the kidney and transdifferentiate into mature tubular epithelial cells. Further studies to define the precise contribution and timing and role of each of these processes to restoring tubule integrity after injury are likely to be particularly important.

Increased renal DNA synthesis following injury is preceded by prominent changes in gene expression, and these changes can be grouped in at least three major categories (Table 33-2). Many of the genes that are expressed after renal injury are involved in cell cycle regulation and are similar to those expressed when growth factors are

TABLE 33-2   Molecular Responses to Renal Ischemia

Increased gene expression
  Genes involved in cell fate determinations: regeneration, apoptosis
    Transcription factors: c-jun, c-fos
    Cyclin-dependent kinase inhibitors: p21
  Genes involved in inflammation
    Chemokines: MCP-1, IL-8
    Adhesion molecules: ICAM-1, integrins

Decreased gene expression—loss of mature phenotype
  Prepro epidermal growth factor
  Tamm-Horsfall protein
  Aquaporin-2

ICAM-1, intercellular adhesion molecule 1; IL-8, interleukin-8; MCP-1, monocyte chemotactic protein 1; NHE3, sodium-proton exchanger 3.

added to cells to stimulate them to enter the growth cycle. Although the endogenous growth factors that serve this response have not been identified with certainty, administration of growth factors exogenously has been shown to ameliorate and hasten recovery from ARF (see Treatment of ARF). Another group of genes are proinflammatory and chemotactic and may be responsible for the apparent inflammatory aspects of ARF. Depletion of leukocytes and blockade of leukocyte adhesion both reduce renal injury following ischemia, indicating that the inflammatory response is in part responsible for some features of ARF. This mechanism may be especially prominent in ARF subsequent to transplant. This proinflammatory state may also be an important variable in predicting outcome, in that recent evidence in a large study of seriously ill patients with ARF demonstrated that plasma cytokine levels predict mortality in patients with ARF.

These two aspects of the renal molecular response to injury (the increases in protooncogene and chemokine expression) resemble what is observed in cells exposed to adverse environmental conditions such as ionizing radiation, oxidants, and hypertonicity. This response to adversity has been termed the *stress response* and is a major determinant of whether cells survive the insult or not. In some circumstances, the stress response leads to apoptosis rather than survival. Whether a cell survives or not is probably a function of the duration of the stress response, its degree, and the specific cell in which the response takes place.

A summary of these important features of the renal stress pathway and their possible consequences is given in Figure 33-2. It can be seen that initiation of the stress response may ultimately determine much of the proinflammatory, reparative, cytoreductive, and functional aspects of renal failure. Particular limbs of the response can be targeted for up- or down-regulation to limit injury or improve function. Experiments using growth factors (presumably to tip the balance between cell gain and cell loss), as well as the use of antiadhesion molecules to reduce inflammation, support the notion that the renal stress response is an appropriate target for therapy (see Treatment of ARF).

The third group of molecular responses to renal ischemia involves an apparent loss of the mature phenotype of the kidney; many of the changes in gene expression involve the loss of proteins that are only expressed maximally during the maturation of the kidney. These proteins include the prepro epidermal growth factor and Tamm-Horsfall protein genes, whose functions are unknown in the kidney, but also include important membrane transporter genes, such as Aquaporin-2 and NHE3 (sodium-proton exchanger 3). The loss of these latter proteins may be responsible, in part, for the tubular reabsorptive defects typical of ARF (see later).

Pathophysiology of the Cell Injury

The mechanisms of the changes in cell viability during renal injury are complex and incompletely understood. Most of the experimental data have been derived from the ischemia-reperfusion model of ARF and have focused on necrotic cell death. Because as many as 50% of patients have ischemia-induced ARF, the observations should be relevant to a large portion of the patients at risk.

As previously mentioned, different stresses initiate common biochemical events, so that an understanding of the relevant pathways of one stress will most likely shed light on others. Such studies have focused on several biochemical pathways: defects in energy metabolism, reactive oxygen species, lipotoxicity, and executioners of cell death.

The mechanism of the depletion of intracellular ATP stores that accompanies renal failure has increasingly focused on the mitochondria. Reduced aerobic production of ATP from glucose and fatty acid oxidation is a hallmark of postischemic and cytotoxic ARF. Hyperglycemia and hyperlipidemia often accompany ARF, and renal cells accumulate lipids after ischemia and nephrotoxic insults. A decrease in energy production causes, among other processes, a collapse of electrolyte gradients and increases the cytosolic concentration of several solutes including calcium. Such increases in intracellular calcium can damage epithelial cells by activating proteases and phospholipases, and can further disrupt cellular integrity. The mechanism for this inhibition of aerobic metabolism is not known, but the salutary effect of insulin and newer hypoglycemic agents such as the peroxisome proliferator-activated receptor-α ligands on the course of ARF in experimental models suggest that understanding these changes in fuel choice is fundamental to our understanding of ARF.

Restoration of renal blood flow (RBF) after ischemia produces a burst of reduced oxygen species from a variety of processes. Resultant lipid, protein, and DNA damage could lead to cell death. As recently demonstrated, inter-

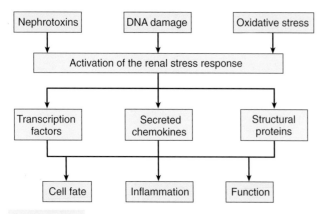

FIGURE 33-2 The stress response and its consequences.

action between the nitric oxide system and superoxide anion to form a damaging peroxynitrite species may be an important mediator of tubular and vascular injury following ischemia. Understanding the specific mechanism involved in their generation and the specific oxygen radical species responsible for cell injury under different conditions are areas of intense research interest.

Members of the phospholipase family, which hydrolyze membrane lipids, could contribute to ischemic renal injury as they appear to do in other organs injured by ischemia. Products of phospholipid breakdown themselves, as well as those converted by cytoplasmic oxidases, are vasoconstrictive and chemotactic, and could participate in the functional and cytotoxic events of renal failure. Adequate assessment of their role in the cytotoxicity of ischemia awaits the availability of effective inhibitors of the various members of these lipid mediators of cell function.

Activation of endonucleases, which cleave DNA, and caspases, which are cysteine proteases that activate endonucleases to induce cell death, each serve apoptosis and necrosis during cell stress. The use of specific inhibitors of these executioners of cell death shows promise in mitigating the effects of oxidant injury in renal cells. Future studies of the regulation of these pathways are likely to reveal new insights into mechanisms of cell death during ARF.

PATHOPHYSIOLOGY OF ABNORMAL FUNCTION

Reduced Glomerular Filtration Rate

By considering the forces and flows at the glomerular capillary vascular bed, it is possible to form a conceptual framework in which to analyze the causes of reduced GFR in ARF.

Glomerular filtration rate may decrease because of reduced renal flood flow, reduced glomerular capillary pressure, increased intratubular pressure, reduced glomerular capillary ultrafiltration coefficient (K_f), or some combination of these.

Intrarenal vasoconstriction is the dominant mechanism for the reduced GFR in ARF. Increased preglomerular vascular resistance will have especially devastating effects, in that glomerular capillary pressure will fall along with the decrease in renal blood flow. The reduction in RBF also reduces glomerular filtration by increasing the rate of rise of glomerular oncotic pressure along the length of glomerular capillaries, thus further reducing net ultrafiltration pressure. The mediators of this vasoconstriction are unknown, but tubule injury seems to be an important concomitant finding. There is some experimental evidence that a low ultrafiltration coefficient may also play a role in reducing GFR during ARF, presumably as a result of mesangial cell contraction and consequent

reduction in the area available for filtration. Although obstruction to the outflow of urine into the collecting system is an obvious cause of reduced net ultrafiltration, less obvious is the intratubular obstruction that results from sloughed cells and cellular debris that evolves in the course of renal failure. The importance of this mechanism is highlighted by the improvement in renal function that follows relief of such intratubular obstruction. Also, when obstruction is prolonged (longer than a few hours), intrarenal vasoconstriction is prominent. Damaged renal epithelium is also abnormally permeable to markers of glomerular filtration, such as inulin; thus, back-leak of glomerular filtrate may be an additional mechanism of renal failure. Each of these mechanisms—vasoconstriction, mesangial cell contraction, tubular obstruction, and back-leak—contribute individually or in combination to the reduction in GFR during the course of ARF.

Apart from the increase in basal renal vascular tone observed during ARF, it is also true that the stressed renal microvasculature is more sensitive to the introduction of potentially vasoconstrictive drugs and otherwise tolerated changes in systemic blood pressure. For example, the use of nonsteroidal anti-inflammatory drugs in patients with severe liver disease may precipitate ARF. As a result, a prerenal state may progress to an intrinsic form of renal failure and thus reduce GFR further. Prolonged vasoconstriction may evolve into intrinsic ARF, especially when there is concomitant large-vessel arterial disease. This latter form of renal failure is often induced by the use of angiotensin-converting enzyme inhibitors and/or diuretics. The vasculature of the injured kidney has an impaired vasodilatory response and loses its autoregulatory behavior. This latter phenomenon has important clinical relevance, because the frequent reduction in systemic pressure during intermittent hemodialysis may provoke additional damage that could delay recovery of ARF.

PATHOPHYSIOLOGY OF THE CONCENTRATING DEFECT

Another physiologic hallmark of intrinsic ARF is the failure to concentrate urine maximally. The defect is not responsive to pharmacologic doses of vasopressin and is postreceptor in nature. The injured kidney fails to generate and maintain a high medullary solute gradient. Because the accumulation of solute in the medulla depends on normal distal nephron function, this is yet another example of the role of the distal nephron in the pathophysiology of ARF. The mechanism of this defect is not simply a function of lethally injured cells, because necrosis is not prominent in the distal nephron, but rather may involve more subtle effects on function, such as the observed loss of Aquaporin 2 expression following renal ischemia. The loss of Aquaporin 2 function would not only limit the reabsorption of water from the collecting ducts but also limit the deposition of urea from the terminal portion of the collecting ducts and limit medullary solute content. The failure to excrete a concentrated urine even in the face of oliguria is a helpful diagnostic tool to distinguish prerenal from intrinsic renal disease.

INDICES OF GLOMERULAR AND TUBULAR FUNCTION IN THE DIFFERENTIAL DIAGNOSIS OF ACUTE RENAL FAILURE

A rapid rise in serum creatinine, sometimes associated with a reduced urine volume, defines ARF. Given the conceptual framework previously discussed, determination of whether the cause of the renal failure is prerenal, intrinsic, or postrenal usually requires only a few noninvasive tests, in addition to detailed history and a thorough physical examination.

If a prerenal cause of ARF is suggested by history, confirmation of the adaptive nature of the response can be obtained by examining the urine and searching for evidence of enhanced renal water and solute reabsorption. The findings of a highly concentrated urine with a low pH in the absence of cellular elements are suggestive of an adaptive response to volume depletion. These findings, combined with a disproportionate rise of blood urea nitrogen as compared with creatinine and an elevated serum uric acid concentration, all point to prerenal causes. A widely used aid to discriminate between prerenal and intrinsic ARF is the determination of the fractional excretion of sodium ion:

$$FE_{Na} = (U_{Na}/P_{Na})/(U_{Cr}/P_{Cr}) \times 100$$

Low (less than 1%) fractional excretion indicates salt and water avidity and is consistent with prerenal causes of renal failure. The fractional excretion of other substances such as urea and uric acid has also been used (Table 33-3). Lethal and sublethal renal cell injury, on the other hand, would lead to diminished salt reclamation and failure to reach maximum urine concentration, and, as a result, FE_{Na} rises and exceeds 1%. This index is most helpful when the patient is oliguric, and the finding of high FE_{Na} under such circumstances is indicative of intrinsic causes of ARF.

A reliance on any of these determinations alone is hazardous, because the regulation of salt and water metabolism is complex and other variables that affect salt and water reabsorption may override those involved in ARF. For example, the fractional excretion of sodium may be low in intrinsic ARF when there are other comorbid events that enhance salt reabsorption. Coexistent heart and liver disease enhance renal sodium absorption even in the diseased kidney. An accurate history and thorough physical examination are a great help in this regard.

TABLE 33-3 Urinary Findings in Acute Renal Failure

Measure*	Prerenal	Intrinsic
BUN/Cr	>20/1	<20/1
U_{OSM} (mOsmol/kg)	>500	<350
U_{Na}	<20	>40
U_{urea}/P_{urea}	>8	<3
U_{Cr}/P_{Cr}	>40	<20
FE_{Na} (%)	<1	>1
FE_{urea} (%)	<35	>50
$FE_{uric\ acid}$ (%)	<7	>15
Urine microscopy	Nonspecific	May show muddy-brown granular casts, tubular cell casts

*Fractional excretion (FE) of substance X is given by the formula

$$(U_x/P_x)/(U_{Cr}/P_{Cr}) \times 100$$

where U_x and P_x represent the urine and plasma concentration of X in the same units.

Postrenal causes are detected by renal sonography. Renal perfusion scans do not usually help distinguish among the various causes of reduced renal perfusion except when there is asymmetric perfusion suggestive of renal vascular lesions. In this case, the presence of such lesions should be corroborated by magnetic resonance imaging angiography and ultimately confirmed by renal angiography.

TREATMENT OF ACUTE RENAL FAILURE: IMPLICATIONS DERIVED FROM NEWER UNDERSTANDING OF ITS PATHOPHYSIOLOGY

The mortality of ARF is still high, especially in those patients who require dialysis. This high mortality is in part due to a sicker and older population of patients receiving potentially nephrotoxic medical and surgical therapies. Recent insights into the pathophysiology of ARF have provided newer targets for therapy with the hope of improving outcome in these patients. Such approaches are summarized in Table 33-4.

Renal Vasodilation

A variety of therapeutic approaches have been used to limit the fall in RBF and renal vasoconstriction. Calcium channel blockade to relax the renal vasculature and ameliorate renal failure may be useful in ARF seen after kidney transplantation, cyclosporine administration, or radiocontrast dye exposure. It has not been effective in most other forms of renal failure. Dopamine, which vasodilates the normal renal vasculature and increases sodium excretion, is not effective clinically and is associated with significant side effects, especially in the critically ill patient. Atrial natriuretic peptide may improve

TABLE 33-4 Therapeutic Targets of Treatment of Acute Renal Failure

Offsetting vasoconstriction	Calcium channel blockage Atrial natriuretic factor Endothelin blockade Adenosine receptor blockade Nitric oxide regulation

Limiting inflammation	α-MSH
	Antiadhesion strategies
	    Anti-ICAM
	      Anti-integrins
	Biocompatible membranes
	Cytokine-absorbing
	    biomembranes

Altering cell outcome	Growth factors and "survival" factors
Dialysis prescription	High-flux membranes CAVHD CVVHD CVVH

CAVHD, Continuous arteriovenous hemodialysis; CAVVHD, Continuous venovenous hemodialysis; CVVH, Continuous venovenous hemofiltration; ICAM, intracellular adhesion molecule; α-MSH, α-melanocyte-stimulating hormone.

renal function in oliguric ARF patients but not in those who are nonoliguric. Isotonic saline infusion at relatively modest rates has been shown to ameliorate radiocontrast-induced ARF in patients with modest reduction of renal function before exposure. Newer studies documenting amelioration of experimental ischemic renal failure using specific antagonists of the renal adenosine system also show early promise. Modifying nitric oxide production has also been shown to protect kidneys experimentally. Finally, high-dose *N*-acetylcysteine, which ameliorates ischemia-reperfusion injury experimentally, may do so by its vasodilatory effects. Whether its use at lower dose in humans to prevent dye-induced renal failure will prove to be effective remains controversial. In every case, these strategies have been used to prevent rather than treat renal failure, so their use in established renal failure is unwarranted. Identification of the effector pathways responsible for the renal vasoconstriction offers the hope of more successful therapy targeted to the mechanism for the intense vasoconstriction observed during renal failure.

Modifying the Inflammatory Aspects of Acute Renal Failure

Several aspects of the renal stress response are proinflammatory in nature, including the increased expression of the potent monocyte and neutrophil chemotactic chemokines, monocyte chemotactic protein 1, and interleukin-8, respectively. Overproduction of cytokines may be an influence in many aspects of renal failure, including vasoconstriction and leukocyte invasion. The salutary

effect of α-melanocyte-stimulating hormone may be mediated by inhibition of chemokine production. Blockade of intracellular adhesion molecule I and integrin-mediated adhesion is a promising approach, which is mediated perhaps by interfering with inflammation. Strategies directed against the integrins may also operate by reducing intratubular obstruction, as stated earlier. Additional insight into how these chemokines affect kidney function will most likely yield additional approaches.

As indicated earlier, peroxisome proliferator-activated receptor-α ligands, such as etomoxir, protect the kidney from a variety of nephrotoxic insults, including ischemic and cisplatin-induced renal failure. The mechanism of this protection is not precisely known, but of special interest is the relationship of these observations to the salutary effects of insulin therapy in prevention of the need for renal replacement therapy in patients with sepsis in the ICU. Hyperglycemia, hyperlipidemia, and insulin resistance are common features of severe ARF. It would appear that the development of insulin resistance and lipid toxicity may be a consequence of the stress response in renal cells that is reversible by administration of these newer hypoglycemic agents.

Survival Factors

As previously discussed, renal stress initiates a transcriptional program that is intimately involved in cell fate. Some cells participating in this response will survive and repair, whereas others will die by apoptosis. What determines whether a cell will recover from such injury or undergo cell death by necrosis or apoptosis is probably a function of the severity of the stress, specific changes in gene regulation, and the availability of survival factors in the cell's external milieu. For example, cells may be made more vulnerable to otherwise tolerated doses of radiation by disabling a critical DNA repair enzyme or pathway. The survival of bone marrow cells damaged by cancer chemotherapeutic agents may be prevented by addition of growth factors essential to their survival even under normal conditions. Manipulation of the signal transduction pathways responsive to renal ischemia ameliorates cell death and improves renal function. Figure 33-3 provides the conceptual framework for this approach. The provision of survival factors, such as trophic cytokines and growth factors, in addition to accelerating entry of cells into replicative phases of the cell cycle and hence increasing the rate at which cells reline injured tubules, may also alter an apoptotic or even necrotic outcome to one of survival and repair. Early success with exogenously administered growth factors such as epidermal growth factor and insulin-like growth factor (among others), however, has not yet been successful in broadly applied strategies in diverse ARF settings. Survival factors identified during early morphogenesis of the kidney are also likely to be used in treatment of the injured kidney or be

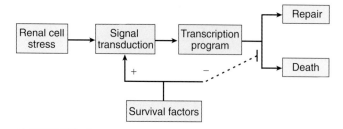

FIGURE 33-3 Survival factors and cell fate during renal cell stress.

used before exposure to mitigate the injury. It is highly likely that the vulnerability of a patient to the development of ARF after exposure to a nephrotoxic insult could be predicted by changes in the levels or activities of such response genes based on their DNA structure. Efforts to identify single-nucleotide polymorphisms and other polymorphisms in the stress pathway that correlate with outcome and response to treatment of ARF will be closely watched to see if they yield such predictive information.

Given the complex interaction among different tissues of the injured kidney, including vascular, epithelial, and interstitial components such as invading cells activated by secreted mediators of inflammation, it is not surprising that single strategies have failed so consistently to improve outcome especially in critically ill patients. It may be that multiple pathways will have to be targeted simultaneously in a therapeutic paradigm reminiscent of that used in the chemotherapy of cancer.

Renal Replacement Therapy

The decision to offer renal replacement therapy should be made cautiously, closely adhering to the indications for such therapy as outlined in other chapters of this text, because of the instability of the renal vasculature, the hypotension that acute intermittent hemodialysis can provoke, and the proinflammatory state of the injured kidney. For these reasons, modifications in the hemodialysis prescription to limit the frequency of hypotensive episodes and diminish cytokine production are currently being pursued.

BIBLIOGRAPHY

Basile DP: Rarefaction of peritubular capillaries following ischemic acute renal failure: A potential factor predisposing to progressive nephropathy. Curr Opin Nephrol Hypertens 13:1–7, 2004.

Burne-Tancy MJ, Rabb H: The role of adhesion molecules and T cells in ischemic renal injury. Curr Opin Nephrol Hypertens 12:85–90, 2003.

Chertow GM, Christiansen CL, Cleary PD, et al: Prognostic stratification in critically ill patients with acute renal failure requiring dialysis. Arch Intern Med 155:1505–1511, 1995.

Conger J, Rohinette JB, Hammond WS: Differences in vascular reactivity in models of ischemic acute renal failure. Kidney Int 39:1087–1097, 1991.

DiMari J, Megyesi J, Udvarhelyi N, et al: N-acetyl cysteine ameliorates ischemic renal failure. Am J Physiol 272:F292–F298, 1997.

Di Mari JF, Saggi S, Aronson P, Safirstein R: Renal ischemia reperfusion injury reduces Aquaporin-2 and NHE3 expression. J Am Soc Nephrol 7:1823, 1996.

Gobe Glenda C, Endre ZH: Cell death in toxic nephropathies. Semin Nephrol 23: 416–424, 2003.

Goligorsky MS, Lieberthal W, Racusen LC, Simon EE: Integrin receptors in renal tubular epithelium: New insights into pathophysiology of acute renal failure. Am J Physiol 264: F1–F8, 1993.

Gupta S, Verfaillie C, Chmielewski D, et al: A role for extrarenal cells in the regeneration following acute renal failure. Kidney Int 62:1285–1290, 2002.

Hakim RM: Clinical implications of hemodialysis membrane bio-compatibility. Kidney Int 44:484–494, 1993.

Kelly KJ, Williams LWW, Colvin RB, Bonventre JN: Antibody to intracellular adhesion molecule-I protects the kidney against ischemic injury. Proc Natl Acad Sci USA 91:812–816, 1994.

Morigi M, Imberti B, Zoja C, et al: Mesenchymal stem cells are renotropic, helping to repair the kidney and improve function in acute renal failure. J Am Soc Nephrol 15:1794–1804, 2004.

Noiri E, Peresleni T, Miller F, Goligorsky MS: In vivo targeting of inducible NO synthase with oligodeoxynucleotides protects rat kidney against ischemia. J Clin Invest 97:2377–2383, 1996.

Nouwen E, Verstrepen W, Buyssens N, et al: Hyperplasia, hypertrophy, and phenotypic alterations in the distal nephron after acute proximal tubular injury in the rat. Lab Invest 70:479–493, 1994.

Oliver JA, Barasch J, Yang J, et al: Metanephric mesenchyme contains embryonic renal stem cells. Am J Physiol Renal Physiol 283:F799–F809, 2002.

Safirstein R, Miller P, Dikman S, et al: Cisplatin nephrotoxicity in rats: Defect in papillary hypertonicity. Am J Physiol 241: F175–F185, 1981.

Safirstein R, Bonventre JV: Molecular response to ischemic and nephrotoxic acute renal failure. In Schlondorff D, Bonventre JV (eds): Molecular Nephrology: Kidney Function in Health and Disease. New York, Dekker, 1995, pp. 839–854.

Simmons EM, Himmelfarb J, Sezer MT, et al, for the PICARD Study Group: Plasma cytokine levels predict mortality in patients with acute renal failure. Kidney Int 65:1357–1365, 2004.

Solez K, Finckh ES: Is there a correlation between morphologic and functional changes in human acute renal failure? Data of Finckh, Jeremy, and Whyte re-examined twenty years later. In Solez K, Whelton A (eds): Acute Renal Failure: Correlations between Morphology and Function. New York, Dekker, 1984, pp. 3–12.

Star RA: Treatment of acute renal failure. Kidney Int 54: 1817–1831, 1998.

Tepel M, van der Giet M, Schwarzfeld C, et al: Prevention of radiographic-contrast-agent-induced reductions in renal function by acetylcysteine. N Engl J Med 20:180–184, 2000.

Van Bommel E, Bowry N, So K, et al: Acute dialytic support for the critically ill: Intermittent hemodialysis versus continuous arteriovenous hemodiafiltration. Am J Nephrol 15:192–200, 1995.

Van Den Berghe G, Wouters P, Weekers F, et al: Intensive insulin therapy in critically ill patients. N Engl J Med 345:1359–1367, 2001.

CHAPTER 34

Clinical Approach to the Diagnosis of Acute Renal Failure

Jean L. Holley

Acute renal failure (ARF) is a sudden reduction in glomerular filtration rate (GFR) that is expressed clinically as the retention of nitrogenous waste products (urea, creatinine) in the blood. The accumulation of these nitrogenous waste products is termed azotemia. In most cases of ARF, the serum creatinine rises 1 to 2 mg/dL/day. Depending on the clinical circumstances and the patient's symptoms, renal replacement therapy (dialysis) may be required. Despite the widespread availability of dialysis, the mortality of patients who develop ARF remains high, from 10% to 50% depending on the patient's comorbidities and the medical setting in which the kidney dysfunction occurs (e.g., intensive care unit, obstetric, surgical). At least half of all episodes of ARF are iatrogenic and related to medications or procedures. In most cases, by following a basic algorithm that focuses on the patient's history, physical exam, urinalysis, review of basic laboratory results, and, in some instances, radiologic imaging of the kidneys and determination of urine sodium and fractional excretion of sodium and urea, the cause of ARF can be determined. The patient's history (especially medications, procedures, changes in blood pressure), findings on physical exam (particularly assessment of volume status), blood urea nitrogen (BUN)/creatinine ratio, and urinalysis results will usually provide the information necessary to determine if the ARF is a prerenal, intrinsic renal, or postrenal event. In some cases, a spot urine sodium concentration or ultrasound of the kidneys may also be needed in the initial evaluation. Once the appropriate classification (prerenal, intrinsic renal, or postrenal) has been determined, the need for additional diagnostic tests as well as therapeutic interventions will be clear.

ACUTE VERSUS CHRONIC KIDNEY DISEASE

Because ARF usually resolves and chronic kidney disease often progresses to endstage renal disease and the need for chronic dialysis, it is useful to determine if a patient's elevated creatinine is the result of an acute insult or a progressive loss of functioning nephrons. When past serum creatinine values are not available, it may be difficult to distinguish acute from chronic kidney disease. In such cases, a kidney ultrasound to document the size of the kidneys may be helpful. The kidneys will often be small (less than 10 cm longitudinally in a person of normal stature) and echogenic if the kidney disease is chronic and slowly progressive. Normal-sized kidneys on ultrasound do not absolutely exclude chronic kidney disease, but small, echogenic kidneys are not consistent with ARF. Clearly an individual may have concomitant ARF and chronic kidney disease, and in such cases of ARF superimposed on chronic kidney disease, the kidney size is less helpful. Laboratory features suggestive but not diagnostic of chronic kidney disease include a normocytic anemia, hyperphosphatemia, and hypocalcemia. The presence of nonspecific symptoms of uremia (e.g., nausea and vomiting, pruritus, fatigue) may also suggest chronic rather than ARF, but there is no single variable other than kidney size or serial elevated creatinine values over time that conclusively establishes that the kidney function impairment is chronic and not acute. Patients with chronic kidney disease may also develop episodes of ARF. In such cases, the kidneys are usually small and the baseline creatinine is elevated. An abrupt and unexpected rise in the baseline creatinine in such patients should prompt an evaluation for superimposed, potentially reversible ARF.

CLASSIFICATION OF ACUTE RENAL FAILURE

All cases of ARF can be classified into prerenal, intrinsic (or intrarenal), and postrenal causes (Table 34-1). Classifying each episode of ARF directs appropriate diagnostic and therapeutic strategies. ARF is also clinically described as oliguric (less than 400 mL urine output/24 hours), nonoliguric (greater than 400 mL urine output/24 hours), or anuric (less than 100 mL urine/24 hours). These categories are helpful to establish cause and predict prognosis. Anuria is uncommon and suggests either complete obstruction or a major vascular event such as bilateral renal infarction, renal vein thrombosis, cortical necrosis, or high-grade ischemic acute tubular necrosis (ATN). Prerenal, intrinsic renal, and postrenal ARF can each present

TABLE 34-1   Classification of Acute Renal Failure

Prerenal (Reduced renal perfusion)
  Volume depletion
    Renal loss—diuretics, osmotic diuresis (DKA),
      addisonian crisis
    Extrarenal loss—vomiting, diarrhea, skin losses (burns,
      Sweating)
  Hypotension (regardless of cause)
  Cardiovascular
    Congestive heart failure, reduced myocardial function,
      arrhythmias
  Hemodynamic (intense intrarenal vasoconstriction)
    Radiographic contrast
    Prostaglandin inhibition (NSAIDs)
    Cyclosporine and tacrolimus
    ACE inhibitors
    Amphotericin B
  Hypercalcemia
  Hepatorenal syndrome (bland urinary sediment, oliguria,
    low urine sodium, not reversed with volume repletion,
    reversible with successful liver transplant)

Intrinsic or intrarenal
  Vascular
    Renal infarction, renal artery stenosis, renal vein
      thrombosis
    Malignant hypertension, scleroderma renal crisis,
      atheroemboli
  Tubular
    Ischemic—prolonged prerenal state, sepsis syndrome,
      systemic hypotension
    Nephrotoxic—aminoglycosides, methotrexate, cisplatin,
      myoglobin (rhabdomyolysis), hemoglobin
  Glomerular
    Acute glomerulonephritis
    Vasculitis (Wegener's granulomatosis, polyarteritis)
    Thrombotic microangiopathy (hemolytic uremic
      syndrome, TTP)
  Interstitium
    Medications—penicillins, cephalosporins, ciprofloxacin,
      NSAIDs, phenytoin
    Tumor infiltration (lymphoma, leukemia)

Postrenal (obstruction)
  Prostate hypertrophy, neurogenic bladder
  Intraureteral obstruction—crystals (uric acid, acyclovir,
    indinavir), stones, clots, tumor
  Extraureteral obstruction—tumor (cervical, prostate),
    retroperitoneal fibrosis

ACE, angiotensin converting enzyme; DKA, diabetic ketoacidosis;
NSAIDs, nonsteroidal anti-inflammatory drugs; TTP, thrombotic
thrombocytopenic purpura.

clinically with oliguria or nonoliguria. Nonoliguric ARF is common in intrarenal ARF (e.g., nephrotoxin-induced ATN, acute glomerulonephritis, and acute interstitial nephritis). Oliguria more commonly characterizes obstruction and prerenal azotemia. Regardless of the cause of decreased kidney function, the patient who is oliguric is more difficult to manage because volume overload will occur earlier. Moreover, patients with nonoliguric ARF have a more favorable prognosis and reduced mortality.

PRERENAL ACUTE RENAL FAILURE

Prerenal abnormalities are physiologic responses that lead to decreased kidney function (decreased GFR). These manifest clinically as an elevated BUN and creatinine because of decreased perfusion of the kidney. The reduced renal perfusion that results in prerenal ARF may occur as a consequence of inadequate volume (e.g., due to blood loss or overly aggressive diuresis), inadequate cardiac output due to impaired myocardial function (e.g., cardiogenic shock following an acute myocardial infarction or, more commonly, progressive cardiomyopathy), or marked vasodilatation as may occur with sepsis. In each of these situations, the underlying kidney is normal but ARF occurs because the primary disorder (volume depletion or reduced cardiac output) compromises renal blood flow enough to reduce GFR. In cases of depleted intravascular fluid volume and congestive heart failure (the two most common causes of prerenal azotemia), the kidney will initially compensate for the diminished perfusion to preserve filtration function. Mechanisms of self-preservation include autoregulatory afferent arteriolar dilation and attenuation of afferent vasoconstriction by intrarenal prostaglandin-mediated vasodilatation. These and other physiologic maneuvers compose renal compensation or autoregulation and are ultimately an attempt by the kidney to maintain the GFR in the face of hypoperfusion. When the renal compensation is maximized and the conditions causing the hypoperfusion remain uncorrected, renal compensation becomes decompensation and ARF occurs. The development of ARF after ingestion of a nonsteroidal anti-inflammatory drug (NSAID) by a patient who has congestive heart failure is a common clinical example of this type of hemodynamic insult. In this situation, the protaglandin-mediated compensatory renal vasodilatation that occurs because the kidneys are hypoperfused from poor cardiac output is inhibited by the NSAID and a consequent reduction in GFR occurs, manifested by a rising BUN and creatinine.

Intense intrarenal vasoconstriction may result in ARF, causing reduced renal blood flow and subsequent reduction of glomerular perfusion. This hemodynamically mediated form of ARF resembles prerenal azotemia and is seen with exposure to radiographic contrast, cyclosporine and tacrolimus, amphotericin, and NSAIDs (see Table 34-1). Uncorrected, such episodes of prerenal azotemia may progress to ischemic ATN. Like other forms of prerenal azotemia, the urinalysis in cases of vasoconstrictor or hemodynamically mediated prerenal azotemia is bland and urinary sodium is often low.

Evidence of preserved renal functional ability and the kidney's attempt to compensate for the reduced perfusion in prerenal states is the maximum tubular sodium reabsorption that occurs and is reflected in a low urine sodium (less than 20 mEq/L) and/or low fractional excretion of sodium or urea (less than 1% and 35%, respectively; Table 34-2). The fractional excretion of sodium, unlike the simpler urine sodium, evaluates only the fraction of filtered sodium that is excreted and is therefore not affected by changes in water reabsorption that can affect the simple urine sodium concentration. The filtered sodium is the product of the GFR (estimated by creatinine clearance) and the concentration of plasma sodium. Thus, the fractional excretion of sodium, FE_{Na} (where U_x is the urinary concentration of x, P_x is the plasma concentration of x, and V is urine volume) is defined as:

$$FE_{Na} = \frac{\text{Na excreted}}{\text{Na filtered}} \times 100$$

$$= \frac{U_{Na} \cdot V}{P_{Na} \cdot GFR} \times 100$$

$$\text{Since } GFR = \frac{U_{Creat} \cdot V}{P_{Creat}}$$

$$FE_{Na} = \frac{U_{Na} \cdot V}{P_{Na} \cdot \dfrac{U_{Creat} \cdot V}{P_{Creat}}} \times 100$$

$$= \frac{\dfrac{U_{Na}}{P_{Na}}}{\dfrac{U_{Creat}}{P_{Creat}}} \times 100$$

Although the urine sodium and fractional excretion of sodium are typically low in ARF as a result of prerenal causes, and high (greater than 40 mEq/L and greater than or equal to 1%, respectively) in the setting of ATN, occasionally, a fractional excretion of sodium less than 1% may be seen with nonoliguric ATN, ARF due to radiographic contrast, and sepsis. In addition, diuretics are often given as part of the treatment of prerenal conditions (e.g., congestive heart failure) so as to increase urine output. In such settings, the fractional excretion of urea may be a more sensitive and specific indicator of a prerenal state. The fractional excretion of urea is calculated by substituting urea nitrogen for sodium in the equation just given. A result less than or equal to 35% is consistent with a prerenal state (see Table 34-2).

With prerenal azotemia, the renal insult, which results from hypoperfusion, is indirect. The kidney's intrinsic ability to function is preserved. Glomeruli and glomerular basement membrane are intact, and there is no tubular or interstitial damage. The urine is generally concentrated, with a high specific gravity and osmolality, but otherwise unremarkable. The dipstick shows no proteinuria or blood, and the microscopic examination is bland, with no red blood cells (RBCs), white blood cells (WBCs), or cellular casts. Hyaline casts may be present. Mild qualitative proteinuria (e.g., trace or 1+ on dipstick) may sometimes be seen in highly concentrated urines. The history will suggest volume loss or cardiac failure (Tables 34-1 and 34-3). The most important aspect of the physical exam is to assess the patient's volume status. In terms of renal perfusion, intravascular volume overload with a decrease in effective arterial volume (congestive heart failure, cirrhosis) and intravascular volume depletion are identical; each leads to renal hypoperfusion. Thus, in these situations that are clinically quite different, the renal response is the same: maximal sodium retention in an attempt to compensate for the reduced perfusion. Clearly, the appropriate treatment for ARF in this situation is to increase the renal perfusion, and, indeed, rapid reversal of the prerenal azotemia occurs if appropriate treatment is given (e.g., volume repletion). Unlike creatinine, urea diffuses across membranes and active urea reabsorption occurs when there is reduced urine flow. Therefore, prerenal azotemia is characterized by an

TABLE 34-2 Urinalysis, U_{Na}, FE_{Na}, FE_{UN}, and BUN/Creatinine Ratio in Acute Renal Failure

Type of Acute Renal Failure	Urinalysis	U_{Na} (mEq/L)	FE_{Na} (%)	FE_{UN} (%)	BUN/Creatinine Ratio
Prerenal	High specific gravity Normal or hyaline casts	<20	<1	≤35	>20:1
Intrarenal					
Acute tubular necrosis	Low specific gravity Muddy-brown casts Renal tubular epithelial cells	>40	≥1	>50	≤20:1
Vascular disorders	Normal or hematuria	>20	Variable		
Glomerulonephritis	Proteinuria, hematuria RBC casts	<20	<1		
Interstitial nephritis	Mild proteinuria, hematuria WBCs, WBC casts, eosinophils	>20	≥1		
Postrenal	Normal or hematuria WBCs, occasional granular casts	>20	Variable		≥20:1

FE_{Na}, fractional excretion of sodium; FE_{UN}, fractional excretion of urea; U_{Na}, urinary sodium.
U_{Na}, FE_{Na}, and FE_{UN} are variable with postrenal, interstitial nephritis, and glomerulonephritis.

TABLE 34-3 Using the History and Physical Exam as Tools to Categorize Acute Renal Failure

Type of Acute Renal Failure	History	Physical Exam
Prerenal	Volume loss (vomiting, diarrhea, diuretics, burns)	Weight, supine and standing blood pressure and pulse
	Past weights, daily intake/output values	
	Cardiac disease, liver disease	Mucous membranes, axillary moisture
	Thirst	Neck veins, S3, lung exam, edema
	Medications (NSAIDs, ACE inhibitors, cyclosporine)	
	Radiographic contrast (CT, angiography)	
Inrarenal		
ATN	Medications (aminoglycosides)	Same as above—volume status
	Alcohol abuse, trauma, muscle necrosis (rhabdomyolysis)	Compartment syndrome—extremities
	Episode of hypotension	
Vascular	Trauma, known nephrotic syndrome, flank pain	BP, livedo reticularis
	Vessel catheterization, anticoagulation (atheroemboli)	Funduscopic exam (malignant hypertension)
	Progressive systemic sclerosis	Thickened skin, sclerodactyly, telangiectasia
Glomerular	Systemic disease (SLE, vasculitis)—arthritis, rash	Oral ulcers, arthritis, skin lesions, foot drop
	Uveitis, weight loss, fatigue, intravenous drug use (hepatitis C)	Pleural and pericardial rubs
	Cough, hemoptysis (Goodpasture's), foamy urine	Edema—periorbital, leg, presacral
Interstitial	Medications (antibiotics, allopurinol, phenytoin)	Fever, drug rash
	Arthralgias	
Postrenal	Urinary urgency, hesitancy, gross hematuria	Bladder distention, pelvic masses, prostate
	Intermittent polyuria, history of stones	
	Medications (indinavir, acyclovir, anticholinergics)	

ACE, angiotensin converting enzyme; CT, computed tomography; NSAIDs, nonsteroidal anti-inflammatory drugs; SLE, systemic lupus erythematosus.

elevated BUN/creatinine ratio (greater than 20:1). Other causes of a BUN/creatinine ratio greater than 20:1 include postrenal ARF, gastrointestinal blood loss (digested protein from an upper gastrointestinal bleed is absorbed and metabolized by the liver), high-dose corticosteroid therapy, and intense catabolism.

POSTRENAL ACUTE RENAL FAILURE: OBSTRUCTIVE UROPATHY

The extent of pathology in postrenal ARF (obstructive uropathy) is determined by the level at which the obstruction occurs (see Chapter 51). However, the endpoint of all obstructive lesions is the potential destruction of functioning kidney parenchyma. The elevated pressures in obstructed conduits results in adaptive dilatation (hydroureter, hydronephrosis), which ultimately progresses to nephron destruction (atrophy of the tubular epithelium, interstitial fibrosis, and ultimately glomerular scarring) if unrelieved. Postrenal causes of ARF necessarily involve obstruction of both kidneys or both ureters, unless the patient has only a single functioning kidney. In patients with two functioning kidneys, unilateral obstruction (e.g., an obstructing kidney stone) will rarely cause ARF because the glomerular filtration of the unobstructed kidney is not reduced. In postrenal azotemia, the history can identify predisposing factors and symptoms (see Tables 34-1 and 34-3). Reduced urine output (oliguria) and/or anuria are common in postrenal ARF. The

physical exam, like the history, should focus on the possibility of obstruction (pelvic masses, distended bladder, prostatic enlargement). Because there is reduced urine flow with obstruction, the BUN/creatinine ratio is usually elevated, as is the case in prerenal azotemia. Development of a type IV renal tubular acidosis may sometimes be a diagnostic clue in obstructive uropathy. The urine sediment and concentration are variable and generally not helpful in the diagnosis of obstruction, except that hematuria may be seen with stones or tumor and gross hematuria due to urothelial tumors may obstruct the collecting system with clots. A renal ultrasound will usually show hydronephrosis when obstruction is causing the ARF. Bladder catheterization with marked urine volume or a postvoid residual of greater than 100 mL confirm the presence of postrenal ARF. Rarely, despite the presence of obstruction, hydronephrosis may not be demonstrated on ultrasound. Retroperitoneal fibrosis is often seen in such cases and may be confirmed by computed tomography (CT) scan or magnetic resonance imaging (MRI). When the clinical suspicion of obstruction is high and hydronephrosis is not seen on ultrasound, additional kidney imaging such as a CT scan, MRI, or retrograde nephrograms should be done.

Like the external obstruction that occurs with tumor or prostate enlargement, intraureteral obstruction may also cause azotemia (see Table 34-1). Kidney stones, endogenous (uric acid as in acute tumor lysis) or exogenous crystals (medications such as indinavir, acyclovir), or other material (blood clots, renal papillae as in papillary necrosis, or uroepithelial tumors of the ureter or renal pelvis) can cause postrenal ARF by intraureteral obstruction. The ARF caused by obstruction will usually resolve with relief of the obstruction (by placement of a bladder catheter or nephrostomy tube). However, prolonged obstruction may cause irreversible nephron destruction and lead to chronic kidney disease.

INTRINSIC OR INTRARENAL ACUTE RENAL FAILURE

Intrinsic ARF can be categorized anatomically by the area of the kidney parenchyma involved: vascular, glomerular, tubular, or interstitial areas. Differences in the clinical setting and presentation, particularly in the history, physical exam, and urinalysis, will distinguish between these types of ARF. Determining if a patient has ATN, acute interstitial nephritis, or acute glomerulonephritis as the cause of ARF is necessary because the treatment and prognosis of each may differ. With all types of intrarenal ARF, the kidney itself is the site of the abnormality. Unlike prerenal and postrenal ARF, the decrement in GFR is directly linked to kidney damage and not the result of reduced renal perfusion or elevated pressures in the renal conduits. Since urea reabsorption is not preferentially increased, urea and creatinine concentrations rise in parallel and the BUN/creatinine ratio is usually preserved (10–20:1). Similarly, because the impaired kidney function results from direct kidney injury, the urinalysis is usually abnormal. Specific findings on dipstick and microscopic examination of the urine provide important clues to the location of the parenchymal injury responsible for the kidney dysfunction (see Table 34-2). In some cases, despite a careful history, physical exam, urinalysis, and additional specific tests (see Table 34-3), the type of the kidney disorder (tubular, vascular, glomerular, interstitial) remains undefined and a percutaneous kidney biopsy will be needed to determine the cause.

Acute tubular necrosis is the most common type of acute intrinsic ARF seen in hospitalized patients. Unfortunately, the term ATN is sometimes used interchangeably with ARF. As illustrated in Table 34-1, ATN is only one form of intrinsic ARF.

Acute Tubular Necrosis as a Cause of Intrinsic Acute Renal Failure

At least 45% of the cases of ARF are caused by ATN. Since the two major causes of ATN are ischemia and nephrotoxins, ATN can be characterized as ischemic or nephrotoxic. Important clues to these kidney insults are in the patient's history. Ischemia is the most common cause of ATN and often follows a prolonged prerenal state with its associated renal hypoperfusion. The history may reveal systemic hypotension, marked volume depletion,

or reduced effective circulating volume. Distinguishing between ongoing prerenal azotemia that is reversible and ATN may be difficult. However, the hallmark of prerenal ARF is its reversibility with restoration of renal perfusion (e.g., appropriate volume repletion); ATN does not improve simply with volume repletion. The point at which a patient moves from prerenal azotemia to ischemic ATN will vary depending on the patient and the clinical situation. Unless the patient is clearly volume overloaded, a fluid challenge to exclude a prerenal state will usually be an integral part of the diagnosis as well as the therapy of suspected ischemic ATN.

Clinical features that may help to distinguish ischemic ATN from prerenal azotemia include the urinalysis and urinary sodium and fractional excretion of sodium and urea (see Table 34-2). As already discussed, because the kidney is essentially normal in prerenal ARF, the urinalysis is unremarkable. In contrast, with ATN, evidence of the damaged tubules is usually seen in the urinary sediment; renal tubular epithelial cells and granular casts characterize ATN. The hallmark of ATN is the presence of dirty (or muddy) brown casts, a urinalysis finding that is pathognomonic of ATN. Because the tubules are the only site of renal injury in ATN, urinary findings that typify glomerular (proteinuria, RBCs, RBC casts) or interstitial injury (hematuria, WBCs, WBC casts) are not seen. Prerenal azotemia is characterized by intact tubular function, reduced renal blood flow, and, therefore, maximal tubular reabsorption of sodium and urea (see Table 34-2). With ATN, in contrast, there is direct tubular damage and a loss of tubular function manifested by a high urine sodium and fractional excretion of sodium and urea. These characteristic findings on urinalysis and urinary sodium determination occur with both ischemic and nephrotoxic forms of ATN.

Aminoglycosides are among the most common causes of nephrotoxic ATN (see Chapter 35). With aminoglycoside-induced ATN, the creatinine usually begins to rise 5 to 10 days after administration. Other nephrotoxins that may cause ATN include methotrexate, cis-platinum, and endogenous pigments such as hemoglobin and myoglobin (as seen with rhabdomyolysis). As discussed earlier, the fractional excretion of sodium and urea are usually high in ATN. In most cases, both nephrotoxic and ischemic ATN resolve. However, depending on the level of kidney dysfunction that occurs, temporary dialysis may be necessary.

Vascular Damage Resulting in Intrinsic Acute Renal Failure

Acute events involving the main renal arteries or veins can cause ARF. As with obstruction, bilateral involvement is required for acute azotemia to develop, unless at baseline the patient has a solitary functioning kidney. Bilateral kidney infarction, renal vein thrombosis, or acute occlusion of the renal arteries may lead to acute intrinsic renal failure. Because the kidney parenchyma itself may not be initially directly injured, some would classify these forms of ARF as prerenal azotemia rather than as cases of intrinsic ARF. Involvement of smaller blood vessels may also cause intrinsic ARF. Examples of this kind of ARF include malignant hypertension, scleroderma renal crisis, and cholesterol atheroembolic disease. In some systems of classification, ARF due to vasculitis will also be included among the vascular types of intrinsic ARF. However, because glomerular involvement with its associated proteinuria and active urinary sediment is common with vasculitis, here vasculitides are classified under glomerular causes of intrinsic ARF (see Table 34-1).

Historical data that suggest an acute vascular event as the cause of ARF include trauma, underlying nephrotic syndrome with significant proteinuria (a predisposition to renal vein thrombosis), or acute flank pain with hematuria. Microscopic hematuria, with or without proteinuria, is the most common finding on urinalysis in intrinsic ARF caused by vascular problems. Disease of the renal arteries or veins that results in ARF will generally require imaging to confirm the diagnosis. For example, MRI may reveal renal vein thrombosis or renal artery stenosis, CT scan may show renal infarction, and a radionuclide renal scan or Doppler ultrasound study may confirm the presence or absence of renal blood flow. Atheroemboli are the most common vascular problem causing intrinsic ARF. Important historical features of atheroembolic ARF include catheterization of the arterial system and anticoagulation. The physical exam in atheroembolic ARF may suggest widespread atheroemboli by demonstrating livedo reticularis in the skin of the toes and feet, and Hollenhorst plaques in the retina (see Chapter 37).

Glomerular Type of Intrinsic Acute Renal Failure

Acute inflammation of vessels and/or glomeruli causing ARF may reflect renal involvement of a systemic illness (e.g., systemic lupus erythematosus, Wegener's granulomatosis, polyarteritis nodosa) that will be suggested by the medical history and physical exam (see Table 34-3; Chapters 16 and 26). Because proteinuria occurring with glomerular involvement is often in the nephrotic range (greater than 3 g/24 hours), volume overload, and especially edema and hypertension on physical exam, will be common with acute glomerulonephritis. The urinalysis provides the most important clues to intrinsic ARF due to glomerulonephritis. Proteinuria and blood on urine dipstick and microscopic hematuria and RBC casts are characteristic (see Table 34-2). Probably because renin, and thus, aldosterone is stimulated in the setting of glomerulonephritis, the urine sodium may be low. However, the urinalysis and supporting history and physical exam are the diagnostic keys to acute glomerulonephritis. The abnormal urinalysis in acute glomerulonephritis essentially excludes prerenal azotemia and ATN, and thus urine sodium is rarely a diagnostic key to ARF caused by glomerulonephritis.

Interstitial Type of Intrinsic Acute Renal Failure

Involvement of the interstitium can also cause ARF on an intrarenal basis (see Chapter 48). Acute interstitial nephritis is associated with a variety of medications (penicillin antibiotics, allopurinol). Thus, the history of exposure to a new medication is the key to the diagnosis of this kind of intrinsic ARF. In about a third of the cases of acute interstitial nephritis, a systemic illness may occur that is characterized by fever, a maculopapular erythematous rash, arthralgias, and eosinophilia. These clinical features have led some to refer to this entity as allergic interstitial nephritis. The urinalysis with acute interstitial nephritis usually shows mild proteinuria, microscopic hematuria, WBCs, and sometimes WBC casts. Eosinophiluria may be present on Hansel or Wright stain of the urine. However, eosinophiluria is not pathognomonic of acute interstitial nephritis, because urine eosinophils may also be seen in cholesterol atheroembolic ARF, glomerulonephritis, and prostatitis. Percutaneous kidney biopsy may sometimes be needed to distinguish between interstitial nephritis and other forms of acute intrinsic renal failure (notably ATN).

BIBLIOGRAPHY

Carvounis CP, Nisar S, Guro-Razuman S: Significance of the fractional excretion of urea in the differential diagnosis of acute renal failure. Kidney Int 62:2223–2229, 2002.

Esson ML, Schrier RW: Diagnosis and treatment of acute tubular necrosis. Ann Intern Med 137:744–752, 2002.

Hou SH, Bushinsky DA, Wish JB, et al: Hospital-acquired renal insufficiency: A prospective study. Am J Med 74:243–248, 1983.

Klahr S, Miller SB: Acute oliguria. N Engl J Med 338:671–675, 1998.

Liano F, Pascual J: Epidemiology of acute renal failure: A prospective, multicenter community-based study. Madrid Acute Renal Failure Study Group. Kidney Int 50:811–818, 1996.

Miller TR, Anderson RJ, Linas SL, et al: Urinary diagnostic indices in acute renal failure: A prospective study. Ann Intern Med 89:47–50, 1978.

Nolan CR, Anderson RJ: Hospital-acquired acute renal failure. J Am Soc Nephrol 9:701–718, 1998.

CHAPTER 35

Kidney Failure Due to Therapeutic Agents

Thomas M. Coffman

Compounds used for diagnostic and therapeutic purposes are a major cause of acute renal failure (ARF) and chronic kidney disease. Because it is a major route of excretion for a variety of drugs, the kidney is a frequent target for injury by therapeutic agents. As a part of the excretory process, these materials are greatly concentrated in the urinary space and within renal tubular cells, enhancing their potential to cause local toxicity. Also, the rate of blood flow per gram of tissue weight in the kidney is relatively high, resulting in exaggerated exposure of renal endothelial cells and glomeruli to circulating substances. Since most kidney functions are dependent on tightly regulated blood flow patterns, agents that impair these hemodynamic relationships may interfere with the ability of the kidney to maintain normal homeostasis.

Drug toxicity in the kidney is manifested through the prototypical clinical syndromes that are associated with kidney diseases of other causes. As depicted in Table 35-1, these include ARF, chronic kidney disease, and nephrotic syndrome. Moreover, a single agent may cause more than one of these clinical syndromes. The particular clinical manifestation of nephrotoxicity is determined by the chemical properties of the agent, the dose and duration of exposure, and individual patient variables such as age, volume status, and genetic background. This chapter describes a general approach to nephrotoxicity and reviews the renal effects of some common causative agents. More detailed discussions of individual agents or syndromes associated with toxic kidney injury can be found in other chapters (see Chapters 38, 40, and 48, for example).

DIAGNOSIS OF DRUG-INDUCED NEPHROTOXICITY

The possibility of drug-induced nephrotoxicity should be considered when the serum creatinine concentration rises during administration of a therapeutic agent. Because of the nonlinear relationship between serum creatinine and glomerular filtration rate (GFR), a substantial reduction in GFR is necessary before toxic injury can be appreciated clinically. This point is particularly important

to consider in the context of agents that may cause chronic nephropathy. In this case, kidney injury may not be detected until 40% to 50% of kidney function has been irreversibly lost. A number of diagnostic markers, such as urinary excretion of tubular enzymes, have been evaluated as indicators of kidney toxicity that might be more sensitive and specific than serum creatinine. However, none of these has yet found widespread clinical application.

The clinical syndromes caused by drugs mimic those associated with kidney diseases of other causes. Thus, when the etiology of renal failure is being investigated, the possible role of therapeutic agents should always be considered, and a detailed medication history is an essential component of the clinical evaluation. Accordingly, temporal associations between the appearance of a kidney abnormality and medication changes must be documented. In patients who are receiving compounds known to be nephrotoxic, the plan for clinical management should include avoidance of clinical risk factors, careful monitoring of kidney function, and, when appropriate, monitoring of serum drug levels. Also, the role of nephrotoxins in exacerbating renal failure from other causes should be considered. For example, in the hospitalized patient with acute tubular necrosis (ATN), the potential aggravating consequences of aminoglycosides, radiocontrast, or other nephrotoxins must be recognized. Renal clearance of certain drugs will also be substantially reduced in such patients, and dosing must be adjusted appropriately (see Chapter 41).

ACUTE RENAL FAILURE FROM THERAPEUTIC AGENTS

In approaching any patient with acute kidney dysfunction, a potential causative role for therapeutic agents should always be considered. As illustrated in Table 35-1, mechanisms of ARF related to drugs can be roughly categorized as prerenal/hemodynamic, intrarenal, or postrenal/obstructive syndromes. As described in Chapter 34, this separation can be extremely helpful in identifying the etiology and directing management of patients with ARF from any cause.

TABLE 35-1 Kidney Syndromes Caused by Therapeutic Agents*

Clinical Syndrome	Causative Agents
Acute renal failure	
Prerenal/hemodynamic	Cyclosporine, tacrolimus, radiocontrast, ACE inhibitors, amphotericin B, ARBs, NSAIDs, IL-2
Intrarenal	
Acute tubular necrosis	Aminoglycosides, amphotericin B, cisplatin, certain cephalosporins
Acute interstitial nephritis	Penicillins, cephalosporins, sulfonamides, rifampin, NSAIDs, interferon, IL-2
Postrenal/obstructive	Acyclovir, analgesic abuse, methysergide, methotrexate, indinavir, sulfadiazine
Chronic kidney disease	Lithium, analgesic abuse, cyclosporine, tacrolimus, cisplatin, nitrosoureas
Nephrotic syndrome	Gold, NSAIDs, penicillamine, captopril, interferon

ACE, angiotensin-coverting enzyme; ARBs, angiotensin receptor blockers; IL-2, interleukin-2; NSAIDs, nonsteroidal anti-inflammatory drugs.
*This is a representative, but not exhaustive list of etiologic agents. Please refer to individual chapters for more complete listings.

PRERENAL AZOTEMIA: HEMODYNAMICALLY MEDIATED REDUCTION IN KIDNEY FUNCTION ASSOCIATED WITH DRUGS

As shown in Table 35-1, several classes of therapeutic agents, including cyclosporine, tacrolimus, radiocontrast, nonsteroidal anti-inflammatory drugs (NSAIDs), angiotensin-converting enzyme (ACE) inhibitors, and angiotensin receptor blockers (ARBs), can cause a syndrome of abnormal kidney function that resembles prerenal azotemia. Similar to prerenal azotemia from other causes, hemodynamic renal dysfunction caused by drugs can be associated with low urine sodium excretion. Generally, kidney dysfunction rapidly remits when the offending agent is discontinued, but persistent injury may result if exposure is prolonged or if aggravating conditions are present.

Drugs cause hemodynamically mediated kidney dysfunction through several mechanisms. Agents such as cyclosporine, tacrolimus, radiocontrast, and amphotericin B cause intense vasoconstriction in the kidney, reducing renal blood flow and glomerular perfusion. These compounds do not seem to affect vascular tone directly but may stimulate production of other vasoconstrictors such as endothelin or thromboxane A_2. Cyclosporine, tacrolimus, and amphotericin B can produce kidney dysfunction in normal subjects with no underlying kidney abnormalities.

In contrast, hemodynamic kidney dysfunction associated with NSAIDs generally occurs in patients with pre-existing impairment of renal perfusion. NSAIDs inhibit the cyclooxygenase isoenzymes, turning off the synthesis of prostaglandins. In normal subjects, renal prostaglandin production is low and administration of NSAIDs has little effect on kidney function. However, as an adaptive mechanism, production of vasodilator prostaglandins increases when renal perfusion is threatened. In these circumstances, inhibiting production of these vasodilator compounds by NSAIDs can cause precipitous declines in renal blood flow and GFR. This syndrome is most often seen in patients with volume depletion, heart failure, and pre-existing kidney disease (see Chapter 40).

Similarly, ARF following administration of ACE inhibitors or ARBs is seen almost exclusively in patients with underlying abnormalities of the renal vasculature and circulation. This syndrome is most commonly seen in patients with congestive heart failure on diuretics, patients with severe bilateral renal artery stenosis, patients with critical renal artery stenosis in a single functioning kidney, and patients with vascular disease and nephrosclerosis. ACE inhibitors lower blood pressure by inhibiting the conversion of angiotensin I to angiotensin II. ARBs block the actions of angiotensin II at the type I (AT_1) angiotensin receptor. Activation of AT_1 receptors by angiotensin II causes potent vasoconstriction, increasing peripheral resistance. Within the glomerular circulation, angiotensin II preferentially constricts efferent arterioles to preserve glomerular transcapillary pressure and maintain GFR when renal blood flow is compromised. In the clinical settings described previously, ACE inhibitors cause ARF by reducing systemic blood pressure while simultaneously reducing glomerular transcapillary pressure due to the fall in postglomerular, efferent arteriolar resistance. As with other forms of drug-induced hemodynamic reductions in GFR, kidney function usually returns to baseline when the ACE inhibitor or ARB is discontinued.

INTRARENAL ACUTE RENAL FAILURE: ACUTE TUBULAR NECROSIS AND ACUTE INTERSTITIAL NEPHRITIS CAUSED BY DRUGS

Drug-induced ARF from intrarenal mechanisms can be classified into two entities with distinct clinical and pathophysiologic characteristics: ATN and acute interstitial nephritis (AIN). ATN associated with drug administration shares many of the clinical features of ATN from other causes. This form of ARF can be seen following administration of agents that are primarily excreted by the kidney, such as aminoglycoside antibiotics, amphotericin B, and chemotherapeutic agents such as cisplatin. Nephrotoxicity generally reflects direct toxic effects of the compound on renal tubular cells, although hemo-dynamic mechanisms may play a role. In this setting, the onset of ARF is often nonoliguric and may be slow to develop. If nephrotoxicity is not detected and adminis-tration of the causative agent is continued, oliguric ARF may develop. The urinalysis is characteristically bland and may show modest proteinuria, tubular epithelial cells, and noncellular casts. Tubular toxicity will generally abate when the offending agent is discontinued, although there may be a lag before complete recovery of kidney function occurs. However, irreversible chronic kidney disease may result from repetitive exposure to tubular toxins.

In AIN, drug exposure causes ARF through a syndrome of intrarenal inflammation. This disorder is described in detail in Chapter 48 and is characterized by inflammatory cell infiltration of the renal interstitium with reduced GFR and renal blood flow. Systemic signs of hypersensi-tivity, including rash, arthralgias, and fever may also occur. The urinalysis reflects active renal inflammation and usually contains red cells, white cells, and occasional cellular casts with nonglomerular levels of proteinuria. Eosinophiluria can also be observed but is not pathogno-monic. Common causative agents include penicillins, cephalosporins, sulfonamide analogues, rifampin, and NSAIDs. AIN usually resolves after the offending agent is removed.

URINARY TRACT OBSTRUCTION ASSOCIATED WITH THERAPEUTIC AGENTS

Drug-associated obstructive uropathy may be caused by intratubular obstruction, intraureteral obstruction, or extrinsic ureteral obstruction from retroperitoneal fibro-sis. These obstructive syndromes have been associated with specific causative agents. For example, the antiviral agent acyclovir can cause ARF as a result of the precipita-tion of the drug, which is relatively insoluble, within renal tubular lumina. In analgesic-associated nephropa-thy (discussed in Chapter 40), patients may present with symptoms of acute ureteral obstruction due to sloughing of necrotic renal papillary tissue (see also Chapter 50). Methysergide has been associated with retroperitoneal fibrosis causing obstructive nephropathy. However, in one survey of patients with retroperitoneal fibrosis, drugs were identified as a cause in less than 3% of cases. Obstructive uropathy has also been reported with the anti-HIV drug indinavir. Although the incidence of this disorder is not clear, indinavir treatment has been as-sociated with crystalluria and nephrolithiasis. Affected patients present with colic and signs of acute urinary tract obstruction. A more chronic and asymptomatic clin-ical course has also been observed. In both settings, the kidney abnormalities regress when the drug is discontin-ued (also discussed in Chapter 32).

CHRONIC KIDNEY DISEASE FROM THERAPEUTIC AGENTS

Chronic kidney disease caused by drugs is usually mani-fested as tubulointerstitial injury. This syndrome of chronic interstitial nephropathy has been associated with a number of structurally diverse agents including lith-ium, analgesics, cyclosporine, cisplatin, and nitrosureas. Chronic interstitial disease caused by a drug most often presents as an elevation in serum creatinine, which may be slowly progressive. However, abnormalities of tubular function may be a predominant feature. Such abnormal-ities include renal tubular acidosis, concentrating defects, defective potassium secretion, and tubular proteinuria. On histologic examination, interstitial fibrosis, tubular atrophy, and infiltration of the renal interstitium with chronic inflammatory cells are observed. The urinalysis may contain white cells and red cells with modest levels of proteinuria. Although patients with drug-induced chronic interstitial nephropathy may progress to end-stage renal disease requiring renal replacement therapy, the course of the disease can usually be stabilized or reversed if the offending agent is identified and dis-continued.

NEPHROTIC SYNDROME ASSOCIATED WITH THERAPEUTIC AGENTS

Glomerulopathy with proteinuria may be caused by several drugs, including gold, penicillamine, and NSAIDs. Affected patients often present with proteinuria, edema, and hypoalbuminemia. Pathologically, membranous nephropathy has been associated with all of the agents just listed, whereas minimal-change nephropathy has been seen in patients taking certain NSAIDs and penicil-lamine. In addition, interferon-α may cause focal seg-mental glomerulosclerosis. In most cases, proteinuria remits when the agent is discontinued. However, in a few cases, renal injury has progressed after the drug is stopped.

SPECIFIC AGENTS THAT CAUSE RENAL FAILURE

Antibiotics

As a class of drugs, antibiotics are the most common cause of clinically recognized drug-induced renal failure. Within this group, aminoglycosides are responsible for the majority of episodes of nephrotoxicity in hospitalized patients. Aminoglycosides most commonly cause ATN, whereas other antibiotics such as penicillins, rifampin, and sulfonamides more commonly produce AIN. In prac-tice, antibiotics are often administered to patients who are severely ill with other coexistent disorders that can independently affect kidney function or aggravate and potentiate nephrotoxicity. Thus, in an individual patient, a causative role for an antibiotic may be difficult to establish precisely.

Aminoglycosides

Aminoglycosides are amphophilic, cationic antibiotics that are used to treat serious gram-negative bacterial infections. They are by far the most common cause of antibiotic-associated reductions in kidney function in hospitalized patients. Depending on the criteria used for defining nephrotoxicity, the reported incidence of nephrotoxicity ranges between 7% and 36% of patients receiving aminoglycosides. The incidence increases with the duration of drug administration and may approach 50% with more than 14 days of therapy. Serum protein binding of aminoglycosides is minimal, they are freely filtered at the glomerulus, and renal excretion is the major route of elimination. Aminoglycosides accumulate in the renal cortex, reaching saturation within the first 3 days of treatment. Accumulation of drug in cortical tubular cells probably causes toxicity, although the specific cellular mechanisms of aminoglycoside-induced ARF have not been completely defined. Evidence of tubular cell abnormalities and injury may be seen by both light and electron microscopy.

The usual clinical presentation of aminoglycoside nephrotoxicity is a rising creatinine concentration that typically appears 5 to 7 days into the antibiotic course, but reduced GFR may occur earlier in the presence of risk factors. Frank azotemia is often preceded by the development of a concentrating defect manifested as polyuria. The urinalysis most commonly shows minimal proteinuria with noncellular casts and occasional tubular epithelial cells. Fractional excretion of sodium is usually increased (greater than 1%), often accompanied by urinary potassium, calcium, and magnesium wasting. Characteristically, kidney function deteriorates progressively, but the process is reversible if the diagnosis is suspected and the aminoglycoside is discontinued. However, there may be a lag time before kidney function begins to improve, with patients often requiring several weeks for complete recovery. This lag time is probably related to the kinetics of accumulation of aminoglycosides in renal cortical tissue, since urinary excretion of aminoglycosides has been detected for days to weeks after drug administration is stopped.

Even though virtually every patient who receives aminoglycosides is at some risk of developing kidney toxicity, there is a positive association between the dose and duration of therapy and the risk of developing renal failure. Tailoring aminoglycoside doses to maintain drug levels within a defined therapeutic range minimizes the risks of toxicity while maintaining bactericidal concentrations of antibiotic. When calculating aminoglycoside doses, it is important to recognize that changes in serum creatinine may underestimate reduction in GFR in elderly

TABLE 35-2 Risk Factors for the Development of Aminoglycoside Nephrotoxicity

Prolonged course of treatment (>10 days)
Volume depletion
Sepsis
Pre-existing kidney disease
Hypokalemia
Elderly patient
Combination therapy with certain cephalosporins (particularly cephalothin)
Concomitant exposure to other nephrotoxins (e.g., radiocontrast, amphotericin B, cisplatin)
Gentamicin > amikacin > tobramycin

patients, those with substantial muscle wasting, or patients with liver disease. Single daily-dose regimens have been advocated by some authors as an approach to avoid aminoglycoside nephrotoxicity, but the benefits of these regimens have not been clearly demonstrated. Because aminoglycosides are primarily excreted by the kidney, increased aminoglycoside levels can be both a cause and a marker of nephrotoxicity. Monitoring peak and trough drug levels along with serum creatinine every 2 to 3 days is prudent, but daily monitoring may be required in the unstable patient with a serious infection and fluctuating level of kidney function.

Several risk factors for aminoglycoside nephrotoxicity have been identified and are illustrated in Table 35-2. When aminoglycoside therapy is being initiated, these characteristics identify patients at high risk of developing toxicity who require more intensive monitoring and modification of risk factors such as volume status and electrolyte abnormalities. When possible, alternative antibiotic choices should also be considered in high-risk patients. All members of the aminoglycoside family can cause nephrotoxicity, but compared with gentamicin, tobramycin exhibits less nephrotoxicity in animal models. Amikacin's potential for nephrotoxicity is intermediate between gentamicin and tobramycin.

Cephalosporins

Cephalosporins are semi-synthetic β-lactam derivatives that have broad-spectrum bactericidal activity. Although they are generally tolerated well by patients, diminished kidney function is an infrequent but well-defined complication of cephalosporin therapy. Two forms of renal failure have been described with cephalosporins: ATN and AIN. A profile of tubular toxicity has been best documented with cephaloridine and cephalothin, especially when higher doses are used. A rank order potential for cephalosporins to produce proximal tubular toxicity has been defined in animal studies as cephaloglycin > cephaloridine >> cefaclor > cephazolin > cephalothin >>> cephalexin and ceftazidime. Combination therapy with aminoglycosides or furosemide may increase the risk for cephalosporin-associated ATN.

Amphotericin B

Amphotericin B is a polyene antibiotic that is the treatment of choice for many serious fungal infections. Unfortunately, this agent produces a number of side effects, with nephrotoxicity being the most clinically problematic. The degree of nephrotoxicity is roughly proportional to the total cumulative dose received. At least two mechanisms mediate the adverse effects of amphotericin in the kidney. First, amphotericin is highly bound to cell membranes and causes damage that affects membrane integrity and permeability. In the kidney, this membrane injury is thought to be the basis for characteristic clinical syndromes of potassium and magnesium wasting, inability to maximally concentrate urine, and distal tubule acidification defects. These abnormalities, along with abnormal urine sediment, usually precede the development of clinically apparent azotemia. In addition, the drug produces acute renal vasoconstriction causing reduction in GFR that is hemodynamically mediated. The mechanism of amphotericin-associated renal vasoconstriction is not clear, but a role for tubulo-glomerular feedback (TGF) has been suggested. This may be due to membrane toxicity in macula densa cells, leading to altered sodium permeability thereby triggering TGF.

Renal failure is frequently nonoliguric and progressive, but will slowly abate when the amphotericin is discontinued. However, high doses and repetitive exposure to amphotericin can cause permanent kidney damage and chronic kidney disease. Volume depletion potentiates nephrotoxicity, whereas sodium loading and volume expansion can prevent or ameliorate kidney injury; it has been suggested that one of the benefits of sodium loading is to abrogate TGF-dependent vasoconstriction. Risk factors for amphotericin nephrotoxicity include: male gender, high daily dose, prolonged duration of therapy, hospitalization in the ICU when therapy is initiated, and concomitant cyclosporine therapy. Several formulations of amphotericin in lipid vehicles, including liposomes, are available for clinical use. These newer formulations are significantly more expensive than conventional amphotericin. Nonetheless, they appear to be effective at eradicating invasive fungal infections, and kidney toxicity, indicated by increases in serum creatinine, appears to be lower than with conventional amphotericin B.

Acyclovir

Acyclovir is an effective and relatively nontoxic antiviral agent that is widely used to treat herpesvirus infections. When given by the oral route, acyclovir is essentially devoid of significant kidney toxicity. However, nephrotoxicity has been described in a small number of patients who have received intravenous courses of acyclovir, particularly at high doses (greater than $500\,mg/m^2$). Acyclovir undergoes tubular secretion in the kidney, and renal tissue levels increase substantially during treatment. The mechanism of ARF is thought to be precipitation of the relatively insoluble drug within tubular lumina, causing obstruction. The urine sediment may contain red cells and white cells with needle-shaped birefringent crystals. Renal failure generally resolves when the acyclovir is discontinued. Risk factors for toxicity are volume depletion and bolus administration of drug, but ARF has been observed even with adequate fluid repletion and the use of continuous-infusion protocols.

Pentamidine

Approximately 25% of patients treated with pentamidine may experience a reversible fall in GFR. Nephrotoxicity with pentamidine may be more common in AIDS patients and has been associated with significant hyperkalemia. Although the incidence of kidney problems is reduced with inhaled preparations, renal failure has also been reported with aerosolized pentamidine use. Nonetheless, a specific role for pentamidine is often difficult to identify because of the presence of other drugs or comorbid conditions that might also affect kidney function.

Drugs Used to Treat HIV

As discussed in Chapter 32, patients infected with HIV have increased risk for developing ARF. This is related in part to HIV infection and its secondary infectious complications. In addition, several of the drugs commonly used to control HIV infection can cause ARF, either directly or indirectly. For example, ritonavir and adefovir have been associated with the development of ATN. The mechanism of toxicity seems to involve depletion of mitochondrial DNA. In addition, the antiretroviral drug zidovudine has been associated with severe myopathy and rhabdomyolysis. Finally, as discussed earlier, crystal nephropathy with obstruction caused by deposition of insoluble crystals in the kidney has been observed with indinavir.

Radiocontrast

The administration of radiocontrast is a frequent cause of nephrotoxic ARF accounting for up to 10% of ARF cases in hospitalized patients. Although the reported incidence of contrast nephropathy from published studies is somewhat variable, this variation seems to be related to differences in criteria for defining the syndrome, the period of observation after the contrast administration, and the prevalence of risk factors in the population studied. The major risk factors are listed in Table 35-3. A pre-existing reduction in kidney function is the most important and best-documented risk factor, and significant contrast-induced nephropathy is rare in patients with normal kidney function.

The vasoactive effects of radiocontrast contribute to the pathogenesis of nephropathy. In animals, contrast injection initially causes vasodilatation of the renal

TABLE 35-3   Risk Factors for the Development of Acute Renal Failure Following Radiocontrast Administration

Pre-existing renal dysfunction
Diabetic nephropathy
Severe congestive heart failure
Volume depletion
Elderly patient
Multiple myeloma
Large volumes of radiocontrast
Concomitant treatment with ACE inhibitors, NSAIDs, or exposure to other nephrotoxins

ACE, angiotensin-converting enzyme; NSAIDs, nonsteroidal anti-inflammatory drugs.

circulation, followed by intense and persistent vasoconstriction. The etiology of this vasoconstrictive phase is not clear but may include reduced production of vasodilator prostaglandins, enhanced endothelin release, or changes in intracellular calcium. Patients with contrast nephrotoxicity typically develop a rise in their serum creatinine within 24 hours after radiocontrast administration that peaks within 7 to 10 days. Radiocontrast nephropathy is typically nonoliguric but can be associated with oliguria in severe cases. The urinary sediment is unremarkable and, unlike many other forms of drug-induced ARF, the fractional excretion of sodium is typically very low (less than 1%), reflecting the hemodynamic component of kidney function impairment.

The typical patient with radiocontrast nephropathy will develop a mild, transient reduction in kidney function. Clinically significant kidney dysfunction is less common, but occasionally patients will require acute dialysis. Because radiographic studies are generally planned in advance, the clinician's efforts should be directed toward prevention of contrast nephropathy by avoiding unnecessary studies, particularly in patients with risk factors. In the high-risk patient, alternate approaches to imaging should be considered. If contrast administration is unavoidable, the amount of contrast used during the study should be kept to a minimum and concomitant administration of other nephrotoxic agents should be avoided. Low-osmolality radiocontrast agents may help to reduce the risks for nephrotoxicity in patients with a pre-existing abnormal kidney function. In addition, hypovolemia should be corrected, and medications such as NSAIDs should be discontinued. Current recommendations suggest that saline should be infused intravenously at a rate of 1 mL/kg body weight/hour beginning 12 hours before the procedure and continued for an additional 12 hours afterward. In this circumstance, 0.9% saline appears to provide more benefit than 0.45% saline. Saline infusion regimens provide better protection against acute impairment of kidney function than hydration plus mannitol or furosemide. Moreover, a recent study, which may alter current practice if confirmed, suggests that isotonic bicarbonate may be even more effective than hydration with sodium chloride for prophylaxis of contrast-induced renal failure.

A number of other agents have been tested for potential value in preventing radiocontrast nephropathy. In two randomized clinical studies, N-acetylcysteine ameliorated the rise in serum creatinine after radiocontrast but did not alter the development of severe ARF. Other studies have failed to show even this modest benefit, but the drug is now widely used because it is relatively inexpensive and nontoxic. Likewise, clinical trials of other agents such as dopamine, fenoldopam, and atrial natriuretic peptide have failed to demonstrate clear-cut benefits in preventing severe radiocontrast nephropathy. Similarly, prophylactic hemodialysis or hemofiltration do not appear to be beneficial.

Calcineurin Inhibitor Immunosuppressive Drugs

Cyclosporine and tacrolimus are immunosuppressive agents that inhibit the early events involved in T-cell activation effectively suppressing transplant rejection. These agents have distinct chemical structures; cyclosporine is a cyclic peptide, whereas tacrolimus is a macrolide. Despite these marked structural differences, they have identical mechanisms of action. Both compounds produce potent inhibition of calcineurin, an intracellular phosphatase that plays a central role in coordinating T-cell activation by foreign antigens. On the basis of their efficacy as antirejection therapies, calcineurin inhibitors are the cornerstone of immunosuppressive regimens for patients with virtually every type of organ graft. However, the frequent occurrence of nephrotoxicity and, especially, concern over the potential for developing chronic, irreversible kidney injury have complicated their clinical use.

The clinical manifestations of nephrotoxicity are similar for cyclosporine and tacrolimus, consisting of acute reversible kidney dysfunction and chronic interstitial nephropathy. Acute nephrotoxicity is the predominant kidney abnormality seen within the first 6 to 12 months after initiating treatment and is characterized by an acute or subacute reduction in kidney function that is often dose dependent. Generally, kidney dysfunction is nonprogressive and remits when the dose is lowered or the drug is discontinued. Virtually every patient who receives therapeutic doses of a calcineurin inhibitor will experience a component of persistent, reversible reduction in GFR and renal blood flow. The mechanism of this acute nephrotoxicity is hemodynamic and results from the ability of these agents to induce intense renal vasoconstriction. Calcineurin inhibitors do not cause renal vasoconstriction directly but may act by stimulating production of other vasoconstrictor compounds such as thromboxane A_2, endothelin, and leukotrienes.

In kidney transplant recipients within the first year after transplant, it is often difficult to distinguish acute nephrotoxicity from acute rejection. A stable or slowly progressive increase in serum creatinine that reverses when the cyclosporine or tacrolimus dose is reduced suggests nephrotoxicity. Kidney biopsy can be helpful in this setting, since aggressive inflammatory cell infiltrates are usually absent in acute nephrotoxicity and their presence in a biopsy specimen would suggest ongoing rejection. Isometric tubular vacuolization may be observed with calcineurin toxicity. Although serum drug levels are frequently used to monitor therapeutic efficacy and to prevent toxicity, there is only a rough correlation between serum levels and clinical events.

Chronic nephrotoxicity is defined by the development of interstitial fibrosis with reduced levels of GFR in patients receiving long-term treatment with calcineurin inhibitors. The clinical features of the chronic cyclosporine nephrotoxicity are better characterized, although chronic nephropathy also occurs with tacrolimus. Generally, 6 to 12 months of treatment are required before signs of chronic nephropathy become apparent. Because of the irreversible nature of the morphologic abnormalities, this form of toxicity is more ominous than the acute form. Histologically, chronic nephrotoxicity is characterized by focal or striped medullary interstitial fibrosis. Often these changes are accompanied by tubular atrophy and obliterative arteriolar changes. In more advanced cases, diffuse interstitial fibrosis with focal and segmental glomerular sclerosis can be seen. In kidney transplant patients, these changes may be difficult to differentiate from the typical features of chronic allograft nephropathy. Although the mechanism of chronic nephrotoxicity is not known, it is likely that cumulative dose, arterial hypertension, and immunologic injury contribute to the development of the lesion. Animal studies suggest that severe sodium depletion may potentiate the development of renal fibrosis associated with administration calcineurin inhibitors.

Cyclosporine is metabolized primarily through the action of hepatic P450 microsomal enzymes. Thus, agents that influence the activity of this enzyme system can cause significant changes in cyclosporine metabolism. Generally, drugs that reduce the rate of cyclosporine metabolism, such as erythromycin, ketoconazole, and verapamil, produce increased serum levels and potentiate toxicity. On the other hand, agents that increase the rate of cyclosporine metabolism, such as phenytoin, phenobarbital, and rifampin, may reduce serum levels and thus may blunt therapeutic efficacy.

Antineoplastic Drugs

A number of compounds used in the treatment of cancer may be toxic to the kidney. As with other nephrotoxic drugs, recognizing and anticipating the potential for kidney injury is crucial so that appropriate preventative measures may be implemented. A representative list of antineoplastic agents that affect the kidney is provided in Table 35-4. The renal effects of three commonly used antitumor drugs are discussed in detail here.

Cisplatin

Cis-diamminedichloroplatinum (cisplatin) is a very effective antineoplastic agent with a broad range of activity against a number of malignancies. However, cisplatin also has a substantial capacity for nephrotoxicity. Cisplatin is primarily excreted by the kidney, where it is concentrated in glomerular ultrafiltrate accumulating in renal tubular epithelium. Tubular injury seems to be mediated by direct effects on epithelial cell metabolism and through generation of free oxygen radicals. The development of cisplatin nephrotoxicity is dose-related and cumulative. Although the drug can cause reversible ARF, irreversible decline of kidney function associated with repeated cisplatin administration is the most problematic clinical manifestation of toxicity. The development of chronic cisplatin injury may be associated with dense interstitial fibrosis. Another common sequela of cisplatin-induced tubular injury is renal magnesium wasting that often produces clinically significant hypomagnesemia. Hypomagnesemia may be exacerbated by concomitant administration of aminoglycoside antibiotics, and it may persist for months after cisplatin has been discontinued.

Maneuvers that increase urine volume during cisplatin administration reduce the risk of nephrotoxicity. Thus, vigorous intravenous fluid administration is indicated for

TABLE 35-4   Nephrotoxicity of Selected Antineoplastic Agents

Drug	Clinical Syndrome
Alkylating agents	
Cisplatin	Tubular injury, acute and chronic renal failure, renal Mg^{2+} wasting
Carboplatin	Less nephrotoxicity than cisplatin
Cyclophosphamide	Hemorrhagic cystitis, hyponatremia
Streptozotocin	ARF, tubular dysfunction
Antibiotics	
Mitomycin C	Hemolytic uremic syndrome
Mithramycin	ATN
Antimetabolites	
Methotrexate	ARF with high-dose therapy
Ara-C	Interstitial nephritis
5-FU	ARF
Biological response modifiers	
IL-2	Hemodynamically mediated ARF
Interferon-α	Focal segmental glomerulosclerosis, ATN

Ara-C, cytosine arabinoside; ARF, acute renal failure; ATN, acute tubular necrosis; 5-FU, 5-fluorouracil; IL-2, interleukin-2.

prophylaxis. Increasing urine flow may prevent cisplatin toxicity by limiting the duration of contact between the drug and the renal epithelium. In addition, since increasing the extracellular chloride concentration may inhibit the conversion of cisplatin to a more toxic metabolite, inclusion of isotonic sodium chloride in hydration protocols has been advocated. Infusions of mannitol also seem to be effective. Fluids should be administered to maintain urine flows of at least 100 mL/hour and preferably above 200 mL/hour for 12 hours before and 12 to 18 hours after cisplatin is administered. Second-generation platinum compounds such as carboplatin appear to have a reduced potential for nephrotoxicity, but both renal failure and hypomagnesemia have also been observed with carboplatin.

Cyclophosphamide

Cyclophosphamide is widely used for treating lymphomas and other hematologic malignancies. Its common adverse effects are bone marrow suppression, gastrointestinal toxicity, and hemorrhagic cystitis. With high doses of cyclophosphamide (greater than or equal to 50 mg/kg), hyponatremia has been observed. High doses of cyclophosphamide inhibit renal water excretion, causing increased urine osmolality in the presence of reduced plasma osmolality. Since vasopressin levels are not elevated, the defective water handling appears to be a direct effect of the drug on the distal nephron. This defect generally resolves within 24 hours after drug administration, and hypotonic fluids should be avoided during this period. Accordingly, when intravenous fluids are used to maximize urine flow for preventing cyclophosphamide-induced bladder hemorrhage, isotonic fluids should be used.

Methotrexate

Methotrexate is an antimetabolite used to treat a variety of cancers and leukemias. In the absence of pre-existing kidney dysfunction, nephrotoxicity is uncommon with standard doses of methotrexate. However, significant nephrotoxicity has been observed with high-dose methotrexate regimens. Intratubular precipitation of the drug causing obstruction may contribute to kidney dysfunction. In addition, methotrexate has direct toxic effects on renal epithelial cells. Fluid administration to achieve urine volumes of more than 3 l/day reduces the potential for nephrotoxicity. Because the solubility of methotrexate and its metabolites is increased in alkaline solutions, alkalinization of urine during drug administration is also recommended.

BIBLIOGRAPHY

Bates DW, Su L, Yu DT, et al: Correlates of acute renal failure in patients receiving parenteral amphotericin B. Kidney Int 60:1452–1459, 2001.

DeMattos AM, Olyei AJ, Bennnett WM: Nephrotoxicity of immunosuppressive drugs: Long term consequences and challenges for the future. Am J Kidney Dis 35:333–346, 2000.

Deray G: Amphotericin B nephrotoxicity. J Antimicrob Chemother 49(suppl 1):37–41, 2002.

Fishbane S, Durham JH, Marzo, et al: N-acetylcysteine in the prevention of radiocontrast induced nephropathy. J Am Soc Nephrol 15:251–260, 2004.

Kaloyanides GJ: Antibiotic-related nephrotoxicity. Nephrol Dial Transplant 9(suppl 4):130–134, 1994.

Kintzel PE: Anticancer drug-induced kidney disorders. Drug Saf 24:19–38, 2001.

Merten GJ, Burgess WP, Gray LV, et al: Prevention of contrast-induced nephropathy with sodium bicarbonate: A randomized control trial. JAMA 291:2328–2334, 2004.

Meyer KB, Madias NE: Cisplatin nephrotoxicity. Miner Electrolyte Metab 20:201–213, 1994.

Murphy SW, Barrett BJ, Parfrey PS: Contrast nephropathy. J Am Soc Nephrol 11:177–182, 2000.

Parfrey PS, Griffiths SM, Barrett BJ, et al: Contrast-material induced renal failure in patients with diabetes mellitus, renal insufficiency, or both: A prospective controlled study. N Engl J Med 320:143–149, 1989.

Perazella MA: Acute renal failure in HIV-infected patients: A brief review of common causes. Am J Med Sci 319:385–391, 2000.

Reis F, Klastersky J: Nephrotoxicity induced by cancer chemotherapy with special emphasis on cisplatin. Am J Kidney Dis 8:368–379, 1986.

Rihal CS, Textor SC, Grill DE, et al: Incidence and prognostic importance of acute renal failure after percutaneous coronary intervention. Circulation 105:2259–2264, 2002.

Robinson RF, Nahata MC: A comparative review of conventional and lipid formulations of amphotericin B. J Clin Pharmacol Ther 24:249–257, 1999.

Rudnick MR, Goldfarb S, Wexler L, et al: Nephrotoxicity of ionic and non-ionic contrast media in 1196 patients. A randomized trial. Kidney Int 47:254–261, 1995.

Sawyer MH, Webb DE, Balow JE, Straus SE: Acyclovir-induced renal failure. Am J Med 84:1067–1071, 1988.

Solomon R, Werner C, Mann D, et al: Effects of saline, mannitol, and furosemide on acute decreases in renal function induced by radiocontrast agents. N Engl J Med 331:1416–142, 1994.

Swan SK. Aminoglycoside nephrotoxicity. Semin Nephrol 17:27–33, 1997.

Tanji N, Tanji K, Kambham N, et al: Adefovir toxicity: Possible role of mitochondrial DNA depletion. Hum Pathol 32:734–740, 2001.

Tepel M, van der Giet M, Schwazfeld C, et al: Prevention of radiographic contrast agent-induced reductions in renal function by acetylcysteine. N Engl J Med 343:180–184, 2000.

Tune BM, Hsu C-Y, Fravert D: Cephalosporin and carbacephem nephrotoxicity: Roles of tubular cell uptake and acylating potential. Biochem Pharmacol 51:557–561, 1996.

CHAPTER 36

Acute Uric Acid Nephropathy

F. Bruder Stapleton

In humans, uric acid is the end product of purine metabolism. Although uric acid provides an efficient means of eliminating nitrogen (containing twice the nitrogen per mole as does urea), uric acid has been retained as the principal source of urinary nitrogen excretion only by birds and some reptiles, most likely because of the low solubility of uric acid in biological fluids. The insoluble nature of uric acid is of particular importance to humans, who, unlike most other mammals, lack hepatic uricase and have a high concentration of uric acid in plasma; therefore, modest alterations in urate homeostasis may lead to severe impairment of kidney function.

URIC ACID HOMEOSTASIS

Uric acid is a weak organic acid with a pK_a of 5.75. At physiologic pH, uric acid is present almost entirely as monosodium urate. The solubility of monosodium urate is nearly 15 times that of uric acid in aqueous solution. In human plasma, saturation occurs at a monosodium urate concentration of approximately 7 mg/dL. The proton concentration of a solution containing uric acid determines not only the relative amount of monosodium urate but also the solubility of urate. Thus, in maximally acidified urine, uric acid predominates, with minimal solubility. In addition to pH, the concentrations of other cations affect the solubility of uric acid. Sodium and ammonium decrease urate solubility, whereas potassium increases solubility.

The elimination of uric acid by the kidney involves four components: glomerular filtration, tubular reabsorption, tubular secretion, and reabsorption beyond secretory sites. Uric acid is nearly completely filtered by the glomerular membrane; tubular reabsorption, secretion, and further reabsorption occur along the proximal tubule. Excessive excretion of uric acid, to the extent that glomerular filtration is impaired, may be the result of hyperuricemia or altered renal tubular reabsorption or secretion. Fractional excretion of uric acid is less than 10% in healthy adults; however, it is much higher in young children.

URINARY URIC ACID EXCRETION

Urate is primarily excreted by the kidneys, although some urate is disposed through the gastrointestinal tract. Normal urinary uric acid excretion, in individuals ingesting an unrestricted diet, is less than 700 mg/day in men and less than 600 mg/day in women. In children, uric acid excretion per kilogram of body weight is greater than in adults, with mean values exceeding 20 mg/kg/day in term neonates. In children 3 years of age, the mean urate excretion is 13.5 mg/kg/day and declines during childhood to adult mean values of 6 mg/kg/day. The measurement of uric acid excretion per glomerular filtration rate (GFR) may be a more physiologically relevant assessment of urate elimination. Normal values are less than 0.6 mg/dL GFR in adults and less than 0.56 mg/dL GFR in children. This value is calculated as (urine uric acid [mg/dL] × serum creatinine [mg/dL])/urine creatinine (mg/dL).

ACUTE RENAL FAILURE

Acute uric acid nephropathy is an important etiology of oliguric acute renal failure (ARF) in selected groups of patients in whom the serum urate concentration becomes markedly elevated or in whom a massive uricosuria develops. The most common clinical setting for acute urate nephropathy occurs with rapid turnover of nucleoproteins in patients with leukemia, lymphoma, or other neoplasms, especially during cytotoxic therapy. Called tumor lysis syndrome, ARF with hyperuricemia during therapy for leukemia or lymphomas is associated with hyperkalemia, acidosis, hypocalcemia, and hyperphosphatemia. These metabolic complications develop rapidly and may be life threatening. Rarely, spontaneous acute urate nephropathy may precede cytotoxic therapy in patients with leukemia or lymphoma. Renal failure from increased serum uric acid and uric aciduria also may complicate inherited disorders of purine metabolism (e.g., Lesch-Nyhan syndrome or hypoxanthine-guanine phosphoribosyl transferase deficiency), hemolysis, rhabdomyolysis, perinatal asphyxia, extreme exercise, and prolonged muscle contractions from status epilepticus. Important risk factors for ARF from hyperuricemia are dehydration and acidemia. Many pharmacologic agents increase uric acid excretion. Some, such as the diuretic, ticrynafen, have produced ARF. Radiographic contrast agents also markedly increase uric acid excretion and should be avoided, or used with caution, during hyperuricemia. Urinary flow drops dramatically in patients with acute uric acid nephropathy. Oliguria results from renal tubular obstruction by the precipitation of uric acid

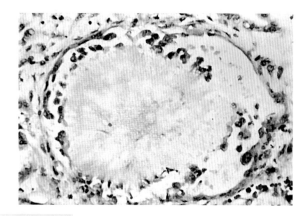

FIGURE 36-1 Uric acid crystals are shown obstructing a renal tubule from a child with lymphoma, acute renal failure, and hyperuricemia.

in collecting tubules (Fig. 36-1). As a result of intraluminal obstruction of the distal nephron, dilatation of proximal tubules occurs. As discussed earlier, uric acid is least soluble in highly concentrated urine of low pH and, predictably, uric acid precipitation occurs in the renal medulla and papilla in acute uric acid nephropathy (Fig. 36-2). Uric acid precipitation may also occur in the vasa recti supplying the distal nephron. Histologic studies of kidneys during acute urate nephropathy show minimal

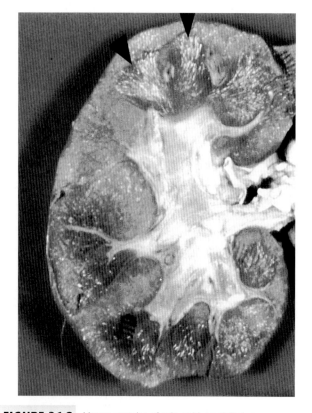

FIGURE 36-2 Linear streaks of uric acid precipitates (*arrowheads*) are seen within the renal medulla in a patient with acute renal failure and a serum uric acid concentration of 34 mg/dL.

interstitial cellular infiltration; the pathologic changes of acute urate nephropathy are reversible.

Kidney function in acute uric acid nephropathy correlates with the rate of urinary excretion of urate, rather than the serum urate level. In patients with hyperuricemia and leukemia, inulin clearance (C_{IN}), a measure of GFR, and para-amino hippurate clearance (C_{PAH}), a measure of renal plasma flow, are decreased. The filtration fraction (C_{IN}/C_{PAH}) is also decreased. Studies of acute hyperuricemia in laboratory animal models have shown similar alterations in C_{IN} and renal blood flow. Urinary flow is almost always markedly diminished. Precipitation of uric acid in the distal renal tubules and distal renal microvasculature results in increased proximal tubule and distal tubule pressure, and a marked increase in peritubular capillary vascular resistance.

DIAGNOSIS

The clinical diagnosis of acute urate nephropathy should be suspected in high-risk populations when oliguria and decreased kidney function (azotemia, hyperkalemia, acidosis, and/or hyperphosphatemia) develop with either an elevated serum uric acid concentration or with copious uric acid or urate crystals in the urinary sediment. Uric acid crystals in the urinary sediment, however, are not a constant finding. Determination of the ratio of urinary uric acid to urinary creatinine concentration may be helpful in the diagnosis of acute urate nephropathy. In adults with ARF, a urinary uric acid/urine creatinine (mg/mg) ratio of greater than 1.0 is found in patients with urate nephropathy. This test cannot be applied to infants or children, since the urinary uric acid/urine creatinine ratio normally exceeds 1.0 during childhood. Uric acid excretion is routinely decreased in ARF from etiologies other than urate nephropathy. Serum uric acid concentrations alone are not predictive for acute urate nephropathy.

THERAPY

Although the mortality in acute urate nephropathy was once nearly 45%, current dialysis therapies have dramatically improved survival, so that mortality is now related almost exclusively to the underlying disease process. Medical therapy for patients at risk for urate nephropathy is directed toward reducing intrarenal precipitation of uric acid by maintaining a high urine flow rate with as much hydration as the level of kidney function allows. To prevent acute uric acid nephropathy in patients undergoing induction antineoplastic therapy, intravenous fluid administration is begun at 3000 mL/m² body surface area per day in both children and adults, when extracellular fluid volume allows. In patients with extracellular fluid volume depletion, replacement of fluid deficits must precede high-volume maintenance. An alkaline urine is maintained with intravenous sodium bicarbonate infusions. When the urine pH cannot be maintained above a value of 7.0, acetazolamide may also be given orally (provided systemic acidosis is not present). The relative protective roles of urinary flow rate, urine osmolality, and urine pH in the prevention of acute urate nephropathy have been examined in laboratory settings. These studies suggest that a high tubular fluid flow rate, regardless of urine pH or osmolality, offers the maximal protection against urate nephropathy. As mentioned earlier, use of uricosuric drugs, especially radiographic contrast agents, should be avoided in patients with hyperuricemia.

During cytotoxic therapy or in patients with a sustained source of urate overproduction, the filtered urate load is reduced by administering either intravenous or oral allopurinol. Allopurinol is an inhibitor of xanthine oxidase and is effective in reducing the concentration of uric acid in the serum. Urinary oxypurine excretion is increased during allopurinol therapy, however. Renal failure secondary to xanthine precipitation has been observed rarely during allopurinol therapy.

Dialysis or hemofiltration is effective in reducing the serum uric acid concentration and in treating the metabolic consequences of ARF. The clearance of uric acid by hemodialysis is 10 times greater than with peritoneal dialysis; therefore, hemodialysis is the dialysis treatment of choice for ARF from uric acid nephropathy. Hemodialysis should be the initial treatment if oliguria or life-threatening hyperkalemia are present when renal failure is discovered. Occasionally, ARF resolves after one or two dialysis treatments. Because of the tremendous production of uric acid with initial cytotoxic therapy, frequent hemodialysis therapies may be required. When time and the initial metabolic derangements allow, continuous arteriovenous or venovenous hemofiltration or hemodiafiltration has been shown to be advantageous as renal replacement therapy for patients with acute tumor lysis syndrome. Continuous hemodiafiltration allows for the provision of intravenous nutrition and more flexibility in management. Allopurinol is removed by hemodialysis, and a dose should be given at the conclusion of dialysis treatment.

Uricolysis therapy with the intravenous administration of the enzyme, uricase (uric acid oxidase), is an exciting advance in the treatment and prevention of urate nephropathy during cytotoxic therapies. Uric acid is degraded to allantoin in the presence of uricase. Allantoin is extremely soluble, is filtered by the glomerular membrane, and has no known nephrotoxicity. Intravenous administration of uricase in doses of 0.15 mg/kg to 0.2 mg/kg, diluted in saline, is administered over 1 to 2 hours during the first 5 to 7 days of chemotherapy. This regimen is superior to allopurinol in reducing serum uric acid concentrations and preventing oliguric ARF in children with leukemia. Some patients (less than 5%) receiving the nonrecombinant uricase develop bronchospasm, hives, and other hypersensitivity reactions. Uricase should not be administered to patients with G6PD deficiency. Enzymatic uricolysis therapy may replace the initial use of allopurinol and dramatically reduce the need for dialysis therapies in patients with tumor lysis syndrome.

BIBLIOGRAPHY

Agha-Razil M, Amyot SL, Pichette V, et al: Continuous venovenous hemodiafiltration for the treatment of spontaneous tumor lysis syndrome complicated by acute renal failure and severe hyperuricemia. Clin Nephrol 54:59–63, 2000.

Baldree LA, Stapleton FB: Uric acid metabolism in children. Pediatr Clin North Am 2:391–418, 1990.

Cameron JS, Maro F, Simmonds HA: Gout, uric acid and purine metabolism in paediatric nephrology. Pediatr Nephrol 7:105–118, 1993.

Conger JD, Falk SA: Intrarenal dynamics in the pathogenesis and prevention of acute urate nephropathy. J Clin Invest 59:786–793, 1977.

Conger JD, Falk SA, Guggenheim SJ, et al: A micropuncture study of the early phase of acute urate nephropathy. J Clin Invest 58:681–689, 1976.

Jeha S: Tumor lysis syndrome. Semin Hematol 38(suppl):4–8, 2001.

Jones DP, Stapleton FB, Kawinsky D, et al: Renal dysfunction and hyperuricemia at presentation and relapse of acute lymphoblastic leukemia. Med Pediatr Oncol 18:283–286, 1990.

Maesaka JK, Fishbane S: Regulation of renal urate excretion: A critical review. Am J Kidney Dis 32:917–933, 1998.

Pui CH: Urate oxidase in the prophylaxis or treatment of hyperuricemia: The United States experience. Semin Hematol 38(suppl 10):13–21, 2001.

Rieselbach RE, Steele TH: Influence of the kidney upon urate homeostasis in health and disease. Am J Med 56:665–675, 1974.

Spencer HW, Yarger WE, Robinson RR: Alterations of renal function during dietary-induced hyperuricemia in the rat. Kidney Int 9:489–500, 1976.

Stapleton FB: Urate nephropathy. In Edelmann CM, Bernstein J, Meadow R, et al (eds): Pediatric Kidney Disease, 2nd ed. Boston, Little, Brown, 1992, pp 1647–1661.

Stapleton FB, Strother DR, Roy III S, et al: Acute renal failure at onset of therapy for advanced stage Burkitt lymphoma and B cell acute lymphoblastic lymphoma. Pediatrics 82:863–869, 1988.

Tsokos GC, Balow JE, Speigel RJ, et al: Renal and metabolic complications of undifferentiated and lymphoblastic lymphomas. Medicine 67:218–227, 1981.

CHAPTER 37

Cholesterol Atheroembolic Kidney Disease

Arthur Greenberg

Cholesterol atheroembolic kidney disease results when cholesterol crystals and other debris separate from atheromatous plaques, flow downstream, and lodge in small renal arteries, producing luminal occlusion, ischemia, and kidney dysfunction. Depending on the source and distribution of emboli, kidney disease may be the sole or predominant manifestation or simply one feature of a systemic illness characterized by multiorgan ischemia or infarction. Early, autopsy-derived descriptions of renal atheroembolism overemphasized a catastrophic presentation with irreversible kidney failure, intestinal infarction, and death from intra-abdominal sepsis. Atheroembolism is now recognized as a cause of occult or reversible declines in kidney function. Recovery of function may follow extended survival on renal replacement therapy.

PATHOLOGY

The initial lesion in cholesterol atheroembolism is obstruction of a medium-sized or small artery by atheromatous debris. Arterioles and capillaries are less commonly affected. Lesions may occur in any organ. Cholesterol dissolves during routine processing of tissue for histologic examination; crystals are not seen in tissue sections unless special fixatives are used. However, a characteristic cleft marks the space formerly occupied by the needle-like crystals (Fig. 37-1). The size of the artery affected is typically around 200 μm but may range from 55 to 900 μm. The earliest lesion consists of cholesterol crystals and thrombi. After dissolution of the thrombi, macrophages engulf the cholesterol, but the predominant reaction is endothelial. New endothelium covers the crystals. If the vessel wall is eroded by the crystals, an intense perivascular inflammatory response with giant cells is established (see Fig. 37-1). Concentric fibrosis, particularly involving the adventitia, occurs later. Finally, there is recanalization of small vascular channels. Crystal dissolution in vivo is slow; in experimental models, cholesterol clefts persist as long as 9 months after embolization. Although crystals may reach the glomerular capillary loops (Fig. 37-2), the principal glomerular finding is ischemia with glomerular collapse and basement membrane wrinkling. Focal segmental glomerulosclerosis with glomerular collapse and epithelial cell prominence may occur. This finding accounts for some of the cases associated with nephrotic range proteinuria. Antineutrophil cytoplasm antibody–positive (ANCA–positive) pauci-immune crescentic glomerulonephritis has been reported in a few patients who also had biopsy evidence of atheroembolism.

PATHOGENESIS

The classic autopsy description by Flory noted cholesterol atheroembolism solely in patients with erosive plaques. The prevalence of atheroembolism paralleled the severity of aortic disease. Less severe atherosclerotic lesions or plaques covered by thrombus do not pose a risk of atheroembolism.

Embolization may be spontaneous, particularly with severe aortic disease, but mechanical disruption of plaque during angiographic or surgical procedures usually precedes it. Table 37-1 lists predisposing factors. Irrespective of the area primarily targeted for imaging, passage of a catheter along the ascending or descending aorta proximal to the renal arteries confers a risk of embolization to the kidneys. Renal artery angioplasty or revascularization may pose a particular risk, and patients who develop atheroembolism in this setting have a worsened outcome. The site of any concurrent nonrenal embolization depends on the path of the catheter.

Thrombus overlying atheromatous plaque can bind and immobilize friable debris. Anticoagulation or thrombolysis removes this protective covering. Atheroembolism has been reported after heparin, warfarin, or thrombolytic therapy without angiography.

CLINICAL FEATURES

As expected of a process that complicates severe atherosclerosis, risk factors for atherosclerosis as well as evidence of disseminated atherosclerotic disease are commonly present. Most patients have a history of tobacco abuse, and the incidence is higher in tobacco users. Up to 75% of patients are male. The mean age at diagnosis is in the mid-seventh decade. Fewer than 5% of patients are below age 50. Table 37-2 lists other

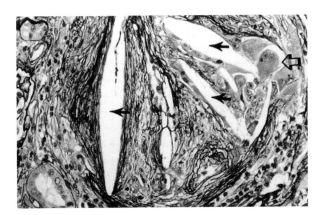

FIGURE 37-1 Cholesterol atheroembolus occluding the lumen of an interlobular renal artery. Needle-like clefts (*solid arrows*) are present, along with a macrophage–multinucleated giant cell reaction (*open arrow*). (Methenamine silver–trichrome stain, magnification ×450.) (Courtesy of Dr. S.I. Bastacky. Reproduced with permission from Greenberg A, Bastacky SI, Iqbal A, et al: Focal segmental glomerulosclerosis associated with nephrotic syndrome in cholesterol artheroembolism: Clinicopathologic correlations. Am J Kidney Dis 29:334–344, 1997.)

accompanying or predisposing features. Notably, diabetes mellitus is a feature of only 2.5% to 31% of reported cases. In a large prospective study of patients undergoing cardiac catheterization, among the 1.4% of patients who developed cholesterol atheroembolism, multivariate analysis identified an increased C-reactive protein level, presence of an aortic aneurysm, smoking, hypertension, multivessel coronary artery disease, and acute coronary syndrome as predisposing factors.

The severity of cholesterol atheroembolism is highly variable, and manifestations of the disorder depend on both the extent of renal involvement and the extrarenal sites affected. The frequency of organ involvement is summarized in Table 37-3. Massive and widespread embolization, in the multiple cholesterol emboli syndrome, presents catastrophically with fever, stroke, acute

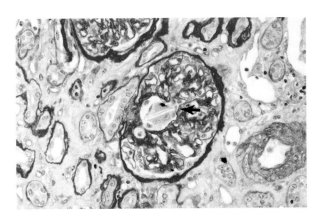

FIGURE 37-2 Glomerulus with cholesterol clefts at hilum (*arrow*). The remainder of the glomerulus shows capillary loop thickening and wrinkling due to ischemia. Adjacent tubules show acute ischemic injury. (Hematoxylin-eosin stain, magnification ×250). (Courtesy of Dr. S.I. Bastacky.)

TABLE 37-1 Risk Factors for Cholesterol Atheroembolic Kidney Disease

Iatrogenic
  Manipulation of the aorta proximal to the renal arteries
    Angiography or angioplasty
    Aortic aneurysm repair
    Aortic aneurysm or other endovascular stenting
    Coronary artery bypass grafting
    Cardiac valve surgery
    Intra-aortic balloon pump circulatory augmentation
    Other
  Anticoagulation, thrombolytic, or antiplatelet therapy
    Heparin
    Low-molecular-weight heparin
    Warfarin
    Tissue plasminogen activator
    Streptokinase
    Urokinase

Spontaneous
  Severe ulcerating atherosclerosis

TABLE 37-2 Associated Findings in 221 Patients with Cholesterol Atheroembolism

Associated Findings	Percentage of Cases
Hypertension	61
Coronary artery disease	44
Aortic aneurysm	25
Cerebrovascular disease	21
Congestive heart failure	21
Diabetes mellitus	11

Modified from Fine MJ, Kapoor W, Falanga V: Cholesterol crystal embolization: A review of 221 cases in the English literature. Angiology 38:769–784, 1987.

TABLE 37-3 Histologic Involvement at Autopsy in Cholesterol Atheroembolic Kidney Disease

Organ	Percentage of Cases
Kidney	75
Spleen	52
Pancreas	52
Gastrointestinal tract	31
Adrenal glands	20
Liver	17
Brain	14
Skin	6

renal failure, abdominal pain, and gastrointestinal bleeding due to bowel infarction, intra-abdominal sepsis, and death. In contrast, spontaneous embolization can have an indolent course.

Autopsy reports are skewed toward patients with severe involvement. In milder disease, kidney and cutaneous involvement predominate. Typically, the renal course is characterized by slowly deteriorating kidney function. The daily increase in serum creatinine may be as little as 0.1 to 0.2 mg/dL, and progression to endstage disease may occur over a period of 30 to 60 days or longer. Patients may also present with an insidious deterioration of kidney function occurring over many months. Occasional patients present with heavy proteinuria, with or without associated clinical features of atheroembolism.

The severity of skin involvement is highly variable. In some patients, digital necrosis and gangrene with pain is a prominent feature. The classic "blue toes" lesion comprises livedo reticularis of the lower extremities, due to occlusion of small arteries, together with cyanosis of the toes. The distal pulses are typically preserved. In other patients, cutaneous involvement may be overlooked unless specifically sought. Livedo that is very subtle when the patient is supine can be made more conspicuous by asking the patient to dangle the feet below the bed or to stand. Features of gastrointestinal involvement include abdominal pain, anorexia, weight loss, and bleeding that can range from a positive stool test for occult blood to brisk hemorrhage. Pancreatitis and acalculous cholecystitis may occur if emboli reach these organs. Bowel infarction and sepsis may also follow an episode of embolization. Central nervous system involvement includes stroke or diffuse cortical dysfunction due to widespread embolization and spinal cord lesions as well as the scotomata, field cuts, or blindness that accompany the classic, but rare, retinal Hollenhorst plaque.

DIAGNOSIS

The diagnosis of atheroembolism relies on a high index of suspicion in patients at risk. During the acute phase, leukocytosis and an elevated erythrocyte sedimentation rate may be present. Eosinophilia is observed in 25% to 50% of affected individuals; hypocomplementemia occurs rarely. However, all of these findings are transient, and reports of their prevalence vary widely. Their absence cannot be taken as evidence against the diagnosis. Hyperamylasemia suggests pancreatic involvement. Although nephrotic range proteinuria may occur, proteinuria is typically modest and the urine sediment nonspecific.

Cholesterol atheroembolism is often confused with radiocontrast nephropathy (see Chapter 35). The course of the latter is much more rapid, a feature that permits the two to be readily distinguished. In dye nephropathy, renal failure occurs immediately, kidney function reaches a nadir within 3 to 4 days, and substantial recovery usually occurs over a similar period. In atheroembolism, the onset of renal failure may be delayed and progression is slower. Recovery occurs after many weeks or months, if at all. Thus, a protracted episode of "radiocontrast nephropathy" occurring after an arteriogram is quite likely due to cholesterol atheroembolism rather than dye-induced. Other disorders that can be mimicked by atheroembolic disease include ischemic acute tubular necrosis, systemic vasculitis, allergic interstitial nephritis, cryoglobulinemia, myeloma, hypertensive nephrosclerosis, and renal artery stenosis.

Most instances of cholesterol atheroembolism are diagnosed clinically, and it is usually not necessary to obtain biopsy confirmation. If a tissue diagnosis is deemed necessary, biopsy of an area of livedo reticularis is the least invasive approach. A muscle biopsy may also be employed. A kidney biopsy showing cholesterol atheroemboli is definitive, but alternative means of diagnosis should be considered first.

PREVENTION

Because cholesterol atheroembolism is so rare, data from controlled trials are unavailable. Conventional measures to limit development of atherosclerosis, including smoking cessation and treatment of hypercholesterolemia with diet, statins, and other drugs, are of presumed benefit. Where possible, manipulation of the vasculature and use of anticoagulants and thrombolytic drugs should be avoided. This is particularly important for secondary prevention in patients who have already sustained an episode of cholesterol atheroembolism. Preliminary studies suggest benefit of downstream filter devices to protect organs at risk during aortic manipulation or catheterization.

THERAPY AND OUTCOME

Spontaneous atheroembolism occurs only in patients with more severe vascular involvement. Shedding of atheromatous debris often continues with a progressive downhill course. In patients with atheroembolism after vascular surgery or angiography, embolization may be limited to the initial episode. Stabilization and gradual improvement may follow as small-vessel inflammation subsides and recanalization with restoration of blood flow occurs. A typical patient who recovers will have gradually lessening anorexia and abdominal and digital pain with subsequent healing of digital ischemic lesions. Not surprisingly, patients with pre-existing kidney function impairment had a worse prognosis for dialysis-free survival and mortality. Recent series note 1-year survivals of 62% to 87% in contrast to historical controls with 19% to 36% 1-year survival. To some extent, this striking improvement is due to meticulous supportive care. However, some of the improvement is due simply to the availability of renal replacement therapy. The changing etiology of cholesterol atheroembolism has also resulted in ascertainment bias. Current cases are mainly provoked by angiography, whereas older series reported spontaneous cases with a fulminant course.

Management focuses on several issues. Patients require local care of digital ischemia, analgesia for pain, and digital amputation if tissue is not viable. Anticoagulation should be stopped and repeat angiographic procedures scrupulously avoided. Careful attention to supplemental nutrition is beneficial for patients with anorexia due to gastrointestinal tract involvement. Hemodialysis or peritoneal dialysis may be successfully employed, and up to one third of patients recover sufficient kidney function to permit discontinuation of dialysis. Use of statins is associated with improved survival. Glucocorticoids and cytotoxic agents have been employed for patients with ANCA-positive glomerulonephritis. Low-dose glucocorticoids have been used in some patients with the rationale of diminishing vascular inflammation and improving tissue blood flow. Vasodilator prostaglandin infusions have also been used to increase blood flow. Controlled trials are lacking, and the benefit of such treatments is unproven. Although abdominal or transesophageal ultrasonography may be used to localize diseased areas of aorta, cholesterol atheroembolism occurs in an elderly population with extensive atherosclerotic disease and a high prevalence of hypertensive cardiovascular disease. Such patients present a formidable surgical risk. The roles of endarterectomy, resection of diseased aortic segments, and use of endovascular stents to cover affected endothelial segments have not been established.

BIBLIOGRAPHY

Aviles B, Ubeda I, Blanco J, Barrientos A: Pauci-immune extra-capillary glomerulonephritis and atheromatous embolization. Am J Kidney Dis 40:847–851, 2002.

Belenfant X, Meyrier A, Jacquot C: Supportive treatment improves survival in multi visceral cholesterol crystal embolism. Am J Kidney Dis 33:840–850, 1999.

Elinav E, Chajek-Shaul T, Stern M: Improvement in cholesterol emboli syndrome after iloprost therapy. BMJ 324:268–269, 2002.

Fine MJ, Kapoor W, Falanga V: Cholesterol crystal embolization: A review of 221 cases in the English literature. Angiology 38:769–784, 1987.

Flory CM: Arterial occlusions produced by emboli from eroded aortic atheromatous plaques. Am J Pathol 21:549–565, 1945.

Fukumoto Y, Tsutsui H, Tsuchihashi M, et al, for the Cholesterol Embolism Study (CHEST) Investigators: The incidence and risk factors of cholesterol embolization syndrome, a complication of cardiac catheterization: A prospective study. J Am Coll Cardiol 42:211–216, 2003.

Greenberg A, Bastacky SI, Iqbal A, et al: Focal segmental glomerulosclerosis associated with nephrotic syndrome in cholesterol atheroembolism: Clinicopathologic correlations. Am J Kidney Dis 29:334–344, 1997.

Kasinath BS, Corwin HL, Bidani AK, et al: Eosinophilia in the diagnosis of atheroembolic renal disease. Am J Nephrol 7:173–177, 1987.

Kassirer JP. Atheroembolic renal disease. N Engl J Med 280:812–818, 1969.

Krishnamurthi V, Novick AC, Myles JL: Atheroembolic renal disease: Effect on morbidity and survival after revascularization for atherosclerotic renal artery stenosis. J Urol 161:1093–1096, 1999.

McGowan JA, Greenberg A: Cholesterol atheroembolic renal disease. Report of 3 cases with emphasis on diagnosis by skin biopsy and extended survival. Am J Nephrol 6:135–139, 1986.

Modi KS, Rao VK: Atheroembolic renal disease. J Am Soc Nephrol 12:1781–1787, 2001.

Parodi JC, Mura RL, Ferreira LM: Safety maneuvers to prevent embolism complicating endovascular aortic repair. J Vasc Surg 36:1076–1078, 2002.

Saleem S, Lakkis FG, Martinez-Maldonado M: Atheroembolic renal disease. Semin Nephrol 16:309–318, 1996.

Scolari F, Tardanico R, Zani R, et al: Cholesterol crystal embolism: A recognizable cause of renal disease. Am J Kidney Dis 36:1089–1109, 2000.

Scolari F, Ravani P, Pola A, et al: Predictors of renal and patient outcomes in atheroembolic renal disease: A prospective study. J Am Soc Nephrol 14:1584–1590, 2003.

Thadhani RI, Carmago CA, Xavier RJ, et al: Atheroembolic renal failure after invasive procedures: Natural history based on 52 histologically proven cases. Medicine 74:350–358, 1995.

Tunick PA, Perez JL, Kronzon I: Protruding atheromas in the thoracic aorta and systemic embolization. Ann Intern Med 115:423–427, 1991.

CHAPTER 38

Myoglobinuric and Hemoglobinuric Acute Renal Failure

Narayana S. Murali   Karl A. Nath

The exposure of the kidney to heme proteins such as myoglobin (as occurs in myoglobinuria) or hemoglobin (as occurs in hemoglobinuria) may lead to acute kidney failure, or oliguric acute tubular necrosis (ATN) and the need for hemodialysis. However, kidney function may be entirely unperturbed in myoglobinuria and hemoglobinuria, and not all forms of kidney function impairment occurring in such states reflect myoglobin-induced or hemoglobin-induced pigment nephropathy.

RHABDOMYOLYSIS

Rhabdomyolysis describes the syndrome arising from the loss of integrity of skeletal muscle and the release of contents of muscle into the extracellular fluid (ECF). The clinical manifestations of this disorder occupy a diverse spectrum, including, at one end, asymptomatic elevation in creatine kinase (CK), and at the other, acute oliguric ATN and multiorgan failure. Rhabdomyolysis is responsible for 5% to 20% of all cases of acute kidney failure. An early and critical contribution to the current understanding of this disorder was provided by Bywaters and Beall in their description of the crush syndrome in four patients who were injured and succumbed during the blitz of London in 1940. Bywaters and colleagues noted that the pathologic changes in the kidneys of these patients resembled changes previously described in patients who died from mismatched blood transfusions, and in a series of clinical and experimental studies, they provided strong evidence for the role of myoglobin, especially in aciduric states, to induce kidney damage following crush injury. A diverse array of traumatic and medical conditions is now recognized as causes for rhabdomyolysis (Table 38-1).

Pathogenesis of Rhabdomyolysis

Most if not all causes of rhabdomyolysis listed in Table 38-1 involve one or a combination of the following mechanisms occurring in the muscle cell: (1) a demand for adenosine triphosphate (ATP) that outstrips the supply of ATP, (2) increased permeability of the plasma membrane (sarcolemma), and (3) sustained increments in calcium concentrations in the cytoplasm (sarcoplasm). As

compared with the ECF, the sarcoplasm is hyperoncotic and electronegative, and exhibits significantly lower concentrations of sodium and calcium, and markedly higher concentrations of potassium. This profile of the sarcoplasm is punctuated by intermittent elevations in cytosolic calcium during muscle contraction, and is continually threatened by the tendency of sodium and calcium to move down their electrochemical gradient from the ECF into the sarcoplasm. The composition of the sarcoplasm is maintained, at least in part, by an adequate supply of ATP, and by the relative impermeability of the sarcolemma. ATP serves to lower the sarcoplasmic concentration of calcium by sequestering calcium in the sarcoplasmic reticulum and by extruding calcium from the cell; ATP also facilitates the extracellular extrusion of sodium. When ATP is depleted, the attendant increase in cellular concentrations of calcium can activate a variety of proteolytic and other cytotoxic enzymes; additionally, the accretion of sodium in the sarcoplasm due to depletion of ATP is accompanied by the intracellular movement of water, cell swelling, and cell injury. Such intracellular flux of calcium, sodium, and water can also occur when the impermeability of the sarcolemma is impaired by physical trauma or toxic substances (such as alcohol). Cell swelling is also driven by the osmotic effect of an increasing number of protein products generated as cellular proteins are degraded. Swelling of muscle is restricted by the surrounding fascia and other structures, thereby leading to increased compartmental pressures, and thus predisposing to muscle ischemia and necrosis, and the compartment syndrome. This pathogenetic sequence also accounts for the "second wave" of elevation of CK after the initial peak of CK following rhabdomyolysis. Other mechanisms contributing to muscle injury following the original insult include the ischemia-reperfusion pathway and inflammatory processes, either of which can generate reactive oxygen species, reactive nitrogen species, and diverse cytokines.

Causes of Rhabdomyolysis

Although the differential diagnosis of rhabdomyolysis is extensive (see Table 38-1), the more common causes of rhabdomyolysis include alcohol abuse, physical exertion,

TABLE 38-1   Differential Diagnosis of Rhabdomyolysis

Physical trauma to muscle
  Crush injury
  Contact sports
  Physical abuse
  Compression (e.g., immobilization, restraint, or
    confinement)
 	
Inordinate/aberrant muscular activity
  Exercise and sports
  Seizures, ECT
  Delirium tremens
  March myoglobinuria
  Movement disorders
 	
Compromised blood flow to muscle
  Arterial thrombus, embolus, dissection, or clamping
  Compartment syndrome
  Shock
  DIC
  Capillary leak syndrome
  Sickle cell disease
 	
Electrolyte and metabolic disturbances
  Hypokalemia
  Hypophosphatemia
  Hyponatremia/hypernatremia
  Hyperosmolar states
  Hypothyroidism/thyroid storm
  Diabetic ketoacidosis
  Diabetic muscle infarction
  Pheochromocytoma
 	
Drugs (Prescribed and illicit)
  HMG CoA reductase inhibitors
  Fibrates
  Isoniazid
  Colchicine
  Diphenhydramine
  Phenytoin
  Propofol
  Antimalarials
  Zidovudine
  Cocaine
  Amphetamines
  Heroin
  Methadone
  Phencyclidine
	Toxins
	  Ethanol
	  Carbon monoxide
	  Hydrocarbons
	  Solvents
	  Toluene
	  Fish poisoning (Haff disease, Buffalo fish)
	  Venom (snakes, bees, spiders)
	  Quail poisoning
	  Mushroom poisoning
	
	Deranged temperature
	  Heat stroke
	  Hyperthermia
	  Burns
	  Electrical injury and lightning
	  Malignant hyperthermia
	  Neuroleptic malignant syndrome
	  Serotonergic syndrome
	  Hypothermia
	  Frostbite
	
	Deficiencies in metabolic enzymes
	  Glycogenolysis (e.g., myophosphorylase)
	  Glycolysis (e.g., phosphofructokinase)
	  Fat metabolism (e.g., carnitine palmityltransferase)
	  Mitochondrial metabolism (e.g., respiratory chain enzymes)
	
	Inflammatory conditions
	  Dermatomyositis and polymyositis
	  Vasculitis
	  Systemic inflammatory response syndrome
	
	Infectious causes
	  Bacterial infections (e.g., Legionnaire's disease, tularemia,
	    toxic shock syndrome, streptococcal or staphylococcal
	    infections, *Clostridium*, *Salmonella* infection)
	  Viral infections (e.g., influenza, parainfluenza, coxsackie,
	    HIV, EBV, herpes, CMV)
	  Protozoal (e.g., falciparum malaria)
	  Septicemia

CMV, cytomegalovirus; DIC, disseminated intravascular coagulation; EBV, Epstein-Barr virus; ECT, electroconvulsive therapy.

compression due to immobilization, seizures, and the use of illicit drugs; additionally, rhabdomyolysis is often multifactorial in origin.

Trauma and Exertion

Muscle trauma may be readily apparent (e.g., after motor vehicle accidents or disasters) or may be less obvious, as occurs following compression due to immobilization or restraints. Muscle compression during anesthesia and surgical procedures can result in rhabdomyolysis and postoperative ATN, and has recently been recognized as a significant complication after bariatric surgery for morbid obesity.

Conditioning by regular exercise avoids the rise in CK that may occur after severe exercise in healthy individuals unaccustomed to exercise. A lack of conditioning contributes to "white-collar" rhabdomyolysis, which occurs in otherwise healthy individuals who undergo exhaustive, protracted, or closely repetitive bursts of exercise, especially after exercise that involves eccentric (e.g., downhill running) rather than concentric (e.g., uphill running) muscular activity. White-collar rhabdomyolysis is more likely to occur in men rather than women, in inadequately hydrated or fasting individuals, and following physical exertion in humid and hot conditions. Concomitant or resolving viral infections also predispose to exertional rhabdomyolysis even after seemingly mild exertion such as described in a patient recovering from a viral syndrome who developed myolysis after typing at a computer keyboard for an extended period. A major and common predisposing factor for rhabdomyolysis is potassium deficiency. During muscular contraction, intracellular potassium is normally released into the extracellular space, and by its vasorelaxant effects, such increased potassium concentrations in the interstitium maintain blood flow to exercising muscle. Additionally, potassium stimulates glycogen synthesis, the latter providing a rapid supply of ATP. Exercise-induced rhabdomyolysis is also more likely to occur in individuals with enzyme deficiencies in ATP-generating pathways such as anaerobic glycolysis and oxidative phosphorylation. Two of the more common enzyme deficiencies include deficiency of carnitine palmityl transferase (an enzyme that facilitates the import of fatty acids into mitochondria) and deficiency of myophosphorylase (an enzyme that breaks down glycogen).

Drugs, Toxins, and Other Causes

HMG CoA reductase inhibitors (statins) may induce asymptomatic elevations in CK, myalgia without an elevation in CK, and frank rhabdomyolysis. Although the risk of rhabdomyolysis with cerivastatin (Baycol) led to its withdrawal from the market, the risk of muscle injury and rhabdomyolysis with currently prescribed statins is quite low and is overwhelmingly outweighed by the benefit of these agents. Statins may induce muscle injury by decreasing cholesterol content in the sarcolemma; additionally, by decreasing mitochondrial content of ubiquinone (coenzyme Q10), statins may impair mitochondrial oxidative phosphorylation. Any of the following conditions increase the risk for statin-induced muscle injury: larger doses of statins, kidney disease, hepatic disease, hypothyroidism, and the concomitant use of drugs such as gemfibrozil, erythromycin, warfarin, cyclosporine, and itraconazole. The potentiating effects of these compounds reflect, at least in part, their inhibition of metabolism of statins via the CYP 3A4 system and glucuronidation; for example, cyclosporine and erythromycin may inhibit the cytochrome P450-3A4 (CYP-3A4) system, whereas gemfibrozil inhibits the glucuronidation pathway.

Ethanol induces rhabdomyolysis through direct and indirect effects: direct myotoxicity, malnutrition and poor caloric intake, potassium and phosphate depletion, hyperactivity and delirium tremens, associated trauma, and muscle compression due to coma. Illicit drugs, in particular cocaine and derivatives of amphetamines, also commonly provoke rhabdomyolysis. Cocaine-induced muscle injury arises from direct myotoxicity, vasoconstriction, seizures, agitation and delirium, hyperthermia, and muscle compression in obtunded patients.

Rhabdomyolysis occurs in hyperthermic states such as heat stroke, sepsis, neuroleptic malignant syndrome (inducible by butyrophenones and phenothiazines), and malignant hyperthermia. Malignant hyperthermia may be precipitated by anesthetics in patients with a genetic abnormality involving the calcium channel in the sarcoplasmic reticulum; the clinical features of this syndrome include hyperthermia, muscular rigidity, tachycardia, hypotension, and acidosis. Hyperthermia predisposes to myolysis because of direct myotoxicity and increased metabolic demand in conjunction with an inability to adequately supply ATP due to uncoupling of oxidative phosphorylation. Infectious processes induce myolysis by direct muscle involvement, by toxins generated by the infectious agent, or by cytokines and other toxic species elaborated in response to the infectious process.

Consequences of Rhabdomyolysis

The pathophysiologic consequences of rhabdomyolysis largely reflect the release of cellular contents of muscle into the ECF and the uptake of ECF into muscle (Fig. 38-1). Hyperkalemia, often severe, commonly occurs since 70% of total body stores of potassium reside in muscle, and at concentrations some 30-fold higher than plasma potassium. Hyperphosphatemia promotes the deposition of calcium phosphate in injured muscle, thereby contributing to hypocalcemia. Hyperuricemia reflects the generation of uric acid from purines derived from damaged muscle, whereas lactic acid and other organic acids contribute to a metabolic acidosis with an increased anion gap. The movement of large amounts of ECF into muscle induces ECF contraction and predisposes to a compartment syndrome. Hypoalbuminemia may occur, at least in part, from the leakage of plasma albumin across injured capillaries in muscle, whereas disseminated intravascular coagulation may be induced by thromboplastin from damaged muscle.

At least three mechanisms resulting from rhabdomyolysis converge on the kidney to induce pigment nephropathy: the release of myoglobin, ECF depletion, and systemic acidosis/aciduria; the role of hyperuricemia in pigment nephropathy is uncertain.

Pathogenesis of Pigment Nephropathy

The kidney is particularly vulnerable to the toxicity of heme proteins (such as myoglobin and hemoglobin) for several reasons. First, renal blood flow is dependent on the availability of nitric oxide, and the latter is avidly scavenged by heme proteins. Second, heme proteins stimulate the production of potent renal vasoconstrictors (endothelin and isoprostanes). Third, the kidney concentrates and internalizes heme proteins. Fourth, hydrogen peroxide present in urine oxidizes heme proteins, thereby increasing their toxicity. Fifth, reduced urinary pH also denatures heme proteins as well as facilitates the interaction of heme proteins and Tamm-Horsfall protein to form urinary casts.

ECF depletion, acidosis, and sepsis all increase the nephrotoxicity of heme proteins, and thus the likelihood

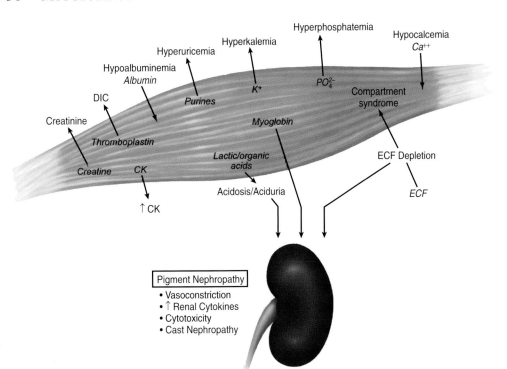

FIGURE 38-1
Complications of rhabdomyolysis. This figure summarizes the complications of rhabdomyolysis occurring as a consequence of either the release of muscle contents into the extracellular fluid (ECF) or the uptake into muscle of ECF. Ca^{++}, calcium; CK, creatine kinase; DIC, disseminated intravascular coagulation; K^+, potassium; PO_4^{2-}, phosphate. For detailed discussion, see text.

of pigment nephropathy following rhabdomyolysis. Pigment nephropathy involves the following major mechanisms: (1) renal vasoconstriction, (2) renal cytokine production (e.g., endothelin-1 and monocyte chemoattractant protein-1), (3) cytotoxic effects of heme proteins, and (4) cast formation. Renal vasoconstriction and attendant ischemia predispose toward cell injury and the sloughing of cellular debris into the nephron, thereby promoting cast formation. Not only do tubular casts occlude nephrons, but by inhibiting the urinary excretion of heme proteins, these casts also prolong the exposure of renal epithelial cells to denatured heme proteins, thereby fostering cellular uptake of heme proteins and the risk of cytotoxicity. When incorporated within renal epithelial cells, heme proteins are split into their heme and protein moieties, and heme, either directly or through its released iron, can damage cells and their organelles; additionally, heme proteins can directly promote oxidant stress. In this manner, vasoconstriction, cell injury, and cast formation interact in the pathogenesis of pigment nephropathy.

Diagnosis

Patients with rhabdomyolysis may present with features of the underlying disease, the inciting cause, or a systemic process. Patients may also present with such localizing symptoms and signs as muscle pain, swelling, stiffness, weakness, bruising, features of a compartment syndrome, or a neurologic deficit. However, a significant number of patients with rhabdomyolysis do not exhibit such clinical findings, and thus rhabdomyolysis should

be considered even in largely asymptomatic patients presenting with dark urine, decreased urinary output, abnormalities in serum electrolytes, an acid-base disorder, or an acute decline in kidney function.

Myoglobinuria may cause the urine to appear dark in color, and in approximately 50% of patients, the urinalysis reveals the presence of heme proteins on dipstick in the absence of red blood cells (less than 5 RBCs/high-power field). The urinalysis may also show an acid pH, tubular epithelial cells, granular casts, or dark pigmented casts. Proteinuria is present in 50% of cases and may attain nephrotic range. The fractional excretion of sodium may be low (less than 1%), especially in the early stages of the disease.

Myoglobinuria is transient, and the demonstration of myoglobin in urine by specific assays is rarely required to make the diagnosis. The diagnosis of rhabdomyolysis is readily confirmed by measuring plasma CK, since CK peaks within 48 hours after rhabdomyolysis, and with a half-life of 48 hours, CK noticeably declines thereafter in the absence of ongoing muscle damage. This decline in CK assists in differentiating rhabdomyolysis from other myopathic conditions. Whereas values of CK of 100,000 IU/L or greater are not infrequently seen, rhabdomyolysis also occurs with lesser elevation in CK values (1000–10,000 IU/L). There is a lack of consensus regarding the extent to which CK should be elevated to diagnose rhabdomyolysis; plasma CK values that are fivefold greater than the upper limit of normal, or greater than 500 IU/L, are employed in the literature. Mild elevations in CK may result from cardiac and neurologic disorders, and these diseases should be excluded by appropriate tests including troponins for suspected cardiac disease. A "second-wave" CK profile should raise the suspicion of an evolving compartment syndrome. The extent and severity of rhabdomyolysis can be visualized by magnetic resonance imaging scan.

Other helpful diagnostic features in rhabdomyolysis include a pentad of alterations in the electrolyte/acid-base profile (hyperkalemia, hyperphosphatemia, hypocalcemia, hyperuricemia, and increased anion gap metabolic acidosis), and a low blood urea nitrogen (BUN)/creatinine ratio (less than 10). Following rhabdomyolysis, the rate of rise in serum creatinine may outstrip that of BUN, a finding ascribed to enhanced conversion of creatine (from damaged muscle) to creatinine. However, it has been suggested that the low BUN/creatinine ratio observed in rhabdomyolysis simply reflects that patients with greater mass muscle (such as younger men) are more susceptible to rhabdomyolysis. Eventually, the BUN/creatinine ratio increases as the rate of generation of urea increases as a result of the catabolism of protein from damaged muscle.

Management of Rhabdomyolysis and Pigment Nephropathy

Patients with rhabdomyolysis, or suspected rhabdomyolysis, require vigorous hydration with isotonic saline begun as soon as possible after muscle injury. Such administration of isotonic saline expands the ECF, improves glomerular filtration rate (GFR), increases urinary flow rate, and may diminish the risk of cast nephropathy. For example, intravenous hydration should be initiated in patients with the crush syndrome even before these patients are extricated from the debris, with as much as 1 to 1.5 L of 0.9% saline given within the first hour; within the first 24 hours, up to 10 L or more of total intravenous fluid may be given to monitored patients with the crush syndrome in whom there is adequate urinary output. Clinical observations suggest that such high rates of infusion are beneficial in traumatic rhabdomyolysis and have been used to suggest therapy in nontraumatic rhabdomyolysis. Although the optimal rate of intravenous hydration in nontraumatic rhabdomyolysis is currently uncertain, hydration in these patients, at a minimum, should be prompt, and sufficiently vigorous to rapidly and completely correct ECF depletion and any volume-dependent impairment in systemic hemodynamics. Alkalinization of urine (achieving a urinary pH greater than 6.5) may also reduce the risk of pigment nephropathy and may be achieved in several ways including the use of 0.45% saline containing 75 mmol sodium bicarbonate/L. Mannitol provides an additional approach that may decrease the risk of pigment nephropathy. Mannitol may improve renal hemodynamics, increases urinary flow rate, scavenges reactive oxygen species, and diminishes the risk of urinary cast formation; mannitol may also decrease the

sequestration of ECF in injured muscle. One commonly used regimen for coadministering mannitol and bicarbonate utilizes isotonic fluid prepared by adding sodium bicarbonate (100 mL of 100 mEq NaHCO$_3$) and mannitol (100 mL of 25% mannitol) to 800 mL of 5% dextrose. One liter of this solution can be infused over 4 hours; if urinary flow rate significantly improves, then the rate of infusion of this solution can be adjusted to match urinary flow rate. If urinary flow rate remains low (urine output less than 20 mL/hour), mannitol should not be administered. Initiation of hemodialysis may be required for persisting oligoanuria and increasing uremia, hyperkalemia not readily responsive to conservative treatment (e.g., insulin/glucose, β$_2$-agonists, sodium polystyrene sulfonate exchange resin), and systemic acidosis. The administration of alkali may worsen hypocalcemia, which is generally asymptomatic and does not require treatment. Intravenous calcium salts, however, may be required to treat symptomatic hypocalcemia, hypocalcemia-induced seizures, or hyperkalemia. In the recovery phase of ATN, hypercalcemia may occur and reflects, mainly, the mobilization of calcium deposited in muscle during the oliguric phase; plasma levels of 1,25-dihydroxyvitamin D may be elevated for unclear reasons in some patients during the recovery phase and may contribute to such hypercalcemia.

Measurement of compartmental pressure in muscle by manometry may aid in the diagnosis of a compartment syndrome, the latter likely to occur when such pressures exceed 30 to 40 mm Hg (normal values: 0–10 mm Hg) or attain values 20 to 30 mm Hg less than the diastolic blood pressure. The indications for fasciotomy to decompress a compartment syndrome are generally more stringent now than previously because of the high risk of bleeding and sepsis. In nonoliguric patients there is renewed emphasis on the use of mannitol to decrease intracompartmental pressures and thereby relieve the compartment syndrome.

HEMOGLOBINURIC ACUTE KIDNEY FAILURE

Hemoglobinuria describes the presence in urine of hemoglobin that is filtered by the kidney and has escaped uptake and degradation by the renal tubular epithelium. Hemoglobin released from lysed RBCs is avidly bound to haptoglobin, and this hemoglobin-haptoglobin complex is sufficiently large so as to preclude renal filtration. In contrast, myoglobin (MW 18 kD) released from injured muscle, lacks a specific binding protein in plasma, and is rapidly cleared by renal filtration; myoglobin thus does not accumulate in plasma following rhabdomyolysis. The retention in serum of hemoglobin imparts a pink color to serum, and this finding aids in distinguishing hemoglobinuria from myoglobinuria.

The release of hemoglobin from lysed erythrocytes in quantities that swamp the binding capacity of haptoglobin leads to the presence in serum of free hemoglobin, the latter existing not only as a tetramer (2α and 2β chains, MW 68 kD) but also as a dimer (1α and 1β chain, MW 32 kD). Dimeric hemoglobin readily undergoes renal filtration and contributes substantially to hemoglobin found in urine in hemoglobinuria. Filtered hemoglobin is taken up by the renal tubules and split into the heme and globin moieties. The heme moiety is degraded by heme oxygenase (HO), leading to the release of iron, which either enters the cellular iron pool or is stored as ferritin/hemosiderin. In hemoglobinuria, hemosiderin may be detected in tubular epithelial cells shed into urine, and such hemosiderinuria is used as a diagnostic aid. When extravascular hemolysis occurs, hemoglobin so released is readily metabolized by HO in the reticuloendothelial system such that the kidney is not exposed to large amounts of hemoglobin. In contrast, intravascular hemolysis, of sufficient severity, may impose such a large burden of hemoglobin that the binding capacity of haptoglobin and the degradative capacity of HO are both overwhelmed: large amounts of hemoglobin are thus presented to the kidney. Kidney function impairment from hemoglobinuria usually reflects intravascular, and not extravascular, hemolysis.

The pathogenesis of hemoglobin-induced pigment nephropathy is broadly similar to myoglobin-induced pigment nephropathy, and is described earlier in this chapter.

Differential Diagnosis of Hemoglobinuria

Hemoglobinuria may originate from stresses intrinsic or extrinsic to the RBC (Table 38-2). In paroxysmal nocturnal hemoglobinuria, the abnormal erythrocyte is unduly sensitive to complement-mediated lysis, which occurs spontaneously, after infections, or following blood transfusions. Deficiencies in erythrocyte enzymes such as glucose-6-phosphate dehydrogenase promote the oxidation of hemoglobin to methemoglobin, and ultimately the release of the heme moiety; the buildup of oxidatively denatured hemoglobin and heme can induce hemolysis. Thus, individuals deficient in glucose-6-phosphate dehydrogenase are prone to hemoglobinuria, especially when exposed to oxidizing drugs (quinine) or conditions (sepsis).

Immune-mediated processes include acute transfusion reactions due to intravascular hemolysis of transfused cells by preformed antibodies in the recipient. Autoimmune hemolytic anemia may be caused by warm- or cold-associated antibodies, the former induced by hematologic malignancies, connective tissue diseases, or medications. Viral or mycoplasma infections may lead to a cold-reacting antibody and paroxysmal cold hemoglobinuria.

Drugs and chemicals used in clinical practice can induce hemoglobinuria, and these include antibiotics (penicillin, cefotetan, rifampicin, minocycline), non-steroidal anti-inflammatory agents, ribavirin, γ-interferon, intravenous immunoglobulin, fluorescein, and ethanolamine oleate (used for sclerotherapy of varicose veins). Hemolysis may be induced by chemicals in industrial and other uses (e.g., benzene, phenol, naphthalene, copper, and mercuric salts). Hypotonic solutions used to irrigate the genitourinary tract, or inadvertently employed in plasmapheresis may cause hemolysis. Conversely, hypertonic stress and attendant hemolysis may arise from the use of contrast agents in dehydrated patients, hypertonic saline as an abortifacient, hypertonic glycerol to reduce intracranial pressure, or propylene glycol employed as a vehicle for medications.

TABLE 38-2 Differential Diagnosis of Hemoglobinuria

I. Mechanisms intrinsic to red blood cells	
Abnormalities in erythrocyte membrane/cytoskeleton (e.g., paroxysmal nocturnal hemoglobinuria)	
Abnormalities in erythrocyte metabolism (e.g., glucose-6-phosphate dehydrogenase deficiency)	
Abnormalities in hemoglobin (e.g., sickle cell disease)	
II. Mechanisms extrinsic to red blood cells	
Immune-mediated	Transfusion reactions
	Autoimmune hemolytic anemia
Drugs/chemicals	Oxidant stressors
	Immune injury
	Other agents
Osmotic stressors	Hypotonic solutions
	Hypertonic solutions
Mechanical injury	Heart valves, extracorporeal circulation/device
	Transcatheter coil embolization, mechanical thrombectomy
	March hemoglobinuria, conga drumming, karate
	Physical abuse
Thermal injury	Burns
	Radiofrequency ablation
Microangiopathies	Disseminated intravascular coagulation
	TTP/HUS
	Vasculitides
Severe hypophosphatemia	
Bone marrow transplantation	
Infections	Parasitic
	Bacterial
Venoms/toxins	
Hemoglobin-based red blood cell substitute	

TTP/HUS, thrombotic thrombocytopenic purpura and hemolytic uremic syndrome.
Modified from Nath KA: Hemoglobinuria. In Molitoris B, Finn WF (eds): Acute Renal Failure: A Companion to Brenner and Rector's The Kidney. Philadelphia, WB Saunders, 2001, pp 214–219. With permission.

Infectious causes of hemoglobinuria include falciparum malaria, in which extravascular hemolysis of parasitized and nonparasitized cells can occur in conjunction with intravascular hemolysis, especially in the setting of glucose-6-phosphate dehydrogenase deficiency, and antimalarial agents that are pro-oxidant. Fulminant hemolysis in malaria leading to hemoglobinuria and dark urine is described as blackwater fever. Hemoglobinuria may also result from hemolysins produced by bacteria (e.g., *Clostridium perfringens*), and venoms derived from certain species of snakes, spiders, scorpions, and jellyfish.

Diagnosis and Treatment

Evidence of hemolysis usually accompanies hemoglobinuria. Thus, elevations in serum lactate dehydrogenase and unconjugated bilirubin occur in conjunction with reduced serum levels of haptoglobin and elevated free hemoglobin concentrations; reticulocytosis may be apparent, and the peripheral smear may demonstrate, depending on the underlying cause, fragmented erythrocytes, spherocytes, and other abnormalities in RBC morphology. In addition to acute kidney failure, hyperkalemia and acidosis may also occur.

A spun urinary sample may aid in differentiating hemoglobinuria from other causes of red or dark urine, in that a red sediment following centrifugation is suggestive of hematuria whereas a supernatant that is red and is heme-positive by dipstick is indicative of myoglobinuria or hemoglobinuria. Pink discoloration of serum occurs in hemoglobinuria but not in myoglobinuria.

The underlying approach to the treatment of hemoglobin-induced pigment nephropathy is similar to the therapeutic approach in myoglobin-induced pigment nephropathy, namely, vigorous hydration and forced mannitol-alkaline diuresis. In certain instances, hemodialysis may temporarily be required over several days or weeks, after which recovery of kidney function usually occurs. Specific therapies should target, whenever possible, the underlying mechanism accounting for the destruction of RBCs, for example, cessation of exposure to the offending drug or agent, employing appropriate protocols for transfusion reactions, and surgical correction for cardiac/vascular prostheses.

BIBLIOGRAPHY

Baliga R, Ueda N, Walker PD, et al: Oxidant mechanisms in toxic acute renal failure. Am J Kidney Dis 29:465–477, 1997.

Better OS, Rubinstein I, Reis DN: Muscle crush compartment syndrome: Fulminant local edema with threatening systemic effects. Kidney Int 63:1155–1157, 2003.

Better OS, Stein JH: Early management of shock and prophylaxis of acute renal failure in traumatic rhabdomyolysis. N Engl J Med 322:825–829, 1990.

Bywaters EG, Beall D: Crush injuries with impairment of renal function. BMJ 1:427–432, 1941.

Gabow PA, Kaehny WD, Kelleher SP: The spectrum of rhabdomyolysis. Medicine (Baltimore). 61:141–152, 1982.

Knochel JP: Nontraumatic rhabdomyolysis. In Molitoris B, Finn WF (eds): Acute Renal Failure: A Companion to Brenner and Rector's The Kidney. Philadelphia, WB Saunders, 2001, pp 227–235.

Knochel JP: Mechanisms of rhabdomyolysis. Curr Opin Rheumatol 5:725–731, 1993.

Knochel JP: Catastrophic medical events with exhaustive exercise: "White collar rhabdomyolysis." Kidney Int 38:709–719, 1990.

Moore KP, Holt SG, Patel RP, et al: A causative role for redox cycling of myoglobin and its inhibition by alkalinization in the pathogenesis and treatment of rhabdomyolysis-induced renal failure. J Biol Chem 273:31731–31737, 1998.

Nath KA: Hemoglobinuria. In Molitoris B, Finn WF (eds): Acute Renal Failure: A Companion to Brenner and Rector's The Kidney. Philadelphia, WB Saunders, 2001, pp 214–219.

Nath KA, Balla G, Vercellotti GM, et al: Induction of heme oxygenase is a rapid, protective response in rhabdomyolysis in the rat. J Clin Invest 90:267–270, 1992.

Nath KA, Grande JP, Croatt AJ, et al: Intracellular targets in heme protein-induced renal injury. Kidney Int 53:100–111, 1998.

Slater MS, Mullins RJ: Rhabdomyolysis and myoglobinuric renal failure in trauma and surgical patients: A review. J Am Coll Surg 186:693–716, 1998.

Thompson PD, Clarkson P, Karas RH: Statin-associated myopathy. JAMA 289:1681–1690, 2003.

Vanholder R, Sever MS, Erek E, et al: Rhabdomyolysis. J Am Soc Nephrol 11:1553–1561, 2000.

Warren JD, Blumbergs PC, Thompson PD: Rhabdomyolysis: A review. Muscle Nerve 25:332–347, 2002.

Zager RA: Rhabdomyolysis and myohemoglobinuric acute renal failure. Kidney Int 49:314–326, 1996.

CHAPTER 39

Management of Acute Renal Failure

Kerry C. Cho   Glenn M. Chertow

Despite many advances in nephrology, renal replacement therapy and intensive care medicine, the mortality and morbidity of acute renal failure (ARF) remain high. Mortality rates of 50% to 80% for ARF requiring kidney support are commonly cited in observational studies. Although mortality rates have not changed significantly since the advent of hemodialysis, evidence suggests that comorbidities and illness severity have increased, masking real improvements in the care and outcomes of ARF. Successful management of ARF requires early recognition, management of uremic complications, timely renal replacement therapy, prevention of ongoing kidney injury, aggressive supportive care, and correction of the primary disorder(s). For the purposes of this discussion, we focus primarily on acute tubular necrosis (ATN), one of the most common causes of ARF in hospitalized patients.

Acute renal failure is usually diagnosed by nonnephrologists such as internists, intensivists, and surgeons. Unfortunately, recognition of ARF and its severity is often missed or delayed. Increases in the serum creatinine may not be noted for 24 to 48 hours after the onset of ARF. The serum creatinine concentration is deceptive in patients with malnutrition, cachexia, or decreased muscle mass; small absolute changes in serum creatinine may reflect large changes in glomerular filtration rate (GFR). Predictive formulas for creatinine clearance, such as the Cockcroft-Gault formula, may be used inappropriately in ARF, potentially delaying diagnosis and therapy. Changes in urine output, especially oliguria and anuria, may reflect kidney dysfunction prior to changes in serum creatinine concentration, but some physicians may mistake nonoliguria for preserved kidney function. A response to diuretics may be interpreted as recovering kidney function or the absence of kidney failure. The misperception that nephrologists have little to offer therapeutically except renal replacement therapy may also delay appropriate consultation, allowing uremic complications and further kidney injury to occur. A recent study suggested that delayed nephrology consultation was associated with increased mortality and increased length of hospital and ICU stays. A low serum creatinine and nonoliguria were the two conditions significantly associated with delayed consultation.

Once ARF has been identified, management begins with prompt diagnosis and correction of the underlying cause (see Chapter 34). Correction of prerenal or postrenal causes often leads to rapid recovery. Prerenal ARF resolves with restoration of normal hemodynamics and kidney perfusion by fluid resuscitation, cardiovascular support, and withdrawal of offending medications. The lack of complete or even partial recovery following restoration of perfusion requires a re-examination of other potential diagnoses. Postrenal ARF results from urinary obstruction; relief of obstruction may lead to kidney recovery and profound diuresis (see Chapter 51). Early involvement of urologists and interventional radiologists for stone removal, ureteral stents, or nephrostomy tube placement may prevent the development of intrinsic kidney disease from longstanding obstruction. With prerenal and postrenal ARF, nephrologists may cautiously withhold dialytic support in anticipation of imminent kidney recovery. However, the diagnosis of intrarenal (or intrinsic) ARF portends a less favorable prognosis, longer time to recovery, and a higher likelihood for dialysis or continuous renal replacement therapy.

NONDIALYTIC KIDNEY SUPPORT

The goals of nondialytic management of ARF are prevention of further kidney injury and supportive care to allow potential functional recovery. Successful management requires meticulous attention to many details: volume status, hemodynamics, fluid and electrolyte management, acid-base status, nutrition, and medication dose adjustment or discontinuation (Table 39-1). Adjuvant therapy for concomitant sepsis, shock, and the systemic inflammatory response may also be required.

In general, the kidneys in ARF have impaired autoregulation; they are unable to maintain perfusion and GFR over a range of mean arterial pressures. Maintaining adequate hemodynamics and kidney perfusion is essential for functional recovery. Successful volume management requires a careful physical examination, attention to daily weights and overall fluid balance, recognition of insensible losses, correct interpretation of hemodynamic parameters (including central pressure measurements), and selection of appropriate fluids. The goal is to achieve and maintain euvolemia while restoring effective circulating volume to allow adequate tissue and kidney perfusion. The physician may use crystalloids, colloids, blood

TABLE 39-1 Nondialytic Management of Acute Renal Failure

Treat or reverse underlying cause(s) of acute renal failure.
Achieve and maintain normal hemodynamics and euvolemia, avoiding, hypovolemia and prerenal states.
Adjust medication dosages and frequency for level of kidney function.
Avoid nephrotoxic agents if possible, including aminoglycosides, radiocontrast, NSAIDs, ACE inhibitors, and angiotensin receptor blockers.
Provide adjuvant therapy, including antibiotics, mechanical ventilation, enteral or parenteral nutrition, intensive insulin therapy, and adrenal corticosteroid replacement as indicated.
Enlist the assistance of nephrologists and/or intensivists for supportive care and to determine the need for, and timing of, renal replacement therapy.

ACE, angiotensin-converting enzyme; NSAIDs, nonsteroidal anti-inflammatory drugs.

products, vasopressors, or inotropes, incorporating information from the physical examination and central venous and pulmonary artery catheters as necessary toward this goal. Except possibly in the case of hepatic cirrhosis, colloids have not been found superior to crystalloids for volume expansion and ARF prevention. Identification and correction of hypovolemia may rapidly reverse prerenal ARF.

Unfortunately, precise recommendations for volume and hemodynamic management are not available. Despite its importance in the prevention and treatment of ARF, fluid resuscitation has not been adequately tested. Optimal hemodynamic targets for resuscitation are not well defined. A trial of goal-oriented hemodynamic therapy (i.e., using specific hemodynamic and physiologic parameters as resuscitation end points) in critically ill patients (with and without ARF) to raise cardiac index and oxygen delivery failed to improve survival, decrease ICU length of stay, or decrease the number of dysfunctional organs. However, another trial of early goal-directed therapy in patients with severe sepsis or septic shock used a protocol algorithm to maintain hemodynamic parameters (central venous pressure, mean arterial pressure, and central venous oxygen saturation) at specified targets using fluid resuscitation, inotropes, vasoactive agents, and red cell transfusions. Instituted before ICU admission, this protocol therapy reduced in-hospital mortality and organ dysfunction, although ARF was not specifically mentioned. Finally, a prospective cohort study of ICU patients showed increased mortality, length of stay, and costs in those who received pulmonary artery catheterization compared with those who did not.

Large randomized clinical trials of fluid composition, hemodynamic targets, and invasive monitoring specifically in ARF have not been conducted, and there is no consensus on optimal strategies. However, adequate hydration to correct possible hypovolemia is generally recommended to diagnose and treat prerenal ARF. Invasive monitoring with central venous pressures or pulmonary artery catheterization may be helpful to guide volume management with fluid resuscitation, diuretics, or ultrafiltration. The management of shock may require vasopressors and inotropic agents.

Often preceded or exacerbated by the oliguria of ARF, hypervolemia may complicate patient mobility, mechanical ventilation, extubation, wound healing, central venous access, and abdominal compartment syndrome. Total parental nutrition and intravenous medications (in either bolus or continuous forms) are often overlooked sources of fluid intake. Fluid restriction, diuretics, and dopamine are potentially helpful, but should be used cautiously. Nutrition and blood products should not be restricted solely for volume concerns. Indeed, renal replacement therapy may be necessary in patients with relatively preserved or recovering kidney function to provide maximal nutritional therapy or blood products, such as continuous infusions of fresh-frozen plasma in patients with liver failure and coagulopathy.

Diuretics may be useful to manage volume overload in ARF, but they have toxicities and potential pitfalls. Loop diuretics are ototoxic in high doses; concomitantly administered aminoglycosides may increase the ototoxicity. Continuous infusions of loop diuretics may reduce drug toxicity by reducing cumulative dose requirements and peak serum concentrations. It is important to recognize that although oliguria has been established as a poor prognostic sign in ARF, conversion of oliguria to nonoliguria (with diuretics or vasoactive substances) has not been shown to reduce mortality or facilitate kidney recovery. Conversion of oliguria to nonoliguria with diuretics may simply reflect less severe ARF. Ultimately, a trial of diuretics should not delay the initiation of dialysis when otherwise required in a nonoliguric patient.

Dopamine has been shown in animal and human trials to increase renal blood flow, GFR, and urine output. Some investigators have argued that low doses of dopamine (less than 3 µg/kg/minute) provide selective renal vasodilation with few inotropic and vasoactive effects. Despite these theoretical physiologic benefits, meta-analyses and randomized clinical trials of dopamine in ARF have failed to demonstrate any benefit on outcomes, including prevention or treatment of ARF. The most recent meta-analysis concluded that dopamine did not decrease the incidence of ARF, the need for dialysis, or mortality. Although some may recommend a brief trial of diuretics and low-dose dopamine, it is important to note that dopamine commonly leads to arrhythmias, tachycardia, and myocardial ischemia. Furthermore, there is evidence that dopamine may cause intestinal ischemia, anterior pituitary dysfunction, and decreased T-cell function. Thus, aggressive attempts to restore urine output with fluids, diuretics, and vasoactive drugs may result in complications (hypervolemia, drug toxicity, and arrhythmias) and unnecessarily postpone nephrology consultation and kidney support.

Since renal water and sodium handling may be abnormal in ARF, dysnatremias are common. Unfortunately, hypo- and hypernatremia in hospitalized patients with ARF are often iatrogenic; improper volume management and fluid composition unmasks the kidney's inability to maintain sodium and water homeostasis. Hyponatremia usually results from excess free water relative to sodium and solute intake. Hypernatremia may result from hypotonic fluid losses via nasogastric suctioning, stool output, osmotic diuresis (including glucose, mannitol, and urea), and insensible losses. Overly aggressive normal saline resuscitation and inadequate free water intake are iatrogenic causes. Hypernatremia is usually seen in association with hypovolemia. Hypervolemic hypernatremia is rare, typically the result of hypertonic solute administration (e.g., sodium bicarbonate or hypertonic saline).

Metabolic acidosis is commonly seen in ARF due to reduced renal acid excretion. Dietary protein restriction to 0.6 to 0.8 g/kg/day may reduce acid production and improve the metabolic acidosis, but may not be desirable in hypercatabolic patients. Alkaline intravenous fluids such as sodium bicarbonate will correct acidosis, especially if concomitant hypovolemia allows large-volume resuscitation with isotonic sodium bicarbonate. An alternative buffer is sodium acetate found in parenteral nutrition. However, the exogenous sodium load with the potential for complications of hypervolemia, including pulmonary edema, often limits the capacity for aggressive alkali replacement. Hemodialysis or continuous renal replacement therapy should be employed in refractory or severe cases of acidemia, especially in the setting of shock, multiorgan dysfunction, and other indications for kidney support.

Hyperkalemia associated with electrocardiographic changes and/or clinical manifestations requires emergent therapy (see Chapter 12). Exogenous sources of potassium should be discontinued immediately, including nutrition (oral, enteral, or parenteral), potassium supplements, and intravenous fluids. The medical management of hyperkalemia includes immediate temporizing measures such as intravenous calcium gluconate, insulin, sodium bicarbonate, and the inhaled β-agonist albuterol. Unless kidney function can be restored quickly (as in cases of acute obstruction), therapy to remove potassium should be initiated. Administered either orally or rectally, sodium polystyrene sulfonate is an exchange resin that binds and removes potassium. However, its onset of action is measured in hours. It is relatively contraindicated in postoperative patients, including those recovering from kidney transplantation, because of the risk of bowel necrosis and perforation. Hemodialysis is the definitive treatment for hyperkalemia, rapidly correcting the serum potassium and electrocardiographic changes. Unfortunately, electrolyte testing, nephrology

consultation, dialysis catheter placement, activation of a dialysis nurse and technician, and preparation of a dialysis machine can delay the initiation of hemodialysis by hours. Although continuous renal replacement therapies (e.g., continuous venovenous hemodiafiltration) may be initiated soon after line placement, these therapies are less efficient per unit time and may not rapidly correct acute hyperkalemia.

Hyperphosphatemia and hypermagnesemia may occur in the course of ARF, particularly with direct tissue injury (e.g., rhabdomyolysis). Exogenous phosphorus in the diet, tube feedings, and parenteral nutrition should be reduced. Oral phosphorus binders, including calcium acetate and calcium carbonate, reduce phosphorus absorption from the intestinal tract. Aluminum hydroxide is an effective phosphorus binder, but its use should be limited to short courses (less than 2 to 3 weeks) to decrease the possibility of aluminum toxicity. Citrate salts increase aluminum absorption and should never be used with aluminum hydroxide. Sevelamer hydrochloride is a noncalcium, nonaluminum-containing phosphate binder frequently used in endstage renal disease (ESRD); its physical structure as a hydrogel (expanding within a feeding tube) makes its use with forced enteral feeding problematic. Hypermagnesemia is often iatrogenic, from either overzealous magnesium replacement or magnesium-containing medications.

Bleeding diatheses may complicate ARF. Synthetic analogues of arginine vasopressin may be used acutely to correct uremic platelet dysfunction, but repeated doses result in tachyphylaxis. Estrogens and cryoprecipitate have also been used for treatment of uremic bleeding. Unfortunately, estrogens have an onset of action measured in hours, whereas cryoprecipitate must be given repeatedly for a sustained effect. Hemodialysis is the definitive therapy for uremic bleeding. Patients with intracranial, gastrointestinal, retroperitoneal, or surgical bleeding should receive prompt dialytic support. Anticoagulation for hemodialysis or continuous renal replacement therapy can be reduced or withheld for these patients. Heparin-induced thrombocytopenia is a real concern for patients requiring either intermittent hemodialysis or continuous therapy. Other anticoagulants such as citrate and prostacyclin may be used. When this diagnosis is being considered, all heparin products, including flushes used to lock dialysis catheters between treatments, should be withheld.

Medications, especially antimicrobials, should be appropriately dosed for the level of kidney dysfunction or the modality of renal replacement (see Chapter 41). A rapidly changing serum creatinine concentration or oligoanuria suggests markedly diminished kidney function; dosing medications for an assumed GFR of less than 10 mL/minute is prudent. Drug levels for vancomycin and aminoglycosides should be monitored to avoid toxicity and to guarantee therapeutic levels. The doses of most penicillins (including extended-spectrum penicillins used against *Staphylococcus* and *Pseudomonas* spp.) and many cephalosporins and quinolones require adjustment. Imipenem should be avoided if other alternatives exist; imipenem metabolites can lead to seizures. If acute interstitial nephritis is a diagnostic possibility, the offending agent and other culprits should be discontinued. Narcotic analgesics and their metabolites generally have prolonged half-lives in ARF, potentially exacerbating uremic encephalopathy. Like imipenem, meperidine should be avoided in severe ARF given its epileptogenic primary metabolite (normeperidine).

Potentially nephrotoxic agents should be avoided entirely if possible. Medications that adversely affect renal and systemic hemodynamics should be avoided. Nonsteroidal anti-inflammatory drugs reduce kidney perfusion and GFR. Angiotensin-converting enzyme inhibitors and angiotensin receptor blockers tend to reduce GFR (although kidney perfusion is generally maintained); the use of these drugs in ARF may confound the severity of injury or rate of potential recovery. To decrease the possibility of hypotension and prerenal ARF, antihypertensive agents should be carefully titrated. Intravenous radiocontrast may be required for either diagnostic or therapeutic purposes. Other diagnostic modalities such as ultrasonography, magnetic resonance imaging, and nuclear medicine should be explored in consultation with radiologists. In cases where there are no alternatives to intravascular radiocontrast, physicians should consider gentle volume expansion prior to radiocontrast administration, if tolerated. The use of agents to further reduce the rate of radiocontrast-associated nephropathy, including *N*-acetylcysteine, should be considered, recognizing that clinical trial results have been mixed. Any prophylactic strategy should not delay imaging studies in critically ill patients.

NUTRITION, ERYTHROPOIETIN, AND THERAPEUTIC AGENTS

Acute renal failure that occurs in the setting of multiorgan dysfunction is a hypercatabolic state with muscle and visceral protein wasting and negative nitrogen balance. Isolated ARF, however, has not been conclusively proven to be a catabolic state. Moreover, although total parenteral nutrition (TPN) is commonly used, clear evidence of its benefits in critically ill patients is lacking. A recent meta-analysis concluded that TPN may have a positive effect on nutritional end points and possibly minor complications, but there was no evidence for decreased mortality or major complication rates (including organ failure). Randomized and nonrandomized trials of TPN specifically in the setting of ARF have been largely inconclusive. Nonetheless, it is axiomatic that nutrition is superior to no nutrition. General recommendations for TPN include a calorie intake of 30 to 35 kcal/kg/day and a maximum protein intake of 1.5 g/kg body weight/day

for hypercatabolic patients and 0.6 g/kg/day for noncatabolic patients. Potassium, phosphorus, and magnesium are typically withheld from parenteral nutrition solutions in patients with ARF. If electrolyte deficiencies develop, they can be quickly corrected with supplements. Energy and protein requirements should be estimated (often by an experienced registered dietitian), adjusting for dialysis-related losses of amino acids where appropriate. Continuous renal replacement therapies are associated with the largest dialytic losses of amino acids, often necessitating the administration of an additional 10 to 30 g protein per day.

Experimental models of ARF have shown decreased synthesis and secretion of erythropoietin. Decreased circulating levels combined with bone marrow hyporesponsiveness to erythropoietin produce the anemia of ARF and critical illness. Recombinant human erythropoietin (rHuEpo) in rat models of ARF reverses anemia and leads to earlier recovery of kidney function. However, investigators have only begun to study rHuEpo in patients with ARF and critical illness. A recent trial of critically ill patients found that weekly rHuEpo (40,000 U subcutaneously) increased hemoglobin and reduced red cell transfusions. Unfortunately, clinical outcomes such as mortality and organ failure were not studied; a subgroup analysis in ARF patients was not performed. Thus the risk-benefit and cost-benefit of rHuEpo in human ARF remain undefined.

The search for effective therapeutic agents for ARF has been frustrating. Despite encouraging results in experimental models, many agents with favorable phase II study results have shown no benefit in randomized clinical trials: atrial natriuretic peptide, thyroxine, insulin-like growth factor I, loop diuretics, and dopamine. Other biologic agents have no benefit in either experimental or human sepsis trials: antibodies to tumor necrosis factor-α, nitric oxide synthase inhibitors, tissue factor pathway inhibitor, endothelin antagonists, epidermal growth factor, inhibitors of arachidonic acid metabolism, and antithrombin. Other agents currently under study are platelet-activating factor inhibitors and leukocyte adhesion inhibitors.

However, some interventions have recently been shown to be effective in the treatment of critically ill patients, a population at risk for the development of ARF. These interventions include activated protein C, intensive insulin therapy, hemodynamic goal-directed therapy, the combination of hydrocortisone and fludrocortisone, and low-tidal-volume mechanical ventilation. Although these interventions have not been tested directly in an ARF population, they should be considered the standard of care and adjuvant therapy for ARF patients with critical illness. Recombinant activated protein C is the first drug approved by the U.S. Food and Drug Administration for the treatment of sepsis, decreasing mortality in a large randomized trial of patients with known or suspected infection, organ failure, and signs of systemic

---

TABLE 39-2 Uremic Complications

Platelet dysfunction and uremic bleeding
Pericarditis and pleuritis
Neuropathy including asterixis, myoclonus, and wrist or
foot drop
Encephalopathy
Seizures

---

inflammation. Intensive insulin therapy to maintain a glucose concentration between 80 and 110 mg/dL increased survival compared with conventional glucose control in a randomized trial of mechanically ventilated patients in a surgical ICU. Intensive insulin reduced both ICU and in-hospital mortality, while also reducing the incidence of ARF and the need for renal replacement therapy. The combination of hydrocortisone and fludrocortisone reduced mortality in adult septic shock patients identified with relative adrenal insufficiency. Low-tidal-volume mechanical ventilation improved survival in acute respiratory distress syndrome. Unless there are specific contraindications, patients with ARF and other complications should enjoy the potential benefits of these recent advances in critical care medicine.

KIDNEY SUPPORT

Traditional indications for renal replacement therapy in ARF include acid-base disturbances, electrolyte abnormalities, volume overload refractory to diuretics, and uremic complications (Tables 39-2 and 39-3). Urgent

---

TABLE 39-3 Renal Replacement Therapy in Acute Renal Failure

Traditional indications
Acid-base disturbances, most commonly metabolic acidosis
Electrolyte imbalances, especially hyperkalemia (serum
  potassium ≥6.0 mEq/L) with or without ECG abnormalities
Volume overload refractory to diuretics, especially with
  pulmonary edema and respiratory compromise
Uremia, including encephalopathy, pericarditis,
  coagulopathy

Proactive indications
Impending acid-base or electrolyte disturbances
Oligoanuria with large obligate fluid intake for medications
  and nutrition
Moderate to severe ARF with poor prognosis for immediate
  kidney recovery
ARF in the setting of sepsis or systemic inflammatory
  response syndrome

Goals of renal replacement therapy
Acid-base, electrolyte, and volume homeostasis
Prevention of uremia and its complications
Maintenance of optimal cardiopulmonary performance and
  normal hemodynamics
Maximum nutritional support

---

hemodialysis should be considered in all cases of ARF with serum potassium concentrations of 6.0 mEq/L and above, especially if nondialytic treatment is unsuccessful, kidney recovery is not imminent, the patient is oligoanuric, or the electrocardiogram (ECG) shows evidence of hyperkalemia (peaked T waves, PR prolongation, QRS widening, and ventricular arrhythmias). However, electrocardiographic manifestations correlate poorly with the severity of hyperkalemia. A patient with severe hyperkalemia and a normal EKG still requires cardiac monitoring, immediate conservative treatment for hyperkalemia, and possibly emergent hemodialysis.

The development of uremic complications correlates poorly with serum markers such as creatinine and blood urea nitrogen. Moreover, delay of renal replacement while attempting conservative management may be detrimental to the patient. Waiting for uremic complications to develop before initiating dialysis does not make intuitive sense. Some nephrologists feel that the initiation of kidney support should be anticipatory—that is, starting support before uremic complications arise to allow optimal care, especially if prolonged or delayed kidney recovery is expected. Unfortunately, there are few data on early or prophylactic initiation of renal replacement and its effects on outcomes such as survival and kidney recovery. The optimal timing of initiation of kidney support is unknown and varies widely, often depending on local practice patterns.

There are two major types of renal replacement therapy for ARF. Continuous renal replacement therapy (CRRT) includes hemodialysis, hemofiltration, and hemodiafiltration modalities. Intermittent hemodialysis includes standard hemodialysis and alternative forms such as sustained low-efficiency dialysis (SLED). Alternative forms are usually used when continuous therapies are not available or undesirable (possibly because of patient immobility or the requirement for continuous anticoagulation). The extended treatment times allow more gradual ultrafiltration rates and improved solute clearance. Peritoneal dialysis is uncommonly used for ARF in the United States, but it may be the only available modality in other areas or under certain emergency circumstances. External variables such as modality availability and the training and expertise of the physician prescribing kidney support will often determine the selection of support modality.

Regardless of hemodialysis modality, vascular access must be achieved, usually via a dual-lumen dialysis catheter placed in a central vein. The femoral vein is suitable for ventilated, immobilized, and sedated patients in the ICU, but the internal jugular vein may be preferred for ambulatory patients, especially if prolonged dialytic support is anticipated. The subclavian vein should be avoided because of the high incidence of venous stenosis that precludes using the ipsilateral extremity for future arteriovenous fistulae and grafts. Vein preservation from subclavian venous catheters, unnecessary phlebotomy, and intravenous access is important for patients with ARF who may require permanent vascular access for end-stage renal disease (ESRD). Patients requiring permanent or indefinite dialysis should have long-term vascular access prior to hospital discharge. Peritoneal catheter insertion or internal jugular tunneled catheter placement are relatively minor procedures. Vascular surgical consultation for creation of an arteriovenous fistula and graft should be considered for suitable candidates.

Continuous therapy has several advantages and disadvantages, both real and theoretical, compared with intermittent hemodialysis. The advantages include hemodynamic stability, continuous correction of electrolyte and acid-base disorders, volume homeostasis, improved solute clearance, and the ability to provide maximal nutrition therapy. For example, TPN often requires large fluid volumes, which may be difficult or impossible to manage with intermittent hemodialysis. Other investigators have suggested that continuous therapies remove and/or adsorb cytokines and other important biological agents in the inflammatory state of sepsis and ARF. It remains controversial whether removal and absorption of these agents by continuous therapies is significant relative to their production, or whether CRRT has a therapeutic role in critical illness among patients without ARF.

The potential disadvantages of CRRT include limited availability, patient immobilization, continuous anticoagulation, and hypocalcemia with hemofiltration or citrate extracorporeal anticoagulation. CRRT is also heavily resource dependent, requiring ICU monitoring and labor-intensive nursing care, which may be temporarily unavailable even in centers that offer CRRT therapy. Some investigators have argued that CRRT is more expensive than intermittent hemodialysis, although it is difficult to calculate infrastructure expenses and other embedded costs of hemodialysis. Others have suggested that CRRT may facilitate kidney recovery, resulting in fewer days of kidney support and potentially lower costs. Ultimately, patient outcomes, not cost considerations, should determine the selection of one modality over another.

Unfortunately, neither intermittent hemodialysis nor continuous renal replacement has been conclusively shown to be superior in terms of survival and kidney recovery. Unbalanced randomization plagued the one randomized clinical trial comparing CRRT and intermittent hemodialysis, which may also have been underpowered. It is difficult to draw firm conclusions from the numerous retrospective studies because of selection bias. In general, patients who received CRRT were sicker and had higher illness severity scores compared with patients who received intermittent hemodialysis. The advent of alternative hemodialysis modalities such as SLED and high-filtration hemodialysis will make future nonrandomized comparisons of hemodialysis and hemofiltration even more difficult. The final selection of dialysis

modality depends on several variables: patient variables (hemodynamic stability, fluid balance, nutritional requirements, indication for kidney support), hospital variables (modality availability, nursing and ICU availability), and physician variables (training, expertise, and modality preference).

The dose of renal replacement therapy has not been as well defined in ARF as in ESRD. Research has shown that the prescribed dose of dialysis in ARF patients often fails to reach the minimum recommended dose of dialysis for ESRD patients. Furthermore, the delivered dose of dialysis often fails to meet the prescribed dose for several reasons: catheter dysfunction, treatment failure, and early termination for diagnostic and therapeutic procedures. Most nephrologists would agree that ARF patients should receive at minimum the recommended dose of dialysis for chronic ESRD patients. Given the hypercatabolic state found in many ARF patients, one would assume that the dialysis dose should be increased relative to the dose for stable ESRD patients. Recent trials have found that higher doses of dialysis improve outcomes such as mortality and kidney recovery in ARF. Compared with conventional alternate day treatment, daily hemodialysis decreased mortality (28% vs 46%). Daily dialysis also produced better azotemic control, fewer episodes of intradialytic hypotension, and more rapid kidney recovery. Another trial demonstrated that high-volume ultrafiltration (minimum of 35 mL/kg/hour) during continuous hemofiltration improved survival in ICU patients with ARF compared with low-volume ultrafiltration (20 mL/kg/hour).

KIDNEY RECOVERY AND PROGNOSIS

Increased urine production is the first sign of kidney recovery in oliguric and anuric patients. A 12- or 24-hour urine collection for creatinine clearance can confirm recovery. The serum creatinine concentration will stabilize and then decrease. Kidney support can be stopped if kidney function and urine output are adequate for solute clearance, electrolyte and acid-base homeostasis, and volume management. However, precise indications for stopping kidney support in the recovery phase of ARF remain undefined. The overall prognosis of ARF is poor; up to 30% of patients requiring kidney support for ARF will require long-term dialysis following hospital discharge.

FUTURE DIRECTIONS

Progress in ARF management can proceed along many fronts. The identification of patient characteristics, co-morbidities, and possibly genetic polymorphisms that are risk factors for the development of ARF is crucial. Prophylactic agents, such as *N*-acetylcysteine for contrast nephropathy, and preventive strategies are the next step for critically ill and other high-risk patients. Improved techniques for the early detection and more precise diagnostic classification of ARF are being developed using urinary markers of tubular injury. The search continues for effective therapeutic agents for established ATN. Long-standing questions such as the timing of initiation of support or the superiority of one dialysis modality remain unanswered. Although recent trials have estab-

lished minimum doses, the optimal amount of kidney support required for ARF is not known. The accurate identification of patients who are unlikely to benefit from renal replacement therapy would be clinically useful. The effects of new critical-care interventions (e.g., activated protein C, early goal-directed therapy, intensive insulin therapy, and steroid replacement) in ARF patients are unknown. Clearly, further work in the biology of ARF and additional clinical trials are needed.

BIBLIOGRAPHY

Annane D, Sebille V, Charpentier C, et al: Effect of treatment with low doses of hydrocortisone and fludrocortisone on mortality in patients with septic shock. JAMA 288:862–871, 2002.

Bernard GR, Vincent JL, Laterre PF, et al: Efficacy and safety of recombinant human activated protein C for severe sepsis. N Engl J Med 344:699–709, 2001.

Brady HR, Singer GG. Acute renal failure. Lancet 346:1533–1540, 1995.

Corwin HL, Gettinger A, Pearl RG, et al: Efficacy of recombinant human erythropoietin in critically ill patients: A randomized controlled trial. JAMA 288:2827–2835, 2002.

De Vriese AS: Prevention and treatment of acute renal failure in sepsis. J Am Soc Nephrol 14:792–805, 2003.

Esson ML, Schrier RW: Diagnosis and treatment of acute tubular necrosis. Ann Intern Med 137:744–752, 2002.

Heyland DK, MacDonald S, Keefe L, Drover JW: Total parenteral nutrition in the critically ill patient: A meta-analysis. JAMA 280:2013–2019, 1998.

Kellum JA, Decker JM: Use of dopamine in acute renal failure: A meta-analysis. Crit Care Med 29:1526–1531, 2001.

Leverve X, Barnoud D: Stress metabolism and nutritional support in acute renal failure. Kidney Int Suppl 66:S62–S66, 1998.

Mehta RL, McDonald B, Gabbai F, et al: Nephrology consultation in acute renal failure: Does timing matter? Am J Med 113:456–461, 2002.

Mehta RL, Pascual MT, Soroko S, Chertow GM: Diuretics, mortality, and nonrecovery of renal function in acute renal failure. JAMA 288:2547–2553, 2002.

Rivers E, Nguyen B, Havstad S, et al: Early goal-directed therapy in the treatment of severe sepsis and septic shock. N Engl J Med 345:1368–1377, 2001.

Ronco C, Bellomo R, Homel P, et al: Effects of different doses in continuous veno-venous haemofiltration on outcomes of acute renal failure: a prospective randomised trial. Lancet 356:26–30. 2000.

Schiffl H, Lang SM, Fischer R: Daily hemodialysis and the outcome of acute renal failure. N Engl J Med 346:305–310, 2002.

Sponsel H, Conger JD: Is parenteral nutrition therapy of value in acute renal failure patients? Am J Kidney Dis 25:96–102, 1995.

Thadhani R, Pascual M, Bonventre JV: Acute renal failure. N Engl J Med 334:1448–1460, 1996.

van den Berghe G, Wouters P, Weekers F, et al: Intensive insulin therapy in the critically ill patients. N Engl J Med 345:1359–1367, 2001.

SECTION *VI*

Drugs and the Kidney

CHAPTER 40

Analgesics and the Kidney

Biff F. Palmer   William L. Henrich

Nonsteroidal anti-inflammatory drugs (NSAIDs) are some of the most widely utilized therapeutic agents in clinical practice today. Although the gastrointestinal toxicity of these medications is well known, it is also apparent that the kidney is also an important target for untoward clinical events. The kidney toxicity associated with the use of NSAIDs can be classified into several distinct clinical syndromes (Table 40-1). These include a form of vasomotor acute renal failure, nephrotic syndrome associated with interstitial nephritis, chronic kidney disease, and abnormalities in sodium, water, and potassium homeostasis. The common link in these syndromes is a disruption in metabolism of prostaglandins, the class of compounds whose synthesis is inhibited by these agents.

PROSTAGLANDIN BIOSYNTHESIS AND COMPARTMENTALIZATION

Nonsteroidal anti-inflammatory drugs act by inhibiting cyclooxygenase, which is the rate-limiting enzyme in the metabolic conversion of arachidonic acid into prostanoids. The cyclooxygenase enzyme exists as two isoforms termed cyclooxygenase-1 (COX-1) and cyclooxygenase-2 (COX-2). The COX-1 enzyme is constitutively expressed in most tissues and is responsible for producing prostaglandins involved in maintaining normal tissue homeostasis. The COX-2 enzyme is principally an inducible enzyme that is rapidly up-regulated in response to a variety of stimuli such as growth factors and cytokines typically found in the setting of inflammation. In the kidney both the COX-1 and COX-2 enzymes are constitutively expressed and are up-regulated in response to various physiologic stimuli. As a result, the kidney toxicity of both nonselective and selective COX-2 inhibitors is similar. The very similar renal physiologic effects of specific COX-2 inhibitors and nonselective NSAIDs support the idea that COX-2 inhibition is the crucial pharmacologic effect underlying kidney toxicity. This topic is discussed in more detail later.

Prostacyclin (PGI_2) is the most abundant prostaglandin produced in the cortex and is primarily synthesized in cortical arterioles and glomeruli. This location corresponds to the known effects of PGI_2 in regulating renal vascular tone, glomerular filtration rate (GFR), and renin release. The most abundant prostaglandin found in the tubules is prostaglandin E_2 (PGE_2). This location

provides the anatomic basis for PGE_2 to modulate sodium and chloride transport in the loop of Henle, arginine vasopressin-mediated (AVP-mediated) water transport, and vasa recta blood flow.

BIOLOGIC ACTIONS OF PROSTAGLANDINS IN THE KIDNEY

Prostaglandins play an important role in the maintenance of kidney function primarily in the setting of a systemic or intrarenal circulatory disturbance. The role of prostaglandins is best illustrated when examining kidney function under conditions of volume depletion (Fig. 40-1). In this setting, renal blood flow is decreased while sodium reabsorption, renin release, and urinary concentrating ability are increased. To a large extent, these findings are mediated by the effects of increased circulating levels of angiotensin II, AVP, and catechols. At the same time, these hormones stimulate the synthesis of renal prostaglandins, which in turn act to dilate the renal vasculature, inhibit salt and water reabsorption, and further stimulate renin release. Prostaglandin release under these conditions serves to dampen and counterbalance the physiologic effects of the hormones that elicit their production. As a result, kidney function is maintained near normal despite the systemic circulation being clamped down. Predictably, inhibition of prostaglandin synthesis will lead to unopposed activity of these hormonal systems, resulting in exaggerated renal vasoconstriction and magnified antinatriuretic and antidiuretic effects. In fact, many of the renal syndromes that are associated with the use of NSAIDs can be explained by the predictions of this model.

VASOMOTOR ACUTE RENAL FAILURE INDUCED BY NONSTEROIDAL ANTI-INFLAMMATORY DRUGS

Acute renal failure induced by NSAIDs occurs under conditions where maintenance of kidney function is critically dependent on vasodilatory prostaglandins (Table 40-2). Under conditions of decreased absolute or effective circulatory volume (diarrhea, congestive heart failure, cirrhosis), prostaglandins act to oppose the vasoconstrictive input of circulating effectors such as angiotensin II,

TABLE 40-1   Renal Syndromes Associated with Use of Nonsteroidal Anti-inflammatory Drugs

Vasomotor acute renal failure
Nephrotic syndrome with tubulointerstitial nephritis
Chronic kidney disease
NaCl retention
Hyponatremia
Hyperkalemia

TABLE 40-2   Risk Factors for Acute Vasomotor Renal Failure Induced by Nonsteroidal Anti-inflammatory Drugs

Decreased EABV	Normal or Increased EABV
Congestive heart failure	Chronic kidney disease
Cirrhosis	Glomerulonephritis
Nephrotic syndrome	Elderly
Sepsis	Contrast-induced nephropathy
Hemorrhage	Obstructive uropathy
Diuretic therapy	Cyclosporine, tacrolimus
Postoperative patients with "third space" fluid	
Volume depletion/ hypotension	

EABV, effective arterial blood volume.

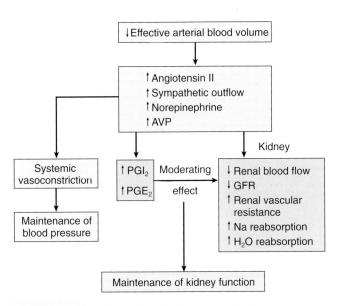

FIGURE 40-1   In the setting of absolute or effective volume depletion, a number of effectors are activated that serve to defend the circulation and at the same time stimulate the synthesis of renal prostaglandins. In turn, renal prostaglandins function to moderate the effects of these hormonal systems such that kidney function is maintained in the setting of systemic vasoconstriction. AVP, arginine vasopressin; GFR, glomerular filtration rate; PGE$_2$, prostaglandin E$_2$; PGI$_2$, prostacyclin.

sympathetic nerves, and circulating catecholamines. A similar dependency can occur when effective circulatory volume is normal or expanded but there is increased production of intrarenal vasoconstrictors (urinary obstruction, radiocontrast administration, and acute glomerulonephritis). In these conditions prostaglandins act to oppose the vasoconstrictive effect of substances such as endothelin, leukotrienes, thromboxane, and platelet-activating factor.

Acute renal failure induced by NSAIDs is most commonly an oliguric form of renal failure that begins within several days after initiation of the drug. The urinalysis is unremarkable in the majority of cases. Unlike other causes of acute oliguric renal failure, the fractional excretion of sodium is often less than 1%. This low fractional excretion of sodium reflects the underlying hemodynamic nature of the kidney function impairment. Hyperkalemia out of proportion to the decrement in kidney function is also a typical feature of this lesion. If recognized early, the renal functional impairment is reversible with discontinuation of the NSAID. As a result, dialysis is usually not required.

ARE SPECIFIC COX-2 INHIBITORS RENAL SPARING?

It was anticipated that specific COX-2 inhibitors would be renal sparing, since COX-2 is primarily an inducible enzyme. However, observations in both experimental animals and humans have shown that COX-2 is constitutively expressed in renal tissue and plays an important role in maintaining kidney function in states of prostaglandin dependency.

Clinical observations comparing specific COX-2 inhibitors with nonselective NSAIDs are consistent with an important role of the COX-2 enzyme in maintenance of normal kidney function. In data presented at the U.S. Food and Drug Administration advisory committee, celecoxib was reported to increase blood pressure and decrease urinary sodium excretion similar to traditional NSAIDs. A similar antinatriuretic effect has also been reported with rofecoxib in a study of elderly patients on a high sodium intake. In salt-depleted normal subjects, celecoxib and naproxen were found to produce similar reductions in GFR, urine output, and sodium and potassium excretion. In elderly patients with a creatinine clearance ranging from 30 to 80 mL/minute, administration of rofecoxib or indomethacin both reduced GFR to a similar extent, which was significantly greater than placebo. A number of cases have now been reported linking the use of COX-2 inhibitors to the development of reversible acute renal failure.

Thus, both experimental and clinical studies suggest that the specific COX-2 inhibitors may not offer any distinct advantage over traditional NSAIDs with respect to kidney toxicity. As with other NSAIDs, these agents should be used with caution and require close monitoring of kidney function in those patients at high risk for adverse renal outcomes.

GLOMERULAR AND INTERSTITIAL DISEASE INDUCED BY NONSTEROIDAL ANTI-INFLAMMATORY DRUGS

The use of NSAIDs can be associated with the development of a distinct syndrome characterized by the development of interstitial nephritis and nephrotic range proteinuria. Although virtually all NSAIDs have been reported to cause this syndrome, the vast majority of cases have been reported in association with use of the propionic acid derivatives (fenoprofen, ibuprofen, and naproxen). Of these, fenoprofen has been implicated in more than 60% of cases. Interstitial nephritis with and without nephrotic syndrome has also been reported with the COX-2 inhibitors, rofecoxib and celecoxib.

Unlike hemodynamically mediated acute renal failure, there are no clear-cut risk factors that serve to identify those at risk for development of this syndrome. The mean age of patients is 65 years. The presence of an underlying kidney disease before exposure to the NSAID has been notably absent. This syndrome has generally been referred to as an example of acute interstitial nephritis. There are, however, a number of features that distinguish this form of interstitial kidney disease from that observed with other pharmacologic agents (Table 40-3). First, the average duration of exposure prior to the onset of disease is typically measured in months and can be as long as a year. By contrast, allergic interstitial nephritis due to other drugs usually presents within several days to weeks after exposure to the drug. Second, nephrotic range proteinuria is found in more than 90% of cases of NSAID-induced interstitial disease, a degree of proteinuria that is distinctly uncommon in acute allergic interstitial nephri-

tis due to other drugs. Third, symptoms of hypersensitivity that are commonly seen in acute allergic interstitial nephritis, such as rash, fever, arthralgias, or peripheral eosinophilia, are uncommon in NSAID-associated disease. Fourth, the vast majority of cases associated with NSAIDs have been reported in older patients. On the other hand, allergic interstitial nephritis is seen in all age groups.

Renal biopsy findings typically show a diffuse or focal lymphocytic infiltrate. The number of eosinophils in the infiltrate is variable but generally is not marked. The glomerular changes are most commonly those seen in minimal-change disease, although a few patients have been described with changes typical of membranous glomerulopathy. In particular, the glomeruli are normal by light microscopy, whereas fusion of the podocytes is seen with electron microscopy. In some cases there is evidence of glomerulosclerosis. Since most patients who develop this syndrome are older, this latter finding may simply represent the normal age-related increase in glomerulosclerosis. Immunofluorescence studies are typically nonspecific. There has been an occasional report of weak and variable staining for immunoglobulin G (IgG) and C3 along the tubular basement membrane. Electron microscopy typically shows diffuse fusion of the podocytes in cases with heavy proteinuria. Mesangial electron-dense deposits have been observed in only three patients, suggesting that this is not an immune-mediated disease.

The clinical course of patients is to develop a spontaneous remission after removal of the offending NSAID. The time until resolution is variable but can range from a few days to several weeks. In some patients, the degree of kidney function impairment can be severe enough that dialytic support is required. Steroid therapy has been used in many of the reported cases; however, the efficacy and necessity of this therapy are unknown. It should be noted that relapses have been reported after inadvertent exposure to the same NSAID or after exposure to a different NSAID.

NONSTEROIDAL ANTI-INFLAMMATORY DRUGS AND SODIUM BALANCE

Sodium retention is a characteristic feature of virtually all NSAIDs, occurring in as many as 25% of patients who use them. The physiologic basis of this effect is directly related to the natriuretic properties of prostaglandins (Fig. 40-2).

It would at first seem paradoxical that under conditions of volume depletion the kidney would elaborate a compound that would have further natriuretic properties. The role of prostaglandins in this setting, however, is to moderate the avid salt retention that would otherwise

TABLE 40-3 Clinical Characteristics of Tubulointerstitial Nephritis Induced by Nonsteroidal Anti-inflammatory Drugs and of the Typical Drug-Induced Form

Characteristic	NSAID-Induced TIN	Typical Drug-Induced TIN
Duration of exposure	5 days to >1 year	5–26 days
Hypersensitivity symptoms	7%–8%	80%
Eosinophilia	17%–18%	75%–80%
Proteinuria >3.5 g/24 hr	>90%	<10%
Eosinophiluria	0–5%	80%–85%
Peak serum creatinine	1.5–>10 mg/dL	3.7–>10 mg/dL

NSAIDs, nonsteroidal anti-inflammatory drugs; TIN, tubulointerstitial nephritis.

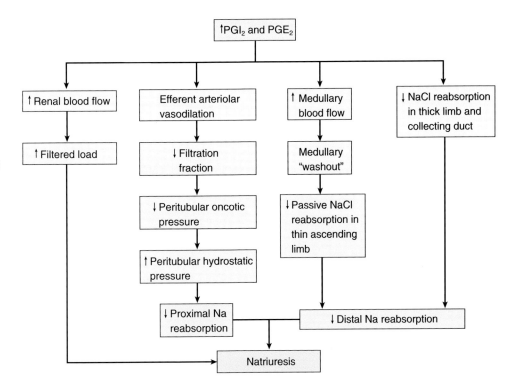

FIGURE 40-2 The direct and indirect mechanisms by which renal prostaglandins exert a natriuretic effect. PGE_2, prostaglandin E_2; PGI_2, prostacyclin.

occur in the setting of unopposed activation of the renin-angiotensin-aldosterone and adrenergic systems. By virtue of their natriuretic properties, prostaglandins play a role in ensuring adequate delivery of filtrate to more distal nephron segments under conditions in which distal delivery is threatened (e.g., renal ischemia, hypovolemia). In addition, diminished NaCl reabsorption in the thick ascending limb of Henle reduces the energy requirements of this segment. This reduction in thick limb workload in conjunction with a prostaglandin-mediated reallocation in renal blood flow helps to maintain an adequate oxygen tension in the medulla under conditions that would otherwise have resulted in substantial hypoxic injury.

In considering the natriuretic and vasodilatory properties of prostaglandins, it is not surprising that administration of NSAIDs has been shown to interfere with blood pressure control. In pooled studies, administration of NSAIDs has been associated with an average increase in blood pressure of between 5 and 10 mm Hg. Of the various subgroups examined, this effect is most pronounced in patients who are already hypertensive and much less so in those who are normotensive. Of the hypertensive patients, those treated with beta blockers seem to be the most vulnerable to the hypertensive effect of NSAIDs. Less interaction occurs with diuretics and angiotensin-converting enzyme inhibitors, whereas no effect is seen with calcium channel blockers. Further subgroup analysis shows that patients with low-renin hypertension (elderly and blacks) are also at higher risk for this hypertensive effect. The pathogenesis of NSAID-induced

hypertension is not known with certainty. In a recent meta-analysis, NSAIDs were found not to alter body weight or urinary sodium excretion significantly, implying that mechanisms other than salt retention were responsible for the increased blood pressure. In this regard, elimination of the vasodilator PGI_2 from the resistance blood vessels is believed to play some role in the development of hypertension in individuals at risk.

RENIN RELEASE, HYPERKALEMIA, AND NONSTEROIDAL ANTI-INFLAMMATORY DRUGS

The use of NSAIDs has been associated with the development of hyperkalemia in the setting of chronic kidney disease as well as normal kidney function. The physiologic basis for this effect is primarily due to inhibition of prostaglandin-mediated renin release with subsequent development of hypoaldosteronism. The development of hyperkalemia in patients receiving NSAIDs is most likely to occur in the setting of impaired kidney function or those with baseline abnormalities in the renin-angiotensin-aldosterone system. Diabetic patients are at risk due to the increased incidence of hyporeninemic hypoaldosteronism that occurs in this patient population. Diabetics are also prone to hyperkalemia because of insulin lack. Similarly, the elderly are at higher risk by virtue of the normal age-related decrease in circulating renin and aldosterone levels. Particular caution should be used when NSAIDs are combined with other pharmacologic agents known to interfere with the renin-angiotensin-aldosterone cascade. Examples would include beta blockers, the calcineurin inhibitors, angiotensin-converting enzyme inhibitors, heparin, ketoconazole, high-dose trimethoprim, and potassium-sparing diuretics.

WATER METABOLISM AND NSAIDs

Prostaglandins have important modulatory effects on renal water metabolism. Their primary effect is to impair the ability to maximally concentrate the urine by interfering with two processes that are central in the elaboration of a concentrated urine—namely, the generation of a hypertonic interstitium and maximal collecting-duct water permeability. AVP is known to stimulate PGE_2 synthesis in collecting-duct cells; by doing so, AVP induces its own antagonist. This interaction is another example in which prostaglandins exert a moderating effect on an effector mechanism that elicited their synthesis. In this case, prostaglandins play an important role in minimizing the water retention that would otherwise occur if the activity of AVP were unopposed. In most circumstances hyponatremia does not develop with use of NSAIDs, since a decrease in serum osmolality would result in inhibition of vasopressin release. This complication typically occurs in the setting of nonsuppressible vasopressin release. Removing the counterbalancing effect of renal prostaglandins allows for any given level of vasopressin to exert a greater hydro-osmotic effect resulting in hyponatremia (Fig. 40-3). Patients at risk for this complication would include those with high circulating levels of vasopressin driven by a decreased effective arterial blood volume such as congestive heart failure or cirrhosis. Patients with syndrome of inappropriate antidiuretic hormone (SIADH) or those taking medications capable of stimulating vasopressin secretion or impairing urinary dilution by other mechanisms are also at risk for the development of hyponatremia.

CHRONIC KIDNEY DISEASE AND ANALGESIC NEPHROPATHY INDUCED BY NONSTEROIDAL ANTI-INFLAMMATORY DRUGS

The most common form of drug-induced chronic kidney disease is analgesic nephropathy. This lesion has most commonly been linked to the chronic ingestion of compound analgesics containing aspirin, phenacetin, and caffeine. A still unresolved question is whether long-term use of NSAIDs alone can similarly result in a progressive and irreversible form of chronic kidney disease. In this regard, a number of observations have emerged that would appear to substantiate the belief that long-term use of NSAIDs can lead to a chronic form of kidney injury. Furthermore, the clinical characteristics of NSAID-induced chronic kidney disease are sufficiently different from those in analgesic nephropathy to suggest that this is a distinct clinical entity (Table 40-4). Before reviewing the data linking chronic NSAID use and chronic kidney disease, analgesic nephropathy will be discussed.

Analgesic nephropathy is a chronic kidney disease characterized by renal papillary necrosis and chronic interstitial nephritis. The early reports linking analgesics and kidney disease were generally found in patients who consumed combination products containing phenacetin. This fact focused attention on phenacetin as the primary cause of the syndrome and prompted many countries to remove the drug officially from nonprescription analgesics. Importantly, the removal of phenacetin has not been uniformly followed by the expected reduction in the incidence of the syndrome. Given that other agents such as acetaminophen or salicylamide have been substituted for phenacetin in many combination products, the lack of decline in incidence of analgesic nephropathy suggests that the use of combination products is

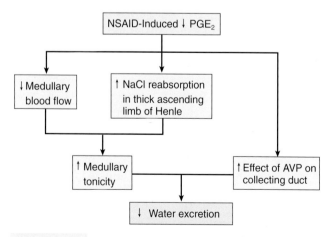

FIGURE 40-3 The mechanisms by which NSAIDs lead to decreased water excretion. AVP, arginine vasopressin; PGI_2, prostacyclin.

TABLE 40-4 Clinical Characteristics of Patients with Analgesic Nephropathy versus Chronic Kidney Disease Induced by Nonsteroidal Anti-inflammatory Drugs

Characteristic	Analgesic Nephropathy	NSAID-Induced Chronic Kidney Disease
Age (years)	40–50	>60
Female/male	6:1	1:1
Psychiatric disorder	Common	Not a feature
Papillary necrosis (%)	90	30
Creatinine clearance (mL/min)	<20	40–60
Urinary tract infection	Common	Not a feature
Uroepithelial tumors	Increased risk	Not a feature
Ischemic heart disease	Common	Not a feature

NSAIDs, nonsteroidal anti-inflammatory drugs.

as important as whether the compound contains phenacetin. This conclusion is further supported by the experience in Belgium, where a strong geographic correlation exists between the prevalence of analgesic nephropathy and sales of analgesic mixtures containing a minimum of two analgesic components.

Numerous epidemiologic studies performed in the past demonstrated a wide variation in the geographic incidence of analgesic nephropathy. Much of this variability could be explained by differences in the annual per capita consumption of phenacetin. In those countries with the highest consumption, such as Australia and Sweden, analgesic nephropathy was found to be responsible for up to 20% of cases of endstage renal disease (ESRD). In Canada, which had the lowest per capita consumption, analgesic nephropathy accounted for only 2% to 5% of ESRD patients. It has been estimated that between 2% and 4% of all ESRD cases in the United States can be attributable to habitual analgesic consumption. Within the United States, there are also regional differences in the reported incidence of analgesic nephropathy, which are thought to be reflective of differences in analgesic consumption. For example, the use of combination analgesics is more common in the southeastern United States, and the incidence of analgesic nephropathy is three to five times as common a cause of ESRD in North Carolina as in Philadelphia.

The development of analgesic nephropathy is associated with a number of well-defined clinical characteristics. The disease is more common in women by a factor of 2 to 6 and has a peak incidence at age 53 years. Patients typically consume compound analgesics on a daily basis, often for chronic complaints such as headache, dyspepsia, or to improve work productivity. It has been estimated that nephropathy occurs after the cumulative ingestion of 2 to 3 kg of the index drug. Often patients will exhibit a typical psychiatric profile characterized by addictive behavior. Gastrointestinal complications such as peptic ulcer disease are common. The patients are frequently anemic as a result of gastrointestinal blood loss as well as chronic kidney disease. Ischemic heart disease and renal artery stenosis have both been reported to occur with higher frequency in these patients. In fact, regular use of analgesic drugs containing phenacetin is associated with an increased risk of hypertension and mortality and morbidity due to cardiovascular disease. Finally, long-term use of analgesics is known to be a risk factor for the subsequent generation of uroepithelial tumors.

Patients with analgesic nephropathy have predominantly tubulomedullary dysfunction characterized by impaired concentrating ability, acidification defects, and occasionally a salt-losing state. Proteinuria tends to be low to moderate in quantity. Interestingly, the pattern of proteinuria is typically a mixture of glomerular and tubular origin. Pyuria is common and is often sterile. Occasionally hematuria is noted, but if persistent should raise the possibility of a uroepithelial tumor.

There are several features of analgesic nephropathy that make it difficult to diagnose. The disease is slowly progressive, and the symptoms and signs are nonspecific. Patients are often reluctant to admit to heavy usage of analgesics and therefore are either misdiagnosed or not diagnosed at all until the chronic kidney disease is far advanced. In addition, the lack of a simple and noninvasive test that reliably implicates analgesics as the cause of the renal injury has been an important limiting factor. Noncontrast abdominal computed tomography may emerge as a useful diagnostic tool in this setting, given its usefulness in the diagnosis of papillary necrosis. Characteristic findings using computed tomography include small kidneys with irregular contours and intrarenal calcifications particularly in the medulla.

As mentioned earlier, there are a number of reports that suggest that chronic use of NSAIDs alone may also lead to renal injury. In this regard, several NSAIDs have been associated with the development of papillary necrosis, either when administered alone or in combination with aspirin. In addition to inhibiting prostaglandin synthesis, the ability of these agents to redistribute blood flow to the cortex, rendering the renal medulla ischemic, may underlie this association. Although the reports linking papillary necrosis and NSAIDs are predominantly anecdotal in nature, more recent observations would suggest that chronic kidney disease resulting from long-term use of NSAIDs may be more prevalent than once thought. In a multicenter case control study, daily use of NSAIDs was associated with a twofold increase in the risk for chronic kidney disease. Chronic kidney disease was newly diagnosed and was defined as a serum creatinine concentration of 1.5 mg/dL or greater. This increased risk was primarily limited to older men. An additional report linking chronic use of NSAIDs with development of chronic kidney disease described 56 patients from Australia. These patients had taken only NSAIDs over a period of 10 to 20 years for treatment of a variety of rheumatic diseases. In 19 patients (34%), radiographic evidence of papillary necrosis was found. In 37 patients, kidney biopsy material was available that disclosed evidence of chronic interstitial nephritis. The clinical characteristics of these patients were quite different from those with analgesic nephropathy, suggesting that NSAID-induced chronic kidney disease is indeed a distinct entity. In particular, patients with NSAID-associated kidney disease were older, had an equal female/male ratio, had a lower incidence of papillary necrosis, had less severe kidney functional impairment, and had a lower incidence of urinary tract infections. In addition, an increased risk of uroepithelial tumors has not been described in these patients.

Further evidence of chronic toxicity has been reported in a preliminary communication in which patients treated with NSAIDs for rheumatoid arthritis and osteoarthritis were compared to a matched control arthritis population. In this study, the NSAID-treated patients had a rise in the serum creatinine concentration from 1.28 mg/dL to 2.58 mg/dL over a mean period of 47.5 months. The control group not taking NSAIDs had stable kidney function. In a prospective study of 259 heavy analgesic abusers, 69 patients developed radiographic evidence of papillary necrosis. Of these, 29 used NSAIDs either singularly (17 patients) or in combination with another NSAID (12 patients). Another 9 patients used NSAIDs in combination with acetaminophen, aspirin, caffeine, or a traditional herbal medicine. Chronic kidney disease (serum creatinine concentration of 1.4 to 8.8 mg/dL) was noted in 26 of the 38 patients who had used an NSAID chronically. Similar to the patients from Australia, this disorder was more common in males (1.9:1), distinguishing this disorder from classic analgesic nephropathy, which typically occurs in females. Similarly, these patients did not exhibit the usual psychological profile associated with analgesic abuse.

Thus, although further studies are needed to definitely assess the question of cumulative toxicity, it appears that some chronically treated patients may develop a change in kidney function over a long term. Given the abuse potential of powerful NSAIDs and the fact that ibuprofen, naproxen, and ketoprofen are now available on an over-the-counter basis, it is possible that chronic NSAID abuse may become a more common cause of chronic kidney disease in the future.

In considering the definite association of compound analgesic abuse and the possible linkage of chronic NSAID use to the development of chronic kidney disease, it has become common clinical practice to recommend acetaminophen whenever possible for analgesia. In this regard, a recent case control study examining the use of over-the-counter analgesics as a risk factor for ESRD found that acetaminophen may also cause chronic kidney disease when used on a continual basis. In this study, heavy average use of acetaminophen (more than 1 pill/day) and medium to high cumulative intake (1000 or more pills in a lifetime) each doubled the odds of ESRD. It was concluded that reduced consumption of acetaminophen could decrease the overall incidence of ESRD approximately 8% to 10%. The findings in this study confirmed an earlier report that also concluded that long-term daily use of acetaminophen is associated with an increased risk of chronic kidney disease. Although these studies do not establish a cause-and-effect relationship between acetaminophen ingestion and chronic kidney disease, the data do suggest that ingestion of acetaminophen on a continual and chronic basis should be discouraged.

A recent organized review by a consensus panel of the National Kidney Foundation (NKF) surveyed more than 600 articles and studied the implications of several different kinds of analgesic ingestion and chronic kidney disease risks. The highlights of the recommendations from the NKF consensus panel were that ingestion of aspirin and nonsteroidal combinations were not encouraged because of an increased risk of chronic kidney disease when those combinations were ingested together; that habitual consumption of analgesics was discouraged, and monitoring was recommended when such use was mandatory; that combination analgesics were recommended to be available by prescription only with an explicit warning to physicians that the habitual consumption of these combination products could lead to the insidious development of chronic kidney disease; and that there should be an explicit warning to consumers regarding NSAID ingestion. The panel concluded that there was negligible clinical evidence to suggest that habitual use of acetaminophen alone causes the clinical entity of analgesic nephropathy and that there was no evidence that occasional use of acetaminophen causes kidney injury. Finally, the panel pointed out that there was no risk from the regular use of aspirin in the relatively small doses recommended for prevention of cardiovascular events.

BIBLIOGRAPHY

Catella-Lawson F, McAdam B, Morrison B, et al: Effects of specific inhibition of cyclooxygenase-2 on sodium balance, hemodynamics, vasoactive eicosanoids. J Pharmacol Exp Ther 289: 735–741, 1999.

Elseviers M, De Broe M: A long-term prospective controlled study of analgesic abuse in Belgium. Kidney Int 48:1912–1919, 1995.

Henrich WL, Anderson RJ, Berns AS, et al: The role of renal nerves and prostaglandins in control of renal hemodynamics and plasma renin activity during hypotensive hemorrhage in the dog. J Clin Invest 61:744–750, 1978.

Henrich WL, Agodoa L, Barrett B, et al: Analgesics and the kidney: Summary and recommendations to the Scientific Advisory Board of the National Kidney Foundation from an Ad Hoc Committee of the National Kidney Foundation. Am J Kidney Dis 27:162–165, 1996.

Palmer BF: Renal complications associated with use of nonsteroidal antiinflammatory agents. J Invest Med 43:516–533, 1995.

Palmer BF, Henrich WL: Clinical acute renal failure secondary to non-steroidal antiinflammatory drugs. Semin Nephrol 15: 214–227, 1995.

Perneger TV, Whelton PK, Klag MJ: Risk of kidney failure associated with the use of acetaminophen, aspirin, and nonsteroidal antiinflammatory drugs. N Engl J Med 331:1675–1679, 1994.

Rossat J, Maillard M, Nussberger J, et al: Renal effects of selective cyclooxygenase-2 inhibition in normotensive salt-depleted subjects. Clin Pharmacol Ther 66:76–84, 1999.

Sandler DP, Smith JC, Weinberg CR, et al: Analgesic use and chronic renal disease. N Engl J Med 320:1238–1243, 1989.

Schlondorff D: Renal complications of nonsteroidal antiinflammatory drugs. Kidney Int 44:643–653, 1993.

Segasothy M, Samad SA, Zulfigar A, et al: Chronic renal disease and papillary necrosis associated with the long-term use of nonsteroidal anti-inflammatory drugs as the sole or predominant analgesic. Am J Kidney Dis 24:17–24, 1994.

CHAPTER 41

Principles of Drug Therapy in Kidney Failure

Gary R. Matzke

Reductions in kidney function can be associated with disease states, drug effects (e.g., drug-induced nephrotoxicity), or the result of age-related diminution of kidney function. In adults, age-related declines in kidney function combined with the increased use of medications make this patient group particularly susceptible to toxic effects secondary to the accumulation of a drug or its active metabolite. Clinicians must understand that drug disposition is altered in the presence of diminished kidney function and the appropriate methods to individualize drug therapy.

Diminished kidney function is accompanied by progressive alterations in the bioavailability, plasma protein binding, distribution volume, and metabolism of many drugs. Individualization of therapy for those agents that are predominantly eliminated by the kidney can be accomplished with a simple proportional dose adjustment based on the fractional reduction in creatinine clearance (CrCl). However, a more complex adjustment scheme will usually be required for medications that are extensively metabolized by the liver or for which changes in protein binding and/or distribution volume have been noted as a result of kidney failure. Patients with diminished kidney function may also respond to a given dose or serum concentration of a drug differently than those with normal kidney function because of the physiologic and biochemical changes associated with progressive chronic kidney disease (CKD).

General pharmacokinetic principles and the knowledge of disposition characteristics of a drug, combined with the degree of pathophysiologic alterations associated with CKD make it possible for the clinician to design an individualized therapeutic regimen. This chapter describes the influence of acute renal failure (ARF) and CKD on drug absorption, distribution, metabolism, and elimination, and provides a practical approach for drug dosage individualization for patients with reduced kidney function as well as those receiving continuous renal replacement therapy, continuous ambulatory peritoneal dialysis, or hemodialysis.

EFFECT ON DRUG ABSORPTION

There is little quantitative information about the influence of impaired kidney function on drug absorption. Several variables, including changes in gastrointestinal transit time and gastric pH, edema of the gastrointestinal tract, vomiting and diarrhea (frequently seen in those with severe reductions in kidney function or diabetes), and antacid administration have been associated with alterations in absorption. Most of the drug absorption studies, which determine the fraction of a drug that reaches the systemic circulation after oral administration compared to intravenous administration, in patients with renal failure have documented alterations in the peak concentration (C_{max}), time at which the peak concentration was attained (t_{max}), or in the amount of drug recovered in the urine in a finite time period. Although the bioavailability of some drugs, such as furosemide and pindolol, has been reported to be reduced, there are no consistent findings in patients with CKD that absorption is impaired. An increase in bioavailability as the result of a decrease in metabolism during the drug's first pass through the gastrointestinal tract and liver, however, has been noted for some beta blockers, dextropropoxyphene, and dihydrocodeine.

EFFECT ON DRUG DISTRIBUTION

The volume of distribution of many drugs is significantly altered in patients with endstage renal disease (Table 41-1) and changes in patients with oliguric ARF have also been reported. This may be the result of changes in plasma protein binding, tissue binding, or body composition; volume expansion or contraction; or an artifact of the calculation method used to determine the volume term. The plasma protein binding of acidic drugs such as warfarin and phenytoin is decreased in CKD patients, whereas the binding of basic drugs (e.g., quinidine) is usually decreased or unchanged. The plasma concentration of the principal binding protein for several basic drug compounds, α_1-acid glycoprotein, is increased in kidney transplant patients and hemodialysis patients. Thus the fraction of these drugs principally bound to α_1-acid glycoprotein may be significantly increased in these patients. The decrease in binding of acidic drugs has been attributed to changes in the binding sites, accumulation of endogenous inhibitors of binding, and decreased concentrations of albumin. In addition, the high concentrations of metabolites of some drugs that accumulate in CKD patients may interfere with the protein binding of the parent compound. Although the fraction of drug not

TABLE 41-1   Volume of Distribution of Selected Drugs*

Drug	Volume of Distribution (L/kg)	
	Normal	**Chronic Dialysis**
Increased in chronic dialysis patients		
Amikacin	0.20	0.29
Azlocillin	0.21	0.28
Cefazolin	0.13	0.16
Cefoxitin	0.16	0.26
Cefuroxime	0.20	0.26
Clofibrate	0.14	0.24
Cloxacillin	0.14	0.26
Dicloxacillin	0.08	0.18
Erythromycin	0.57	1.09
Furosemide	0.11	0.18
Gentamicin	0.20	0.29
Isoniazid	0.60	0.80
Naproxen	0.12	0.17
Phenytoin	0.64	1.40
Trimethoprim	1.36	1.83
Vancomycin	0.64	0.85
Decreased in chronic dialysis patients		
Digoxin	7.30	4.10
Ethambutol	3.70	1.60
Methicillin	0.45	0.30

*A change of greater than 25% was considered clinically significant.

bound to plasma proteins may be increased, the concentration of drug that is not bound to plasma proteins is usually unaltered. Thus the net effect of changes in protein binding is an alteration in the relationship between unbound and total drug concentrations, an effect frequently encountered with phenytoin. The increase in unbound fraction to values as high as 20% to 25%, from the normal of 10%, results in increased hepatic clearance and decreased total concentrations. Although the unbound concentration therapeutic range is unchanged, the therapeutic range for total phenytoin concentration is reduced to 4 to 10 µg/mL (normal, 10–20 µg/mL) as the degree of kidney impairment increases. Thus unbound concentration measurements (normal, 1–2 µg/mL) provide the best means for individualizing phenytoin therapy in CKD patients.

Altered tissue binding may also affect the apparent volume of distribution of a drug. For example, the distribution volume of digoxin has been reported to be reduced by 30% to 50% in patients with severe CKD. This reduction in the distribution volume may be the result of competitive inhibition by endogenous or exogenous digoxin-like immunoreactive substances that bind to and inhibit membrane ATPase or acidosis. The absolute amount of digoxin bound to the receptor is reduced, and the resultant serum digoxin concentration observed after the administration of any dose would be greater than expected.

Thus, in patients with CKD, a "normal" total drug concentration may be associated with either serious adverse reactions secondary to elevated unbound drug concentrations or subtherapeutic responses because of an altered plasma-to-tissue drug concentration ratio. Therefore, the monitoring of unbound drug concentrations is suggested for those drugs that have a narrow therapeutic range, are highly protein bound (greater than 80%), or for which marked variability in the fraction bound has been reported (e.g., phenytoin and disopyramide).

EFFECT ON METABOLISM

The relationship of ARF and CKD to cytochrome P450–mediated (CYP-mediated) metabolism in the liver and other organs has recently been reviewed. In rat models of CKD, protein expression in the liver of several CYP enzymes, including CYP3A1 and CYP3A2 (equivalent to human CYP3A4), is reduced by as much as 75%: CYP2C11 and CYP3A2 activity is significantly reduced, whereas CYP1A2 activity is unchanged in animals. In humans, CYP2C19 and CYP3A4 activity is reduced, whereas CYP2D6 and CYP2E1 is not affected by the presence of CKD. The reduction of nonrenal clearance (CL_{NR}) of several drugs in patients with severe CKD supports this premise (Table 41-2).

The effect of CKD on the metabolism of a particular drug is, however, difficult to predict even for drugs within the same pharmacologic class. The reductions in CL_{NR} for those with CKD have frequently been noted to be proportional to the reductions in glomerular filtration rate (GFR). In the small number of studies that have evaluated CL_{NR} in critically ill patients with ARF, residual CL_{NR} was higher than the values reported in patients with CKD who had a similar CrCl. Since a patient with ARF may

TABLE 41-2   Influence of Severe CKD on the Nonrenal/Metabolic Clearance of Selected Drugs*

Decreased in CKD

Acyclovir	Cilastatin	Minoxidil
Aztreonam	Cimetidine	Moxalactam
Bufuralol	Ciprofloxacin	Nicardipine
Captopril	Cortisol	Nitrendipine
Cefmenoxime	Encainide	Nimodipine
Cefmetazole	Guanadrel	Procainamide
Cefonicid	Erythromycin	Quinapril
Cefotiam	Imipenem	Roxithromycin
Cefotaxime	Isoniazid	Verapamil
Cefsulodin	Methylprednisol	Zidovudine
Ceftizoxime	Metoclopramide	

Increased in CKD

Bumetanide	Fosinopril	Phenytoin
Cefpiramide	Nifedipine	Sulfadimidine

CKD, chronic kidney disease.
*A change of greater than 40% was considered to be clinically significant.

have a higher CL_{NR} than a CKD patient, the resultant plasma concentrations will be lower than expected and possibly subtherapeutic if classic CKD-derived dosage guidelines are followed.

EFFECT ON EXCRETION BY THE KIDNEY

Renal clearance (CL_R) is the net result of glomerular filtration of unbound drug plus tubular secretion minus tubular reabsorption. An acute or chronic progressive reduction in GFR thus results in a decrease in CL_R. The degree of change in the total body clearance of a drug is dependent on the fraction of the dose eliminated unchanged by the normal kidney, the intrarenal pathways for drug transport, and the degree of functional impairment of each of these pathways. Secretion and reabsorption involve carrier-mediated renal transport systems as well as passive diffusion. The primary renal transport systems of clinical significance include the organic anionic (OAT), organic cationic (OCT), and P-glycoprotein transporters. β-Lactam antibiotics, diuretics, nonsteroidal anti-inflammatory drugs, and several glucuronide metabolites are eliminated by OAT transporters. The OCT transporters contribute to the secretion and excretion of cimetidine, famotidine, and quinidine, whereas the P-glycoprotein transport system in the kidney is involved in the secretion of cationic and hydrophobic drugs (e.g., digoxin and *Vinca* alkaloids). The limited data regarding these and other renal transport systems have been recently reviewed. The clearance of drugs that are extensively secreted by the kidney (CL_R greater than 300 mL/minute) may be significantly reduced in the presence of normal kidney function as well as mild to moderate CKD as a result of drug and or disease interactions with one of these renal transporters.

Despite the different mechanisms involved in the elimination of drugs by the kidney, the clinical measurement or estimation of CrCl or GFR remains the guiding principle for drug dosage regimen design. The importance of an alteration in kidney function on drug elimination thus depends primarily on two variables: the fraction of drug normally eliminated by the kidney unchanged and the degree of kidney functional impairment. Serial estimates or measurements of kidney function are routinely recommended to guide individualization of drug dosage regimens to optimize clinical outcomes. The calculation of CrCl from a timed urine collection with creatinine measurement in serum and urine has been the standard clinical measure of kidney function for decades. Urine is difficult to collect accurately in most clinical settings, and the interference of many commonly utilized medications with creatinine measurement limits the utility of this approach. The administration of radioactive ([^{125}I]iothalamate, ^{51}Cr-EDTA, or ^{99m}Tc-DTPA) or non-radioactive (aminoglycosides, iohexol, iothalamate, and inulin) markers of GFR, though scientifically sound, is clinically impractical, because intravenous or subcutaneous administration of the marker and the collection of multiple timed blood and urine collections makes the procedures expensive and cumbersome.

Estimation of CrCl or GFR, however, requires only routinely collected laboratory and demographic data. The Cockroft and Gault method for CrCl and the MDRD (modification of diet in renal disease) method for GFR estimation correlate well with CrCl and GFR measurements in individuals with stable kidney function (see Chapter 2). CrCL is still the standard for drug dosing, because most of the primary literature used this method to derive the relationship between kidney function and actual plasma drug levels or total body clearance of a drug. These methods, however, are extremely poor predictors of kidney function in individuals with liver disease, and their use is not recommended for such patients. Although several methods for CrCl estimation in patients with unstable kidney function have been proposed, the accuracy of these methods has not been rigorously assessed, and at the present time their use cannot be recommended.

STRATEGIES FOR DRUG THERAPY INDIVIDUALIZATION

The design of the optimal dosage regimen for the individual patient is dependent on the availability of an accurate characterization of the relationship between the pharmacokinetic parameters of the drug and kidney function and an accurate assessment of the patient's kidney function (CrCl). Secondary references such as the *AHFS Drug Information, Drug Prescribing in Renal Failure: Dosing Guidelines for Adults* by Aronoff and colleagues, Goodman and Gilman's *The Pharmacological Basis of Therapeutics*, and computer databases (e.g., Micromedex or Clinical Pharmacology) are excellent sources for the pharmacokinetic characteristics of drugs in subjects with normal and impaired kidney function. However, if they do not provide the explicit relationships of CrCl with the kinetic parameters of interest such as total body clearance (CL), elimination rate constant (k), and distribution volume (V_D), one may have to identify an original research publication or use the estimation approach outlined here later. The patient's kinetic parameters can be predicted and an individualized therapeutic regimen formulated to attain the desired therapeutic outcome if the patient's kidney function and the relationship between CrCl and the drug's kinetic parameters are known.

If specific literature recommendations and/or the relationship of kinetic parameters to CrCl are not available, then the pharmacokinetic parameters of a given drug in a particular patient can be estimated using the method of Rowland and Tozer, provided that the fraction of the drug that is eliminated unchanged by the kidney (f_e) in subjects with normal kidney function is known. These approaches assume that the change in CL and k are proportional to CrCl, that kidney disease does not alter the drug's metabolism, that the metabolites if formed are inactive and nontoxic, that the drug obeys first-order (linear) kinetic principles, and that it is adequately described by a one-compartment model. If these assumptions are true, the kinetic parameter/dosage adjustment factor (Q) can be calculated as $Q = 1 - [f_e(1 - KF)]$, where KF is the ratio of the patient's CrCl to the assumed normal value of 120 mL/minute. Thus, the Q factor for a patient who has a CrCl of 10 mL/minute and a drug that is 85% eliminated unchanged by the kidney would be:

$$Q = 1 - [0.85(1 - (10/120))]$$
$$= 1 - [0.85(0.92)]$$
$$= 1 - 0.78$$
$$= 0.22$$

The estimated CL and k for this patient would then be calculated as $CL_{PT} = CL_{norm} \times Q$, and $k_{PT} = k_{norm} \times Q$, where CL_{norm} and k_{norm} are the respective values in patients with normal kidney function derived from the literature. If there is a significant relationship between peak concentration and clinical response (e.g., aminoglycosides) or toxicity (e.g., quinidine, phenobarbital, and phenytoin), then attainment of the target peak value is critical. If a specific peak (C_{peak}) or trough (C_{trough}) concentration is desired, then the adjusted dosage interval (τ_f) and the maintenance dose (D_f) for the CKD patient can be calculated as follows if the drug's disposition is adequately characterized with a one-compartment linear model and it is administered by intermittent intravenous infusion with infusion duration (tinf):

$$\tau_f = ([1/k_{PT}] \times \ln[C_{peak}/C_{trough}]) + tinf$$
$$D_f = [k_{PT} \times V_D \times C_{peak}][1 - e^{-(k_{PT})(\tau f)}/1 - e^{-(k_{PT})(tinf)}]$$

For antihypertensive agents, cephalosporins and many other drugs for which there are no target values for peak or trough concentrations, attainment of an average steady-state concentration similar to normal subjects is appropriate. The principal means to achieve this goal are to decrease the dose or prolong the dosing interval. If the dose is reduced and the dosing interval is unchanged, the desired average steady-state concentration will be similar; however, the peak will be lower and the trough higher. Alternatively, if the dosing interval is increased and the dose remains unchanged, the peak and trough concentrations will be similar to those in the patients with normal kidney function. This dosage adjustment method is often preferred because it is likely to yield significant cost savings. Finally, the dose and dosing interval may both need to be changed to attain a desired peak or trough serum concentration time profile.

If a loading dose is not administered, it will take four to five half-lives for the desired steady-state plasma con-

centrations to be achieved in any patient; this may require days rather than hours because of the prolonged half-life of many drugs in CKD patients. To achieve the desired concentration rapidly, a loading dose (D_L), which can be calculated as follows, may need to be administered: $D_L = (C_{peak}) \times (V_D) \times$ (body weight). The loading dose is usually the same for CKD patients as it is for patients with normal kidney function. However, if the V_D in CKD patients is significantly different from the V_D in patients with normal kidney function, then that value should be utilized to calculate the D_L.

The maintenance dose (D_f) for the patient or the adjusted dosing interval (τ_f) can then be calculated from the following relationships, where D_n is the normal dose and τ_n is the normal dosing interval:

$$D_f = D_n \times Q$$
$$\tau_f = \tau_n/Q$$

If these approaches yield an interval or a dose that is impractical, a new dose can be calculated using a fixed, prespecified dose interval (τ_{CKD}) such as 24 or 48 hours, as follows:

$$D_f = \frac{D_n \times Q \times \tau_{CKD}}{\tau_n}$$

PATIENTS RECEIVING CONTINUOUS RENAL REPLACEMENT THERAPY

Continuous renal replacement therapy (CRRT) is used for the management of fluid overload and the removal of uremic toxins in patients with ARF. Drug therapy individualization for the patient receiving CRRT must take into account that patients with ARF may have a higher residual CL_{NR} of a drug than CKD patients who have a similar CrCl. In addition to patient-specific differences, there are marked differences in the efficiency of drug removal between the three primary types of CRRT: continuous arteriovenous or venovenous hemofiltration (CAVH/CVVH), continuous arteriovenous or venovenous hemodialysis (CAVHD/CVVHD), and continuous arteriovenous or venovenous hemodiafiltration (CAVHDF/CVVHDF). The primary variables that influence drug clearance during CRRT are the ultrafiltration rate, blood flow rate, dialysate flow rate, and the type of hemofilter used. For example, clearance during CAVH/CVVH is directly proportional to the ultrafiltration rate (UFR) as a result of convective transport of drug molecules from plasma water into the ultrafiltrate. The clearance of a drug in this situation is thus a function of the membrane permeability for the drug, which is called the sieving coefficient (SC), and the UFR. The SC can be approximated by the fraction unbound to plasma proteins (f_u), and thus the clearance can be calculated as $CL_{CVVH} = UFR \times SC$ or $CL_{CVVH} = UFR \times f_u$.

Clearance during CAVHD/CVVHD depends on the dialysate flow rate and the SC of the drug. If UFR is negligible (less than 3 mL/minute), as is often the case with CAVHD/CVVHD, CL_{CVVHD} can be estimated as the product of DFR and f_u or SC. Clearance of a drug by CAVHDF/CVVHDF (CL_{CAVHDF}/CL_{CVVHDF}) is generally greater than by CAVHD/CVVHD, because drug is removed by diffusion as well as convection/ultrafiltration. The CL_{CVVHDF} in many clinical settings can be mathematically approximated as CL_{CVVH} = (UFR + DFR) × SC, provided that the DFR is less than 33 mL/minute and blood flow rate is at least 75 mL/minute. Changes in blood flow rate generally have only a minor effect on drug clearance by any mode of CRRT, because blood flow rate is usually much larger than the dialysate flow rate and is therefore not the limiting factor for drug removal.

Individualization of therapy for a patient receiving CRRT therapy is dependent on the patient's residual kidney function and the clearance of the drug by the mode of CRRT they are receiving. The patient's residual drug clearance can be predicted as described in the previous section of this chapter. The CRRT clearance can also be ascertained from published literature reports. The SCs of frequently used drugs are summarized in Table 41-3. These data can be used to design initial dosage regimens for patients receiving CRRT with the mathematical

TABLE 41-3 Measured Sieving Coefficients of Selected Drugs

Drug	Measured SC
Amikacin	0.88
Amphotericin	0.32–0.4
Ampicillin	0.6–0.69
Cefoperazone	0.27–0.69
Cefotaxime	0.55–1.1
Cefoxitin	0.32
Ceftazidime	0.38–0.78
Ceftriaxone	0.71–0.82
Clindamycin	0.49–0.98
Digoxin	0.96
Erythromycin	0.37
5-Fluorocytosine	0.98
Gentamicin	0.81–0.75
Imipenem	0.78
Metronidazole	0.80
Mezlocillin	0.68
Nafcillin	0.47
N-acetyl procainamide	0.92
Netilmicin	0.85
Oxacillin	0.02
Phenobarbital	0.86
Phenytoin	0.45
Procainamide	0.86
Theophylline	0.85
Tobramycin	0.78–0.86
Vancomycin	0.5–0.8

SC, sieving coefficient.
Adapted from Joy MS, Matzke GR, Armstrong DK, et al: A primer on continuous renal replacement therapy for critically ill patients. Ann Pharmacother 32:362–375, 1998.

approaches described earlier. When feasible, plasma drug level monitoring for certain drugs such as aminoglycosides is highly recommended.

CHRONIC HEMODIALYSIS PATIENTS

Although many new hemodialyzers have been introduced in the past 20 years and the efficiency of the hemodialysis procedure has increased, the effect of hemodialysis on drug disposition is rarely re-evaluated after initially reported. Thus, most of the literature probably represents an underestimation of the impact of hemodialysis on drug disposition. The effect of hemodialysis on a patient's drug therapy is dependent on the molecular weight, protein binding, and distribution volume of the drug, the composition of the dialyzer membrane, its surface area, blood and dialysate flow rates, and whether or not the dialysis unit reuses the dialyzer. Drugs that are small molecules but are highly protein bound are also not well dialyzed, because both of the principal binding proteins (α_1-acid glycoprotein and albumin) have a very high molecular weight. Finally, those drugs that are widely distributed throughout the body are poorly removed by hemodialysis.

Low-flux dialyzers are relatively impermeable to drugs with a molecular weight over 1000 D, and the clearance declines dramatically (by up to 60%) as molecular weight increases from 100 to 500 D. High-flux hemodialyzers allow the passage of most drugs that have a molecular weight of 20,000 D or less. The effect of reuse of dialyzers on clearance has been reported for very few drugs (cefazolin, ceftazidime, tobramycin, and vancomycin). Minimal to no change was observed with a low-flux cellulose acetate dialyzer. Ceftazidime and vancomycin clearance decreased by up to 13% with reused high-flux polysulfone dialyzers. In contrast, significant decreases (24% to 43%) in clearance were observed with reused high-flux cellulose triacetate dialyzer for all four drugs.

The determination of drug concentrations at the start and end of dialysis, with the subsequent calculation of the half-life during dialysis ($\tau_{1/2,onHD}$), has frequently been used as an index of drug removal by dialysis. A more accurate means of assessing the effect of hemodialysis is to calculate the dialyzer clearance (CL_D) of the drug. Because drug concentrations are generally determined in plasma, the CL_D can be calculated as: $CL^p_D = Q_p([A_p - V_p]/A_p)$, where p represents plasma and Q_p is plasma flow calculated as Q_b (1 − hematocrit). This clearance calculation accurately reflects dialysis drug clearance only if the drug does not penetrate or bind to formed blood elements. Because of potential problems in accurately determining Q_b or Q_p, the dialysate collection method is widely used as the gold standard for the determination of CL_D. The hemodialysis clearance values reported in the literature may vary significantly depending on which method was used to calculate CL_D and whether compartmentalization into blood cells is taken into account.

For patients receiving hemodialysis, the usual objective is to restore the amount of drug in the body at the end of dialysis to the value that would have been present if the patient had not been dialyzed. Here, the supplementary dose ($D_{post-HD}$) is calculated as:

$$D_{post-HD} = V_D \times C(e^{-k \cdot t} - e^{-k_{HD} \cdot t})$$

where ($V_D \cdot C$) is the amount of drug in the body at the start of dialysis, $e^{-k \cdot t}$ is the fraction of drug remaining as a result of the patient's residual total body clearance during the dialysis procedure, and $e^{-k_{HD} \cdot t}$ is the fraction of drug remaining as a result of elimination by the dialyzer ($k_{HD} = CL_{HD}/V_D$). Values for CL_{HD} can be obtained for specific dialysis procedures from literature cited in the bibliography.

The impact of hemodialysis on drug therapy can thus not be viewed as a "generic procedure" that will result in the removal of a fixed percentage of the drug in the body with each dialysis session; neither should simple "yes/no" answers on the dialyzability of drug compounds be considered sufficient information for therapeutic decisions. Compounds considered nondialyzable with low-flux dialyzers may in fact be significantly removed by high-flux hemodialyzers.

PATIENTS RECEIVING CHRONIC AMBULATORY PERITONEAL DIALYSIS

Peritoneal dialysis, like other dialysis modalities, has the potential to affect drug disposition; however, drug therapy individualization is often less complicated in these patients because of the continuous nature and relative inefficiency of the procedure per unit time. Variables that influence drug removal in peritoneal dialysis patients include drug-specific characteristics such as molecular weight, solubility, degree of ionization, protein binding, and volume of distribution, as well as peritoneal membrane characteristics such as blood flow, pore size, and surface area. There is an inverse relationship between peritoneal drug clearance and molecular weight, protein binding, and volume of distribution. The contribution of peritoneal dialysis to total body clearance is often low and, for most drugs, markedly less than the contribution of hemodialysis. Anti-infective agents are the most commonly studied drugs because of their primary role in the treatment of peritonitis. Most other drugs can generally be dosed according to the residual kidney function of the patient, because clearance by peritoneal dialysis is so small.

CONCLUSIONS

The adverse outcomes associated with inappropriate drug use and dosing are largely preventable if the pharmacokinetic principles illustrated in this chapter are used by the clinician in concert with reliable population pharmacokinetic estimates to design a rational initial drug dosage regimen for the patient with impaired kidney function. Subsequent individualization of therapy should be undertaken whenever clinical therapeutic monitoring tools are available.

BIBLIOGRAPHY

Aronoff GR, Berns JS, Brier ME, et al: Drug Prescribing in Renal Failure: Dosing Guidelines for Adults, 4th ed. Philadelphia, American College of Physicians–ASIM, 1999.

Joy MS, Matzke GR, Armstrong DK, et al: A primer on continuous renal replacement therapy for critically ill patients. Ann Pharmacother 32:362–375, 1998.

Lee W, Kim RB: Transporters and renal drug elimination. Annu Rev Pharmacol Toxicol 44:137–166, 2004.

Matzke GR, Millikin SP: Influence of renal disease and dialysis on pharmacokinetics. In Evans WE, Schentag JJ, Jusko WJ (eds): Applied Pharmacokinetics: Principles of Therapeutic Drug Monitoring, 3rd ed. Applied Therapeutics, Spokane, Washington, 1992, pp 8.1–8.49.

Matzke GR, Frye RF: Drug administration in patients with renal insufficiency: Minimising renal and extrarenal toxicity. Drug Safety 16:205–231, 1997.

Matzke GR: Status of hemodialysis of drugs in 2002. J Pharm Practice 15:405–418, 2002.

McEvoy GK, Litvak K, Welsh OH, et al: American Hospital Formulary Service, Drug Information. Bethesda, Md, American Society of Hospital Pharmacists, 2004.

Mueller BA, Pasko DA, Sowinski KM: Higher renal replacement therapy dose delivery influences on drug therapy. Artif Organs 27:808–814, 2003.

Nolin TD, Frye RF, Matzke GR: Hepatic drug metabolism and transport in patients with kidney disease. Am J Kidney Dis 42:906–925, 2003.

Rowland M, Tozer TN: Clinical Pharmokinetics: Concepts and Applications, 3rd ed. Philadelphia, Lea and Febiger, 1995.

St Peter WL, Halstenson CE: Pharmacologic approach in patients with renal failure. In Chernow B (ed): The Pharmacologic Approach to the Critically Ill Patient. Baltimore, Md, Williams & Wilkins, 1994, pp 41–79.

Taylor CA, Abdel-Rahman E, Zimmerman SW, Johnson CA: Clinical pharmacokinetics during continuous ambulatory peritoneal dialysis. Clin Pharmacokinet 31:293–308, 1996.

Thummel KE, Shen DD: Design and optimization of dosage regimens: Pharmacokinetic data. In Hardman JG, Limbird LE, Goodman GA (eds): Goodman & Gilman's the Pharmacological Basis of Therapeutics, 10th ed. New York, McGraw-Hill, 2001, pp 1917–2024.

Veltri MA, Neu AM, Fivush BA, et al: Drug dosing during intermittent hemodialysis and continuous renal replacement therapy: Special considerations in pediatric patients. Pediatr Drugs 6:45–65, 2004.

Hereditary Kidney Disorders

CHAPTER 42

Genetic Basis of Glomerular and Structural Kidney Disorders

Ali Gharavi

Diseases of the glomerulus are diverse disorders that have traditionally been distinguished on the basis of renal histology. Interindividual variation in clinical presentation, progression, and therapeutic response among patients with similar renal pathologies has, however, suggested additional heterogeneity among histologic classes. In the past decade, genetic studies have identified primary molecular mechanisms underlying several familial glomerular disorders, delineating novel biological pathways that resolve histologic subsets. The success of these studies emanates from the recognition that most glomerular disorders comprise Mendelian subtypes amenable to genetic investigation using linkage analysis and positional cloning techniques. The identification of genes underlying Mendelian forms of glomerular disease has diagnostic and therapeutic implications, enabling genetic counseling, identification of individuals at risk, and implementation of appropriate therapies. Mutations in genes causing Mendelian syndromes are also responsible for some fraction of sporadic (nonfamilial) disease.

FAMILY HISTORY AMONG PATIENTS WITH GLOMERULAR DISEASE

Depending on the ethnic group surveyed, 5% to 30% of patients with endstage renal disease (ESRD) have an affected first- or second-degree relative, suggesting a hereditary contribution to disease. This familial aggregation of kidney failure is frequently observed for complex traits that are not normally considered to be hereditary, such as diabetic, hypertensive, or human immunodeficiency virus (HIV)-associated nephropathy. Hence, a positive family history of kidney disease, even among distant relatives of a patient, should not be simply attributed to shared environment or chance occurrence. More importantly, most glomerular disorders include Mendelian subtypes that require proper diagnosis (Table 42-1). The exact prevalence of Mendelian forms of glomerular disease is not known, but they are usually discernible once a thorough family history has been obtained. A good-quality family history should document disease occurrence in first- and second-degree relatives, any history of spontaneous abortion or childhood deaths, age of onset of disease in all affected cases, gender distribution, ethnic origin, presence of consanguinity, and potential environmental exposure. Variables such as age, gender, ethnicity, and environment may influence the penetrance and expressivity of disease, complicating initial detection of a clear Mendelian pattern. Recessive inheritance is suggested by parental consanguinity but may be difficult to recognize in small sibships, because there may only be a single affected individual. In addition to a positive family history, clues suggestive of a genetic disorder include associated syndromic abnormalities, early-onset disease, and ethnic/geographic origin from an isolated population.

NEPHROTIC SYNDROME AND FOCAL SEGMENTAL GLOMERULOSCLEROSIS

This category encompasses the pathologic diagnoses of minimal-change disease and focal segmental glomerulosclerosis (FSGS), disorders that often overlap in clinical presentation and subsequent course. In addition to idiopathic forms, these disorders (particularly FSGS) can occur in association with infections, drugs, or tumors, and are therefore considered as end manifestations of diverse forms of glomerular injury. The characteristic pathologic feature in nephrotic syndrome is fusion of podocyte foot processes; more advanced lesions display segmental sclerosis in some or all glomeruli. More recently, systematic investigations have identified familial subtypes for nephrotic syndrome, with dominant, recessive, and mitochondrial transmission documented. Family members of probands can have classic nephrotic syndrome and impaired kidney function, or more subtle abnormalities such as microalbuminuria. To date, most defects identified in familial nephrotic syndromes involve genes that are primarily expressed in the glomerular podocyte (Fig. 42-1), implicating injury or structural defects in this cell as the initiating influence.

Two genes for recessive disease have been identified to date. Congenital nephrotic syndrome (also known as Finnish congenital nephrosis) presents in utero or perinatally with massive proteinuria and no extrarenal manifestations. The disease affects 1 in 10,000 newborns in Finland, but has been reported worldwide. It is not responsive to steroid therapy and usually leads to ESRD by 2 years of age, necessitating kidney transplantation. Congenital nephrotic syndrome is due to inactivating

TABLE 42-1   Mendelian Forms of Glomerular Disease

Syndrome	Transmission	Locus	Gene
Nephrotic syndrome	AD	19q, 13	α-Actinin 4
	AD	6p12	CD2AP
	AR	19q13	Nephrin
	AR	1q24	Podocin
	AD	11p13	*WT1*
	AD	9q34	*LMX1B*
	Mit	–	tRNA
	Other AD, AR	11q21–11q22, 9q31, 2p12–2p13, 14q24	?*
Alport's syndrome	AD	2q36	Collagen type IV, α3 and α4
	AR	2q36	Collagen type IV, α3 and α4
	XL	Xq22	Collagen type IV, α5
TBMD	AD	2q36	Collagen type IV, α3 and α4
IgA nephropathy	AD	6q22–6q23	?
Membranous nephropathy	AR in mother of affected offspring	1q32	Neutral endopeptidase
Lipoprotein glomerulopathy	AD	19q13	Apolipoprotein E
Membranoproliferative glomerulonephritis	AR	1p36, 6p21	Complement c1q, 2, 3, 4
	AR	1q32	Complement H
	AD	1q32	?
Amyloidosis	AD	18q11	Transthyretin
	AD	4q28	Fibrinogen A α-chain
	AD	12q14	Lysozyme
	AD	11q23, 1q21	Apolipoprotein AI or AII
	AR	16p13	*MEFV* (FMF)
	AD	12p13	*TNFRSF1A* (TRAPS)

AD, autosomal dominant; AR, autosomal recessive; FMF, familial Mediterranean fever; MEFV, familial Mediterranean fever gene; Mit, mitochondrial transmission; TBMD, thin basement membrane disease; TNFRSF1A, tumor necrosis factor receptor superfamily member 1A; TRAP, tumor necrosis factor receptor-associated periodic syndrome.
*Identity of gene unknown.

mutations in the *NPHS1* gene, encoding nephrin, a podocyte-specific transmembrane protein of the immunoglobulin superfamily. The extracellular domain of nephrin proteins extend from adjacent podocyte foot processes and interdigitate to form the zipper-like structure observed at the glomerular slit diaphragm by electron microscopy. Mutations in nephrin disrupt the glomerular filtration barrier with consequent proteinuria and reduced kidney function. Disease recurrence after transplantation can occur in patients with null mutations (that lead to absence of nephrin in the native kidney) and is due to production of antibodies against nephrin.

Steroid-resistant nephrotic syndrome, a second form of recessive disease, is characterized by proteinuria, lack of response to steroid therapy, and progression to ESRD. There are no extrarenal manifestations, and recurrence after transplantation is rare. This syndrome is due to mutations in the *NPHS2* gene, encoding podocin, another podocyte-specific protein that interacts with nephrin and enhances nephrin signaling. Patients with podocin mutations generally present in childhood or young adulthood, a later onset than patients with nephrin mutations. Significantly, mutations in podocin account for 10% to 20% of sporadic steroid-resistant nephrotic syndrome in European children and young

adults, suggesting a relatively high carrier rate. One variant (an arginine-to-glutamine substitution at position 229) is particularly common in the general population (approximately 3%) and may cause disease when inherited with a second mutant allele. The lack of response to steroid therapy in these patients can be explained by the structural nature of the primary defect.

There are three genes known to cause dominant forms of nephrotic syndrome. Mutations in α-actinin 4 cause FSGS without extrarenal manifestations. α-Actinin 4 is a ubiquitously expressed filament-binding protein that localizes to podocyte foot processes in the kidney. It serves to maintain cytoskeletal architecture by enabling attachment of microfilaments to the cell membrane at adherens-type junctions. Patients with α-actinin 4 defects generally have adult-onset disease and progress to ESRD.

Heterozygous mutations in CD2-associated protein (CD2AP) have also been reported in a few patients with FSGS. CD2AP is an adaptor protein that serves as scaffolding for the actin cytoskeleton and also anchors the T-lymphocyte surface CD2 antigen. CD2AP is highly expressed in the podocyte and interacts with podocin and other nephrin-like proteins.

Dominant, syndromic forms of nephrosis include Frasier's and Denys-Drash syndromes. These are both

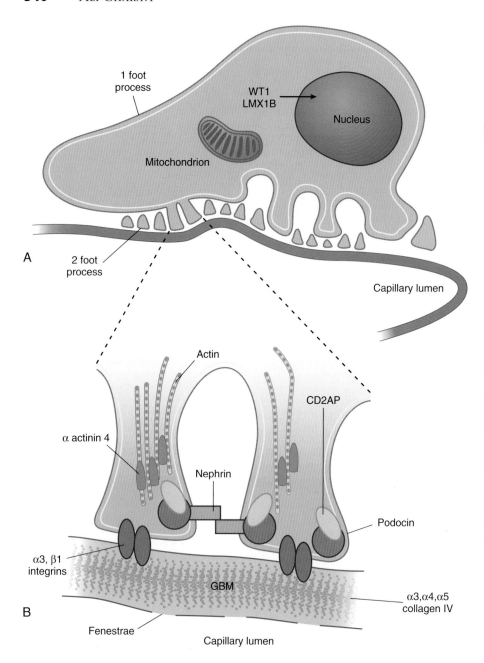

A

1 foot process

WT1
LMX1B

Nucleus

Mitochondrion

2 foot process

Capillary lumen

Actin

CD2AP

α actinin 4

Nephrin

Podocin

α3, β1 integrins

GBM

α3,α4,α5 collagen IV

B

Fenestrae

Capillary lumen

FIGURE 42-1   Podocyte proteins implicated in nephropathy. *A,* Schematic view of a podocyte resting on a capillary loop. Primary foot processes give rise to interconnected secondary processes that cover the glomerular basement membrane (GBM) at the filtration barrier. WT1 and LMX1B are transcription factors that regulate expression of proteins at the filtration barrier. Some mitochondrial mutations cause focal segmental glomerulosclerosis. *B,* Magnified view of secondary foot processes, which are anchored on the GBM by α3, β1 integrin complexes. Nephrin proteins extend from adjacent foot processes and interdigitate to form the zipper-like structure at the slit diaphragm. Nephrin is anchored onto the cell membrane by podocin and CD2AP. CD2AP interacts with actin filaments, thereby linking proteins at the filtration barrier to the cytoskeleton. α-Actinin type IV serves to connect actin filaments to various cellular structures such as adherens junctions. α3, α4, and α5 collagen type IV chains are components of the GBM and are mutant in Alport's syndrome.

caused by mutations in the *WT1* gene, the gene mutated in Wilms tumor. WT1 is a transcription factor that has tumor suppressor activity and is required for the development of the genitourinary system. It is highly expressed in early nephrogenesis but down-regulated in the mature kidney, with exclusive expression in podocytes. Frasier's syndrome presents as male pseudohermaphroditism, streak gonads, and nephrotic syndrome leading to ESRD. It is caused by mutations in intron 9 of the *WT1* gene, changing the balance of WT1 splice isoforms. Denys-Drash syndrome is caused by *WT1* coding mutations leading to mesangial sclerosis, male pseudohermaphroditism, and Wilms' tumor. Finally, mutation in another transcription factor, *LMX1B,* causes the nail-patella syndrome, characterized by dysplastic nails and patellae, reduced elbow motility, and nephropa-

thy. LMX1B was recently found to regulate podocin and CD2AP expression. Hence, the mechanism of glomerulosclerosis postulated in these syndromes is altered expression of the WT1- or LMXB1-regulated podocyte proteins such as nephrin, podocin, or CD2AP.

Finally, mitochondrial transmission of FSGS has also been documented. Mutations in mitochondrial genes interfere with cellular energy metabolism, resulting in dysfunction in a variety of organs. Mitochondrial disease may be recognized by maternal transmission of disease (mitochondria are transmitted by the ovum) and the presence of extrarenal features such as deafness, diabetes, or cardiomyopathy. Mitochondrial mutations are associated with considerable interindividual variability in the phenotypic manifestation and course of disease, such that the prediction of complications is difficult even among patients with identical mutations. For example, the same point mutation in the mitochondrial *tRNA(Leu)* gene (i.e., the tRNA that adds the amino acid leucine to the growing protein) can present as encephalomyopathy, diabetes/deafness, cardiomyopathy, ophthalmoplegia, or FSGS in different patients.

Genes causing familial nephrotic syndrome remarkably converge on the glomerular podocyte, delineating a biologic pathway responsible for maintaining the glomerular filtration barrier, cytoskeletal architecture, and cell-cell signaling. Following these findings, other studies have now demonstrated physical interaction between proteins implicated in familial nephrotic syndromes, while homology searches have resulted in the discovery of additional components of the glomerular filtration barrier. These data provide a rational pathway for investigation of sporadic forms of disease, for which the podocyte now represents the most probable site of initial injury. On the clinical side, these discoveries now permit identification of patients who will likely be unresponsive to corticosteroid therapy, sparing them from treatment side effects. How disruptions of podocyte proteins evolve from proteinuria to glomerulosclerosis and impaired kidney function is still not fully understood. However, genetically engineered mice lacking the WT1, LMX1B, nephrin, podocin, α-actinin 4, and CD2AP proteins have now been generated, and they recapitulate the human phenotypes, providing tools for further investigation of the mechanisms of nephrotic syndrome. There is also additional heterogeneity among familial syndromes, with several other recessive and dominant loci mapped to date. For example, a locus for steroid-sensitive nephrotic syndrome has been mapped to chromosome 2p12–2p13. The identification of these additional genes will further clarify the mechanisms underlying renal injury and nephrosis.

ALPORT'S SYNDROME AND THIN BASEMENT MEMBRANE DISEASE

Alport's syndrome (see also Chapter 46) is characterized by progressive kidney disease with hematuria and proteinuria, in association with sensorineural deafness and variable ocular changes. Renal lesions include characteristic splitting and laminated appearance of the glomerular basement membrane (GBM). Eighty-five percent of cases are X-linked and due to mutations of the collagen type IV, α5 gene (*COL4A5*). A subtype of X-linked Alport's syndrome features diffuse leiomyomatosis and is due to deletions in *COL4A5* and the first two exons of the adjacent collagen type IV, α6 gene. Autosomal-dominant or -recessive disease (15%) occurs as a result of inheritance of mutations of the collagen type IV, α3 or α4 genes on chromosome 2. These collagens are essential constituents of the GBM, their absence resulting in structural impairment of the filtration barrier. Their expression in the eyes and ears explains the extrarenal manifestations of

disease. Several other clinical points are noteworthy. As many as 15% of affected patients have de novo mutations in *COL4A5*, such that absence of a family history should not exclude the diagnosis in a patient with suggestive symptoms. Females carrying the mutations can also be affected but generally have a milder phenotype. Finally, a subset of transplanted patients develops anti-GBM nephritis resulting in graft loss, but this and other clinical outcomes cannot be reliably predicted by the nature of the germline mutation. Adverse prognostic clinical findings include development of deafness and worsening proteinuria.

Thin basement membrane disease (TBMD, also known as benign familial hematuria) is an autosomal-dominant trait presenting with hematuria and, rarely, late-onset renal impairment. It is identified by attenuation of the GBM on electron microscopy. Heterozygous mutations in the collagen type IV, α3 and α4 genes are present in 50% of TBMD cases, suggesting that in some cases, TBMD constitutes a mild presentation in the phenotypic spectrum of autosomal Alport's syndrome.

LIPOPROTEIN GLOMERULOPATHY

Lipoprotein glomerulopathy (LPG) is a rare cause of nephrotic syndrome that is mostly reported in the Japanese and Chinese populations. Its histologic profile is characterized by lipoprotein thrombi that occlude glomerular capillaries. Patients present with proteinuria and nephrotic syndrome with progression to ESRD and also often have type III hyperlipoproteinemia. LPG is caused by rare mutations in the *APOE* gene that are thought to increase binding of lipoprotein to capillary endothelial cells. An Arg145Pro variant, apolipoprotein E (ApoE) Sendai, accounts for a large portion of Japanese cases. Anecdotal reports suggest that aggressive lipid-lowering therapy is effective in this disorder.

MEMBRANOUS NEPHROPATHY

Membranous nephropathy (see Chapter 20) is generally an adult-onset disease presenting with nephritic-range proteinuria and variable progression of impaired kidney function; familial forms have rarely been reported. It is characterized by subepithelial deposition of immune complexes in GBM, imparting a thickened appearance of the basement membrane on light microscopy. A few cases of neonatal membranous glomerulopathy that also include familial aggregation have been reported. In one situation, the mother was shown to lack neutral endopeptidase, a glycoprotein enzyme that is highly expressed on epithelial cells in the glomerulus and proximal tubular cells. Although absence of neutral endopeptidase did not have any phenotypic consequences in the mother, it resulted in alloimmunization during pregnancy and production of neutralizing antibodies that caused podocyte injury and transplacental membranous nephropathy in the child. This finding presents a novel mechanism of glomerular disease and suggests that neutral endopeptidase may be a target of injury in sporadic or secondary forms of membranous nephropathy.

IMMUNOGLOBULIN A NEPHROPATHY

Immunoglobulin A (IgA) nephropathy (see Chapter 21) is characterized by mesangial proliferation with deposition of IgA. It presents with gross or microscopic hematuria and proteinuria, commonly after a viral infection, and leads to ESRD in 25% of cases. Like nephrotic syndrome, IgA nephropathy probably encompasses heterogeneous disorders that are not distinguishable on the basis of renal histology. The disease also aggregates with Henoch-Schönlein purpura, a childhood disorder featuring kidney disease identical to IgA nephropathy together with abdominal pain, palpable purpura, and arthritis. Familial aggregation of IgA nephropathy has been reported and conforms to autosomal-dominant inheritance with reduced penetrance. Family members present with a wide range of abnormalities, ranging from classic IgA nephropathy, to mesangial proliferative glomerulonephritis without IgA deposition, to microscopic hematuria not warranting kidney biopsy. Linkage analysis has mapped one locus for familial disease on chromosome 6q22–6q23 but the identity of the gene is not yet known.

MEMBRANOPROLIFERATIVE GLOMERULONEPHRITIS

Membranoproliferative glomerulonephritis (MPGN; see Chapter 18) is characterized by immune complex deposition in the GBM, and hypercellularity and lobulation of the glomerular tufts. Patients can present with a full-blown nephritic syndrome or with hematuria/proteinuria similar to IgA nephropathy. Some forms can be caused by hereditary deficiencies in complements, particularly complement factor H. Recessive mutations in factor H, which normally down-regulates the alternative and classic complement pathways, cause uncontrolled activation of complement leading to immune complex formation. Interestingly, mutations in factor H more commonly cause dominant and recessive hemolytic uremic syndrome, but the basis for this variation in phenotypic expression is not known. Another autosomal-dominant familial type of MPGN and a variant with fibronectin deposits both show linkage to chromosome 1q32.

GENETICALLY DETERMINED SYSTEMIC DISORDERS RESULTING IN GLOMERULAR DISEASE

Several genetically determined systemic disorders present with kidney disease as their principal manifestation. Proper diagnosis is important for genetic counseling and identification of presymptomatic individuals; moreover, there may be specific therapies available to ameliorate or reverse these diseases.

Fabry's disease is caused by mutations of the α-galactosidase A gene on chromosome X. Deficiency of the α-galactosidase A enzyme causes accumulation of glycosphingolipids in all body fluids and tissues, resulting in organ dysfunction. The severity of symptoms correlates with residual α-galactosidase A enzyme activity. Patients with no residual enzyme have the classical presentation of pain and paresthesias in their extremities, anhydrosis, angiokeratomas, and corneal opacities. Later manifestations include cerebrovascular disease, cardiomyopathy, and ESRD. Renal histology demonstrates characteristic vacuolization and foamy appearance of glomerular epithelial cells due to accumulation of glycosphingolipids. Like other X-linked traits, heterozygote females have a mild phenotype and rarely present with severe disease. In patients without the full spectrum of disease manifestations, the diagnosis may be missed or delayed, typically for a mean of 13 years from the first onset of symptoms. In particular, recent data indicate that there may be a "renal variant" of Fabry's disease, characterized by ESRD as the sole disease manifestation: in one series, 1.2% of 500 Japanese males on dialysis who were screened for α-galactosidase A activity had previously undiagnosed Fabry's disease renal variant. Other recent studies among male dialysis patients in Europe show a prevalence of 0.1% to 0.5%, a 10- to 50-fold higher prevalence than previously reported in registries. Identification of such patients is important, since clinical trials have now shown that α-galactosidase A replacement therapy, usually administered intravenously at 2-week intervals, reduces glycosphingolipid accumulation in tissues. Small, short-term trials now suggest that replacement therapy results in symptomatic improvement in end-organ damage, but the effectiveness of this therapy in reversing established cardiac and kidney dysfunction is currently under testing in large-scale clinical trials.

The amyloidoses (see Chapter 30) are increasingly being recognized as disorders of protein misfolding, whereby normally soluble protein precursors accumulate as β-pleated fibrils, forming extracellular tissue deposits that are identified by Congo red staining. The accumulation of amyloidogenic material can result from (1) mutations that perturb native protein conformation and facilitate misfolding (e.g., transthyretin in hereditary forms), (2) overproduction of precursors (serum amyloid A in inflammatory conditions, immunoglobulins in multiple myeloma), or (3) reduced clearance (e.g. β_2-microglobulin in dialysis patients; see Chapter 64). The kidney is often the target of amyloid deposition, resulting in nephrotic syndrome. Associated findings include polyneuropathy, hepatosplenomegaly, and congestive heart failure.

Hereditary forms can be caused by mutations in a growing list of proteins, including transthyretin, fibrinogen A α-chain, lysozyme, apolipoprotein AI or AII. Patients with transthyretin mutations present with neurologic and cardiac involvement, whereas mutations in other genes present primarily with kidney complications. Mutations in these genes were found in 10% of patients referred with a diagnosis of AL amyloidosis, a finding with important therapeutic implications: AL amyloidosis (formerly, primary amyloidosis) is due to plasma-cell dyscrasias producing immunoglobulin light chains and can respond to chemotherapy, whereas hereditary amyloidoses are unresponsive to this therapy. Some forms can potentially be treated with liver transplantation.

Secondary amyloidosis (also known as amyloidosis AA or reactive amyloidosis) occurs in patients with chronic inflammatory conditions, such as chronic infection or inflammatory bowel disease. The elevation of acute-phase inflammatory response proteins, including serum amyloid A, promotes amyloidogenesis. Familial forms include the periodic fever syndromes such as familial Mediterranean fever or tumor necrosis factor (TNF) receptor-associated periodic syndrome (TRAPS), caused by mutations in the *MEFV* and TNF receptor superfamily, member 1A genes, respectively. Mutations in these genes may change the inflammatory response threshold, with characteristic episodes of fever, rash, serositis, and arthritis. Familial Mediterranean fever responds to colchicine therapy, whereas TRAPS may respond to antibodies specific to the TNF receptor.

ENDSTAGE RENAL DISEASE AS AN INHERITED TRAIT

Diabetes and hypertension are the most common causes of ESRD worldwide, but only a subset of patients with these systemic conditions develop kidney failure; epidemiologic data suggest that genetic variables contribute to the development of ESRD. For example, chronic kidney disease affects one third of the diabetic population, independent of the duration, severity, or therapy of diabetes. Relatives of index cases with diabetic or hypertensive nephropathy show an increased prevalence of ESRD from all causes, with the highest risks reported in Pima Indians and African Americans. This familial aggregation has been documented for other disorders such as systemic lupus erythematosus nephritis or even HIV nephropathy, indicating shared inherited factors that increase the risk of development or progression of kidney function impairment from a variety of insults. Although this may initially seem surprising, the existence of pathways common to different nephropathies is also intimated by the clinical observation that systemic disorders such as diabetes or lupus can be associated with diverse renal lesions and that blockade of the renin-angiotensin system is beneficial in a variety of nephropathies. In human families with ESRD, the pattern of inheritance is most consistent with multifactorial determination (i.e., does not conform to Mendelian patterns), suggesting that many genetic and environmental variables contribute to the development of the trait through additive and/or epistatic interactions. Although a number of studies have attempted to localize the gene(s) predisposing to kidney functional impairment, the identity of these putative genetic risk factors has not yet been determined and there are no loci confirmed to date. It is likely, however, that more success will be achieved in the near future as advancing genomic technologies will improve analytic power in the investigation of complex traits.

BIBLIOGRAPHY

Boute N, Gribouval O, Roselli S, et al: *NPHS2*, encoding the glomerular protein podocin, is mutated in autosomal recessive steroid-resistant nephrotic syndrome. Nat Genet 24:349–354, 2000.

Debiec H, Guigonis V, Mougenot B, et al: Antenatal membranous glomerulonephritis due to anti-neutral endopeptidase antibodies. N Engl J Med 346:2053–2060, 2002.

Desnick RJ, Iannou YA, Eng CM: Alpha-galactosidase deficiency: Fabry disease. In Beaudet AL, Sly WS, Valle D (eds): The Metabolic and Molecular Basis of Inherited Disease, 8th ed. New York, McGraw-Hill, 2001, pp 3733–3774.

Gharavi AG, Yan Y, Scolari F, et al: IgA nephropathy, the most common cause of glomerulonephritis, is linked to 6q22–23. Nat Genet 26:354–357, 2000.

Kaplan JM, Kim SH, North KN, et al: Mutations in ACTN4, encoding α-actinin-4, cause familial focal segmental glomerulosclerosis. Nat Genet 24:251–256, 2000.

Kestila M, Lenkkeri U, Mannikko M, et al: Positionally cloned gene for a novel glomerular protein—nephrin—is mutated in congenital nephrotic syndrome. Mol Cell 1:575–582, 1998.

Kim JM, Wu H, Green G, et al: CD2-associated protein haploinsufficiency is linked to glomerular disease susceptibility. Science 300:1298–1300, 2003.

Lachmann HJ, Booth DR, Booth SE, et al: Misdiagnosis of hereditary amyloidosis as AL (primary) amyloidosis. N Engl J Med 346:1786–1791, 2002.

Neary JJ, Conlon PJ, Croke D, et al: Linkage of a gene causing familial membranoproliferative glomerulonephritis type III to chromosome 1. J Am Soc Nephrol 13:2052–2057, 2002.

Online Mendelian Inheritance in Man, OMIM (TM). McKusick-Nathans Institute for Genetic Medicine, Johns Hopkins University (Baltimore) and National Center for Biotechnology Information, National Library of Medicine (Bethesda, Maryland), 2000. Available at http://www.ncbi.nlm.nih.gov/omim/

Pollak MR: Inherited podocytopathies: FSGS and nephrotic syndrome from a genetic viewpoint. J Am Soc Nephrol 13:3016–3023, 2002.

Siamoopoulos KC: Fabry disease: Kidney involvement and enzyme replacement therapy. Kidney Int 65:744–753, 2004.

Tryggvason K, Martin P: Alport syndrome and basement membrane collagen. In Beaudet AL, Sly WS, Valle D (eds): The Metabolic and Molecular basis of Inherited Disease, 8th ed. New York, McGraw-Hill, 2001, pp 5453–5466.

CHAPTER 43

Genetic Basis of Renal Transport Disorders

Steven J. Scheinman

The coming of age of clinical chemistry in the latter half of the twentieth century, bringing with it the routine measurement of electrolytes and minerals in patient samples, produced descriptions of a variety of distinct inherited syndromes of abnormal renal tubular transport. Clinical investigation led to speculation, often quite ingenious and in some cases controversial, about the underlying causes of these syndromes. In the past decade, the tools of molecular biology have made possible the cloning of genes found to be mutated in patients with these monogenic disorders of renal tubular transport. In a sense, these diseases represent experiments of nature, and the discoveries they have revealed are exciting. Some of these provided gratifying confirmation of our existing knowledge of transport mechanisms along the nephron. Examples include mutations in diuretic-sensitive transporters in Bartter's and Gitelman's syndromes. In other cases, positional cloning led to the discovery of previously unknown proteins, often surprising ones, that appear to play important roles in epithelial transport. The voltage-gated chloride channel ClC-5 and the tight-junction protein paracellin-1, for example, were not known to exist until they were discovered through positional cloning in Dent's disease and inherited hypomagnesemic hypercalciuria, respectively.

Genetic diseases of renal tubular transport for which the molecular basis is known are summarized in Table 43-1. The diseases listed are each explained by abnormalities in the protein indicated. Such monogenic conditions tend to be uncommon or rare. Common conditions can often have important genetic components but are usually polygenic. In those settings, inheritance is often complex and involves polymorphisms in several genes, each of which contributes to the disease phenotype. Some genes responsible for the rare monogenic diseases may also contribute in subtle ways to the common polygenic conditions, but determining the contributions of these genes, and presumably others yet to be identified, for complex conditions such as hypertension will be the next major challenge for genetics.

DISORDERS OF PROXIMAL TUBULAR TRANSPORT FUNCTION

Selective Proximal Transport Defects

Sodium reabsorption in the proximal tubule occurs through secondary active transport processes in which entry of sodium is coupled to entry of glucose, amino acids, or phosphate, or coupled to the exit of protons. Autosomal-recessive conditions of impaired transepithelial transport of glucose and dibasic amino acids have been shown to be caused by mutations in sodium-dependent transporters that are expressed both in kidney and in the intestine, resulting in urinary losses and intestinal malabsorption of these solutes. Other disorders with renal selective transport defects are also thought, but not yet proven, to result from mutations in transporters expressed specifically in the kidneys.

X-linked (dominant) hypophosphatemic rickets (XLH) is characterized by impaired sodium-dependent phosphate reabsorption, in which the maximal transport capacity for phosphate is reduced, and this is reflected in a reduced number of units of the sodium-dependent phosphate transporter NaPi2 in the apical membrane of proximal tubular cells. This is the most common form of hereditary rickets. Mutations involve not the gene encoding NaPi2 but rather a neutral endopeptidase, designated "PHEX," that is expressed in bone and is thought to be involved in processing of a circulating phosphate transport-regulating hormone designated "phosphatonin." The more rare autosomal-dominant form of hypophosphatemic rickets (ADHR) is associated with mutations in a gene encoding a member of the fibroblast growth factor family, FGF-23, which protect FGF-23 from proteolytic cleavage. Physiologic effects of FGF-23 are consistent with its being the presumed phosphatonin that is the substrate for the PHEX enzyme, and serum

TABLE 43-1   Molecular Bases of Genetic Disorders of Renal Transport

Inherited Disorder	Defective Protein
Proximal tubule	
Glucose-galactose malabsorption syndrome	Sodium-glucose transporter 1
Dibasic aminoaciduria (lysinuric protein intolerance)	Basolateral dibasic amino acid transporter
XLH	Phosphate-regulating gene with homologies to endopeptidases on the X chromosome (PHEX)
ADHR	Fibroblast growth factor 23 (FGF-23)
Hereditary hypophosphatemic rickets with hypercalciuria	Unknown
Fanconi's syndrome (hereditary fructose intolerance)	Aldolase B
Oculocerebrorenal syndrome of Lowe	Inositol polyphosphate-5-phosphatase (OCRL1)
Cystinuria	Apical cystine-dibasic amino acid transporter
Dent's disease (X-linked nephrolithiasis)*	Voltage-gated chloride channel (ClC-5)
Proximal RTA	Basolateral sodium-bicarbonate cotransporter (NBC1)
Thick ascending limb of Henle's loop	
Bartter's syndrome	Bumetanide-sensitive Na-K-2Cl cotransporter (NKCC2)
	Apical potassium channel (ROMK)
	Basolateral chloride channel (ClC-Kb)
	Barttin (ClC-Kb-associated protein)
	CaSR (activation)
Familial hypomagnesemia with hypercalciuria	Paracellin-1
Familial benign hypercalcemia[†]	CaSR (inactivation)
Neonatal severe hyperparathyroidism[†]	CaSR (inactivation)
Familial hypercalciuric hypocalcemia[†]	CaSR (activation)
Familial juvenile hyperuricemic nephropathy	Uromodulin (Tamm-Horsfall protein)
Distal convoluted tubule	
Gitelman's syndrome	Thiazide-sensitive NaCl cotransporter (NCCT)
Pseudohypoparathyroidism type Ia[‡]	Guanine nucleotide-binding protein (Gs)
Familial hypomagnesemia with secondary hypocalcemia	TRPM6 cation channel[§]
Isolated renal Mg loss	γ Subunit of Na$^+$ K$^+$-ATPase
Collecting duct	
Liddle's syndrome	β and γ subunits of epithelial Na channel (ENaC)
Pseudohypoaldosteronism	
Type 1	
Autosomal recessive	α, β, γ Subunits of ENaC
Autosomal dominant	Mineralocorticoid (type I) receptor
Type 2 (Gordon's syndrome)	WNK1 and WNK4 kinases
Glucocorticoid-remediable aldosteronism	11β-Hydroxylase and aldosterone synthase (chimeric gene)[‖]
Syndrome of apparent mineralocorticoid excess	11β-Hydroxysteroid dehydrogenase type II
Distal renal tubular acidosis	
Autosomal recessive (with hearing deficit)	B1 subunit of proton-ATPase
Autosomal recessive (no hearing deficit)	a4 isoform of α subunit of proton ATPase
Autosomal dominant	Basolateral anion exchanger (AE1)
Carbonic anhydrase II deficiency[¶]	Carbonic anhydrase type II
Nephrogenic diabetes insipidus	
X-linked	Arginine vasopressin 2 (V2) receptor
Autosomal	Aquaporin-2 water channel

ADHR, autosomal-dominant hypophosphatemic rickets; CaSR, calcium-sensing receptor; RTA, renal tubular acidosis; XLH, X-linked hypophosphatemic rickets.
*Gene also expressed in medullary thick ascending limb and collecting duct.
[†]Gene also expressed in collecting duct and elsewhere.
[‡]Gene also expressed in proximal tubule, where functional abnormalities are clinically apparent.
[§]Gene also expressed in intestine.
[‖]Gene expressed in adrenal gland.
[¶]Clinical phenotype can be of proximal RTA, distal RTA, or combined.

levels of uncleaved FGF-23 are excessive in XLH, AHDR, and also tumor-induced hypophosphatemic osteomalacia, all of which are characterized by impaired renal phosphate reabsorption.

Hereditary hypophosphatemic rickets with hypercalciuria differs from XLH and ADHR, which are associated with reduced urinary calcium excretion. Although it had been speculated that this condition resulted from inacti-

vation of the sodium-phosphate transport protein NaPi2, current evidence excludes that gene.

The rare condition of familial proximal renal tubular acidosis (RTA) is associated with mutations that inactivate the basolateral sodium-bicarbonate cotransporter NBC1. These patients also suffer ocular abnormalities leading to blindness, probably as a consequence of impaired bicarbonate transport in the eye.

Inherited Fanconi's Syndrome

Several inherited forms of Fanconi's syndrome are associated with generalized impairment in reabsorptive function of the proximal tubule. These include hereditary fructose intolerance, caused by mutations in the gene for aldolase B, as well as Lowe's syndrome and Dent's disease.

Hereditary fructose intolerance results from deficiency of the aldolase B enzyme that cleaves fructose-1-phosphate. Symptoms are precipitated by intake of sweets. Massive accumulation of fructose-1-phosphate occurs, leading to sequestration of inorganic phosphate and deficiency of adenosine triphosphate (ATP). Acute consequences can include hypoglycemic shock, severe abdominal symptoms, and impaired function of the Krebs cycle producing metabolic acidosis, and this is exacerbated by impaired renal bicarbonate reabsorption. ATP deficiency leads to impaired proximal tubular function in general, including the full expression of Fanconi's syndrome, with consequent rickets and stunted growth. ATP breakdown can be so dramatic as to produce hyperuricemia, and also hypermagnesemia from dissolution of the Mg-ATP complex. Acute symptoms, as well as chronic consequences such as liver disease, can be minimized by avoiding dietary sources of fructose.

Characteristic features of the oculocerebrorenal syndrome of Lowe include congenital cataracts, mental retardation, muscular hypotonia, and renal Fanconi's syndrome. In contrast, Dent's disease is confined to the kidney. In both syndromes, low-molecular-weight (LMW) proteinuria is a prominent feature, together with other evidence of proximal tubulopathy such as glycosuria, aminoaciduria, and phosphaturia. One important difference is that proximal RTA, with growth retardation, can be severe in patients with Lowe's syndrome but is not a part of Dent's disease. Rickets occurs in both, though not in all patients, and is thought to be a consequence of hypophosphatemia (and, in Lowe's, of acidosis). Hypercalciuria is a characteristic feature of Dent's disease, associated with nephrocalcinosis in most or kidney stones in many patients, but these are less evident in Lowe's syndrome. Kidney failure is common in both, progressing to endstage renal disease in young adulthood in Dent's disease and even earlier in patients with Lowe's syndrome.

Dent's disease is caused by mutations that inactivate the voltage-gated chloride channel ClC-5. This chloride channel is expressed in the proximal tubule, medullary thick ascending limb (mTAL) of Henle's loop, and the α-intercalated cells of the collecting tubule. In the cells of the proximal tubule, ClC-5 colocalizes with the proton ATPase in subapical endosomes. These endosomes are important in the processing of proteins that are filtered at the glomerulus and taken up by the proximal tubule through adsorptive endocytosis. The activity of the proton ATPase acidifies the endosomal space, releasing the proteins from membrane binding sites and making them available for proteolytic degradation. Chloride flow through channels into the endosome appears to be necessary to dissipate the positive charge generated by proton entry. Thus, mutations that inactivate ClC-5 in patients with Dent's disease would interfere with the mechanism for reabsorption of LMW proteins and explain the consistent finding of LMW proteinuria. Glycosuria, aminoaciduria, and phosphaturia are less consistently seen and may be secondary consequences of ClC-5 inactivation, possibly through alterations in membrane trafficking. Lowe's syndrome is associated with mutations in *OCRL1*, which encodes a phosphatidylinositol 4,5-bisphosphate 5-phosphatase. In renal epithelial cells, this phosphatase is localized to the trans-Golgi network, which plays an important role in directing proteins to the appropriate membrane. Thus, the similarities in the renal features of these two syndromes may be the result of a final common consequence of the two molecular defects.

DISORDERS OF TRANSPORT IN THE MEDULLARY THICK ASCENDING LIMB OF HENLE

Bartter's Syndrome

Solute transport in the mTAL involves the coordinated functions of a set of transport proteins depicted in Figure 43-1. These are the bumetanide-sensitive Na-K-2Cl cotransporter (NKCC2) and the renal outer medullary potassium channel (ROMK) on the apical surface of cells of the mTAL, and the chloride channel ClC-Kb on the basolateral surface. Optimal function of the ClC-Kb chloride channel requires interaction with a subunit called barttin. Mutations in any of the genes encoding these four proteins lead to the phenotype of Bartter's syndrome. In addition, activation of the epithelial calcium-sensing receptor (CaSR) inhibits activity of the ROMK potassium channel. Mutations producing constitutive activation of the CaSR cause familial hypocalcemic hypercalciuria, which is discussed later. Some patients with hypocalcemic hypercalciuria have the phenotype of Bartter's syndrome, and thus mutations in the CaSR must be considered a fifth molecular cause of Bartter's. Together these five genes still do not account for all patients with Bartter's syndrome.

The ClC-Kb basolateral chloride channel provides the route for chloride exit to the interstitium. Flow of potassium through the ROMK channel is important in assuring that potassium concentrations in the tubular lumen will not be limiting for the activity of the Na-K-2Cl cotransporter, and also maintains a positive electrical potential in the lumen of this nephron segment. This positive charge is the driving force for paracellular reabsorption of calcium and magnesium.

Bartter's syndrome presents in infancy or childhood, often as failure to thrive. It is characterized by hypokalemic metabolic alkalosis, typically with hyper-

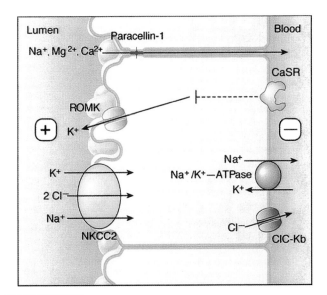

FIGURE 43-1 Transport mechanisms in the thick ascending limb (TAL) of Henle's loop indicating transport proteins affected by mutations in genetic diseases. Reabsorption of sodium chloride occurs through the electroneutral activity of the bumetanide-sensitive Na$^+$-K$^+$-2Cl$^-$ cotransporter NKCC2. Activity of the basolateral Na$^+$ K$^+$-ATPase provides the driving force for this transport and also generates a high intracellular concentration of potassium, which exits through the ATP-regulated apical potassium channel ROMK. This assures an adequate supply of potassium for the activity of the NKCC2 transporter and also produces a lumen-positive electrical potential, which itself is the driving force for paracellular reabsorption of calcium, magnesium, and sodium ions through the tight junctions and involving the protein paracellin-1. Chloride transported into the cell by NKCC2 exits the basolateral side of the cell through the voltage-gated chloride channel ClC-Kb. Activation of the extracellular calcium-sensing receptor CaSR inhibits solute transport in the TAL by inhibiting activity of the ROMK potassium channel and possibly other mechanisms. Mutations that inactivate NKCC2, ROMK, and ClC-Kb occur in patients with Bartter's syndrome, resulting in salt wasting, hypokalemic metabolic alkalosis, and hypercalciuria. Mutations that inactivate the CaSR are associated with enhanced calcium transport and hypocalciuria in familial benign hypercalcemia, and mutations that activate the CaSR occur in patients with familial hypercalciuria with hypocalcemia. (Adapted from Scheinman SJ, Guay-Woodford LM, Thakker RV, Warnock DG: Genetic disorders of renal electrolyte transport. N Engl J Med 340:1177–1187, 1999, with permission. Copyright © 1999, Massachusetts Medical Society. All rights reserved.)

calciuria, and these patients thus resemble patients chronically taking loop diuretics that inhibit the activity of NKCC2 pharmacologically. Defective function of NKCC2, ROMK, ClC-Kb, or barttin leads to impaired salt reabsorption in the mTAL, resulting in volume contraction and activation of the renin-angiotensin-aldosterone axis, which stimulates distal tubular secretion of potassium and protons and produces hypokalemic metabolic alkalosis. Despite impaired reabsorption of magnesium, serum magnesium levels are usually normal in patients with Bartter's syndrome, but occasionally are mildly depressed. The hypercalciuria often leads to nephrocalci-

nosis, particularly in those patients with mutations in genes encoding NKCC2 and ROMK.

Inherited Hypomagnesemic Hypercalciuria

Reabsorption of calcium and magnesium in the mTAL occurs through the paracellular route driven by the positive electrical potential in the tubular lumen. Selective movement of cations (calcium, magnesium, and sodium) is determined by the tight junctions between the epithelial cells. Disturbance of this selective paracellular barrier would be expected to produce parallel disorders in the reabsorption of calcium and magnesium.

A familial syndrome of hypomagnesemia with substantial renal magnesium losses, and associated with hypercalciuria, has been reported to be inherited in an autosomal-recessive fashion. Patients develop nephrocalcinosis, kidney failure, and kidney stones. These patients also have a variety of ocular abnormalities. Through investigation of these families by positional cloning, a gene encoding a protein designated paracellin-1 was discovered. Paracellin-1 is homologous to the claudin family of tight-junction proteins. It is expressed at the tight junction between cells of the mTAL (see Fig. 43-1), as well as in the distal convoluted tubule. A range of mutations in this gene have been identified and segregate with disease in families with this syndrome. This is the first instance of a disease shown to result from mutations that alter a tight-junction protein. It is thought that paracellin-1 either itself constitutes the pore in the tight junction that permits selective conductance of cations, or is a regulator of the conductance. It is not clear, however, why this defect in tight junctions would be associated with hyperuricemia, a consistent finding in this disease.

Familial Hypomagnesemia with Secondary Hypocalcemia

These patients have severe hypomagnesemia, often with neonatal seizures and tetany. If not recognized and treated early, the hypomagnesemia can be fatal. Serum magnesium levels fall to levels low enough to impair parathyroid hormone (PTH) release or responsiveness, and this is presumed to be the mechanism of the hypocalcemia that commonly accompanies the hypomagnesemia in these patients. The primary defect appears to be in intestinal magnesium absorption, although renal magnesium conservation is also deficient. These patients have mutations in a gene encoding the TRPM6 protein. TRPM6 is a member of the long transient receptor potential channel family and is expressed in both the intestine and the distal convoluted tubule. It may function as both a cation channel and a kinase, although this speculation requires confirmation.

Familial Hypocalciuric Hypercalcemia

The extracellular CaSR is expressed in many tissues where ambient calcium concentration triggers cellular responses. In the parathyroid gland activation of the CaSR suppresses synthesis and release of PTH. In the kidney the CaSR is expressed on the basolateral surface of cells of the TAL (cortical more than medullary), on the luminal surface of the cells of the papillary collecting duct, and in other portions of the nephron. Activation of the CaSR in the TAL probably mediates the known effects of hypercalcemia to inhibit the transport of calcium, magnesium, and sodium in this nephron segment. For example, CaSR activation inhibits activity of the ROMK potassium channel (see Fig. 43-1). This would be expected to reduce the positive electrical potential in the lumen and thereby suppress the driving force for reabsorption of calcium and magnesium. In the papillary collecting duct, activation of the apical CaSR could explain the effects of hypercalciuria to impair the hydro-osmotic response to vasopressin.

In familial hypocalciuric hypercalcemia (FHH), loss-of-function mutations of the CaSR increase the set point for calcium sensing, resulting in hypercalcemia with relative elevation of PTH levels. Urinary calcium excretion is low because of enhanced calcium reabsorption in the TAL and PTH-stimulated calcium transport in the distal convoluted tubule. FHH occurs in patients heterozygous for such mutations, and is benign, since tissues are resistant to the high serum calcium levels. A family history is very useful in distinguishing FHH from primary hyperparathyroidism, and parathyroidectomy should not be performed. Infants of consanguineous parents with FHH can be homozygous for these mutations, resulting in a syndrome of severe hypercalcemia with marked hyperparathyroidism, fractures, and failure to thrive known as neonatal severe hyperparathyroidism.

Other mutations result in constitutive activation of the CaSR, and this produces hypocalcemia with hypercalciuria, without elevation in PTH concentrations. As discussed earlier, this can also produce the phenotype of Bartter's syndrome. It has been speculated that such mutations, if they produce mild gain of function of the CaSR without frank hypocalcemia, could be responsible for some cases of idiopathic hypercalciuria, but this has not been demonstrated.

Familial Juvenile Hyperuricemic Nephropathy

Mutations in the *UMOD* gene encoding uromodulin (also known as the Tamm-Horsfall protein) occur in families in which children present with hyperuricemia and gout. This syndrome overlaps with medullary cystic kidney disease type 2, also associated with *UMOD* mutations. Cytosolic inclusions seen on electron microscopy in the epithelial cells of the mTAL appear to be crystallized uro-

modulin. A physiologic explanation for the hyperuricemia has not been offered. The occurrence of hyperuricemia in this disease and in the syndrome associated with mutations in paracellin-1 indicates that our understanding of the role of the mTAL in uric acid transport is not fully understood.

DISORDERS OF TRANSPORT IN THE DISTAL CONVOLUTED TUBULE

Gitelman's Syndrome

Reabsorption of sodium chloride in the distal convoluted tubule occurs through electroneutral transport mediated by the thiazide-sensitive sodium chloride cotransporter (NCCT). Mutations in the NCCT gene are associated with Gitelman's syndrome, another condition of hypokalemic metabolic alkalosis. Gitelman's syndrome was formerly viewed as a variant of Bartter's syndrome. An essential distinction between these two conditions is the hypocalciuria in Gitelman's syndrome, in contrast to the hypercalciuria that occurs in Bartter's syndrome or in patients taking loop diuretics. Hypocalciuria in Gitelman's syndrome resembles the reduction in calcium excretion that occurs in patients taking thiazide diuretics. These findings are satisfying in that they connect nicely the clinical physiology with molecular physiology. However, our current understanding of renal transport does not yet allow us to explain why significant hypomagnesemia with renal magnesium wasting is typical of Gitelman's syndrome, whereas in Bartter's syndrome it is much less common and, when it does occur, milder.

DISORDERS OF TRANSPORT IN THE COLLECTING TUBULE

Liddle's Syndrome

Sodium reabsorption by the principal cells of the cortical collecting duct is under physiologic regulation by aldosterone. As in other cells, low intracellular sodium concentrations are maintained by the basolateral $Na^+ K^+$-ATPase, and this drives sodium entry through amiloride-sensitive epithelial sodium channels (ENaCs) on the apical surface. Mutations that render ENaCs persistently open produce, as would be predicted, a syndrome of excessive sodium reabsorption and low-renin hypertension known as Liddle's syndrome. This is an autosomal-dominant condition often presenting in children with severe hypertension and hypokalemic alkalosis. It resembles primary hyperaldosteronism, but serum aldosterone levels are quite low, and for this reason the disease has also been termed pseudohyperaldosteronism. In their original description of the syndrome, Liddle and colleagues demonstrated that aldosterone excess was not responsible for this disease and that whereas spironolactone had no effect on the hypertension, patients did respond well to triamterene or dietary sodium restriction. They proposed that the primary abnormality was excessive renal salt conservation and potassium secretion independent of mineralocorticoid. This proved to be correct and is explained by the excessive sodium channel activity. Kidney transplantation in Liddle's original proband led to resolution of the hypertension, consistent with the defect being intrinsic to the kidneys.

In Liddle's syndrome, gain-of-function mutations in the gene encoding ENaC produce channels that are resistant to down-regulation by physiologic stimuli such as volume expansion. ENaC is formed by three homologous subunits designated αENaC, βENaC, and γENaC. Missense or truncating mutations in patients with Liddle's syndrome alter the carboxyl-terminal cytoplasmic tail of the β or γ subunits in a domain that is important for interactions with the cytoskeletal protein that regulates activity of ENaC. In addition to the severe phenotype of Liddle's syndrome resulting from these mutations, it has been proposed that polymorphisms in the ENaC sequence that have less dramatic effects on sodium channel function could contribute to the much more common low-renin variant of essential hypertension.

Pseudohypoaldosteronism Types 1 and 2

These are referred to as "pseudohypoaldosteronism" because they feature hyperkalemia and metabolic acidosis without aldosterone deficiency. Type 1 disease is associated with salt wasting and results from mutation that inactivates either the mineralocorticoid receptor (autosomal recessive) or the epithelial sodium channel ENaC (autosomal dominant). Type 2 disease, however, is a hypertensive condition, and in this respect patients differ substantially from those with hypoaldosteronism. Type 2 pseudohypoaldosteronism, also known as Gordon's syndrome, is a mirror image of Gitelman syndrome, with hyperkalemia, metabolic acidosis, and hypercalciuria, although serum magnesium levels are normal. Gordon's syndrome is caused by mutations in two kinases known as WNK1 and WNK4. WNK4 down-regulates the activity of the NCCT sodium chloride cotransporter, and inactivating mutations in WNK4 result in increased NCCT activity and thereby enhanced sodium reabsorption. WNK1 seems to be a negative regulator of WNK4, and gain-of-function WNK1 mutations indirectly increase NCCT activity.

Two other hereditary conditions produce hypertension in children with clinical features resembling primary hyperaldosteronism. The syndrome of apparent mineralocorticoid excess (AME) is an autosomal-recessive disease in which the renal isoform of the 11β-hydroxysteroid dehydrogenase enzyme is inactivated by mutation. This is in a sense a genetic analogue of ingestion of black licorice, which contains glycyrrhizic acid that inhibits this enzyme. Inactivation of the enzyme results in failure to convert cortisol to cortisone locally in the collecting duct, allowing cortisol to activate mineralocortoicoid receptors and produce a syndrome resembling primary hyperaldosteronism but, like Liddle's syndrome, with low circulating levels of aldosterone. As in Liddle's syndrome, kidney transplantation has been reported to result in resolution of hypertension in AME. The autosomal-dominant condition glucocorticoid-remediable aldosteronism (GRA) is caused by a chromosomal rearrangement that produces a chimeric gene in which the regulatory region of the gene encoding the steroid 11β-hydroxylase (which is part of the cortisol-biosynthetic pathway and normally is regulated by adrenocorticotropic hormone [ACTH]) is fused to distal sequences of the aldosterone synthase gene. This results in production of aldosterone that responds to ACTH rather than normal regulatory stimuli. Patients with GRA may have variable elevations in plasma aldosterone levels, and are often normokalemic. Aldosterone levels are suppressed with glucocorticoid therapy. Elevated urinary levels of 18-oxacortisol and 18-hydroxy cortisol are characteristic of GRA.

Hereditary Renal Tubular Acidosis

Secretion of acid by the α-intercalated cells of the collecting duct is accomplished by the apical proton ATPase. Cytosolic carbonic anhydrase catalyzes the formation of bicarbonate from hydroxyl ions, and this bicarbonate then exits the cell in exchange for chloride through the basolateral anion exchanger AE1. Mutations affecting each of these proteins have been documented in patients with hereditary forms of RTA. Autosomal-recessive distal RTA is associated with mutations in the B1 subunit of the proton ATPase. This form of RTA is often severe, presenting in young children, and can be associated with hearing loss, consistent with the expression of this ATPase in the cochlea and endolymphatic sac of the inner ear as well as in kidney tissue. Other patients with autosomal-recessive distal RTA have mutations in the gene encoding a noncatalytic a4 isoform of the α accessory subunit of the ATPase, and these patients have no hearing deficit. Autosomal-dominant RTA, a milder disease often undetected until adulthood, is associated with mutations in the basolateral anion exchanger AE1. Other genetic loci appear to be responsible for additional familial cases of distal RTA. Familial deficiency of carbonic anhydrase II is also characterized by cerebral calcification and osteopetrosis, the latter reflecting the important role of carbonic anhydrase in osteoclast function. The acidification defect in carbonic anhydrase II deficiency affects bicarbonate reabsorption in the proximal tubule as well as collecting duct.

Nephrogenic Diabetes Insipidus

Reabsorption of water across the cells of the collecting duct occurs only when arginine vasopressin (AVP) is present. AVP activates V2 receptors on the principal cells and cells of the inner medullary collecting duct, initiating a cascade that results in fusion of vesicles containing Aquaporin-2 (AQP-2) water channel pores into the apical membranes of these cells. The V2 receptor is encoded by a gene on the X chromosome, and the most common form of nephrogenic diabetes insipidus (NDI) is caused by inactivating mutations in the V2 receptor gene. This results in vasopressin-resistant polyuria that is typically more severe in males and is also associated with impaired responses to the effects of AVP that are mediated by extrarenal V2 receptors, specifically vasodilatation and endothelial release of von Willebrand's factor. Less commonly, families have been described with autosomal-recessive inheritance of NDI, and these patients have mutations in the gene encoding AQP-2 that result in either impaired trafficking of water channels to the plasma membrane or defective pore function. Rare autosomal-dominant occurrence of NDI with mutation in the AQP-2 gene has also been reported.

BIBLIOGRAPHY

Ali M, Rellos P, Cox TM: Hereditary fructose intolerance. J Med Genet 35:353–365, 1998.

Guay-Woodford LM: Bartter syndrome: Unraveling the pathophysiologic enigma. Am J Med 105:151–162, 1998

Hebert S, Brown E, Harris H: Role of the Ca^{2+}-sensing receptor in divalent mineral ion homeostasis. J Exp Biol 200:295–302, 1997.

Jonsson KB, Zahradnik R, Larsson T, et al: Fibroblast growth factor 23 in oncogenic osteomalacia and X-linked hypophosphatemia. N Engl J Med 348:1656–1663, 2003.

Karet FE: Inherited distal renal tubular acidosis. J Am Soc Nephrol 13:2178–2184, 2002.

Knoers NV, Monnens LL: Nephrogenic diabetes insipidus. Semin Nephrol 19:344–352, 1999.

Reilly RF, Ellison DH: Mammalian distal tubule: Physiology, pathophysiology, and molecular anatomy. Physiol Rev 80:277–313, 2000.

Scheinman SJ: X-linked hypercalciuric nephrolithiasis: Clinical syndromes and chloride channel mutations. Kidney Int 53:3–17, 1998.

Scheinman SJ, Guay-Woodford LM, Thakker RV, Warnock DG: Genetic disorders of renal electrolyte transport. N Engl J Med 340:1177–1187, 1999.

Simon DB, Bindra RS, Mansfield TA, et al: Mutations in the chloride channel gene, *CLCNKB*, cause Bartter's syndrome type III. Nat Genet 17:171–178, 1997.

Simon DB, Lu Y, Choate KA, et al: Paracellin-1, a renal tight junction protein required for paracellular Mg resorption. Science 285:103–106, 1999.

Torres VE, Scheinman SJ: Genetic diseases of the kidney. NephSAP 3:54–70, 2004.

Walder RY, Landau D, Meyer P, et al: Mutation of *TRPM6* causes familial hypomagnesemia with secondary hypocalcemia. Nat Genet 31:171–174, 2002.

Warnock DG: Liddle syndrome: An autosomal dominant form of human hypertension. Kidney Int 53:18–24, 1998.

Warnock DG: Hypertension. Semin Nephrol 19:374–380, 1999.

Wilson FH, Kahle KT, Sabath E, et al: Molecular pathogenesis of inherited hypertension with hyperkalemia: The Na-Cl cotransporter is inhibited by wild-type but not mutant WNK4. Proc Natl Acad Sci USA 100:680–684, 2003.

CHAPTER 44

Sickle Cell Nephropathy

Antonio Guasch

The sickle hemoglobinopathies are caused by the homozygous (Hb SS disease) or heterozygous (Hb AS or sickle cell trait) inheritance of the sickle β-globin gene. The substitution of valine for glutamic acid at the 6 position of the β-chain of hemoglobin leads to production of an unstable isoform that, when slowly deoxygenated, can polymerize, leading to the production of sickle cells. These cells lack the fluidity of normal erythrocytes and can impede or block capillary flow, resulting in tissue ischemia. Other hemoglobin variants (Hb C, D, E, or β-thalassemia) may coexist with sickle cell anemia (SCA), producing double heterozygosity. In the United States, the sickle cell trait occurs in about 8% of individuals of African-American origin, and SS disease is present in about 1 in 500 African-American newborns.

Because the kidney is a highly vascular organ and there is a low pO_2 in the renal medullary interstitium, the kidney is one of the sites vulnerable to vaso-occlusive events. Renal involvement in SCA is very common and is summarized in Table 44-1.

RENAL HEMODYNAMICS IN SICKLE CELL ANEMIA

Children with SCA have a high glomerular filtration rate (GFR) (glomerular hyperfiltration) and high renal plasma and blood flows (renal hyperperfusion), both consequences of renal vasodilation. A marked glomerular hypertrophy, present histologically in individuals with no clinical disease, also contributes to the glomerular hyperfiltration. The hypertrophy can be observed in individuals as young as 2 years of age. The elevated GFR is presumed to be a compensation for hypoxia. The supernormal GFR returns to "normal" values after the second or third decade, but renal blood flow rates continue to be higher than in healthy individuals. The mechanisms mediating the renal vasodilation are not known, but some evidence supports a role for vasodilatory prostaglandins or enhanced activity of the nitric oxide system. Treatment of SCA patients with a dose of indomethacin that does not affect GFR or renal plasma flow in normal individuals normalizes GFR and decreases renal plasma flow toward but not completely to normal.

BLOOD PRESSURE IN SICKLE CELL ANEMIA

Despite a higher prevalence of hypertension in the African-American population, hypertension is uncommon in SCA. Blood pressure values are, on average, 5 to 15 mm Hg lower in SS patients than in healthy African Americans matched for age and gender, probably as a consequence of a low systemic vascular resistance. A higher mortality rate due to vascular events occurs in SCA individuals with blood pressure values higher than the 90th percentile of the blood pressure distribution for the SCA population. In patients with SS disease, this increase in mortality occurs when blood pressure values are higher than 130/84 mm Hg. Therefore, blood pressure values higher than 130/84 mm Hg should be considered abnormal in SCA patients and should be treated.

SICKLE CELL GLOMERULOPATHY

Glomerular involvement, manifested by proteinuria and/or progressive loss of kidney function, occurs commonly in SCA. Dipstick-positive proteinuria occurs in 25% to 30% of adult SCA patients, and 14% have proteinuria of 2+ or more. The proteinuria results from enhanced glomerular passage of albumin and larger proteins (glomerular origin) and is not the result of tubular failure to reabsorb low-molecular-weight proteins. Proteinuria occurs more frequently in patients with SS disease than in other sickle hemoglobinopathies (SC or Sβ-thalassemia) and is uncommon in sickle cell trait.

Albuminuria in Sickle Cell Anemia

Abnormal albumin excretion rates may occur in children with SCA. In recent series, microalbuminuria was present in 19% of children and dipstick proteinuria in 6%. In older teenagers, the prevalence of dipstick clinical proteinuria was 12%. The development of albuminuria is age-dependent, so that microalbuminuria was present in 24% of children ages 7 to 14 years and in 29% of children older than 15 years. In children, the development of abnormal albuminuria is inversely correlated with hemoglobin levels and is associated with other complications

TABLE 44-1 Kidney Involvement in Sickle Cell Anemia

Glomerular
Glomerular hyperfiltration and hyperperfusion
Sickle cell glomerulopathy (focal segmental glomerulosclerosis)
    Microalbuminuria and Macroalbuminuria
    Progressive reduction in GFR
    Endstage renal disease
Membranoproliferative glomerulonephritis

Medullary
Concentrating defects with preserved diluting capacity
Renal papillary necrosis
Hematuria

Tubular dysfunction
Incomplete distal RTA
Hyperkalemic hyperchloremic acidosis
    Type IV RTA
    Distal RTA with hyperkalemia
    Selective aldosterone deficiency
Decreased potassium excretion without aldosterone deficiency
Increased sodium, phosphate reabsorption
Increased urate secretion

Malignancy

Renal medullary carcinoma

GFR, glomerular filtration rate; RTA, renal tubular acidosis.

such as stroke, episodes of acute chest syndrome, and hospitalizations.

The prevalence of abnormal albuminuria in adults is higher than in the pediatric population. In a recent series, 27% of adults with SS disease had macroalbuminuria and 41% had microalbuminuria, for a combined prevalence of abnormal albuminuria of 68%. The clinical significance of microalbuminuria in SCA patients is unknown, but those individuals could be at risk for progression to macroalbuminuria or even loss of kidney function. However, the presence of macroalbuminuria in SCA patients indicates the presence of a glomerulopathy (see later). In other sickle hemoglobinopathies (SC, Sβ-thalassemia), abnormal albuminuria is much less frequent than in SS disease, with prevalences of macroalbuminuria and microalbuminuria of 6% and 36% of adult patients, respectively. A lower prevalence of glomerular involvement occurs in SS disease patients with coinheritance of α-thalassemia.

Pathophysiology

Some SCA patients may develop chronic kidney disease with progressive loss of kidney function associated with worsening proteinuria. Detailed studies of glomerular filtration using neutral dextrans of graded size as filtration markers show an increase in glomerular pore size in SCA patients with proteinuria, indicative of impaired membrane permselectivity. Initially, the glomerular capillary ultrafiltration coefficient, K_f, is increased, in keeping with the increase in membrane surface area associated with the glomerular hypertrophy observed. With progression of disease, GFR and renal plasma flow fall to normal and then subnormal values. Proteinuria increases and K_f falls. At this stage, the histologic findings consist of focal glomerulosclerosis (see later section on Pathology). As sclerosis progresses, glomerular membrane surface area decreases, accounting for the decrease in K_f.

Clinical Presentation

Sickle cell glomerulopathy occurs more frequently in SS disease than in other sickle hemoglobinopathies and is usually detected by the finding of proteinuria at the time of a routine urinalysis. In the initial stages, the only clinically evident abnormality is proteinuria; serum creatinine and the creatinine clearance are in the normal range. As disease progresses, kidney function begins to decline. Proteinuria is usually between 0.5 and 2.5 g/day but can be in the nephrotic range. Urinalysis usually reveals no hematuria or pyuria. The presence of hematuria or red blood cell casts should alert the physician to the possibility of other causes for the glomerulonephritis. Because of the long-term exposure of these patients to blood products and higher incidence of infections, other glomerulopathies such as hepatitis-associated glomerulonephritis or human immunodeficiency virus (HIV) nephropathy should be ruled out. Acute glomerulonephritis has been reported in association with parvovirus infection. Because of the lower values of systemic blood pressure in the SCA population, relative hypertension (see earlier) should be identified in patients with SCA and appropriately treated.

The prevalence of impaired kidney function in adult patients with SCA has been reported to be between 4% and 7%, based on abnormal serum creatinine values. Reduced GFR is more common in hemoglobin SS patients than in patients with hemoglobin SC disease. Caution should be exercised, however, when the assessment of kidney function in SCA patients is based on the serum creatinine norms for healthy individuals. SCA patients have a lower muscle mass than healthy individuals, and serum creatinine values are lower in SCA than in healthy controls. Therefore, serum creatinine values above 1.0 to 1.1 mg/dL could be abnormal in this population. The determination of the creatinine clearance from a 24-hour urine collection or the estimation of the creatinine clearance from the Cockroft-Gault formula or MDRD equation (see Chapter 2) could be extremely valuable in this population.

Pathology

Early descriptions of the pathological features of SCA individuals with heavy proteinuria emphasized the occurrence of a membranoproliferative glomerulonephritis, possibly a reflection of an unrecognized infection-related glomerulonephritis. Current reports indicate that focal segmental glomerulosclerosis (FSGS) rather than membranoproliferative glomerulonephritis predominates in proteinuric SCA individuals. Quantitative morphometric analysis of biopsy specimens obtained in this population show a significant increase in glomerular diameter and cross-sectional area compared with age-matched autopsy controls. These observations are in accord with the conventional histologic findings of FSGS in SCA, which include hypertrophy of unaffected glomeruli, segmental sclerotic lesions that are more prominent in juxtamedullary nephrons and in the perihilar region, global nephrosclerosis, and tubular atrophy with interstitial fibrosis in regions downstream from the affected glomeruli. As with other cases of FSGS, minor deposits of immunoglobulin M (IgM), Clq, and C3 may be found in sclerotic areas on immunofluorescence, but immune complex deposits are absent on electron microscopy. Electron-lucent subendothelial expansion with mesangial interposition is observed in some cases.

Treatment

Because of the findings of proteinuria and focal glomerulosclerosis, angiotensin-converting enzyme (ACE) inhibitors are a logical choice in patients with sickle cell glomerulopathy. In proteinuric patients with mild to moderate impairment of kidney function, low-dose enalapril (5–10 mg/day), given over a 2-week period, has been observed to produce a 50% reduction in proteinuria, without lowering GFR or reducing systemic blood pressure. The efficacy of ACE inhibitors over the long term has not been studied. In patients with microalbuminuria, ACE inhibitors also reduce albumin excretion when given short term, but the long-term use of ACE inhibition in microalbuminuric patients has not been studied.

Hypertension, even in relative terms, should be treated to achieve blood pressure levels below 130/80 mm Hg. Diuretics should be avoided as initial antihypertensive agents, because they may cause volume depletion and precipitate sickle cell crises. Patients may also benefit from moderate protein restriction, 0.7 to 0.8 g/kg/day, although the benefit of protein restriction has not been proved (see Chapters 58 and 63). In patients with more advanced chronic kidney disease, potassium levels should be followed closely. Many SCA patients have selective tubular excretion defects for potassium, which can be worsened by ACE inhibitor therapy. Other potentially nephrotoxic drugs such as nonsteroidal anti-inflammatory drugs should be avoided. Metabolic acidosis can be treated with alkali supplementation. Erythropoietin has been used with moderate success to correct worsening anemia and reduce the need for transfusions.

Patients who develop kidney failure and endstage renal disease can be successfully treated with dialysis or transplantation. The reported survival of SCA patients on dialysis is very poor, with a median survival of only 2 years, although there is a clinical impression that survival has improved lately. In transplanted patients, data from the United States Renal Data System (USRDS) database (see Chapter 62) indicate that the 1-year kidney allograft survival of SCA individuals is similar to that of non-SCA African-American recipients (78% versus 77%), but their 3-year allograft survival is lower (48% versus 60%, respectively). SCA recipients tolerate immunosuppressive treatment relatively well, but the frequency of sickle pain crises is higher after successful transplantation. Caution should be used with antilymphocyte preparations to prevent or treat acute rejections, because they could precipitate acute vaso-occlusive episodes or the acute chest syndrome. Despite these potential drawbacks, USRDS data indicate a trend toward better survival in transplanted patients, as compared with patients who remain on the transplant waiting list. Quite apart from survival data, quality of life is better with transplantation. Thus, patients with SCA-related kidney failure should be fully informed of the risks but encouraged to undergo transplant evaluation. A high level of panel-reactive antibodies due to repeated prior blood transfusions may significantly prolong the wait time for transplantation. The high prevalence of stroke, iron overload, and other disorders, however, makes careful screening essential.

RENAL CONCENTRATING DEFECTS

One of the most common renal abnormalities in SCA is an inability to maximally concentrate the urine. The hypertonic and relatively hypoxic environment in the renal medulla is conducive to sickling in the vasa recta. Obstruction of flow and the associated concentration defect can be reversed by early transfusion, which reduces the number of sickled cells. By age 15, however, the concentration defect is fixed and associated with fibrosis and obliteration of the medullary vasa recta with papillary shortening, as shown by microangiographic studies. Impairment of vasa recta flow interferes with the formation of the medullary urea and sodium gradient necessary for water reabsorption along those segments of the nephron. Patients with SCA cannot achieve urinary osmolalities above 400 mOsm/kg and have obligatory water losses of 1.5 to 2.0 L/day. A less severe defect occurs in patients with sickle cell trait. Maximal urinary concentration in older children and young adults with Hb AS is 800 mOsm/kg and reaches 450 to 500 mOsm/kg in older individuals. Therefore, SCA patients should drink 2 to 3 liters of water daily to prevent dehydration that could precipitate sickle cell pain crises. The free-water clearance and urinary diluting ability is preserved in SCA.

HEMATURIA

Hematuria is a relatively common manifestation of SCA and may occur in both sickle cell trait and Hb SS disease. Hematuria is usually painless and originates from the left kidney in about 70% to 80% of cases, but can be bilateral in about 10% of cases. It results from sickling in the vasa recta, causing microinfarctions or severe stasis in peritubular capillaries with extravasation into the renal parenchyma and collecting system. The differential diagnosis includes glomerulonephritis, nephrolithiasis, renal papillary necrosis, urinary tract infections, and urological malignancies. Initial episodes should be evaluated thoroughly to rule out malignancies. Once the initial workup has been negative, subsequent episodes may be treated without performing imaging studies, but periodic reevaluation may be necessary because of the longer life expectancy of SCA patients and the possibility of a higher frequency of renal medullary carcinoma in this population.

The treatment is bed rest and forced diuresis with hypotonic intravenous fluid administration to decrease the tendency to clot formation in the urinary system. Alkalinization of the urine or diuretics can also be used to reduce medullary sickling. The benign nature and the possible relapsing nature of the condition should be explained to patients to avoid unnecessary procedures. In persistent cases, ε-aminocaproic acid (EACA) at a dose of 4 to 12 g/day in four divided doses can be administered. When EACA is used, a high urinary flow rate should be maintained to avoid clot formation in the renal collecting system. Chronic relapsing hematuria can be treated with exchange transfusion, EACA administration, iron supplementation, and the avoidance of strenuous physical activity. Severe cases may require selective embolization, but nephrectomy is only warranted in case of life-threatening hemorrhage because of the tendency to recurrence in the contralateral kidney.

RENAL PAPILLARY NECROSIS

Renal papillary necrosis is a very common manifestation of SCA, because intravenous pyelography demonstrates unilateral or bilateral papillary necrosis in as many as 67% of unselected patients without a prior history of urinary symptoms. Papillary necrosis is usually asymptomatic but may present with microscopic hematuria or renal colic. It results from localized medullary ischemia and necrosis of the medullary tip as a result of obliteration of the medullary vessels from sickling. The diagnosis is made with intravenous pyelography or ultrasound. Radiographically, there are irregularities in the renal calyces, with formation of a sinus tract that with time progresses to complete sequestration of the affected area, producing the radiographic "ring sign." In late stages, there is "clubbing" due to the sloughing or reabsorption of the papillae. By ultrasound, there is increased echogenicity of the inner medulla. In more advanced cases, a filling defect in the area of the medullary tip can be seen. In symptomatic patients with renal papillary necrosis, an associated urinary tract infection should be ruled out. In contrast to other forms of renal papillary necrosis, the prognosis for long-term renal function is good (see also Chapter 50). Nonsteroidal anti-inflammatory drugs should be avoided.

ACIDIFICATION AND POTASSIUM EXCRETION DEFECTS

Under normal conditions, most SCA patients have normal acid-base balance or a mild respiratory alkalosis. Metabolic acidosis can occur when SCA patients are given an acute acid load or when they are stressed by intercurrent illness such as diarrhea that results in gastrointestinal bicarbonate loss. This incomplete form of distal renal tubular acidosis (RTA) results from an inability to lower the urinary pH below 5.3 (normal response less than 5.0), with a resultant decrease in titratable acid and ammonium excretion. Proximal tubular bicarbonate reabsorption is normal.

Other variants have been described. Some patients with SCA, including sickle cell trait, may develop a hyperkalemic hyperchloremic metabolic acidosis. In some patients, selective aldosterone deficiency or hyporeninemic hypoaldosteronism leads to hyperkalemia, impaired ammoniagenesis, and proton retention despite a normal ability to lower urine pH. Other patients have hyperkalemic distal RTA, an inability to generate the tubular transepithelial electrical gradient that permits normal potassium or proton secretion. Treatment is with sodium bicarbonate, a low-potassium diet, mineralocorticoids, and loop diuretics.

OTHER TUBULAR ABNORMALITIES

Proximal tubular transport processes are typically increased in patients with SCA, but usually with little clinical significance. In some patients, hyperphosphatemia may occur as a result of increased proximal tubular phosphate reabsorption. Uric acid excretion is increased as a result of an increased red blood cell turnover rate and an increase in uric acid production. Even so, gout is uncommon in SCA.

RENAL MEDULLARY CARCINOMA

Recent reports suggest an increased incidence of renal medullary carcinoma in SCA patients. This rare, highly aggressive tumor occurs in young people; the reported age at diagnosis ranges from the second to the fifth decade. The tumor arises in the medulla, but in the reported series, it had already extended beyond the capsule, and metastases were present at diagnosis. Presenting findings are hematuria, abdominal pain, flank mass, or weight loss. Diagnosis requires demonstration by renal imaging studies such as a computed tomography (CT) scan followed by excision. Chromosomal abnormalities in the tumor tissue have been localized to chromosome 11 and, less often, to chromosome 3. Interestingly, the former is the locus of the gene encoding the hemoglobin β-chain. The latter is the site of the mutation for von Hippel-Lindau syndrome, which is also associated with renal cell carcinoma. Renal medullary carcinoma has a poor prognosis. In one study, mean survival after excision was only 15 weeks (range 2 to 52 weeks). Neither radiotherapy nor chemotherapy has proven useful. The available studies are retrospective, and clinical details were not available for all patients. Thus, these findings require confirmation in more carefully conducted studies. Nevertheless, a urologic evaluation should be performed in patients with SCA presenting with hematuria or abdominal pain, but screening asymptomatic SCA patients with CT or ultrasonography to uncover urologic malignancies is not indicated.

BIBLIOGRAPHY

Allon M, Lawson L, Eckman JR, et al: Effects of nonsteroidal anti-inflammatory drugs on renal function in sickle cell anemia. Kidney Int 34:500–506, 1988.

Batlle D, Itsarayoungyuen K, Arruda JA, Kurtzman NA: Hyperkalemic hyperchloremic metabolic acidosis in sickle cell hemoglobinopathies. Am J Med 72:188–192, 1982.

Falk RJ, Scheinman J, Phillips G, et al: Prevalence and pathologic features of sickle cell nephropathy and response to inhibition of angiotensin-converting enzyme. N Engl J Med 326:910–915, 1992.

Figenshau RS, Easier JW, Ritter JH, et al: Renal medullary carcinoma. J Urol 159:711–713, 1998.

Guasch A, Cua M, Mitch WE: Extent and the course of glomerular injury in patients with sickle cell anemia. Kidney Int 49:786–791, 1996.

Guasch A, Cua M, You W, Mitch WE: Sickle cell anemia causes a distinct pattern of glomerular dysfunction. Kidney Int 51:826–833, 1997.

Guasch A, Zayas CF, Eckman JR, Elsas L: Evidence that microdeletions in the α globin gene protect against the development of sickle cell glomerulopathy, J Am Soc Nephrol 10:1014–1019, 1999.

McBurney PG, Hanevold CD, Hernadez CM, et al: Risk factors for microalbuminuria in children with sickle cell anemia. J Pediatr Hematol Oncol 24:473–477, 2002.

Ojo AO, Govaerts TC, Schmouder RL, et al: Renal transplantation in endstage sickle cell nephropathy. Transplantation 67:291–295, 1999.

Pandya KK, Koshy M, Brown N, Presman D: Renal papillary necrosis in sickle cell hemoglobinopathies. J Urol 115:497–501, 1976.

Pegelow CH, Colangelo L, Steinberg M, et al: Natural history of blood pressure in sickle cell disease: Risks for stroke and death associated with relative hypertension in sickle cell anemia. Am J Med 102:171–177, 1997.

Pham PT, Pham PC, Wilkinson AH, Lew SQ: Renal abnormalities in sickle cell disease. Kidney Int 57:1–8, 2000.

Powars DR, Elliot-Mills DD, Chan L, et al: Chronic renal failure in sickle cell disease: Risk factors, clinical course, and mortality. Ann Intern Med 115:614–620, 1991.

Saborio P, Scheinman JI: Sickle cell nephropathy. J Am Soc Nephrol 10:187–192, 1999.

Statius van Eps LW, Pinedo-Veels C, Vries GH, de Koning J: Nature of concentrating defect in sickle-cell nephropathy. Micro-radioangiographic studies. Lancet 1:450–452, 1970.

Wigfall DR, Ware RE, Burchinal MR, et al: Prevalence and clinical correlates of glomerulopathy in children with sickle cell disease. J Pediatr 136:749–753, 2000.

Zayas CF, Platt J, Eckman JR, et al: Prevalence and predictors of glomerular involvement in sickle cell anemia [Abstract]. J Am Soc Nephrol 7:1401, 1996.

CHAPTER 45

Polycystic and Other Cystic Kidney Diseases

Dana Rizk   Arlene B. Chapman

Significant advances have been made in our understanding of the genetics and molecular pathogenesis of inherited cystic disorders of the kidney (Table 45-1). Genes responsible for all but one of these diseases have now been identified. Final common pathways are involved in the formation and development of a variety of kidney cysts.

AUTOSOMAL-DOMINANT POLYCYSTIC KIDNEY DISEASE

Autosomal-dominant polycystic kidney disease (ADPKD) is the most common inherited kidney disease, affecting 1 in 400 to 1000 live births. Although the proportion of cases of endstage renal disease (ESRD) resulting from this disease differs among races, the prevalence of ADPKD is similar in all ethnic groups. ADPKD accounts for 5% of the ESRD population in the United States and Europe.

Pathogenesis

At least two responsible genes (*PKD1* and *PKD2*) have been identified in the heterogenetic disorder of ADPKD. Whether ADPKD in a given family is due to mutations in *PKD1* or *PKD2* has prognostic implications, in that PKD2 patients develop renal cysts, hypertension, and ESRD at a later age than do PKD1 patients.

Families with ADPKD not linked to *PKD1* or *PKD2* have been reported, but a third locus for ADPKD has not yet been identified. In 85% of affected families, the disorder is linked to a mutation in the *PKD1* gene located on the short arm of chromosome 16 (16p13.3). *PKD1* codes for an integral membrane protein (polycystin 1) made up of 4304 amino acids with as yet an incompletely defined function. Currently, its known properties are those of a ligand with extracellular interactions and cell cycle regulation. It is localized in the membrane, specifically in the base and tip of the cilia of epithelial cells. Mutations in the *PKD2* gene located on the long arm of chromosome 4 (4q.21.2) account for 15% of affected families. *PKD2* codes for a 968–amino acid protein (polycystin 2), structurally similar to polycystin 1. It colocalizes with poly-

cystin 1 in cilia and independently in the membrane of the endoplasmic reticulum. Polycystin 2 belongs to the family of voltage-activated calcium channels and is involved in intracellular calcium regulation through multiple pathways. The physical interaction of polycystins 1 and 2 is required for the normal functioning of the calcium channel. Polycystin 1 and 2 in the primary cilium of renal epithelial cells functions as mechanical sensors. Primary cilia create a transmembrane calcium current in the presence of stretch or luminal flow. The pathophysiologic role of both polycystins in the development of cysts remains speculative. One model suggests that polycystin 1 and 2 interacts to raise intracellular calcium, which initiates a signaling cascade leading to vesicle fusion and change in gene transcription. Another model suggests that the two polycystins affect cell proliferation, differentiation, and fluid secretion through either a G protein– or JAK-STAT–mediated signaling pathway.

The clinical hallmark of ADPKD is massive cystic enlargement of the kidneys. Renal cysts are lined by epithelial cells and arise from the renal tubules and collecting system. A small portion of all nephrons is affected (less than 5%). Approximately 75% of cysts detach from the parent nephron. This is more common when cyst size exceeds 2 cm. The renal cysts are clonal, with somatic mutations in both *PKD1* and *PKD2* genes present, indicating that a "second hit" is involved in cyst growth and development.

Diagnosis

Autosomal-dominant polycystic kidney disease is diagnosed in at-risk individuals by ultrasonography. The presence of enlarged kidneys with multiple cysts is required for the diagnosis. Age-specific recommendations for a positive diagnosis have been developed with reference to patients from PKD1 families. The presence of two cysts bilaterally in an at-risk individual under 30 years of age demonstrates 99% specificity and sensitivity for the presence of ADPKD. For those over 30 and under 60 years of age, four cysts bilaterally are necessary for the same level of diagnostic precision. For those over 60 years of age,

TABLE 45-1 Demographic Characteristics of Inherited Cystic Diseases of the Kidney

Disease	Frequency	Chromosome	Gene Locus	Protein	Function
ADPKD	1:400	16p13.3	*PKD1*	Polycystin 1	Receptor?
	1:1000	4q21.2	*PKD2*	Polycystin 2	Cation channel
ARPKD	1:20,000	6q24.2	*PKHD*	Fibrocystin/polyductin	Receptor
VHL	1:35,000	3p25	*VHL*	VHL	Tumor suppressor
TSC	1:6000	9p34.3	*TSC1*	Hamartin	Tumor suppressor
		16p13.3	*TSC2*	Tuberin	

ADPKD, autosomal-dominant polycystic kidney disease; ARPKD, autosomal-recessive polycystic kidney disease; TSC, tuberous sclerosis complex; VHL, von Hippel-Lindau.

more than four cysts bilaterally are needed for a positive diagnosis. In the 10% to 15% of ADPKD individuals who do not have a family history, more strict criteria are required for a diagnosis. At least five cysts bilaterally and a phenotype consistent with ADPKD (see later) must be present. A negative ultrasound by the age of 20 implies a likelihood of disease inheritance below 10%, whereas a negative ultrasound at age 30 implies a likelihood below 5%. When disease status must be determined with greater certainty (i.e., evaluation of a donor for living related transplantation), computed tomography (CT) scans or magnetic resonance imaging (MRI) are often more informative. Genetic testing may be required.

Gene linkage analysis can be performed if DNA from at least three affected family members is available. Mutation screening in a single individual is commercially available to determine if mutations are present in *PKD1* or *PKD2* genes. Currently, the success rate of detecting mutations in the *PKD2* and *PKD1* genes in previously diagnosed ADPKD individuals is 90% and 75%, respectively. Direct sequencing is the most accurate and reliable method to screen for the presence of mutations; however, expense is a limiting factor.

Renal Manifestations and Complications

Because kidney enlargement is always a feature of ADPKD, individuals with multiple cysts and small kidneys do not have this disorder. Significant progression of cyst growth and development precedes loss of kidney function (Fig. 45-1). The volume of ADPKD kidneys usually exceeds 1000 mL (normal, 150 mL) before a drop in glomerular filtration rate (GFR) is detectable. Cyst expansion leads to stretching and narrowing of neighboring intrarenal vessels, causing ischemia and activation of the renin-angiotensin-aldosterone system. Interstitial fibrosis may also be related to the release of cytokines from the cysts, causing inflammation.

Flank and back pain are common complaints in affected individuals, usually from massive enlargement of the kidneys and/or liver. The etiology of chronic pain is complicated and multifactorial. Cyst hemorrhage is common as kidneys enlarge. Site-specific pain is common with cyst hemorrhage and may be associated with hematuria or fever. This diagnosis is usually a clinical one. However, if needed, a CT scan can be helpful by revealing a hyperdense cyst. Pain related to cyst hemorrhage is treated with analgesics, bed rest, and hydration, which may shorten the duration of hemorrhage. There may be benefit to aggressive management of cyst hemorrhage, since hematuria in general is associated with a poorer renal outcome.

Renal cyst infection may also present with pain and requires prolonged courses of treatment (up to 4 weeks) with antibiotics that penetrate cysts adequately, such as trimethoprim-sulfamethoxazole, a fluoroquinolone such as ciprofloxacin, chloramphenicol, or vancomycin. Other antibiotics such as cephalosporins or aminoglycosides used to treat pyelonephritis will not adequately penetrate renal cysts. Blood cultures identify the infecting organism more often than urine cultures.

Hematuria, whether gross or microscopic, is associated with increased kidney size and is a negative predictor for renal outcome in ADPKD. Hematuria may be due to cyst hemorrhage, cystitis, cyst or kidney infection, and

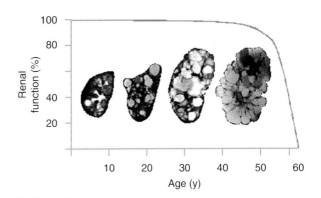

FIGURE 45-1 Demonstration of age-dependent progression in autosomal-dominant polycystic kidney disease in individuals with intact kidney function. Kidney volume increases tremendously over 4 decades with no loss of glomerular filtration rate.

nephrolithiasis. Nephrolithiasis affects as many as 20% of patients, with the presence of calcium oxalate and urate stones being the most common. Medullary deformities secondary to cysts and hypocitraturia (present in two thirds of patients) may contribute to stone formation.

A decrease in renal concentrating ability is one of the earliest manifestations of ADPKD and has direct treatment implications (see later) The concentrating defect is mild and declines with age and level of kidney function in ADPKD. Proteinuria occurs in one third of patients and is usually less than 1 g/24 hours, consistent with other tubulointerstitial disorders. In individuals whose urine protein excretion exceeds 2 g/24 hours, evaluation for other kidney diseases is warranted. Although low levels are present in ADPKD, albuminuria and proteinuria are independent predictors of poor renal outcome.

Hypertension is a common and early manifestation of ADPKD, occurring in 60% of patients with normal kidney function. The mean age of onset is 31, with men demonstrating higher blood pressure than women. Polycystin expression is present in vascular smooth muscle cells, and PKD mutations may contribute directly to the hypertensive state or vasculopathy. The renin-angiotensin system is activated early in the course of ADPKD, presumably secondary to cyst expansion, resulting in bilateral intrarenal ischemia. Hypertension contributes to an accelerated loss of kidney function and should be treated aggressively. Currently there is no evidence that angiotensin-converting enzyme (ACE) inhibitors or angiotensin receptor blockers (ARBs) are more effective than other antihypertensive agents in retarding progression to ESRD in ADPKD; however, ACE inhibitors increase renal blood flow and are more effective than calcium channel blockers in reversing left ventricular hypertrophy in ADPKD.

The mean age of onset of ESRD in ADPKD is 53 years for PKD1 patients and 69 years for PKD2 patients. Importantly, ADPKD individuals maintain normal GFR for decades with significant cyst and kidney enlargement occurring before loss of kidney function (see Fig. 45-1). Once kidney function is impaired, progression is universal, with an average decline in GFR of 4.0 to 5.0 mL/minute/year. Negative prognostic indicators for the progression to ESRD include male gender in PKD2 individuals, the presence of hypertension, increased kidney size or volume, and increased urinary protein or albumin excretion.

No contraindications to kidney transplantation are specific to ADPKD, and transplanted patients with ESRD due to ADPKD survive longer than patients transplanted due to other causes of ESRD. Potential transplant recipients are screened for the possible presence of an intracranial aneurysm. Native polycystic kidneys do not have to be removed before transplantation unless chronic infections are present or their large size interferes with nutrition or quality of life.

Extrarenal Manifestations

Polycystic Liver Disease

Hepatic cysts are the most common extrarenal manifestation in ADPKD. Liver cysts are usually detected approximately 10 years after renal cysts first appear. Hepatic function is preserved even in the presence of massive cystic disease, and biochemical tests are normal except for a mild elevation in serum alkaline phosphatase. Hepatic enlargement is the predominant complication of polycystic liver disease (PKLD), resulting in symptoms of shortness of breath, pain, early satiety, decreased mobility, ankle swelling, and, rarely, inferior vena cava compression. This severe form of PKLD predominantly affects women and may require surgical cyst deroofing, fenestration and resection, or transplantation. Isolated autosomal-dominant PKLD independent of ADPKD has been reported and linked to a gene mutation on chromosome 19.

Cardiovascular Manifestations

Intracranial aneurysms (ICA) occur in 4% to 8% of asymptomatic ADPKD patients. Other vascular abnormalities, including intracoronary aneurysms, may also be present. ICA cluster in ADPKD families and occur in 10% of individuals with a family history of a nonruptured ICA and 20% of individuals with a family history of a ruptured ICA. The aneurysms occur most often in the anterior circulation, similar to the general population; however, multiple ICA are common in ADPKD, similar to non-ADPKD familial ICA. Individuals who underwent screening with magnetic resonance angiography (MRA) and were aneurysm-free did not demonstrate new ICA when screened 7 years later.

Rupture of an ICA is associated with more than 50% immediate mortality and more than 80% permanent morbidity. Screening is indicated in asymptomatic patients with a positive family history for ICA, previous history of intracranial hemorrhage, those with high-risk occupations, or before major elective surgery that would affect intracranial hemodynamics. The imaging modality of choice for screening is time-of-flight three-dimensional MRA.

Although rupture of an ICA is associated with significant morbidity and mortality, only 50% of individuals with ICA will have a rupture during their lifetimes. Postoperative complications related to surgical clipping are common, and recovery from elective surgery can be prolonged. For larger aneurysms (greater than 10 mm), the risk of rupture is significant and elective surgical intervention is recommended. In those individuals with ICA smaller than 5 mm, longitudinal studies have not demonstrated significant growth of the ICA and the risk of rupture is relatively small. At present, the specific indications for repair of these smaller ICA are unclear. With the development of less invasive and safer therapies (coiling or stenting), potential approaches to successful treatment of small asymptomatic ICA may become available. Mitral valve prolapse (MVP) and regurgitation is common in ADPKD, occurring in 26% of individuals as compared with 3% of the general population. Aortic insufficiency also occurs more frequently (11%) in ADPKD.

Pregnancy

Overall, fertility rates in ADPKD men and women are similar to those in the general population despite a higher incidence of ectopic pregnancies, congenital absence of the seminiferous tubules, and amotile spermatozoa. Affected women with normal GFR and normal blood pressure have pregnancy outcomes similar to those of the general population. Hypertensive ADPKD women have a higher incidence of worsening hypertension, preeclampsia, and prematurity. Those with decreased GFR before pregnancy are at high risk for midtrimester fetal loss.

Autosomol-Dominant Polycystic Kidney Disease in Children

Renal manifestations of ADPKD in children are similar to adults. Typically 40% of at-risk individuals are diagnosed asymptomatically as part of a family screening program. Children present more often with diffuse abdominal pain as opposed to flank or back pain. Hypertension is common, occurring in 10% to 15% of affected children, and loss of nocturnal decline in blood pressure occurs in approximately one third of affected children. Cerebral aneurysms have been described, albeit rarely, in this age group. At-risk offspring should have their blood pressure and urinalysis monitored regularly. However, there are as yet no recommendations for a presymptomatic diagnosis for ADPKD.

Therapy

Treatment of ADPKD individuals with ACE inhibitors, rigorous blood pressure control, and dietary protein restriction have failed to demonstrate renoprotection. However, studies have thus far been inadequately designed or powered to definitely determine if these therapies are ineffective. Therefore, current recommendations for target blood pressure level and the initial drug of choice are based on the Seventh Joint National Committee (JNC7) recommendations for other kidney disease patients with hypertension: below 130/80 mm Hg and an ACE inhibitor or angiotensin receptor blocker. Recently, promising therapy aimed at reducing intracellular cyclic adenosine monophosphate (cAMP) accumulation by blocking the vasopressin V2 receptor has successfully retarded renal cyst progression in four distinct genetic forms of cystic disease: the PKD2 transheterozygote mouse, the Han:SPRD rat (acquired cystic disease), the

pcy mouse (homologous to human FJN 3), and the pck rat (homologous to human ARPKD). These results suggest that therapies may soon be available for individuals with ADPKD.

AUTOSOMAL-RECESSIVE POLYCYSTIC KIDNEY DISEASE

Autosomal-recessive polycystic kidney disease (ARPKD) affects approximately 1 in 20,000 individuals. At-risk offspring have a 25% chance of being affected. ARPKD has been linked to a mutation in the *PKHD1* gene on the short arm of chromosome 6 (6p21.1). The protein product is a 4074–amino acid protein called polyductin or fibrocystin, characterized by a single transmembrane segment and a short cytoplasmic C terminal. No other causative gene has been identified. This protein is thought to act as a membrane receptor involved in transducing intracellular signals. Similar to the PKD1 and PKD2 gene products, polyductin colocalizes to primary epithelial cilia usually at its base.

Autosomal-recessive polycystic kidney disease is characterized by ectatic dilatation of the distal collecting ducts leading to renal "cysts." Mutations have been identified in the *PKHD1* gene in approximately 60% of affected individuals. The majority of mutations are heterogeneic, with the most severe disease associated with homozygous mutations that predict immediate stop codons. Congenital hepatic fibrosis is a universal feature of ARPKD and often predominates in children who survive the perinatal period.

Clinical Features

Prenatally, the disease is diagnosed by the presence of echogenic, enlarged kidneys. Poor prognostic indicators for survival include oligohydramnios, with resultant lung hypoplasia and compressed (Potter) facies. Perinatal death is usually due to respiratory failure secondary to delayed pulmonary development and difficulties with ventilation due to large kidneys. In a contemporary series from 34 centers of 166 ARPKD infants born after 1990, 50% of whom were diagnosed prenatally, 74.7% survived the neonatal period. Among those children who died, respiratory failure and sepsis were the most common causes of death.

In infancy, affected children present with pneumomediastinum, pneumothorax, hypertension, cardiac hypertrophy, congestive heart failure from endomyocardial fibrosis, and impaired kidney function. In the most recent series, 40% required mechanical ventilation at birth and 12% developed chronic lung disease. Beyond infancy, a number of clinical features are present. Growth retardation occurs in approximately 25% of patients. Hypertension is common, occurring in more than 60% of individuals. Chronic kidney disease is present in 42%, with an additional 21% requiring dialysis or transplantation. Hepatic fibrosis, as well as portal hypertension and its complications (ascending cholangitis and variceal bleeding), predominate as ARPKD individuals become older.

Treatment

Hypertension should be treated with salt restriction and ACE inhibitors, aiming for a blood pressure below the 75th percentile for age and gender. Adequate anemia and growth management should be addressed in all ARPKD children with decreased kidney function. Dialysis should be offered when needed. Liver involvement rarely leads to hepatocellular damage or synthetic dysfunction, but portal hypertension usually develops between the ages of 5 and 10. Therapy includes portosystemic shunts for severe varices, and ARPKD children are candidates for liver or combined liver and kidney transplantation in advanced cases.

TUBEROUS SCLEROSIS COMPLEX

Tuberous sclerosis complex (TSC) affects 40,000 Americans and about 2 million people worldwide and has a prevalence of up to 1 in 6000 individuals. It is an autosomal-dominant disorder with a high rate of spontaneous mutations (65% to 75% of patients), particularly in those with mutations in the *TSC2* gene. Patients with defects in the *TSC1* gene seem to demonstrate less severe disease and a lower rate of spontaneous mutations.

Two genes leading to the tuberous sclerosis clinical phenotype have been identified. *TSC1* is located on the long arm of chromosome 9 (9q34) and is responsible for the protein product hamartin. *TSC2* is on the short arm of chromosome 16 (16p13.3), and its protein product is tuberin. This gene is only 48 base pairs away from the *PKD1* gene, and a contiguous deletion of both *TSC2* and *PKD1* genes leads to the severe phenotype of very early onset polycystic kidney disease. The *TSC* genes are tumor suppressor genes that coassemble and interact with each other. No phenotypic features distinguish TSC1 from TSC2 patients. Many of the tumors in TSC show a loss of heterozygosity, suggesting a "two-hit" process. Genetic mosaicism has been documented and includes somatic mutations (not found in all cell lines) or germline mutations (found only in gonadal cells and hence transmitted to all offspring while parents are spared from any disease manifestation). The hamartin-tuberin complex appears to antagonize an insulin signaling pathway that may play an important role in the regulation of cell size, cell number, and organ size. Activation of the mTOR metabolic pathway is associated with the growth of tuberous sclerosis lesions, suggesting that rapamycin or their analogues might be useful in the treatment of this disease.

In July 1998, the National Institutes of Health sponsored a consensus conference of international experts to review the literature on TSC and to determine diagnostic criteria. Major skin manifestations included facial angiofibromas (adenoma sebaceum), ungal or periungal fibromas, hypomelanotic macules, and shagreen patches (connective tissue nevi). Retinal hamartomas are the most common ocular manifestation. Central nervous system findings include cortical tubers, subependymal nodules, or giant cell astrocytomas. Epilepsy is the most common neurologic manifestation, and when it starts early, carries a poor prognosis marking cognitive impairment.

Cardiac rhabdomyoma is a rare manifestation that can be detected prenatally by ultrasonography. Lymphangiomyomatosis is a progressive lung pathology seen almost exclusively in females of reproductive age. Renal angiomyolipomas occur in 70% to 80% of affected individuals and are detected based on their fat content by CT or MRI. The significant complication from these lesions is bleeding, especially when they reach 4 cm in size. A definite diagnosis of TSC entails the presence of any two of the major features just mentioned.

VON HIPPEL-LINDAU DISEASE

Von Hippel-Lindau (VHL) disease is a rare autosomal-dominant disorder affecting 1 in 35,000 individuals. VHL disease is clinically characterized by the development of benign and malignant tumors in multiple organs. Benign cysts of the kidneys, pancreas, and epididymis are common and rarely lead to renal and/or pancreatic dysfunction or infertility, respectively. The lifetime risk of renal cell carcinoma (RCC) is greater than 70%. These are clear-cell silent tumors that are widely metastatic by the time patients have symptoms. Therefore, the management strategy includes annual screening of patients with CT, ultrasonography, or both. The treatment of choice remains parenchymal-sparing renal surgery. Other common manifestations are hemangioblastomas, which are highly vascular, nonmetastatic, noninvading tumors that occur almost exclusively in the cerebellum, the spinal cord, or the brain stem. They affect 21% to 72% of VHL patients and are often multiple. Compression of adjacent neurologic structures determines the presenting symptoms. Surgical intervention is the treatment of choice, with or without radiation therapy. Patients should be screened annually for these tumors using gadolinium-enhanced MRI. Other common tumors include retinal angiomas (50%) that can lead to retinal detachment and blindness. These are treated by laser photocoagulation. Endolymphatic sac tumors (10%) that arise from the membranous labyrinth of the inner ear are usually bilateral, leading to vertigo, tinnitus, and hearing loss. Current therapeutic recommendations are surgical. Pheochromocytomas are seen in 7% to 20% of patients, tend to occur at a younger age, and are often bilateral, multiple, and extra-adrenal. Patients with suggestive symptoms should be screened biochemically and radiologically for pheochromocytomas. Asymptomatic patients scheduled for any elective surgery also should be screened, to prevent fatal complications associated with anesthesia.

Von Hippel-Lindau disease is due to the inactivation of the *VHL* (tumor suppressor) gene located on chromosome 3 (3p25). Affected individuals do not develop the disease without a somatic mutation (second hit). Genetic screening of at-risk family members is considered standard of care. There now appears to be a genotype phenotype relationship in VHL whereby the development of RCC is correlated with a specific missense mutation.

The wild-type *VHL* gene encodes for the VHL protein (pVHL), which, under normoxic conditions, is involved in the degradation of hypoxia-inducible factors such as vascular endothelial growth factor and erythropoietin. In the absence of functional pVHL, these factors accumulate, despite the presence of oxygen, which may explain the vascular nature of the tumors in VHL and the presence of polycythemia as a paraneoplastic syndrome in some cases.

ACQUIRED CYSTIC KIDNEY DISEASE

Acquired cystic kidney disease (ACKD) refers to the development of cysts during a period of chronic kidney disease or ESRD. A finding of three to five cysts in each kidney in the setting of chronic kidney disease is required to make the diagnosis in patients who have small kidneys and lack a family history of ADPKD. Cysts tend to be bilateral, multiple, and usually less than 3 cm in diameter. Between 8% and 13% of patients initiating renal replacement therapy have ACKD, and the prevalence increases with years of renal replacement therapy. The dialysis modality (hemodialysis versus peritoneal dialysis) does not affect the prevalence; however, gender and race do, with African-American men more frequently affected.

Cyst microdissection and analysis suggest that acquired cysts arise from the proximal tubules secondary to epithelial hyperplasia and hypertrophy after nephron loss. Two murine models of proximal cyst formation similar to ACKD exist including the HAN:sprd rat and the cpk mouse. The risk of RCC increases slightly in ACKD, possibly as a result of mutations and dysregulation of proto-oncogenes.

Most patients with ACKD are asymptomatic; however, cyst rupture can lead to hematuria or perinephric hematomas with flank pain. The most feared complication from ACKD is the development of RCC, estimated at 2% to 7%. Whereas most sporadic cases are clear-cell or granular carcinomas, papillary tumors are the most common histologic variety arising in the setting of ACKD.

Ultrasonography is a good screening tool for the diagnosis of ACKD; however, CT and MRI should be performed in patients who develop symptoms suggestive of carcinoma (such as hematuria, unexplained anemia, or back pain), since these modalities are more sensitive in detecting small tumors. Irregular appearance and enhancement with dye usually suggest the presence of a neoplasm. When detected, tumors larger than 3 cm should be treated surgically with total nephrectomy.

Screening of ESRD patients for ACKD is a controversial issue. A decision analysis model revealed that screening provided significant benefits only to patients with a life expectancy of at least 25 years. It may, however, be beneficial to screen high-risk individuals, namely, male African-American patients in good medical condition, who have been on dialysis for more than 3 years, or who have signs and symptoms of ACKD. For transplant candidates, this screening strategy should be considered, although the American Society of Transplantation does not officially recommend either pre- or post-transplant screening for ACKD and/or RCC.

BIBLIOGRAPHY

Belz MM, Fick-Brosnahan GM, Hughes RL, et al: Recurrence of intracranial aneurysms in autosomal dominant polycystic kidney disease. Kidney Int 63:1824–1830, 2003.

Chapman AB, Guay-Woodford LM, Grantham JJ, et al: Renal structure in early autosomal dominant polycystic kidney disease (ADPD): The Consortium for Radiologic Imaging Studies of Polycystic Kidney Disease (CRISP) cohort. Kidney Int 64:1035–1045, 2003.

Choyke PL: Acquired cystic kidney disease. Eur Radiol 10:1716–1721, 2000.

Couch V, Lindor NM, Karnes PS, et al: Von Hippel-Lindau disease. N Engl J Med 75:265–272, 2000.

Dabora SL, Jozwiak S, Franz DN, et al: Mutational analysis in a cohort of 224 tuberous sclerosis patients indicates increased severity of TSC2 compared to TSC1, disease in multiple organs. Am J Hum Genet 68:64–80, 2001.

El-Hashemite N, Zhang H, Henske EP, Kwiatkoski DJ: Mutation in *TSC2* and activation of mammalian target of rapamycin signaling pathway in renal angiomyolipoma. Lancet 361:1348–1349, 2003.

Gattone VH II, Wang X, Harris PC, et al: Inhibition of renal cystic disease development and progression by a vasopressin V2 receptor antagonist. Nat Med 9:1323–1326, 2003.

Guay-Woodford LM, Desmand RA: Autosomal recessive polycystic kidney disease: The clinical experience in North America. Pediatrics 111:1072–1080, 2003.

Hes FJ, McKee S, Taphoorn MJ, et al: Cryptic von Hippel Lindau disease: Germline mutations in patients with hemangioblastoma only. J Med Genet 37:939–943, 2000.

Hyman MH, Whittemore VH: National Institutes of Health consensus conference: Tuberous sclerosis complex. Arch Neurol 57:662–665, 2000.

Kaelin WG Jr: Molecular basis of VHL hereditary cancer syndrome. Nat Rev Cancer 2:673–682, 2002.

Kaplan BS, Kaplan P, Rosenberg HK, et al: Polycystic kidney diseases in childhood. J Pediatr 115:867–880, 1989.

O'Callaghan FJ, Osborne JP: Advances in the understanding of tuberous sclerosis. Arch Dis Child 83:140–142, 2000.

Potter CJ, Huang H, Xu T: Drosophila Tsc1 functions with Tsc2 to antagonize insulin signaling in regulating cell growth, cell proliferation and organ size. Cell 105:357–368, 2001.

Pirson Y, Chauveau D, Torres V: Management of cerebral aneurysms in autosomal dominant polycystic kidney disease. J Am Soc Nephrol 13:269–276, 2002.

Ravine D, Gibson RN, Walker RG, et al: Evaluation of ultrasonographic diagnostic criteria for autosomal dominant polycystic kidney disease 1. Lancet 343:824–827, 1994.

Rossetti S, Turca R, Coto E, et al: A complete mutation screen of *PKDH1* in autosomal recessive polycystic kidney disease (ARPKD) pedigrees. Kidney Int 64:391–403, 2003.

Schrier R, McFann K, Johnson A, et al: Cardiac and renal effects of standard versus rigorous blood pressure control in autosomal dominant polycystic kidney disease: Results of a seven-year prospective randomized study. J Am Soc Nephrol 13:1733–1739, 2002.

Tantravahi J, Steinman TI: Acquired cystic kidney disease. Semin Dial 13:330–334, 2000.

Wiesener MS, Eckardt KU: Erythropoietin, tumours and the von Hippel-Lindau gene: Towards identification of mechanisms and dysfunction of oxygen sensing. Nephrol Dial Transplant 17:356–359, 2002.

Wilson PD: Polycystic kidney disease. N Engl J Med 350:151–162, 2004.

Zhang MJ, Mai W, Li C, et al: PKHD1 protein encoded by the gene for autosomal recessive polycystic kidney disease associates with basal bodies and primary cilia in renal epithelial cells. Proc Natl Acad Sci USA 101:2311–2316, 2004.

CHAPTER 46

Alport's Syndrome and Related Disorders

Martin C. Gregory

Alport's syndrome is a disease of collagen that affects the kidneys always, the ears often, and the eyes occasionally. Cecil Alport described the association of hereditary hematuric nephritis with hearing loss in a family whose affected males died in adolescence. Genetic advances have broadened the scope of the condition to include optical defects, platelet abnormalities, late-onset kidney failure, and normal hearing in some families. At least 85% of kindreds are X-linked, and most or all of those result from a mutation of *COL4A5*, the gene located at chromosome Xq22 that codes for the α5-chain of type IV collagen, or α5(IV). Autosomal-recessive inheritance occurs in perhaps 15% of cases, and autosomal-dominant inheritance has been shown in a few kindreds with associated thrombocytopathy and in rare kindreds without platelet defects.

JUVENILE AND ADULT FORMS

This distinction is fundamental to the understanding of Alport's syndrome. Kidney failure tends to occur at a similar age in all males in a kindred, but this age can differ widely between kindreds. Uremia in males occurs in childhood or adolescence in some families, and in adulthood in others. The familial forms with early onset of kidney failure in affected males are termed "juvenile," and those with kidney failure in middle age are called "adult"-type nephritis. Extrarenal manifestations tend to be more prominent in the juvenile kindreds. Moreover, because males in juvenile kindreds do not commonly survive to reproduce, these kindreds tend to be small and frequently arise from new mutations. Adult-type kindreds are typically much larger, and new mutations occur infrequently.

BIOCHEMISTRY

The open mesh of interlocking molecules of type IV collagen that forms the framework of glomerular basement membrane (GBM) is composed of heterotrimers of α-chains. In fetal life these heterotrimers consists of two α1(IV)-chains and one α2(IV)-chain, but early in postnatal development a switch of production toward α3(IV)-, α4(IV)-, and α5(IV)-chains occurs. The primary chemical defect in Alport's syndrome most commonly involves the α5(IV)-chain, but faulty assembly of the α3,4,5 heterotrimer produces similar pathology in glomerular, aural, and ocular basement membranes regardless of which α-chain is defective. As an illustration of failure of normal heterotrimer formation, most patients whose genetic defect is in the gene coding for the α5(IV)-chain lack demonstrable α3(IV)-chains in GBMs.

CLASSICAL GENETICS

In most kindreds inheritance of Alport's syndrome is X-linked. This was suggested by classical pedigree analysis, strengthened by tight linkage to restriction-fragment-length polymorphism markers (RFLPs), and proven by identification of mutations.

MOLECULAR GENETICS

Causative mutations of *COL4A5*, the gene coding for α5(IV), appear consistently in many kindreds. Deletions, point mutations, and splicing errors occur. There is poor correlation between mutation type and clinical phenotype, but deletions and some splicing errors cause severe kidney disease and early hearing loss. Missense mutations may cause juvenile disease with hearing loss or adult disease with or without hearing loss. Deletions involving the 5' end of the *COL4A5* gene and the 5' end of the adjacent *COL4A6* gene occur consistently in families with esophageal and genital leiomyomatosis.

Homozygotes or mixed heterozygotes for mutations of the *COL4A3* or *COL4A4* genes (chromosome 2) develop autosomal-recessive Alport's syndrome. Heterozygotes for these mutations account for many cases of benign familial hematuria (familial thin basement membrane disease, or TBMD). Patients with autosomal-dominant Alport's syndrome, usually with thrombocytopenia and giant platelets, have mutations of the nonmuscle myosin heavy chain 9 (*MYH9*) gene on chromosome 22.

IMMUNOCHEMISTRY

Males with X-linked Alport's syndrome and patients with autosomal-recessive Alport's syndrome frequently lack the α3-, α4-, and α5-chains of type IV collagen in the GBM, and hemizygous males with X-linked Alport's syndrome often lack α5(IV)-chains in the epidermal basement membrane (EBM). Monoclonal antibodies specific to the α2-chain and α5-chain of type IV collagen are commercially available and can be used to assist in the diagnosis of Alport's syndrome. GBM and EBM of normals and all Alport's patients react with the α2 antibody, but most males and females with autosomal-recessive Alport's syndrome and most males hemizygous for a *COL4A5* mutation show no staining of the GBM with the α5 antibody. X-Linked males also commonly show no staining of EBM with antibody to α5; females heterozygous for a *COL4A5* mutation show interrupted staining of GBM and EBM, consistent with mosaicism.

After transplantation, about 10% of Alport's males develop anti-GBM nephritis, presumably because they are exposed for the first time to normal collagen chains including a normal 26-kD monomer of the α3(IV)-chain to which tolerance has never been acquired. Recurrences of anti-GBM nephritis are usual but not inevitable after retransplantation. The antibodies to GBM developing after transplantation are heterogeneous; all stain normal GBM and some stain EBM.

PATHOLOGY

In young children light microscopy of the kidneys may be normal or near normal. Glomeruli with persisting fetal morphology may be seen. As disease progresses, interstitial and tubular foam cells, which arise for unclear reasons, may become quite prominent, although they can also be found in many other conditions (Fig. 46-1). Eventually progressive glomerulosclerosis and interstitial scarring develop. Routine immunofluorescence examination for immunoglobulins and complement components is negative, but staining for the α5(IV)-chain may be informative (see earlier section on Immunochemistry). The GBM is thickened up to two or three times its normal thickness, split into several irregular layers, and frequently interspersed with numerous electron-dense granules about 40 nm in diameter (Fig. 46-2). In florid cases of juvenile types of disease the lamellae of basement membrane may branch and rejoin in a complex "basket weave" pattern. Early in the development of the lesion, thinning of the GBM may predominate or may be the only abnormality visible. The abnormalities in children or adolescents with adult-type Alport's syndrome may be unimpressive or indistinguishable from those of TBMD disease. See later for further details on thin TBMD disease.

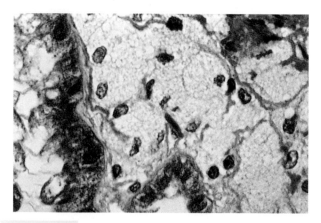

FIGURE 46-1 High-power photomicrograph of foam-filled tubular and interstitial cells in a renal biopsy specimen from a patient with Alport's syndrome. Relatively normal proximal tubular cytoplasm stains red in the tubules on the left and at the bottom. The remaining cells appear "foamy" because of the spaces left where lipids have been eluted during processing.

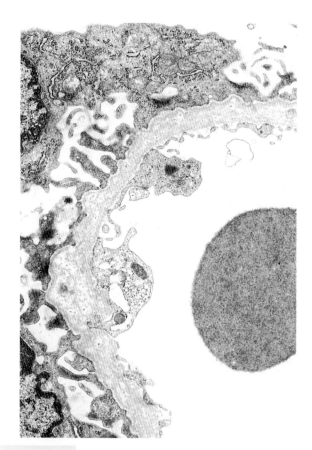

FIGURE 46-2 High-resolution electron micrograph of a glomerular basement membrane (GBM) from a patient with Alport's syndrome. The GBM varies in thickness. It is split into a number of layers, which in some areas are separated by lucent areas containing small, dense granules. (Courtesy of Dr. Theodore J. Pysher.)

CLINICAL FEATURES

Renal Features

Uninterrupted microscopic hematuria occurs from birth in affected males. Hematuria may become visible after exercise or during fever; this is more common in juvenile kindreds. Microscopic hematuria has a penetrance of approximately 90% in heterozygous females in adult-type kindreds. In juvenile kindreds, the penetrance of hematuria in females has been studied less extensively, but it appears to be common. Urinary erythrocytes are dysmorphic, and red cell casts can usually be found in affected males. Proteinuria is very variable; but occasionally it reaches nephrotic levels.

Hemizygous males inevitably progress to endstage renal disease (ESRD). This occurs at widely variable ages that are fairly constant within each family. Heterozygous females are generally much less severely affected. Around one quarter of them will develop ESRD, usually after the age of 50 years, but ESRD in girls in their teens and even younger does occur.

In families with autosomal inheritance, females are affected as severely and as early as males. Kidney failure often occurs before the age of 20 years in homozygotes for autosomal-recessive Alport's syndrome.

Extrarenal Features

Hearing Loss

Bilateral high-frequency cochlear hearing loss is present in many kindreds. X-Linked nephritis progressing to ESRD can occur, however, in families without overt hearing loss. Expectation of hearing loss causes many missed diagnoses. In families with juvenile-type disease, hearing loss is almost universal in male hemizygotes and common in severely affected female heterozygotes.

Patterns of hearing loss are variable. Often the most severe loss is at 2 to 6 kHz but may be at a higher frequency if there has been superimposed noise damage. The loss is also severe at 8 to 20 kHz, but these frequencies are not covered by conventional audiometry. In adult-type Alport's syndrome with hearing loss, there is typically no perceptible deficit until age 20 years, but loss progresses to 60 to 70 dB at 6 to 8 kHz at ages over 40 years. Hearing loss occurs earlier in juvenile kindreds. The rate at which hearing is lost is not well established in juvenile kindreds, but many children of grade-school age or adolescents require hearing aids.

Ocular Defects

Ocular defects appear to be confined to juvenile kindreds. Myopia, arcus juvenilis, and cataracts occur but lack diagnostic specificity. Three changes that are present in a minority of kindreds but that are nearly diagnostic are anterior lenticonus, posterior polymorphous corneal dystrophy, and retinal flecks. Anterior lenticonus is a forward protrusion of the anterior surface of the ocular lens. It results from a weakness of the type IV collagen forming the anterior lens capsule. The resulting irregularity of the surface of the lens causes an uncorrectable refractive error. The retina cannot be clearly seen by ophthalmoscopy, and with a strong positive lens in the ophthalmoscope, the lenticonus can often be seen through a dilated pupil as an "oil drop" or circular smudge on the center of the lens. Retinal flecks are small yellow or white dots scattered around the macula or in the periphery of the retina. If sparse, they may be difficult to distinguish from small, hard exudates. Macular holes occur rarely but can severely affect sight.

Leiomyomatosis

Several X-linked families show the precocious development of striking leiomyomas of the esophagus and female genitalia in association with Alport's syndrome. These tumors are frequently large and multiple. They may bleed or obstruct, and their resection can be difficult. All families described so far have had a deletion at the 5' ends of the contiguous COL4A5 and COL4A6 genes.

DIAGNOSIS

No single clinical feature is pathognomonic. The diagnosis is made by finding hematuria in multiple family members, together with a history of kidney failure in related males, and reinforced by biopsy showing characteristic ultrastructural changes in the proband or a relative. Immunofluorescence examination of the biopsy should include staining with antibodies specific to GBM or to α5(IV); this will help distinguish Alport's syndrome from familial thin GBM disease. In large families without a known mutation, segregation analysis can decide whether a particular individual carries a defective gene. If family members are known to show negative immunofluorescence staining with antibodies to α5(IV), then a skin biopsy examined with these antibodies may be diagnostic.

In families with a previously defined mutation, molecular diagnosis of affected males and gene carrying females is possible. Molecular diagnosis is nearly 100% sensitive and specific but only after a mutation has been found in the family. Sequencing the COL4A5 gene is at least 80% sensitive for mutations, but it is not widely available and will not find mutations in the other causative genes.

The key to diagnosis is to suspect the possibility of Alport's syndrome in any patient with otherwise unexplained hematuria, glomerulopathy, or kidney failure. In many cases, the familial nature of the condition will not be immediately apparent. Inquiry into the family must be detailed and insistent. The patient is usually a young male. Chances are that he knows little of his distant relatives, but his mother will probably know more of the family details. Male relatives linked to the patient through one or more females may have kidney failure. Check urine samples from both the patient's parents, particularly his mother, for microscopic hematuria. Hearing loss is a helpful clue, but it is crucial to remember that hearing loss is neither a sensitive nor a specific marker of Alport's syndrome; it is neither necessary nor sufficient for the diagnosis. Most patients with hearing loss and kidney disease do not have Alport's syndrome but instead a variety of other renal disorders, most often glomerulonephritis, and a more common cause for hearing loss, such as noise exposure, aminoglycoside therapy, or inherited hearing loss unrelated to Alport's syndrome.

TREATMENT

There is no specific treatment for Alport's syndrome. General measures to retard the progression of kidney failure, such as effective treatment of hypertension and modest protein restriction, appear warranted but are unproved. As for other forms of progressive kidney disease, angiotensin-converting enzyme inhibitors and angiotensin receptor blockers may offer a specific advantage, but this has yet to be demonstrated in Alport's syndrome. An unconfirmed report claims benefit from cyclosporine in reducing proteinuria and retarding the progression of kidney disease.

Males should wear hearing protection in noisy surroundings. Hearing aids improve but do not completely correct the hearing loss. Tinnitus is generally resistant to all forms of therapy; hearing aids may make it less disruptive by amplifying ambient sounds. Retinal lesions do not commonly affect vision and require no therapy. The serious impairment of vision caused by lenticonus or cataract cannot be corrected with spectacles or contact lenses. Lens removal with reimplantation of an intraocular lens is standard and satisfactory treatment.

RELATED DISORDERS

Alport's Syndrome with Thrombocytopathy (Epstein's Syndrome)

This uncommon autosomal-dominant variant of Alport's syndrome associates moderate thrombocytopenia with severe hearing loss and kidney failure in both males and females. The platelets (about $7\,\mu m$ in diameter) are much larger than normal ($1-1.5\,\mu m$), and there is a mild or moderate bleeding tendency. In some families there are inclusion bodies (Fechtner bodies) in leukocytes. These syndromes are caused by a mutation in the *MYH9* gene on chromosome 22q12.3–22q13.1.

Autosomal-Recessive Alport's Syndrome

A few children who develop kidney disease before the age of 10 years have homozygous or mixed heterozygous mutations of the genes for the α3(IV)- or α4(IV)-chains of type IV collagen. Boys and girls are equally affected. The heterozygous parents may or may not show hematuria.

Familial Thin Basement Membrane Disease

TBMD or benign familial hematuria is an autosomal-dominant basement membrane glomerulopathy. Many cases result from mutations of the *COL4A3* or *COL4A4* gene at chromosome 2q35–2q37. Ultrastructurally, the GBM is uniformly thinned to about half its normal thickness. There is no disruption or lamellation of the GBM, nor are any other abnormalities of the glomeruli, tubules, vessels, or interstitium visible by light, immunofluorescence, or electron microscopy. Kidney failure does not occur. Longevity is unaffected by this condition, and survivors into the ninth decade are recorded. Minor degrees of lamellation of the GBM and hearing loss have been described in some families, but these families could have had unrecognized Alport's syndrome.

Once the precise diagnosis is established, the patient and family can be spared further invasive tests and an appropriate prognosis given to them and to insurers. Unfortunately, the distinction between Alport's syndrome and benign familial hematuria is not always easy to make. Ascertainment of the pattern of inheritance requires a large pedigree with accurate diagnoses in all the family members. A single mistaken diagnosis from incidental kidney disease, inaccurate urinalysis, or incomplete penetrance may vitiate conclusions about the pattern of inheritance in the entire pedigree. Even biopsy evidence is fallible. Early cases of Alport's syndrome may show ultrastructural changes indistinguishable from those of benign familial hematuria. This is particularly likely to occur if a child from an adult-type Alport's kindred undergoes biopsy examination. Stability of serum creatinine for several years in a child does not exclude adult-type Alport's syndrome. The interpretation is further clouded because members of families with TBMD may present with autosomal-recessive Alport's syndrome. In these families, autosomal-dominant TBMD and autosomal-recessive Alport's syndrome are caused by the same mutations (see earlier section on Autosomal-Recessive Alport's Syndrome).

APPROACH TO THE PATIENT WITH HEREDITARY NEPHRITIS

Although Alport's syndrome is less common than polycystic kidney disease, it is probably more common than is generally appreciated. Important differential diagnoses of hematuria in young persons are immunoglobulin A (IgA) nephropathy or other glomerulonephritis, renal calculi, or medullary sponge kidney. The differential diagnosis of familial kidney disease with hematuria includes TBMD, familial IgA nephropathy, and, of course, polycystic disease. Familial kidney diseases without hematuria that might be confused with Alport's syndrome include polycystic kidney disease, medullary cystic disease, and rare forms of inherited glomerular and tubulointerstitial kidney disease.

If a patient with unexplained hematuria or kidney failure has a family history of hematuria or kidney failure, the family history should be extended, concentrating particularly on the mother's male relatives. Finding hearing loss strengthens suspicion for Alport's syndrome, and finding a specific ocular lesion intensifies this suspicion. Kidney biopsy would generally be indicated in one family member, but once the diagnosis of a basement membrane nephropathy is established in a family, it is difficult to justify additional biopsies unless there are features that suggest another diagnosis. The extent of investigation will be guided by clinical judgment and will relate inversely to the strength of the family history. For example, a young man on the line of descent of a known Alport's family whose urine contains dysmorphic erythrocytes requires minimal investigation. He may require nothing more than an assessment of glomerular filtration rate and urine protein measurement unless there are additional clinical features suggesting a systemic disease. A patient with hematuria and an uncertain family history may merit the standard nephrologic workup for hematuria. If available, and if suspicion of Alport's syndrome is moderate or high, a skin biopsy with staining for the $\alpha5(IV)$-chain might be considered. Genetic testing is presently of limited applicability in sporadic cases and small kindreds, because most families have unique mutations. For a few hundred small families and two very large kindreds in the United States, specific mutation tests are available. In these families, direct mutation analysis can quickly establish whether an individual is a gene carrier and spare the need for a kidney biopsy. It is not yet clear whether the two common mutations are sufficiently widespread to justify screening for them in adults with unexplained kidney failure or before undertaking a kidney biopsy in an adult or child with hematuria.

Patients with any hereditary nephropathy should be informed of the nature of the disease and perhaps given a copy of the genetic analysis or kidney biopsy report to avoid unnecessary further investigation. Similar conclusions apply to family members who are potentially gene carriers. Those with Alport's syndrome should be followed regularly for elevation of blood pressure and serum creatinine. The frequency of follow-up will depend on the anticipated age of onset of kidney function deterioration in the family and will become more often as this age is approached. Those with familial TMBD should be checked about every 2 years, because some may ultimately turn out to have Alport's syndrome.

BIBLIOGRAPHY

Barker DF, Hostikka SL, Zhou J, et al: Identification of mutations in the *COL4A5* collagen gene in Alport's syndrome. Science 248:1224–1227, 1990.

Gleeson MJ: Alport's syndrome: Audiological manifestations and implications. J Laryngol Otol 98:449–465, 1984.

Govan JA: Ocular manifestations of Alport's syndrome: A hereditary disorder of basement membranes? Br J Ophthalmol 67:493–503, 1983.

Gregory MC: Alport's syndrome. In Schrier RW, Gottschalk CW (eds): Diseases of the Kidney, 7th ed. Boston, Little Brown, 2001, pp 589–619.

Gregory MC: Alport's syndrome and thin basement membrane nephropathy: Unraveling the tangled strands of type IV collagen. Kidney Int 65:1109–1110, 2004.

Heath KE, Campos-Barros A, Toren A, et al: Nonmuscle myosin heavy chain IIA mutations define a spectrum of autosomal dominant macrothrombocytopenias: May-Hegglin anomaly and Fechtner, Sebastian, Epstein, and Alport-like syndromes. Am J Hum Genet 69:1033–1045, 2001.

Jais JP, Knebelmann B, Giatras I, et al: X-Linked Alport syndrome: Natural history in 195 families and genotype-phenotype correlations in males. J Am Soc Nephrol 11:649–657, 2000.

Jais JP, Knebelmann B, Giatras I, et al: X-Linked Alport syndrome: Natural history and genotype-phenotype correlations in girls and women belonging to 195 families. A "European Community Alport Syndrome Concerted Action" study. J Am Soc Nephrol 14:2603–2610, 2003.

Kashtan CE, Kleppel, MM, Gubler M-C: Immunohistologic findings in Alport's syndrome. In Tryggvason K (ed): Molecular Pathology and Genetics of Alport's syndrome. Basel, Karger, 1996, pp 142–153.

Lemmink HH, Nielsson WN, Mochizuki T, et al: Benign familial hematuria due to mutation of the type 4 collagen gene. J Clin Invest 98:1114–1118, 1996.

Tiebosch TA, Frederik PM, van Breda Vriesman PJ, et al: Thin basement membrane nephropathy in adults with persistent hematuria. N Engl J Med 320:14–18, 1989.

CHAPTER **47**

Nephronophthisis and Medullary Cystic Kidney Disease

John F. O'Toole   Friedhelm Hildebrandt

Nephronophthisis (NPHP) and medullary cystic kidney disease (MCKD) represent a set of rare genetic kidney diseases with a similar renal histopathology, which includes interstitial fibrosis with tubular atrophy, changes in the tubular basement membrane, and cyst formation. These two diseases can be distinguished clinically by their inheritance pattern and, usually, by age of onset. NPHP has an autosomal-recessive inheritance pattern and results in endstage renal disease (ESRD) within the first 3 decades of life. MCKD has an autosomal-dominant inheritance pattern and generally results in ESRD between the fourth and seventh decades of life (Table 47-1).

EPIDEMIOLOGY

Nephronophthisis has long been recognized as a rare cause of ESRD worldwide, but it is the most common genetic cause of ESRD in the pediatric population. Historically, the incidence of NPHP alone has been quoted as between 1 in 50,000 and 1 in 1 million live births. Because NPHP slowly progresses to ESRD, we have used the dialysis population to obtain more current data regarding the incidence and prevalence of the NPHP-MCKD diagnosis in this population as representative of these diagnoses in the general population. Data from the U.S. Renal Data System (USRDS) between 1997 and 2001 reported 189 new cases of ESRD from NPHP or MCKD in patients starting dialysis, implying an annual incidence of 0.05%. The number of patients with NPHP or MCKD in the prevalent dialysis population can be estimated from the Dialysis Outcomes and Practice Patterns Study (DOPPS) data sampling 16,238 dialysis patients from six countries in North America, Europe, and Asia. Patients were asked their primary renal diagnosis, and from this sample 22 reported either NPHP or MCKD, giving a prevalence of 0.14%. This suggests that at least 0.14% of all hemodialysis patients have ESRD secondary to either NPHP or MCKD.

The incidence and prevalence of these diseases from these sources may be an underestimate of the disease frequency, since patients will often come to clinical attention only after developing ESRD. In addition, urinalysis in these disorders is typically bland, without significant proteinuria or hematuria, making aggressive diagnostic procedures such as biopsy less likely to be pursued. Finally, the only way to diagnose these disorders definitively is through genetic testing, which until recently has been unavailable.

PATHOLOGY

The similar appearance of the kidney histology between NPHP and MCKD led to the historical association of these two disorders. The classic triad of kidney pathology, which is shared by NPHP1, NPHP3, and NPHP4 disease, includes tubular basement membrane (TBM) disruption, interstitial fibrosis with tubular atrophy, and corticomedullary cysts. This triad is characteristic of NPHP, but it is not diagnostic. Periglomerular fibrosis and sclerosis have also been noted. Cysts range in size from 1 to 15 mm and generally arise from the distal convoluted tubule or medullary collecting duct. The kidney size is normal to reduced in these types of NPHP, and the cysts may not be apparent by imaging early in the course of the disease. In contrast to autosomal-dominant polycystic kidney disease (ADPKD), cysts have not been observed in other organs.

Infantile nephronophthisis (NPHP2) is caused by mutations in the gene for inversin, *INVS*, and has a kidney pathology and clinical course distinct from the other types of NPHP. NPHP2 results in ESRD in the first decade of life, often within the first 2 years, and is characterized by the cystic enlargement of the kidneys bilaterally. Kidney pathology is characterized by more remarkable cyst formation, which appears more prominent in the cortex but can also be present in the medulla. Cysts seem to arise from the proximal and distal tubules, and cystic enlargement of the glomerulus has also been noted. Tubulointerstitial nephritis is another prominent finding in NPHP2, which it shares with the other forms of NPHP. TBM disruption is a less consistent finding in the setting of NPHP2. Whereas the classic kidney pathology of NPHP consists of a triad, individual biopsies may not demonstrate all three features. Therefore, in the proper clinical setting (i.e., kidney function impairment in the first 3 decades of life with a prominent tubulointerstitial process on biopsy), the diagnosis of NPHP

TABLE 47-1 Genetic Causes and Extrarenal Manifestations of Nephronophthisis and Medullary Cystic Kidney Disease

Disease	Gene	Protein	Inheritance Pattern	ESRD Median Yr	Chromosomal Location	Extrarenal Manifestations
NPHP1	*NPHP1*	Nephrocystin-1	AR	13	2q13	Retinitis pigmentosa Oculomotor apraxia, Cogan type
NPHP2	*INVS*	Inversin	AR	2.7	9q31	Retinitis pigmentosa Situs inversus
NPHP3	*NPHP3*	Nephrocystin-3	AR	19	3q22.1	Retinitis pigmentosa Liver fibrosis
NPHP4	*NPHP4*	Nephrocystin-4	AR	20	1p36.22	Retinitis pigmentosa Oculomotor apraxia, Cogan type
MCKD1	Unknown	Unknown	AD	62	1q21	Hyperuricemia, gout
MCKD2	*UMOD*	Uromodulin	AD	32	16p13.11	Hyperuricemia, gout

AD, autosomal dominant; AR, autosomal recessive; HP, nephronophthisis; MCKD, medullary cystic kidney disease.

should be entertained. At present the only definitive diagnostic modality is genetic testing.

The gross appearance of the kidney in MCKD is normal to slightly reduced in size, as in NPHP. Histologically, the kidney pathology of MCKD is virtually indistinguishable from that of NPHP, a situation that has led to the historical nomenclature of these diseases as the NPH-MCKD disease complex.

PATHOGENESIS

Four genes have been identified that cause NPHP (see Table 47-1). All four genes have a broad tissue expression pattern. Mutation in any one of these genes has been shown to result in the corresponding NPHP type, consistent with an autosomal-recessive inheritance pattern.

Approximately 85% of mutations in nephrocystin-1, the protein product of *NPHP1*, consist of large deletions, which typically include the whole gene. Nephrocystin-1 has been found to localize to sites of cell-cell contact in polarized epithelial cells. Disruption of the src-homolgy 3 (SH3) domain of nephrocystin-1 results in an impaired ability of cells to form normal cell-cell junctions. Additional studies have demonstrated that nephrocystin-1 contains a unique conserved domain in its C-terminal region called the nephrocystin homology domain (NHD), which may be important for targeting to the sites of cell-cell junctions. The following proteins have been shown to bind to nephrocystin-1 either directly or as part of a complex: focal adhesion kinase 2 (PYK2), p130^{Cas}, tensin, and filamins, a family of actin-binding proteins. These proteins all have prominent roles at sites of cell-cell contact. Interestingly, the tensin knockout mouse also demonstrates a kidney phenotype strikingly similar to NPHP.

The recent localization of nephrocystin-1 to the primary cilia has suggested that it plays a more complex functional role. Nephrocystin-1, inversin, and nephrocystin-4 have all been identified in the primary cilia, an organelle present on most mature polarized

cell types. The subcellular localization of nephrocystin-3, the protein product for *NPHP3*, has not yet been identified. Additionally, nephrocystin-1 has been shown to bind to inversin, nephrocystin-3, and nephrocystin-4, consistent with these proteins being components of a functional complex. The function of these proteins in the primary cilia is unknown, but it is tempting to speculate that it may have some role in cystogenesis, since other proteins responsible for cystic kidney diseases, such as polycystin-1 and polycystin-2, have also been localized to this organelle.

Mutations in inversin result in the clinical phenotype of NPHP2, infantile nephronophthisis. A knockout mouse model (inv) has been described that has a phenotype, including cystic kidneys and situs inversus. Inversin has been localized to primary cilia and functions in left-right axis determination as demonstrated in this mouse model. A 125-kD isoform has been shown to localize to sites of cell-cell contact, and a 90-kD isoform has been demonstrated in the nucleus in a complex with β-catenin. Additionally, inversin has been shown to interact with Apc2, a member of the anaphase-promoting complex. Inversin plays a role in the cell cycle and has a cell cycle–dependent subcellular expression pattern. It is localized to the centrosome during prophase and the spindle poles during metaphase and anaphase. Additionally, inversin contains two IQ domains, which have been shown to bind calmodulin. This may suggest a calcium-mediated link between inversin and other proteins responsible for cystic kidney diseases, notably polycystin-2, which forms a mechanically stimulated calcium channel in conjunction with polycystin-1.

Two gene loci have been identified for MCKD: *MCKD1* on 1q21 and *MCKD2* on 16p12. The causative gene for MCKD1 has not yet been identified. Mutations in uromodulin, the Tamm-Horsfall protein, have been shown to cause MCKD2, familial juvenile hyperuricemic nephropathy (FJHN), and glomerulocystic kidney disease (GCKD). Uromodulin is expressed in the thick ascending limb of the nephron and is the most abundant protein found in the urine. The excretion of uromodulin is reduced in these patients, and pathologic intracellular accumulation of uromodulin occurs in the tubular epithelial cells of the thick ascending limb.

CLINICAL FEATURES AND DIAGNOSIS

Nephronophthisis and medullary cystic kidney disease differ in the age of onset of renal impairment and the pattern of inheritance in familial cases (see Table 47-1). Renal impairment in NPHP will occur early, resulting in a slow decline in kidney function toward ESRD within the first 3 decades of life. The earliest clinical manifestation of NPHP is a urinary concentrating defect and results in the clinical symptoms of polyuria, secondary enuresis, and consistently drinking throughout the night. These findings may precede the onset of kidney functional impairment. A family history of affected siblings with an autosomal-recessive inheritance pattern is strongly suggestive of the diagnosis, but given the rarity of the disease sporadic cases are more common.

Age of onset is the strongest clinical distinction between the different types of nephronophthisis, leading to the historical definition of the disease as infantile (NPHP2), juvenile (NPHP1 and NPHP4), or adolescent (NPHP3). With the exception of NPHP2, which leads to ESRD in the first decade of life, it is not clear that there is truly a predictable difference in the age of onset for the other types of NPHP.

The extrarenal manifestations of NPHP (see Table 47-1) include retinitis pigmentosa, which can be present in any of the types of NPHP. Oculomotor apraxia type Cogan is associated with mutations in *NPHP1* and *NPHP4*. Situs inversus can occur with NPHP2. Liver fibrosis, progressing to endstage liver disease, has been associated with NPHP3. A number of other recognized clinical syndromes have been identified that can include a kidney phenotype similar to NPHP; these include Joubert's, Jeune's, COACH, Arima's, Sensenbrenner's, and Bardet-Biedl syndromes.

Physical findings related to nephronophthisis include growth retardation related to chronic kidney disease. High blood pressure is less prevalent than would be expected from the degree of kidney dysfunction.

The laboratory evaluation of nephronophthisis patients includes a urinalysis from first morning void, which is generally normal except for a low specific gravity reflecting a urinary concentrating defect; it is not known if they also have a diluting defect. The absence of proteinuria or hematuria may serve to distinguish NPHP from other heritable kidney diseases such as focal segmental glomerulosclerosis and Alport's syndrome, respectively. Anemia is another clinical feature commonly noted at the time of presentation that is probably related to interstitial infiltration and a resultant erythropoietin deficiency. Other laboratory abnormalities can be seen

commensurate with the degree of kidney function impairment.

The most relevant diagnostic test is renal ultrasound examination, which demonstrates normal to slightly reduced kidney size with increased echotexture and a loss of the corticomedullary border. Cysts, when present, may be observed at the corticomedullary junction, but cysts visible on imaging are not required for the diagnosis of NPHP. The imaging findings for patients with NPHP2 are substantially different from those of other types of NPHP as noted earlier.

Medullary cystic kidney disease generally presents in the fourth to seventh decades of life. Two exceptions to this are FJHN and GCKD, which are allelic (i.e., caused by mutations in the same gene) to MCKD2, but present within the first 3 decades of life. MCKD, FJHN, and GCKD are inherited in an autosomal-dominant pattern. The only extrarenal manifestations associated with these diseases aside from those attributable to declining kidney function are hyperuricemia and gouty arthritis, which can occur with MCKD, FJHN, or GCKD but is not universally present.

There are no other distinctive findings on physical examination associated with MCKD. Laboratory evaluation is notable for a urinary concentrating defect, with a reduced fractional excretion of uric acid, but the urinalysis is otherwise unremarkable. Ultrasound examination demonstrates normal to slightly reduced kidney size, increased echogenicity, loss of corticomedullary differentiation, and medullary cysts, but again, these may be too subtle for detection with ultrasound or computed tomography scanning. Ultrasonographic exam of GCKD patients may reveal normal to small kidney size and cortical cysts.

Although biopsy findings in conjunction with the appropriate clinical and historical presentation can be suggestive of a diagnosis of NPHP or MCKD, the only definitive diagnostic modality is genetic testing. Most genetic testing is done on a research basis, but recently commercial testing has also become available. A list of research and clinical laboratories offering genetic testing is available online at http://www.genetests.org.

Nephronophthisis should be suspected in the setting of kidney function impairment within the first 3 decades of life. The urine sediment is bland and is associated with minimal proteinuria, distinguishing NPHP from glomerular diseases. Renal ultrasonography demonstrates normal to small kidney sizes, except in the case of NPHP2, which may demonstrate cystic enlargement of the kidneys. NPHP2 can be distinguished from autosomal-recessive polycystic kidney disease (ARPKD), because NPHP2 lacks liver pathology. MCKD occurs later in life and also presents with kidney function impairment and bland urine sediment. Because it is autosomal dominant, careful questioning will often reveal affected family members. MCKD can be distinguished from ADPKD by renal ultrasonography. The ultrasonogram in MCKD will show normal to small-sized kidneys, whereas ADPKD will show cystic enlargement.

TREATMENT

No systematic trials have been undertaken to examine different treatment regimens for NPHP or MCKD in human subjects. Some studies have been done on the effect of treatment in a mouse model of NPHP. The *pcy* mouse is a model of *NPHP3*. A missense mutation has been identified in the murine homolog of *NPHP3*, which when present homozygously results in renal cystic disease and ESRD at around 40 weeks of age. In various studies these mice have been treated with soy proteins, glucocorticoids, probucol, and a vasopressin-2 receptor antagonist. All of these treatments demonstrated a reduction in cyst formation and slower progression of chronic kidney disease in this mouse model. In the same trial the vasopressin-2 receptor antagonist was also tested on a rat model of ARPKD and demonstrated efficacy. The mechanism by which vasopressin-2 receptor antagonism inhibits cystic changes in the renal parenchyma remains incompletely understood, but decreased levels of cyclic adenosine monophosphate (cAMP) were observed in the renal tubules of both animal models, suggesting that cAMP is functioning as a second messenger in the abnormal proliferation of renal epithelial cells in cystic kidney diseases.

Until human trials become available for the treatments, which look promising in rodent models of cystic kidney diseases, no disease-specific therapies can be recommended. At present, conservative therapies known to slow progression of kidney disease in general or those appropriate to treat the attendant systemic manifestations of reduced kidney function, including anemia, acidosis, and hyperparathyroidism, remain the standard of care. The role of angiotensin-converting enzyme inhibitors or angiotensin receptor blockers has not been studied specifically in these disease entities, and it is not known what impact they have on disease progression. Patients with NPHP and MCKD have successfully undergone kidney transplantation without evidence of recurrent disease.

BIBLIOGRAPHY

Benzing T, Gerke P, Hopker K, et al: Nephrocystin interacts with Pyk2, p130(Cas), and tensin and triggers phosphorylation of Pyk2. Proc Natl Acad Sci USA 98:9784–9789, 2001.

Dahan K, Devuyst O, Smaers M, et al: A cluster of mutations in *UMOD* gene causes familial hyperuricemic nephropathy with abnormal expression of uromodulin. J Am Soc Nephrol 14:2883–2893, 2003.

Donaldson JC, Dise RS, Ritchie MD, Hanks SK: Nephrocystin-conserved domains involved in targeting to epithelial cell-cell junctions, interaction with filamins and establishing cell polarity. J Biol Chem 277:29028–29035, 2002.

Gattone VH, Wang X, Harris PC, Torres VE: Inhibition of renal cystic disease development and progression by a vasopressin V2 receptor antagonist. Nat Med 9:1323–1326, 2003.

Hart TC, Gorry MC, Hart PS, et al: Mutations of the *UMOD* gene are responsible for medullary cystic disease 2 and familial hyperuricemic nephropathy. J Med Genet 39:882–892, 2002.

Hildebrandt F: Nephronophthisis-medullary cystic kidney disease. In Avner ED, Harmon WE, Niaudet P (eds): Pediatric Nephrology, 5th ed. Philadelphia, Lippincott, Williams & Wilkins, 2004, pp 665–673.

Hildebrandt F, Otto E, Rensing C, et al: A novel gene encoding an SH3 domain protein is mutated in nephronophthisis type 1. Nat Genet 17:149–153, 1997.

Mollet G, Salomon R, Gribouval O, et al: The gene mutated in juvenile nephronophthisis type 4 encodes a novel protein that interacts with nephrocystin. Nat Genet 32:300–305, 2002.

Morgan D, Eley L, Sayer J, et al: Expression analyses and interaction with the anaphase-promoting complex protein Apc2 suggest a role for inversin in primary cilia and involvement in the cell cycle. Hum Mol Genet 11:3345–3350, 2002.

Morgan D, Goodship J, Essner JJ, et al: The left-right determinant inversin has highly conserved ankyrin repeat and IQ domains and interacts with calmodulin. Hum Genet 110:377–384, 2002.

Olbrich H, Fliegauf M, Hoefele J, et al: Mutations in a novel gene, *NPHP3*, cause adolescent nephronophthisis, tapeto-retinal degeneration and hepatic fibrosis. Nat Genet 34:455–459, 2003.

Otto E, Hoefele J, Ruf R, et al: A gene mutated in nephronophthisis and retinitis pigmentosa encodes a novel protein, nephroretinin, conserved in evolution. Am J Hum Genet 71:1161–1167, 2002.

Otto EA, Schermer B, Obara T, et al: Mutations in *INVS* encoding inversin cause nephronophthisis type 2, linking renal cystic disease to the function of primary cilia and left-right axis determination. Nat Genet 34:413–420, 2003.

Rampoldi L, Caridi G, Santon D, et al: Allelism of MCKD, FJHN and GCKD caused by impairment of uromodulin export dynamics. Hum Mol Genet 12:3369–3384, 2003.

Wolf MT, Mucha BE, Attanasio M, et al: Mutations of the uromodulin gene in MCKD type 2 patients cluster in exon 4, which encodes three EGF-like domains. Kidney Int 64:1580–1587, 2003.

Tubulointerstitial Nephropathies and Disorders of the Urinary Tract

CHAPTER 48

Acute and Chronic Tubulointerstitial Disease*

Catherine M. Meyers

Primary interstitial nephropathies make up a diverse group of diseases that elicit interstitial inflammation associated with renal tubular cell damage. Traditionally, interstitial nephritis has been classified morphologically and clinically into acute and chronic forms. Acute interstitial nephritis (AIN) generally induces rapid deterioration in kidney function and elicits marked interstitial inflammatory responses characterized by interstitial edema with varying degrees of tubular cell damage, as well as mononuclear cell infiltrates consisting primarily of lymphocytes (Fig. 48-1). This process typically spares both glomerular and vascular structures. Eosinophils, macrophages, plasma cells, and neutrophils may also be apparent within these infiltrates. In some cases of AIN, interstitial granuloma formation is also observed. Most commonly, this form of granulomatous interstitial nephritis is associated with either drug- or infection-induced renal inflammation. AIN is not an uncommon cause of kidney dysfunction and should always be considered in the differential diagnosis of acute renal failure (ARF). Moreover, estimates from large clinical studies suggest that AIN accounts for approximately 10% to 15% of reported cases of ARF.

By contrast, chronic interstitial nephritis (CIN) follows a more indolent course and is characterized by tubulointerstitial fibrosis and atrophy, associated with interstitial mononuclear cell infiltration. Over time, glomerular and vascular structures are involved, with progressive fibrosis and sclerosis within the kidney. Recent studies suggest that more than 15% of endstage renal disease (ESRD) cases occur as a result of primary CIN.

ACUTE TUBULOINTERSTITIAL NEPHRITIS

Histopathology

Despite the varied inciting factors of acute tubulointerstitial nephritis in humans (Table 48-1), the striking similarity of induced interstitial lesions, which consist primarily of T-cell lymphocytes, suggests that immune-mediated mechanisms are important either in initiating the interstitial damage or in amplifying primary intersti-

tial injury from nonimmune causes. Studies from experimental models of interstitial disease suggest that both humoral and cell-mediated immune mechanisms are relevant effector pathways for inducing interstitial injury. Cell-mediated events probably play a prominent role in most forms of human disease, in view of the preponderance of T-cell lymphocytes (CD4+ and CD8+) present within interstitial infiltrates, generally in the absence of antibody deposition. Circulating or deposited antibodies against tubular basement membrane (TBM) have also been reported in some settings (e.g., rifampin-induced lesions and systemic immune disorders).

Immunohistochemical studies conducted on biopsy specimens obtained in drug-induced AIN also indicate the importance of cell-cell interactions in intrarenal inflammation, since there is a significant increase in interstitial expression of cellular adhesion molecules. In AIN, increased expression of leukocyte function antigen-1 and very late antigen-4 cell surface receptors, as well as their respective ligands, intercellular adhesion molecule-1 and vascular cell adhesion molecule-1, is generally observed in areas of mononuclear cell infiltration. Recent studies have extended these observations by examining the role of chemokines, a family of proinflammatory chemotactic mediators, in a number of kidney disease models associated with marked tubulointerstitial infiltration. RANTES, osteopontin, and monocyte chemotactic peptide-1, chemoattractants for inflammatory cells, have been best characterized, and studies demonstrate that their expression is markedly up-regulated in AIN, correlating directly with the level of monocyte infiltration and interstitial damage.

Clinical Features

Acute interstitial nephritis occurs in four distinct clinical settings (see Table 48-1). It may occur as a result of drug or toxin exposure, systemic or local infection, as a consequence of immunologic disease, or as an idiopathic lesion without an apparent precipitating cause. AIN is observed in all age groups; however, older patients appear more predisposed to developing ARF. Systemic manifestations of a hypersensitivity reaction, such as fever, rash, and arthralgias, are nonspecific findings that may

---

*This chapter is in the public domain.

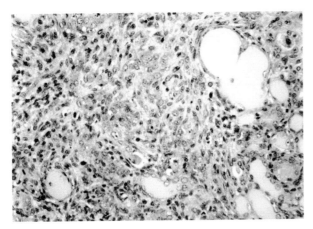

FIGURE 48-1 Acute interstitial nephritis. Light microscopic findings demonstrate the loss of normal tubulointerstitial architecture with a dense mononuclear cell infiltrate and some evidence of tubular dilation and atrophy. Note that the renal tubules are displaced by infiltrating mononuclear cells, edema, and mild interstitial fibrosis. (Magnification ×100.)

TABLE 48-2 Laboratory Findings in Acute Interstitial Nephritis

Parameter	Finding
Urinary sediment	Erythrocytes, leukocytes (eosinophils), leukocyte casts
Urinary protein excretion	<1 g/day, rarely >1 g/day (NSAIDs)
Fractional excretion of sodium	Usually >1%
Proximal tubular defects	Glucosuria, bicarbonaturia, phosphaturia, aminoaciduria, proximal RTA
Distal tubular defects	Hyperkalemia, sodium wasting, distal RTA
Medullary defects	Sodium wasting, urine-concentrating defects

NSAIDs, nonsteroidal anti-inflammatory drugs; RTA, renal tubular acidosis.

accompany AIN. In such cases, an erythematous maculopapular rash involves the trunk and proximal extremities. Hypertension and edema are not characteristic of AIN but have been reported in specific drug-induced lesions. Other nonspecific constitutional symptoms, as well as flank pain with gross hematuria, have been variably reported.

The spectrum of urinary abnormalities (Table 48-2) consists primarily of microscopic hematuria that at times may be macroscopic, sterile pyuria, and white blood cell casts. Red blood cell casts have also been reported, albeit rarely, in AIN. Eosinophiluria, with greater than 1% of urinary leukocytes positive by Hansel's stain, is suggestive of AIN but can be seen in other forms of renal injury and inflammation, such as rapidly progressive glomerulonephritis and renal atheroemboli. A recent review of four retrospective patient series suggested that the sensitivity of eosinophiluria for AIN overall was 67%, and

TABLE 48-1 Acute Interstitial Nephritis

Drugs
Antibiotics (most commonly penicillin analogues, cephalosporins, sulfonamides, and rifampin)
Nonsteroidal anti-inflammatory drugs
Diuretics (most commonly thiazides and furosemide)

Infections
Direct infection of renal parenchyma
Associated with a systemic infection

Immunologic disorders
Systemic lupus erythematosus
Sjögren's syndrome
Sarcoidosis
Mixed essential cryoglobulinemia
Acute allograft rejection

Idiopathic

the specificity was 82%. Because considerable variability was apparent between series and not all diagnoses were biopsy-confirmed, the presence of eosinophiluria is best considered consistent with, but not diagnostic of, AIN.

Mild proteinuria, generally less than 1 g/day, is frequently observed in AIN. Nephrotic-range proteinuria with acute disease has been reported, however, with nephropathies induced by nonsteroidal anti-inflammatory drugs (NSAIDs), and rarely by ampicillin, rifampin, and α-interferon therapy. Serologic studies in AIN, such as anti-DNA antibodies, antinuclear antibodies, and complement levels, are typically normal, except when AIN occurs in the setting of a systemic autoimmune disorder. Case reports also relate antineutrophil cytoplasmic antibody (ANCA) positivity, a serologic marker for systemic vasculitis, in some patients during the acute phase of interstitial nephritis. Elevated perinuclear ANCA (pANCA) titers have been observed in drug-induced AIN (omeprazole, ciprofloxacin, and cimetidine), and cytoplasmic ANCA (cANCA) in the tubulointerstitial nephritis and uveitis (TINU) syndrome, although the clinical relevance of ANCA titers in AIN is unclear.

Urinary fractional excretion of sodium is greater than 1% in many patients with AIN, but it is not a reliable diagnostic indicator. Biochemical abnormalities (see Table 48-2) reflective of the tubular damage induced by the inflammatory process are also observed in these patients. The pattern of tubular dysfunction will vary depending on the principal site of injury. Lesions affecting the proximal tubule result in renal glucosuria, aminoaciduria, phosphaturia, uricosuria, and proximal renal tubular acidosis (type 2 RTA). Distal tubular lesions result in an inability to acidify urine (type 1 RTA), secrete potassium, and regulate sodium balance. Medullary lesions will interfere with maximal urinary concentration and promote polyuria. A considerable degree of overlap in these proximal and distal abnormalities, however, may be apparent clinically. Kidney ultrasonography in affected patients typically reveals normal or enlarged kidneys, depending on the degree of interstitial edema. Renal gallium scanning has been advocated in some centers to distinguish AIN from other causes of ARF, primarily acute tubular necrosis, but this test lacks both sensitivity and specificity. In view of the nonspecific nature of many of these clinical features of AIN, a definitive diagnosis can therefore only be made through kidney biopsy.

Clinical Course and Therapy

The spectrum of kidney dysfunction in AIN ranges from mild, self-limited disease to oliguric renal failure requiring dialysis therapy. Because this kidney lesion is generally reversible, even despite initial severe renal functional impairment, the overall prognosis is quite favorable. Recovery of kidney function may occur over weeks to several months. Some patients have persistent tubular defects and/or residual renal functional impairment. Progression to ESRD, however, has been reported with all forms of AIN.

Clinical studies suggest that a less favorable prognosis in AIN correlates with extensive interstitial infiltrates, interstitial fibrosis, tubular atrophy, and interstitial granuloma formation on kidney biopsy. Other variables that correlate with chronic kidney disease are advanced patient age, pre-existing kidney disease, and a protracted course of oliguric ARF (more than 3 weeks). In general, chronic kidney disease following a bout of AIN is most commonly induced by NSAIDs.

The therapy of AIN consists primarily of supportive measures, after eliminating possible inciting influences such as drugs or infections. Patients with mild renal functional impairment and evidence of recovery of kidney function a few days after discontinuing the inciting drug do not require further therapy. The role of corticosteroids in treating more severe cases of AIN has not been clearly elucidated. Rapid improvement and complete recovery of kidney function following steroid therapy in several drug-induced lesions, however, have suggested their therapeutic usefulness in AIN. Two empirically derived steroid regimens have been implemented in drug (primarily antibiotic)-induced AIN, generally when biopsy findings have confirmed the diagnosis. One protocol, for patients with severely impaired kidney function, consists of parenteral methylprednisolone (0.5–1.0 g) administration for 1 to 3 days, followed by daily high-dose oral prednisone (1 mg/kg/day). The other more commonly used regimen consists only of high-dose daily oral prednisone therapy or alternate-day oral prednisone (2 mg/kg every other day), administered for approximately 2 to 3 weeks, with gradual tapering initiated after plasma creatinine levels return to near baseline levels. Anecdotal reports have indicated that steroid-unresponsive patients (after 2–3 weeks of therapy) may respond to cyclophosphamide (2 mg/kg/day). Recognizing that interstitial fibrosis, a lesion unresponsive to current immunotherapy, can begin occurring in AIN as soon as 10 to 14 days after disease induction, many clinicians are reluctant to expose patients to more potent reagents after steroid treatment failure.

Some clinical reports have not corroborated the steroid responsiveness of this kidney lesion, however, particularly for NSAID-induced cases. It should also be noted that prospective randomized studies have not been conducted. Steroids are not used in infection-related AIN, but may be helpful in the treatment of nephritogenic responses in systemic immunologic disorders. Although experimental models have suggested a disease-protective role for cyclophosphamide and cyclosporine in interstitial nephritis, similar studies have not been conducted in human disease. Anecdotal reports have also suggested efficacy of adjunctive plasmapheresis therapy, with immunosuppressant therapy, for the rare occurrence of AIN associated with circulating or deposited antibodies against TBM.

DISTINCT CAUSES OF ACUTE INTERSTITIAL NEPHRITIS

Drug-Induced Acute Interstitial Nephritis

The list of drugs that reportedly induce AIN is quite extensive (Table 48-3). Many of these are reports of single cases, however, and have developed in patients exposed to a number of different medications. Drug-induced AIN is a rare idiosyncratic reaction that occurs in a small subset of patients exposed to a particular medication. It is not dose-dependent, and it typically recurs on repeat exposure to the same or closely related drug. As seen in Table 48-3, implicated drugs have diverse chemical structures, although within a class of related drugs, structural similarity can lead to cross-reactive sensitivities. This has been observed particularly with β-lactam drugs, in that penicillin-induced nephropathies have been exacerbated with cephalosporin therapy. A few drugs, most notably penicillins, rifampin, NSAIDs, and sulfonamide derivatives, account for the majority of reported cases of AIN, and their characteristic features will be specifically discussed.

Penicillins

β-Lactam antibiotics, predominantly penicillins, are the most common cause of drug-induced AIN. The largest number of cases has occurred with methicillin, which is no longer used in clinical practice. AIN has been reported with most of the penicillin analogues more routinely prescribed (see Table 48-3), though with much lower inci-

TABLE 48-3   Drug-Induced Acute Interstitial Nephritis*

Antibiotics
  Penicillin analogues
    Methicillin, ampicillin, penicillin, nafcillin, carbenicillin, oxacillin, amoxicillin, mezlocillin, flucloxacillin
  Cephalosporins
    Cephalothin, cefotetan, cephradine, cephalexin, cefoxitin, cefazolin, cefaclor, cefotaxime
  Sulfonamide derivatives
    Sulfamethoxazole, cotrimoxazole
  Other antibiotics
    Rifampin, ciprofloxacin, gentamicin, kanamycin, vancomycin, acyclovir, indinavir, aztreonam, erythromycin, azithromycin, ethambutol, tetracyclines, nitrofurantoin

Nonsteroidal anti-inflammatory drugs
  Fenoprofen, ibuprofen, indomethacin, piroxicam, tolmetin, naproxen, zomepirac, diflunisal, sulindac, *phenylbutazone,* aspirin, phenacetin, mefenamic acid, 5-aminosalicylates

Diuretics
  Thiazides, furosemide, triamterene, chlorthalidone

Miscellaneous medications
  Phenytoin, allopurinol, cimetidine, omeprazole, ranitidine, famotidine, phenobarbital, azathioprine, cyclosporine, α-methyldopa, carbamazepine, diazepam, phenylpropanolamine, captopril, clofibrate, α-interferon, interleukin-2, anti-CD4 monoclonal antibodies, ticlopidine, quinine, propylthiouracil, streptokinase, Chinese herbs, clozapine, phentermine/phendimetrazine, pranlukast, lansoprazole

*Drugs reported with greatest frequency are shown in *italics.*

dence than with methicillin. Marked impairments in kidney function in this setting have been observed most commonly in older children and young adults. The classic hypersensitivity triad of fever, rash, and eosinophilia in the setting of ARF may occur in up to 30% of patients with β-lactam-induced AIN. Oliguric renal failure has been reported in approximately 30% of these patients. Clinical studies have suggested a beneficial role for steroids in this patient population, although as already stated, randomized controlled studies have not been performed. AIN has developed during treatment of a variety of infections, although an underlying infection is clearly not requisite for inducing this reaction, since several patients given prophylactic antibiotics have subsequently developed AIN.

NSAIDs

NSAIDs are among the most widely prescribed medications in clinical practice. They mediate a number of adverse renal side effects, largely as a result of their inhibition of renal prostaglandin synthesis, and are extensively discussed in Chapter 40. AIN is a less commonly observed side effect of these medications. Propionic acid derivatives appear to cause a disproportionate number of

cases (two thirds of cases have been attributed to fenoprofen, ibuprofen, and naproxen), although AIN has been reported with most NSAIDs currently available (see Table 48-3). Unlike other drug-induced reactions, AIN occurs after long-term exposure to the medication, and has been reported 2 weeks to 18 months after initiating therapy. Patients tend to be nonoliguric females older than 60 years of age, generally lack systemic manifestations of a hypersensitivity reaction, and may present with hypertension, edema, and nephrotic-range proteinuria (up to 80% of cases). Histologic features of induced interstitial lesions are the associated minimal-change glomerulopathy and occasional interstitial granuloma formation apparent on kidney biopsy. Kidney disease generally improves after discontinuing the drug, with or without steroid therapy, although chronic kidney disease and ESRD are not infrequent complications.

Rifampin

Numerous cases of rifampin-induced AIN have occurred during treatment of tuberculosis. Most of these cases have developed with intermittent therapy or on restarting rifampin after a lapse in uneventful daily therapy. Patients typically complain of flulike symptoms such as fever, chills, malaise, and headache. Unlike other drug-induced lesions, flank pain and hypertension are common in this form of AIN. Moreover, oliguric ARF occurs frequently, and dialysis is required in approximately two thirds of affected patients. In many cases, this reaction has occurred within hours of a single dose of rifampin. Some patients have developed thrombocytopenia, hemolysis, or abnormalities in liver function in addition to AIN. Histologically, evidence of acute tubular necrosis may be apparent in addition to AIN. In a few cases, an associated proliferative glomerulonephritis has also been observed. Circulating rifampin-specific antibodies, as well as immunoglobulin G (IgG) deposition along the TBM have been reported in some affected patients. Since AIN has developed in patients receiving concurrent rifampin and prednisone therapy, there is no evidence to suggest that steroids play a therapeutic role in this disease.

Sulfonamide Derivatives

Drug-induced AIN was first described in the setting of sulfonamide administration. The majority of cases of sulfonamide derivative–induced AIN are reported with combination sulfamethoxazole and trimethoprim therapy. Thiazides and furosemide have also been associated with a few cases of AIN, some of which have developed in patients with pre-existing kidney disease. The associated hypersensitivity triad of fever, rash, and eosinophilia with kidney dysfunction is variably present in affected patients. In addition to the characteristic histologic features of AIN, some biopsy specimens have revealed a predominance of eosinophils within interstitial infiltrates, as well as interstitial granuloma formation. Isolated case reports have suggested beneficial effects of steroid therapy in treating this drug-induced AIN.

Infections Associated with Acute Interstitial Nephritis

Acute interstitial nephritis was first described in the pre-antibiotic era in the setting of diphtherial and streptococcal infections. It is now apparent that AIN complicates the clinical course of a number of bacterial, viral, fungal, and parasitic infections, as listed in Table 48-4. This inflammatory response within the kidney may occur as a result of direct renal infection, that is, pyelonephritis, or as a reaction to a systemic infection. Pyelonephritis, the most common cause of acute infectious interstitial nephritis, typically presents with fever, costovertebral tenderness, dysuria, pyuria, bacteriuria, and leukocytosis. Kidney function is unimpaired unless complicated by urinary tract obstruction. Characteristic renal parenchymal lesions consist of focal areas of neutrophils throughout the interstitium. Pyelonephritis responds well to antibiotic therapy and is discussed more extensively in Chapter 54.

Of note, transplant centers have more recently observed human polyoma (BK and JC viruses)-associated interstitial nephritis occurring in kidney allografts. Human polyoma viruses, predominantly BK virus, induce interstitial nephritis in immunosuppressed patients after reactivation of latent virus in renal epithelium. Histologic features of this lesion are interstitial inflammatory cell infiltration with extensive tubulitis, basophilic or amphophilic intranuclear inclusions, and in situ evidence of virally infected cells on kidney biopsy. Distinguishing polyoma virus interstitial nephritis from acute rejection is critical in this setting, because therapeutic intervention in these disorders is vastly different. Viral

---

TABLE 48-4 Infections Associated with Acute Interstitial Nephritis*

Bacterial infections
Streptococcus, diphtheria, brucella, legionella, pneumococcus, *tuberculosis*

Viral infections
Epstein-Barr virus, *cytomegalovirus, polyomavirus, Hantaan virus,* measles (rubeola), human immunodeficiency virus, herpes simplex virus type 1

Fungal infections
Candidiasis, histoplasmosis

Other infections
Toxoplasmosis, leishmaniasis, schistosomiasis, *Rocky Mountain spotted fever,* ehrlichiosis, malaria, mycoplasma, *leptospirosis,* syphilis, ascaris lumbricoides

*Infections associated with direct renal infection are shown in *italics.*

---

infection–associated graft dysfunction dictates a prudent decrease in immunosuppression, whereas acute rejection requires more intensive immunosuppression. Specific BK virus diagnostic testing and therapy are not currently available, although some centers have reported anecdotal experience with molecular diagnostic techniques and antiviral agents. Further discussion of kidney allograft therapeutics can be found in Chapter 69.

In contrast to pyelonephritis, other infection-associated interstitial processes occur in the absence of urinary tract infection. Interstitial infiltrates are frequently perivascular and composed of mononuclear cells, predominantly T-cell lymphocytes. As already discussed, the pathogenesis of such immune targeting in these infections is not well understood, although cross-reactive determinants may play a role in immune recognition of interstitial structures.

Infection-associated interstitial nephritis is generally transient, and kidney function improves with appropriate therapy of the systemic illness; however, chronic kidney disease has been reported.

Immune Disorders Associated with Acute Interstitial Nephritis

Although glomerulonephritis is the most common renal manifestation of systemic immunologic disorders, predominant interstitial pathology can be seen in systemic lupus erythematosus, sarcoidosis, Sjögren's syndrome, and mixed essential cryoglobulinemia. Most affected patients present with nonoliguric renal failure and biochemical evidence of tubular dysfunction. In addition to the typical pathologic features of AIN, biopsy samples from many of these patients also reveal immune-complex and complement deposition along the TBM, and occasionally within interstitial vessels. Concurrent glomerular pathology may also be apparent. Interstitial inflammation and granuloma formation associated with uveitis are observed in Sjögren's syndrome, sarcoidosis, and the TINU syndrome (see section on Idiopathic Acute Interstitial Nephritis), and such patients require further evaluation to distinguish these disorders. Standard therapeutic modalities in these immunologic disorders consist of corticosteroids and/or cytotoxic agents. Such therapy is beneficial unless irreversible tubulointerstitial damage has occurred. Acute kidney allograft rejection, a distinct subset of immunologic disorders, also induces acute interstitial inflammation and is discussed further in Chapter 69.

Idiopathic Acute Interstitial Nephritis

In approximately 10% to 20% of biopsy-proven cases of AIN, no precipitating cause is detected. Systemic manifestations of a hypersensitivity reaction are generally absent in the majority of these idiopathic cases, which often present with nonoliguric renal failure. A subset of these apparently idiopathic lesions is probably associated with the TINU syndrome, which has been reported in approximately 130 patients, with a median age of 15 years at presentation. Cases in adults and the elderly have also been reported. A 3:1 female-to-male predominance has been observed. TINU is associated with a variety of systemic complaints such as fever, malaise, rash, arthralgias, and weight loss. Anterior uveitis can precede, accompany, or follow AIN. Although the cause of TINU syndrome is not known, an autoimmune nature is suggested by occasional positive serologies, such as cANCA, rheumatoid factor, and ANA, in affected patients. Diminished cellular immune responses have also been observed. Kidney disease is frequently reversible and typically responds to a brief course of corticosteroid therapy, although a few patients have developed chronic kidney disease. Relapse of ocular problems has been commonly reported.

CHRONIC TUBULOINTERSTITIAL NEPHRITIS

Histopathology

Histopathology of CIN is remarkably consistent among a variety of apparent causes (Table 48-5). In addition to tubular cell damage and predominantly mononuclear cell inflammation, CIN is characterized by the development of tubulointerstitial fibrosis and scarring. Interstitial granulomatous disease has also been observed in certain forms of CIN (sarcoidosis). Glomerular and vascular structures may be relatively preserved early in the course of disease, but ultimately become involved in progressive fibrosis and sclerosis. Observations from the experimental literature recently suggested that renal tubular epithelial-myofibroblast transition (TEMT) may play a pivotal role in initiation and progression of tubulointerstitial fibrosis. Although the processes relevant for primary CIN in humans have not been elucidated, experimental models of injury have implicated a large role for transforming growth factor-β and other fibrogenic mediators such as fibroblast growth factor-2, advanced glycation end products, and angiotensin II in regulating renal TEMT, and thereby propagating chronic interstitial damage and fibrosis.

Similar to AIN, mononuclear cell infiltrates generally accompany CIN, further suggesting a pathogenic immune-mediated mechanism for disease progression. One hypothesis concerning immune recognition of the interstitium suggests that portions of infectious particles or drug molecules may cross-react with or alter endogenous renal antigens. An immune response directed against these inciting agents would theoretically therefore also target the interstitium. Intriguing results of a study examining a series of kidney biopsy samples

TABLE 48-5 Chronic Interstitial Nephritis

Drugs/toxins
Analgesics
Heavy metals (lead, cadmium)
Lithium
Chinese herbs
Calcineurin inhibitors (cyclosporine, tacrolimus)
Cisplatin
Nitrosoureas

Hereditary disorders
Polycystic kidney disease
Medullary cystic disease–juvenile nephronophthisis
Hereditary nephritis

Metabolic disturbances
Hypercalcemia/Nephrocalcinosis
Hypokalemia
Hyperuricemia
Hyperoxaluria
Cystinosis

Immune-mediated disorders
Renal allograft rejection
Systemic lupus erythematosus
Sjögren's syndrome
Sarcoidosis
Wegener's granulomatosis
Vasculitis

Hematologic disturbances
Multiple myeloma
Light chain disease
Dysproteinemias
Lymphoproliferative disease
Sickle cell disease

Infections
Renal
Systemic

Obstruction/mechanical disorders
Tumors
Stones
Vesicoureteral reflux

Miscellaneous disorders
Endemic nephropathy
Radiation nephritis
Aging
Hypertension
Renal ischemia

obtained over 8 years at a single center suggest a prominent role of Epstein-Barr virus (EBV) in cases of CIN previously deemed idiopathic. Investigators detected EBV DNA, and its receptor CD21, primarily in proximal tubular cells of all 17 patients with primary idiopathic interstitial nephritis. These findings were not apparent in 10 control kidney biopsy specimens. Such observations imply a more prominent role than previously appreciated for EBV infections in eliciting chronic deleterious immune responses that target the interstitium.

Clinical Features

As shown in Table 48-5, CIN occurs in a variety of clinical settings, most commonly following exposure to drugs or toxins, or in the setting of hereditary disorders, metabolic disorders, immune-mediated diseases, hematologic disturbances, infections, or obstruction. Because CIN tends to occur as a slowly progressive disease, most patients diagnosed with CIN present with systemic complaints of the primary underlying disease, if there is one, or with symptoms of chronic kidney disease. Laboratory findings in these patients include non-nephrotic-range proteinuria, microscopic hematuria, and pyuria. As listed in Table 48-2, other urinary abnormalities such as glucosuria, phosphaturia, and sodium wasting, reflective of tubular defects are frequently reported. Affected patients may also have elevated urinary excretion of low-molecular-weight proteins that are commonly associated with tubular injury and damage, such as lysozyme, β_2-microglobulin, and retinol-binding protein, and increased enzymuria with N-acetyl-β-D-glucosaminidase, alanine aminopeptidase, and intestinal alkaline phosphatase. Routine assessment of urinary low-molecular-weight proteins and enzymes is not typically conducted, however, since it is of little diagnostic or prognostic use. Hypertension is another common clinical feature of CIN, although in many forms of CIN it is not apparent until the patient approaches ESRD. With progressive CIN, kidney ultrasonography in patients without significant structural abnormalities (e.g., cystic kidney disease) typically reveals shrunken kidneys. Irregular renal contours as well as renal calcifications are seen in some forms of CIN.

Clinical Course and Therapy

In view of the slowly progressive loss of kidney function observed in most cases of CIN, general therapeutic considerations include treating an underlying systemic disorder (sarcoidosis), avoiding the drug or toxin exposure (analgesics, lead), or eliminating the condition that has induced the chronic interstitial lesion (obstruction). The interstitial fibrosis and scarring, and resultant impairment in kidney function, in CIN are not currently amenable to therapeutic intervention. Although definitive diagnosis of CIN requires kidney biopsy, it is probably of limited usefulness in patients with kidney failure. Therapy for CIN is therefore largely supportive, with renal replacement therapy initiated in patients who develop ESRD. More specific therapies for interstitial lesions associated with lead exposure or sarcoidosis will be discussed in the following section.

DISTINCT CAUSES OF CHRONIC TUBULOINTERSTITIAL NEPHRITIS

Many causes of CIN listed in Table 48-5 are more fully described in other chapters of this text. This section will focus on a few common causes of CIN.

Lead

Chronic exposure to high levels of lead, over several years to decades, is associated with a progressive CIN. Most such chronic exposures are occupational, and seen in the manufacturing or use of lead-containing paints, ammunitions, radiators, batteries, wires, ceramic glazes, solder, and metal cans. In addition, environmental lead exposure can occur in several settings, such as using lead pipes and solder joints in drinking-water lines, consuming crops grown in lead-contaminated soil, or ingesting lead-based paint scraps or moonshine generated in lead-lined car radiators. Recent population-based studies have also noted a trend of increased blood lead levels in the general population and a related inverse trend in creatinine clearance. It is unclear, however, whether these population-based observations reflect an increase in chronic lead nephropathy, or an increase in kidney disease that induces lead retention.

Because an early histologic lesion observed with chronic lead exposure is proximal tubular intranuclear inclusion bodies composed of a lead-protein complex, the early stage of lead-induced kidney damage probably results from proximal reabsorption with subsequent intracellular lead accumulation. Early clinical manifestations reflect proximal tubular dysfunction with hyperuricemia, as well as aminoaciduria and glucosuria. Because the kidney disease is slowly progressive, affected patients typically present with symptoms of chronic kidney disease, and with hypertension, hyperuricemia, and gout. This symptom complex might, however, suggest the diagnosis of either chronic urate nephropathy or hypertensive nephrosclerosis. Chronic urate nephropathy with tophaceous gout is currently an uncommon condition; moreover, some studies suggest that previously reported cases were actually associated with chronic lead exposure. By contrast, hypertensive nephrosclerosis is not typically associated with hyperuricemia and gout. Patients presenting with hypertension, hyperuricemia, and chronic kidney disease should therefore be questioned about lead exposure.

The diagnosis of chronic lead intoxication is generally established with a lead mobilization test, performed by measuring urinary lead excretion after administering ethylenediaminetetraacetic acid (EDTA). X-ray fluorescence can also be used to determine bone lead levels. The diagnosis of lead nephropathy, however, is frequently made on the basis of a history of lead exposure in the setting of hyperuricemia, hypertension, and slowly progressive kidney disease consistent with CIN. Treatment of lead intoxication consists of chelation therapy, with EDTA or oral succimer. Although chronic lead nephropathy has generally been considered an irreversible process, recent studies from Taiwan have suggested that chelation therapy may slow progression of kidney disease in patients with excessive total body lead levels.

Chinese Herb Nephropathy

Rapidly progressive fibrosing interstitial nephritis has been described in clusters of patients in weight loss programs who ingested Chinese herbal preparations tainted with a plant nephrotoxin derived from *Aristolochia fangchi* (aristolochic acid). Approximately 100 cases have been reported in the literature, although some cases were observed in patients that ingested herb preparations not containing aristolochic acid. Kidney disease in all affected individuals was progressive and irreversible despite withdrawal of toxin exposure, with many patients requiring dialysis therapy or transplantation within 1 year of presentation. The mechanism of herb-induced nephrotoxicity, however, has not been delineated. The observation that some patients exposed to toxic herbs do not develop kidney disease further suggests variability in patient susceptibility to kidney injury. A frequent association of cellular atypia and urothelial cell malignancies of the genitourinary tract has also been reported in some patient series.

Endemic Nephropathy

Endemic or Balkan nephropathy is a form of CIN endemic to the areas of Bulgaria, Romania, Serbia, Croatia, Bosnia, and Herzegovina. It occurs most commonly along the confluence of the Danube River and has been reported almost exclusively in farmers. Although the disease etiology has not been elucidated, several environmental toxins (plant nephrotoxins, trace metals) have been explored. The tendency for clustering of cases in families has also suggested that genetic variables play a role in disease susceptibility. Like many forms of CIN, endemic nephropathy is a slowly progressive kidney disease, and patients present with blood and urinary evidence of tubular dysfunction. It is typically observed in the fourth, or later, decade of life, and rarely affects patients younger than 20 years of age. Patients generally present with normal blood pressure and either normal-sized, or slightly reduced, kidney size on ultrasonography. A specific diagnostic test has not been developed for endemic nephropathy, and there is not currently a specific treatment or preventive regimen for the disorder. Similar to Chinese herb nephropathy, endemic nephropathy is associated with urothelial tumors. Studies have reported a wide range of tumor incidence, from 2% to 47% of patients with endemic nephropathy.

Sarcoidosis

The most common renal manifestation of sarcoidosis is mediated through disordered calcium metabolism resulting in hypercalcemia and hypercalciuria. Although interstitial disease, at times with noncaseating granuloma formation, is relatively common in sarcoidosis (15% to 30%), autopsy series indicate that it is unusual for the interstitial abnormalities to result in clinically significant kidney dysfunction. Moreover, it is also unusual to observe interstitial disease in the absence of extrarenal involvement in sarcoidosis. Although most patients with impaired kidney function respond well to corticosteroid therapy (1 mg/kg/day), recovery of kidney function is frequently incomplete because of chronic interstitial inflammation and fibrosis. Relapse of renal functional impairment during steroid taper has been reported, and progression to ESRD is rare.

BIBLIOGRAPHY

Becker JL, Miller F, Nuovo GJ, et al: Epstein-Barr virus infection of renal proximal tubule cells: Possible role in chronic interstitial nephritis. J Clin Invest 104:1673–1681, 1999.

Brause M, Magnusson K, Degenhardt S, et al: Renal involvement in sarcoidosis—a report of 6 cases. Clin Nephrol 57:142–148, 2002.

De Vriese AS, Robbrecht DL, Vanholder RC, et al: Rifampicin-associated acute renal failure: Pathophysiologic, immunologic, and clinical features. Am J Kidney Dis 31:108–115, 1998.

Kannerstein M: Histologic kidney changes in the common acute infectious diseases. Am J Med Sci 203:65–73, 1942.

Kim R, Rotnitsky A, Sparrow D, et al: A longitudinal study of low-level lead exposure and impairment of renal function. The Normative Aging Study. JAMA 275:1177–1181, 1996.

Kleinknecht D: Interstitial nephritis, the nephrotic syndrome, and chronic renal failure secondary to nonsteroidal anti-inflammatory drugs. Semin Nephrol 15:228–235, 1995.

Lin JL, Lin-Tan DT, Hsu KU, et al: Environmental lead exposure and progression of chronic renal diseases in patients without diabetes. N Engl J Med 348:277–286, 2003.

Liu Y: Epithelial to mesenchymal transition in renal fibrogenesis: Pathologic significance, molecular mechanism, and therapeutic intervention. J Am Soc Nephrol 15:1–12, 2004.

Magil AB, Tyler M: Tubulointerstitial disease in lupus nephritis: A morphometric study. Histopathology 8:81–87, 1984.

Meyers CM: New insights into the pathogenesis of interstitial nephritis. Curr Opin Nephrol Hypertens 8:287–292, 1999.

Michel DM, Kelly CJ: Acute interstitial nephritis. J Am Soc Nephrol 9:506–515, 1998.

Neilson EG: Pathogenesis and therapy of interstitial nephritis. Kidney Int 35:1257–1270, 1989.

Nortier JL, Martinex M-C, Schmeiser HH, et al: Urothelial carcinoma associated with the use of a Chinese herb (*Aristolochia fangchi*). N Engl J Med 342:1686–1692, 2000.

Randhawa PS, Finkelstein S, Scantlebury V, et al: Human polyoma virus–associated interstitial nephritis in the allograft kidney. Transplantation 67:103–109, 1999.

Rossert J: Drug-induced interstitial nephritis. Kidney Int 60:804–817, 2001.

Simon AHR, Alves-Filho G, Ribeiro-Alves MAVF: Acute tubulointerstitial nephritis and uveitis with antineutrophil cytoplasmic antibody. Am J Kidney Dis 28:124–127, 1996.

Takemura T, Okada M, Hino S, et al: Course and outcome of tubulointerstitial nephritis and uveitis syndrome. Am J Kidney Dis 34:1016–1021, 1999.

Vanherweghem JL, Depierreux M, Tielemans C, et al: Rapidly progressive interstitial renal fibrosis in young women: Association with slimming regimen including Chinese herbs. Lancet 341:387–391, 1993.

CHAPTER 49

Lithium-Induced Kidney Disease

Gregory L. Braden

Lithium is an important treatment for bipolar disorders, but therapy with this drug has been associated with side effects in many body systems including the kidneys. Lithium is freely filtered at the glomerulus, reabsorbed like sodium at several tubular sites, and concentrated in the renal medulla, circumstances that might favor lithium-induced kidney disease. Although lithium was initially thought to produce only functional kidney disorders, such as nephrogenic diabetes insipidus (NDI), additional disorders now attributed to lithium include renal tubular acidosis, chronic interstitial nephritis, and nephrotic syndrome.

NEPHROGENIC DIABETES INSIPIDUS

Polydipsia occurs in up to 40% and polyuria greater than 3 L/day occurs in up to 20% of patients treated with lithium. Despite the high prevalence of polyuria, urine volume is rarely increased enough to require cessation of lithium therapy. Most humans with lithium-induced polyuria are unresponsive to the administration of exogenous antidiuretic hormone (ADH). This could occur as either a result of abnormalities in the medullary osmotic gradient that drives ADH-mediated water reabsorption or through direct inhibition of the tubular hydro-osmotic effects of ADH. Chronic administration of lithium diminishes the medullary and papillary osmolar gradients as a result of depletion of urea without affecting sodium chloride concentrations. However, lithium-induced polyuria is largely due to direct inhibition of the ADH-dependent aspects of water conservation. Only one lithium-treated patient has been reported to have a defect in the pituitary release of ADH indicative of central diabetes insipidus.

Lithium impairs the hydro-osmotic response to ADH by several mechanisms. Normally, ADH binds to its V2 receptor in collecting tubules and activates adenylate cyclase associated with guanine nucleoside regulatory proteins, which catalyze the production of cyclic adenosine 3,5-monophosphate (cAMP). Enhanced water permeability normally occurs as cAMP activates protein kinase A, which phosphorylates the water channel protein, aquaporin-2, leading to insertion of these water channels from intracellular vesicles into the apical membrane of collecting duct cells. There is abundant physiological and biochemical evidence that lithium directly inhibits the adenylate cyclase system in the mammalian distal nephron, leading to decreased generation of the second messenger, cAMP. In addition, lithium inhibits transepithelial water movement after the administration of exogenous cAMP, suggesting inhibition of water flow at a site distal to the generation of cAMP. Indeed, chronic lithium administration can down-regulate the expression of aquaporin-2 water channels in collecting ducts, leading to impaired water reabsorption and polyuria.

Although lithium-induced NDI usually improves after lithium withdrawal, some patients have persistent concentrating defects lasting for years. Amiloride reduces urinary volume and enhances the concentrating ability of patients with lithium-induced NDI. This inhibitor of the epithelial sodium channel blocks distal tubular reabsorption of lithium, thus lowering the kidney tissue lithium level. In addition, amiloride has diuretic activity, and the combination of dietary salt restriction and the natriuretic effect of the diuretic induces mild extracellular fluid volume depletion, which decreases the glomerular filtration rate (GFR) and lessens urinary volume. Thiazide diuretics have also been utilized for this purpose, but they may raise serum lithium levels. Notably, amiloride has been shown to be effective without inducing any changes in creatinine clearance or serum lithium levels, suggesting that the inhibition of lithium uptake in the distal nephron may be the most important influence for its efficacy. Indomethacin has been effective in a few patients, presumably by inducing a significant fall in the GFR, which, similar to diuretics, may lower urinary volume. In addition, indomethacin inhibits synthesis of urinary prostaglandins that inhibit the tubular action of ADH. Finally, a few patients with severe NDI will require cessation of lithium and the substitution of either carbamazepine or valproic acid to treat their bipolar disorder.

RENAL TUBULAR ACIDOSIS

Lithium impairs distal hydrogen ion secretion in at least 50% of treated patients. During administration of intravenous sodium bicarbonate, distal nephron bicarbonate delivery is increased. In normal humans, this stimulates hydrogen ion excretion by the distal nephron proton pumps. The additional protons are buffered by bicarbonate; the carbonic acid formed then dissociates and raises the urinary pCO_2 from 40 mm Hg to 80 mm Hg or greater. This distal nephron response is impaired in lithium-treated patients; however, there is no evidence for renal bicarbonate wasting, such as in proximal renal tubular acidosis, and the excretion of the urinary buffer, ammonium, is normal. Despite this defect in urinary acidification, the serum bicarbonate and pH remain normal. Taken together, these studies indicate that lithium induces incomplete distal renal tubular acidosis. Thus, patients treated with lithium are prone to systemic acidosis during stressful conditions, such as sepsis or catabolic states.

ACUTE RENAL FAILURE AND LITHIUM INTOXICATION

Acute renal failure due to biopsy-proven acute tubular necrosis may occur in lithium-intoxicated patients. Nephrotic syndrome due to minimal-change disease may occur concomitantly with acute tubular necrosis. Whether lithium can directly cause tubular necrosis or whether tubular necrosis in these patients is secondary to hemodynamic factors is unknown.

Lithium intoxication is classified into three grades of severity based on the blood level (mild, less than 2.5 mEq/L; moderate, 2.5 to 3.5 mEq/L; severe, more than 3.5 mEq/L). Toxic effects include nausea, ataxia, tremors, twitching, muscle rigidity, disordered consciousness, seizures, coma, and the neuroleptic-malignant syndrome characterized by high fever, rhabdomyolysis, and acute tubular necrosis. The pathophysiology of lithium intoxication may be due to its ability to induce dehydration and salt depletion secondary to its inhibitory effect on ADH action and the acute effects of lithium to induce a natriuresis leading to extracellular fluid volume depletion, activation of the serum-angiotensin system, decreased GFR, and, in turn, increased serum lithium levels. In addition, angiotensin-converting enzyme inhibitors, angiotensin receptor blockers, and nonsteroidal anti-inflammatory drugs may cause kidney dysfunction leading to lithium intoxication, especially in patients on high therapeutic doses. Patients who require treatment with these drugs should have serum lithium levels, electrolytes, blood urea nitrogen, and creatinine monitored 7 to 10 days after initiation of therapy and frequently thereafter. A lithium dosage reduction may be needed.

Patients with lithium intoxication should be admitted to the hospital, because seizures can occur at any time. The drug should be discontinued and, if there is an acute ingestion, either gastric lavage or ipecac should be given. Restoration of depleted extracellular fluid volume should occur with the administration of intravenous 0.9% normal saline if there is no hypernatremia present. For those patients with mild intoxication with a serum level of 2.5 mEq/L or less, saline diuresis may be enough to enhance renal lithium clearance. If there is no history to preclude vigorous volume expansion, then up to 6 liters of saline can be given daily until the lithium level decreases to the nontoxic range. With this therapy, the lithium level should fall approximately 1 mEq/day. However, patients who are euvolemic usually do not respond to saline or forced diuresis. For those patients with a blood level greater than 2.5 mEq/L and neurotoxic symptoms or acute renal failure, hemodialysis is the therapy of choice and may need to be repeated if serum lithium levels rebound after the first hemodialysis treatment. Continuous venovenous hemodiafiltration also effectively removes lithium and can prevent post-therapy rebound.

NEPHROTIC SYNDROME

Lithium causes nephrotic syndrome in a small number of patients. Kidney biopsy has demonstrated focal segmental glomerulosclerosis in the majority of patients and minimal-change disease in a smaller number. Several patients with focal segmental glomerulosclerosis and serum creatinine levels greater than 2.0 mg/dL have progressed to endstage renal disease, requiring dialysis. Patients with minimal-change disease often have complete remission of the nephrotic syndrome upon withdrawal of lithium. However, minimal-change disease may occur after readministration of lithium.

CHRONIC INTERSTITIAL NEPHRITIS

Lithium was first associated with chronic interstitial nephritis in 1977 when a kidney biopsy study described an increase in interstitial fibrosis, focal nephron atrophy, or both, in lithium-treated patients compared with age-matched controls. In this study, 80% of the lithium-treated patients had decreased creatinine clearances. Subsequently, a number of retrospective and uncontrolled studies found the prevalence of chronic kidney disease to be 3% to 20% in patients treated long-term with lithium, but other disorders causing chronic kidney disease were not always excluded. In contrast, additional studies compared lithium-treated patients to a more suitable control group made up of psychiatric patients not receiving lithium, and found no differences in serum creatinine or creatinine clearance, but kidney biopsies were not performed.

Prospective studies have shown that chronic lithium therapy in psychiatric patients can significantly impair the GFR compared with similarly matched psychiatric patients who never received lithium. Kidney biopsies in lithium-treated patients have demonstrated increased interstitial fibrosis and a unique tubular lesion consisting of microcyst formation due to cystic dilation of the distal tubules lined with enlarged columnar epithelium. Renal microcysts measuring 1 to 2 mm may be detected by magnetic resonance imaging.

Taken together, these studies indicate that a small number of patients treated with lithium develop chronic kidney disease associated with chronic interstitial nephritis. In those patients with mild to moderate chronic kidney disease from lithium, withdrawal of lithium may be associated with gradual improvement in GFR. However, several patients have been reported to develop endstage renal disease requiring dialysis therapy despite withdrawal of lithium, particularly if they were treated with lithium for more than 20 years. Baseline kidney function studies, including serum creatinine, blood urea nitrogen, and creatinine clearance, should be performed prior to the initiation of lithium therapy and thereafter measured yearly. Patients who demonstrate deterioration in kidney function should have lithium therapy withdrawn and either carbamazepine or valproic acid initiated. For those patients who can only be managed on lithium because of psychological dependence on this drug, lithium therapy can probably be continued with careful monitoring of kidney function by creatinine clearance over time while maintaining the serum lithium level within the lower therapeutic range.

BIBLIOGRAPHY

Allen HM, Jackson RL, Winchester MD, et al: Indomethacin in the treatment of lithium-induced nephrogenic diabetes insipidus. Arch Intern Med 149:1123–1126, 1989.

Batlle D, Gaviria M, Grupp M, et al: Distal nephron function in patients receiving chronic lithium therapy. Kidney Int 21:477–485, 1982.

Batlle DC, von Riotte AB, Gaviria M, Grupp M: Amelioration of polyuria by amiloride in patients receiving long-term lithium therapy. N Engl J Med 312:408–414, 1985.

Farres MT, Ronco P, Saadoun D, et al: Chronic lithium nephropathy: MR imaging for diagnosis. Radiology 229:570–574, 2003.

Hestbech J, Hansen HE, Amdisen A, Olsen S: Chronic renal lesions following long-term treatment with lithium. Kidney Int 12:205–213, 1977.

Jorkasky DK, Amsterdam JD, Oler J, et al: Lithium-induced renal disease: A prospective study. Clin Nephrol 30:293–302, 1988.

Kwon TH, Laursen UH, Marples D, et al: Altered expression of renal AQPs and Na$^+$ transporters in rats with lithium-induced NDI. Am J Physiol Renal Physiol 279:F552–F564, 2000.

Leblanc M, Raymond M, Bonnardeaux A, et al: Lithium poisoning treated by high-performance continuous arteriovenous and venovenous hemodiafiltration. Am J Kidney Dis 27:365–372, 1996.

Lehmann K, Ritz E: Angiotensin-converting enzyme inhibitors may cause renal dysfunction in patients on long-term lithium treatment. Am J Kidney Dis 25:82–87, 1995.

Poindexter AE, Braden GL, Honeyman D, et al: Lithium-induced chronic renal failure: Improved renal function after discontinuing lithium vs progression to endstage renal disease with long-term continued use. J Am Soc Nephrol 10:86A, 1999.

Presne C, Fakhuri F, Noel LH, et al: Lithium-induced nephropathy: Rate of progression and prognostic factors. Kidney Int 64:585–592, 2003.

Rimmer RT, Sands JM: Lithium intoxication. J Am Soc Nephrol 10:666–674, 1999.

Tam VKK, Green J, Schwieger J, Cohen AH: Nephrotic syndrome and renal insufficiency with lithium therapy. Am J Kidney Dis 27:715–720, 1996.

Walker RG, Bennett WM, Davies BM, Kincaid-Smith P: Structural and functional effects of long-term lithium therapy. Kidney Int 21:513–519, 1982.

CHAPTER **50**

Renal Papillary Necrosis

Garabed Eknoyan

Necrosis of the renal parenchyma may affect the cortex or the medulla. Unlike cortical necrosis, which is a rare, acute, and often catastrophic event, necrosis of the medulla is a relatively common, chronic event, which generally pursues an insidious course and is often localized to the inner zone of the medulla and, more specifically, the papilla. Renal papillary necrosis (RPN) is a distinct clinicopathologic entity that occurs in a relatively limited number of individuals afflicted with an apparently disparate group of diseases (Table 50-1).

PATHOGENESIS

Restriction of the necrotic lesions to the papilla can be ascribed to the unique structural and functional features of this region (Fig. 50-1). The first is the blood supply to the papilla. The rich vascular plexus formed by the descending and ascending vasa rectae is principally devoted to the countercurrent exchange mechanism necessary to maintain medullary hypertonicity. The relatively small fraction of medullary blood flow that serves a nutrient function is provided by capillaries that branch off for this purpose. Hence, total medullary blood flow cannot be equated with medullary tissue nutrient supply. Additionally, the number and size of the vasa rectae and their intercommunications and that of their branching nutrient capillaries gradually decrease during the course of their descent to the inner zone such that the tip of the papilla has only small terminal vessels with sparse intercommunications. Since there is a three- to fourfold increase in interstitial mass in the inner zone of the medulla compared with that of the cortex and medulla, the net effect is a relatively poor blood supply to the parenchyma of the papilla compared with the remainder of the kidney. Conditions associated with occlusive lesions of the small vasculature of the kidney (diabetes mellitus, sickle hemoglobinopathy, transplanted kidney) or compromised blood flow to the kidneys (shock or hypovolemia in neonates) therefore predispose to ischemic necrosis of the renal papilla. The propensity of the elderly to arteriosclerosis has been implicated as an additional cause of reduced medullary blood flow. More than 50% of RPN cases are observed in individuals older than 60 years of age (except in sickle hemoglobinopathies). Another important feature of the papillary vasculature that predisposes it to necrosis is its greater

dependence on vasodilator prostanoids. On a mole-per-tissue-weight basis, the ratio of prostaglandin synthetase activity of the papilla to that of the medulla and cortex is 100:10:1. Agents that inhibit cyclooxygenase (COX) activity (nonsteroidal anti-inflammatory drugs, or NSAIDs, be they selective or nonselective COX-2 inhibitors) will compromise blood flow sufficiently to result in ischemia of this relatively underperfused region. Patients with chronic arthralgias (rheumatoid arthritis, gouty arthritis, osteoarthritis) who use NSAIDs chronically (more than a cumulative dose of 1000 tablets) have a 12% risk of developing RPN.

A second variable predisposing the papilla to necrosis is the ability of the tubule to concentrate solutes in this region. Though necessary to promote water reabsorption, this has a deleterious effect when potentially nephrotoxic agents are concentrated in the medulla, with their greatest accumulation being in the papillary tip. This explains the prevalence of RPN in individuals who abuse analgesics (phenacetin, acetaminophen, salicylates). Whereas the coadministration of these agents provides a biochemical basis of their cytotoxicity, by producing an oxidant stress and blocking its reduction, it is their concentration in the medulla that localizes the initial and major injury caused by analgesic abuse to the papilla. Abolition of medullary hypertonicity by water diuresis results in a reduction in the concentration of analgesics in the papilla and provides protection from RPN.

Another aspect of medullary hypertonicity relevant to papillary necrosis may be its detrimental effect on the normal phagocytic function of polymorphonuclear leukocytes, which would predispose it to infection. Urinary tract infection was once considered a principal cause of papillary necrosis. However, although urinary tract infection is present in most patients with papillary necrosis, it is not a uniform finding. It is more likely a secondary complication superimposed on necrotic foci, particularly when the necrotic tissue causes obstruction. Independent of infection, obstruction of the urinary tract can cause RPN because of reduced medullary blood flow. Following obstruction, an initial brief period of vasodilatation is followed by significant and persistent vasoconstriction. That this vasoconstriction should exert its most detrimental effect in the papilla is not unexpected given the sparse blood flow of this region and its dependence on vasodilatory prostanoids.

TABLE 50-1 Clinical Conditions Associated with Renal Papillary Necrosis

Conditions	Frequency (%)*
Diabetes mellitus	50–60
Urinary tract obstruction	10–40
Analgesic abuse	15–20
Sickle hemoglobinopathy	10–15
Kidney allograft rejection	<5
Pyelonephritis	<5

*Frequency with which each cause has been noted at autopsy in major reviews of RPN cases.

In the clinical conditions that have been associated with RPN, more than one causative factor (obstruction, infection, diabetes, chronic analgesic or NSAID use) is present in more than half of the patients who develop papillary necrosis. As such, although each of these clinical conditions (see Table 50-1) alone may cause papillary necrosis, the coexistence of more than one predisposing condition increases the risk of papillary necrosis. Thus, a diabetic patient who uses analgesics chronically would be more prone to develop medullary injury, since the papilla injured by diabetic vasculopathy produces a smaller amount of vasodilatory prostanoids at a time that the sclerotic vessels are less responsive to them, thereby making the papilla more prone to ischemic injury due to NSAIDs. Additionally, the resultant necrotic focus can

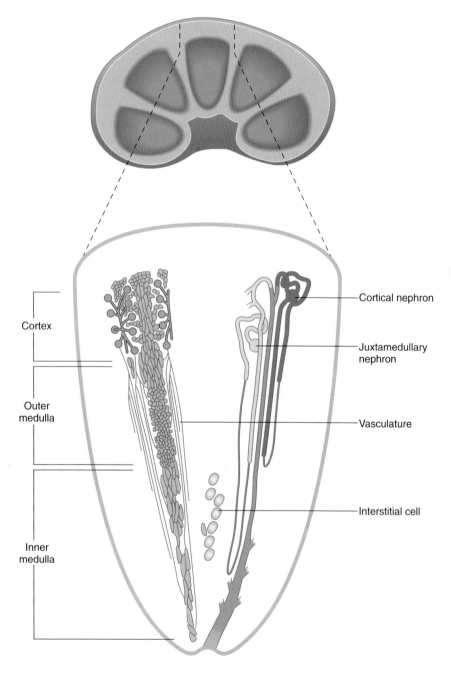

Cortex

Outer medulla

Inner medulla

Cortical nephron

Juxtamedullary nephron

Vasculature

Interstitial cell

FIGURE 50-1 Schematic representation of the multilobular kidney. The magnified lobule at the bottom shows on the right the different termination in the medulla of the cortical and juxtamedullary nephrons, and on the left the vascular supply to the various regions of the kidney. Note the diminishing vasculature of the vasa rectae in the course of their descent to the medulla and papillary tip.

become the nidus of an infection, and should it slough, it could cause obstruction. Thus, it is usually a vicious cycle of vascular occlusion, vasospasm, infection, and obstruction that leads to full-blown papillary necrosis, whereby RPN would result from the overlap of several detrimental influences operating in concert.

COURSE AND CLINICAL MANIFESTATIONS

The necrotic process may be localized to one or involve several papillae (see Fig. 50-1). Both kidneys are involved in 65% to 70% of cases. Patients who have a unilateral lesion at the time of initial diagnosis will often develop papillary necrosis in the other kidney as well. The process begins with foci of coagulative necrosis, consistent with ischemic necrosis, which coalesce and extend to involve the rest of the papillary tissue. Depending on the localization of the initial necrotic process it may assume the medullary form, in which the necrosis is found in the innermost medullary region while the fornices and papillary tip are viable, or the papillary form, in which the fornices and papillary tip are destroyed. The medullary form is more common in sickle cell hemoglobinopathies.

The necrotic lesions have a well-demarcated sharp border and proceed to form a sequestrum that may calcify, slough, or be resorbed, leaving a sinus tract or cavity at its site. Cavity and sinus formation are more common in the medullary form, whereas calcification and sloughing are more common in the papillary form. Sloughing is generally associated with hematuria, which can be gross and massive. The passage of sloughed necrotic tissue may be associated with lumbar pain and ureteral colic, which are clinically similar to that of nephrolithiasis. This can be confusing if the sloughed tissue is calcified and mimics a stone on imaging studies. The necrotic tissue or the stagnant urine in the cavities may be the nidus of a urinary tract infection that either can be chronic, smoldering, and recurrent, or may present in an acute, fulminant form. With the advent of antibiotics and improved management of superimposed urinary tract infection, the central role once attributed to infection in the development and course of RPN has diminished considerably.

The course of papillary necrosis is variable. Occasionally, it will present as an acute disease with septicemia and rapidly progressive loss of kidney function. Sometimes, it will pursue a protracted but symptomatic course with recurrent episodes of urinary infection or renal colic. Much more commonly, the lesions remain totally asymptomatic, with RPN detected as an incidental finding on urinary tract imaging or an unexpected discovery at postmortem examination as in more than one half of diabetics, two thirds of patients with sickle cell disease, and one tenth of arthritic patients who consume analgesics.

The magnitude of lost kidney function that develops depends on the number of papillae involved. Although some loss of functional reserve is expected to result from any parenchymal necrosis, kidney failure does not always occur. Even when several papillae are affected, localization of the necrosis to the papillary tips results in the loss of only the juxtamedullary nephrons whose loops descend to the papillary tip while the cortical nephrons, which terminate in the outer zone of the medulla, are spared (see Fig. 50-1). Consequently, a sufficient number of functioning nephrons remain to maintain homeostasis. As a greater number of the papillae are affected and cortical scarring develops, progressive loss of kidney function and kidney failure will ultimately occur. Patients with kidney failure due to any of the conditions in Table 50-1 can develop de novo RPN while on maintenance dialysis. Therefore, the diagnosis of RPN should be entertained when hematuria or severe urinary tract infection occur in dialysis patients.

Because it is the deep nephrons that are primarily affected, an inability to concentrate the urine maximally is an early manifestation. Consequently, polyuria and nocturia are common and may be a presenting complaint, elicited in the history, or demonstrated by appropriate testing.

Proteinuria is common (70% to 80% of cases) but is usually only modest (less than 2 g/day). Pyuria is also common (60% to 80% of cases). Microscopic hematuria (20% to 40%) and gross hematuria (20%) are less common, except during episodes of acute necrosis.

DIAGNOSIS

In symptomatic patients, the diagnosis can be made on finding portions of necrotic tissue in the urine, the pathologic examination of which establishes their papillary origin. A deliberate search for papillary fragments should be made by straining the urine through a filter.

In the absence of tissue diagnosis, excretory or retrograde urography has been the best method to establish a diagnosis. Unfortunately, the radiologic changes do not become apparent until the lesions are advanced and the papillae are shrunken or sequestered (Fig. 50-2). Ultrasonography, technetium scintigraphy, and computerized tomography are less sensitive but can be helpful, especially in patients with poor kidney function.

THERAPY

In the absence of a causative influence that can be readily avoided (analgesics) or surgically corrected (obstruction), therapy is directed toward associated complications. Control and/or eradication of urinary infection are essential. The blood glucose of diabetics should be well controlled. Analgesic mixtures and NSAIDs should be avoided. Increased fluid intake should be encouraged to

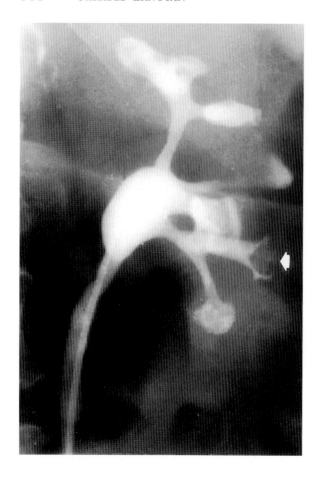

FIGURE 50-2   Retrograde pyelogram of a diabetic patient with papillary necrosis. The calyces are all blunted. One (*arrow*) demonstrates a sloughed papilla nearly encircled by contrast—the "ring" sign. (Courtesy of Dr. William L. Campbell.)

avoid the medullary concentration of these potentially nephrotoxic agents if their continued use is necessary to relieve pain. Control of hypertension, as in any other kidney disease, is important. Antihypertensive agents that reduce blood flow to the kidneys (beta blockers, thiazides) are best avoided. Conversely, angiotensin-converting enzyme inhibitors can provide protection. Volume depletion, which compromises blood flow to the kidneys and increases blood viscosity, should be prevented.

BIBLIOGRAPHY

Bach PH, Nguyen TK: Renal papillary necrosis. 40 years on. Toxicol Pathol 26:73–91, 1998.

Delzell E, Shapiro S: A review of epidemiologic studies of nonnarcotic analgesics and renal disease. Medicine 77:102–121, 1998.

Eknoyan G, Qunibi WY, Grissom RT, et al: Renal papillary necrosis: An update. Medicine 61:55–73, 1982.

Garber SL, Mirochnik Y, Arruda JA, et al: Differential effect of enalapril and irbesartan in experimental papillary necrosis. Kidney Blood Press 24:39–43, 2001.

Griffin MD, Bergstralh EJ, Larson TS: Renal papillary necrosis—a sixteen year clinical experience. J Am Soc Nephrol 6:248–256, 1995.

Groop L, Laasonen L, Edgren J: Renal papillary necrosis in patients with IDDM. Diabetes Care 12:198–202, 1989.

Sabatini S, Eknoyan G (eds): Renal papillary necrosis. Semin Nephrol 4:1–106, 1984.

Segasothy M, Sansad SA, Zulfigar A, Bennett WM: Chronic renal disease and papillary necrosis associated with long-term use of nonsteroidal anti-inflammatory drugs as the sole or predominant analgesic. Am J Kidney Dis 24:17–24, 1994.

CHAPTER 51

Obstructive Uropathy

William L. Whittier Stephen M. Korbet

Obstructive uropathy refers to the structural or functional interference with normal urine flow anywhere along the urinary tract from the renal tubule to the urethra. The resultant increase in pressure within the urinary tract proximal to the obstruction contributes to a number of structural and physiologic changes. Hydronephrosis, dilatation of the calyces and renal pelvis, is the anatomic outcome of an obstructive process that affects the collecting system distal to the renal pelvis (Fig. 51-1). Hydroureter, the term applied to ureteral dilatation, often accompanies hydronephrosis when the level of obstruction is distal to the ureteropelvic junction. The functional and pathologic changes of the kidney that can ensue are termed obstructive nephropathy.

In the United States, approximately 400,000 patients a year are hospitalized with problems related to obstructive uropathy. The overall prevalence of obstructive uropathy as diagnosed at autopsy by the presence of hydronephrosis is approximately 3%, with men and women affected equally. This obviously underestimates the true prevalence of the disorder, since temporary conditions such as nephrolithiasis would not be included. Differences in the frequency and causes of obstruction occur between males and females when evaluated at different times of life. The frequency of obstruction is similar between males and females up to the age of 20 years. Strictures of the urethra or ureter and neurologic abnormalities account for most causes of obstruction identified at autopsy in those patients 10 years of age and younger. The rate of obstruction in women is greatest between the ages of 20 and 60 years, primarily as a result of obstruction from pregnancy and gynecologic cancers. When obstructive uropathy occurs over the age of 60 years, it is more common in males due to benign prostatic hypertrophy or prostate cancer.

Urinary tract obstruction, if left untreated, can result in progressive, irreversible loss of kidney function and endstage renal disease if both kidneys are affected or only a solitary kidney is present. However, obstructive uropathy represents one of the few potentially curable forms of kidney disease and should therefore be considered in the differential diagnosis of any patient presenting with unexplained acute renal failure or chronic kidney disease. Since the overall success of therapeutic intervention is directly linked to the duration and degree of obstruction, early identification is crucial.

CLASSIFICATION AND CLINICAL AND LABORATORY MANIFESTATIONS

Urinary tract obstruction is often classified on the basis of duration, location, and degree of the obstructive process. The duration of obstruction is described as acute (hours to days), subacute (days to weeks), and chronic (months to years). The location of the obstruction (Tables 51-1 through 51-3) can be anywhere from the renal tubule to the urethral meatus and thus can affect one (unilateral obstruction) or both (bilateral obstruction) collecting systems. Finally, the degree of obstruction may be partial or complete.

These basic attributes of the obstructive process ultimately determine the clinical and laboratory manifestations with which a patient presents. The clinical presentation of patients with an acute obstruction is typically that of abrupt pain. If the process is unilateral and at the level of the renal pelvis or ureter, severe flank pain results, often described as colicky in nature when due to an intraluminal process such as nephrolithiasis or papillary necrosis. If this occurs at the level of the bladder outlet, then suprapubic pain and fullness may be experienced. This may be accompanied by urinary frequency and urgency if the outlet obstruction is partial, or anuria if the obstruction is complete. On physical examination, hypertension as well as flank pain on percussion or a suprapubic mass may be demonstrated in patients with outlet obstruction. In patients with two kidneys, laboratory manifestations of unilateral obstruction will often be limited to abnormalities of the urinalysis. With intrinsic forms of obstruction, microscopic or gross hematuria may be observed, and with either intrinsic or extrinsic processes, secondary infection may result in pyuria and bacteriuria. In conditions leading to bilateral obstruction (or unilateral obstruction in patients with a solitary kidney), laboratory features of acute renal failure will be observed.

The presenting clinical features associated with subacute or chronic obstruction are generally more subtle and insidious in nature. Instead of severe pain, the development of vague symptoms such as flank or suprapubic fullness may be described depending on the location of the obstruction. In addition, patients may experience frequency, polyuria, or nocturia, and may also have difficulty initiating or stopping urination, as well urgency if

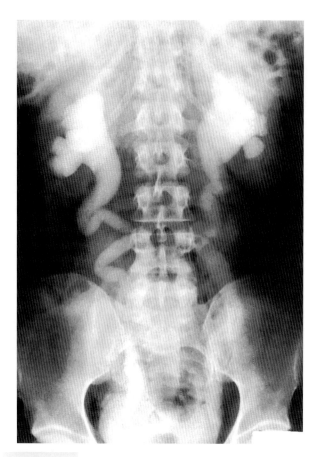

FIGURE 51-1   Intravenous pyelogram demonstrating bilateral, severe dilatation of the renal calyces, pelvis, and ureter. (Courtesy of Dr. Suresh K. Patel, Rush Medical College.)

TABLE 51-2   Extrinsic Causes of Obstructive Uropathy

Reproductive disorders
   Female
      Uterus (pregnancy, prolapse, tumors)
      Ovary (abscess, cysts, tumor)
      Fallopian tubes (pelvic inflammatory disease)
   Male
      Prostate (benign hyperplasia, adenocarcinoma)

Gastrointestinal disorders
   Appendicitis
   Crohn's disease
   Diverticulitis
   Pancreatitis
   Colorectal carcinoma

Vascular disorders
   Aneurysms (abdominal aortic, iliac)
   Venous (ovarian vein thrombophlebitis, retrocaval ureter)

Retroperitoneal disorders
   Fibrosis (idiopathic, drug related, inflammatory)
   Infection
   Radiation therapy
   Tumor (primary or metastatic)
   Iatrogenic complication of surgery

bladder outlet obstruction is present. In addition to elevated blood pressure, the physical findings may include a flank mass from a hydronephrotic kidney or a suprapubic mass, extending to the umbilicus, due to a greatly distended bladder. Laboratory evaluation of the urine can be similar to that seen in acute obstruction but may include proteinuria (often less than 2 g/day). Impairment in kidney function will also be observed in patients with bilateral disease, as indicated by laboratory features of chronic kidney disease, hyperkalemia, renal tubular acidosis, and an inability to concentrate the urine.

The differential diagnosis of obstructive uropathy is extensive (see Tables 51-1 through 51-3). In addition to the features already described, clinical and laboratory characteristics unique to the individual disorders should

TABLE 51-1   Intrinsic Causes of Obstructive Uropathy

Intraluminal
   Intrarenal
      Tubular precipitation of proteins or crystals
         Bence Jones proteins
         Uric acid
         Medications
   Extrarenal
      Nephrolithiasis, blood clots, papillary necrosis, fungus balls

Intramural
   Anatomic
      Tumors (renal pelvis, ureter, bladder, urethra)
      Strictures (ureteral or urethral)
         Infections
         Granulomatous disease
         Instrumentation or trauma
         Radiation therapy
   Functional disorders of the bladder
      Diabetes mellitus
      Multiple sclerosis
      Spinal cord injury
      Anticholinergic agents

TABLE 51-3   Congenital Causes of Obstructive Uropathy

Ureter
   Ureteropelvic junction obstruction
   Ureteroceles
   Ectopic ureter
   Ureteral valves
   Megaureter

Bladder
   Myelodysplasias
   Bladder diverticula

Urethra
   Prune-belly syndrome
   Urethral diverticula
   Posterior urethral valves

be considered and pursued in the evaluation of a patient with obstructive uropathy.

ETIOLOGY

Acquired-Intrinsic

The acquired forms of obstructive uropathy (see Tables 51-1 and 51-2) are often classified according to the location of the obstructive process as intrinsic (obstruction occurring within the urinary tract) or extrinsic (obstruction resulting from external compression of the urinary tract). Intrinsic disorders leading to obstruction are divided into intraluminal and intramural processes.

Intraluminal obstruction may be the result of renal tubular obstruction, otherwise called intrarenal obstruction. This is most often identified with acute renal failure in multiple myeloma from the precipitation of Bence Jones proteins in the tubules (myeloma kidney), and in the tumor lysis syndrome in which the chemotherapeutic treatment of a malignancy (generally a lymphoma) or the spontaneous lysis of the tumor leads to the massive production and subsequent precipitation of uric acid crystals within the tubules. Several drugs are also associated with intrarenal obstruction due to precipitation or crystal formation within the renal tubules, and these include sulfadiazine, sulfamethoxazole, ciprofloxacin, cephalexin, ampicillin, foscarnet, acyclovir, indinavir, nelfinavir, triamterene, primidone, aspirin, vitamin C, xylitol, allopurinol, and methotrexate. The predisposition for obstruction in most of these conditions is enhanced in the setting of volume contraction with the excretion of a concentrated, acidic urine. Of the extrarenal causes of obstruction, nephrolithiasis is the most common, particularly in young men. The most common form of stone contains calcium, most often calcium oxalate (see Chapter 53). Papillary necrosis can lead to ureteral obstruction and may be seen in sickle cell disease, diabetes mellitus, amyloidosis, and analgesic abuse (see Chapter 50). In addition, gross hematuria with blood clots resulting from any cause, but including kidney trauma, polycystic kidney disease, immunoglobulin A (IgA) nephropathy, or sickle cell trait may lead to extrarenal obstruction.

Intramural obstruction can be divided into anatomic and functional causes. Of the anatomic abnormalities that lead to urinary obstruction (tumors and strictures), transitional-cell carcinomas of the renal pelvis and ureter account for the highest proportion. Of particular note, patients with analgesic nephropathy are at increased risk for the development of transitional-cell carcinoma of the urinary tract. Ureteral or urethral strictures may result from infection, trauma, or postradiation therapy for pelvic tumors. Worldwide, schistosomiasis infection (caused by the blood fluke *Schistosomiasis haematobium*) is a considerable problem that affects nearly 100 million people. The parasites deposit their ova in the walls of the distal ureter and bladder, causing inflammation that leads to ureteral stricture, and fibrosis and contracture of the bladder in 50% of chronically infected patients. The incidence of bladder cancer is also increased. Rarely, obstructive uropathy may result from ureteral strictures from granulomatous disease or urethral stricture due to gonococcal and nongonococcal infections. Functional obstruction results from an abnormality (neuromuscular) leading to an alteration in the normal dynamic response of the urinary tract. In neurologic disorders resulting in injury to upper motor neurons, involuntary bladder contraction (spastic bladder) results, whereas with lower motor neuron injury the bladder becomes flaccid and atonic. Either condition may lead to abnormalities in the forward flow of urine and an increase in residual urine volume that can result in obstructive uropathy with vesicoureteral reflux. Almost 90% of patients with multiple sclerosis develop bladder dysfunction. This disorder is also common in patients with long-standing diabetes mellitus, and it may complicate Parkinson's disease as well as cerebrovascular accidents. Several medications are known to alter the neuromuscular activity of the bladder, resulting in decreased contractility or tone and thus urinary retention, with an incidence of greater than 10% in some instances (levodopa and disopyramide). The use of these agents may be particularly problematic in patients with a pre-existing obstructive condition, such as benign prostatic hyperplasia in men.

Acquired-Extrinsic

The most common cause of extrinsic obstruction in women is pregnancy. In as many as 90% of pregnant women, some degree of ureteral dilatation will be observed by the third trimester. This has been attributed to pressure by the gravid uterus on the pelvic rim and affects the right ureter more than the left. However, ureteral dilatation may be seen as early as the first trimester, and it has been suggested that this may be the result of hormonal (progesterone) effects on peristalsis. This process is often asymptomatic and resolves spontaneously after delivery. Rarely, bilateral ureteral obstruction during pregnancy can lead to acute renal failure (see Chapter 56). The second most common cause of urinary obstruction in women is carcinoma of the cervix, with obstruction seen in 30% of patients, usually a result of direct extension. In older women, uterine prolapse can lead to hydronephrosis, and this may occur in as many as 80% of patients if there is total prolapse. In these women, the ureters are trapped between the levator muscles and the fundus of the prolapsed uterus. Endometriosis occasionally leads to pelvic inflammation with fibrosis and ureteral obstruction. Pelvic inflammatory disease may result in obstruction in as many as 40% of patients if associated with a tubo-ovarian abscess.

Benign prostatic hyperplasia is the most common cause of obstructive uropathy in older men, with symptoms of outlet obstruction in 50% to 75% of males over 50 years of age and significant hydronephrosis in 10% of cases. Overall, adenocarcinoma of the prostate is second only to carcinoma of the cervix as the leading form of extrinsic obstruction due to tumors. Obstruction from prostate cancer (or any pelvic malignancy) can be due to either direct extension of tumor to the bladder outlet or ureters, or metastases to the ureters or surrounding lymph nodes.

In addition to colorectal carcinomas (ureteral metastases), a number of gastrointestinal disorders are associated with obstruction (often unilateral) resulting from local infection and/or inflammatory processes. Vascular diseases, the most common of which is abdominal aortic aneurysm, will lead to ureteral obstruction from retroperitoneal fibrosis (inflammatory aneurysms) or from direct pressure of the expanding aneurysm. Rarely, systemic diseases associated with vasculitis (e.g., systemic lupus erythematosus, polyarteritis nodosa, Wegener's granulomatosis, and Henoch-Schönlein purpura) have been associated with obstruction.

Several conditions involving the retroperitoneal space may result in ureteral obstruction by fibrosis or direct invasion and compression. Periureteral fibrosis can be a consequence of radiation therapy, trauma, surgery, granulomatous disease, malignancy, autoimmune diseases, or infection. Retroperitoneal fibrosis has been linked to the use of several drugs, including methysergide, bromocriptine, phenacetin, ergotamines, hydralazine, methyldopa, and beta blockers. Patients in whom an obvious cause for retroperitoneal fibrosis cannot be identified have idiopathic retroperitoneal fibrosis, which is predominantly a disease of men (3:1) in the fifth and sixth decade of life. Flank pain that is insidious in onset, dull, and not colicky, is the presenting symptom in 80% of patients. This may be accompanied by fever, weight loss, and nonspecific gastrointestinal complaints. On intravenous pyelography (IVP), medial deviation of the ureters is a characteristic feature. The fibrous tissue appears to extend from the aorta, encasing and drawing the ureters medially, and can be up to 6 cm thick. Hydroureteronephrosis is typically visualized on kidney ultrasonography (US) but may be absent in as many as 2.5% of patients. Although the etiology of this entity is unknown, there are theories that the fibrosis is a result of a localized inflammatory reaction to ceroid, an oxidized low-density lipoprotein. The histologic findings are those of an inflammatory process involving collagen and fibrosis. Surgical release of the ureters (ureterolysis) is often successful in relieving obstruction and pain symptoms, and in cases in which the etiology is truly idiopathic, long-term steroid therapy has been used in addition to surgery.

Primary tumors, such as lymphomas, can involve the retroperitoneal space and can lead to obstruction. In addition, metastatic spread to the retroperitoneum of a number of carcinomas, most commonly the cervix (30%) and bladder (20%), but including the breast, prostate, colon, and ovary, can also result in ureteral obstruction. The most likely cause of obstruction after pelvic irradiation for malignancy is recurrent tumor if obstruction occurs within 2 years of therapy. Radiation fibrosis is the more common cause after 2 years.

Congenital

Of the congenital causes of obstructive uropathy (see Table 51-3), ureteropelvic junction obstruction (UPJ) and posterior urethral valves are the most common. If severe enough, obstruction may have its onset in utero and may lead to major renal abnormalities in the developing fetus. Early in development, obstruction results in a kidney that appears dysplastic. Obstruction later on leads to a kidney with cortical cysts and a reduced nephron mass. Those fetuses in whom obstruction develops late in gestation have features similar to those seen postnatally, such as hydronephrosis and renal parenchymal thinning. Occasionally, obstruction may not manifest itself until childhood.

Ureteropelvic junction obstruction is the most common cause of hydronephrosis in infancy and early childhood. In childhood, the majority of patients are males, whereas in adults, females predominate. In infancy, UPJ obstruction is bilateral in 30% of cases, an uncommon finding in adults. The presentation in children is that of an abdominal mass with flank pain or abdominal pain and failure to thrive. In adults, the pain is episodic and is often precipitated by high urine flow rates. Abnormal peristalsis due to a derangement in the smooth muscles of the renal pelvis has been proposed as the primary mechanism for UPJ obstruction. Additionally, a hyperdistensible renal pelvis that is incapable of draining completely has been suggested as the cause in some cases. Less often, UPJ obstruction may result from crossing blood vessels, fibrous bands, or strictures.

Posterior urethral valves, leading to outlet obstruction, are seen strictly in males and are best diagnosed by a voiding cystourethrogram. Presentation in infancy is with a palpable bladder and kidneys along with marked renal functional impairment. Older children will often present with urgency or enuresis. One of the more unusual causes of obstructive uropathy is the prune-belly syndrome. Predominantly seen in males, this consists of the triad of deficiency of abdominal muscles (resulting in loose, wrinkled, redundant skin over the abdomen appearing like a "prune"), cryptorchidism, and hydroureteronephrosis. The obstruction is bilateral, with abnormal ureteral peristalsis and prostatic hypoplasia implicated as possible mechanisms.

Nonobstructive Urinary Tract Dilatation

In a number of situations, dilatation of the urinary tract may occur without evidence of obstruction. However, these conditions, if chronic, may also result in impaired kidney function and atrophy of renal parenchyma. This can be seen with vesicoureteral reflux, acute pyelonephritis, and high-flow states (such as diabetes insipidus or primary polydipsia). As already mentioned, ureteral dilatation can be observed in 90% of women during pregnancy, but it usually resolves within a few weeks of delivery and therefore does not result in any functional or pathologic renal impairment unless complicated by infection.

PATHOPHYSIOLOGY

Our understanding of the consequences of urinary tract obstruction on kidney function is primarily derived from the effects of short-term (24 hours) complete obstruction in experimental animals. The alterations in kidney function that result are divided into those that affect either glomerular or tubular function.

Glomerular Function

Glomerular filtration rate (GFR) declines progressively after complete obstruction. Within the first few hours of acute ureteral obstruction, there is an increase in proximal tubular pressure, the magnitude of which is partially dependent on hydration status (greater with increased hydration). This results in a decrease in net glomerular filtration pressure (net glomerular filtration pressure = glomerular filtration pressure – intratubular pressure) and thus a decrease in GFR. Simultaneously, an increase in the production of prostacyclin and prostaglandin E_2 leads to afferent arteriolar dilatation (vasodilative phase) and an increase in renal blood flow, which increases glomerular filtration pressure. However, since the increase in glomerular filtration pressure is not as great as that in intratubular pressure, the decrease in net glomerular filtration pressure persists, resulting in a GFR that is 80% of the preobstruction value.

At 4 to 5 hours after obstruction, intratubular pressure begins to decline due to ongoing reabsorption of sodium and water by the nephron, dilatation of the collecting system, and lymphatic removal of solute and water. A decrease in renal blood flow due to an increase in afferent arteriolar resistance (vasoconstrictive phase) also ensues, leading to a decrease in glomerular filtration pressure. Since glomerular filtration pressure declines at a faster rate than the intratubular pressure, a further decrease in net glomerular filtration pressure occurs and GFR continues to decline. Thus, the relatively higher intratubular pressure continues to contribute significantly to the

ongoing decrease in GFR, which can be as low as 20% of normal by 24 hours.

The vasoconstrictive phase is mediated by angiotensin II (AII), thromboxane A_2, antidiuretic hormone (ADH), and a decrease in endothelium-derived relaxing factor or nitric oxide production. The increase in intrarenal production of AII is a consequence of decreased delivery of sodium and chloride to the macula densa and the effects of vasodilating prostaglandins on renin release. The source for the increased synthesis of thromboxane A_2 in the obstructed kidney includes intrinsic glomerular cells and leukocytes (macrophages and T lymphocytes), which infiltrate soon after obstruction. In addition to their effects on vascular resistance, AII and thromboxane A_2 alter GFR by producing mesangial contraction, which leads to a decrease in the ultrafiltration coefficient. Pretreatment with angiotensin-converting enzyme (ACE) inhibitors and inhibitors of thromboxane A_2 synthesis has been shown to counteract the effects of obstruction on GFR and renal plasma flow in experimental models.

The degree of improvement in GFR after release of obstruction in animals is related to the duration of obstruction. Complete recovery of GFR is observed after obstruction of up to 7 days, 70% recovery with 14 days of obstruction, 30% recovery with 28 days of obstruction, and essentially no recovery of kidney function after obstruction of 56 days.

Tubular Function

Abnormalities in reabsorption of sodium and water are characteristic of obstructive nephropathy. In the acute phases of obstruction, there is an initial increase in sodium and water reabsorption secondary to underperfusion of the distal nephron. This is shown by reductions in urinary sodium concentration, fractional excretion of sodium, and free-water clearance. In clinical practice, this results in urinary indices that can have a prerenal pattern, with a urinary sodium of less than 20 mEq/L, a fractional excretion of sodium of less than 1%, and a urine osmolality of greater than 500 mOsmol (see Chapter 34). With more prolonged or chronic obstruction, subsequent alterations in tubular function result in a decrease in sodium and water reabsorption and indices similar to those seen with acute tubular necrosis.

After the release of chronic obstruction, there is decreased sodium reabsorption by the nephrons, leading to an increased fractional excretion of sodium. The decrease in sodium reabsorption results from a reduction in Na^+ K^+-ATPase activity in the nephron. Additionally, there is an associated increase in excretion of calcium, phosphate, and magnesium that parallels sodium excretion. The ability to concentrate urine is also impaired after release of obstruction and results in an increased fractional excretion of water. The concentrating defect is due to several influences, including: (1) decreased medullary tonicity from washout of solute due to an increase in medullary blood flow and decreased sodium chloride reabsorption at the thick ascending limb of Henle, (2) decreased response to ADH, and (3) a decrease in the number of functional juxtamedullary nephrons. The greater natriuresis and diuresis observed after release of bilateral ureteral obstruction (BUO) as compared with unilateral ureteral obstruction (UUO) is attributed to the accumulation of sodium and water, urea retention, retention of other impermeable solutes, and higher levels of atrial natriuretic peptide, which occur in BUO but not UUO.

Abnormalities in potassium and hydrogen ion excretion are also common in obstructive uropathy. Hyperkalemia results, since the fractional excretion of potassium is less in obstructive uropathy than in other forms of kidney disease with similar reductions in kidney function. The decrease in potassium secretion is attributed to a reduction in the secretion or response of the distal tubule to aldosterone, or a combination of both. Hyperkalemic-hyperchloremic acidosis is also frequently seen in patients with obstructive uropathy. This may be explained by a defect in hydrogen ion secretion and maximal urine acidification (distal renal tubular acidosis), and/or a defect in secretion of aldosterone secondary to a decrease in renin production (hyporeninemic hypoaldosteronism or type IV renal tubular acidosis). Furthermore, a decrease in sodium reabsorption in the distal nephron has been suggested as an additional influence, which by reducing the degree of intraluminal negativity would decrease the voltage-dependent secretion of both potassium and hydrogen. Finally, reduced levels of H^+-ATPase (a major transport pathway) in the cortical and medullary collecting ducts have been observed in obstructive uropathy and may further explain the problem with hydrogen ion excretion. The acidifying defect is often reversible, but it may persist in some cases.

RENAL PATHOLOGY

The pathology of hydronephrosis is similar irrespective of the underlying cause of obstruction. In early hydronephrosis, the kidney is enlarged and edematous with an increase in the renal pelvic cavity and blunting of the renal papilla. Later on there is retraction and dimpling of the papilla, and this is most evident at the upper and lower poles. Microscopically, the renal cortex appears normal, but the tubules may be dilated, and Tamm-Horsfall protein is seen in Bowman's space (characteristic of obstruction or reflux). The principal lesion in the medulla and papilla is ischemic atrophy associated with flattening and atrophy of tubular epithelium and interstitial fibrosis. As the hydronephrosis advances, the atrophy becomes even more pronounced. The kidney transforms into essentially a fluid sac with loss of papillae and marked thinning of the cortex and medulla. The pro-

gressive sclerosis and fibrosis results in few renal features that are recognizable.

The morphologic changes in obstructive uropathy are primarily attributed to the ischemia from the marked reduction in renal blood flow. However, another contributing feature that has gained interest is the role played by macrophages and T lymphocytes, which invade the interstitium early during obstruction. Within 4 to 12 hours after obstruction, there is an increase in interstitial macrophages that continues thereafter. Chemoattractants, such as monocyte chemoattractant peptide-1 and osteopontin, appear to be released from tubular epithelial cells in response to the increase in intratubular pressure from ureteral obstruction. Fibrogenic cytokines, such as transforming growth factor-β (TGF-β), produced by the invading macrophages and T lymphocytes become central in the progressive fibrosis observed in obstructive nephropathy. TGF-β increases matrix synthesis by interstitial fibroblasts and decreases matrix degradation by down-regulating the production of matrix degradation proteins and promoting the generation of proteinase inhibitors. Other factors that have been linked to the progressive fibrosis include tumor necrosis factor-α (TNF-α), growth factors such as interleukin-6 and platelet-activating factor, nuclear factor κB, adhesion proteins, and matrix or basement membrane proteins. A reduction in levels of bone-morphogenic protein-7 (BMP-7) and hepatocyte growth factor have also been shown to contribute to fibrosis in animal models of obstruction. Finally, it has been shown that vasoactive compounds such as angiotensin II (which is increased in obstruction) may directly stimulate the production of TGF-β by tubular epithelial cells or macrophages. In experimental obstructive uropathy, the use of ACE inhibitors significantly reduces the messenger RNA (mRNA) levels of TGF-β and type IV collagen, resulting in a marked decrease in the degree of tubulointerstitial fibrosis and preventing further progression of kidney disease. The beneficial effects of ACE inhibitors were observed even when initiated 1 week after the onset of obstruction. Antifibrotic effects are even more striking with the use of the tubular developmental morphogen BMP-7. Although clinical data are as yet lacking, these experimental insights suggest a potentially important role for ACE inhibitors as well as other inhibitors of fibrosis in the medical management of patients with obstructive uropathy.

DIAGNOSIS

Dilatation of the urinary tract is the radiographic feature characteristically used to confirm the presence of obstruction (see Fig. 51-1). When the diagnosis of obstructive uropathy is suspected, a careful history, physical examination, and laboratory evaluation (measurement of kidney function, electrolytes, and urinalysis and culture) are essential in developing a differential diagnosis and diagnostic approach (Fig. 51-2).

Obstructive uropathy should always be a consideration in patients presenting with markedly impaired kidney function (acute or chronic), especially when the nature of the kidney dysfunction is unexplained. Reduced kidney function in obstructive uropathy may come as a result of either bilateral upper tract obstruction or, more commonly, outlet or lower tract obstruction. In the presence of clinical clues to obstruction of the bladder outlet (i.e., difficulty urinating, suprapubic pain, or fullness and a palpable bladder), a postvoid bladder catheterization is initially beneficial both diagnostically and therapeutically. Additional diagnostic evaluation with US allows a quick, noninvasive way to confirm and assess the cause and severity of obstruction and avoids the possibility of nephrotoxic insult from the use of intravenous contrast required in other imaging procedures such as the IVP.

The use of US to diagnose chronic obstruction when sufficient time has elapsed for the urinary tract to dilate has a sensitivity of 98% and a specificity of 75%. False-positive results (up to 26%) are often due to normal variants such as blood vessels in the renal sinuses, and these can be discerned with the use of duplex Doppler evaluation. The use of duplex Doppler evaluation in determining the resistive index is also helpful in distinguishing true obstruction (elevated resistive index) from nonobstructive causes (having a normal resistive index of 50% to 60%) of urinary tract dilatation. A false-negative ultrasonographic evaluation is extremely rare in the evaluation of chronic obstruction. Computerized tomography (CT) is also an accurate technique for the detection of urinary tract dilatation and may be more likely than US to identify the obstructing lesion. However, to enhance structural identification with conventional CT, contrast is often required. Whether or not unenhanced spiral CT will prove beneficial, over and above conventional CT or US, in the evaluation of chronic obstruction is yet to be seen. Magnetic resonance imaging (MRI) is another option for detection of urinary tract dilation, particularly in the patient with abnormal kidney function or pregnancy, since it avoids potentially nephrotoxic contrast administration as well as ionizing radiation. However, MRI is more expensive and has no proven benefit over the conventional US or unenhanced spiral CT. Ultimately, with upper tract obstruction, antegrade or retrograde pyelography may be required to further define the site and cause of obstruction. The use of retrograde pyelography may be of particular value in the situation in which a nondilated obstructive uropathy due to retroperitoneal fibrosis or an infiltrating malignancy is suspected. Although these studies can be useful when it is not possible to do an IVP or when the use of intravenous contrast is contraindicated (allergy to contrast or impaired kidney function), the risk of urinary tract infection is of concern particularly with retrograde pyelography. To further evaluate (and treat) causes of lower urinary tract obstruction, cystoscopy and urodynamic studies may be indicated. Urodynamic studies are most worthwhile when a functional abnormality of the bladder (neurogenic bladder) is suspected.

In patients with symptoms of acute, unilateral obstruction (renal function is often normal), such as in nephrolithiasis, sufficient time for identifiable dilatation of the collecting system may not have elapsed, and therefore the IVP has been considered the "gold standard." Whether or not the use of less invasive technology such as US can replace the IVP in detecting acute urinary tract obstruction has been an area of intense interest

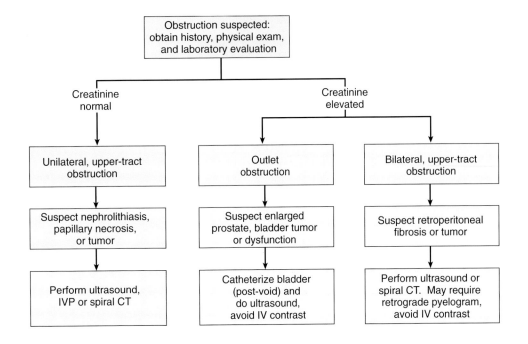

FIGURE 51-2 Initial diagnostic approach when obstructive uropathy is suspected.

(Fig. 51-3A, B). This stems primarily from the small but definite morbidity and mortality associated with the use of radiographic contrast. The success of US in diagnosing acute obstruction varies substantially (sensitivity reported to be as low as 50% and as high as 90%). In part, the variable success of US is attributed to its subjective nature, making it highly operator dependent, with most false negatives due to cases of grade 1 hydronephrosis (mild dilatation of the renal sinus central-echo complex) or nondilated obstructive uropathy (i.e., retroperitoneal fibrosis). Because nephrolithiasis is the leading cause of acute renal colic and obstruction, and more than 90% of renal stones are radiopaque, combining plain abdominal radiography (kidney, ureter, bladder, or KUB) with US increases the sensitivity of detecting obstruction to greater than 95%. Finally, the use of duplex Doppler ultrasound, to demonstrate the presence of a high resistive index (greater than 70%) from increased vascular resistance in unilateral obstruction, has been shown to reduce further the false-negative results associated with US (this is helpful in either acute or chronic obstruction). Thus, the combination of US and KUB may be a viable alternative to studies requiring radiographic contrast. A limitation of US remains its inability to determine the level and the cause of obstruction as compared with IVP. Enthusiasm is mounting for the use of unenhanced spiral CT in the evaluation of acute renal colic. The scan takes less than 20 seconds to obtain images from the top of the kidneys to the base of the bladder and does not require contrast. Furthermore, it is more sensitive than combined KUB and US in identifying causes of renal colic, and it allows visualization of the obstructive lesion, including radiolucent stones not detectable on KUB.

Though a chronic condition, UPJ obstruction is often associated with symptoms that are acute in nature and reproduced only during periods of high urine flow rates. Often a diagnosis of UPJ obstruction requires the use of diuresis urography, which combines the administration of intravenous furosemide with an IVP to evaluate for dilatation and abnormal emptying of the upper urinary tract during a state of high urine flow. A similar evaluation can be obtained with diuresis renography using radionuclides (see later).

NONOBSTRUCTIVE URINARY TRACT DILATATION

Nonobstructive urinary tract dilatation may be differentiated from that due to obstruction with diuresis renography or diuresis urography. Diuresis renography utilizes radionuclide imaging and evaluates the pattern of radionuclide elimination by each kidney before and after administration of intravenous furosemide. Prolonged retention of radioactivity after diuresis is consistent with obstruction. In nonobstructive dilatation, there is a rapid "washout" of radioactivity with diuresis. Similar findings can be demonstrated with the use of diuresis urography.

TREATMENT

The treatment of obstructive uropathy is dictated not only by the underlying cause but also by the location. It should be obvious that evidence for impaired kidney function (acute or chronic) resulting from urinary tract obstruction warrants emergency attention, since the potential for permanent kidney damage increases with the duration of obstruction. The urgency and aggressiveness with which obstructive uropathy must be treated is also determined by the severity of symptoms (flank pain, dysuria, frequency, etc.) as well as the presence of infection.

Nephrolithiasis, the most common cause of acute unilateral obstruction, can most often be treated with conservative measures such as intravenous fluids and pain medications. Because 90% of stones smaller than 5

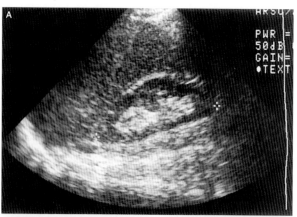
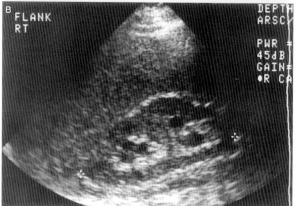

FIGURE 51-3 *A,* Ultrasonogram of the right kidney, long axis, demonstrating the normal echo-dense central area, the renal sinus central echo complex. *B,* Repeat ultrasonogram of the right kidney, long axis, in the same patient 3 weeks later after presenting with a 3-day history of right flank pain. Note hydronephrosis (pyelocalyceal dilatation) as demonstrated by a marked separation of the renal sinus central echo complex.

mm pass spontaneously with increased urine flow alone, no additional treatment is required. However, with increasing stone size, the likelihood of spontaneous passage diminishes and the possible need for more aggressive measures arises. These are discussed in detail in Chapter 53. In extreme situations of chronic or recurrent unilateral obstruction of any cause, the obstructive process may lead to advanced hydronephrosis associated with severe pain, recurrent pyelonephritis, or pyonephrosis, in which case a nephrectomy may be indicated, especially if the remaining function of the affected kidney is minimal.

The initial treatment approach for patients presenting with bilateral urinary tract obstruction and impaired kidney function is primarily dictated by the location of the obstruction. In patients with a neurogenic bladder or disorders involving the bladder outlet (i.e., prostatic hyperplasia or cancer), the placement of a urethral catheter will often suffice. For patients in whom a urethral catheter cannot be passed into the bladder, a suprapubic cystostomy may be required. Lesions obstructing the ureters require cystoscopy and stent placement. If a stent cannot be passed beyond the ureteral obstruction in a retrograde fashion, a percutaneous nephrostomy tube can be placed and antegrade placement of a stent can be attempted. Placement of a percutaneous nephrostomy is successful in over 90% of patients, resulting in clinical improvement in up to 70% of cases. Major complications (abscess, sepsis, hematomas) occur in less than 5% of patients.

Once an acute solution to relieve the obstruction has been initiated, then specific treatment of the underlying disease becomes the primary focus. For example, in neurogenic disorders of the bladder, timed voiding and pharmacologic agents (in patients with a spastic bladder, anticholinergic agents: oxybutynin or propantheline bromide) may be useful, but in many patients, particularly those with bladder atony, intermittent catheterization of the bladder (four times daily) is necessary. For men with prostatic hyperplasia, the long-term treatment approach is dependent on the severity of the outlet obstruction. If symptoms are minimal and are not associated with infection or upper urinary tract abnormalities, close observation is appropriate. Cases with mild to moderate symptoms of prostatism can be managed medically with either alpha antagonists or 5α-reductase inhibitors. Alpha antagonists (doxazosin or terazosin) act by relaxing the smooth muscle of the prostate and bladder neck, thus decreasing urethral pressure and outlet obstruction. Hormonal therapy with a 5α-reductase inhibitor (finasteride) inhibits the conversion of testosterone to the active dihydrotestosterone and thereby leads to a reduction in prostate size. The combined use of these agents may be beneficial in some patients, since they are felt to act synergistically. In patients with hyperplasia of the prostate resulting in signs and symptoms of severe obstruction (significant urinary retention or impaired kidney function), surgical intervention (i.e., transurethral resection of the prostate, transurethral incision of the prostate, or laser ablation) is generally required.

In disease processes that lead to irreparable damage of the lower urinary tract (as in bladder, cervical, or prostate cancer) or ureters, a diversion procedure such as an ileal conduit or percutaneous nephrostomy will be needed. In patients with obstructive nephropathy secondary to malignancy, percutaneous nephrostomy can relieve the obstruction in more than 75% of cases and results in a significant increase in survival (more than 6 months in 50%) as well as an increase in number of days spent at home as compared with patients in whom the procedure was not performed. Thus, patients with apparently terminal diseases can benefit from this aggressive approach.

Postobstructive Diuresis

Release of bilateral obstruction can result in marked polyuria (postobstructive diuresis). Several physiologic and pathologic influences lead to development of this condition. Physiologic influences contributing to the diuresis include excess sodium and water retention, accumulation of urea and other nonreabsorbable solutes, and accumulation of atrial natriuretic peptide. Pathologic factors include decreased tubular reabsorption of sodium, inability to maximally concentrate urine due to a decreased medullary concentrating gradient and decreased response to ADH, and increased tubular flow reducing equilibration time for absorption of sodium and water. Once the accumulated excess of sodium and water has been excreted, the potential exists for severe volume contraction as well as hypokalemia if patients are not carefully monitored and given appropriate fluid and solute replacement. Urinary output should be measured frequently during the diuresis (at least every 6 hours and in cases with large urine outputs, hourly). Once the patient has diuresed to the point of euvolemia, fluid replacement (intravenous plus oral) should be administered as needed to prevent volume contraction based predominantly on clinical and laboratory parameters. This is often accomplished by replacement of 75% of the urine losses with intravenous fluids having a solute composition similar to what is excreted (0.45% normal saline). Serum electrolyte levels should also be monitored closely during the diuresis, at least daily if not more often, and replaced as needed. The postobstructive diuresis is self-limited, resolving over several days to a week. Persistence of the polyuria is often due to overzealous hydration (in excess of urinary output), which perpetuates the solute and water diuresis.

Recovery of Kidney Function

The likelihood of regaining kidney function postobstruction is dependent on the degree and duration of obstruction. The longer the process goes untreated, the less likely it is that significant recovery in kidney function will occur. In general, the majority of improvement in kidney function should be apparent within 2 weeks after the obstruction. Complete recovery of kidney function is anticipated in patients with acute uncomplicated obstruction of short duration (less than 1 to 2 weeks), and little to no improvement in severe, complete, or partial obstruction that persists for a prolonged period of time (more than 12 weeks). However, recovery of kidney function in patients has been recorded after obstruction for as long as 70 days. The use of radionuclide renography has been suggested as one way to predict or assess recovery of kidney function. This is usually done several weeks after a temporary procedure to relieve the obstruction (such as a percutaneous nephrostomy) has been performed.

BIBLIOGRAPHY

Better OS, Arieff AI, Massry SG, et al: Studies on renal function after relief of complete unilateral obstruction of three months duration in man. Am J Med 54:234–240, 1973.

Cronan JJ: Contemporary concepts for imaging urinary tract obstruction. Urol Radiol 14:8–12, 1992.

Davidson AJ, Hartman DS: The dilated pelvocalyceal system. In Davidson AJ, Hartman DS (eds): Radiology of the Kidney and Urinary Tract, 2nd ed. Philadelphia, WB Saunders, 1994, pp 571–780.

Demko T, Diamond J, Groff J: Obstructive nephropathy as a result of retroperitoneal fibrosis: A review of its pathogenesis and associations. J Am Soc Nephrol 8:684–688, 1997.

Diamond JR: Macrophages and progressive renal disease in experimental hydronephrosis. Am J Kidney Dis 26:133–140, 1995.

Haddad MC, Sharif HS, Shahed MS, et al: Renal colic: Diagnosis and outcome. Radiology 184:83–88, 1992.

Harrington KJ, Pandha HS, Kelly SA, et al: Palliation of obstructive nephropathy due to malignancy. Br J Urol 76:101–107, 1995.

Hill GS: Calcium and the kidney, hydronephrosis. In Jennette JC, Olson JL, Schwartz MM, Silva FG (eds): Heptinstall's Pathology of the Kidney, 5th ed. Philadelphia, Lippincott-Raven, 1998, pp 891–936.

Hoffman LM, Suki WN: Obstructive uropathy mimicking volume depletion. JAMA 236:2096–2097, 1976.

Hruska K: Treatment of chronic tubulointerstitial disease: A new concept. Kidney Int 61:1911–1922, 2002.

Ishidoya S, Morrissey J, McCracken R, Klahr S: Delayed treatment with enalapril halts tubulointerstitial fibrosis in rats with obstructive nephropathy. Kidney Int 49:1110–1119, 1996.

Perazella MA: Crystal-induced acute renal failure. Am J Med 106:459–465, 1999.

Katz DS, Lane MJ, Sommer FG: Unenhanced helical CT of ureteral stones: Incidence of associated urinary tract findings. Am J Radiol 166:1319–1322, 1996.

Klahr S: Pathophysiology of obstructive nephropathy: A 1991 update. Semin Nephrol 11:156–168, 1991.

Klahr S: New insight into the consequences and mechanisms of renal impairment in obstructive nephropathy. Am J Kidney Dis 18:689–699, 1991.

Klahr S, Purkerson ML: The pathophysiology of obstructive nephropathy: The role of vasoactive compounds in the hemodynamic and structural abnormalities of the obstructed kidney. Am J Kidney Dis 23:219–223, 1994.

Klahr S, Ishidoya S, Morrissey J: Role of angiotensin II in the tubulointerstitial fibrosis of obstructive nephropathy. Am J Kidney Dis 26:141–146, 1995.

Klahr S, Morrissey J: Obstructive nephropathy and renal fibrosis: The role of bone morphogenic protein-7 and hepatocyte growth factor. Kidney Int 64(suppl 87):S105–S112, 2003.

Klahr S, Morrissey J, Hruska K, et al: New approaches to delay the progression of chronic renal failure. Kidney Int 61(suppl 80):S23–S26, 2002.

Spital A, Spataro R: Nondilated obstructive uropathy due to a ureteral calculus. Am J Med 98:509–511, 1995.

Suki W, Eknoyan G, Rector FC Jr, Seldin DW: Patterns of nephron perfusion in acute and chronic hydronephrosis. J Clin Invest 45:122–131, 1966.

Vehmas T, Kivisaari L, Mankinen P, et al: Results and complications of percutaneous nephrostomy. Ann Clin Res 20:423–427, 1988.

Webb JA: Ultrasonography in the diagnosis of renal obstruction. BMJ 301:944–946, 1990.

Zeidel ML, Pirtskhalaishvili G: Urinary tract obstruction. In Brenner BM (ed): The Kidney, 7th ed. Philadelphia, WB Saunders, 2004, pp 1867–1893.

CHAPTER 52

Vesicoureteral Reflux and Reflux Nephropathy

Billy S. Arant, Jr.

The urine that emerges from the papillary collecting ducts through the ducts of Bellini is collected in the calyces and flows into the renal pelvis and down the ureter to enter the bladder via the ureteral orifice located in the trigone. The intravesical pressure is usually maintained low (less than 20 cm H_2O) as the smooth muscle of the bladder wall relaxes while the bladder gradually fills with urine. During micturition, the intravesical pressure rises, but it usually does not exceed 35 cm H_2O as the bladder smooth muscle contracts, because the external sphincter relaxes to permit urine to exit the bladder via the urethra. In the normal bladder, urine does not re-enter the ureter, because the distal end of the ureter forms a flap valve by penetrating the bladder wall in an oblique fashion and following a submucosal course of about 5 cm in the adult before reaching the bladder lumen. The contraction of the bladder smooth muscle and flattening of the mucosa by the increased intravesical pressure assure competence of the ureterovesical junction during micturition.

An incompetent ureterovesical junction permits urine to flow retrogradely from the bladder into the ureter, an occurrence termed vesicoureteral reflux (VUR). Often, a shortened submucosal portion does not permit the flap valve to occlude the ureter during micturition—one explanation for the more frequent presence of VUR in infants, since their submucosal ureter may be only 2 cm long. When intravesical pressure is high enough, refluxing urine can fill the ureter and renal pelvis, actually re-enter the ducts of Bellini, and even traverse the entire course of the nephron to reach Bowman's space—intrarenal reflux. When there is no other abnormality of the bladder, VUR is primary and may be observed in the fetus or at birth, in which case it is congenital. If identified only at some time after birth, it is considered acquired. However, in the presence of functional or anatomic obstruction, VUR is considered secondary. When VUR is associated with unusually high intravesical pressure or pyelonephritis, any resulting renal parenchymal injury is termed reflux nephropathy.

PREVALENCE

The actual incidence of VUR in the general population has never been described. When individuals with no history of a urinary tract infection (UTI) underwent voiding cystourethrography, VUR was identified in fewer than 0.5%. On the other hand, VUR could be demonstrated in 20% to 60% of infants and children but in only 4% of adults when they were investigated after their first recognized UTI. In children under 6 years of age, the cumulative incidence rate for a first-time symptomatic UTI is 6.6% for girls and 1.8% for boys. Although girls have more UTIs than boys, there is no gender difference in the incidence of VUR after a first UTI. VUR seems to occur equally among races, except for African-American children who, in most reports, have had VUR associated with UTI in fewer than 4%. Therefore, based on a current U.S. population of approximately 25 million children under 6 years of age, just over 1 million will have a symptomatic UTI, and 40% (460,000) will have VUR.

When asymptomatic siblings of children with VUR were screened, VUR was found in about 35% to 45%. Although a common gene has not been identified, VUR does occur in several generations of the same family, suggesting that hereditary factors predispose to primary VUR. Screening of siblings of a child with VUR who are under 5 years old and asymptomatic or are newborns is recommended to identify patients at risk of kidney injury before the first episode of UTI. There is no such familial pattern or screening recommendation among children with secondary VUR.

DIAGNOSTIC STUDIES TO IDENTIFY VESICOURETERAL REFLUX

A voiding cystourethrogram (VCUG) is the only diagnostic imaging technique in current use that is reliable in identifying VUR (Fig. 52-1). To perform this study, a catheter is inserted through the urethra or a suprapubic needle is used to fill the urinary bladder with radiographic contrast material or with a solution containing a radionuclide. Observations are made before, during, and after micturition. VUR will be identified most often at peak intravesical pressure generated during micturition. The reported incidence of VUR is based mostly on studies that used contrast VCUG data. This technique is dependent on the skill of the examiner and may fail to detect VUR in as many as 40% of patients with UTI, including some with dilated collecting systems. Although the increased sensitivity of radionuclide testing is desirable, neither the grading of VUR nor identification of

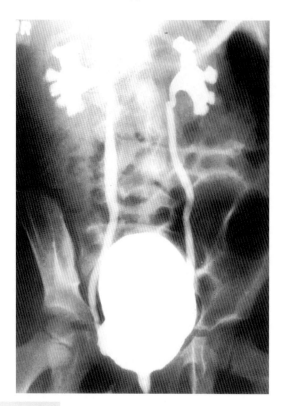

FIGURE 52-1 Contrast voiding cystourethrogram demonstrates vesicoureteral reflux when intravesical pressure is highest. Both collecting systems are filled completely and dilated with mild tortuosity of the ureters and blunting of the calyces: grade III VUR (international classification).

anatomic abnormalities can be accomplished by this method. Ultrasonography is of no value in detecting VUR but can identify dilatation of the renal collecting system.

The grading of VUR has had an important role when clinical decisions are considered. In general, higher grades of VUR are associated more often with kidney injury and, in the past, were grounds for early recommendation of surgical correction. The five-grade classification proposed by the International Study of Reflux in Children has been adopted almost universally. When contrast enters the ureter but does not reach the renal pelvis, grade I is assigned. If the entire collecting system is filled but not dilated, grade II is assigned. In grades III, IV, and V, progressive dilatation and tortuosity of the ureter are observed. Such a classification is useful when a prospective study is conducted or an individual patient is followed with serial studies to confirm any change in VUR, but its reproducibility depends heavily on the VCUG being conducted in a standardized fashion. Although it is relatively easy for anyone to assign a grade of VUR on any static image, VUR is an active urodynamic process that depends not only on the competence of the ureterovesical junction but also on the intravesical pressure, the elasticity of the collecting system, the rate of antegrade flow of urine, and the timing of the study. The international classification depends on the grade of VUR being assigned at peak voiding pressure, which usually occurs within 30 to 60 seconds of initiating the urinary stream. Although the grading system has been relied on heavily, there is probably no clinical relevance to grading VUR other than nondilating (grades I and II) or dilating (grades III, IV, and V), because the resolution rate and the prevalence of kidney injury are similar among grades in these two groups.

RENAL SCARRING

Vesicoureteral reflux may predispose to UTI but does not cause it. When VUR is associated with UTI and pyelonephritis develops, kidney injury can result in parenchymal scarring, which may also be termed reflux nephropathy. Similar scarring that follows acute pyelonephritis without VUR has always been termed chronic pyelonephritis. Kidney ultrasonography can detect only gross parenchymal scarring but can provide accurate measurements of kidney size; a discrepancy in length of the two kidneys should raise suspicion of renal scarring. Intravenous urography will not identify acute renal injury, but when it is performed carefully, established renal scars or parenchymal thinning overlying an abnormal calyx can be identified (Fig. 52-2). A radionuclide scan using intravenous ^{99}Tc-dimercaptosuccinic acid (DMSA) is the imaging study that may detect both pyelonephritis during acute infection and renal scars 3 to 6 months after the infection has subsided. The isotope attaches to the proximal tubular epithelium located in the renal cortex and is detected in the scan. In nephrons not functioning because of acute inflammation or scarring, the isotope is not attached and a paucity of radioactivity is detected in the affected cortex. The DMSA scan is expensive. It delivers considerable radiation to the renal parenchyma, where the isotope remains attached for many hours, in close proximity in females to the ovaries. Therefore, the study does not represent standard of care but rather a useful tool for clinical research.

Renal scarring will occur in about 6% of kidneys after the first episode of pyelonephritis with or without VUR and irrespective of the grade of VUR. With each subsequent episode, the likelihood of scarring increases, reaching 58% after the fourth episode. Although renal scarring has been observed most often (25% to 50%) when severe dilating VUR (grades IV to V) is present at the time of diagnosis, only 25% of refluxing ureters exhibit this much dilatation. The total number of kidneys with renal scarring and severe dilating VUR, therefore, is relatively small. A much larger total number of children with UTI have lesser grades of VUR (grades I to III) with normal-appearing kidneys at diagnosis and a lower incidence of renal scarring (10% to 28%) identified in follow-up studies. Only half of the children with acute pyelonephritis will exhibit VUR, but many without VUR will also develop renal scarring. Therefore, the total number of

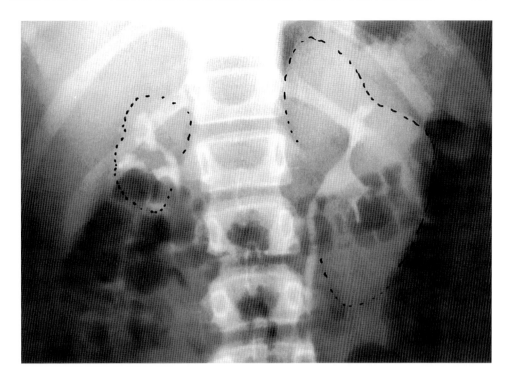

FIGURE 52-2 Intravenous urography demonstrates a small right kidney with extensive scarring but prompt excretion of contrast material into deformed calyces. The left kidney is larger than normal (compensatory hypertrophy) but has a cortical depression overlying a deformed calyx in the upper pole.

kidneys scarred by pyelonephritis is larger when VUR is absent or grades I to III. The fraction of kidneys scarred with severe dilating VUR is higher, but the total number of kidneys actually exposed to dilating reflux is less. Previously, there has been a strongly held opinion that renal scarring occurs only in infants and young children. One study, however, reported new renal scarring in previously normal kidneys in 80% of older children and adolescents with acute pyelonephritis; this was nearly identical to the incidence in younger patients. Similar findings of new scars in children after the age of 10 years have been observed by others.

PATHOLOGY

The gross appearance of a renal scar, either from pyelonephritis or reflux nephropathy, is a cortical depression overlying a calyx. The characteristic histopathologic findings include atrophy of both cortex and medulla in which glomerular remnants and thyroidization of tubular structures (tubules that have atrophied and dilated after injury and that have a histopathologic appearance similar to thyroid tissue) may still be identified. Failure to identify glomeruli in segmental scars was once interpreted as renal hypoplasia—the kidney did not develop normally, and, therefore, glomeruli were never formed in the segment. Subsequent studies, however, demonstrated that segmental scarring in a previously normal kidney was produced by parenchymal injury that heals by segmental atrophy with progressive glomerular sclerosis. Deterioration of kidney function after cessation of further acute renal injury is probably caused by hyperfiltration, as with any other remnant kidney or untreated arterial

hypertension. In fact, focal segmental glomerulosclerosis may be seen in both the scarred as well as the contralateral unscarred kidney. This finding suggests a substance produced by the scarred kidney, angiotensin perhaps, circulated to produce similar glomerular changes in the normal kidney.

CONSEQUENCES OF RENAL SCARRING

The morbidities associated with renal scarring of any degree are hypertension, and, when scarring is more extensive and involves both kidneys, chronic kidney disease. In fact, a common cause of hypertension in women under 30 years of age is renal scarring from VUR. The hypertension from renal scarring is mediated by angiotensin. Such hypertension is observed most often in females at puberty, when birth control pills are prescribed, and during pregnancy. This suggests a role for estrogen in raising blood pressure. Since hypertension may go undetected for years in this age group, it may follow a malignant course and can be responsible for further renal parenchymal destruction, especially during pregnancy. Once renal scarring is detected, blood pressure must be serially measured and glomerular filtration rate must be regularly assessed. Proteinuria is a sign of kidney injury and may be minimal or heavy, even in the nephrotic range when focal glomerulosclerosis is present.

PREVENTING KIDNEY INJURY

Because kidney injury is associated with acute pyelonephritis and because scarring occurs rarely in adults, prevention of kidney damage must be directed at aggressive management of UTIs in children with or without associated VUR. Prompt treatment of acute pyelonephritis with an effective antibiotic can prevent renal scarring. Every clinician should understand that although most children with acute pyelonephritis will have fever, some will not. Moreover, a urinalysis is not sufficient to confirm the presence of a UTI. A urine culture is required. Once a diagnosis of UTI has been made in a child, with or without a urine culture, there is an obligation to follow through with a complete radiologic evaluation and plan of follow-up if not done before. Controversy exists over what to do about asymptomatic bacteriuria. Without VUR, most recommendations are not to introduce antibiotic therapy. The dilemma comes when the patient has VUR and one is determined to prevent another episode of acute pyelonephritis. There are studies that detected no differences in renal scarring with or without antibiotic treatment of asymptomatic bacteriuria. One must understand, however, that acute pyelonephritis may not always be associated with fever, and clinical symptoms, especially in infants, may be related more to the gastrointestinal than to the urinary tract.

When patients with a UTI and VUR were treated medically for more than 30 years using a regimen that included daily antibiotic prophylaxis, additional renal scarring was prevented in all patients who remained free of UTI. In contrast, episodic treatment of UTI without prophylaxis was associated with renal scarring in more than 21% of patients. Therefore, prophylaxis should be considered as part of conservative treatment efforts to maintain the urine sterile as long as VUR persists. The drugs recommended most often for antibiotic prophylaxis are trimethoprim, trimethoprim-sulfamethoxazole, or nitrofurantoin. Equally important are good perineal hygiene, establishing a normal pattern of micturition to empty the bladder regularly and completely, and avoiding constipation. These efforts will reduce the number of bacteria that gain transurethral access to the bladder, particularly in females. Alternative treatments when medical management is unsatisfactory may include submucosal injection by cystoscopy of a compatible material such as collagen or surgical reimplantation of refluxing ureters. Indications of failed medical management include inability to prevent breakthrough UTI and perhaps, on some occasions, parental choice when there is either inability or unwillingness to comply with medical management. Well-designed, prospective studies comparing patients allocated randomly to surgery or medical management alone demonstrated no advantage of one over the other for long-term outcome. When children were managed

medically, 80% of nondilating VUR resolved within 5 years, whereas dilating VUR required as long 10 years to resolve.

Clinical guidelines for managing UTI in infants and young children have been established more recently by the American Academy of Pediatrics, and recommendations for managing VUR have been made by the American Urological Association. Together, these reports suggest more vigilance in detecting UTI, imaging studies after the first UTI in all infants and in children with UTI and fever, and more consistent follow-up of patients with UTI and VUR—more or less setting a conservative standard of care aimed toward preventing kidney injury that is based on the best information and opinion available.

Children with abnormal urodynamics or dysfunctional micturition not only have recurrent UTIs but also may generate high intravesical pressures, which may lead to or worsen VUR, risking acute pyelonephritis. Surgical correction of the VUR in these patients is usually unsuccessful. These patients require special attention and management that may include antibiotic prophylaxis, bladder training to develop coordination between bladder contraction and sphincter relaxation using biofeedback techniques, and anticholinergic drugs.

When scarring is bilateral and glomerular filtration rate is decreased below normal, consideration should be given to initiating treatment to reduce angiotensin effects, glomerular hyperfiltration, and deterioration of kidney function even if blood pressure is normal, in keeping with JNC7 guidelines (less than 125/80 mm Hg for adults). A common approach to limiting the progressive loss of kidney function, controlling hypertension, and reducing proteinuria in the focal segmental glomerulosclerosis of reflux nephropathy, like that of a primary glomerulopathy, is the use of angiotensin-converting enzyme inhibitors or angiotensin receptor blockade. Glucocorticoid therapy is not recommended to reduce proteinuria in focal segmental glomerulosclerosis secondary to reflux nephropathy. Surgical correction of VUR does not prevent further deterioration of kidney function due to prior parenchymal injury but, as discussed earlier, may be indicated to prevent or reduce subsequent episodes of acute pyelonephritis.

The overall prognosis is quite good for a child with VUR to resolve spontaneously without significant kidney injury when consistent clinical oversight is provided along established guidelines by the well-informed primary care physician. Kidney injury will occur more often when a clinician departs from the established consensus of recommendations or fails to critically appraise any new approach to managing UTI or VUR.

BIBLIOGRAPHY

American Academy of Pediatrics: Practice parameter: The diagnosis, treatment, and evaluation of the initial urinary tract infection in febrile infants and young children. Pediatrics 103:843–852, 1999.

Arant BS Jr: Vesicoureteric reflux and renal injury. Am J Kidney Dis 17:491–511, 1991.

Arant BS Jr: Medical management of mild and moderate vesicoureteral reflux: Follow-up studies of infants and young children. A preliminary report of the Southwest Pediatric Nephrology Study Group. J Urol 148:1683–1687, 1992.

Arar MY, Arant BS Jr, Hogg RJ, et al: Etiology of sustained hypertension in children in the Southwestern United States. Pediatr Nephrol 8:186–189, 1994.

Benador D, Benador N, Slosman D, et al: Are younger children at highest risk of renal sequelae after pyelonephritis? Lancet 149:17–19, 1997.

Bernstein J, Arant BS Jr: Morphologic characteristics of segmental renal scarring in vesicoureteral reflux. J Urol 148:1712–1714, 1992.

Chobanian AV, Bakris GL, Black HR, et al: The seventh report of the Joint National Committee on Prevention, Detection, Evaluation and Treatment of High Blood Pressure: The JNC 7 report. JAMA 289:2560–2572, 2003.

Elder JS, Peters C, Arant BS Jr, et al: Pediatric Vesicoureteral Reflux Guidelines Panel summary report on the management of primary vesicoureteral reflux in children. J Urol 157:1846–1851, 1997.

Jacobson SH, Eklof O, Eriksson CG, et al: Development of uraemia and hypertension after pyelonephritis in childhood—27 year follow-up. BMJ 299:703–706, 1989.

Jodal U: The natural history of bacteriuria in childhood. Infect Dis Clin North Am 1:713–729, 1987.

Marild S, Jodal U: Incidence rate of first-time symptomatic urinary tract infection in children under 6 years of age. Acta Paediatr 87:549–552, 1998.

Martinell J, Jodal U, Lidin-Janson G: Pregnancies in women with and without renal scarring after urinary infections in childhood. BMJ 300:840–844, 1990.

Noe HN: The long-term results of prospective sibling reflux screening. J Urol 148:1739–1742, 1992.

Rushton HG, Majd M, Jantausch B, et al: Renal scarring following reflux and nonreflux pyelonephritis in children. Evaluation with 99m-technetium dimercaptosuccinic acid scintigraphy. J Urol 147:1327–1332, 1992.

Smellie JM, Jodal U, Lax H, et al: Outcome at 10 years of severe vesico-ureteric reflux managed medically. Report of the International Reflux Study in Children. J Pediatr 139:656–663, 2001.

Wennerstrom M, Hansson S, Jodal U, et al: Primary and acquired renal scarring in boys and girls with urinary tract infection. J Pediatr 136:30–34, 2000.

CHAPTER 53

Nephrolithiasis

Gary Curhan

SCOPE OF THE PROBLEM

Nephrolithiasis is a major cause of morbidity involving the urinary tract. The prevalence of nephrolithiasis in the U.S. population increased from 3.8% in the late 1970s to 5.2% in the early 1990s. The increase in prevalence was observed in men and women, and whites and blacks. There were nearly 2 million physician office visits for stone disease in 2000. Surprisingly, the estimated annual costs have remained at approximately $2 billion, probably as a result of the shift from inpatient to outpatient procedures.

The lifetime risk of nephrolithiasis is about 12% in men and 6% in women. In men, the first episode of renal colic is most likely to occur in the third to sixth decade. The incidence for men who have never had a stone is about 0.3% per year between the ages of 30 and 60 years and then falls with age. For women, the rate is about 0.2% per year between the ages of 20 and 30 years and then declines to 0.1% for the next 4 decades.

The risk of the first recurrent stone after the incident stone in untreated patients remains controversial. Reported frequencies of stone recurrence from uncontrolled studies ranged from 30% to 50% at 5 years. However, data from the control groups of recent randomized controlled trials suggest much lower rates of first recurrence after an incident calcium oxalate stone, ranging from 2% to 5% per year. Sex-specific rates are not available from the randomized trials.

ACUTE RENAL COLIC

With the passage of a stone from the renal pelvis into the ureter resulting in partial or complete obstruction, there is sudden onset of unilateral flank pain of sufficient severity that the individual usually seeks medical attention. Despite the use of the misnomer "colic," the pain does not completely remit but rather waxes and wanes. Nausea and vomiting may accompany the pain. The pattern of pain depends on the location of the stone: when the stone is in the upper ureter, pain may radiate anteriorly to the abdomen; when in the lower ureter, pain may radiate to the ipsilateral testicle in men or labium in women; if lodged at the ureterovesical junction (UVJ), the primary symptoms may be urinary frequency and urgency. A less common acute presentation is gross hematuria without pain.

The symptoms from a ureteral stone may mimic several other acute conditions. A stone lodged in the right ureteropelvic junction can mimic acute cholecystitis. A stone lodged in the lower right ureter as it crosses the pelvic brim can mimic acute appendicitis. A stone lodged at the UVJ can mimic acute cystitis. A stone lodged in the lower left ureter as it crosses the pelvic brim can mimic diverticulitis. An obstructing stone with proximal infection can mimic acute pyelonephritis. Note that infection in the setting of obstruction is a medical emergency ("pus under pressure") that requires emergent drainage, either by placement of a ureteral stent or a percutaneous nephrostomy tube. However, because nephrolithiasis is common, the simple presence of a kidney stone does not confirm the diagnosis of renal colic in a patient presenting with acute abdominal pain.

Other conditions to consider in the differential diagnosis of suspected renal colic include muscular or skeletal pain, herpes zoster, duodenal ulcer, abdominal aortic aneurysm, gynecologic causes, ureteral obstruction due to other intraluminal factors, such as a blood clot or sloughed papilla, and ureteral stricture. Extraluminal factors causing compression tend not to present with symptoms of renal colic.

The physical examination alone will rarely make the diagnosis, but clues guide the evaluation. The patient will typically be in obvious pain and unable to achieve a comfortable position. There may be ipsilateral costovertebral angle tenderness or, in cases of obstruction with infection, signs and symptoms of sepsis may be present.

Although serum chemistries are typically normal, there might be a leukocytosis due to stress or infection. The serum creatinine is typically normal but may be elevated in the setting of volume depletion, bilateral ureteral obstruction, or unilateral obstruction in a patient with a solitary kidney. The urinalysis classically reveals red blood cells and white blood cells and may occasionally show crystals. If there is complete ureteral obstruction due to the stone, it is possible that there will be no red blood cells, since no urine will be flowing through that ureter into the bladder.

Because of the often nonspecific physical exam and laboratory findings, imaging studies play a crucial role in making the diagnosis. The imaging modality of choice is helical (spiral) computed tomography, because it does not require radiocontrast and can allow detection of stones as small as 1 mm, even pure uric acid stones (traditionally considered "radiolucent"). Typically, the study will show a ureteral stone or evidence of recent passage (e.g., perinephric stranding or hydronephrosis). A plain abdominal x-ray of the kidney, ureter, and bladder (KUB) can miss a stone in the ureter or kidney, even if radiopaque, and provides no information on obstruction. Although KUB is often used to follow the progress of a ureteral stone or growth of asymptomatic kidney stones, the sensitivity is limited. An intravenous pyelogram (IVP) requires contrast and can miss small stones, thus should only rarely be ordered for the evaluation and treatment of patients with nephrolithiasis. Although there is a general belief that the osmotic diuresis induced by the radiocontrast may facilitate stone passage, there is insufficient confirmatory evidence. Ultrasonography, while avoiding radiation, can only image the kidney and proximal ureter.

Renal colic is one of the most excruciating types of pain; therefore, pain control is essential. Narcotics and parenteral nonsteroidal anti-inflammatory drugs are effective, and the latter are preferable because they cause fewer side effects. Other treatments that may be effective include antispasmodics and alpha blockers. Urinary alkalinization may be effective for a uric acid stone, but this type is relatively rare and there must be adequate urine flow past the stone.

TYPES OF STONES

Nearly 90% of stones in men and 70% in women contain calcium, most commonly as calcium oxalate (Fig. 53-1). Other types of stones, such as cystine, pure uric acid, and struvite, are much less common. However, these types of stone also deserve careful attention, because recurrences are common. No information is available on the frequencies from first-time stone formers, in part because the first stone is typically not retrieved or sent for analysis.

PATHOGENESIS

The urinary concentrations of calcium, oxalate, and other solutes that influence stone formation are high enough that they should result in crystal formation in the urine of most individuals, but this is clearly not the case. This condition is termed supersaturation. However, substances in the urine—termed inhibitors—prevent crystal formation. The most common inhibitor is citrate, which works by chelating calcium cations in the urine, decreasing the free calcium available to bind with oxalate or phosphate anions. If the supersaturation is sufficiently high or there are insufficient inhibitors, precipitation occurs with resulting crystalluria.

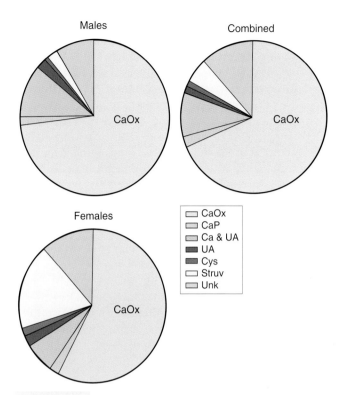

FIGURE 53-1 Types of stones and frequency in adults. Ca & UA, calcium and uric acid; CaOx, calcium oxalate; CaP, calcium phosphate; Cys, cystine; Struv, struvite; UA, uric acid; Unk, unknown. (Reprinted with permission from Coe F, Parks J [eds]: Nephrolithiasis: Pathogenesis and Treatment. Chicago, Year Book Medical, 1988.)

The causes of stone formation differ for different stone types. Cystine stones form only in individuals with the autosomal-recessive disorder of cystinuria. Uric acid stones form only in individuals with persistently acid urine with or without hyperuricosuria. Struvite stones form only in the setting of an upper urinary tract infection with a urease-producing bacterium. These stones are seen in individuals with recurrent urinary tract infections, particularly those with abnormal urinary tract anatomy such as patients who have urinary diversions or who require frequent catheterization. Stones may occasionally result from precipitation of medications such as acyclovir and indinavir in the urinary tract.

Calcium-based stones have a multifactorial etiology. Traditionally, stone formation was believed to occur from the following: (1) crystal formation in the renal tubule, (2) attachment of the crystal to the tubular epithelium, usually at the tip of the papilla, and (3) growth of the attached crystal by deposition of additional crystalline material. However, a recent study's results may change the way we view the initial steps in the process of stone formation. New evidence suggests that the initial crystal forms in the medullary interstitium and is composed of calcium phosphate. This may then erode through the papilla, on which calcium oxalate is subsequently deposited. Several medical conditions increase the likelihood of calcium oxalate stone formation. With primary hyperparathyroidism, urinary calcium is increased. Crohn's disease and other malabsorptive states in which the colon is intact are associated with increased urinary oxalate excretion. With fat malabsorption, calcium is bound in the small bowel to free fatty acids, leaving a smaller amount of free calcium to bind to oxalate. An increased amount of unbound oxalate is then available for absorption in the colon. The accompanying low urine volume presents an additional risk factor. Citrate reabsorption is increased by metabolic acidosis, leaving less urinary citrate to serve as a calcium chelator. Thus, distal renal tubular acidosis predisposes to stone formation as well.

Calcium phosphate stones are more likely to form in the presence of high urine calcium, low urine citrate, and alkaline urine. Systemic conditions that are present more frequently in patients with calcium phosphate stones include renal tubular acidosis and primary hyperparathyroidism. The remainder of this chapter will focus on calcium oxalate stones except where noted.

Urinary variables that increase the risk of calcium oxalate stone formation are higher levels of calcium, oxalate, and uric acid, and those that decrease the risk are the presence of citrate and total volume (Table 53-1). The traditional approach to urinary abnormalities is based on 24-hour urinary excretion. There are generally accepted definitions of "abnormal" values: hypercalciuria is defined as 250 mg/day or more for women and 300 mg/day or more for men; hyperoxaluria is defined as 45 mg/day or more for both women and men; hyperuricosuria exists in women excreting 750 mg/day or more and in men excreting 800 mg/day or more; hypocitraturia is defined as 320 mg/day or more for both women and men. After being evaluated, patients have typically been classified into categories according to their urinary abnormalities, and treatment and advice have been directed at correcting the abnormalities.

Although this approach has been used successfully for decades, it has several limitations that should be discussed. Stone formation is a disease of concentration. Thus, it is not just the absolute amount of the substances that determines likelihood of stone formation. Therefore, the traditional definitions of "abnormal" excretion must be applied cautiously for several reasons. First, there are insufficient data supporting the cutoff points used regarding the risk of actual stone formation. For example, the traditional definition of hypercalciuria is 50 mg/day higher in men than women. However, there is no justification with respect to stone formation for allowing the urine of a man to contain more calcium than that of a woman. Similarly, another common definition of hypercalciuria is urinary calcium excretion in excess of 4 mg/kg body weight/day. However, this definition "allows" an individual who is heavier or gains weight to excrete more calcium than someone who is thinner. Second, an individual could have "normal" excretion of calcium but still have high urinary calcium concentration of urinary calcium due to low urine volume. This situation has therapeutic implications, because the goal is to modify the concentration of the lithogenic factors. Finally, the risk of stone formation is a continuum, thus using a specific cutoff point may give the false impression that a patient with "high normal" urinary calcium excretion is not at risk for stone recurrence. Just as cardiovascular risk increases with increasing blood pressure (even in the "normal" range), the risk of stone formation increases with increasing urine calcium.

Pak and colleagues advocate subdividing individuals with elevated urinary calcium into three categories: (1) absorptive (increased gastrointestinal absorption of ingested calcium), (2) resorptive (increased bone resorption), and (3) renal (increased urinary excretion of filtered calcium). However, there is not general agreement on the clinical importance of this approach. A substantial proportion of patients cannot be classified, and there is evidence that individuals may change categories when studied years later. Thus, most clinicians do measure 24-hour urine chemistries as part of the metabolic evaluation but do not subclassify patients. The underlying mechanisms for idiopathic hypercalciuria remain unknown, although 1,25-dihydroxyvitamin D and the vitamin D receptor probably play important roles.

Increased urinary oxalate may result from either increased gastrointestinal absorption, due to high dietary oxalate intake or increased fractional oxalate absorption, or increased endogenous production. The relative contribution of exogenous and endogenous oxalate sources to urinary oxalate remains controversial but is probably close to 50% from each.

Purines are metabolized to uric acid. Increased urinary uric acid is the result of higher purine intake and higher endogenous production from purine turnover.

TABLE 53-1 Risk Factors for Calcium Oxalate Stone Formation

High Levels	Low Levels
Urinary risk factors	
Calcium	Citrate
Oxalate	Total volume
Uric acid	
Dietary risk factors	
Purines	Calcium, dietary
Animal protein	Potassium
Sodium	Phytate
Sucrose	Fluid
Calcium, supplemental	
Vitamin C	
Other risk factors	
Obesity	
Gout	
Hypertension	
Anatomic abnormalities	

Low urine citrate is typically seen in the setting of a systemic metabolic acidosis, such as from a renal tubular acidosis or excessive gastrointestinal bicarbonate losses with diarrhea. Because citrate is a potential source of bicarbonate, it is actively reclaimed in the proximal tubule after being filtered by the glomerulus.

Dietary variables associated with decreased risk of incident stone formation include dietary calcium, potassium, and fluid intake, whereas those associated with increased risk include supplemental calcium, animal protein, sodium, and sucrose (see Table 53-1). Although dietary oxalate intake is generally believed to be important for stone formation, data are limited. Many foods contain small amounts of oxalate, whereas foods that are high in oxalate are less common. Unfortunately, measurements of the oxalate content of foods have varied widely on account of differences among laboratories and analytic methods. In addition, little is known about the bioavailability of dietary oxalate.

Data from observational and randomized controlled studies support the concept that dietary calcium intake is inversely associated with risk of stone formation. The mechanism by which dietary calcium may reduce the risk of stone formation is unknown but may be related to calcium binding to oxalate in the intestine, thereby blocking oxalate absorption. It is also quite possible that there is some other protective substance in dairy products, the major source of dietary calcium.

Differences in timing of ingestion may explain the apparent contradiction between the protective effect of dietary calcium and the detrimental effect of supplemental calcium. If the calcium supplement were not taken with meals containing oxalate, a protective effect would not be expected. Rather the observed increase in risk might be due to increased urinary calcium excretion without any change in urinary oxalate excretion.

Nondietary factors that increase the risk for kidney stone formation include genitourinary anatomic abnormalities, medical conditions such as medullary sponge kidney, primary hyperparathyroidism, gout and hypertension, and larger body size.

CLINICAL EVALUATION

There is lack of agreement on the appropriate evaluation after the first kidney stone, although such an evaluation appears to be cost effective. The decision to proceed with an evaluation depends on several variables. First, what is the stone burden? Even though the episode that brought the patient to medical attention may have been the first symptomatic event, an appreciable proportion of patients will have remaining kidney stones and thus could be considered "recurrent" stone formers. Thus, if the patient had only a KUB or even an IVP during the acute evaluation, either of which could miss small stones, it seems prudent to obtain a computed tomography scan or kidney ultrasonogram to determine if there are residual kidney stones. Second, if the initial stone was large (e.g., greater than 10 mm) or required an invasive intervention to remove, an evaluation would be indicated. Finally, and most importantly, are the patient's preferences.

A detailed history will provide information crucial for treatment recommendations. The following points should be covered: total number of stones, evidence of residual stones, number and types of procedures, types and success of previous preventive treatments, family history of stone disease, and dietary intake and medication use before the stone event. After having experienced acute renal colic, a patient may attribute a variety of types of chronic back or flank pain to the kidney or a residual stone. However, further questioning often reveals other causes, particularly musculoskeletal. The physical examination may reveal findings of systemic conditions associated with stone formation.

LABORATORY (METABOLIC) EVALUATION

Retrieving the stone for chemical analysis is an often overlooked but essential part of the evaluation, because treatment recommendations vary by stone type. The decision to proceed with a metabolic evaluation should be guided by the patient's willingness to make life-style changes to prevent recurrent stone formation. Some experts advocate proceeding with an evaluation only after the second stone. However, safe and inexpensive interventions (such as modifying fluid intake) can be prescribed according to the relatively inexpensive 24-hour urine collection. If a metabolic evaluation is pursued, the evaluation should be identical for the first-time and recurrent stone formers. Serum chemistries that should be measured include electrolytes, kidney function, and calcium and phosphorus. The decision to measure parathyroid hormone or vitamin D levels is based on the results of the serum and urine chemistries. If the patient has high serum calcium, low serum phosphorus, or high urine calcium, then a parathyroid hormone level should be measured. The cornerstone of the evaluation is the 24-hour urine collection. Two 24-hour urine collections should be done while the patient is consuming his or her usual diet. Because individuals often change their dietary habits soon after an episode of renal colic, a patient should wait at least 6 weeks before carrying out the collections. Two collections are needed because there is substantial day-to-day variability in the values.

The variables that should be measured in the 24-hour urine collections are: total volume, calcium, oxalate, citrate, uric acid, sodium, potassium, phosphorus, pH, and creatinine. Some laboratories calculate the relative supersaturation from the measurements of the urine factors, which can be used to gauge the impact of therapy.

MEDICAL TREATMENTS

Stones can remain asymptomatic for years; thus, the actual time of formation of the stone that brought the patient to medical attention is usually unknown. Therefore, the current metabolic evaluation may be completely normal, and no changes in life-style would be needed. Whether the patient is an active stone former influences the decision to treat. The likelihood of recurrence cannot be definitely predicted from the urine chemistries; therefore, a repeat imaging study 1 year later will help determine if the patient is an active stone former. For patients at risk for stone recurrence, life-style modification should be attempted first, tailoring the recommendation according to stone type and urine chemistries. Life-long changes are needed to prevent recurrence of this chronic condition. In addition, the supersaturation required for an existing stone to grow is lower than that needed for a new stone to form; thus, recommendations may be more aggressive to prevent stone growth rather than just new stone formation.

Dietary Recommendations

Dietary recommendations useful in preventing nephrolithiasis are listed in Table 53-2. There is no evidence that dietary calcium restriction is helpful in preventing stone formation and substantial evidence that it is harmful. Decreasing purine intake (meat, chicken, and seafood) will reduce urine uric acid. For low urine citrate, the patient should increase intake of potential alkali (fruits and vegetables) and decrease intake of acid-producing foods such as animal protein. The role of calcium supplements deserves comment, because their use is common. In someone who has never had a kidney stone, the attributable risk due to the supplement is low. For a patient who has had a calcium-containing stone and wishes to continue taking the supplement, 24-hour urine chemistries should be measured on and off the supplement. Increased fluid intake decreases the risk of stone

formation and recurrence. On the basis of the urine volume, the patient should be instructed on how many additional 8-oz glasses of fluid to drink each day with the goal of producing approximately 2 liters of urine daily.

For patients with high urine oxalate, the benefit of a low-oxalate diet is less clear on account of the previously addressed issues regarding the oxalate content of food. There is no accepted definition of a low-oxalate diet. An increase in dietary calcium with meals may reduce oxalate absorption, thereby reducing urine oxalate excretion. In addition, higher vitamin C intake may increase urine oxalate excretion.

Pharmacologic Options

The use of medication is indicated if dietary recommendations are unsuccessful in adequately modifying the urine composition. The three most commonly used classes of medications for stone prevention are: (1) thiazides, which are used to reduce urine calcium excretion (e.g., chlorthalidone, hydrochlorothiazide); (2) alkali, which is used to increase urine citrate excretion (e.g., potassium citrate); (3) allopurinol, which is used to reduce urine uric acid excretion.

For patients who have elevated urinary calcium but do not have an excessive calcium intake (more than 2 g/day), a thiazide diuretic has been demonstrated to reduce the likelihood of stone recurrence and also to help maintain bone density. The dosages required to reduce urinary calcium adequately are substantially higher than those typically used for treatment of hypertension (at least 25 mg/day and often 50 to 100 mg/day). Randomized trials of at least 3 years' duration have consistently shown a 50% reduction in the risk of recurrence. Adequate sodium restriction (less than 3 g/day) is necessary to achieve maximum benefit from the thiazides; a higher sodium intake leads to a greater distal sodium delivery, which minimizes or negates the beneficial effect of the thiazides. For patients who are unable to increase their fluid intake, a thiazide may be helpful even if the total

TABLE 53-2 Dietary and Pharmacologic Treatments According to Urinary Abnormality

Urinary Abnormality	Dietary Changes	Medication
High calcium	Avoid excessive intake of calcium supplements Adequate dietary calcium intake Reduce animal protein intake Reduce sodium intake <3 g/day Reduce sucrose intake	Thiazide
High oxalate	Avoid high-oxalate foods Adequate dietary calcium intake	Oxabsorb? High-dose pyridoxine?
High uric acid	Reduce purine intake (i.e., meat, chicken, fish)	Allopurinol
Low citrate	Increase fruit and vegetable intake Reduce animal protein intake	Alkali (e.g., K citrate)
Low volume	Increase total fluid intake	Not applicable

urine calcium excretion is not high, because it will reduce their urinary calcium concentration. In addition, a thiazide may be more readily prescribed if there is evidence of low bone density.

For patients with low urine citrate, any form of alkali will increase the urine citrate. However, citrate is the base of choice because it is better tolerated than bicarbonate. Potassium salts are preferred over sodium because of the potential effect on urinary calcium excretion. The alkali preparations must be taken at least twice daily to maintain adequate citrate levels. Randomized trials suggest a greater than 50% reduction in risk of recurrence with alkali supplementation.

In one randomized trial, allopurinol reduced the recurrence rate by 50% among individuals with a history of recurrent calcium oxalate stones and isolated hyperuricosuria.

NONCALCIUM STONES

For the less common types of stones (uric acid, struvite, and cystine), there is little or no information on the influence of dietary factors on actual stone formation (and not simply changes in urine composition). Thus, the following recommendations are based on our current understanding of the pathophysiology of these stone types, but caution is warranted because these are based on studies of urine composition rather than actual stone formation.

Uric Acid Stones

A higher intake of animal protein intake may increase the risk of uric acid stone formation. Consumption of meat, chicken, and seafood increases uric acid production, on account of the purine content of animal flesh. Animal protein is composed of more sulfur-containing amino acids, the metabolism of which leads to increased acid production with a subsequent lowering of the urinary pH. Both increased uric acid excretion and the lower urine pH increase the risk of uric acid crystal formation. Higher intake of fruits and vegetables, which are high in potential base such as citrate, may raise the urine pH, thereby reducing the risk of uric acid crystal formation.

Alkali supplementation is the most effective treatment of existing uric acid stones. If the urine pH is maintained at or above 6.5 (often requiring 90 to 120 mEq of supplemental alkali per day), pure uric acid stones will actually dissolve. Slightly lower doses can be used to prevent new uric acid stone formation. Allopurinol is the second-line choice if the patient has marked hyperuricosuria and/or is unable to maintain a urine pH of 6.5 or higher.

Cystine Stones

Higher sodium intake may increase urine cystine excretion. Because the solubility of cystine increases as pH

rises, a higher consumption of fruits and vegetables may have a beneficial effect by increasing urine pH. Although the restriction of proteins high in cystine (e.g., animal protein) seems advisable, there is little evidence to support this recommendation for directly lowering urinary cystine; however, reducing animal protein intake may be beneficial by raising urine pH.

Medications such as tiopronin and penicillamine increase the solubility of the filtered cystine. The effectiveness of these drugs is limited by the amount of cystine excreted daily and the high side effect profile. If adequate amounts of the medication enter the urine, cystine stones can be dissolved. Supplemental potassium alkali salts may also provide some additional benefit by increasing the urine pH.

Struvite Stones

Because struvite stones form only in the setting of an infection in the upper urinary tract with urease-producing bacteria, it is very unlikely that dietary factors directly influence struvite stone formation. Struvite stones are almost always quite large and may fill the renal pelvis (referred to as "staghorn calculi"); these stones should be removed by an experienced urologist. In addition to complete removal of all residual fragments, prevention of urinary tract infections is the cornerstone for preventing recurrence. Acetohydroxamic acid is the only drug available that inhibits urease; however, this should be used with extreme caution on account of the very common and serious side effects.

Calcium Phosphate Stones

Information on dietary issues related to actual calcium phosphate stone formation is limited. However, on the basis of the known physicochemical aspects, nutrients that might stimulate calcium phosphate crystal formation include higher calcium intake (resulting in higher urinary calcium excretion), higher phosphate intake (resulting in higher urinary phosphate excretion), and higher intake of fruits and vegetables resulting in a higher urinary pH. Nonetheless, caution is advised, since these "theoretical" benefits may not be realized and there are, of course, other reasons to maintain an adequate intake of calcium, fruits, and vegetables.

Reduction in urine calcium can be achieved by thiazides using a similar approach to that recommended for calcium oxalate stones. Because patients who form calcium phosphate stones may also have low urine citrate, alkali supplementation may be used with caution. Alkali supplementation often increases urine pH and thus could increase the risk of calcium phosphate crystal formation.

SURGICAL MANAGEMENT OF STONES

In the acute setting, the urologist will assist in the management. If the stone does not pass rapidly, the patient can be sent home with appropriate oral analgesics and instructions to return for fever or uncontrollable pain. Most urologists wait several days before intervening for a ureteral stone unless one of the following exists: urinary tract infection, stone greater than 6 mm in size, presence of an anatomic abnormality that would prevent passage, or intractable pain. A cystoscopically placed ureteral stent is typically used but requires anesthesia. The stent can be quite uncomfortable and not infrequently causes gross hematuria. Although it is debatable whether a stent helps with stone passage, the cystoscopy or stent placement may push the stone back up into the renal pelvis, thus relieving the obstruction and permitting its management on a nonemergent basis.

Stone size, location, and composition, urinary tract anatomy, availability of technology, and experience of the urologist determine the method of stone removal. Extracorporeal shock wave lithotripsy (ESWL) is the least invasive. Cystoscopic stone removal, either by basket extraction or fragmentation, is invasive but effective, and newer instruments allow removal of stones even in the kidney. Percutaneous nephrostolithotomy, an approach requiring the placement of a nephrostomy tube, is more invasive but is necessary for large stone burdens or kidney stones that cannot be removed cystoscopically; this is the gold standard for freeing a patient of stones. Fortunately, open procedures such as ureterolithotomy or nephrolithotomy are rarely needed.

The surgical treatment of asymptomatic stones is controversial. The availability of ESWL has lowered the threshold for treating asymptomatic stones; most urologists consider treating only asymptomatic stones that are at least 1 cm in size.

With the increasing prevalence of obesity in the United States, the treatment of existing stones in morbidly obese individuals deserves mention. The ability to image the urinary tract may be limited if the patient's size prohibits access to scanning by computed tomography. ESWL may not be an option, because morbid obesity may impede stone localization and the ability of the shock waves to reach the calculus; thus, more invasive approaches, such as ureteroscopy, are used.

LONG-TERM FOLLOW-UP

The nephrologist or primary care provider should assume responsibility for the long-term prevention program and refer back to the urologist as needed for further surgical interventions. The plan should include recommendations for prevention based on the evaluation and repetition of the metabolic measurements after interventions are initiated to assess the success of the intervention, adjustment of recommendations, and follow-up imaging.

Adherence to recommendations frequently declines over time. In addition, the long-term sequelae of the treatments and the underlying abnormalities may have other implications for the health of the patient. For example, individuals with higher urine calcium excretion on average have lower bone density and are at increased risk for osteoporosis. With appropriate attention and evaluation, the morbidity and cost of recurrent stone disease can be dramatically reduced.

BIBLIOGRAPHY

Coe FL, Favus MJ, Pak CY, et al (eds): Kidney Stones: Medical and Surgical Management. Philadelphia, Lippincott Williams & Wilkins, 1996.

Curhan GC, Willett WC, Rimm EB, Stampfer MJ: A prospective study of dietary calcium and other nutrients and the risk of symptomatic kidney stones. N Engl J Med 328:833–838, 1993.

Curhan GC, Willett WC, Speizer FE, Stampfer MJ: Beverage use and the risk for kidney stones in women. Ann Intern Med 128:534–540, 1998.

Evan AP, Lingeman JE, Coe FL, et al: Randall's plaque of patients with nephrolithiasis begins in basement membranes of thin loops of Henle. J Clin Invest 111:607–616, 2003.

Teichman JMH: Acute renal colic from ureteral calculus. N Engl J Med 350:684–693, 2004.

CHAPTER 54

Urinary Tract Infection

Lindsay E. Nicolle

Urinary infection is the presence of microbial pathogens within the normally sterile urinary tract. Infections are overwhelmingly bacterial, although fungi, viruses, and parasites are also occasionally pathogens (Table 54-1). Urinary infection is the most common bacterial infection in humans and can be either symptomatic or asymptomatic. Symptomatic infection is associated with a wide spectrum of morbidity, from mild irritative voiding symptoms to bacteremia, sepsis, and, occasionally, death. Asymptomatic urinary infection is isolation of bacteria from urine in quantitative counts consistent with infection, but without localizing genitourinary signs or symptoms, and with no systemic symptoms attributable to the infection.

The term bacteriuria simply means bacteria present in the urine, although it is generally used to imply isolation of a significant quantitative count of organisms. This term is often used interchangeably with asymptomatic urinary infection. Recurrent urinary infection is common in individuals who experience an initial infection. It may be either relapse (i.e., recurrence subsequent to therapy with the pretherapy isolate) or reinfection (i.e., recurrence with a different organism). An important consideration in the management of urinary infection is whether the patient has a functionally or structurally normal (uncomplicated urinary infection or acute nonobstructive pyelonephritis) or abnormal (complicated urinary infection) genitourinary tract.

The microbiologic diagnosis of urinary infection requires isolation of a pathogenic organism in sufficient quantitative amounts from an appropriately collected urine specimen. A quantitative bacterial count of 10^5 cfu/mL or higher is the usual standard to discriminate infection from organisms present as contaminants. The use of the quantitative urine culture has been important in the diagnosis of urinary infection and description of natural history, but this single quantitative standard is not currently considered valid for all potential clinical presentations.

ACUTE UNCOMPLICATED URINARY INFECTION

Acute uncomplicated urinary infection, or acute cystitis, is infection occurring in individuals with a normal genitourinary tract and no prior instrumentation. It is a common syndrome that occurs virtually entirely in women. As many as 30% to 50% of young, sexually active women experience at least one urinary infection, and 1% to 2% will have frequent recurrent infection. Risk factors for infection in these women are both genetic and behavioral. First-degree female relatives of women with recurrent acute uncomplicated urinary infection also have an increased frequency of urinary infection, and women who are nonsecretors of blood group substances are more likely to have urinary infection. Sexual activity is strongly associated with infection, and the frequency of infection increases with frequency of intercourse. The use of spermicides or a diaphragm for birth control also increase the risk of infection, but not use of the birth control pill or condoms without spermicide.

Escherichia coli are the most common infecting organisms and are isolated from 80% to 85% of episodes. *Staphylococcus saprophyticus*, a coagulase-negative staphylococcus, occurs in 5% to 10% of episodes. This organism is seldom identified as a pathogen outside the urinary tract or isolated from individuals with complicated urinary infection. It also has a unique seasonal variation, with increased occurrence in the late summer and early fall. *Klebsiella pneumoniae* and *Proteus mirabilis* are each isolated in 2% to 3% of cases. Organisms that cause infection originate from the normal gut flora, colonize the vagina and periurethral area, and ascend to the bladder. Women who experience this syndrome frequently have alterations in vaginal flora. The normal lactobacilli, which maintain an acid pH, are decreased or absent, and the pH is increased with *E. coli* and other uropathogens present.

The clinical presentation, diagnosis, and recommended treatment for acute uncomplicated urinary infection are summarized in Table 54-2. A quantitative bacterial count of 10^5 cfu/mL or greater is no longer considered the diagnostic microbiologic standard for this syndrome, since 30% to 50% of women with symptoms have lower quantitative counts of uropathogens isolated. Any quantitative count of a potential uropathogen with pyuria is considered sufficient for diagnosis in the presence of consistent clinical symptoms. Since the bacteriology is predictable and quantitative microbiology is not definitive, it is often recommended that routine pretherapy urine culture not be obtained, and empiric antimicrobial therapy be given. A urine specimen for culture

TABLE 54-1   Nonbacterial Pathogens Causing Urinary Tract Infection

Fungi	Viruses	Parasites
Candida albicans	JC, BK viruses	Schistosoma hematobium
Candida parapsolosis	Adenovirus types 11, 21	
Candida glabrata	Mumps	
Candida tropicalis	Hantavirus[†]	
Blastomyces dermatitidis*		
Aspergillus fumigatus*		
Cryptococcus neoformans*		
Histoplasma capsulatum*		

*With disseminated infection.
[†]Hemorrhagic fever and renal syndrome.

before antimicrobial treatment is recommended, however, if there is uncertainty about the diagnosis, or failure of or early recurrence subsequent to therapy. The differential diagnosis includes urethritis due to sexually transmitted diseases such as *Neisseria gonorrheae* or *Chlamydia trachomatis*, yeast vulvovaginitis, or herpes genitalis.

Antimicrobial therapy is selected according to patient tolerance, documented efficacy for treating urinary infection, and local prevalence of resistance of community-acquired *E. coli*. Although trimethoprim-sulfamethoxazole has been recommended empiric therapy for many years, resistance to this antimicrobial in community *E. coli* has reached a prevalence of over 20% in some areas, and alternate empiric regimens may need to be considered. Fluoroquinolones are effective as 3-day therapy, but there are concerns about the potential for promoting resistance with widespread use of this class of antimicrobials. Fosfomycin trometemol and pivmecillinam are antimicrobials with indications virtually limited to treatment of this syndrome, whereas nitrofurantoin is used only for treatment of lower urinary infection. A 3-day course of antimicrobial therapy is usually effective. However, a longer course of 7 days may be preferable for individuals treated with nitrofurantoin or a β-lactam antibiotic, for postmenopausal women, for women with symptoms longer than 7 days, or for women with an early recurrence of symptomatic infection (less than 30 days) following prior antimicrobial therapy.

Frequent recurrence of acute cystitis is a disruptive and distressing problem for many women. Antimicrobial prophylaxis, given either as a long-term low-dose regimen or after intercourse, will prevent recurrent infection (Table 54-3). Continuous low-dose prophylaxis is recommended to be taken at bedtime, and initially courses of 6 to 12 months are given. It remains effective when continued for as long as 2 to 5 years. When prophylactic therapy is discontinued, urinary infection occurs with a frequency similar to that observed before prophylaxis.

Approximately 50% of women will have recurrent infection within 3 months. Postintercourse prophylaxis is obviously most appropriate for women who identify sexual intercourse as a precipitating factor for recurrent symptomatic episodes. An alternate approach preferred by some women is self-treatment. This has been shown to be effective with single-dose trimethoprim-sulfamethoxazole therapy, or 3-day ciprofloxacin or ofloxacin. It is appropriate for compliant women who can reliably identify their symptomatic episodes and wish a role in self-management. Nonantimicrobial management of recurrent urinary infection includes avoidance of spermicide use. One study reported a decreased frequency of reinfection with daily intake of cranberry juice. Vaccines to prevent recurrent uncomplicated urinary infection remain investigational.

ACUTE NONOBSTRUCTIVE PYELONEPHRITIS

Acute nonobstructive pyelonephritis is symptomatic kidney infection occurring in women with an otherwise normal genitourinary tract. Women who experience acute uncomplicated urinary infection are also at risk of nonobstructive pyelonephritis, with the frequency of episodes of cystitis relative to pyelonephritis reported to be 18 to 29 to 1. The bacteriology is similar to that of acute uncomplicated urinary infection, with *E. coli* isolated in about 85% of episodes. Strains of *E. coli* isolated from pyelonephritis are characterized by almost uniform expression of a specific virulence factor, the p fimbria. This surface antigen attaches to uroepithelial cells within the urinary tract and induces an inflammatory response. Additional organism virulence factors include hemolysin and acrobactin production. Bacteremia, which occurs in about 10% of episodes, is more frequent in diabetic and elderly women.

Acute pyelonephritis presents classically with fever with costovertebral angle pain and tenderness. There may be associated lower urinary tract symptoms. Fever may be low grade or, occasionally, absent. A urine specimen for culture and susceptibility testing should be obtained before the initiation of antimicrobial therapy from every woman with a suspected diagnosis of pyelonephritis. Growth of 10^4 cfu/mL or more of a uropathogen with pyuria and consistent clinical findings are sufficient for diagnosis. The majority of women can be treated as outpatients with oral antimicrobial therapy (see Table 54-2). Hospitalization and initial parenteral antimicrobial therapy are recommended for women in whom oral medication may not be tolerated because of severe gastrointestinal symptoms, where there is hemodynamic instability, or when there are significant systemic signs of illness and concerns about compliance. If parenteral therapy is initiated, it can usually be replaced by oral therapy once clinical improvement has occurred, usually

TABLE 54-2 Diagnosis and Management of Common Symptomatic Syndromes of Urinary Infection

Clinical Presentation	Microbiologic Diagnosis	Treatment
Acute uncomplicated urinary infection (acute cystitis) Lower-tract irritative symptoms: dysuria, frequency, urgency, suprapubic discomfort, hematuria	$\geq 10^3$ cfu/mL of uropathogen with pyuria	First line TMP/SMX 160/180 mg bid, 3 days TMP 100 mg bid, 3 days Nitrofurantoin 50–100 mg qid, 7 days Fosfomycin trometamol 3 g, one dose Pivmecillinam 400 mg bid*, 3 or 7 days Second line Norfloxacin 400 mg bid, 3 days Ciprofloxacin 250 mg bid, 3 days Ciprofloxacin extended release 500 mg od, 3 days Ofloxacin 400 mg bid, 3 days Levofloxacin 400 mg od, 3 days Gatifloxacin 400 mg od, 3 days Amoxicillin/clavulanic acid 500 mg bid, 3 or 7 days Cephalexin 500 mg qid, 7 days Cefixime 400 mg od, 7 days Cefuroxime axetil 500 mg bid, 7 days
Acute nonobstructive pyelonephritis Costovertebral angle pain and tenderness; ± fever, ± lower-tract symptoms	$\geq 10^4$ cfu/mL	First line TMP/SMX 160/800 mg bid[†] TMP 100 mg bid[†] Norfloxacin 400 mg bid Ciprofloxacin 500 mg bid Ofloxacin 400 mg bid Gentamicin 3–5 mg/kg/24 hr in one or two doses[‡] ± ampicillin 1 g q4–6 hr Second line Amoxicillin/clavulanic acid 500 mg tid Cephalexin 500 mg qid[‡] Cefotaxime 1 g tid[‡] Ceftriaxone 1–2 g od[‡] Levofloxacin 500 mg od Gatifloxacin 400 mg od
Complicated urinary infection Variable symptoms, including lower-tract symptoms; pyelonephritis; systemic symptoms (fever, shock)	$\geq 10^5$ cfu/mL	TMP/SMX 160/800 mg bid Norfloxacin 400 mg bid Ciprofloxacin 250–500 mg bid Ciprofloxacin extended release, 1 g od Ofloxacin 400 mg bid Levofloxacin 500 mg od Gatifloxacin 400 mg od Amoxicillin/clavulanic acid 500 mg tid Cephalexin 500 mg qid Gentamicin 3–5 mg/kg/24 hr in one or two doses[‡] ± ampicillin 1 g q4–6 hr or piperacillin 3 g q4hr Piperacillin/tazobactam 3.375 g q6hr Ceftazidime 1 g tid[‡] Cefotazime 1 g tid[‡]

TMP/SMX, trimethoprim/sulfamethoxazole.
*Not licensed in United States.
[†]If organism known to be susceptible.
[‡]Parenteral therapy.

by 48 to 72 hours. The urine culture results are also available by this time and can direct optimal selection of the oral antimicrobial for continuing therapy.

By 48 to 72 hours following initiation of effective antimicrobial therapy, there should be evidence of clinical improvement, including decreased costovertebral discomfort and a decrease in or resolution of fever. If there has been no improvement, an abnormality within the genitourinary tract causing urinary obstruction or abscess formation should be excluded. Women with early symp-

tomatic recurrence following therapy should also be evaluated for a potential complicating abnormality of the genitourinary tract. An initial ultrasonographic examination is helpful to exclude obstruction, although it may not identify small stones. Computed tomography scanning is superior to ultrasonography for identifying small stones or an intrarenal abscess. The selection of an imaging approach should be individualized according to initial presentation, clinical course, and access to diagnostic testing.

TABLE 54-3 Prophylactic Antimicrobial Therapy for Women with Frequent Recurrence of Acute Uncomplicated Urinary Infection

| Agent | Regimen | |
	Long Term	Postcoital (One Dose)
TMP/SMX*	80/400 mg daily or 3× weekly	80/400 mg
TMP*	100 mg daily	100 mg
Nitrofurantoin*	50 mg daily	50–100 mg
Cephalexin	125 mg daily	250 mg
Norfloxacin	200 mg every other day	200–400 mg
Ciprofloxacin	–	250 mg

TMP/SMX, trimethoprim/sulfamethoxazole.
*Recommended first-line agents.

COMPLICATED URINARY TRACT INFECTION

The most important host defense preventing urinary infection is intermittent, unobstructed voiding of urine. Any abnormality of the genitourinary tract that impairs voiding may increase the frequency of urinary infection. Urinary infection in individuals with structural or functional abnormalities of the urinary tract, including those who have undergone instrumentation, including indwelling urethral catheters, is considered "complicated urinary infection" (Table 54-4). The frequency of infection is determined by the underlying abnormality and is independent of gender or age. For some abnormalities, infection is infrequent but difficult to manage, such as infected cysts with polycystic kidney disease. In others, such as indwelling catheters, where the infection rate is 5% per day, infection is very frequent.

The clinical presentation of symptomatic complicated urinary infection varies along a spectrum from mild lower tract irritative symptoms to systemic manifestations such as fever, and even septic shock. Individuals with complete obstruction of urine flow or with mucosal bleeding are at greatest risk of the more severe clinical presentations. The quantitative count of organisms in the urine of 10^5 cfu/mL or greater remains the standard for diagnosis of complicated urinary infection. The microbiology of complicated urinary infection is characterized by a greater diversity of organisms and increased prevalence of antimicrobial resistance when compared with uncomplicated infection. Organisms isolated are less likely to express virulence factors, because the host abnormality of impaired voiding is sufficient for infection to develop. Increased antimicrobial resistance is common in infecting organisms because of nosocomial acquisition or repeated prior courses of antimicrobial therapy for recurrent infection. Where broad-spectrum antimicrobial therapy has been given for prolonged periods, reinfection

may occur with yeast species or highly resistant strains, such as some *Pseudomonas aeruginosa* strains.

Antimicrobial treatment is based on the known or suspected susceptibilities of the infecting organism, as well as patient tolerance. If possible, antimicrobial therapy should be delayed until urine culture results are available. Patients with moderate to severe symptoms, however, may require empiric therapy before culture results become available. The recent history of antimicrobial use and prior urine culture results in the individual patient are helpful in directing the choice of empiric therapy. Parenteral therapy may initially be required for ill patients with severe systemic manifestations, where oral therapy is not tolerated, or when the infecting organism is suspected or known to be resistant to any available oral therapy. When the clinical presentation is of lower tract symptoms, 7 days of therapy are generally adequate. Where fever or other systemic symptoms are present, 10 to 14 days of therapy are recommended.

Complicated urinary infection can be prevented if the underlying abnormality can be corrected. There is a high probability of recurrence when the underlying genitourinary abnormality cannot be corrected. For instance, 50% of patients with a neurogenic bladder and voiding managed by intermittent catheterization will experience recurrent infection by 4 to 6 weeks after antimicrobial therapy. Prophylactic antimicrobials are not recom-

TABLE 54-4 Abnormalities of the Genitourinary Tract Consistent with Complicated Urinary Tract Infection

Abnormality	Examples
Metabolic or structural	Medullary sponge kidney Nephrocalcinosis Malakoplakia Xanthogranulomatous pyelonephritis Diabetes mellitus
Congenital	Cystic disease Duplicated drainage system with obstruction Urethral valves
Obstruction	Vesicoureteral reflux Pelvicalyceal obstruction Papillary necrosis Urethral fibrosis/stricture Bladder diverticulum Neurogenic bladder Prostatic hypertrophy Tumors Urolithiasis
Instrumentation	Indwelling catheter Intermittent catheterization Cystoscopy Ureteric stent
Other	Nephrostomy tube Immunocompromised Subsequent to renal transplant Neutropenic

mended, since long-term antimicrobial therapy has not been shown to decrease infections, and reinfection will be with organisms resistant to the antimicrobial given. In selected cases with severe recurrences and an abnormality that cannot be corrected, long-term suppressive therapy may be considered. This therapy is individualized in every case. Full therapeutic antimicrobial doses are initiated and subsequently decreased to one half the regular dose if the urine culture remains negative and the clinical course is satisfactory.

ASYMPTOMATIC URINARY INFECTION

Asymptomatic bacteriuria is isolation of uropathogens in quantitative counts consistent with urinary infection (10^5 cfu/mL or greater) in a patient with no signs or symptoms local to the genitourinary tract. Pyuria is common, being present in 50% to 90% of patients. Asymptomatic bacteriuria occurs with increased frequency in persons who also experience symptomatic urinary infection, suggesting that the biologic defect promoting urinary infection is similar. Asymptomatic infection, with or without pyuria, does not usually require treatment. Long-term cohort studies do not document adverse effects attributable to bacteriuria, and prospective randomized trials do not report clinical benefits of treatment. In fact, adverse antibiotic effects and reinfection with organisms of increased resistance are observed with treatment. The important exception to the recommendation for nontreatment is pregnant women. Identification and treatment of asymptomatic bacteriuria in early pregnancy prevents pyelonephritis and negative fetal outcomes. Antimicrobial therapy is also indicated before an invasive genitourinary procedure—in this situation, however, as prophylaxis to prevent perioperative sepsis rather than as treatment of asymptomatic bacteriuria.

SPECIAL POPULATIONS

Urinary Tract Infection in Children

Urinary infection occurs more frequently in boys than girls in the first year of life. Infection in boys often occurs within 3 months of birth and may be associated with congenital anomalies of the urinary tract or lack of circumcision. The clinical presentation is usually of neonatal sepsis without localizing signs to the genitourinary tract, and these episodes are treated as neonatal sepsis. Subsequent to the first year of life, urinary infection occurs more frequently in girls than boys, and the clinical presentation is of genitourinary symptoms. Most episodes in girls are acute uncomplicated urinary infection, and these girls will also experience urinary infection more frequently as adults. For girls with recurrent urinary infection, vesicoureteral reflux, which may lead to impaired kidney function, must be excluded. Imaging studies including voiding cystourethrogram, ultrasonography, and ^{99}Tc-dimercaptosuccinic acid (DMSA) scan are indicated for any child presenting with pyelonephritis, for a first urinary infection in a boy of any age or a girl under 3 years, for a second urinary infection in a girl older than 3 years, and for a first urinary infection at any age with a family history of urinary tract abnormalities, with abnormal voiding, hypertension, or poor growth.

Treatment of acute lower tract infection in young girls consists of 3 to 7 days of therapy. Pyelonephritis should be treated for 10 to 14 days. Generally, the antimicrobials used are similar to those in adults, with appropriate dose adjustments for weight. The quinolones are not recommended for children under the age of 16 years because of potential adverse effects on cartilage. Long-term low-dose prophylactic therapy is indicated for young girls with vesicoureteral reflux and recurrent urinary infection or frequent symptomatic recurrence.

Asymptomatic urinary infection is common in schoolgirls. Treatment of asymptomatic urinary infection does not alter the natural history of kidney disease in young girls and does not influence renal scarring. In fact, treatment of asymptomatic bacteriuria with antimicrobials appears to increase the frequency of symptomatic infection. Thus, it is not recommended to screen for or treat asymptomatic bacteriuria in girls.

Urinary Infection in Pregnancy

Hormonal changes in pregnancy produce hypotonicity of the autonomic musculature, leading to urine stasis. In addition, obstruction at the pelvic brim, more marked on the right than the left side, occurs with the enlarging fetus. These changes are maximal at the end of the second trimester and beginning of the third trimester, and they probably explain the increased risk of pyelonephritis at this stage of gestation. Acute pyelonephritis may precipitate premature labor and delivery, as may any febrile illness in later pregnancy. Women who have asymptomatic bacteriuria in early pregnancy have as much as a 30% risk of developing acute pyelonephritis later in the pregnancy. From 75% to 90% of episodes of acute pyelonephritis in pregnancy are prevented by identification and treatment of asymptomatic bacteriuria early in pregnancy. Premature delivery and low birth rate are also prevented with treatment.

Because of these benefits of treatment of asymptomatic bacteriuria in pregnancy, all pregnant women should be asked to provide a urine specimen for culture at 12 to 16 weeks' gestation. If significant bacteriuria is identified, it should be confirmed with a second urine culture and, if confirmed, treated. The antimicrobial is selected according to the susceptibilities of the infecting organism. A 3-day course of amoxicillin, nitrofurantoin, or cephalexin is usually sufficient. Trimethoprim-sulfamethoxazole has been widely used and is effective, but it may be associated with increased fetal abnormalities when used in the first trimester and should be avoided early in pregnancy. Quinolones are contraindicated. Women with either symptomatic or asymptomatic infection treated in early pregnancy should be followed with monthly urine cultures throughout the remainder of the pregnancy to identify recurrent infection. If a second episode occurs, it should be treated, and low-dose prophylactic therapy with nitrofurantoin or cephalexin should be continued until delivery.

Urinary Infection in Men

Men rarely present with acute uncomplicated urinary infection or acute nonobstructive pyelonephritis. Lack of circumcision, acquisition of infection from a sexual partner, and men who have sex with men are potential risk factors in the few cases that do occur. *Escherichia coli* are the usual infecting organisms. Uncomplicated infection, however, is so uncommon in men that any man presenting with urinary infection should be investigated for the possibility of an underlying abnormality. Pelvic and kidney ultrasonography is the most useful initial test.

Elderly men have an increased frequency of urinary infection due to prostatic hypertrophy leading to obstruction and turbulent urine flow. These men also develop bacterial prostatitis. Once bacteria are established in the prostate, poor diffusion of antibiotics into the prostate and formation of prostatic stones mean infection is often impossible to eradicate. The prostate then serves as a nidus for recurrent symptomatic or asymptomatic bladder infection. If recurrent symptomatic infection occurs, suggesting prostatic infection, a repeat course of 6 to 12 weeks of therapy can increase the likelihood of long-term cure.

Urinary Tract Infections in the Elderly

Urinary infection is the most common infection occurring in either ambulatory or institutionalized elderly populations. The prevalence of bacteriuria is 5% to 10% for women and 5% in men over 65 years of age living in the community, and increases further with advancing age. In long-term care facilities, 25% to 50% of all elderly residents have asymptomatic bacteriuria at any time. The prevalence increases with increasing functional impairment, including dementia and bladder and bowel incontinence. Asymptomatic bacteriuria in elderly patients should not be treated with antimicrobials. Antimicrobial treatment does not decrease morbidity or mortality but is associated with increased adverse drug effects, cost, and increasing antimicrobial resistance. It follows that asymptomatic elderly populations should not be screened for bacteriuria.

Symptomatic infection in the elderly may have a clinical presentation similar to younger populations. However, the diagnosis may not be straightforward, particularly in the institutionalized or functionally impaired population. Difficulties in communication, comorbid illnesses with chronic symptoms, and the high frequency of asymptomatic bacteriuria may all impair diagnostic acumen. A decreased fever response and lower frequency of leukocytosis characterize infection in the elderly, and acute confusion may be a prominent presenting symptom.

Antimicrobial selection for therapy is similar to younger populations. The dosage should be adjusted for kidney function but not for age per se. The duration of treatment is also similar to that recommended for younger populations, although cure rates with 3-day therapy for older women are lower. It has been suggested that 7 days of therapy are preferable to treat postmenopausal women presenting with cystitis. Post-treatment urine cultures to document microbiologic cure are not recommended unless symptoms persist or recur. Some women with frequent, recurrent, symptomatic infection may have a decreased number of infections with use of topical intravaginal estradiol. Systemic estrogen therapy, however, does not prevent infections, and topical estrogen is less effective for prevention than prophylactic antimicrobials.

Urinary Infection in Patients with Impaired Kidney Function

Treatment of urinary infection requires high concentrations of effective antimicrobials in the urine. There is decreased excretion of antimicrobials into the urine when kidney function is decreased, and adequate urinary antimicrobial levels may not be achieved. With severe bilateral kidney functional impairment, it is difficult to cure urinary infection. Antimicrobials such as nitrofurantoin and tetracyclines other than doxycycline are toxic in the presence of impaired kidney function and should be avoided. Aminoglycosides may not penetrate nonfunctioning kidneys sufficiently to provide effective therapy. The penicillins and cephalosporins, as well as quinolones, constitute effective treatment for most individuals with impaired kidney function. Obviously, dosage adjustments appropriate for the level of kidney function are necessary. In some situations, such as infected native kidneys in transplant recipients, infection cannot be eradicated and long-term suppressive therapy may be necessary to prevent frequent symptomatic recurrences.

If renal functional impairment is unilateral, the better functioning kidney will preferentially excrete the antimicrobial. Antimicrobial levels may be high in bladder urine but may not achieve therapeutic levels in the nonfunctioning kidney. If the nonfunctioning kidney is infected, effective antimicrobial levels may not be achieved at the site of infection despite adequate levels in the excreted urine. This may explain relapsing infection in some individuals.

Fungal Urinary Tract Infection

Fungal urinary infection has been increasing in frequency. It is primarily a nosocomial infection and occurs in the setting of diabetes, indwelling urethral catheters, and intense broad-spectrum antimicrobial therapy. *Candida albicans* is the species most frequently isolated, but other *Candida* species, such as *C. glabrata*, *C. krusei*, *C. parapsolosis*, and *C. tropicalis* also occur. The clinical importance of fungal urinary infection is often difficult to assess, in part because these patients have complex, multiple medical problems. If there are no symptoms, treatment is not necessary. An indwelling urethral catheter, if present, should be discontinued where possible. Fungus balls may lead to obstruction and should be excluded in individuals with obstructive uropathy and candiduria or candidemia.

Where repeated cultures have grown yeast organisms at 10^4 cfu/mL or more, and there are symptoms referable to the genitourinary tract, funguria should be treated. Fluconazole 100 to 400 mg/day for 7 days is recommended, because it is well excreted in the urine and may be given as oral therapy. However, itraconazole (100 to 400 mg/day), 5-fluorocytosine (50 to 150 mg/kg/day for 7 days), and amphotericin B have also been effective. There is as yet limited experience with newer antifungal drugs such as caspofungin and voriconazole. The *Candida* species other than *C. albicans* are more likely to be resistant to the azole antifungals, and amphotericin B may be necessary for treatment. Amphotericin B bladder irrigation (50 mg/L continuous for 5 days) is no longer considered first-line therapy, because it requires urethral catheterization and is no more effective than other therapeutic options. In selected situations, however, particularly in subjects with markedly impaired kidney function and bladder infection, the washout method may still be useful. The cure rate with any treatment is only 70% to 75%, but assessment of outcome is often limited by serious accompanying illnesses.

BIBLIOGRAPHY

Cardenas DD, Hooton TM: Urinary tract infection in persons with spinal cord injury. Arch Phys Med Rehab 76:272–280, 1995.

Collins TR, Devries CR: Recurrent urinary tract infections in children: A logical approach to diagnosis, treatment, and long-term management. Compr Ther 23:44–48, 1997.

Foxman B: Epidemiology of urinary tract infections: Incidence, morbidity, and economic costs. Am J Med 113(suppl 1A): 5S–11S, 2002.

Gupta K, Scholes D, Stamm WE: Increasing prevalence of antimicrobial resistance among uropathogens causing acute uncomplicated cystitis in women. JAMA 281:736–738, 1999.

Gupta K, Hooton TM, Roberts PL, Stamm WE: Patient-initiated treatment of uncomplicated recurrent urinary tract infections in young women. Ann Intern Med 135:9–16, 2001.

Lipsky BA: Urinary tract infection in men. Epidemiology, pathophysiology, diagnosis, and treatment. Ann Intern Med 110: 138–150, 1989.

Nickel JC: Prostatitis: Evolving management strategies. Urol Clin North Am 26:789–796, 1999.

Nicolle LE: A practical guide to the management of complicated urinary tract infection. Drugs 53:583–592, 1997.

Nicolle LE: SHEA Long Term Care Committee. Urinary tract infections in long term care facilities. Infect Control Hosp Epidemiol 22:167–175, 2001.

Nicolle LE: Asymptomatic bacteriuria: When to screen and when to treat. Infect Dis Clin North Am 17:367–394, 2003.

Pinson AG, Philbrick JT, Lindbeck GH, Schorling JB: Oral antibiotic therapy for acute pyelonephritis: A methodologic review of the literature. J Gen Intern Med 7:544–553, 1992.

Sobel JD, Kauffman CA, McKinsey D, et al: Candiduria: A randomized, double-blind study of treatment with fluconazole or placebo. The National Institute of Allergy and Infectious Diseases Mycoses Study Group. Clin Infect Dis 30:19–24, 2000.

Stamm WE, Hooton TM: Management of urinary tract infections in adults. N Engl J Med 329:1328–1334, 1993.

Warren JW: Catheter-associated urinary tract infections. Infect Dis Clin North Am 11:609–622, 1997.

Warren JW, Abrutyn E, Hebel JR, et al: Guidelines for antimicrobial therapy of uncomplicated acute bacterial cystitis and acute pyelonephritis in women. Clin Infect Dis 29:745–758, 1999.

The Kidney in Special Circumstances

CHAPTER 55

The Kidney in Infants and Children

R. Ariel Gomez Victoria F. Norwood

ANATOMIC DEVELOPMENT OF THE KIDNEY

In humans, the metanephric, or definitive, kidney appears during the fifth week of gestation and nephrogenesis continues until 32 to 36 weeks. Term infants are therefore born with a full complement of nephrons. Kidney function and urine production begin about 10 weeks into embryonic life. However, because deeper glomeruli develop earliest (centrifugal maturation), juxtamedullary glomeruli are larger and more mature than developing outer cortical glomeruli. Glomeruli become equal in size by the 14th postnatal month and reach adult size (200μm) at 3½ years of age. The proximal tubule continues to increase in length well into adult life.

FUNCTIONAL DEVELOPMENT OF THE KIDNEY

Glomerular Filtration Rate

In newborn babies, glomerular filtration rate (GFR) correlates with gestational age. The GFR increases postnatally, doubling by 2 weeks of age. When corrected for surface area, the GFR reaches adult values at 1 to 2 years of age. The normal values of GFR for infants and children are shown in Table 55-1. Influences responsible for the increase in GFR with maturation include increases in arterial pressure, in renal blood flow, in glomerular permeability, and in filtration surface area.

Creatinine clearance can be used to measure the GFR after 1 month of age, providing that urinary creatinine excretion is between 15 and 25 mg/kg/day. However, it is difficult to obtain 24-hour urine collections in infants, and shorter collections are not adequate because of variations in creatinine excretion throughout the day. The following formula permits estimation of GFR (mL/minute/1.73 m²) without the need for urine collections: $GFR = K \times L/SCr$, where K is a constant (0.33 in preterm, 0.45 in term neonates, 0.55 in children and adolescent girls, and 0.70 in adolescent boys), L is the length of the infant or standing height of the child in centimeters, and SCr is serum creatinine concentration (mg/dL). Although this formula is clinically useful, inulin clearance or iothalamate clearance should be obtained if a more accurate value of GFR is needed. Along with changes in GFR, SCr levels vary with age and degree of maturity. During the first 48 hours after birth, SCr levels are similar to the maternal values. A week after birth, the full-term neonate should have a SCr below 1.0 mg/dL. These levels should continue to decrease to about 0.3 mg/dL by 3 months of postnatal life. In preterm infants, however, SCr levels can be high (about 1.5 mg/dL) during the first few weeks of postnatal life. These levels progressively decrease to 0.4 to 0.8 mg/dL by 3 to 6 months of postnatal life. When evaluating a neonate with a high SCr, serial measurements are more meaningful than a single determination; SCr levels should progressively decrease. An increase in SCr indicates a reduction in GFR, regardless of the gestational age. The normal values for SCr during childhood are shown in Figure 55-1.

Urine Concentration

In human fetuses, urine flow rate increases from 0.1 mL/minute at 20 weeks of gestation to 1.0 mL/minute at 40 weeks of gestation. In neonates, urine flow rate decreases again to around 0.1 mL/minute. Fetal urine flow correlates with (and may be modulated by) fetal arterial pressure. The fetal urine is hypotonic (100 to 200 mOsm/L), unless stress such as hypoxemia or volume depletion develops. Nevertheless, the urinary concentrating ability is lower in the fetus than in the adult. Several conditions contribute to the decreased urinary concentrating ability. In the fetus, the organization and anatomic development of the medulla is delayed with respect to glomerular development. Short loops of Henle and reduced sodium chloride transport in the ascending loops of Henle are also important variables. In addition, preferential blood flow to the inner portions of the cortex dissipates an already low intrarenal concentration gradient. Although arginine vasopressin is secreted properly in response to volume and osmolar challenges, decreased arginine vasopressin receptor number or coupling to cyclic adenosine monophosphate (cAMP) generation probably contribute to the decreased concentrating ability found in infants.

Maximal urinary concentration increases progressively throughout the first year of life (Table 55-2). In premature neonates, maximal urine osmolality is about 400 to 500 mOsm/L. Later in life, infants born prematurely are able to concentrate their urine to levels found in term

TABLE 55-1   Normal Values of Glomerular Filtration Rate (GFR) in Children

Age	Normal GFR (mL/min/1.73 m²)
Preterm (25–28 weeks)	
1 week	11.0 ± 5.4
2–8 weeks	15.5 ± 6.2
Preterm (29–34 weeks)	
1 week	15.3 ± 5.6
2–8 weeks	28.7 ± 13.8
Term	
5–7 days	50.6 ± 5.8
1–2 months	64.6 ± 5.8
3–4 months	85.8 ± 4.8
5–8 months	87.7 ± 11.9
9–12 months	86.9 ± 8.4
2–12 years	133 ± 27

From Schwartz GJ, Brion LP, Spitzer A: The use of plasma creatinine concentration for estimating glomerular filtration rate in infants, children and adolescents. Pediatr Clin North Am 34:571–590, 1987, and Greene MG: The Harriet Lane Handbook. A Manual for Pediatric House Officers, 12th ed. St. Louis, Mosby, 1991, pp 1–434. Adapted from Meites S (ed): Pediatric Clinical Chemistry, 2nd and 3rd eds. Philadelphia, Saunders. The American Association for Clinical Chemistry, 1981; Tietz NW: Textbook of Clinical Chemistry 1986; Lundberg GD, et al: JAMA 260:73, 1988; and Wallach J: Interpretation of Diagnostic Tests, Boston, Little, Brown, 1992.

TABLE 55-2   Maximal Urine Osmolality in Children and Youths*

Age	Osmolality (mOsm/L)
3 days	515 ± 172
6 days	663 ± 133
10–30 days	896 ± 179
10–12 months	1118 ± 154
14–18 years	1362 ± 109

*Means ± SD.
Data from Polacek E: The osmotic concentrating ability in healthy infants and children. Arch Dis Child 40:291, 1965.

About 30% of dietary sodium is retained by a healthy infant receiving formula containing different sodium concentrations. Although sodium intake varies widely, positive sodium balance is usually maintained, thus allowing the necessary conservation of sodium, a requirement for normal somatic growth. However, premature infants excrete more sodium than full-term infants. In fact, sodium excretion is negatively correlated with gestational age. The fractional excretion of sodium at 31 weeks of gestation is approximately 5% and declines to less than 1% by 2 months after birth. Thus, in contrast to full-term healthy newborns who are able to conserve sodium and maintain a positive sodium balance, preterm infants are at risk of developing a negative sodium balance during the first weeks of life. It is believed that the high sodium excretion in the premature neonate is due to a relative inability of the distal tubule to respond to aldosterone. Newly born preterm infants who receive human breast milk or formula with a composition similar to that of breast milk containing relatively low sodium concentrations continue to excrete large amounts of sodium in the urine and eventually develop a negative sodium balance and hyponatremia. The hyponatremia can be prevented by the addition of supplemental sodium chloride to the formula.

infants of similar postnatal age, probably because of rapid maturation of the concentration gradient in the premature infant.

Sodium

Sodium metabolism in the newborn period is characterized by (1) a progressive increase in renal reabsorptive capacity, (2) positive balance in the term infant, and (3) an inability to excrete a solute and volume load promptly.

FIGURE 55-1   Values of plasma creatinine in normal males and females. (From Schwartz GJ, Haycock MB, Chir B, Spitzer A: Plasma creatinine and urea concentration in children: Normal values for age and sex. J Pediatr 88:828–830, 1976. With permission.)

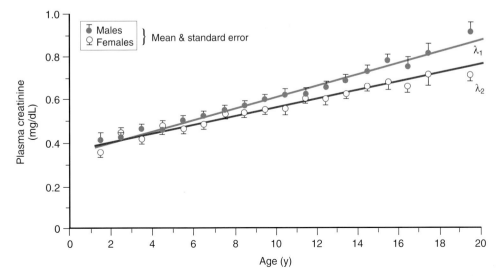

Although sodium retention in the maturing individual is essential for growth, the counterpart of this chronically enhanced sodium reabsorption is that newborns have difficulty in rapidly excreting an acute load of sodium and water. The renal excretory response to a sodium load increases progressively during infancy and is fully developed by the first year of life. In addition to the low GFR, enhanced distal tubular sodium reabsorption is responsible for the retention of sodium.

According to the information already given, the sodium requirements for a term newborn range from 1 to 1.5 mEq/kg/day, whereas the requirements for a preterm neonate range from 3 to 5 mEq/kg/day. The sodium content of breast milk is appropriate for the feeding of the healthy term infant. It should be remembered, however, that if excess sodium is given, such as feeding undiluted cow's milk, there is a risk of inducing sodium and water retention with extracellular volume expansion and sometimes clinically evident edema.

Oliguria

Most neonates void within the first 24 hours after birth. Any newborn baby, whether term or premature, who has not urinated within the first 24 hours of life should be evaluated for kidney disease. Oliguria in infancy is defined as urine flow rate less than 1 mL/kg/hour. This is based on the usual renal solute load (7 to 15 mOsm/kg/day) contributed by feedings and a maximal urinary osmolality of 500 mOsm/kg. To maintain solute balance, the newborn will therefore need to urinate about 30 mL/kg/day (1.25 mL/kg/hour). In infants, oliguria can be easily evaluated by calculating the fractional excretion of sodium (FE_{Na}) (see Chapter 34).

Determination of the FE_{Na} is convenient because it does not require a timed urine collection. The FE_{Na} is particularly helpful in distinguishing oliguria that is due to a prerenal (low FE_{Na}) etiology from that due to a renal (high FE_{Na}) cause. In the oliguric term neonate, a FE_{Na} higher than 2.5% indicates a renal cause (such as acute tubular necrosis), whereas a FE_{Na} of less than 2.5% suggests prerenal causes such as dehydration, hypovolemia, hypoalbuminemia, or decreased effective plasma volume. As previously mentioned, premature babies normally have higher FE_{Na} (around 5%) and, therefore, the cutoff of 2.5% is not useful until after 10 days of postnatal life. In the older child, as in adults, a FE_{Na} of 1% is utilized as the break point (see Chapter 34).

Calcium

Fetal calcium levels are higher than maternal values because of active calcium transport across the placenta toward the fetal side. The fractional reabsorption of calcium by the loop of Henle increases with maturation. Therefore, infants excrete more calcium in the urine than

TABLE 55-3   Calcium Levels According to Age

Age	Calcium Level (mg/dL)
Premature (<1 week)	6–10
Fullterm (<1 week)	7–12
Child	8.0–10.5
Adult	8.5–10.5

From Greene MG: The Harriet Lane Handbook. A Manual for Pediatric House Officers, 12th ed. St. Louis, Mosby, 1991, pp 1–434. Adapted from Meites S (ed): Pediatric Clinical Chemistry, 2nd and 3rd eds. The American Association for Clinical Chemistry, 1981; Tietz NW: Textbook of Clinical Chemistry. 1986; Lundberg GD, et al: JAMA 260:73, 1988; and Wallach J: Interpretation of Diagnostic Tests, Boston, Little, Brown, 1992.

older children. Most commonly, hypercalciuria in the newborn is seen in neonates with bronchopulmonary dysplasia who have received calciuric drugs such as furosemide or glucocorticoids. Hypercalciuria, in turn, can lead to nephrocalcinosis, urolithiasis, and decreased kidney function. When possible, a thiazide diuretic that reduces urine calcium excretion should be used instead of furosemide. Phosphate depletion in preterm infants can also lead to hypercalciuria.

Urine calcium excretion in the neonate can be estimated by calculating the calcium-to-creatinine ratio in a random urine sample. A ratio above 0.8 in preterm and above 0.4 in full-term infants is considered hypercalciuria. In older children, a ratio above 0.2 or a calcium excretion in a timed urine sample of greater than 4 mg/kg/24 hours are used to diagnose hypercalciuria.

Newborn infants are also prone to hypocalcemia, especially when they are sick. Contributing characteristics include decreased responses to parathyroid hormone, high serum phosphate levels, and the rapid bone mineralization characteristic of the newborn period. The normal range for calcium levels in infants and children are shown in Table 55-3.

Phosphate

Serum phosphate concentration is normally higher in the neonate than in the adult (Table 55-4). Any neonate with a serum phosphate below 4 mg/dL should be evaluated for tubular wasting of phosphate. This can be easily done by calculating the tubular reabsorption of phosphate (TRP) after measuring the concentrations of creatinine and phosphate both in urine and plasma. The TRP can be envisioned as the complement of the fractional excretion of phosphate: $TRP = (1 - FE_{PO_4}) \times 100\%$. Since

$$FE_{PO_4} = \frac{U_{PO_4}/P_{PO_4}}{(U_{cr}/P_{cr})}$$

then

$$TRP = \left[1 - \frac{(U_{PO_4}/P_{PO_4})}{(U_{cr}/P_{cr})} \right] \times 100\%$$

TABLE 55-4 Normal Phosphate Levels

Age	Phosphate Level (mg/dL)
Newborn	4.2–9.0
1 year	3.8–6.2
2–5 years	3.5–6.8
Adult	3.0–4.5

From Greene MG: The Harriet Lane Handbook. A Manual for Pediatric House Officers, 12th ed. St. Louis, Mosby, 1991, pp 1–434. Adapted from Meites S (ed): Pediatric Clinical Chemistry, 2nd and 3rd eds. The American Association for Clinical Chemistry, 1981; Tietz NW: Textbook of Clinical Chemistry 1986; Lundberg GD, et al: JAMA 260:73, 1988; and Wallach J: Interpretation of Diagnostic Tests, Boston, Little, Brown, 1992.

where U_{PO_4} and P_{PO_4} are the urinary and plasma concentrations of phosphate (mg/dL), respectively, and P_{cr} and U_{cr} are the plasma and urinary concentrations of creatinine (mg/dL). It should be remembered that the normal TRP varies with age. After the first week of postnatal life, the TRP should exceed 95% in full-term and 75% in preterm neonates. After the first month of postnatal life and throughout adulthood, the TRP should be greater than 85%. Values below those just mentioned should suggest Fanconi's syndrome, hyperparathyroidism, or advanced chronic kidney disease.

Potassium

The total body potassium (K^+) in infants is 40 mEq/kg, compared with the larger quantity found in adults (50 mEq/kg). Growing infants maintain a positive K^+ balance that is necessary for growth. Conservation of K^+ during infancy is reflected also by higher serum K^+ values (Table 55-5). In comparison with the adult, the newborn has a low basal rate of K^+ excretion and a decreased ability to rapidly excrete a K^+ load (see Table 55-5). The fractional excretion of K^+ in the newborn is about half of that in the adult (see Table 55-5), in part because of reduced K^+ secretion by the cortical collecting duct, the main site for K^+ excretion. The characteristics that limit urinary K^+ excretion by the principal cells during early life are (1) unfavorable electrochemical gradient (low cellular K^+ concentration, decreased Na^+ K^+-ATPase activity and transepithelial voltage), (2) limited membrane permeability to K^+, (3) low tubular fluid flow rates, and (4) decreased sensitivity to mineralocorticoids. Also, enhanced K^+ absorption by intercalated cells of the medullary collecting ducts may contribute. In fact, medullary collecting tubules (which reabsorb K^+) mature earlier than the principal cells of the cortical collecting duct (which secrete K^+), a characteristic that may be important in the decreased ability to excrete K^+ during early life. In addition, as GFR increases with maturation, so does fluid delivery to the cortical collecting duct, promoting K^+ secretion. Under normal conditions, the reduced ability of the neonate to excrete K^+ is not manifested clinically. However, hyperkalemia can develop if the neonate is exposed to excessive exogenous or endogenous (i.e., cell breakdown) K^+ loads.

Acid-Base Balance

Infants have lower blood pH and HCO_3^- than older children and adults (Table 55-6). Overall, the newborn kidney is capable of maintaining normal acid-base status. However, infants are prone to the development of acidosis when they are sick or receive inadequate nutrition or in response to an exogenous acid load. The plasma concentration of HCO_3^- increases with age as a result of an increase in the renal threshold of HCO_3^- with maturation. The approximate renal threshold of HCO_3^- is 18 mEq/L in the premature and 21 mEq/L in the term neonate. Adult values (24 to 26 mEq/L) are reached by 1 year of age. Apparently responsible for the low renal HCO_3^- threshold observed in infancy are several conditions: low activity of

TABLE 55-5 Plasma Levels and Excretion of Potassium in Normal Infants and Children

Age (years)	Plasma [K^+] (mEq/L)	K^+ Clearance (mL/min/1.73 m²)	FE_K* (%)
0–0.3	5.2 ± 0.8	5 ± 3	8.5 ± 3.8
0.4–1.0	4.9 ± 0.5	14 ± 6	14.6 ± 5.0
3–10	4.2 ± 0.5	20 ± 11	14.5 ± 8.9
11–20	4.3 ± 0.3	21 ± 8	16.2 ± 8.2

*Fractional excretion of potassium: $FE_K = (U_K/P_K)/(U_{cr}/P_{cr}) \times 100\%$. Modified from Jones DL, Chesney RW: Tubular Function. In Holliday MA, Barrett TM, Avner FD (eds): Pediatric Nephrology, 4th ed. Baltimore, Williams & Wilkins, 1999, pp 59–82.

TABLE 55-6 Acid-Base Measurements in Blood as a Function of Age*

Age	pH	HCO_3^- (mEq/L)
Preterm (1 week)	7.34 ± 0.06	17.2 ± 1.2[†]
Preterm (6 weeks)	7.38 ± 0.02	21.9 ± 4.4[†]
Term (birth)	7.24 ± 0.05	20.0 ± 2.8[†]
Term (1 hour)	7.37 ± 0.05	19.0 ± 2.3[†]
3–6 months	7.39 ± 0.03	22.0 ± 1.9[†]
21–24 months	7.40 ± 0.02	21.8 ± 1.6[†]
3.5–5.4 years	7.39 ± 0.04	22.5 ± 1.3[†]
5.5–12.0 years	7.40 ± 0.03	23.1 ± 1.2[†]
12.5–17.4 years	7.38 ± 0.03	24.0 ± 1.0[†]
Adult males	7.39 ± 0.01	25.2 ± 1.0

*Values are mean ± 1 SD.
[†]Significantly different from adult males ($P < 0.05$) by Tukey's test. Modified from Schwartz GJ: Potassium and acid-base. In Holliday MA, Barratt TM, Avner ED (eds): Pediatric Nephrology, 4th ed. Baltimore, Williams & Wilkins, 1999, p 174.

carbonic anhydrase, extracellular fluid volume expansion contributing to proximal HCO_3^- wasting, immaturity of luminal Na^+-H^+ exchange, and imbalance between filtration and reabsorption of HCO_3^- in newly formed nephrons. Moreover, HCO_3^- reabsorption in the distal nephron may not compensate for HCO_3^- that escapes the proximal tubule.

Infants have a decreased ability to acidify the urine when compared with adults under basal conditions. Maximal titratable acid and ammonium excretion increase with age and achieve adult values (when corrected by GFR) by 2 months of age. Several conditions are responsible for the relative inability of the newborn to excrete an acid load, including a limited availability of urinary buffers such as phosphate and ammonium. The low GFR and high TRP prevailing in the neonatal period markedly limit the phosphate available as a urinary buffer. Before 2 months of age, ammonia generation and secretion are also limited. Immaturity of the collecting ducts (fewer intercalated cells, fewer proton pumps per cell) and immaturity of carbonic anhydrase activity could also limit distal acidification. In addition to this impairment in renal excretion, infants have an increased exogenous and endogenous proton load in comparison with adults. In prematures, endogenous acid production can be as high as 2 to 3 mEq/kg/day. A large amount of acid is generated during the metabolism of proteins. Accretion of calcium into the growing bone also results in the release of 0.5 to 1.0 mEq/kg/day of H^+ that must be excreted by the kidney or neutralized by HCO_3^- absorbed through the gastrointestinal tract. For this reason, during episodes of gastroenteritis, infants are susceptible to metabolic acidosis.

Blood Pressure

The normal blood pressure values vary with age, gender, stature, and degree of maturation. Accepted normal values are based on demographic studies. The reader should consult the report of the Second Task Force on Blood Pressure Control in Children—1987 and its more recent update in 1996 and 2004, which provide normative data and guidelines for detection and treatment of children with hypertension. A child is considered hypertensive if the systolic or diastolic blood pressure is above the 95th percentile for age and sex on at least three occasions. The classification of hypertension by age group is shown in Table 55-7. The most common etiologies of hypertension vary with the age of the patient population. As a rule, the younger the patient, the more likely it is for hypertension to be secondary. In the newborn period, renal artery thrombosis, congenital renal malformations, coarctation of the aorta, and bronchopulmonary dysplasia are the most common causes. In children between infancy and 6 years of age, renal parenchymal diseases, renal artery stenosis, and coarctation of the aorta are leading causes. Between 6 and 10 years of age, renal parenchymal diseases, renal artery stenosis, and essential hypertension are frequently found. In the adolescent, essential hypertension and renal parenchymal diseases are the two most prominent causes, with obesity-related hypertension now the most common etiology in adolescents.

TABLE 55-7 Classification of Hypertension by Age Group

Age Group	Significant Hypertension	Severe Hypertension
Newborn		
7 days	Systolic ≥ 96 mm Hg	Systolic ≥ 106 mm Hg
8–30 days	Systolic ≥ 104 mm Hg	Systolic ≥ 110 mm Hg
Infant (<2 years)	Systolic ≥ 112 mm Hg	Systolic ≥ 118 mm Hg
	Diastolic ≥ 74 mm Hg	Diastolic ≥ 82 mm Hg
Children (3–5 years)	Systolic ≥ 116 mm Hg	Systolic ≥ 124 mm Hg
	Diastolic ≥ 76 mm Hg	Diastolic ≥ 84 mm Hg
Children (6–9 years)	Systolic ≥ 122 mm Hg	Systolic ≥ 130 mm Hg
	Diastolic ≥ 78 mm Hg	Diastolic ≥ 86 mm Hg
Children (10–12 years)	Systolic ≥ 126 mm Hg	Systolic ≥ 134 mm Hg
	Diastolic ≥ 82 mm Hg	Diastolic ≥ 90 mm Hg
Adolescents (13–15 years)	Systolic ≥ 136 mm Hg	Systolic ≥ 144 mm Hg
	Diastolic ≥ 86 mm Hg	Diastolic ≥ 92 mm Hg
Adolescents (16–18 years)	Systolic ≥ 142 mm Hg	Systolic ≥ 150 mm Hg
	Diastolic ≥ 92 mm Hg	Diastolic ≥ 98 mm Hg

From the Report of the Second Task Force on Blood Pressure Control in Children—1987. Pediatrics 79:1–25, 1987.

BIBLIOGRAPHY

Al-Dahhan J, Haycock GB, Nichol B, et al: Sodium homeostasis in term and preterm neonates. III. Effect of salt supplementation. Arch Dis Child 59:945–950, 1984.

Gunn VL, Nechyba C: The Harriet Lane Handbook. A Manual for Pediatric House Officers, 16th ed. St. Louis, Mosby, 2002.

Chevalier RL: Developmental renal physiology of the low birth weight pre-term newborn. J Urol 156:714–719, 1996.

Gomez RA: Postnatal regulation of water and electrolyte excretion. In Brace RA, Ross MG, Robillard JE (eds): Reproductive and Perinatal Medicine. vol XI, Fetal and Neonatal Body Fluids: The Scientific Basis for Clinical Practice. New York, Perinatology Press, 1989, pp 307–318.

Jones DP, Chesney RW: Tubular function. In Holliday MA, Barrett TM, Avner ED (eds): Pediatric Nephrology, 4th ed. Baltimore, Williams & Wilkins, 1999, pp 59–82.

Mathew OP, Jones AS, James E, et al: Neonatal renal failure: Usefulness of diagnostic indices. Pediatrics 65:5760, 1980.

Polacek E: The osmotic concentrating ability in healthy infants and children. Arch Dis Child 40:291, 1965.

Report of the Second Task Force on Blood Pressure Control in Children–1987: Pediatrics 79:1–25, 1987.

Robillard JE, Guillery EN, Petershack JA: Renal function during fetal life. In Holliday MA, Barrett TM, Avner ED (eds): Pediatric Nephrology, 4th ed. Baltimore, Williams & Wilkins, 1999, pp 21–37.

Schwartz GJ, Brion LP, Spitzer A: The use of plasma creatinine concentration for estimating glomerular filtration rate in infants, children and adolescents. Pediatr Clin North Am 34:571–590, 1987.

Update on the 1987 Task Force Report of High Blood Pressure in Children and Adolescents: A Working Group Report from the National High Blood Pressure Education Program. Pediatrics 98(4):649–658, 1996.

Woolf, AS: Embryology. In Holliday MA, Barrett TM, Avner ED (eds): Pediatric Nephrology, 4th ed. Baltimore, Williams & Wilkins, 1999, pp 1–19.

CHAPTER **56**

The Kidney in Pregnancy

Phyllis August

An intriguing aspect of reproduction is the close dependency of reproductive function on normal kidney function. Pregnancy, in the setting of significant maternal kidney disease, is hazardous and frequently unsuccessful. Pregnancy imposes a hemodynamic strain on maternal kidney function such that in some cases kidney function deteriorates irreversibly in women with preexisting kidney disease during or after pregnancy. In general, the closer to normal the glomerular filtration rate (GFR) and blood pressure are, the greater is the chance of successful pregnancy. Management of gravidas with kidney disease may be complicated, and requires an understanding of the physiologic changes associated with pregnancy, as well as close cooperation between obstetrician and nephrologist.

RENAL ANATOMY AND PHYSIOLOGY IN PREGNANCY

Anatomic and Functional Changes in the Urinary Tract

Kidney length increases approximately 1 cm during normal gestation. The major anatomic alterations of the urinary tract during pregnancy, however, are seen in the collecting system, where calyces, renal pelves, and ureters dilate, often giving the erroneous impression of obstructive uropathy. The cause of the ureteral dilation is disputed and has been attributed to hormonal mechanisms as well as mechanical obstruction by the enlarging uterus. These morphologic changes result in stasis in the urinary tract and a propensity of pregnant women with asymptomatic bacteriuria to develop overt pyelonephritis. Because they contain substantial amounts of urine, the dilated ureters may cause an error when a 24-hour urine collection is performed. It has been recommended that pregnant women receive a water load and remain in lateral recumbency for 1 hour before the start of the collection.

Renal Hemodynamics

Pregnancy is characterized by marked vasodilatation, which is detectable early in the first trimester. In fact, recent studies of the menstrual cycle demonstrate that the vasodilatation is also present in the late luteal phase, before conception. There is lower blood pressure throughout gestation, as well as increased renal plasma flow and GFR, and decreased renal vascular resistance. Because renal plasma flow increases slightly more than does GFR, filtration fraction remains constant or slightly lower in pregnancy. The increases in GFR and renal plasma flow reach a maximum during the first trimester, to levels approximately 50% greater than nonpregnant levels. The basis for these increases is unknown. Micropuncture studies performed in the gravid rat are consistent with a major role of renal vasodilatation and increased glomerular plasma flow in these changes. Experimental models of nitric oxide synthesis inhibition suggest that hormonally mediated increased nitric oxide generation may be in part responsible for the renal vasodilatation observed in pregnancy.

Creatinine production is unchanged during pregnancy, thus increments in clearance result in decreased serum levels. One study reported average values of 0.83 mg/dL in nonpregnant women, and 0.74, 0.58, and 0.53 mg/dL in the first, second, and third trimester of pregnancy, respectively. The increased GFR and renal plasma flow also result in increased excretion of glucose, amino acids, calcium, and urinary protein. The clinical consequences of these alterations are an increase in the upper limit of normal for urinary protein excretion (from 150 mg/day to 300 mg/day).

Acid-Base Regulation in Pregnancy

The bicarbonate excretion threshold is shifted to the left, most likely in response to chronic respiratory alkalosis, and early-morning urine specimens are more alkaline than in nonpregnant women. Plasma bicarbonate concentration decreases by approximately 4 mmol/L, averaging 22 mmol/L. The hypocapnia that occurs during pregnancy is probably a result of progesterone-mediated hyperventilation. The pCO_2 averages only 30 mm Hg, and thus, since both pCO_2 and bicarbonate levels are already diminished, pregnant women may be disadvantaged when threatened by acute metabolic acidosis. Finally, it should be appreciated that a pCO_2 of 40 mm Hg signifies considerable carbon dioxide retention in pregnancy.

Water Metabolism

Pregnancy is associated with a decrease in plasma osmolality of 5 to 10 mOsm/kg below that of nongravid women. This decrease in plasma osmolality is associated with appropriate responses to water loading and dehydration, and suggests a resetting of the osmoreceptor system. Clinical studies demonstrating decreased osmotic thresholds for thirst and arginine vasopressin release in pregnant women support this hypothesis. In addition, pregnant women metabolize arginine vasopressin more rapidly as a consequence of increased production of placental vasopressinases. Pregnant women may develop syndromes of transient diabetes insipidus due to the increased metabolism of arginine vasopressin. These syndromes may be treated with DDAVP (desmopressin acetate).

Volume Regulation

Total body water increases by 6 to 8 liters during pregnancy, 4 to 6 liters of which is extracellular. Plasma volume increases 50% during gestation, the largest rate of increment occurring in midpregnancy. There is a gradual cumulative retention of about 900 mEq of sodium during pregnancy, which is distributed between the products of conception and the maternal extracellular space. Despite the increase in plasma volume during pregnancy, there is no evidence for a hypervolemic (i.e., overfilled circulation) state during pregnancy. Indeed, the marked vasodilation that is observed as early as the first trimester may be the stimulus for increased sodium retention and increased plasma volume. The observations that blood pressure is significantly lower, and that the renin-angiotensin system is stimulated during normal pregnancy are consistent with primary vasodilation preceding and causing the increase in plasma volume.

Blood Pressure Regulation

Mean blood pressure decreases early in gestation, with diastolic levels averaging 10 mm Hg less in midpregnancy compared with antepartum levels. Later in pregnancy, blood pressure may increase and reach nonpregnant levels near term. The decrease in blood pressure is due to vasodilation, which may be mediated by the effects of placental hormones on vascular endothelium. Preliminary data suggest that relaxin, a peptide secreted by the corpus luteum and placenta, may also contribute to vasodilation in pregnancy. Several endothelial products associated with vasodilation are increased in pregnancy, including nitric oxide and prostacyclin. Endothelial products associated with vasoconstriction (e.g., endothelin) are decreased. In response to the vasodilation and lower blood pressure, the renin-angiotensin system is markedly stimulated in pregnancy. Increases in plasma renin activity are apparent early in pregnancy, and levels increase to reach a maximum of about four times nonpregnant values by midpregnancy. The increase in plasma renin activity is accompanied by increases in aldosterone secretion. Angiotensin II levels have not been studied extensively, but they are probably increased as well. Despite the increased renin and aldosterone levels, blood pressure and electrolytes are normal during pregnancy. Indeed, normotensive gravidas demonstrate exaggerated responses to acute converting-enzyme inhibition, suggesting that the stimulated renin-angiotensin system is an important defense against hypotension during pregnancy.

Mineral Metabolism

Serum calcium levels decrease in pregnancy, as does serum albumin concentration. Ionized calcium remains normal. There are significant increases in circulating levels of $1,25(OH)_2$ vitamin D_3 during pregnancy, as a result of increased renal production as well as increased placental production. Gastrointestinal absorption of calcium increases, and there is an "absorptive hypercalciuria," with 24-hour urine excretion often exceeding 300 mg/day. Intact parathyroid hormone levels are lower during pregnancy compared with nonpregnant values.

KIDNEY DISEASE IN PREGNANCY

Kidney disease during pregnancy may be due to (1) preexisting kidney disease that was diagnosed before conception, (2) chronic kidney disease that was unappreciated before pregnancy and diagnosed for the first time during pregnancy, or (3) kidney disease that develops for the first time during pregnancy. There is some overlap with respect to the different diseases that are typical of the three categories. For example, lupus nephritis may be a chronic condition, or it may develop for the first time during pregnancy.

Chronic Kidney Disease: General Principles

Fertility and the ability to sustain an uncomplicated pregnancy are related to the degree of kidney function impairment, rather than to the specific underlying disorder. The greater the functional decrement and the higher the blood pressure are, the less likely it is that the pregnancy will be successful. Patients are arbitrarily considered in three categories: preserved or mildly impaired kidney function (serum creatinine less than or at 1.4 mg/dL), moderately impaired kidney function (creatinine 1.5 to 3.0 mg/dL), and severe impairment of kidney function (creatinine higher than or equal to 3 mg/dL). Table 56-1 summarizes the maternal and fetal prognosis in each category. Women with moderate or severe renal dysfunction should be discouraged from conceiving, because as many

TABLE 56-1   Pregnancy and Kidney Disease: Level of Kidney Function and Prospects*

Outcome	Category of Kidney Function		
	Mild (SCr < 1.5 mg/dL)	Moderate (SCr 1.5–3.0 mg/dL)	Severe (SCr > 3.0 mg/dL)
Pregnancy complications	25%	47%	86%
Successful obstetric outcome	96% (85%)	90% (59%)	47% (8%)
Long-term sequelae	<3% (9%)	25% (71%)	53% (92%)

SCr, serum creatinine concentration.

*Estimates are based on 1862 women with 2799 pregnancies (1973–1992) and do not include collagen vascular diseases. Numbers in parentheses refer to prospects when complications develop before 28 weeks' gestation.

From Davison JM, Lindheimer MD: Renal disorders. In Creasy RK, Resnik RK (eds): Maternal Fetal Medicine, 4th ed. Philadelphia, WB Saunders, 1999.

as 40% of these pregnancies are complicated by hypertension or deterioration in kidney function that may be irreversible. The blood pressure at the time of conception is an important variable in pregnancy outcome. In the absence of hypertension, there is significantly less chance of irreversible deterioration in kidney function during pregnancy. When hypertension is present, and especially when it is severe, pregnancy outcome is rarely uncomplicated. Premature delivery and deterioration in kidney function are expected. Urine protein excretion may increase markedly in pregnant women with underlying kidney disease. Although the increments in protein excretion during pregnancy may not necessarily reflect worsening of the underlying kidney disease, increased proteinuria is associated with worse fetal prognosis.

Kidney Diseases Associated with Systemic Illness

Diabetes is one of the most common medical disorders encountered during pregnancy, and the majority of cases are due to gestational diabetes. Preexisting diabetes poses significant risks to pregnancy. Many younger women with pregestational diabetes have type 1 diabetes, and if their disease has been present for 10 to 15 years, they may show early signs of diabetic nephropathy. Women with microalbuminuria, well-preserved kidney function, and normal blood pressure have a good prognosis for pregnancy, although they are at increased risk for preeclampsia and urinary infection. When baseline kidney function and blood pressure are still normal, pregnancy is not likely to accelerate the progression of early diabetic nephropathy, although it is not unusual for urinary protein excretion to increase significantly during pregnancy. Women with non-nephritic-range proteinuria before conception may develop nephritic-range proteinuria during pregnancy that is usually reversible. Women with overt nephropathy before conception, particularly those with impaired kidney function and hypertension, as in any other kidney disease, have a high incidence of premature delivery and deterioration in maternal kidney function. Women with type 1 diabetes with microalbuminuria and normal kidney function and normotension

should be encouraged not to postpone pregnancy, because the prognosis worsens once overt nephropathy develops.

The most important aspect of management of diabetes in pregnancy with or without nephropathy is tight glucose control, because of the clear-cut relationship between glucose control and fetal outcome. Thus all women with diabetes should be managed by physicians experienced with diabetes in pregnancy. Blood pressure control is also important. However, because angiotensin-converting enzyme inhibitors and angiotensin receptor blockers are contraindicated during pregnancy, women should have their medication switched to other agents before conception.

Women with lupus nephritis during pregnancy present unique problems. Although similar considerations apply regarding the relationship between level of kidney function and blood pressure to pregnancy outcome, in general, lupus is a much more unpredictable illness, because of the tendency of the disease to flare. Whether or not pregnancy per se presents risks for lupus flares has been disputed. Recent prospective data from a well-controlled study suggest that pregnancy is in fact associated with a greater chance of disease exacerbation. Women with lupus are advised not to conceive unless their disease has been "inactive" for the preceding 6 months. Additional complications associated with lupus and pregnancy include placental transfer of maternal autoantibodies, which can cause a neonatal lupus syndrome that is characterized by heart block, transient cutaneous lesions, or both. Women with lupus are also more likely to have clinically significant titers of antiphospholipid antibodies and the lupus anticoagulant, which are associated with spontaneous fetal loss, hypertensive syndromes indistinguishable from preeclampsia, and thrombotic events including deep-vein thrombosis, pulmonary embolus, myocardial infarction, and strokes. Thus all women with systemic lupus erythematosus should be screened for antiphospholipid antibodies early in gestation. When titers are elevated (more than 40 GPL), daily aspirin (80 to 325 mg) is recommended. If there is a history of thrombotic events, then heparin in combination with aspirin is recommended. One of the difficulties in managing lupus nephritis during pregnancy is that increased activity of lupus may be difficult to distinguish from preeclampsia. Both are characterized by an increase in proteinuria, a decrease in GFR, and hypertension. Thrombocytopenia may also be observed in both conditions. Hypocomplementemia is not a feature of preeclampsia, whereas abnormal liver function tests may be observed in preeclampsia but are not characteristic of lupus activity. If disease activity is present before 20 weeks of gestation, then preeclampsia is not likely. In the latter half of pregnancy, it may be impossible to distinguish between a renal lupus flare and preeclampsia. In fact, frequently both are present simultaneously, and what starts as increased lupus activity appears to trigger preeclampsia. Unfortunately, delivery may be necessary if immunosuppressive therapy and supportive care fail to stabilize the condition. Appropriate therapy for lupus nephritis during pregnancy includes steroids and azathioprine. Cyclophosphamide is generally not recommended during pregnancy because of potential fetal toxicity and should only be used when the mother's life is in jeopardy. There are no data regarding use of mycophenolate mofetil during pregnancy for treatment of lupus nephritis. Concerns regarding fetal safety are based on animal data, and human use has been too limited to support or refute these data.

Chronic Glomerulonephritis

Childbearing women may be afflicted with any of the forms of chronic glomerulonephritis that are common in this age group. These include immunoglobulin A (IgA) nephropathy, focal segmental glomerulosclerosis, membranoproliferative glomerulonephritis, minimal-change nephritis, and membranous nephropathy. There are insufficient data to suggest that the histologic subtype confers a specific prognosis for pregnancy. Rather, the principles already mentioned are applicable to women with chronic glomerulonephritis; when kidney function is normal and hypertension absent, prognosis is good.

Polycystic Kidney Disease

Young women with autosomal-dominant polycystic kidney disease (ADPKD) are frequently asymptomatic, with normal kidney function and normal blood pressure, and indeed may be unaware of their diagnosis. Older women with progressive disease and functional impairment and hypertension are at risk for preeclampsia and premature delivery. There is an increased incidence of urinary tract infection as well. Estrogen is reported to cause liver cysts to enlarge, and repeated pregnancies may result in symptomatic enlargement of liver cysts. Given the association between cerebral aneurysms and ADPKD in some families, screening for such aneurysms should be considered before natural labor ensues. All affected individuals (male and female) should undergo genetic

counseling to ensure they are aware that their offspring have a 50% chance of being affected.

Chronic Pyelonephritis

Dilation and stasis in the urinary tract make chronic pyelonephritis (nephropathies associated with recurrent urinary tract infection often in association with urinary tract abnormalities, e.g., vesicoureteral reflux) in gravidas more prone to exacerbation. These women should be urged to maintain a high fluid intake and should be screened frequently for bacteriuria. Women with reflux nephropathy have been reported to have an adverse prognosis during pregnancy. These high-risk women should be screened with urine cultures and should be treated promptly when infections are present.

Chronic Kidney Diseases That May Be First Diagnosed During Pregnancy

The presence of chronic kidney disease may first be appreciated during pregnancy, not only because pregnant women are scrutinized more closely but also because the renal hemodynamic alterations during pregnancy may cause proteinuria to increase and be clinically detectable for the first time. Frequent measurement of blood pressure may also lead to diagnosis of kidney diseases accompanied by hypertension. Furthermore, the presence of even mild preexisting kidney disease is associated with an increased risk of preeclampsia. Thus underlying kidney disease may first become apparent after preeclampsia has developed in later pregnancy. Kidney diseases that may have been relatively silent before conception that may "present" during pregnancy include IgA nephropathy, focal segmental glomerular sclerosis, polycystic kidney disease, and reflux nephropathy. Renal diagnostic testing during pregnancy can include blood and urine testing and ultrasonography. Kidney biopsy is usually deferred until after delivery unless there is acute deterioration in kidney function or morbid nephrotic syndrome. The timing of kidney biopsy after delivery depends on the clinical circumstances. If kidney function is normal and only proteinuria is present, it is reasonable to delay biopsy by at least 1 to 2 months, since proteinuria may improve once the hemodynamic alterations associated with pregnancy have resolved. If kidney function is impaired, then biopsy should be considered within a few weeks of delivery.

Kidney Diseases That Develop for the First Time During Pregnancy

Pregnant women are at risk for any of the kidney diseases that occur in women of childbearing age, including pyelonephritis, glomerulonephritis, interstitial nephritis, and acute renal failure. Pyelonephritis in pregnant women is more likely to be associated with significant azotemia compared with nonpregnant women, and should be treated aggressively. Glomerulonephritis and interstitial nephritis are not more likely to develop during pregnancy, although they do occur. Acute renal failure in association with pregnancy is not common. Recent estimates suggest that the incidence of acute renal failure from obstetric causes is less than 1 in 20,000 pregnancies.

When acute renal failure occurs early in pregnancy (12 to 18 weeks), it is usually in association with septic abortion or prerenal azotemia due to hyperemesis gravidarum. Most cases of acute renal failure in pregnancy occur between gestational week 35 and the puerperium, and are primarily due to preeclampsia and bleeding complications. Although most cases of preeclampsia are not usually associated with renal failure, the HELLP syndrome (hemolysis, elevated liver enzymes, low platelet count), which is a variant of preeclampsia, may be associated with significant renal dysfunction, especially if not treated promptly. The important clinical entities causing renal failure during pregnancy are thrombotic microangiopathy, bilateral renal cortical necrosis, acute fatty liver of pregnancy, and urinary tract obstruction.

Thrombotic Microangiopathy

Though rare, thrombotic microangiopathies (thrombotic thrombocytopenic purpura and hemolytic uremic syndrome, or TTP/HUS) are an important cause of pregnancy-associated acute renal failure, because they are associated with considerable morbidity. They also share several clinical and laboratory features of pregnancy-specific disorders such as the HELLP variant of preeclampsia and acute fatty liver of pregnancy; thus distinction of these syndromes is important for therapeutic and prognostic reasons. Features that may be helpful in making the correct diagnosis include timing of onset and the pattern of laboratory abnormalities. Preeclampsia typically develops in the third trimester, with only a few cases developing in the postpartum period, usually within a few days of delivery. TTP usually occurs antepartum, with many cases developing in the second trimester, as well as the third. HUS is usually a postpartum disease. Symptoms may begin antepartum, but most cases are diagnosed postpartum.

Preeclampsia is much more common than TTP/HUS, and it is usually preceded by hypertension and proteinuria. Renal failure is unusual, even with severe cases, unless significant bleeding or hemodynamic instability or marked disseminated intravascular coagulation occurs. In some cases, preeclampsia develops in the immediate postpartum period, and when thrombocytopenia is severe, it may be indistinguishable from HUS. However, preeclampsia spontaneously recovers, whereas HUS only infrequently improves.

In contrast to TTP/HUS, preeclampsia may be associated with mild disseminated intravascular coagulation and prolongation of prothrombin and partial thromboplastin times. Another laboratory feature of preeclampsia/HELLP syndrome that is usually absent in TTP/HUS is a marked elevation in liver enzymes. The presence of fever is more consistent with a diagnosis of TTP than preeclampsia or HUS. The main distinctive features of HUS are its tendency to occur in the postpartum period and the severity of the associated renal failure. Treatment of preeclampsia/HELLP syndrome is delivery and supportive care. More aggressive treatment is rarely indicated. Some centers have reported the use of steroids in cases of severe HELLP syndrome, although this therapy has not been rigorously evaluated in placebo-controlled clinical trials. Treatment of TTP/HUS includes plasma infusion/exchange and other modalities used in nonpregnant patients with these disorders.

Bilateral Renal Cortical Necrosis

Bilateral renal cortical necrosis may be induced by abruptio placenta or other severe complications associated with obstetric hemorrhage. Both primary disseminated intravascular coagulation and severe renal ischemia have been proposed as the initiating events. Affected patients typically present with oliguria or anuria, hematuria, and flank pain. Ultrasonography or computed tomography may demonstrate hyperechoic or hypodense areas in the renal cortex. Most patients ultimately require dialysis, but 20% to 40% have partial recovery of kidney function.

Acute Fatty Liver of Pregnancy

Acute fatty liver of pregnancy (AFLP) is a rare complication of pregnancy that is associated with significant azotemia. One series compared AFLP to HELLP syndrome and observed that acute renal failure was significantly more common with AFLP. The authors hypothesized that, since AFLP is believed to be a disease of mitochondrial dysfunction, it is possible that the kidney dysfunction associated with AFLP reflects inhibition of β-oxidation of fats in the kidney. Autopsy data have demonstrated microvesicular fat in the kidneys of women with AFLP. Women with this disorder often complain of anorexia, nausea, vomiting, and occasionally abdominal pain in the third trimester. Clinical features suggesting preeclampsia including hypertension and proteinuria are not uncommon. Laboratory tests reveal elevations in liver enzymes, hypoglycemia, hypofibrinogenemia, and prolonged partial thromboplastin time. Delivery is indicated, and most patients improve shortly afterward. This disorder was formerly associated with a more ominous outcome, which may have been a consequence of late diagnosis. When AFLP is diagnosed early, long-term morbidity is rare.

Urinary Tract Obstruction

Pregnancy is associated with dilation of the collecting system, which is not usually accompanied by impaired kidney function. Rarely, complications such as large uterine fibroids that enlarge in the setting of pregnancy can lead to obstructive uropathy. Occasionally, acute urinary tract obstruction in pregnancy is caused by a kidney stone. Diagnosis can usually be made by ultrasonography. Often the stone will pass spontaneously, but occasionally cystoscopy is necessary for insertion of a stent to remove a fragment of stone and relieve obstruction, particularly if there is sepsis or a solitary kidney. Extracorporeal shock wave lithotripsy is contraindicated during pregnancy because of the possibility of adverse effects on the fetus.

Management of acute renal failure occurring in pregnancy or immediately postpartum is similar to that in nongravid subjects, although there are several important considerations unique to pregnancy. Uterine hemorrhage near term may be concealed, and blood loss underestimated; thus, any overt blood loss should be replaced early. Both peritoneal dialysis and hemodialysis have been used successfully in patients with obstetric acute renal failure. Neither pelvic peritonitis nor the enlarged uterus is a contraindication to the former method. In fact, this form of treatment is more gradual than hemodialysis and thus less likely to precipitate labor. Because urea, creatinine, and other metabolites that accumulate in uremia traverse the placenta, dialysis should be undertaken early, with the aim of maintaining the blood urea nitrogen at approximately 50 mg/dL. In essence, the advantages of early dialysis in nongravid patients are even more important for the pregnant patient. Excessive fluid removal should be avoided, because it may contribute to hemodynamic compromise, reduction of uteroplacental perfusion, and premature labor. In some cases it may be advisable to perform continuous fetal monitoring during dialysis, particularly after midpregnancy.

THERAPY OF ENDSTAGE RENAL DISEASE DURING PREGNANCY

Dialysis

Fertility is reduced in dialysis patients, and conception is uncommon in women who have had endstage renal disease for several years. Most pregnancies occur within the first few years of starting dialysis. Although in the past the outcomes of such pregnancies were poor, with only approximately 25% resulting in surviving infants, new information suggests that pregnancy in dialysis patients is successful as often as 30% to 50% of the time in pregnancies that reach the second trimester. Considerable problems exist in such pregnancies, however, and

conception should not be encouraged in women on maintenance dialysis. Prematurity is common, and approximately 85% of infants born to women who conceive after starting dialysis are born before 36 weeks' gestation. There is a high incidence of very low birth weight and intrauterine growth restriction. Maternal complications include accelerated hypertension and even death. The approach to dialysis during pregnancy should include increasing dialysis time to minimize the uremic environment. Although there have not been any randomized clinical trials comparing normal with increased dialysis dose in pregnant endstage renal disease patients, several literature reviews, case series, and retrospective reports support the strategy of augmenting dialysis treatments during pregnancy. Both the number of sessions per week and the time per session can be increased to a minimum of 20 hours of hemodialysis. Heparinization should be minimal to prevent obstetric bleeding. If peritoneal dialysis is being used, decreasing exchange volumes and increasing exchange frequency are recommended. Adequate calorie and protein intake should be encouraged. Antihypertensive therapy should be adjusted for pregnancy. Anemia should be treated with supplemental iron, folic acid, and erythropoietin. There is no evidence that one dialysis modality is superior with respect to pregnancy outcome. Complications specific to peritoneal dialysis include peritonitis and mechanical difficulties (i.e., a possible need to reduce dwell volume due to enlarging abdominal girth).

Kidney Transplantation

Several thousand women have undergone pregnancy following kidney transplantation. Living related donor transplant recipients are more likely to have successful pregnancies, particularly human lymphocyte antigen (HLA)-identical transplant recipients in whom graft function is normal and doses of immunosuppressive agents are low. More than 90% of pregnancies that proceed beyond the first trimester succeed, yet there are certain predictable maternal and fetal problems. Maternal difficulties include complications of steroid therapy such as impaired glucose tolerance, hypertension, increased infection rate, ectopic pregnancy, and even uterine rupture. Fetal complications include a higher incidence of premature delivery, intrauterine growth restriction, congenital anomalies, hypoadrenalism, thrombocytopenia, and infection. It is suggested that transplant recipients contemplating pregnancy should meet the following criteria:

- Good health and stable kidney function for 2 years after transplantation
- Absent or minimal proteinuria
- Normal blood pressure or easily managed hypertension

- No evidence of pyelocalyceal distention on ultra-sonography before conception
- Serum creatinine less than 2 mg/dL, and preferably less than 1.5 mg/dL
- Drug therapy: prednisone 15 mg/day or less; azathioprine 2 mg/kg or less; cyclosporine less than 5 mg/kg/day

A transplant registry established at the Department of Surgery, Jefferson Medical College, Philadelphia, has compiled data on pregnancies in the era since the introduction of cyclosporine. The registry data support the recommendation that a creatinine concentration below 1.5 mg/dL and absence of hypertension are associated with the best prognosis. Although cyclosporine levels tend to decrease during pregnancy, there is no information available about whether or not drug dosage should be increased. Tacrolimus has not been used as widely in pregnancy as cyclosporine, although growing experience suggests that it is reasonably safe and similar in side effect profile to cyclosporine. Mycophenolate mofetil has not been widely used in pregnancy and has been reported to be embryotoxic in animals. This drug should be discontinued during pregnancy, and women should be switched to azathioprine if indicated. Because there are insufficient data on sirolimus in pregnancy, this drug should not be considered for pregnant women.

HYPERTENSIVE DISORDERS OF PREGNANCY

Hypertensive disorders are the most common medical disorders complicating pregnancy. Although maternal death is a rare event in most western nations where access to prenatal care is adequate, hypertensive disorders are one of the leading causes of maternal death worldwide, accounting for 15% to 20% of all maternal deaths in the developing as well as the developed world. In the United States, approximately 8% to 10% of all pregnancies are complicated by hypertension, with half of these cases attributable to the pregnancy-specific disorder preeclampsia. In addition to maternal morbidity and mortality, hypertensive disorders in pregnancy are a major cause of fetal morbidity and mortality. Hypertension is one of the leading causes of premature birth, which may be associated with life-long medical complications. Hypertensive disorders are significantly more common than kidney disease in pregnancy, and although they are commonly managed by obstetricians alone, the nephrologist is frequently called as a consultant in cases of severe preeclampsia, especially when multiorgan system involvement is present. The classification schema of hypertensive disorders in pregnancy has been in use for many years in the United States and has been endorsed by the National High Blood Pressure Education Program and the American College of Obstetricians and Gynecologists (Table 56-2).

TABLE 56-2 Classification of Hypertensive Disorders in Pregnancy

Preeclampsia
Chronic hypertension
Chronic hypertension with superimposed preeclampsia
Gestational hypertension

Preeclampsia

Preeclampsia is unique to pregnancy and is not only a systemic maternal syndrome characterized by hypertension, proteinuria, edema, and at times coagulation and liver function abnormalities, but also a fetal syndrome characterized by poor placentation, growth restriction, and at times death. Eclampsia is the convulsive form of preeclampsia. Preeclampsia usually develops in the third trimester, less frequently in the second trimester, and extremely rarely as early as 20 weeks' gestation. The syndrome is more common in nulliparous women. Preexisting kidney disease, hypertension, diabetes, and obesity also increase risk. Additional risk factors include multiple gestations, positive family history, extremes of reproductive age, and hydatiform mole. Thrombophilic disorders, particularly the factor V Leiden mutation, and antiphospholipid antibody syndrome are also associated with an increased risk of preeclampsia.

Hypertension in pregnancy is defined as a blood pressure of 140/90 mm Hg or greater (Korotkoff V). When preeclampsia develops close to term in previously healthy nulliparous women, it is not likely to recur. However, women with early, severe preeclampsia, particularly those who are multiparous, may have a recurrence rate as high as 50%.

The cause of preeclampsia is not known. It is clearly more than a hypertensive disorder, affecting many organ systems including the brain, liver, kidney, blood vessels, and placenta. Thus although the focus may be on hypertension and proteinuria, it is important to recognize that such signs and symptoms may be minimal while other, life-threatening syndromes develop including convulsions and liver failure, both of which are often associated with thrombocytopenia. Current research regarding pathophysiology of the maternal manifestations of preeclampsia has focused on the alterations in maternal endothelial cell function that are present, including reduced nitric oxide and prostacyclin, and increased endothelin. The placenta may be importantly involved in the genesis of preeclampsia, and failure of trophoblastic invasion of the uterine spiral arteries is one of the earliest changes in this disorder. Failure of trophoblast cells to invade these vessels results in more constricted spiral arteries and decreased placental perfusion.

The characteristic renal histologic lesion seen in preeclampsia is called glomerular capillary endotheliosis.

The glomerular capillary endothelial cells are swollen, and the appearance is that of a "bloodless glomerulus." Several alterations in kidney function occur in women with preeclampsia, although as already mentioned (see section on Kidney Diseases that Develop for the First Time during Pregnancy), preeclampsia is rarely associated with significant impairment in kidney function. Both GFR and renal plasma flow decrease in preeclampsia, with decrements on average about 25% in most instances, such that GFR remains above pregravid values in most cases. Changes occur in the renal handling of urate in preeclampsia. There is decreased uric acid clearance that is accompanied by an increase in blood levels, which may in fact precede other clinical signs of the disease. In pregnancy, serum urate levels above 4.5 mg/dL are suspect. The level of hyperuricemia has been observed to correlate with the severity of the preeclamptic renal lesion. Increased proteinuria is an important feature of preeclampsia, and the diagnosis should be strongly questioned in its absence. The magnitude of the proteinuria (which may range from minimal to massive) does not appear to affect maternal prognosis, although severe proteinuria is associated with greater fetal loss. Calcium handling is also altered in preeclampsia. Marked hypocalciuria is often seen in preeclampsia, possibly resulting from increased proximal tubular reabsorption, as well as increased distal tubular reabsorption, which may be mediated by excess parathyroid hormone.

Management

Management of preeclampsia includes accurate early diagnosis, bed rest, judicious use of antihypertensive therapy, close monitoring of both maternal and fetal condition, prevention of convulsions with magnesium sulfate, and appropriately timed delivery. Once the diagnosis of preeclampsia is suspected, hospitalization is advisable in all but the mildest cases. Rest is an important aspect of therapy, because it improves uteroplacental perfusion. Delivery should be considered in all cases at term and in cases remote from term when there are signs of impending eclampsia (hyperreflexia, headaches, epigastric pain) or blood pressure cannot be controlled. Most obstetricians consider the development of significant thrombocytopenia (platelet count less than 100,000 μL) and/or elevated liver enzymes (features of the HELLP syndrome) to be an indication for delivery. The rationale for lowering blood pressure is to prevent the adverse consequences of accelerated hypertension in the mother. Lowering blood pressure does not "cure" preeclampsia, and there is even some concern that aggressive lowering of blood pressure will compromise uteroplacental perfusion, which may be hazardous to fetal well-being. Although there is no consensus as to what level of blood pressure should be treated in women with preeclampsia, levels that exceed 150/100 mm Hg may be hazardous in women who previously had low-normal blood pressures. Parenteral therapy is recommended when delivery is likely to take place in the next 24 hours (Table 56-3). If it appears that delivery can be safely postponed, an oral agent is advisable (see Table 56-3). Magnesium sulfate is an effective agent for the prevention of eclamptic convulsions. Although it is not considered to be an antihypertensive agent, it does in fact lower blood pressure to a mild degree in some women. This agent is usually prescribed immediately after delivery, since convulsions are most likely to occur in the immediate postpartum period. Magnesium is rarely administered antepartum, because not only can it slow the progress of labor, but it can also complicate anesthesia and intraoperative monitoring during cesarean section.

Prevention

Prevention of preeclampsia has not been successful thus far. Although earlier small studies suggested that either low-dose aspirin or calcium supplementation might be beneficial, subsequent large, placebo-controlled trials have all failed to demonstrate a significant benefit of these prophylactic strategies. Women with antiphospholipid antibody syndrome or other thrombophilias (e.g., protein S deficiency, protein C deficiency, factor V Leiden mutation) who may be at risk for early, severe recurrent preeclampsia are an exception. Anticoagulation has been shown to benefit women with antiphospholipid antibody syndrome (heparin and aspirin throughout pregnancy), and these results have led some to recommend treating other thrombophilias with similar approaches, although there are no published data regarding benefits of treatment. Although calcium supplementation was recently shown to be ineffective in preventing preeclampsia in low-risk nulliparous women ingesting a diet containing normal amounts of calcium, data about high-risk women are limited. Moreover, compelling data show that women in developing nations who customarily ingest low-calcium diets experience fewer hypertensive complications in pregnancy after ingesting a calcium-supplemented diet.

TABLE 56-3 Antihypertensive Therapy in Preeclampsia

Imminent Delivery	Delivery Postponed
Hydralazine (intravenous, intramuscular)	Methyldopa
Labetalol (intravenous)	Labetalol, other beta blockers
Calcium channel blockers	Calcium channel blockers
Diazoxide (intravenous; rarely used)	Hydralazine
	Alpha blockers
	Clonidine

Chronic Hypertension

Women with preexisting or chronic hypertension may have either essential or secondary hypertension. Most women with stage 1 or 2 essential hypertension do well during pregnancy, although they are at increased risk for the development of superimposed preeclampsia. This risk may be as high as 25%. Preexisting maternal hypertension is also associated with an increased risk of placental abruption, intrauterine growth restriction, and midtrimester fetal death.

Women with chronic hypertension often have reductions in blood pressure by the end of the first trimester, so that their blood pressures may not exceed that observed in normotensive pregnant women. Either the failure of this decrement to occur, or increases in blood pressure in early or midtrimester pregnancy, indicates a guarded prognosis for the pregnancy. Fetal outcome is certainly worse in hypertensive women with superimposed preeclampsia compared with previously normotensive women who develop preeclampsia. Chronic hypertension with superimposed preeclampsia also seems responsible for most cases of cerebral hemorrhage in pregnancy.

The treatment of chronic hypertension during pregnancy differs from the approach in the nonpregnant individual. In the latter case, the primary concern is reducing long-term cardiovascular risk. In the former case, the concern is the preservation of maternal health during the period of gestation, and the maintenance of a favorable intrauterine environment to allow fetal maturity, while minimizing fetal exposure to potentially harmful drugs. Few data support a specific target level of blood pressure that should be attained during pregnancy. There are also no data that suggest that maintaining blood pressure levels close to normal prevents the development of superimposed preeclampsia. Thus, a reasonable strategy is to treat maternal hypertension when blood pressure exceeds 145 to 150 mm Hg systolic, 95 to 100 mm Hg diastolic. The antihypertensive agents that are currently recommended during pregnancy as well as those that are contraindicated are listed in Table 56-4.

Although secondary hypertension is considerably less common than essential hypertension, failure to recognize the presence of these entities can result in adverse pregnancy outcomes. Kidney disease is the most common form of secondary hypertension and has already been discussed. Both pheochromocytoma and renovascular hypertension are associated with poor maternal and fetal prognosis. Accelerated hypertension, superimposed preeclampsia, and fetal demise are more common. Women with primary aldosteronism may have relatively uncomplicated pregnancies, particularly if hypertension is only stage 1. However, if more severe hypertension is present, then pregnancy may be complicated and dangerous. It is preferable to diagnose secondary hypertension before conception. If women are first seen after conception, then blood and urine tests can be performed to rule out pheochromocytoma and to screen for primary aldosteronism. However, in view of the normal stimulation of the renin-angiotensin-aldosterone system in

TABLE 56-4   **Antihypertensive Drugs and Pregnancy**

Drug Group	Comments
α_2-Adrenergic receptor agonists	Methyldopa is the most extensively used drug in this group. Its safety and efficacy are supported by evidence from randomized trials and a 7.5-year follow-up study of children born to mothers treated with this agent.
β-Adrenergic receptor antagonists	These drugs appear to be safe and efficacious in late pregnancy, but fetal growth restriction has been reported when treatment was started in early or midgestation. Fetal bradycardia can occur, and animal studies suggest that the fetus's ability to tolerate hypoxic stress may be compromised.
α-Adrenergic receptor and β-adrenergic receptor antagonists	Labetolol is as effective as methyldopa, but there is limited information regarding follow-up of children born to mothers given labetolol. Rare cases of hepatotoxicity have been reported.
Arterial vasodilators	Hydralazine is frequently used as adjunctive therapy with methyldopa and β-adrenergic antagonists. Rarely, neonatal thrombocytopenia has been reported. The experience with minoxidil is limited, and this drug is not recommended.
Calcium channel blockers	Small uncontrolled studies and a meta-analysis suggest that these agents are safe and effective in pregnancy. There is limited information regarding follow-up of children exposed to calcium channel blockers in utero.
Angiotensin-converting enzyme inhibitors	Captopril causes fetal death in diverse animal species, and several converting enzyme inhibitors have been associated with oligohydramnios and neonatal renal failure when administered to humans. Do not use in pregnancy.
Angiotensin II receptor blockers	These drugs have not been used in pregnancy. In view of the deleterious effects of blocking angiotensin II generation, angiotensin II receptor antagonists are also considered to be contraindicated in pregnancy.
Diuretics	Many authorities discourage the use of diuretics, but others continue these medications if they were prescribed before conception or there is evidence of salt sensitivity.

pregnancy, plasma renin and aldosterone levels may be difficult to interpret during pregnancy, making diagnosis of hyperaldosteronism extremely difficult. Renovascular hypertension is also difficult to diagnose during pregnancy. Improved technical results with magnetic resonance angiography can aid in anatomic diagnosis of renal artery lesions. Angioplasty has been performed successfully in the early second trimester, and it should be considered in women with severe, poorly controlled hypertension, particularly if previous pregnancies have been complicated by severe preeclampsia in association with fetal complications (e.g., early delivery, growth restriction, demise).

Gestational Hypertension

Gestational hypertension refers to high blood pressure appearing first after midpregnancy and is distinguished from preeclampsia by the absence of proteinuria. This category is broad and includes women who later develop diagnostic criteria for preeclampsia as well as women with chronic hypertension in whom blood pressure decreased in early pregnancy, masking the true diagnosis. Gestational hypertension that resolves postpartum and that was not in retrospect preeclampsia is more likely to occur in women who develop essential hypertension later in life.

BIBLIOGRAPHY

Armenti VT, Ahlswede KM, Ahlswede BA, et al: Variables affecting birthweight and graft survival in 197 pregnancies in cyclosporine-treated female kidney transplant recipients. Transplantation 59:476–479, 1995.

August P, Lindheimer MD: Chronic hypertension in pregnancy. In Lindheimer MD, Roberts JM, Cunningham FG (eds): Chesley's Hypertensive Disorders in Pregnancy, 2nd ed. Stamford, CT, Appleton & Lange, 1999, pp 605–633.

August P, Mueller FB, Sealey JE, Edersheim TG: Role of renin-angiotensin system in blood pressure regulation in pregnancy. Lancet 345:896–897, 1995.

Baylis C: Glomerular filtration and volume regulation in gravid animal models. Clin Obstet Gynecol 1:789–813, 1987.

Bucher HC, Guyatt GH, Cook RJ, et al: Effect of calcium supplementation on pregnancy-induced hypertension and preeclampsia: A meta-analysis of randomized controlled trials. JAMA 275:1113–1117, 1996.

Chapman AB, Johnson AM, Gabow PA: Pregnancy outcome and its relationship to progression of renal failure in autosomal dominant polycystic kidney disease. J Am Soc Nephrol 5:1178–1185, 1994.

CLASP Collaborative Group. CLASP: A randomized trial of low-dose aspirin for the prevention and treatment of preeclampsia among 9364 pregnant women. Lancet 343:619–629, 1994.

Coomarasamy A, Honest H, Papaioannou S, et al: Aspirin for prevention of preeclampsia in women with historical risk factors: A systematic review. Obstet Gynecol 101:1319–1332, 2003.

Davison JM, Shiells EA, Philips PR, Lindheimer MD: Serial evaluation of vasopressin release and thirst in human pregnancy: Role of chorionic gonadotropin in the osmoregulatory changes of gestation. J Clin Invest 81:798–806, 1988.

Fischer MJ, Lehnerz SD, Hebert JR, Parikh CR: Kidney disease is an independent risk factor for adverse fetal and maternal outcomes in pregnancy. Am J Kidney Dis 42:415–423, 2004.

Holley JL, Reddy SS: Pregnancy in dialysis patients: A review of outcomes, complications, and management. Semin Dial 16:384–388, 2003.

Hou S: Pregnancy in chronic renal insufficiency and endstage renal disease. Am J Kidney Dis 33:235–252, 1999.

Jones DC, Hayslett JP: Outcome of pregnancy in women with moderate or severe renal insufficiency. N Engl J Med 335:226–232, 1996.

Jungers P, Chauveau D: Pregnancy in renal disease. Kidney Int 52:871–885, 1997.

Lim VS, Katz AI, Lindheimer MD: Acid-base regulation in pregnancy. Am J Physiol 231:1764–1769, 1976.

Lindheimer MD, Davison JM: Renal biopsy during pregnancy: "To b . . . or not to b . . ." BJOG 94:932–934, 1987.

Lindheimer MD, Richardson DA, Ehrlich EN, Katz AI: Potassium homeostasis in pregnancy. J Reprod Med 32:517–522, 1987.

Moroni G, Ventura D, Riva P, et al: Antiphospholipid antibodies are associated with an increased risk for chronic renal insufficiency in patients with lupus nephritis. Am J Kidney Dis 43:28–36, 2004.

A National High Blood Pressure Education Program Working Group Report on High Blood Pressure in Pregnancy. Am J Obstet Gynecol 183:S1–S22, 2000.

Okundaye IB, Agrinko P, Hou S: A registry for pregnancy in dialysis patients. Am J Kidney Dis 31:766–773, 1998.

Saltiel C, Legendre C, Grunfeld JP, et al: Hemolytic uremic syndrome in association with pregnancy. In Kaplan BS, Trompeter RS, Moake JL (eds): Hemolytic Uremic Syndrome and Thrombotic Thrombocytopenic Purpura. New York, Marcel Dekker, 1992, pp 241–254.

Sibai BM: Drug therapy: Treatment of hypertension in pregnant women. N Engl J Med 335:257–265, 1996.

Sibai BM, Kustermann L, Velasco J: Current understanding of severe preeclampsia, pregnancy-associated hemolytic uremic syndrome, thrombotic thrombocytopenic purpura, hemolysis, elevated liver enzymes, and low platelet syndrome, and postpartum acute renal failure: Different clinical syndromes or just different names? Curr Opin Nephrol Hypertens 3:436–445, 1994.

CHAPTER 57

The Kidney in Aging

Franklin E. Yuan Sharon Anderson

The biologic price of aging includes progressive structural and functional deterioration of the kidney, and the changes in kidney function during normal aging are among the most dramatic of any organ system. This chapter considers the functional and structural changes that occur with normal aging.

AGE-RELATED CHANGES IN KIDNEY FUNCTION AND STRUCTURE

By 2 years of age, glomerular filtration rate (GFR) nears adult levels and remains at 140 mL/minute/1.73 m^2 until the fourth decade. Thereafter, GFR declines by about 8 mL/minute/1.73 m^2 per decade. Acceleration of age-related loss of kidney function has been noted in the setting of systemic hypertension, lead exposure, smoking, atherosclerotic vascular disease, and possibly male gender. Research ranging from the classic inulin clearance studies of Davies and Shock (1950) to recent determinations based on the Third National Health and Nutrition Examination Survey (NHANES) confirm wide variability in the spectrum of loss of kidney function in aging (Fig. 57-1). Surveys such as that used in the NHANES would include both healthy individuals and some with chronic kidney disease. Recently, investigators have reported a large series of healthy potential kidney transplant donors and correlated age with GFR as assessed by iothalamate clearance. Using that method, GFR was noted to decline at an estimated rate of 4.6 mL/minute/decade in men, and by 7.1 mL/minute/decade in women.

The age-related reduction in creatinine clearance (CrCl) is accompanied by a reduction in the daily urinary creatinine excretion due to reduced muscle mass. Accordingly, the relationship between serum creatinine (SCr) and CrCl changes. The net effect is near-constancy of SCr while true GFR (and CrCl) declines, and consequently, substantial reductions of GFR occur despite a relatively normal SCr level. The CrCl in adult males may be estimated from the SCr with the following formula:

$$CrCl = (140 - age)(weight\ in\ kg)/(72 \times SCr)$$

and, in females, by multiplying this value by 0.85. By assuming constancy of SCr and body weight, the major dependence of CrCl upon age is readily apparent using this formula.

Similarly, renal blood flow is well maintained at about 600 mL/minute until approximately the fourth decade, and then declines by about 10% per decade. The decrease in renal blood flow is most profound in the renal cortex; redistribution of flow from cortex to medulla may explain the slight increase in filtration fraction seen in the elderly. Population studies also indicate that the incidence of both microalbuminuria and overt proteinuria increase with advancing age, even in the absence of diabetes, hypertension, or elevated SCr (Fig. 57-2). In the NHANES study, the risk of age-associated microalbuminuria was highest in those of non-Hispanic black and Mexican-American ethnicity.

Renal mass increases from about 50 g at birth to more than 400 g during the fourth decade, after which it declines to less than 300 g by the ninth decade, correlating with the reduction in body surface area. Loss of renal mass is primarily cortical, with relative sparing of the medulla. Glomerular number decreases; studies differ on the size of the remaining glomeruli. The glomerular shape also changes, with the spherical glomerulus in the fetal kidney developing lobular indentations as it matures. With aging, lobulation tends to diminish, and the length of the glomerular tuft perimeter decreases relative to total area. The glomerular basement membrane undergoes progressive folding and thickening. This stage is accompanied by glomerular simplification, with the formation of free anastomoses between a reduced number of glomerular capillary loops. Frequently, dilatation and hyalinization of the afferent arteriole near the hilum is seen at this stage. Eventually, the folded and thickened glomerular basement membrane condenses into hyaline material with glomerular tuft collapse. Degeneration of cortical glomeruli results in atrophy of both afferent and efferent arterioles, with global sclerosis. In the juxtamedullary glomeruli, glomerular tuft sclerosis is accompanied by the formation of direct channels between the afferent and efferent arterioles, resulting in aglomerular arterioles.

The incidence of glomerular sclerosis increases with advancing age, but again, with wide variability. Sclerotic glomeruli make up less than 5% of the total before the age of 40; thereafter, the incidence increases so that sclerosis involves as much as 30% of the glomerular population by the eighth decade. Thus, both diminished glomerular lobulation and sclerosis of glomeruli tend to reduce the surface area available for filtration, and thus contribute to the observed age-related decline in GFR. In addition, age-related changes in cardiovascular

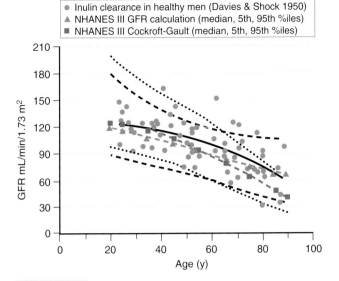

FIGURE 57-1 Percentiles of GFR (estimated using the MDRD equation) and ClCr (by the Cockcroft-Gault equation), by age, plotted on the same graph as data by Davies and Shock (J Clin Invest 29:496–507, 1950) representing measured inulin clearances in healthy men. Dashed lines without symbols show the 5th and 95th percentiles for GFR estimates. (Reproduced from Coresh J, Astor BC, Greene T, et al: Prevalence of chronic kidney disease and decreased kidney function in the adult U.S. population. Am J Kidney Dis 41:1–12, 2003, with permission.)

hemodynamics, such as reduced cardiac output and systemic hypertension, are likely to play a role in the reduced perfusion and filtration of aging.

AGE-RELATED ALTERATIONS IN FLUID AND ELECTROLYTE HOMEOSTASIS

There are no specific age-related changes in serum electrolyte or acid-base parameters in healthy subjects. However, the situation changes markedly when hospitalized or ill elderly subjects are considered. Such patients frequently exhibit elevated values for blood urea nitrogen and creatinine (which correlate with the degree of glomerular sclerosis), whereas alterations in serum electrolyte levels are more prominent (see later). These observations indicate ability of the aging kidney to maintain normal electrolyte homeostasis under steady-state conditions, but impaired ability to respond to perturbations of fluid and electrolyte balance.

Disorders of Sodium Balance

In the absence of acquired kidney disease, the aging kidney is able to adjust sodium handling appropriately in the face of extracellular sodium deficiency or excess; however, the response time is impaired, and management of these disorders accordingly complicated. The renal response to dietary sodium deprivation in the

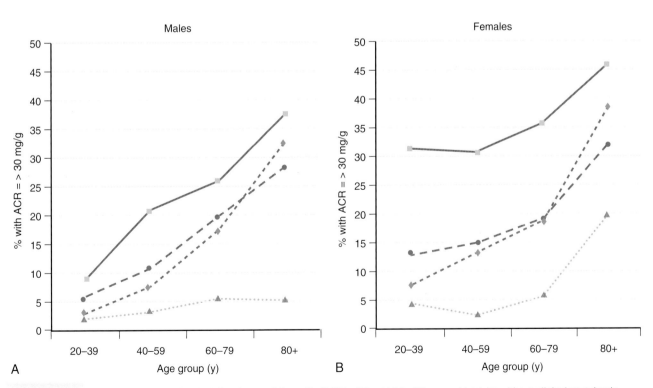

FIGURE 57-2 Prevalence of albuminuria (albumin:creatinine ratio [ACR] > 30 mg/g) in 20+-year-old adults without clinical proteinuria who have diabetes (*yellow squares*), hypertension (*blue circles*), cardiovascular disease (*green diamonds*), and no adverse health conditions (*orange triangles*). (Reproduced from Jones CA, Francis ME, Eberhardt MS, et al: Microalbuminuria in the U.S. population: Third National Health and Nutrition Examination Survey. Am J Kidney Dis 39:445–459, 2002, with permission.)

elderly is blunted. When challenged with an acute reduction in sodium intake (from 100 to 10 mEq/day), elderly subjects can conserve sodium and achieve sodium balance, but at a slower rate than in younger subjects. For example, an acute study of dietary sodium restriction found that as compared with subjects younger than 25 years, those older than 60 years took longer to reduce their urinary sodium excretion rates, and ultimately could not reduce levels down to those achieved by the younger individuals. Studies in elderly patients suggest that sodium handling is fairly normal in the proximal tubule but that the capacity to reabsorb sodium in the ascending limb of the loop of Henle is markedly impaired. The reduced loop capacity to reabsorb sodium has two important consequences: (1) the amount of sodium delivered to the more distal segments increases, and (2) the capacity to concentrate the medullary interstitium is reduced, therefore also contributing to inability to concentrate the urine.

Age-related abnormalities in several hormonal systems controlling sodium excretion play a role in this impaired ability to conserve sodium. Levels of plasma renin and of blood and urinary aldosterone are significantly reduced in the elderly, and responses to appropriate stimuli such as sodium restriction are blunted. The tubular response to aldosterone is also reduced. Mechanisms for suppression of the renin-angiotensin system are not yet well defined. It has been postulated that these age-related changes result from the loss of nephrons; compensatory hyperfiltration in the remaining nephrons leads to increased sodium chloride delivery to the macula densa, with suppression of renin synthesis and release, and therefore reduced formation of angiotensin II and aldosterone. Studies in aging animals indicate that both renal renin synthesis and release in response to volume stimuli are reduced, and that both contribute to the observed fall in plasma renin concentration with aging. Other mechanisms may include the decrease in insulin secretion with aging. Whatever the mechanisms, the impaired response to sodium deprivation (or relative "salt-wasting") makes the elderly patient more susceptible to developing a cumulative sodium deficit and its attendant systemic complications.

Similarly, the renal response to a sodium load is sluggish in elderly patients. Natriuresis is impaired both by the reduced GFR, leading to a diminished delivery of sodium to the nephron, and by abnormalities in tubular handling of sodium. Studies in aging animals indicate a greater fall in renal perfusion and filtration with angiotensin II administration, as well as impaired natriuresis and augmented kaliuresis. Similarly, animal studies indicate impaired natriuretic responses to increased perfusion pressure, mediated in part by the renal nerves. Other vasoactive mediators are also involved, including altered levels of, and/or responsiveness to, various natriuretic stimuli including norepinephrine, atrial natriuretic peptide, kallikrein, and dopamine.

Disorders of Water Balance

Renal concentrating and diluting abilities are also impaired in the aging kidney. In response to water deprivation, the maximal decrease in urine volume and increase in urine osmolality in the healthy elderly are both significantly diminished as compared with responses in younger subjects. For example, one study found that the maximal urine osmolality after dehydration was 1109 mOsm/kg in subjects aged 20 to 39 years, 1051 mOsm/kg in those aged 40 to 59 years, and 882 mOsm/kg in those aged 60 to 79 years. Several conditions may contribute to this deficiency. The reduced number of functioning nephrons may contribute to an obligatory solute diuresis in the remaining intact nephrons. There is altered responsiveness to exogenous antidiuretic hormone (ADH), and the release of endogenous ADH in response to appropriate stimuli is abnormal. In some cases, there is a diminution in thirst perception after rising serum osmolality, so volume depletion or hyperosmolality stimuli are less effective. The increase in plasma ADH levels after infusion of hypertonic saline is greater in elderly than in younger subjects, indicating enhanced osmoreceptor sensitivity. In contrast to the response to an osmolar stimulus, however, the ADH response to volume-pressure stimuli (assumption of upright posture after overnight dehydration) is markedly impaired in some elderly subjects, as is the fall in plasma ADH after drinking water.

Similarly, the aging kidney demonstrates a modest inability to dilute urine appropriately, as determined by the maximal excretion of free water after water loading. This is most likely due to the reduced GFR and renal perfusion, as well as to functional impairment in the diluting segment of the nephron. Studies in aging animals indicate that age-related polyuria is associated with down-regulation of the Aquaporin-2 and -3 receptors in the medullary collecting duct.

Hyponatremia

Serum sodium levels are generally within the normal range in healthy elderly individuals, but the defective sodium and water homeostatic mechanisms render this population markedly susceptible to perturbations. Hyponatremia is the most common electrolyte disorder in the elderly, occurring in as many as one quarter of all hospitalized elderly patients. Numerous mechanisms contribute to the susceptibility to hyponatremia and may generally be deduced after clinical evaluation. The most common underlying mechanisms of geriatric hyponatremia are: (1) decreased ability to excrete water, (2) water intoxication in the setting of diuretic therapy, and (3) oversecretion of ADH. Elderly patients carry a disproportionate burden of illness associated with extracellular fluid volume deficit and excess. Extracellular volume depletion is quite common, particularly after administration of diuretics; in one series of 77 elderly patients, diuretic therapy accounted for two thirds of all cases of hyponatremia. In a survey of 631 hospitalized elderly patients, 11.8% of subjects on thiazides were hyponatremic, with the percentage being higher in elderly women. Several age-related abnormalities probably contribute to this increased susceptibility: volume depletion, potassium depletion, and inhibition of urinary dilution. As compared with younger subjects, elderly patients challenged with a thiazide diuretic exhibit greater impairment of minimum urine osmolality and clearance of free water, possibly associated with lower prostaglandin production. It should also be noted that thiazide diuretics and nonsteroidal anti-inflammatory drugs (NSAIDs) may have an additive effect in causing hyponatremia in the elderly. Hypervolemic hyponatremia is also common in the elderly, with congestive heart failure being the most common etiology of this disorder. Relatively isovolemic hyponatremia is also prominent in the elderly, who may exhibit elevations in plasma ADH levels in the absence of recognizable stimuli for ADH secretion. The presence of excessive levels of ADH, together with impaired ability to excrete free water, render the elderly particularly susceptible to hyponatremia in numerous clinical settings, and particularly in the postoperative setting in the presence of narcotic administration and large amounts of intravenous hypotonic fluids. More recently, the incidence of hyponatremia due to antidepressant medication has been increasingly recognized.

Hypernatremia

Hypernatremia is also prominent in the elderly. A group at particularly high risk is composed of institutionalized older patients with cognitive impairment, who manifest failure to recognize thirst, and/or physical inability to obtain fluids. In a study of hospital-acquired hypernatremia, 86% of the patients lacked free access to water. Additional evidence, while not entirely unequivocal, suggests that hypodipsia, or failure to recognize thirst despite substantial elevations in serum osmolality, may be more common in elderly patients. Cerebrovascular disease may also inhibit thirst, as well as limiting physical ability to gain access to fluids.

Alterations in Potassium Balance

Significant abnormalities in cellular and total body potassium occur with advancing age. Erythrocyte potassium concentration (a reflection of general intracellular potassium content) is decreased, and both total body potassium and total exchangeable body potassium are reduced by about 20% as compared with younger subjects. Mechanisms include decreased muscle mass, alterations of cell membrane characteristics, nutritional deficiencies, and inability of the kidney to conserve potassium.

Hypokalemia is the most prominent potassium abnormality in the elderly population, and in one series was found in 11% of elderly patients visiting an emergency room. The most prominent etiology of hypokalemia in the elderly population is probably diuretic therapy; elderly patients appear to be more susceptible to the hypokalemic effects of these drugs.

In the absence of kidney disease or potassium-raising drugs, hyperkalemia is not usually a problem. The reduction in total body potassium stores may serve to offset the reduced GFR, thus protecting against significant hyperkalemia. However, studies in aging rodent models indicate impaired ability to excrete a potassium load, and studies in aging humans have confirmed that the aldosterone response to hyperkalemia is impaired. These mechanisms, together with reduced activity of the renin-angiotensin-aldosterone system in the elderly, may serve to enhance the risk of hyperkalemia in the presence of excessive potassium intake or potassium-raising drugs. Indeed, hyperkalemia is more prominent in elderly than in younger subjects with administration of potassium supplements or drugs such as NSAIDs and trimethoprim-sulfamethoxazole. Furthermore, the increasing use of angiotensin-converting enzyme inhibitors and aldosterone receptor antagonists for treatment of congestive heart failure is likely to induce further hyperkalemia in the setting of age-related reductions in kidney function.

DISORDERS OF ACID-BASE BALANCE

Abnormalities in both pulmonary and renal acid-base mechanisms may contribute to disorders in the elderly. Acid-base balance is well maintained in the healthy elderly, who are generally able to maintain normal values for serum pH, pCO_2, and bicarbonate concentrations. There is a modest but significant decrease in serum bicarbonate levels (within the normal range) with aging. Although these systems adequately dispose of the normal daily acid load, studies of ammonium loading in elderly patients indicate a reduced ability to excrete an acute exogenous acid load. However, when corrected for the reduced values for GFR, the response of elderly subjects is similar to that in younger subjects, indicating that nephron loss probably accounts for this difference. More chronic acid loading, however, may be associated with delayed normalization, and the response to alkali loading may also be delayed in elderly subjects.

CALCIUM, PHOSPHORUS, AND MAGNESIUM DISORDERS IN AGING

Serum levels of total calcium, ionized calcium, phosphorus, magnesium, and parathyroid hormone generally remain within the normal range in the elderly, although there may be a tendency toward increases in serum parathyroid hormone levels with advancing age. However, calcium metabolism is substantially impaired with aging, as a result of age-related decreases in intestinal calcium absorption, reduced renal 1α-hydroxylase activity, diminished 1,25(OH)$_2$ vitamin D$_3$ activity, and decreased intestinal adaptation to dietary calcium restriction. A decrease in vitamin D levels is frequently seen in elderly patients who are in poor health; contributing influences can include lack of exposure to sunlight, dietary deficiency, and impaired conversion to 1,25(OH)$_2$ vitamin D$_3$. Age-related changes in growth hormone and insulin-like growth factor-1 are among other influences that have also been suggested to affect vitamin D levels in the elderly. However, renal tubular absorption of calcium does not seem to be affected in aging, perhaps contributing to the observed constancy of serum calcium levels. The elderly exhibit decreased renal tubular reabsorption of phosphate, and experimental animals have shown decreased intestinal phosphate absorption and impaired renal tubular adaptation to dietary phosphate restriction. However, as with calcium, these defects do not appear to influence serum levels substantially. Serum magnesium levels do not change with age.

KIDNEY DISEASE IN THE ELDERLY

By itself, age-related kidney disease poses little threat to well-being, since even 50% of the normal GFR is ample for sustaining good renal health. However, the gradual loss of kidney function that accompanies normal aging may be greatly accelerated when acquired kidney disease is superimposed. The incidence of primary kidney disease in the elderly is not significantly different from that in young adults, although the preponderance of specific forms of glomerular injury varies in different age groups.

Several large series of biopsy results in elderly patients have indicated the relative incidence of the major forms of glomerular injury. In published series of elderly patients with nephrotic syndrome, membranous glomerulonephritis is the most frequent etiology, followed in varying degrees by proliferative or rapidly progressive glomerulonephritis and focal glomerular sclerosis. Most studies also found a substantial proportion of minimal-change disease. Thus, the available data indicate that membranous glomerulonephritis remains the most common etiology of nephrotic syndrome in the elderly, whereas rapidly progressive glomerulonephritis is the most common cause of an acute nephritic syndrome in the elderly population. The incidence of kidney disease secondary to systemic illness such as atherosclerosis, hypertension, cardiac failure, diabetes, and malignancy clearly increases with advancing age. Also to be considered are vasculitis and amyloidosis, which are relatively infrequent in younger patients. Particularly prominent in the elderly are deposition diseases, including amyloidosis, light chain deposition disease, and fibrillary glomerulonephritis.

Acute Renal Failure in the Elderly

Elderly patients are at risk for all of the causes of acute renal failure (ARF) seen in the general population, and susceptibility may be enhanced. A wide range of insults can cause ARF. In a study contrasting the etiologies of ARF in 67 young and 298 elderly patients, the older patients, as compared with the younger subjects, had an increased incidence of ARF due to septic shock, volume depletion, nephrotoxins, and obstructive causes. This prevalence of hemodynamic renal failure is echoed in a retrospective study spanning the years 1975 to 1990 in an intensive care unit, where hemorrhagic, septic, or cardiogenic shock was the predominant cause of ARF in the elderly. In the case of treatment-related ARF (Table 57-1), a prospective study found that nephrotoxic drugs (66%, with aminoglycosides, NSAIDs, and angiotensin-converting enzyme inhibitors as the top offenders), sepsis (45.7%), and hypoperfusion (45.7%) were most prominent. Presumably, the elderly are at higher risk for prerenal causes of ARF because of a tendency toward reduced sodium intake, diuretic administration, and inability to conserve sodium, predisposing to dehydration and/or sodium depletion. One representative study found volume depletion to be primarily responsible in 23.4% of cases in elderly patients; preexisting volume depletion would also enhance risk for ARF after administration of contrast agents or nephrotoxic drugs. Older age also increases risk of ARF associated with surgical complications, aminoglycoside nephrotoxicity, NSAIDs, angiotensin-converting enzyme inhibitor therapy, radiocontrast, and postrenal (obstructive) causes. Indeed, more than 80% of reported cases of NSAID-induced ARF are in patients older than 60. Certain other etiologies of ARF are clearly more frequent

TABLE 57-1 Pathologic Diagnoses in Elderly Patients with Acute Renal Failure

Diagnosis	Proportion of Biopsy Specimens (%)
Pauci-immune crescentic GN	31.2
Acute interstitial nephritis	18.6
Acute tubular necrosis with nephrotic syndrome	7.5
Atheroemboli	7.1
Acute tubular necrosis alone	6.7
Light chain cast nephropathy	5.9
Postinfectious GN	5.5
Anti–glomerular basement membrane antibody GN	4.0
IgA nephropathy or Henoch-Schönlein nephritis	3.6
Nondiagnostic for acute renal failure	9.9

GN, glomerulonephritis.
Adapted from Kohli HS, Bhaskaran MC, Muftukumar T, et al: Treatment-related acute renal failure in the elderly: A hospital-based prospective study. Nephrol Dial Transplant 15:212–217, 2000.

in the elderly, including multiple myeloma, carcinoma leading to obstruction, nephrotoxicity from chemotherapeutic interventions, polypharmacy with or without inappropriate drug dosing, obstructive uropathy due to prostatic disease, and atheroembolic renal disease.

Endstage Renal Disease in the Elderly

The number and relative frequency of elderly patients entering endstage renal disease programs and the average age of dialysis patients is increasing each year in the United States, reflecting the aging of the population in general. In recent years, the highest annual increase in the incidence rate of dialysis patients has been in those aged over 75 years. In addition to the direct burden of kidney disease, the presence of this condition greatly increases cardiovascular risk; endstage renal disease at age 75 confers a threefold increase in risk of death, as compared with the population without kidney disease. All projections indicate that these trends will continue, posing a grave challenge for the health-care system the coming years. In recent years, there has been an increase in the number of kidney transplants to elderly recipients. The literature on long-term outcomes of elderly patients after kidney transplantation is inconclusive, but it is clear that long-term survival in the elderly is significantly better in transplanted patients, as compared with those receiving dialysis.

EXPERIMENTAL CONSIDERATIONS AND IMPLICATIONS FOR FURTHER RESEARCH

The potential mechanisms associated with the normal age-related loss of kidney function have been explored in experimental models, and major mechanisms under

TABLE 57-2 Mechanisms of Age-Related Renal Injury

Hemodynamic causes: afferent arteriolar vasodilation, glomerular capillary hypertension, reduction of the glomerular capillary ultrafiltration coefficient
Increased activity of the renin-angiotensin system
Hyperlipidemia
Increased formation of advanced glycosylation end products
Increased oxidative stress
Decreased endothelial nitric oxide synthase
Increased TGF-β and PAI-1
Decreased VEGF with peritubular capillary rarefaction

PAI-1, plasminogen activator inhibitor-1; TGF-β, transforming growth factor-β; VEGF, vascular endothelial growth factor.

investigation are listed in Table 57-2. Many of the disease mechanisms previously identified in other forms of chronic kidney disease now appear to be relevant to age-associated kidney disease, as are potential therapeutic interventions. For example, drugs that block the activity of the renin-angiotensin system have been shown to delay age-associated glomerular sclerosis in animal models, although clinical studies have not been performed. Given the vulnerability of the aging kidney to acceleration of kidney function deterioration after acquired injury, it remains imperative to pay attention to those risk factors (volume depletion, nephrotoxic insults, uncontrolled hypertension, and dietary considerations) that may contribute to loss of kidney function. Although little information is available specifically addressing these interventions in the elderly population, it seems likely that these hemodynamically protective interventions will prove efficacious in this population as well. With the ever-increasing number of elderly patients entering endstage renal disease programs, clinical studies evaluating these therapeutic interventions in this population at risk are certainly warranted.

BIBLIOGRAPHY

Anderson S: Nephrology/fluid and electrolyte disorders. In Cassel CK, Cohen HJ, Larson EB, et al (eds): Geriatric Medicine, 4th ed. New York, Springer-Verlag, 2002.

Anderson S, Rennke HG, Zatz R: Glomerular adaptations with normal aging and with long-term converting enzyme inhibition in the rat. Am J Physiol 267:F35–F43, 1994.

Bleyer AJ, Shemanski LR, Burke GL, et al: Tobacco, hypertension, and vascular disease: Risk factors for renal functional decline in an older population. Kidney Int 57:2072–2079, 2000.

Cameron JS: Nephrotic syndrome in the elderly. Semin Nephrol 16:319–329, 1996.

Choudhury D, Levi M: Renal function and disease in the aging kidney. In Schrier RW (ed): Diseases of the Kidney, 6th ed. Philadelphia, Lippincott Williams & Wilkins, 2001, pp 2387–2420.

Clark BA, Elahi D, Shannon RP, et al: Influence of age and dose on the end-organ responses to atrial natriuretic peptide in humans. Am J Hypertens 4:500–507, 1991.

Coresh J, Astor BC, Greene T, et al: Prevalence of chronic kidney disease and decreased kidney function in the adult US population: Third National Health and Nutrition Examination Survey. Am J Kidney Dis 41:1–12, 2003.

Davies DF, Shock NW: Age changes in glomerular filtration rate, effective renal plasma flow, and tubular excretory capacity in adult males. J Clin Invest 29:496–507, 1950.

Garg AX, Papaioannou Z, Ferko N, et al: Estimating the prevalence of renal insufficiency in seniors requiring long-term care. Kidney Int 65:649–653, 2004.

Haas M, Spargo BH, Wit EJ, Meehan SM: Etiologies and outcome of acute renal insufficiency in older adults: A renal biopsy study of 259 cases. Am J Kidney Dis 35:433–447, 2000.

Hirschberg B, Ben-Yehuda A: The syndrome of inappropriate antidiuretic hormone secretion in the elderly. Am J Med 103: 270–273, 1997.

Jones CA, Francis ME, Eberhardt MS, et al: Microalbuminuria in the US population: Third National Health and Nutrition Examination Survey. Am J Kidney Dis 39:445–459, 2002.

Kohli HS, Bhaskaran MC, Mufhukumar T, et al: Treatment-related acute renal failure in the elderly: A hospital-based prospective study. Nephrol Dial Transplant 15:212–217, 2000.

Luckey E, Parsa CJ: Fluid and electrolytes in the aged. Arch Surg 138:1055–1060, 2003.

Neugarten J, Gallo G, Silbiger S, et al: Glomerulosclerosis in aging humans is not influenced by gender. Am J Kidney Dis 34:884–888, 1999.

Rodrígues-Puyol D: The aging kidney. Kidney Int 54:2247–2265, 1998.

Chronic Kidney Disease and Its Therapy

CHAPTER **58**

Pathophysiology and Management of Chronic Kidney Disease

Arrigo Schieppati   Roberto Pisoni   Giuseppe Remuzzi

MECHANISMS OF PROGRESSION

Stages of Progression

Chronic kidney disease (CKD) is characterized by a progressive course with ongoing loss of kidney function. Once the glomerular filtration rate (GFR) falls below about half of normal, kidney function tends to decline even if the initial insult to the kidney has been eliminated. This phenomenon has been defined as progression of CKD and typically moves through phases from initial diminution of renal reserve to mild, moderate, and severe reductions in GFR, then kidney failure ultimately requiring renal replacement therapy (endstage renal disease, ESRD).

According to the National Kidney Foundation (NKF) Kidney Disease Outcome Quality Initiative (K/DOQI) Clinical Practice Guidelines, CKD is classified in five stages, based on estimated GFR and irrespective of diagnosis (Table 58-1). This staging system for CKD was conceived to provide estimates of disease prevalence, to develop an intervention plan for evaluation and management of each stage of CKD, and to define the characteristics of individuals who are at increased risk for developing CKD.

The stages of CKD reflect gradual adaptation to nephron loss. In the early phase, stages 1 and 2, the patient is asymptomatic, blood urea nitrogen (BUN) and serum creatinine (SCr) are normal or nearly normal, and acid-base, fluid, and electrolyte balance are maintained through an adaptive increase of function in the remaining nephrons. A reduction of GFR to 30 to 59 mL/minute/1.73 m^2 defines stage 3, moderate impairment of GFR. The patient usually has no symptoms; SCr and BUN are increased, and the levels of hormones such as erythropoietin, calcitriol, and parathyroid hormone (PTH) are usually abnormal. Stage 4, severe impairment of GFR, involves a further loss of kidney function. Symptoms, if present, are mild; patients may have anemia, acidosis, hypocalcemia, hyperphosphatemia, and hyperkalemia. The final stage of kidney disease, stage 5, defined by a GFR of less than 15 mL/minute/1.73 m^2, is usually characterized by worsening of all the aforementioned symptoms. At this stage, the institution of renal replacement therapy is required, usually when the true GFR falls below 10 mL/minute or the creatinine clearance (CrCl) is below 15 mL/minute.

Measurement of Progression

The staging of CKD and the assessment of progression are based on GFR measurements or estimates (see Chapters 2 and 58). GFR continues to be the single most useful quantitative index of kidney function in health and disease; it is also used to determine the effectiveness of therapies designed to slow the progression of kidney diseases.

The most reliable assessment of GFR is based on the measurement of renal clearance of a filtration marker such as inulin. This method, however, is not suitable for routine clinical practice.

Radionuclides that are handled by the kidney in a fashion similar to inulin and procedures using nonradioactive contrast agents such as iothalamate and iohexol can provide accurate and precise GFR measurements, but their use is limited and not practical for repeated measurements.

In everyday practice, the most widely utilized method to estimate GFR involves the SCr and CrCl. Unfortunately, since creatinine metabolism is altered in CKD, GFR measurements using CrCl are, at best, gross estimates. Thus other methods have been devised, such as the reciprocal of the SCr. The reciprocal creatinine plotted against time produces a line in most patients, making it possible to predict the course of progression. Limitations of the reciprocal creatinine plot, however, must be kept in mind. When the GFR is greater than 60 mL/minute/1.73 m^2, spontaneous variations in SCr are large relative to the changes that occur as a result of the fall in GFR, and the slope of the reciprocal SCr plot is unreliable.

The level of GFR may also be estimated from prediction equations that take in account the SCr and some variables such as age, gender, body size, and race. The most used equation is the Cockcroft-Gault formula,

TABLE 58-1 Stages of Chronic Kidney Disease

Stage	Description	GFR (mL/min/1.73 m²)
1	Kidney damage* with normal GFR	≥90
2	Kidney damage with mild ↓ GFR	60–89
3	Moderate ↓ GFR	30–59
4	Severe ↓ GFR	15–29
5	Kidney failure	<15

*Kidney damage is defined as pathologic abnormalities or abnormalities in blood or urine tests or imaging studies.
Adapted from K/DOQI Clinical Practice Guidelines for Chronic Kidney Disease: Evaluation, Classification, and Stratification. Part 4. Definition and classification of stages of chronic kidney disease. Am J Kidney Dis 39(Suppl 1):46–75, 2002.

which is simple because it requires only the SCr and body weight:

$$CrCl\,(mL/min) = \frac{[(140 - age\ in\ years) \times (body\ weight\ in\ kg)]}{(Scr, mg/dL \times 72)}$$

This value is multiplied by 0.85 if the patient is female.

More recently, the Modification of Diet in Renal Disease (MDRD) study proposed an equation to calculate GFR. It is more complex because it requires serum albumin, BUN determination, and a calculator:

$$GFR\,(mL/min) = 170 \times (Scr, mg/dL)^{-0.999}$$
$$\times (Age, years)^{-0.176}$$
$$\times (0.762, if\ female)$$
$$\times (1.180, if\ African\ American)$$
$$\times (BUN, mg/dL)^{-0.170} \times (Albumin)^{0.318}$$

An abbreviated, simplified MDRD equation is also in use:

$$GFR\,(mL/min) = 186 \times (Scr, mg/dL)^{-1.154} \times (Age, years)^{-0.203}$$
$$\times (0.74, if\ female)$$
$$\times (1.210, if\ African\ American)$$

Glomerular Hypertension, Hyperfiltration, and the Role of Angiotensin II

In 1982, Brenner and coworkers put forward their hypothesis on the mechanisms of progression of CKD in several seminal papers. They hypothesized that progressive deterioration of kidney function was the result of compensatory glomerular hemodynamic changes in response to nephron loss. In their experimental model of renal mass reduction, the remaining nephrons underwent hypertrophy, with reduced arteriolar resistance and increased glomerular blood flow.

It has been shown that with progression of kidney disease, afferent arteriolar tone decreases more than efferent tone. As a consequence, intraglomerular pressure and the amount of filtrate formed by each single nephron rises (i.e., glomerular hyperfiltration occurs). In this mechanism a central role is played by angiotensin II, which may mediate this process through several mechanisms. In vivo, angiotensin II enhances the vascular tone of both afferent and efferent glomerular arterioles, modulating intraglomerular capillary pressure and GFR. The vasoconstrictor effect of this hormone is predominantly exerted on the postglomerular arterioles, thereby increasing the glomerular hydraulic pressure and the filtration fraction. High glomerular capillary pressure increases the radius of the pores in the glomerular membrane, thus impairing the size-selective permeability of the membrane to macromolecules. Glomerular podocytes have a complex cytoskeleton with contractile properties, and angiotensin II receptors are present on their surface; these findings suggest that in addition to its hemodynamic effects, angiotensin II may directly alter permselective properties of the glomerular barrier by mediating contraction of glomerular foot processes. This would change slit diaphragm architecture and allow proteins to escape more easily into the urinary space. Angiotensin II also modulates renal cell growth, which in turn may contribute to tubulointerstitial injury.

Angiotensin II stimulates the production of plasminogen activator inhibitor-1 (PAI-1) and may therefore further increase the accumulation of the extracellular matrix through inhibition of its breakdown by matrix metalloproteinases, which are converted to their active form by plasmin. By directly stimulating macrophage activation and phagocytosis, angiotensin II may enhance the inflammatory component associated with chronic kidney injury. Angiotensin II up-regulates genes and stimulates secretion of peptides with chemotactic and vasoactive properties in tubular cells.

The Role of Proteinuria

Proteinuria is not merely a consequence of glomerular hyperfiltration, which is a marker of altered glomerular barrier integrity. Abundant experimental evidence supports the notion that proteinuria itself contributes to progressive nephron damage. Filtered proteins are reabsorbed by proximal tubular cells. Moreover, focal breaks of tubular basement membranes and leakage of the tubular contents into the renal interstitium can lead to protein overload in the interstitium, followed by macrophage infiltration and increased production by macrophages of inflammatory mediators such as endothelin-1, monocyte chemoattractant protein-1 (MCP-1), osteopontin, and RANTES (regulated upon activation normal T-cell expressed and secreted), which is a chemotactic cytokine for monocytes and memory T cells (Fig. 58-1).

Complement components may also play a major role in proteinuria-induced interstitial damage. Complement proteins are filtered through the glomerulus, and deposits

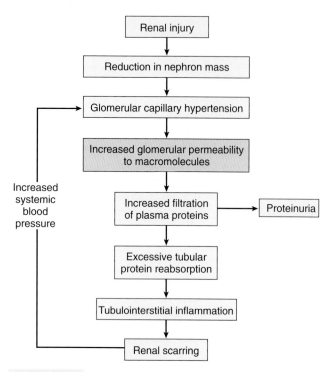

FIGURE 58-1 Schematic representation of the events leading to progressive kidney damage. Excessive reabsorption of proteins as a consequence of increased glomerular permeability results in the accumulation of proteins in proximal tubular cells, which may trigger activation of genes that are dependent and independent on nuclear factor-κB (NF-κB)-dependent and NF-κB-independent genes encoding chemokines, cytokines, and endothelin. Excessive synthesis of inflammatory and vasoactive substances contributes to fibroblast proliferation and interstitial inflammation.

of C3 and C5b-9 are found in proximal tubular cells. Activation of the complement system in tubular cells is associated with alterations of the cytoskeleton, production of reactive oxygen species, and synthesis of proinflammatory mediators. Excessive protein load of the cells can be a condition underlying progressive podocyte injury. Enhanced endocytosis of protein may contribute to the perturbation of podocyte function.

The activation of a variety of molecules, such as cytokines, growth factors, and vasoactive substances deriving from tubular cells, may result in abnormal accumulation of extracellular matrix collagen, fibronectin, and other components that are responsible for interstitial fibrosis. All forms of CKD are associated with marked tubulointerstitial injury (tubular dilatation, interstitial fibrosis), even if the primary process is a glomerulopathy. Furthermore, in almost all chronic progressive glomerular diseases, the degree of tubulointerstitial disease is a better predictor of the GFR and long-term prognosis than is the severity of glomerular injury. It is possible in these settings that tubulointerstitial disease causes tubular atrophy and/or obstruction, eventually leading to nephron loss. The mechanism by which the tubulointerstitial disease occurs is incompletely understood.

Clinical Evidence of the Role of Proteinuria in Progression

The role of proteinuria as a risk factor for progression of CKD is suggested by the strong correlation of the amount of urinary protein with renal outcome. In 840 patients with nondiabetic kidney disease enrolled in the MDRD study, proteinuria was the strongest predictor of kidney disease progression. The Ramipril Efficacy in Nephropathy (REIN) study showed that in 352 patients with chronic nondiabetic proteinuric nephropathies, independent of the nature of the underlying disease, the baseline urinary protein excretion rate was the best single predictor of GFR decline and ESRD. The higher the urinary protein excretion, the faster the subsequent decline in GFR and the quicker the progression to ESRD. Patients with baseline urinary protein excretion less than 1.9 g/24 hours had the lowest rate of GFR decline and kidney failure during 3 years of follow-up. In contrast, patients with proteinuria greater than 3.9 g/24 hours lost more than 10 mL/minute/l.73 m² GFR per year, and 30% developed ESRD at 3 years.

Besides predicting the rate of progression of the decline in kidney function, urinary protein excretion can be used to identify which patients would benefit most from renoprotective treatments. In the MDRD trial, patients with higher baseline proteinuria were those whose rate of GFR decline was reduced most by strict blood pressure control. Among patients with urinary protein excretion greater than 3 g/24 hours in the REIN study, the beneficial effect of ramipril, an angiotensin-converting enzyme (ACE) inhibitor, in slowing the GFR decline and in reducing the risk of ESRD grew as the baseline level of proteinuria increased.

There is also evidence that, in nondiabetic proteinuric chronic nephropathies, the protein-to-creatinine (P/C) ratio in a single spot morning urine sample closely correlates with 24-hour protein excretion and predicts GFR decline and risk progression to ESRD even better than 24-hour protein excretion. A P/C ratio of more than 1.0 g/g distinguishes patients who have progression from those who do not progress. This easy and inexpensive procedure can establish the severity and prognosis of kidney disease and is less time-consuming than 24-hour collection. Furthermore, it avoids any error in urine collection.

In summary, robust experimental evidence and a number of hints from clinical observations indicate that proteinuria is responsible for interstitial inflammation and subsequent fibrosis, thereby contributing to progressive kidney function loss.

Other Factors Associated with Progression

Many studies have shown a direct association between hypertension and the rate of progression that is slowed by lowering blood pressure with antihypertensive agents.

TABLE 58-2   Risk Factors for Kidney Disease Progression

Proteinuria >1.5 g/24 hr or urinary protein-to-creatinine ratio >1 g/g
Hypertension
Type of underlying kidney disease (e.g., polycystic kidney, diabetic nephropathy)
African-American race
Male sex
Obesity
Diabetes mellitus
Hyperlipidemia
Smoking
High-protein diet
Phosphate retention
Metabolic acidosis

In the REIN study, mean arterial pressure was predictive of GFR decline and kidney survival but to a lesser degree than 24-hour urinary protein excretion.

The type of kidney disease also appears to be a risk factor for progression to ESRD: glomerulonephritis, diabetic and hypertensive nephropathies, and polycystic kidney disease tend to progress faster than tubulointerstitial diseases. Finally, other variables such as race, male sex, obesity, high low-density lipoprotein (LDL) cholesterol, cigarette smoking, metabolic acidosis, and phosphate retention may hasten renal disease progression. Variables implicated in the progression of kidney disease are listed in Table 58-2.

PREVENTION OF PROGRESSION OF CHRONIC KIDNEY DISEASE

Early experiments demonstrated that blockade of angiotensin II with an ACE inhibitor could slow the progressive loss of kidney function in several animal models of kidney disease, offering the opportunity to devise a treatment strategy not limited to following patients passively until they reached their destiny of dialysis. Thus, the concept of renoprotection has emerged.

The first statistically robust demonstration of the validity of such an approach was provided by an American collaborative study in patients with type 1 diabetes mellitus who had proteinuria greater than 500 mg/day and SCr concentrations of 2.5 mg/dL or less. Captopril treatment was associated with a 50% reduction in the risk of the combined end points of death, dialysis, and transplantation that was independent of the small disparity in blood pressure between the groups. The role of proteinuria in promoting progression and its impact on kidney outcome was explored by the REIN study. This study was designed to assess the hypothesis that ACE inhibition could be superior to other antihypertensive drugs in reducing proteinuria, limiting the decline in GFR, and preventing ESRD in patients with chronic nephropathies. Patients were randomly assigned to receive ramipril or

conventional antihypertensive therapy to maintain diastolic blood pressure at 90 mm Hg or less.

The study showed that, although blood pressure control was similar in the two treatment groups, ACE inhibitor therapy decreased the progression to ESRD by 50% during 3 years of follow-up. Among patients with proteinuria of 3 g/24 hours or more, those who received the ACE inhibitor had a significantly slower rate of decline in GFR than did patients receiving conventional antihypertensive therapy The study was continued for 2 years (the REIN follow-up study), during which time all patients previously on placebo were switched to ACE inhibitors. In patients continuing to receive ramipril, the rate of GFR decline further decreased to approximately 1 mL/minute per year during follow-up, a figure similar to that associated with normal aging. Patients who switched from conventional therapy to ramipril also benefited from the treatment. This analysis provides evidence that the tendency of GFR to decline with time can be halted and that remission is achievable in some patients with CKD.

Recently, three studies examined the role of drugs in the angiotensin receptor blocker (ARB) class in type 2 diabetic nephropathy. In one study, 1715 patients with nephropathy due to type 2 diabetes mellitus were randomized to receive the ARB irbesartan, the calcium channel blocker amlodipine, or placebo. With irbesartan, the risk of reaching the end point of doubling of SCr, ESRD, or death was 20% lower than with placebo and 23% lower than with amlodipine.

The Reduction of Endpoints in NIDDM with the Angiotensin II Antagonist Losartan (RENAAL) study evaluated the renoprotective effect of losartan versus placebo (in addition to conventional antihypertensive therapy, with the exclusion of ACE inhibitors) in 1513 patients with overt type 2 diabetic nephropathy. The primary composite end point was doubling of SCr, ESRD, or death. Losartan reduced the incidence of doubling SCr by 25% and the risk of ESRD by 28%. The death rate was, however, similar in the two groups, which both attained the same blood pressure level. Proteinuria declined by 35% in the losartan group.

One other study evaluated the renoprotective effect of the ARB irbesartan in hypertensive patients with incipient nephropathy. The end point of the study was the time of onset of overt albuminuria. In 2 years of follow-up, only 5.2% of patients receiving 300 mg of irbesartan reached the end point, as compared with 14.9% of patients on placebo. The groups had similar blood pressure control, a finding that suggests that ARBs are renoprotective independent of their antihypertensive effect. Although these studies have shown that ARBs have a renoprotective effect in type 2 diabetic nephropathy, only small studies have evaluated the role of ACE inhibitors. The results of these studies have shown that, with one exception, no significant difference was found in terms of renoprotection as measured as prevention of

GFR decline over time, between ACE inhibitors and other antihypertensive agents. On the other hand, a very recent study by Canadian investigators has shown that the use of ACE inhibitors was associated with a significant reduction in all-cause and cardiovascular-related mortality in a broad spectrum of patients with type 2 diabetes and no cardiovascular disease.

A head-to-head comparison of the effects of ACE inhibitors and ARBs has not been performed in a large clinical trial, so a direct comparison is lacking. What data are available may make ARBs the first choice for treatment of type 2 diabetic patients, although we would not switch a patient who is already receiving and tolerating an ACE inhibitor to an ARB, if the blood pressure goal is achieved. More likely, a combination of the two classes along with additional agents is required to achieve the target blood pressure.

Other Measures to Prevent Progression

The evidence from both experimental studies and clinical trials suggests that current practice can at best retard development of ESRD for a few years, and cannot avoid dialysis for most patients during their lifetime.

This goal may be attainable with a more complex strategy than with a single pharmacologic intervention. A multidrug intervention may be the strategy needed to delay dialysis significantly. A few trials show that the combination of an ACE inhibitor with an ARB afford greater renoprotection than each drug used alone. The COOPERATE study compared combined treatment with an ACE inhibitor and an ARB with monotherapy with each drug at its maximum dose in patients with nondiabetic kidney disease. Of patients on combination treatment, 11% reached the combined primary end point of doubling of SCr or ESRD, compared with 23% of patients on trandolapril alone and 23% of those on losartan alone at 3 years of follow-up. Although these results are encouraging, they show that other strategies will be needed to achieve complete prevention of progressive nondiabetic kidney disease, because some patients reached the primary end point on combined treatment.

In seeking more effective treatments, the role of lifestyle changes should not be overlooked. Smoking cessation per se may reduce disease progression by 30%, which qualifies it as the single most important renoprotective measure. Physical activity is instrumental to the loss of weight, but activity may have an intrinsic favorable effect, as documented by a small study in 20 patients with CKD who were assigned to 12-week regular aquatic exercise or an armchair. During this short period of time, body mass index did not change in either group. However, proteinuria decreased by 50% in those who performed aquatic exercise, while there was no change in the sedentary group.

A multidrug approach to chronic nephropathies can attain several goals, as summarized in Table 58-3. Patients with CKD and proteinuria greater than 1 g/24 hours are initially treated with a low starting dose of an ACE inhibitor, which is then increased to the maximum dose. Then if the goals of blood pressure under 130/80 and proteinuria less than 0.3 g/24 hours are not achieved, an ARB is added at half-maximum dose. Again, the dose is increased stepwise. Throughout this up-titration of ACE inhibitor, and/or ARB, the addition of a diuretic is usually needed to achieve optimal blood pressure control or prevention of hyperkalemia. If after this titration, target blood pressure and proteinuria are not achieved, the next antiproteinuric drug to be added is usually a nondihydropyridine calcium channel blocker.

To exploit their specific antiproteinuric effect, even if the blood pressure target has been achieved, ACE inhibitors or ARBs may be used at greater doses than usually recommended. ACE inhibitor and ARB use should not be limited by the initial level of GFR, although SCr and potassium should be closely monitored. An increase over baseline of SCr of less than 30% that stabilizes within the first 2 months of treatment is associated with long-term preservation of kidney function and therefore should be considered acceptable. Withdrawal of ACE inhibitor or ARB should be considered only for patients with a rise in SCr that exceeds 30% of baseline, or for development of hyperkalemia greater than 5.5 mmol/L. With such a GFR fall, the presence of renal artery stenosis should be suspected and investigated. The concomitant use of drugs that interfere with kidney function or promote potassium retention, such as nonsteroidal anti-inflammatory drugs, should also be excluded.

Controlled clinical trials show that lipid-lowering therapy, particularly with statins, has an antiproteinuric effect and that treatment is indicated in individuals with serum LDL cholesterol higher than 100 mg/dL. The role of diabetic control in development and progression of CKD has been extensively examined (see Chapter 29). Both interventional and population-based studies link

---

TABLE 58-3   Treatment Goals for Slowing Progression of Chronic Kidney Disease

Tight blood pressure control (<130/80) using stepwise treatment
  Low-sodium diet
  ACE inhibitors
  Angiotensin receptor antagonists
  Diuretics
  Nondihydropyridine calcium channel blockers

Dietary protein restriction

Glycemic control in diabetic patients (HbA1c <7.5%)

Treatment of dyslipidemia (goal LDL cholesterol <100 mg/dL)

ACE, angiotensin-converting enzyme; HbA1c, glycated hemoglobin; LDL, low-density lipoprotein.

hyperglycemia with the risk of development of albuminuria or diabetic nephropathy. Less strong evidence links hyperglycemia with the progression of established diabetic nephropathy to ESRD; the effect of blood pressure control to prevent progression is much greater than the effect of control of blood sugar. Hyperglycemia may play a more decisive role in the initiation of nephropathy, while other variables may be responsible for progression. However, the evidence from randomized trials shows that intensive therapy in patients with type 2 diabetes results in a decreased risk of microvascular complications. Therefore, in patients with diabetic nephropathy, it is recommended that glycemic control be as tight as feasible, although the risk of hypoglycemic complications must be taken into account in individual patients.

COMPLICATIONS OF CHRONIC KIDNEY DISEASE: CLINICAL FEATURES AND TREATMENT

As kidney function declines, the kidney progressively loses its regulatory capacity, so that both excretion and conservation of water and electrolytes are altered. Thus, when sudden loads or losses of fluid or electrolytes occur, decompensation may result. These complications of CKD can be classified into water, electrolyte, acid-base, metabolic, and organ system disorders.

Water

Free-water clearance is maintained until GFR is severely reduced. In advanced stages of CKD, the reduced capacity of the kidney to concentrate or dilute urine may lead to hypernatremia or hyponatremia. The reduced capacity for concentrating the urine is particularly common in patients with diseases affecting the renal medulla, such as interstitial nephritis and pyelonephritis. Patients with a normal thirst mechanism and access to fluid will usually ingest an appropriate amount of fluid to match obligate losses. Dehydration occurs readily in patients with inadequate fluid intake because of persisting diuresis. Attention to the fluid prescription is necessary when access to water is impaired by intercurrent illnesses.

Sodium

Maintaining sodium balance is very important in patients with CKD. Both sodium retention, with signs of volume overload, and sodium depletion, with signs of volume depletion, are common. In most patients with stable CKD, the total body sodium content is already increased but only slightly; more substantial sodium retention is common when GFR falls below 10 mL/minute/1.73 m^2 and in patients with concomitant nephrotic syndrome or cardiac failure. Sodium retention contributes to, or aggravates, hypertension, edema, and

congestive heart failure. A sodium-restricted diet (less than 2 g/day) and loop diuretics are often required. On the other hand, sodium conservation may be impaired early in CKD. In some instances, particularly tubulointerstitial diseases, sodium wasting may be present. For the most part, however, this failure of conservation can be viewed as an adaptation to the need to maintain balance and excrete the daily load of ingested sodium despite a drop in GFR. The diseased kidney may be unable to abruptly reverse this compensatory increase in fractional sodium excretion. Thus, in the setting of CKD, the fractional sodium excretion may be higher than 1% even in the presence of volume depletion.

Extrarenal causes of sodium loss (vomiting, diarrhea, fever) may lead to extracellular fluid volume depletion with thirst, dry mucous membranes, tachycardia, orthostatic hypotension, vascular collapse, dizziness, syncope, and a usually reversible fall in kidney function. Apart from treating the underlying cause of sodium depletion, it may be necessary to give intravenous isotonic saline; diuretics, if used, must be temporarily withdrawn.

Potassium

Because of an adaptive increase in potassium excretion by the remnant nephrons, patients with CKD usually have a normal serum potassium concentration until oliguria occurs. However, in patients with metabolic acidosis, which is characterized by a shift in potassium from intracellular to extracellular fluids, and with hyporeninemic hypoaldosteronism (seen in tubulointerstitial disease and diabetes mellitus), hyperkalemia may develop early. Hyperkalemia can also arise from an acute potassium load or with drugs that alter potassium secretion such as ACE inhibitors, ARBs, potassium-sparing diuretics, beta blockers, aldosterone antagonists, nonsteroidal anti-inflammatory drugs, cyclosporine, and tacrolimus. Acute management of hyperkalemia is discussed in Chapter 12. Dietary restriction is the mainstay of chronic management of hyperkalemia. Loop diuretics and potassium-binding resins can be useful for long-term control, but they are seldom necessary. Spontaneous hypokalemia is uncommon in CKD, but it can be seen in salt-wasting nephropathy, Fanconi's syndrome, hereditary or acquired tubulointerstitial diseases, and renal tubular acidosis. In patients with CKD, hypokalemia is usually due to low dietary potassium intake combined with high doses of diuretics, or to gastrointestinal loss.

Acid-Base Disorders

Acid-base balance is normally maintained by renal excretion of the daily acid load both as titratable acid (primarily phosphate) and as ammonium. With advanced CKD (stage 3 and beyond), hydrogen ion excretion by the kidney is often not sufficient to balance endogenous acid production or exogenous acid loads, and chronic metabolic acidosis develops. As the patient approaches ESRD, the plasma bicarbonate concentration tends to stabilize between 12 and 20 mEq/L and rarely falls below 10 mEq/L. In the early stages of CKD, hyperchloremic renal tubular acidosis with normal anion gap may occur, but with more advanced stages, plasma chloride concentration becomes normal, and a large anion gap may develop. The anion gap is elevated in this setting as a result of the retention of anions such as phosphate, sulfate, urate, and hippurate.

The treatment of mild acidosis (serum bicarbonate between 12 and 18 mEq/L) is desirable to prevent osteopenia and muscle catabolism. In fact, bone buffering of some of the excess hydrogen ions leads to the release of calcium and phosphate from bone, which may worsen bone disease. Moreover, uremic acidosis increases muscle breakdown, which may be exacerbated by a low-protein diet and decreased albumin synthesis, leading to loss of lean body mass and muscle weakness. The muscle breakdown is in part due to the stimulated release of cortisol and reduced release of insulin-like growth factor-1 (IGF-1). These abnormalities in muscle function and albumin metabolism can be reversed by alkali therapy.

Metabolic acidosis may also induce abnormalities in the growth hormone (GH) axis, such as impaired pulsatile GH secretion and decreased secretion of IGF-1, which may contribute to the inhibition of growth in children.

Although there are as yet no definitive studies ascertaining that alkali therapy is definitely beneficial in preventing or delaying osteopenia and hyperparathyroid bone disease, the use of alkali therapy is recommended in patients with CKD with the aim of maintaining a plasma bicarbonate concentration higher than 22 mEq/L. Concern about safety of sodium bicarbonate is probably overstated. Therapy is well tolerated and is usually not associated with signs of sodium retention.

Sodium bicarbonate (in a daily dose of 0.5 to 1 mEq/kg) is the agent of choice; it generally produces little or no sodium retention or increase in blood pressure. Sodium citrate (citrate is rapidly metabolized to bicarbonate) can be used in patients with CKD but should be avoided in patients also receiving phosphate binders containing aluminum, because it increases intestinal aluminum absorption and the risk of aluminum intoxication.

Phosphate, Calcium, and Bone

Phosphate retention begins early in kidney disease. Even during the early stages of CKD, phosphate retention contributes to the development of the secondary hyperparathyroidism that plays an important role in the pathogenesis of bone disease and in other uremic complications. Moreover, the excess phosphate may contribute to CKD progression. This topic is covered in detail in Chapter 64.

THE UREMIC SYNDROME

The uremic syndrome is the clinical manifestation of severe kidney failure. A state of systemic poisoning that affects the cardiovascular, gastrointestinal, hematopoietic, immune, nervous, and endocrine systems, it is partly the result of a reduction in renal excretory function with the retention of toxic substances that impair cell regulatory mechanisms. It is also the consequence of derangements in endocrine and metabolic functions regulated by the kidney. The uremic syndrome is characterized not only by solute accumulation but also by hormonal alterations such as decreased production of erythropoietin and calcitriol, decreased clearance of insulin, end organ resistance to insulin and PTH, and excess production of PTH. The signs and symptoms vary from one patient to another, depending partly on the speed and severity of the loss of kidney function (Table 58-4).

Cardiovascular System

Cardiovascular disorders (see also Chapter 65) are the leading cause of death in patients with ESRD, accounting for over half of the deaths in patients on dialysis. Hypertension and congestive heart failure are common; salt and water retention is very important in the pathogenesis of both. Hypertension is present in more than 80% of patients with ESRD and is presumably a major risk factor for cardiovascular disease, congestive heart failure, and cerebrovascular disease. In addition to salt and water retention, in uremia there are several conditions, such as enhanced activity of the renin-angiotensin system, excess aldosterone secretion, increased sympathetic tone, and reduced production of vasodilatory hormones such as prostaglandins and kinins, that may contribute to the development of hypertension.

Besides the common risk factors for cardiovascular diseases, a number of specific features of uremia can result in enhanced risk. Increased oxidant stress along with the production of complement fragments and cytokines may provide the milieu for the development of accelerated atherosclerosis. In patients on hemodialysis, rapid extracellular fluid volume changes may be associated with episodes of hypotension and electrolyte imbalance. Increased intake of calcium to treat hyperphosphatemia may enhance coronary arterial calcification. In dialysis patients, nitric oxide synthesis is often inhibited, with subsequent vasoconstriction and hypertension.

The introduction of erythropoietin therapy has improved exercise performance and reduced cardiac output and left ventricular mass in dialysis patients. Valvular stenosis and insufficiency, as well as accelerated atherosclerosis are common during the progression to

TABLE 58-4   Major Clinical Abnormalities in Uremia

Fluid and electrolyte abnormalities
    Volume expansion and depletion
    Hypernatremia and hyponatremia
    Hyperkalemia and hypokalemia
    Metabolic acidosis
    Hyperphosphatemia and hypocalcemia
    Hypermagnesemia

Cardiovascular abnormalities
    Hypertension
    Congestive heart failure
    Cardiomyopathy
    Pericarditis
    Accelerated atherosclerosis
    Arrhythmias

Gastrointestinal abnormalities
    Anorexia, nausea, and vomiting
    Uremic fetor
    Stomatitis, gastritis, and enteritis
    Peptic ulcer
    Gastrointestinal bleeding

Hematologic and immunologic abnormalities
    Anemia
    Bleeding
    Phagocyte inhibition
    Lymphocytopenia and lymphocyte dysfunction
    Increased susceptibility to infection and neoplasia

Neurologic abnormalities
    Malaise
    Headache
    Irritability and sleep disorders
    Muscle cramps
    Tremor
    Asterixis
    Seizures
    Stupor and coma
    Peripheral neuropathy
    Restless legs
    Motor weakness

Endocrine and metabolic abnormalities
    Carbohydrate intolerance
    Hypertriglyceridemia
    Protein malnutrition
    Impaired growth
    Infertility, sexual dysfunction, and amenorrhea
    Renal osteodystrophy
    Secondary hyperparathyroidism
    Hyperuricemia

Dermatologic abnormalities
    Pallor
    Hyperpigmentation
    Pruritus
    Ecchymoses
    Uremic frost

ESRD. Serious arrhythmias, as a consequence of electrolyte imbalance, left ventricular dysfunction, or coronary artery disease, occur frequently with uremia. Symptomatic myocardial ischemia usually results from coronary artery disease, but it is nonatherosclerotic in origin in about 25% of patients. Widespread arterial calcification, probably due to secondary hyperparathyroidism and phosphate retention, is a common complication of CKD. Uremic cardiomyopathy, possibly caused by PTH-induced myocardial calcification and fibrosis, has been described, whereas uremic pericarditis has become rare because of earlier initiation of dialytic therapy.

Gastrointestinal System

Gastrointestinal complications are common in CKD and in some cases may be the first or only complaint on presentation. Anorexia, nausea, vomiting, and uremic fetor, with its typical ammoniacal odor on the breath, are common manifestations of uremia. Vomiting may occur without nausea and is often prominent in the early morning. Stomatitis, gastritis, and enteritis can develop with the progression of CKD in patients not treated with dialysis or transplantation. Mucosal ulcerations can occur at any level of the gastrointestinal tract and, with the bleeding tendency of uremia, they largely account for the gastrointestinal bleeding seen in untreated uremia. An altered gastric mucosal barrier may contribute to the development of ulcerative lesions. Peptic ulcer occurs in about one fourth of uremic patients. The parotitis that develops in some patients may be related to the high salivary urea content in the presence of the low salivary flow rates that characterize kidney failure. Pancreatitis is rarely a significant clinical problem. Drugs such as metoclopramide can control nausea and enhance gastric emptying. Ulcerogenic medications, especially nonsteroidal anti-inflammatory drugs, should be avoided.

Red Blood Cells and Hemostasis

Anemia develops early during kidney failure and is one of the major causes of malaise and fatigue as kidney function worsens. In CKD, the management of anemia has radically changed with the advent of recombinant human erythropoietin. Correction of anemia improves cardiac function, central nervous system symptoms, appetite, and sexual function (see Chapter 66).

Immune Response

Functional and phenotypic alterations in both humoral and cellular immunity have been identified at an early stage of CKD. They worsen with the progression of uremia and are exacerbated by the dialysis procedure. The enhanced susceptibility to infection is greater with cellulosic membranes than with synthetic membranes. The antibody response to antigens is impaired, and the serum level of complement may be depressed.

The leukocyte count is normal and increases appropriately in response to infection in uremia, but metabolic and functional abnormalities of polymorphonuclear leukocytes (PMNLs) contribute to an increased susceptibility to infection. They include altered carbohydrate metabolism, adenosine triphosphate (ATP) generation, adherence to endothelial cells, generation of reactive oxygen species, and release of lysosomal enzymes as well as impairment of chemotaxis, phagocytosis, and intracellular killing of bacteria.

Before the introduction of erythropoietin, uremic patients often developed transfusion-related iron overload. Increased ferritin levels correlated with impaired PMNL function, which could be corrected with deferoxamine therapy. Correction of anemia with erythropoietin also improves PMNL function.

Increased intracellular calcium is associated with several alterations of PMNL function and metabolism, which improve by normalization of calcium content by either giving calcium channel blockers or lowering elevated PTH values. Several compounds isolated from uremic serum inhibit the biological activity of PMNLs. Granulocyte inhibitory protein I (GIP I) and II (GIP II) inhibit the uptake of deoxyglucose, chemotaxis, oxidative metabolism, and intracellular killing by PMNLs. GIP I displays homology with immunoglobulin light chain protein and GIP II with β_2-microglobulin. Degranulation inhibitory protein I (DIP I) and II (DIP II) inhibit spontaneous and stimulated PMNL degranulation and are identical to angiogenin and complement factor D. Moderate lymphocytopenia with reduced circulating T cells, increased suppressor cell activity, and reduced helper cell activity may be present in uremic patients. The ratio of T4 to T8 cells may be reduced. The response of lymphocytes to mitogens is reduced. Interferon production is also decreased. Thus, the reduced renal clearance of unknown toxins, in addition to the effects of any concomitant nutritional deficiencies, can lead to aberrant immune regulation in CKD. Typical of uremia are an increased incidence of infections, including tuberculosis and bacteremia, immunologically modulated disorders such as cancer, and inadequate antibody production in response to hepatitis B vaccination. Although impaired humoral and cell-mediated immunity contribute to suboptimal and short-lived antibody responses to vaccines, vaccination still has an important role in attenuating infection risk. Augmented vaccination schedules, increased vaccine dosage, and use of adjuvant immunomodulators have variably improved the defective antibody responses to certain vaccines. Monitoring antibody titers helps to determine the need for booster vaccination. Immunization against hepatitis B virus has significantly decreased the prevalence and incidence of this infection in hemodialysis units. The use of influenza vaccine in uremic patients and of polyvalent pneumococcal vaccine has reduced the morbidity and mortality attributable to these infections.

Neurologic Manifestations

Central nervous system disorders are seen in advanced stages of CKD (see Chapter 67). The early symptoms are those of disturbances of mentation and cognition due to reduced general cerebral activity, such as apathy, fatigue, confusion, impaired memory, and decreased capacity for prolonged intellectual effort. As the disorder progresses, disorientation and irritability may manifest, followed by hallucinations, anxiety, depression, and mania. Finally, lethargy, stupor, and coma occur. Peripheral neuropathy is common in advanced CKD. It is generally symmetric and slowly progressive, and begins distally and spreads proximally. Dialysis can control the progression of peripheral neuropathy.

Metabolic and Endocrine Disorders

Glucose intolerance develops in most patients with CKD, mainly as a result of resistance to the peripheral action of insulin, but release of insulin in response to hyperglycemia may also be impaired. In patients with GFR less than 10 to 15 mL/minute, insulin clearance is reduced so that insulin requirements are lower.

Alterations in lipid metabolism may be present early in the course of CKD. They show only a modest correlation with the severity of the kidney function reduction and respond only slightly to dialysis. Plasma levels of triglycerides are elevated, with a smaller rise in total cholesterol, the so-called type IV hyperlipoproteinemia pattern. Protein synthesis gradually decreases with CKD, and the majority of uremic patients are catabolic, with a negative nitrogen balance. Malnutrition, insulin resistance, metabolic acidosis, and hyporesponsiveness to GH may contribute to the negative nitrogen balance.

Free thyroxine (T4) and serum thyroid-stimulating hormone (TSH, or thyrotropin) are usually normal, whereas serum triiodothyronine (T3) is low because of decreased peripheral conversion of T4 to T3; the majority of these patients are clinically euthyroid and need no treatment. In uremic women, estrogen production is low and prolactin levels are high, leading to disturbances in menstruation and fertility. Men may be impotent, infertile, or oligospermic secondary to low plasma testosterone levels.

Skin Effects

The cutaneous manifestations of uremia include pallor (anemia), ecchymoses (impaired hemostasis), pruritus, pigmentation, and dehydration. Uremic patients have a characteristic sallow pallor due to anemia, retention of urochrome pigments and urea, and increased melatonin. The skin is generally dry and atrophic. In advanced CKD, the precipitation of urea crystals secreted in sweat leads to uremic frost. Several influences have been proposed to have a role in uremic pruritus, including secondary hyperparathyroidism, dry skin, increased calcium phosphate deposition in the skin, anemia, peripheral neuropathy, high aluminum levels, and hypervitaminosis A. Pruritus is probably due to the release of histamines from skin mast cells, although it is not well understood how the previously cited factors induce histamine release. Although many of these abnormalities improve with dialysis, pruritus is not often improved by dialysis and is usually resistant to most systemic and topical therapies. Erythropoietin has been inconsistently reported to improve pruritus, for reasons that are not understood and that appear independent of anemia correction. At present, the best therapy for severe pruritus is a combination of erythropoietin, ultraviolet phototherapy, and, if necessary, an antihistamine.

Uremic Toxins and Hormonal Deficiencies

The retention of a number of organic and inorganic substances contributes to the uremic manifestations. The search for a specific toxin or toxins responsible for all the clinical manifestations of uremia has been largely frustrating, although PTH is receiving renewed attention. Uremic retention substances are classified according to their molecular masses: low-molecular-mass solutes (10 to 3000 Daltons) such as urea and creatinine, middle-mass molecules (3000 to 15,000 Daltons) including PTH and β_2-microglobulin, and large solutes (more than 15,000 Daltons). Protein degradation products and amino acids have received most of the attention.

Urea toxicity has been debated; it causes symptoms only at much higher concentrations than usually found in uremia. Thus urea alone is probably not toxic at the concentrations typical of ESRD. However, urea is an extremely useful marker of uremic retention and elimination in dialysis patients. The U.S. National Cooperative Dialysis Study showed a direct correlation between fractional clearance of urea in body water and patient outcomes such as mortality. This has led to the use of urea kinetic modeling to evaluate dialysis adequacy.

Guanidine compounds are toxic in animals. They may cause gastritis, polyneuritis, reduced calcitriol synthesis, and coagulation abnormalities, but their toxicity in humans has not yet been convincingly demonstrated. Myoinositol (molecular mass 180.2 Daltons) and other polyols are phospholipids that are retained in uremia and are a possible cause of peripheral neuropathy.

In vitro studies have shown that FPA (3-carboxy-4-methyl-5-propyl-2-furanpropanoic acid, molecular mass 236 Daltons), an organic acid derived from the diet and the breakdown of complex lipids, is an inhibitor of erythropoiesis.

Parathyroid hormone, a middle-mass molecule of about 9000 Daltons, is an important uremic toxin; it is oversecreted during ESRD in response to hypocalcemia, hyperphosphatemia, and $1,25(OH)_2$ vitamin D_3 deficiency. Hyperparathyroidism causes intracellular accumulation of calcium, which inhibits mitochondrial oxidative pathways and the generation of ATP. The increased intracellular calcium uptake may affect the brain, myocardium, pancreas, and platelets. Hyperparathyroidism also induces changes in membrane permeability and integrity, as well as phospholipid turnover, stimulation of cyclic adenosine monophosphate (cAMP) production, soft tissue calcification, and protein catabolism. It also contributes to glucose intolerance, inhibition of platelet function and erythropoiesis, and cardiomyopathy.

β_2-Microglobulin is a human leukocyte antigen (HLA) class 1 light chain component present in all mammalian cells. It accumulates in kidney failure and is responsible for amyloid deposition in the carpal tunnel, synovial membrane, and the ends of long bones. Carpal tunnel syndrome, bone cysts, and destructive arthropathy result (see Chapter 64).

Initiation of Renal Replacement Therapy

Uremic patients inevitably progress and require renal replacement therapy in the form of dialysis or transplant. Early identification of patients who will require replacement therapy is important, because adequate preparation may decrease morbidity and also permit the evaluation of the patient and family members for a living related kidney allograft before the start of dialysis. The decision to start dialysis depends more on the severity of uremic complications (uncontrolled hyperkalemia and metabolic acidosis, fluid overload, and gastrointestinal and neurologic symptoms) than on the SCr. However, many nephrologists prefer to start dialysis early to avoid the risk of more serious complications of uremia such as pericarditis and pulmonary edema (see Table 58-4).

There has been no truly randomized study of early versus late initiation of dialysis for ESRD. However, the overall data suggest that early initiation may decrease malnutrition, increase the rate of rehabilitation, and improve long-term survival.

Patients and their families have to be involved in the decision to start renal replacement therapy; the risks and benefits of hemodialytic therapy (at the center or at home), peritoneal dialytic methods (continuous or intermittent), and kidney transplantation (living or cadaveric donor) should be clearly explained (see Chapters 60 and 68). A team approach including nurse clinicians, social workers, and other health professionals to assess the home situation and educate the patient and family may be advantageous in this phase.

454 ARRIGO SCHIEPPATI • ROBERTO PISONI • GIUSEPPE REMUZZI

BIBLIOGRAPHY

Aros C, Remuzzi G: The renin-angiotensin system in progression, remission and regression of chronic nephropathies. J Hypertens 20(suppl 3):S45–S53, 2002.

Brenner BM, Meyer TW, Hostetter TH: Dietary protein intake and the progressive nature of kidney disease: The role of hemodynamically mediated glomerular injury in the pathogenesis of progressive glomerular sclerosis in aging, renal ablation, and intrinsic renal disease. N Engl J Med 307:652–659, 1982.

Brenner BM, Cooper ME, de Zeeuw D, et al: Effects of losartan on renal and cardiovascular outcomes in patients with type 2 diabetes and nephropathy. N Engl J Med 345:861–869, 2001.

Breyer JA, Bain RP, Evans JK, et al: Predictors of the progression of renal insufficiency in patients with insulin-dependent diabetes and overt diabetic nephropathy. Kidney Int 50:1651–1658, 1996.

Dubrow A, Levin NW: Biochemical and hormonal alterations in chronic renal failure. In Jacobson HR, Striker GE, Klahr S (eds): The Principles and Practice of Nephrology. St. Louis, Mosby, 1995, pp 596–603.

Egido J: Vasoactive hormones and renal sclerosis. Kidney Int 49:578–597, 1996.

Eurich DT, Majumdar SR, Tsuyuki RT, Johnson JA: Reduced mortality associated with the use of ACE inhibitors in patients with type 2 diabetes. Diabetes Care 27:1330–1334, 2004.

Fogo AB: The potential for regression of renal scarring. Curr Opin Nephrol Hypertens 12:223–225, 2003.

The GISEN Group (Gruppo Italiano di Studi Epidemiologici in Nefrologia). Randomised placebo-controlled trial of effect of ramipril on decline in glomerular filtration rate and risk of terminal renal failure in proteinuric, non-diabetic nephropathy. Lancet 349:1857–1863, 1997.

Haag-Weber M, Horl WH: Dysfunction of polymorphonuclear leukocytes in uremia. Semin Nephrol 16:192–201, 1996.

Hostetter TH: The next treatments of chronic kidney disease: If we find them, can we test them? J Am Soc Nephrol 13:3024–3026, 2002.

Lakkis FD, Martinez-Maldonado M: Conservative management of chronic renal failure and the uremic syndrome. In Jacobson HR, Striker GE, Klahr S (eds): The Principles and Practice of Nephrology. St. Louis, Mosby, 1995, pp 614–620.

Lewis EJ, Hunsicker LG, Bain RP, et al: The effect of angiotensin-converting-enzyme inhibition on diabetic nephropathy. N Engl J Med 329:1456–1462, 1993.

Lewis EJ, Hunsicker LG, Clarke WR, et al: Renoprotective effect of the angiotensin-receptor antagonist irbesartan in patients with nephropathy due to type 2 diabetes. N Engl J Med 345:851–860, 2001.

Mackenzie HS, Brenner BM: Prevention of progressive renal failure. In Brady HR, Wilcox CS (eds): Therapy in Nephrology and Hypertension. Philadephia, WB Saunders, 1999, pp 463–473.

Nakao N, Yoshimura A, Morita H, et al: Combination treatment of angiotensin-II receptor blocker and angiotensin-converting-enzyme inhibitor in non-diabetic renal disease (COOPERATE): A randomised controlled trial. Lancet 361:117–124, 2003.

Parving H-H: Diabetic nephropathy: Prevention and treatment. Kidney Int 60:2041–2055, 2001.

Parving H-H, Lehnert H, Brochner-Mortensen J, et al: The effect of irbesartan on the development of diabetic nephropathy in patients with type 2 diabetes. N Engl J Med 345:870–878, 2001.

Peterson JC, Adler S, Burkart JM, et al: for the Modification of Diet in Renal Disease (MDRD) Study Group: Blood pressure control, proteinuria, and the progression of renal disease. Ann Intern Med 123:754–762, 1995.

Remuzzi G: Bleeding in renal failure. Lancet 1:1205–1208, 1988.

Remuzzi G, Bertani T: Pathophysiology of progressive nephropathies. N Engl J Med 339:1448–1456, 1998.

Ruggenenti P, Perna A, Remuzzi G, et al: Renoprotective properties of ACE-inhibition in non-diabetic nephropathies with non-nephrotic proteinuria. Lancet 354:359–364, 1999.

Ruggenenti P, Schieppati A, Remuzzi G: Progression, remission, regression of chronic renal diseases. Lancet 357:1601–1608, 2001.

Ter Wee PM: Initial management of chronic renal failure. In Cameron S, Davison AM, Grunfeld JP, et al (eds): Oxford Textbook of Clinical Nephrology. Oxford, Oxford Medical Press, 1992, pp 1173–1191.

UK Prospective Diabetes Study (UKPDS) Group 33: Intensive blood-glucose control with sulphonylureas or insulin compared with conventional treatment and risk of complications in patients with type 2 diabetes. Lancet 352:837–853, 1998.

Weidmann P, Schneider M, Bohlen L: Therapeutic efficacy of different antihypertensive drugs in human diabetic nephropathy: An updated meta-analysis. Nephrol Dial Transplant 10(suppl 9):39–45, 1995.

Zoja C, Corna D, Camozzi D, Cattaneo D, et al: How to fully protect the kidney in a severe model of progressive nephropathy: A multidrug approach. J Am Soc Nephrol 13:2898–2908, 2002.

CHAPTER 59

Chronic Kidney Disease: Staging and Principles of Management

Lesley A. Stevens   Andrew S. Levey

Recently, attention has been directed to the serious public health problem of chronic kidney disease (CKD). The number of persons with kidney failure who are treated with dialysis and transplantation is expected to nearly double, with a projected increase from 340,000 in 1999 to 651,000 in 2010. However, the poor outcomes of CKD are not restricted to kidney failure but also include the morbidity and mortality related to decreased kidney function as well as cardiovascular disease (CVD).

In 2002 the National Kidney Foundation (NKF) sponsored the Kidney Disease Outcomes Quality Initiative (K/DOQI) and published guidelines for the evaluation, classification, and stratification of CKD. The purpose of these guidelines was to create uniform terminology to improve communications among all involved in the care and management of CKD, including patients, physicians, researchers, and policymakers. Previous terms were often imprecisely defined (renal insufficiency, predialysis, progressive renal disease), and it was recognized that consistent language is necessary for the public and medical community to address this problem at all levels. New features of the classification system are that the definition and stages do not depend on identification of the cause of kidney disease, that kidney function is expressed as the level of estimated glomerular filtration rate (GFR), and that higher stages are associated with an increasing prevalence of complications from decreased kidney function and CVD.

The goals of this chapter are to describe the conceptual model for the progression of CKD; the NKF/K/DOQI definition, stages of CKD, and estimated prevalence; an associated clinical action plan; and the role of nephrologists in the care for these patients.

DEFINITION AND STAGING OF CHRONIC KIDNEY DISEASE

Course of Chronic Kidney Disease

A conceptual model for the course of CKD is shown in Figure 59-1. This model describes the natural history of CKD, beginning with antecedent conditions, followed by the stages of CKD, kidney damage, decreased GFR and kidney failure, and other associated outcomes. The model stresses that kidney disease tends to worsen over time by transitions through a defined sequence of stages, regardless of the underlying susceptibility to disease, the specific cause of kidney damage, or the rate of progression through each stage. The earlier stages and the risk factors for progression to higher stages can be identified, permitting improvement in outcome by prevention, earlier detection, and initiation of therapies that can slow progression.

Susceptibility factors are characteristics that put an individual at risk to develop kidney damage (Table 59-1). These factors can be genetic, such as angiotensin-converting enzyme (ACE) polymorphisms, or developmental, such as low birth weight resulting in a reduced nephron mass. Demographic characteristics such as age, race, ethnicity, or low financial income also describe individuals who are at increased risk for the development of kidney damage. The mechanisms underlying all of these associations are not known and have not been definitively proven. Race, for example, may imply an underlying genetic tendency or may be a marker for poor health care. Susceptibility factors may explain why a family history of kidney disease, regardless of the cause, places an individual at an increased risk for development of kidney disease.

Initiation factors are conditions that can directly cause kidney damage, including diabetes, hypertension, autoimmune diseases, and kidney stones (see Table 59-1). Exposure to these conditions, together with the presence of susceptibility factors, determines whether or not an individual develops kidney damage. Individuals with susceptibility or initiation factors for CKD are at increased risk to develop CKD and should be tested for it on a regular basis.

In patients with kidney damage, progression factors influence the risk for and rate of decline in kidney function. Kidney disease may progress because the disorder responsible for inciting damage is continuous or as a result of pathways independent of the initial damage. Progression factors include elevated blood pressure, higher level of proteinuria, poor glycemic control in diabetes, and smoking. Current understanding of the mechanisms of progression; the risks conferred by specific

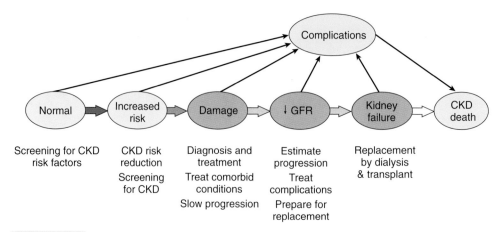

FIGURE 59-1 Conceptual model for stages in the initiation and progression of chronic kidney disease (CKD) and therapeutic interventions. Orange ellipses represent stages of CKD; yellow ellipses represent potential antecedents or consequences of CKD. Thick arrows between ellipses represent "risk factors" associated with initiation and progression of disease that can be affected or detected by interventions: susceptibility factors (*dark blue*); initiation factors (*medium blue*); progression factors (*pale blue*); and endstage factors (*white*) (see Table 59-2). Interventions for each stage are given beneath the stage. Complications refer to all complications of CKD and its treatment. (Reprinted with permission from the National Kidney Foundation.)

progression factors; the interactions between susceptibility, initiation, and progression factors; and the variability of response in individual patients remains limited.

Endstage factors influence the risk for the development of adverse outcomes in patients with kidney failure, and include adequacy of dialysis, type of vascular access, compliance with dialysis prescription, nutritional status, and the presence of CVD.

Outcomes of CKD include loss of kidney function and CVD. Kidney failure is the most visible outcome of CKD. However, more common than kidney failure is decreased kidney function, with a myriad of systemic complications that may result in mortality, morbidity, or decreased quality of life. Similarly, more common than kidney failure is CVD, which deserves special emphasis because CKD per se is a risk factor for CVD. Conversely, CVD is a risk factor for CKD that is treatable and potentially preventable.

Definition of Chronic Kidney Disease

Chronic kidney disease is defined as either kidney damage or a GFR less than 60 mL/minute/1.73 m^2 body surface area that has been present for more than 3 months. CKD can be diagnosed without knowledge of its cause.

Even with normal GFR, kidney damage is defined as CKD, because kidney damage may portend a poor prognosis for the major outcomes related to CKD. Kidney damage is usually ascertained by markers of damage without kidney biopsy. Because most kidney disease in North America is due to diabetes or hypertension, persistent proteinuria (albuminuria) is the principal marker. Numerous studies show that proteinuria is associated with a faster decline in GFR, increased risk of kidney failure, and CVD. Other markers of damage include abnormalities in urine sediment (e.g., tubular cells or

TABLE 59-1 Types of Risk Factors for Chronic Kidney Disease and Its Outcomes

Risk Factors	Definition	Examples
Susceptibility factors	Increase susceptibility to kidney damage	Older age, family history of chronic kidney disease. Reduction in kidney mass, low birth weight, U.S. racial or ethnic minority status, low income or education
Initiation factors	Directly initiate kidney damage	Diabetes, high blood pressure, autoimmune diseases, systemic infections, urinary tract infections, urinary stones, lower urinary tract obstruction, drug toxicity
Progression factors	Cause worsening of kidney damage and faster decline in kidney function	Higher levels of proteinuria, higher blood pressure, poor glycemic control in diabetes, smoking
Endstage factors	Increase morbidity and mortality in kidney failure	Lower dialysis dose (Kt/V), temporary vascular access, anemia, low serum albumin, late referral

Kt/V, urea clearance (K) per unit time (t) related to total body water (V).
Reprinted with permission from the National Kidney Foundation.

casts), abnormal findings on imaging studies (e.g., hydronephrosis, asymmetry in kidney size, polycystic kidney disease, small echogenic kidneys), and abnormalities in blood and urine chemistry measurements (those related to altered tubular function, such as renal tubular acidosis).

Reduced kidney function, specifically a GFR lower than $60 \, mL/minute/1.73 \, m^2$, is also defined as CKD, because decreased GFR is associated with an increased risk of adverse outcome related to CKD. The level of GFR is usually accepted as the best overall index of level of kidney function in health and disease. A GFR level of less than $60 \, mL/minute/1.73 \, m^2$ represents loss of half or more of the adult level of normal kidney function and is associated with an increased prevalence of systemic complications. The normal level of GFR varies according to age, sex, and body size. Normal GFR in young adults is approximately 120 to $130 \, mL/minute/1.73 \, m^2$ and declines with age by approximately $1 \, mL/minute/1.73 \, m^2$ per year after the third decade. More than 25% of individuals aged 70 years and older have GFR less than $60 \, mL/minute/1.73 \, m^2$; this may be due to normal aging or the high prevalence of systemic diseases that cause kidney disease. The definition of CKD does not vary with age. Whatever its cause, a GFR below $60 \, mL/minute/1.73 \, m^2$ in the elderly is an independent predictor of adverse outcomes, such as death and CVD. Just as in younger patients, adjustment of drug doses is required in the elderly with this level of GFR.

Kidney failure is defined as either (1) GFR less than $15 \, mL/minute/1.73 \, m^2$ (which in most cases will be accompanied by signs and symptoms of uremia) or (2) a need to start kidney replacement therapy (dialysis or transplantation). Kidney failure is not synonymous with endstage renal disease (ESRD), the administrative term in the United States that indicates the need for chronic treatment by dialysis or transplantation and confers Medicare eligibility. Thus, ESRD does not include patients with kidney failure who are not treated with dialysis and transplantation.

Stages of Chronic Kidney Disease

The NKF/K/DOQI classification system for stages of CKD is based on the severity of the disease as indicated by the level of GFR, with higher stages representing lower GFR levels, regardless of the specific cause and the rate of progression (Table 59-2). The increased risk of complications with decreased GFR is demonstrated through analyses of the Third National Health and Nutrition Examination Survey (NHANES III), showing an increasing prevalence of complications such as hypertension, anemia, malnutrition, bone disease, neuropathy, and decreased quality of life at higher stages of CKD (Fig. 59-2).

The risk of developing kidney failure is related to the stage of CKD as well as the rate of decline in GFR. The rate of decline of GFR varies between individuals and may even vary within an individual over time. For example, if the rate of decline is $4 \, mL/minute/1.73 \, m^2$ per year, then the interval from a GFR of $60 \, mL/minute/1.73 \, m^2$ to onset of kidney failure (less than $15 \, mL/minute/1.73 \, m^2$) would be 11 to 12 years. This rate of decline is considered fast. By contrast, if the rate of decline in GFR is $1 \, mL/minute/1.73 \, m^2$ per year, an individual with a GFR of $60 \, mL/minute/1.73 \, m^2$ may not reach kidney failure in his or her lifetime.

Prevalence

Table 59-2 shows the prevalence estimates of levels of GFR and albuminuria from the NHANES III. Based on this

TABLE 59-2 National Kidney Foundation–Kidney Disease Outcome Quality Initiative: Classification, Prevalence, and Action Plan for Stages of CKD

Stage	Description	GFR (mL/min/1.73 m²)	Prevalence* n (%)	Clinical Action Plan†
0	Individuals at increased risk	>60		Test for the presence of CKD, CKD risk reduction
1	Kidney damage with normal or ↑ GFR	>90	5,900,000 (3.3)	Diagnosis and treatment, slow progression, CVD risk reduction
2	Kidney damage with mild ↓ GFR	60–89	5,300,000 (3.0)	Estimating progression
3	Moderate ↓ GFR	30–59	7,600,000 (4.3)	Evaluating and treating complications
4	Severe ↓ GFR	15–29	400,000 (0.2)	Preparation for kidney replacement therapy
5	Kidney failure	<15 (or dialysis)	300,000 (0.1)	Kidney replacement therapy (if uremia present and patient wishes)

CKD, chronic kidney disease.
*Prevalence for stage 5 is from the USRDS. Prevalence for stage 1 to 4 is from the NHANES III (1988–1994), population of 177 million adults age 20 years or older.
†National Kidney Foundation. K/DOQI clinical practice guidelines for chronic kidney disease: Evaluation, classification, and stratification. Action plan is cumulative in that each stage incorporates recommendations from the previous stage.
Reprinted with permission from the National Kidney Foundation.

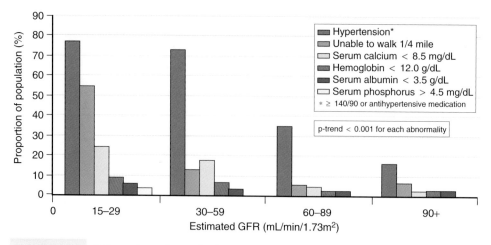

FIGURE 59-2 Estimated prevalence of selected complications, by category of estimated GFR, among participants age 20 years and older in NHANES III 1988–1994. These estimates are not adjusted for age. (Reprinted with permission from the National Kidney Foundation.)

national health survey conducted between 1988 and 1994, approximately 11% of the U.S. adult population of 20 million people have CKD. The prevalence of early stages of disease (stages 1 to 4; 10.8%) is more than 100 times greater than the prevalence of kidney failure (stage 5; 0.1%). Because kidney disease usually begins late in life and progresses slowly, most people in the earlier stages of CKD die before they develop kidney failure. The burden of earlier stages of CKD, in terms of mortality, morbidity, and reduced quality of life, has not been systematically studied; however, it is probably considerable. The systemic complications of decreased GFR begin at levels well above those associated with kidney failure (see Fig. 59-2). In addition, increasing evidence shows that both albuminuria and decreased GFR are independent risk factors for CVD.

Clinical Action Plan

Associated with each stage of CKD is a clinical action plan, as is shown in Table 59-2. The action plan includes care that is recommended for each stage, as well as attention to the progression factors for the transition to a more advanced stage. Three key points must be emphasized. First, the action plan is cumulative in that recommended care at each stage of disease includes care for less severe stages. Second, care for patients with CKD requires multiple interventions, so that providing such care requires the coordinated multidisciplinary effort of primary care physicians (PCPs), allied health-care workers, and other specialists in addition to nephrologists. Third, the management of each stage of disease must take into consideration CKD and CVD, as well as other comorbid conditions. The stage-specific clinical action plan is a

guide, but not a replacement, for the physician's assessment of the needs of a specific patient.

EVALUATION AND MANAGEMENT

Diagnosis

Screening Procedures

As part of routine checkups, all persons should be evaluated to determine whether they are at increased risk for developing CKD because of the presence of susceptibility or initiation factors (see Table 59-1). Individuals at high risk should undergo testing to identify the presence of markers of kidney damage and to estimate GFR. The Joint National Committee (JNC) on Prevention, Detection, Evaluation and Treatment of High Blood Pressure and the American Diabetes Association (ADA) recommend yearly testing for CKD in patients with diabetes and hypertension, respectively. At present, there are few data regarding the optimal frequency of testing for CKD in individuals who have risk factors other than diabetes and hypertension. Until evidence is available, it is reasonable to suggest that individuals at increased risk be tested at least every 3 years.

Assessment of Kidney Function

The National Institute of Diabetes, Digestive and Kidney Diseases (NIDDK), the NKF, and the American Society of Nephrology (ASN) recommend the use of GFR estimated from the serum creatinine concentration (SCr) with an estimating equation as the primary assessment of kidney function in standard clinical practice. CKD is diagnosed when an estimated GFR is found to be less than 60 mL/minute/1.73 m^2 on two occasions more than 3 months apart. Current guidelines focus on estimated GFR rather than SCr alone for a variety of reasons. SCr is affected by influences other than GFR (see Chapter 2). Consequently, there is a wide range of "normal" SCr, and in many patients GFR must decline by approximately 50% before SCr rises above the normal range. This is particularly important in the elderly, in whom the SCr does not reflect the age-related decline in GFR because of a concomitant age-related decline in muscle mass and reduced creatinine production. Thus, it is difficult to use the SCr alone to estimate the level of GFR, especially to detect earlier stages of CKD. Measurement of creatinine clearance (CrCl) can avoid some of the limitations of SCr; however, it requires collection of a timed urine sample, which is inconvenient and frequently inaccurate.

The Modification of Diet in Renal Disease (MDRD) study and Cockcroft-Gault equations provide useful estimates of GFR in adults. The MDRD equation is more accurate and precise than the Cockcroft-Gault equation and measured creatinine clearance for persons with a GFR less than approximately 90 mL/minute/1.73 m^2. However, as indicated in Chapter 2, these and other estimating equations will not perform as well in populations and settings other than those in which they were developed. Thus GFR estimates may be inaccurate in populations that were not included in the original study populations (e.g., diabetes, elderly, other racial groups) or in individuals in whom creatinine production would be expected to differ from the general population (e.g., extremes of body size, with high levels of dietary meat intake, overweight or obesity, malnutrition, amputation, or conditions associated with muscle wasting). Nonetheless, even in these individuals, GFR estimates are likely to be more useful than estimates of the level of kidney function based on SCr alone. If an accurate estimate of GFR is required, a clearance measurement should be obtained, either a 24-hour urine collection for CrCl or clearance of an exogenous filtration marker.

Kidney Damage

Markers of kidney damage include proteinuria, hematuria, other abnormalities of the urinary sediment, or radiologic evidence of damage. The most common causes of CKD in adults are diabetes (see Chapters 28 and 29) and hypertension (see Chapters 70 through 72), and therefore the most common marker for kidney damage is increased protein excretion, specifically albumin.

Urine protein includes albumin, low-molecular-weight proteins that are filtered by the kidney and incompletely reabsorbed, proteins derived from tubular epithelium (e.g., Tamm-Horsfall protein), and proteins derived from the lower urinary tract (see Chapter 4). Healthy, normal persons usually excrete only 50 to 100 mg/day of protein in the urine. However, because of the wide range, the upper limit of normal usually extends to levels as high as 200 to 300 mg/day to avoid false positives. The most common type of protein seen in patients with CKD is albumin, related to glomerular injury. It is the earliest sign of kidney disease secondary to diabetes, glomerular diseases, and hypertension. An elevated albumin excretion rate is a specific sign of kidney damage.

The ratio of concentrations of albumin or total protein to creatinine in an untimed ("spot") urine specimen has replaced 24-hour excretion rates as the preferred method for measuring albuminuria and proteinuria. Using a ratio corrects for variations in urinary protein concentration due to hydration and is far more convenient than timed urine collections. A "positive" result for untimed urine albumin-to-creatinine ratio is greater than 30 mg/g. Values between 30 and 300 mg/g are considered in the microalbuminuria range (i.e., not detectable by standard methods for the detection of total protein), and values greater than 300 mg/g are considered in the macroalbuminuria range. A positive result for urine total protein-to-creatinine ratio is greater than 200 mg/g. Spot urine total protein-to-creatinine ratios greater than 500 to 1000 mg/g generally indicate a glomerular disease (although they may also arise in interstitial and vascular diseases), and at this level of proteinuria, measurement of total protein, instead of albumin, on a spot urine sample is acceptable. Clinical features of the nephrotic syndrome generally arise when the spot urine total protein-to-creatinine ratio is greater than 3000 mg/g (see Chapters 16 through 21).

Proteinuria can be seen intermittently in people without kidney disease secondary to vigorous exercise, fever, and infection. The algorithm for testing for proteinuria shown in Figure 59-3 distinguishes persons with and without risk factors for CKD. A sample of urine from the first voiding after awakening is preferred, but a random specimen is acceptable. Ideally, patients should refrain from vigorous exercise for 24 hours before sample collection. The algorithm for adults at increased risk (see Fig. 59-3) begins with testing of a random untimed urine sample with an albumin-specific dipstick. Patients with a positive result on a dipstick test for albuminuria (20 mg/L, 1+ or greater) should undergo confirmation by measuring the albumin-to-creatinine ratio on an untimed urine sample within 3 months. Alternatively, testing could begin with the albumin-to-creatinine ratio. Patients with two or more positive results on quantitative tests temporally spaced over 3 months have persistent proteinuria and are considered to have CKD irrespective of the level of kidney function.

Urine dipstick or sediment examination (see Chapter 3) should also be performed in all patients who are at high risk for CKD. Imaging studies (see Chapter 5) should be performed in selected individuals, such as those with a family history of polycystic kidney disease or those with history of vesicoureteral reflux in childhood, because these individuals may have chronic scarring from the

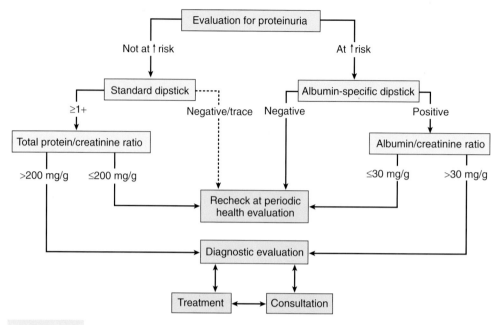

FIGURE 59-3 Evaluation of proteinuria in patients not known to have kidney disease. (Reprinted with permission from the National Kidney Foundation.)

remote injury that increases their risk for ongoing progressive kidney disease.

Evaluation

Starting treatment early in CKD is essential to prevent adverse outcomes. The goals of evaluation are:

1. Identify the stage of CKD.
2. Diagnose the type of kidney disease.
3. Detect reversible causes.
4. Identify risk factors for progression of kidney disease.
5. Identify risk factors for cardiovascular disease.
6. Detect complications of decreased GFR.

Diagnosis of CKD is traditionally based on pathology and etiology. A simplified classification emphasizes diseases in native kidneys (diabetic or nondiabetic in origin) and diseases in transplant kidneys. Diabetic nephropathy is the largest single cause of kidney failure in the United States, accounting for approximately one third of new cases of kidney failure; its earliest manifestation is microalbuminuria with a normal or elevated GFR (CKD stage 1). Nondiabetic kidney disease includes glomerular, vascular, tubulointerstitial, and cystic kidney disorders.

Evaluation of CKD starts with a thorough history and physical examination to detect any signs and symptoms that may be clues to the cause of kidney disease and in particular, any reversible elements or treatable risk factors for progression or CVD. Physical examination should pay particular attention to blood pressure. Laboratory tests should be performed to detect disruptions of other kidney functions besides GFR. These tests include maintenance of the filtration barrier for plasma proteins, reabsorption of water or specific solutes (e.g., sodium, potassium, bicarbonate), and endocrine function. Individuals known to have CKD should undergo quantification of urine protein with spot urine examination for total protein-to-creatinine or albumin-to-creatinine ratio, urine sediment examination, measurement of serum electrolytes, urine specific gravity, urine pH, as well as any indicated imaging studies. Ultrasonography should be done on all patients to detect anatomic abnormalities and to exclude obstruction of the urinary tract. Further testing may be indicated depending on concern about anatomic abnormalities. Individuals with CKD stages 3 through 5 (GFR less than 60 mL/minute/1.73 m^2) should have measurements of hemoglobin, calcium, phosphate, and parathyroid hormone. Laboratory evaluation should also include a search for traditional CVD risk factors, such as a lipid profile, and possibly tests for nontraditional risk factors. Additional studies may be necessary to evaluate symptoms of CVD more fully or to detect asymptomatic CVD in high-risk patients.

Management

The essential features of management are:

1. Treat specific causes of kidney disease.
2. Treat other reversible conditions causing kidney damage or decreased GFR.
3. Treat progression factors.
4. Treat uremic complications and prepare for kidney replacement therapy when appropriate.
5. Treat cardiovascular disease and its risk factors.
6. Avoid exposure to medications that are toxic to the kidneys.

Treatment of progression factors is the cornerstone of care for patients with CKD. The details of their management are described in detail in other chapters (see Chapters 58, 63, 64 and 67). Close attention to returning extracellular fluid volume to normal, achievement of the target blood pressure (see Chapter 71), and blockade of the rennin-angiotensin system are key components of therapy. The target blood pressure for patients with CKD is below 130/80 mm Hg (Table 59-3). ACE inhibitors or angiotensin receptor blockers (ARBs) are recommended for all patients with diabetic kidney disease and in those with nondiabetic kidney disease with spot urine total protein-to-creatinine ratios greater than 200 mg/g. Strong evidence documents the efficacy of these therapies to slow progression of CKD. Most patients will require more than two antihypertensive agents to achieve this blood pressure target. For most diseases, diuretics are preferred as the second agent. Additional therapies may be considered for patients with spot urine total protein-to-creatinine ratios greater than 500 to 1000 mg/g, including a lower blood pressure goal or initiation or increased dosage of agents that reduce proteinuria, including ACE inhibitors, ARBs, and nondihydropyridine calcium channel blockers. Other potential targets of intervention to slow kidney disease progression are dietary protein restriction, lipid-lowering therapy, strict glycemic control in diabetes, and smoking cessation.

Treatment of CVD risk factors are essentially the same as those used to slow progression of CKD. Individuals with CKD should be considered in the group at highest risk for treating traditional cardiac risk factors. Treatment for nontraditional risk factors can also be considered.

Uremic complications should be monitored and treated. These include electrolyte abnormalities (hyperkalemia, metabolic acidosis), anemia, hyperparathyroidism, hyperphosphatemia, bone disease, malnutrition, and nervous system disorders (neuropathy, cognitive changes). The details of their management are discussed in other chapters (see Chapters 63 through 67).

Patient education is a central aspect of the management strategy, particularly in that CKD is a chronic asymptomatic disease and patients may not understand the importance of multidrug regimens and laboratory testing without explicit education. Complete management of chronic disease requires behavior change by the patient, which may include life-style alterations, adherence to medication regimens, self-monitoring of blood pressure, and adherence to plans for medical follow-up. Patient education is also important with respect to avoidance of exposure to medications that are toxic to the kidneys. Patients must be aware that any drugs and herbal remedies either may be directly toxic or may require a dosage adjustment for the level of kidney function.

Health-Care Structure

Nephrology Referral

Chronic kidney disease may be a life-threatening condition. Nephrologists have several functions in the diagnosis and care of patients at all stages of CKD. These functions include determination of the cause of CKD, recommendations for specific therapy, suggestions for treatments to slow progression in patients who have not responded to conventional therapies, identification and treatment for kidney disease–related complications, and preparation for dialysis.

The strongest evidence for the importance of referral to a nephrologist is for management of CKD stages 4 and 5 (GFR less than 30 mL/minute/1.73 m²). Late referral to a nephrologist (i.e., less than 3 months before the start of dialysis therapy) is associated with higher mortality after the initiation of dialysis. It is recommended that all patients with CKD stage 4 be referred to a nephrologist

TABLE 59-3 National Kidney Foundation–Kidney Disease Outcome Quality Initiative: Clinical Practice Guidelines on Hypertension and Antihypertensive Agents in Chronic Kidney Disease

Type of Kidney Disease	Blood Pressure Target (mm Hg)	Preferred Agents for CKD, with or Without Hypertension	Other Agents to Reduce CVD Risk and Reach Blood Pressure Target
Diabetic kidney disease Nondiabetic kidney disease with spot urine total protein-to-creatinine ratio ≥200 mg/g		ACE inhibitor or ARB	Diuretic preferred, then BB or CCBs
Nondiabetic kidney disease with spot urine total protein-to-creatinine ratio <200 mg/g	<130/80		Diuretic preferred, then ACE inhibitor, ARB, BB, or CCB
Kidney disease in the kidney transplant recipient		None preferred	CCB, diuretic, BB, ACE inhibitor, ARB

ACE, angiotensin-converting enzyme; ARB, angiotensin receptor blocker; BB, beta blocker; CCB, calcium channel blocker; CKD, chronic kidney disease; CVD, cardiovascular disease.
Reprinted with permission from the National Kidney Foundation.

for comanagement. During this stage, it is important to prepare the patient for possible onset of kidney failure (CKD stage 5). Preparation involves estimating the risk of progression to kidney failure, discussion regarding kidney replacement therapy (dialysis and transplantation), and conservative therapy for those not willing or unable to undergo kidney replacement therapy. In patients electing replacement therapy, timely creation of vascular access for hemodialysis, home dialysis training, and donor evaluation for preemptive transplantation occur during this stage.

Primary Care and Specialist and Comanagement

Optimal management of chronic disease requires coordination among all physicians, allied health-care workers, and the patient. PCPs and specialists each bring unique skills to patient management and, for many patients, it is important to incorporate both into the care plan. A care delivery model in which PCPs and specialists share responsibility for the care of persons with CKD is recommended.

In this model, most patients with CKD stages 1 through 3 would be under the care of PCPs, generalists, or specialists other than nephrologists, with referral to a nephrologist for assistance in the evaluation and in development and implementation of the clinical action plan. As kidney disease worsens, the need for consultation and comanagement with nephrologists increases (Fig. 59-4). The specific configuration of the comanagement depends not only on the structure of the health-care system and geographic location of the practice but also on the individual patient and physician needs. In rural settings or where there is a shortage of nephrologists or other specialists, comanagement can be done not only with visits, but also by telephone, email, or other forms of electronic information transfer.

Multidisciplinary Clinics

Complex multifaceted disease processes require systematic approaches to care delivery. Optimal management of CKD requires coordination of antihypertensive and antiproteinuric strategies, smoking cessation, lipid-lowering therapies, management of diabetes, and other dietary and life-style modifications; this agenda is best accomplished by coordinated effort among practitioners. Allied health-care workers such as nurse practitioners, nurses, dietitians, pharmacists, and social workers are integral to providing excellent care. Other aspects of chronic care management that can be facilitated in this framework are self-management by patients, decision support by physicians, case management, planned appointments with the multidisciplinary team and nephrologists, and routine laboratory tests.

A small but growing literature demonstrates the benefit of having CKD patients seen by nephrologists in a multidisciplinary clinic. Benefits include delay in need for initiation of kidney replacement therapy, increased rate of seroconversion following hepatitis B vaccination, improved biochemical parameters at hemodialysis start, and decreased left ventricular hypertrophy. In multidisciplinary clinics, patient education can be organized and appropriately delivered. The benefits of patient education was recently shown in a randomized trial of a short patient-directed educational program that led to a prolongation by 17 months of the interval before the need for kidney replacement therapy.

Clinics need not be geographically based. Use of templates or pathways that involve different kinds of care givers may allow for similar delivery of care. The use of information technology is important in coordination of care between multiple care givers but will be particularly important in nongeographically based clinics and in geographically isolated settings.

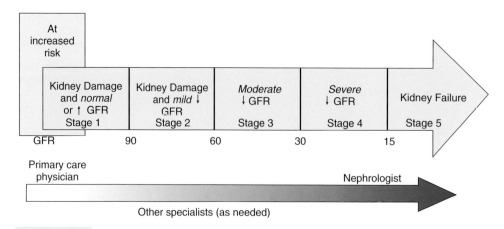

FIGURE 59-4 Primary care physicians and nephrologists are both important in the care of patients with CKD. The relative contribution each makes to the care of a patient shifts as patients reach CKD stage 4.

BIBLIOGRAPHY

Coresh J, Astor BC, Greene T, et al: Prevalence of chronic kidney disease and decreased kidney function in the adult US population: Third National Health and Nutrition Examination Survey. Am J Kidney Dis 41:1–12, 2003.

Coresh J, Astor BC, McQuillan G, et al: Calibration and random variation of the serum creatinine assay as critical elements of using equations to estimate glomerular filtration rate. Am J Kidney Dis 39:920–929, 2002.

The Diabetes Control and Complications Trial/Epidemiology of Diabetes Interventions and Complications Research Group: Retinopathy and nephropathy in patients with type 1 diabetes four years after a trial of intensive therapy. N Engl J Med 342:381–389, 2000.

Eknoyan G, Hostetter T, Bakris G, et al: Proteinuria and other markers of chronic kidney disease: A position statement of the National Kidney Foundation (NKF) and the National Institute of Diabetes and Digestive and Kidney Diseases (NIDDK). Am J Kidney Dis 42:617–622, 2003.

Jafar T, Schmid C, Landa M, et al: Angiotensin-converting enzyme inhibitors and the progression of non-diabetic renal disease: A meta-analysis of patient level data. Ann Intern Med 135:73–87, 2001.

Jafar T, Stark P, Schmid C, et al: Progression of chronic kidney disease: The role of blood pressure control, proteinuria, and angiotensin-converting enzyme inhibition. A patient-level meta-analysis. Ann Intern Med 139:244–252, 2003.

Jungers P, Massy ZA, Nguyen-Khoa T, et al: Longer duration of predialysis nephrological care is associated with improved long-term survival of dialysis patients. Nephrol Dial Transplant 16:2357–2364, 2001.

Kinchen K, Sadler J, Fink N, et al: The timing of specialist evaluation in chronic kidney disease and mortality. Ann Intern Med 137:479–483, 2002.

Klahr S, Levey AS, Beck GJ, et al: The effects of dietary protein restriction and blood-pressure control on the progression of chronic renal disease. N Engl J Med 330:877–884, 1994.

Levey AS, Bosch JP, Lewis JB, et al: A more accurate method to estimate glomerular filtration rate from serum creatinine: A new prediction equation. Modification of Diet in Renal Disease Study Group. Ann Intern Med 130:461–470, 1999.

Levey A, Coresh J, Balk E, et al: National Kidney Foundation practice guidelines for chronic kidney disease: Evaluation, classification, and stratification. Ann Intern Med 139: 137–147, 2003.

Levin A, Lewis M, Mortiboy P, et al: Multidisciplinary predialysis programs: Quantification and limitations of their impact on patient outcomes in two Canadian settings. Am J Kidney Dis 29:533–540, 1997.

Lindeman R, Tobin J, Shock N: Longitudinal studies on the rate of decline in renal function with age. J Am Geriatr Soc 33:278–285, 1985.

National Kidney Foundation. K/DOQI clinical practice guidelines for chronic kidney disease: Evaluation, classification, and stratification. Am J Kidney Dis 39(2 suppl 1):S1–S266, 2002.

National Kidney Foundation: K/DOQI clinical practice guidelines for hypertension and antihypertensive agents in chronic kidney disease. Am J Kidney Dis 43(5 suppl 1):S1–S290, 2004.

Remuzzi G, Ruggenenti P, Perico N: Chronic renal diseases: Renoprotective benefits of renin-angiotensin system inhibition. Ann Intern Med 136:604–615, 2002.

Sarnak M, Levey A, Schoolwerth A, et al: Kidney disease as a risk factor for development of cardiovascular disease: A statement from the American Heart Association Councils on Kidney in Cardiovascular Disease, High Blood Pressure Research, Clinical Cardiology, and Epidemiology and Prevention. Circulation 42:1050–1065, 2003.

UK Prospective Diabetes Study (UKPDS) Group: Intensive blood-glucose control with sulphonylureas or insulin compared with conventional treatment and risk of complications in patients with type 2 diabetes (UKPDS 33). Lancet 352: 837–853, 1998.

USRDS 2000 Annual Data Report: Atlas of End-Stage Renal Disease in the United States. 2001, Bethesda, Maryland, National Institutes of Health, National Institute of Diabetes and Digestive and Kidney Diseases, 2000.

Wright JJ, Bakris G, Greene T, et al: Effect of blood pressure lowering and antihypertensive drug class on progression of hypertensive kidney disease: Results from the AASK trial. JAMA 288:2421–2431, 2001.

CHAPTER 60

Hemodialysis and Hemofiltration*

Alfred K. Cheung

STRUCTURE OF HEMODIALYZERS AND HEMOFILTERS

Extracorporeal therapy for kidney failure refers to the process by which fluid and solutes are removed from or added to the patient's blood outside the body. During this process, blood from the patient is continuously circulated through a hemodialyzer or hemofilter containing an artificial semipermeable membrane, and then returned to the patient. A typical modern hemodialyzer is made up of several thousand parallel hollow fibers. The wall of these fibers is the semipermeable membrane separating the blood in the fiber lumen from the dialysate outside. The total internal surface area of all the fibers is usually between 0.5 and $2.0\,m^2$, although some dialyzers are even larger in order to provide greater solute transport. Less commonly, the membranes are in the form of flat plates rather than hollow fibers. The blood path either in the lumen of the hollow fibers or between the plates converges into a single inlet on one end and a single outlet on the other end of the dialyzer's plastic casing. Also in the dialyzer casing are an inlet and an outlet for the dialysate compartment that are separate from those for the blood. Dialysate is usually circulated in a single-pass fashion, countercurrent to the blood flow. Since hemofiltration does not utilize dialysate, hemofilters that are specifically designed for hemofiltration have an inlet and an outlet for blood but only a single outlet for the ultrafiltrate compartment.

TYPES OF EXTRACORPOREAL THERAPY FOR KIDNEY FAILURE

Hemodialysis removes solutes by diffusion, based on concentration gradients of solutes between the blood and dialysate across the semipermeable membrane (Fig. 60-1A). For example, urea diffuses from the blood to the dialysate compartment, thereby decreasing the total urea mass in the body as well as the urea concentration in the plasma. Conversely, the concentration gradient of bicarbonate usually favors the diffusion of this ion from the dialysate to the blood compartment. Movement of water carrying solutes across the dialysis membrane is not necessary for solute transport in this modality, although removal of fluid from the patient's plasma is often desirable because these patients are usually volume over-loaded. High efficiency in hemodialysis refers to a high rate of removal by diffusion of small-sized solutes, whereas high flux in hemodialysis refers to a high rate of removal by diffusion of "middle molecules" that are substantially larger than urea (Table 60-1).

Hemofiltration is another form of extracorporeal therapy that removes fluid by convection; in other words, movement of solutes across the large-pore hemofiltration membrane into the ultrafiltrate compartment drags along the solutes that are dissolved in the water (Fig. 60-1B). An important distinction between hemodialysis and hemofiltration is that fluid removal, but not a concentration gradient for the solute, is required for solute removal in hemofiltration. Removal of fluid with its accompanying solutes results in a loss in the total body mass of the solute, but not necessarily a decrease in the plasma concentration. To achieve a substantial decrease in the concentration, "clean" replacement fluid devoid of that solute is infused intravenously so as to approximately replace the large volume of plasma fluid removed in the hemofilter. This modality is analogous to glomerular filtration, in which plasma solutes are also removed by convection. In the case of the glomerulus, however, the replacement fluid is the water and electrolytes that are selectively reabsorbed from the renal tubules (Fig. 60-1C). Hemodiafiltration refers to the combination of hemodialysis and hemofiltration operating simultaneously using a large-pore membrane; that is, solutes are removed by both diffusion and convection.

When hemodialysis, hemofiltration, or hemodiafiltration are applied continuously for days to weeks in the setting of acute renal failure, they are referred to as continuous renal replacement therapy (CRRT). The terms are further qualified by the forms of vascular access used. For example, continuous hemofiltration using an artery for blood supply and a vein for blood return for the extracorporeal circuit is called continuous arteriovenous dialysis (CAVH). Continuous hemodiafiltration using veins exclusively for vascular access is called continuous vevovenous hemodiafiltration (CVVHDF). A rather common form of CRRT is slow (or sustained) low-efficiency hemodialysis (SLED).

Hemoperfusion is the removal of solutes (usually toxins) from blood by adsorption onto materials, such as charcoal or resins, in the extracorporeal circuit. Hemoperfusion is primarily used for the treatment of acute

---

*This chapter is in the public domain.

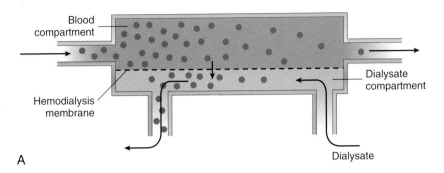

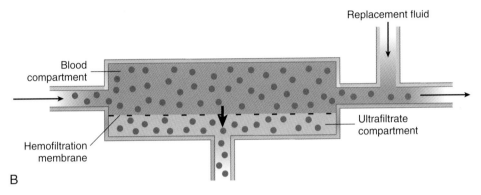

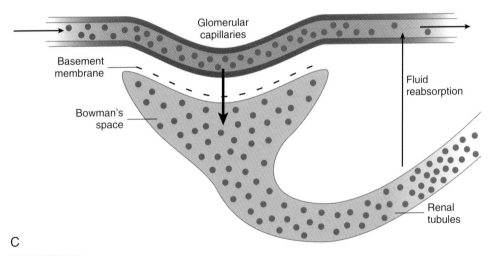

FIGURE 60-1   Schematic representation of solute and fluid transport across the semipermeable artificial membranes and glomerular basement membrane. *A,* Hemodialyzer. Thé plasma concentration of small-sized solutes (*solid circles*) in the blood inlet is high. Because of the diffusive loss across the semipermeable hemodialysis membrane (*broken line*), the plasma concentration in the blood outlet is much lower. The thin arrow across the dialysis membrane represents a small amount of fluid loss (which is not necessary for solute removal). High dialysate flow rate is necessary to maintain the concentration gradient across the dialysis membrane for solute removal. *B,* Hemofilter. Plasma concentrations of small-sized solutes in the blood compartment remain unchanged as blood travels the length of the fiber and are similar to their concentrations in the ultrafiltrate. The hemofiltration membrane (*broken line*) has relatively large pores, which allow the necessary removal of a large volume of fluid (*heavy arrow*). Replacement fluid is infused into the blood outlet to lower the plasma concentration of solutes and compensate for the fluid loss. *C,* Glomerulus. Analogous to hemofiltration, plasma concentration of small solutes remains unchanged throughout the length of the glomerular capillary and is similar to that in Bowman's space. Fluid removal across the glomerular basement membrane (*broken curve*) is large (*heavy arrow*). Reabsorption of fluid from the renal tubules lowers the plasma concentration of the solutes.

TABLE 60-1   Glossary of Various Types of Extracorporeal Therapy for Kidney Failure

A. Hemodialysis (HD)
   1. Conventional hemodialysis uses a conventional low-efficiency, low-flux membrane. Solute removal is primarily by diffusion.
   2. High-efficiency hemodialysis uses a membrane with high efficiency (K_oA) for removal of small-sized solutes, which is typically achieved by a larger surface area and a high blood flow rate.
   3. High-flux hemodialysis uses a membrane with large pore sizes. It is more efficient in removing middle molecules.
   4. Slow or sustained low-efficiency dialysis (SLED) is a continuous low-efficiency hemodialysis using a low blood flow rate and low dialysate flow rate. Continuous venovenous hemodialysis (CVVHD) is practically synonymous with SLED.

B. Hemofiltration (HF)
   1. Continuous arteriovenous or venovenous hemofiltration (CAVH/CVVH) is the removal of small-sized solutes and middle molecules using a high-flux membrane and convection rather than diffusion. Blood is obtained from either an artery using the driving force deriving from the systemic arterial pressure or a vein using an external blood pump, respectively. The blood is returned to a vein in either case. Because it is performed continuously (usually in the intensive care setting), it is also very effective in removing large amounts of fluid.
   2. Intermittent hemofiltration is performed on an intermittent basis for endstage renal disease (ESRD).

C. Hemodiafiltration (HDF)
   1. Continuous arteriovenous hemodiafiltration (CAVHDF/CVVHDF) is similar to CAVH/CVVH in that solutes are removed by convection using a high-flux membrane, usually in the intensive care setting. In addition, dialysate flows continuously through the dialysate compartment to enhance solute removal by diffusion (i.e., it is a combination of hemodialysis and hemofiltration).
   2. Intermittent hemodiafiltration is performed on an intermittent basis for ESRD, often employing a hemodiafiltration machine that also generates sterile pyrogen-free replacement fluid continuously.

D. Hemoperfusion (HP)
   Removal of solutes by adsorption to charcoal or resin, primarily for treatment of acute poisoning.

poisoning. New adsorbents that are effective in removing β_2-microglobulin (β_2M) and other middle molecules are currently in clinical trials in patients with endstage renal disease (ESRD).

HEMODIALYSIS AND HEMOFILTRATION MEMBRANES

Performance and, to a lesser extent, biocompatibility are two characteristics of dialysis membranes that are of interest to clinical nephrologists. Cellulose (a constituent of plants) and synthetic polymers are the two types of material used to fabricate dialysis membranes. Modification of the chemical structure of cellulose results in "modified cellulosic" or "substituted cellulosic" membranes that are more commonly used than unmodified cellulosic membranes. The type of material bears some relationship to biocompatibility and performance, but there are sufficient overlaps such that a dialysis membrane cannot be adequately described only by the material from which it is constructed.

Besides classification according to their composition, dialysis membranes are also classified as low flux or high flux (Table 60-2). Low-flux membranes have small pores that restrict the transport of middle molecules and water, whereas high-flux membranes have large pores that facilitate transport of middle molecules and have high ultrafiltration coefficients, as described later. Modified cellulosic membranes and synthetic membranes can both be fabricated into either high-flux or low-flux dialyzers.

Biocompatibility of dialysis membranes refers to the interactions that occur as a result of contact of blood with the membrane. Examples include the activation of proteins of the coagulation and complement system, as well as various peripheral blood leukocytes and platelets. Biocompatibility is relative, since all dialysis membranes induce reactions to a certain extent; such reactions can manifest, for example, as thrombosis in the dialyzer and rarely as acute anaphylactoid reactions. When in vitro assays of blood collected during hemodialysis are used to determine biocompatibility, unmodified cellulosic membranes appear to be least biocompatible. Epidemiologic

TABLE 60-2   Performance of Different Types of Dialyzers and Hemofilters

	Urea K_oA[*]	Urea Clearance[†]	Ultrafiltration Coefficient	β_2M Clearance[‡]
Dialyzers				
Conventional	<450 mL/min	<150 mL/min	<12 mL/hr/mm Hg	<10 mL/min
High-efficiency	>600 mL/min	>200 mL/min	Variable	Variable
High-flux	Variable	Variable	>12 mL/hr/mm Hg	>20 mL/min
Hemofilters	N.A.[‡]	Variable	>12 mL/hr/mm Hg	>20 mL/min

[*]Product of mass transfer coenefficient × surface area.
[†]Under usual operating conditions.
[‡]Not applicable because the K_oA of a membrane describes its diffusive transport capability, whereas urea clearance in the hemofiltration (convective) mode depends on the filtration rate.

studies also suggest that unmodified cellulosic low-flux membranes are associated with higher patient mortality as compared with synthetic membranes, an adverse outcome that is not shared by modified cellulosic membranes. These studies, however, do not distinguish between the effect of biocompatibility and that of flux. The use of unmodified cellulosic dialysis membrane also appears to be associated with worse recovery in kidney function and patient mortality in acute renal failure. Although they are not definitive, these clinical studies and the plausible biologic basis of membrane incompatibility suggest that membrane materials could indeed affect clinical outcomes. Unmodified cellulosic membranes are rarely used in the United States at present. Hemofiltration membranes are always high flux and are usually made of synthetic materials. Although synthetic membranes are in general considered to be more biocompatible, they are not immune from bioincompatibility reactions.

WATER TRANSPORT AND SOLUTE CLEARANCE PROFILES

The ability of dialysis membranes to transport small-sized solutes, such as urea (molecular mass 60 Daltons) and potassium (31 Daltons), is usually expressed as the mass transfer–area coefficient, which is the product of the mass transfer coefficient (K_o) and membrane surface area (A). High-efficiency dialyzers are those with high K_oA values (greater than 600 mL/minute; see Table 60-2), which are usually achieved using large surface areas, whereas low-efficiency dialyzers are those with low K_oA values (less than 450 mL/minute). The clearance profile of solutes by hemodialysis membranes presented in Figure 60-2 reflects primarily the K_oA of the membranes and only provides a rough estimation of what might be achieved clinically. The actual solute clearance depends also on the rate of blood flow that presents the solute to the dialyzer, the rate of dialysate flow that provides the diffusion gradient, and the rate of fluid removal that supplements the diffusion by convective loss of the solute. The blood flow rate is particularly crucial, since it limits the amount of blood that is available for clearance by the dialyzer at any given time. Diffusive clearance of solutes by hemodialysis decreases rapidly with increasing molecular size. For small solutes such as urea, however, removal per unit time by high-efficiency hemodialysis (180 to 240 mL/minute) is close to two times that achieved by the glomeruli in two native kidneys (90 to 120 mL/minute for adults), which, in turn, is significantly higher than the urinary excretory rate of urea after tubular reabsorption. However, patients spend only 9 to 15 hours per week on hemodialysis, whereas native kidneys function continuously for a total of 168 hours per week. As a result, the total weekly clearance of urea by hemodialysis is far lower than that achieved in a patient with normal functioning kidneys.

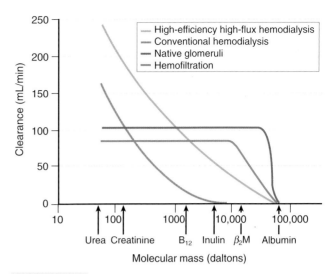

FIGURE 60-2 Solute clearance profile of various modalities. The curves are constructed partially from data and partially from theoretical projection. The actual values may vary depending on the surface area of the membrane and operating conditions, such as blood flow rate. "Native glomeruli" refers to the summation of all the glomeruli in two normal kidneys. "Glomeruli" instead of "kidneys" are used, because tubular reabsorption lowers substantially the renal clearance of certain solutes (e.g., urea and glucose). Clearance of solutes by diffusion (either conventional or high-efficiency, high-flux dialysis) deteriorates rapidly with an increase in the molecular mass of the solute. In contrast, clearance by convection (hemofiltration or glomeruli) remains constant over a wide range of molecular mass. B_{12}, vitamin B_{12}; β_2M, β_2-microglobulin.

The effectiveness of water transport across a dialysis or hemofiltration membrane is measured as the ultrafiltration coefficient, defined as the volume of water transported per unit time, normalized by the transmembrane hydrostatic pressure gradient. Ultrafiltration coefficients for low-flux hemodialysis membranes are usually 2 to 5 mL/hour/mm Hg. With a transmembrane pressure of 200 mm Hg, a dialyzer with a coefficient of 2.5 mL/hour/mm Hg will remove 0.5 L of fluid per hour, or 2 L in 4 hours. Ultrafiltration coefficients for high-flux dialysis or hemofiltration membranes are much higher, at 12 to 60 mL/hour/mm Hg. It should be noted that extracorporeal fluid removal from a patient is usually limited by the rate at which fluid can be mobilized into the intravascular compartment, and is almost never limited by the porosity or flux of the dialysis membrane.

The ability of the membrane to clear middle molecules is governed by the size of the membrane pores and the membrane surface area, and is closely related to the ultrafiltration coefficient. Middle molecules are solutes that are significantly larger than urea but are smaller than albumin (60,000 Daltons); these are often represented by the protein β_2M (11,800 Daltons). Thus, low-flux dialyzers are those with β_2M clearances that have been arbitrarily defined as less than 10 mL/minute and are often close to nil, whereas high-flux dialyzers have β_2M clearances greater than 20 mL/minute under normal operating conditions of the flow rates of blood and dialysate. Diffusive clearance of solutes, however, decreases rapidly with increases in molecular size and is usually only 20 to 60 mL/minute for β_2M, even by high-flux hemodialysis, compared with greater than 150 mL/minute for urea. In contrast to diffusion, solute transport by convection through high-flux membranes is unrestricted and independent of solute size, up to a certain point. Therefore, the clearance of β_2M can be as high as the ultrafiltration rate during intermittent hemofiltration, which is often greater than 100 mL/minute.

The efficiency (i.e., ability to clear small solutes) and flux (i.e., ability to clear middle molecules) are not related to each other. Thus, high-efficiency membranes can be either high flux (large surface area and large pores) or low flux (large surface area but small pores), and low-efficiency membranes can also be either low flux or high flux. Similarly, high-flux membranes can be either high efficiency (large pores and large surface area) or low efficiency (large pores but small surface area). Conventional membranes that were used most commonly in the 1970s and 1980s, are low flux and low efficiency. Although their popularity has significantly declined in the United States, they are still used frequently in other parts of the world.

DIALYSATE

The dialysate creates solute concentration gradients to drive diffusion across the dialysis membrane. The typical composition of dialysate for hemodialysis is shown in Table 60-3. Dialysate sodium is usually kept at concentrations similar to or even slightly higher than that in plasma. Therefore, sodium is removed primarily by convection during hemodialysis. The ultrafiltration of 4 liters of isotonic fluid results in approximately 560 mEq or 13 g of sodium removal without a change in plasma sodium concentration. In contrast, dialysate potassium concentration is often kept low to decrease plasma potassium concentration. Because dialysis patients are generally acidemic, base in the form of either bicarbonate or acetate is offered. Acetate dialysate is slightly less expensive but has the disadvantages of inducing hypoxemia and a transient worsening of metabolic acidosis because of the initial loss of bicarbonate from the plasma. It also causes intradialytic hypotension, cardiac arrhythmias, and an ill sensation in some patients. Proportioning systems in modern machines have made delivery of bicarbonate dialysate a relatively easy task. Dialysates containing primarily acetate are rarely used in the United States, although they are still prevalent in some other countries. Calcium concentration in the dialysate varies depending on the specific need of the patient to gain or lose calcium (see Chapter 64). When citrate is used as the anticoagulant in the extracorporeal circuit (see later), the dialysate must be devoid of calcium to prevent thrombosis. Dialysate magnesium concentration is sometimes lowered so that the patient can tolerate oral magnesium-containing phosphate binders. Glucose is usually provided at 200 mg/dL to maintain the plasma glucose level stable for both diabetic and nondiabetic patients and to avoid hypoglycemia. Minimizing the concentration of trace metals (e.g., aluminum), microorganisms, bacterial products (e.g., endotoxins), disinfectants (e.g., chloramine), and other contaminants in the dialysate is also important.

HEMODIALYSIS AND HEMOFILTRATION MACHINES

The dialysis machine incorporates many important features, such as a pump to deliver blood to the dialyzer at a constant rate up to approximately 500 mL/minute, monitors to ensure that the pressures inside the extracorporeal circuit are not excessive, a detector for leakage of red blood cells from the blood compartment into the dialysate compartment, an air detector and shut-off device to prevent air embolism, a pump to deliver dialysate, a proportioning system for proper dilution of the dialysate concentrates, a heater to warm the dialysate to approximately body temperature, an ultrafiltration controller for precise regulation of fluid removal, and conductivity monitors to check the total ion strength in the dialysate. These devices ensure the proper, safe, and reliable delivery of blood and dialysate to the filter, where exchange of water and solutes takes place. Some modern machines also incorporate more sophisticated features, such as devices that detect changes in the patient's intravascular volume and programs that alter the ultrafiltration rate and dialysate osmolality during the course of the treatment according to individual patient needs so as to maintain the intravascular volume and prevent symptomatic hypotension.

TABLE 60-3 Composition of Dialysate Commonly Used in Clinical Hemodialysis

Ions	Concentrations
Na^+	132–145 mEq/L*
K^+	0–4.0 mEq/L†
Cl^-	103–110 mEq/L
HCO_3^-	0–40 mEq/L
Acetate‡	2–37 mEq/L
Ca^{2+}	0–3.5 mEq/L†
Mg^{2+}	0.5–1.0 mEq/L
Glucose	0–200 mg/dL

*Higher dialysate sodium concentration is sometimes used in "sodium modeling."
†The use of zero concentration of K^+ or Ca^{2+} is rare because of their association with arrhythmia.
‡Either HCO_3^- or acetate is used as the primary buffer; the use of acetate as the primary buffer is uncommon in the United States.

Machines used for intermittent (e.g., three times a week) hemofiltration are similar to those for hemodialysis, with the additional requirements for precise fluid replacement control and online generation of sterile replacement fluids in some machines. In contrast, CAVH does not require any machinery. Blood is delivered to the hemofilter from an artery, such as the femoral artery, via a large-bore (about 14- to 15-gauge) catheter and returned to a large vein, with the driving force derived from the systemic arterial blood pressure rather than a mechanical pump. Unfortunately, blood flow and therefore hemofilter transmembrane pressure and ultrafiltration rates are sometimes erratic in CAVH. Currently, it is more customary to use specially designed machines that pump blood from a vein through the hemofilter and back to a vein, a technique known as continuous venovenous hemofiltration (CVVH). The machines for CVVH are usually simpler in design than conventional hemodialysis machines, since dialysate production and many other features are absent. One disadvantage of CAVH and CVVH is that they are less efficient than hemodialysis in removing urea, potassium, and other small solutes, because there is no dialysate to permit diffusion. To improve solute clearance, continuous dialysate flow is sometimes added to these systems; these techniques are known as continuous arteriovenous hemodiafiltration (CAVHDF) and CVVHDF. Unfortunately, the addition of dialysate also adds complexity to these systems. As a result, CVVHDF machines are in fact quite similar to regular hemodialysis machines.

VASCULAR ACCESS

Maintenance of vascular access is a major challenge for chronic hemodialysis. An adequate vascular access should permit blood flow to the dialyzer of 200 to 500 mL/minute in adults, depending on the size of the patient. In the United States, there is a tendency to use blood pump speeds of 350 to 500 mL/minute, whereas blood pump speeds of 200 to 250 mL/minute are common in Asia. This discrepancy is partly due to the smaller body size in the Asian population, but also because the benefits of very high clearances of small solutes in chronic hemodialysis have not been clearly established. For acute hemodialysis, a large vein, such as the femoral vein, is often cannulated with a double-lumen catheter. One lumen is used to extract the blood from the patient (the "arterial" side, even though it comes from the patient's vein), and the other lumen is used to return blood to the patient ("venous" side). Temporary femoral catheters are seldom left in place for more than one dialysis session unless the patient is confined to bed, because catheters in this location are prone to kinking, dislodgement, and infection.

For usage of several weeks or longer, an indwelling double-lumen catheter or twin single-lumen catheters with a cuff for anchoring are tunneled under the skin and placed in an internal jugular or subclavian vein by a surgeon, an interventional radiologist, or an interventional nephrologist. These catheters allow blood flow rates in excess of 400 mL/minute and are most suitable in the setting of acute renal failure or as an intermediate measure while waiting for the maturation of a permanent arteriovenous (AV) access for chronic dialysis (see later). Unfortunately, they are often used as a form of permanent vascular access because of convenience or poor alternatives. These catheters can become infected, be dislodged, or be occluded by thrombi. In addition, catheters at these sites predispose the vessels to stenosis. Stenosis of these vessels causes obstruction to venous return, which is especially problematic if a permanent arteriovenous fistula, with arterialized venous pressure and augmented blood flow, is present in the ipsilateral arm. Severe swelling, pain, and dysfunction of the arteriovenous access in the ipsilateral arm may result. Stenosis of the superior vena cava sometimes occurs. Subclavian veins appear to be more likely to develop stenosis than internal jugular veins and therefore should be avoided if at all possible. Femoral veins and, very rarely, the hepatic vein and the inferior vena cava, approached from the back, are also used when no other options are available.

The lumina of these catheters are filled with an anticoagulant, most often heparin, in between dialysis sessions. The anticoagulant is removed by aspiration immediately before use of the catheter at the next dialysis session. If thrombosis inside these catheters still occurs, it can sometimes be resolved by the local instillation of thrombolytic agents. Under no circumstances should high pressure with a syringe be applied, because dislodgement of the clot can result in pulmonary embolism.

Long-term vascular access for hemodialysis is usually established by the creation of an AV fistula in an upper extremity, although a lower extremity or even an axillary vessel may sometimes be used. A fistula is established by connecting an artery to a nearby vein, either by direct surgical anastomosis of the native vessels or with a synthetic graft—for example, one made of polytetrafluoroethylene (PTFE). Rarely, a bovine arterial segment is used as the fistula. Native fistulae are preferred over PTFE grafts because of their relative longevity (approximately 80% vs. 50% patency in 3 years) and lower susceptibility to infection. The disadvantages are the requirement for sufficiently large native veins and a 4- to 16-week maturation period during which the wall of the fistula thickens and the lumen enlarges before the fistula can be cannulated with large-bore needles for dialysis. PTFE grafts can be used earlier, occasionally at 1 week or less. However, they tend to elicit acute transient local inflammatory reactions manifested by pain, swelling, and redness that resemble infectious cellulitis but usually subside spontaneously within a few weeks. PTFE grafts are also more prone to thrombosis and infection, but the convenience that they offer has continued to make them a popular choice among many dialysis personnel in the United States. Declotting of AV access can be accomplished surgically, with local infusion of thrombolytic agents or mechanical devices inserted percutaneously to disperse the clot. In general, the reestablishment of blood flow is more successful in a graft than in a native AV fistula.

Stenosis at the outflow tract of AV fistulae, especially PTFE grafts, occurs frequently and represents the major cause of failure of these accesses. The stenosis is almost exclusively caused by neointimal hyperplasia, which comprises proliferating myofibroblasts and deposition of extracellular matrices, very similar to that seen in coronary artery restenosis. Partial obstruction of the dialysis access impedes the flow of cleansed blood from the dialyzer back to the central veins; as a result, the blood recirculates back to the "arterial" (afferent) limb of the fistula and decreases the amount of fresh systemic blood delivered to the dialyzer. Hence, the overall efficiency of the dialysis process is diminished. Obstruction of the fistula outflow tract also leads to an increase in pressure inside the "venous" (efferent) tubing during hemodialysis; such an event has been used as a clue to the presence of fistula outflow stenosis. Techniques involving noninvasive devices and the dilution principle have been developed to assess the total blood flow through AV fistulae. These monitoring techniques are performed during hemodialysis. In fact, the monitoring equipment is sometimes built in as a component of the dialysis machine. Detection of gradual decreases in total blood flow rates through the fistula over time allows earlier detection of stenosis. It is unclear, however, if regular monitoring of flow rates and earlier interventions result in the prolongation of the useful life of vascular accesses. In some centers, Doppler ultrasonography performed outside the dialysis setting is commonly used for the diagnosis of vascular access stenosis. An angiogram (also called "fistulogram" in this context), with the injection of contrast dye (or carbon dioxide for patients who are allergic to contrast), however, remains the gold standard for the confirmation and anatomic definition of AV fistula stenosis. The fistulogram is also helpful in searching for collateral veins, which are impediments for the growth and maturation of native fistulae. Fistula stenosis is treated surgically by replacing or bypassing the stenotic segment. Alternatively, the stenosis may be relieved by percutaneous balloon angioplasty, with or without the placement of a stent to keep the lumen patent. Although it temporarily restores the flow and usefulness of the vascular access, a major problem with angioplasty is that the trauma induced by the balloon actually predisposes the vessel wall to further stenosis, thus establishing a vicious cycle. If left untreated, most stenotic vascular accesses eventually become totally occluded by thrombi. The value of systemic antiplatelet agents to prevent AV graft occlusion is unclear. In a recent study, the combination of aspirin and clopidogrel did not result in longer survival of AV grafts but increased the incidence of systemic bleeding. A large multicenter trial using the combination of aspirin and dipyridamole is currently in progress. Various pharmacologic and radiation strategies are being investigated to prevent dialysis graft stenosis, so as to make synthetic grafts a better option. Until those strategies materialize, the native AV fistula remains the preferred vascular access.

Vascular access infection is common and is particularly prevalent with catheters, where the infection rate is 15 times higher than in native fistulae. Furthermore, bacteremia is frequent with catheter infections. The clinical manifestations of catheter infection, and even the bacteremia, can be indolent. Endocarditis is a detrimental complication of catheter infection and bacteremia when treatment is delayed; therefore, a high index of suspicion is required in these patients. Catheter infection without signs at the exit site is usually diagnosed by blood cultures obtained directly from the catheter. Graft infections are sometimes manifested by gross signs on the overlying skin, such as erythema, fluctuance, or purulent drainage. Deep infections can sometimes be detected using nuclear scans with radiolabeled leukocytes. The infecting organisms for all forms of vascular access are the usual pathogens, such as *Staphylococcus* and Gram-negative bacteria. Mild infection can be treated with antibiotics alone. Although they are more difficult to treat conservatively, infected PTFE grafts do not invariably require surgical removal. Catheter infection complicated by bacteremia is best treated by prompt catheter removal along with antibiotics, unless vascular access is extremely difficult for the patient.

The spontaneous blood flow through an AV fistula or graft often exceeds 1 L/minute and occasionally 2.5 L/minute, accounting for 20% to 40% of cardiac output, although the blood flow through the dialysis needles to the dialyzer is considerably lower. This diversion of cardiac output from the capillary beds by the fistula can cause distal ischemia, also known as steal syndrome. Rarely, it can precipitate or exacerbate congestive heart failure. Surgical ligation or banding to decrease the luminal diameter of the fistula is sometimes necessary.

Early planning and placement of a permanent native AV fistula before the patient requires chronic dialysis should take place when the patient reaches stage 4 chronic kidney disease, so as to avoid the emergency placement of catheters when the patient becomes frankly uremic. The recent popularity of mapping of the arm veins using ultrasound to identify a suitable vessel has increased the use of native fistulae. Nonetheless, in patients with poor veins or inadequate planning to allow time for the maturation of the native fistula, synthetic grafts will need to be used. The tunneled venous catheter should be considered as a temporary measure, until the AV access is ready for use. For patients with a short life expectancy or when sites for AV access are no longer available, these catheters can be used for 2 years or even longer, although infection and obstruction typically require that they be replaced sooner. Percutaneous catheters, which are not tunneled under the skin, must be used only as a temporary access. The internal jugular vein on the contralateral side of the planned AV fistula is preferable to avoid the complications of central vein stenosis. Repeat catheterization of femoral veins for individual dialysis sessions, especially for short periods, is a reasonable alternative.

ANTICOAGULATION

Exposure of blood to the extracorporeal circuit activates the clotting mechanisms. Heparin is the main anticoagulant used for acute and chronic hemodialysis and hemofiltration. It is often given as an intravenous bolus of 1000 to 5000 units at the beginning of the session, followed by continuous infusion at 500 to 2000 units/hour. The monitoring of activated clotting time or partial thrombin time is mandatory for CRRT in the intensive care units but is seldom performed in the clinical dialysis setting. For patients in whom systemic anticoagulation is risky, lower dose heparin (termed by some "tight" or "minimum" heparin) can be used with careful observation of the extracorporeal circuit for clotting. Hemodialysis can sometimes be performed without using any anticoagulants. Underlying coagulation defects, high blood flow rates through the dialyzer, and periodic flushing of the blood compartment with saline are helpful to prevent clotting under these circumstances. This technique is most often indicated in patients who are actively bleeding or who have recently had an intracranial bleeding episode.

Regional heparinization is another technique to minimize systemic anticoagulation. In this technique, heparin is infused into the "arterial" blood entering the dialyzer and is then neutralized by infusion of protamine sulfate into the "venous" line. The beneficial effect of regional heparinization in preventing systemic bleeding has not been convincingly demonstrated. Regional citrate is a similar technique in which calcium-free dialysate is used. The citrate solution infused into the arterial tubing chelates serum calcium, inhibiting activation of the coagulation cascade. Calcium infused into the venous tubing restores the serum calcium concentration before the blood is returned to the patient. Regional citrate anticoagulation is useful not only for patients who are at risk for systemic bleeding but also for patients with heparin-induced thrombocytopenia, in whom heparin cannot be used for extracorporeal anticoagulation. The disadvantages of regional citrate anticoagulation are that the serum concentration of ionized calcium must be carefully monitored, the dosages of citrate and calcium are sometimes difficult to titrate, and the additional volume and alkali associated with the citrate administration have to be accounted for. The antiplatelet agent prostacyclin has also been used successfully, albeit rarely, as a systemic anticoagulant during clinical hemodialysis. Hypotension can be a significant side effect of this medication.

INDICATIONS AND SCHEDULES FOR HEMODIALYSIS AND HEMOFILTRATION

Acute hemodialysis is primarily performed for acute renal failure and drug overdose. Indications for emergency dialysis in the acute renal failure setting include fluid overload (often with pulmonary edema), hyperkalemia (often with serum potassium higher than 7 mEq/L), and uremic signs and symptoms (see Chapter 39 for more details). Depending on the circumstances, the initiation of dialysis before the onset of these problems is preferable. If reversal of the acute renal failure does not appear to be imminent, dialysis is often instituted when the blood urea nitrogen (BUN) is around 70 to 80 mg/dL or estimated glomerular filtration rate is 5 to 10 mL/minute, before overt clinical symptoms occur. On the other hand, when some return of kidney function is immediately expected, for example, upon the relief of urinary tract obstruction, fluid overload and hyperkalemia are not necessarily absolute indications for acute dialysis. Intermittent hemodialysis is usually performed thrice weekly for acute renal failure, although extra sessions are added as needed. Some have also advocated hemodialysis on a daily basis. Beyond the need in some individual patients based on clinical judgment, the benefits of routine daily hemodialysis for acute renal failure are unclear (see later).

Continuous extracorporeal therapies, such as CAVH and CVVH, are particularly useful for patients in the intensive care unit whose cardiovascular status is too unstable for rapid fluid removal, as may occur during intermittent hemodialysis. These therapies are also used for patients from whom removal of substantial amounts of fluid on a continuous basis is desired, for example, patients with multiorgan trauma receiving parenteral nutrition, blood products, and various intravenous medications. Clearances of urea and potassium by CAVH and CVVH are sometimes inadequate to maintain plasma concentrations of these solutes in the desirable range. Under these circumstances, continuous dialysate flow is added to the system using CAVHDF or CVVHDF. The limited available data have not demonstrated a clearly superior clinical outcome associated with continuous therapy compared with intermittent hemodialysis. Peritoneal dialysis is another form of continuous therapy that can be used for patients suffering from acute renal failure with unstable hemodynamics, but for technical reasons it has been largely replaced by extracorporeal modalities in this setting. Rarely, peritoneal dialysis is performed in the United States for acute renal failure accompanying severe pancreatitis or when hemodialysis is not available. The majority of acute renal failure cases are still treated with intermittent hemodialysis, although there is a gradual increase in the use of continuous extracorporeal modalities.

Maintenance dialysis for ESRD is usually started at a glomerular filtration rate of 7 to 10 mL/minute, unless the clinical conditions dictate earlier intervention. Some have advocated the initiation of chronic dialysis even earlier. The optimal timing of initiation of chronic dialysis has not been established and is the objective of an ongoing Australian trial. Hemodialysis is used in approximately 90% of the ESRD patients in the United States, with the remaining 10% using peritoneal dialysis. It is usually conducted in-center in a dialysis unit and far less often at home, with a thrice-weekly schedule and 3 to 5 hours each time. If fluid overload becomes a significant problem, a fourth session is sometimes added. Restrictions on reimbursement have limited more frequent chronic dialysis. In a small number of dialysis programs, hemodialysis is performed for 8 to 10 hours three times a week either in the daytime or at night (nocturnal hemodialysis), or even for a few hours six times a week (daily hemodialysis). A limited literature that is largely anecdotal suggests that these more intense hemodialysis schedules are associated with better control of blood chemistry, lower blood pressure, fewer hospitalizations, and improved nutrition and quality of life. A U.S. multicenter randomized trial examining the intermediate outcomes of nocturnal and daily hemodialysis is underway.

Chronic hemofiltration and hemodiafiltration are practically never used for ESRD in the United States, partly because of the reimbursement structure. The advantage of hemofiltration or hemodiafiltration over hemodialysis is the removal of more middle molecules. Since the clinical benefits of removing more middle molecules have not been clearly established (see later), there are no recommendations on which modality should be employed for the ESRD patient. In Europe and Japan, intermittent hemofiltration or hemodiafiltration is used for ESRD more often than in the United States, but it is still used far less frequently than hemodialysis. In Hong Kong and Mexico, peritoneal dialysis is more prevalent than hemodialysis as chronic therapy.

OUTCOMES OF HEMODIALYSIS

There is no consensus on the best method to quantify hemodialysis and the optimal amount of hemodialysis that should be delivered to patients with acute renal failure or ESRD. Not infrequently, an arbitrary session duration, blood flow rate, and dialyzer are used according to the experience and intuition of the nephrologist. Removal of fluid to maintain the patient euvolemic, or slightly hypovolemic, after dialysis is often desirable, but this "dry weight" for individuals is often defined arbitrarily as the weight below which the patient develops symptomatic hypotension or muscle cramps. There are,

of course, many imprecisions associated with this approach. For example, the likelihood of developing hypotension depends not only on the target weight reached but also on the amount of fluid removed and the rate of its removal. Practice standards for fluid assessment techniques and targets have not been established and are sorely needed.

Normalization of plasma electrolytes, such as potassium and hydrogen ions, is obviously important. Because of the role of phosphorus in the pathogenesis of hyperparathyroidism and vascular calcification (see Chapter 64), extracorporeal removal of phosphorus is usually desirable, although this ion is not seldom used as guide for dialytic therapies. Urea has been widely used as a marker to guide dialysis delivery quantification, since it is an index of the production and accumulation of all nitrogenous waste products derived from protein metabolism. In addition, epidemiologic studies have suggested that the removal of urea by hemodialysis correlates with clinical outcome to some extent. In urea kinetic modeling, the index Kt/V is often used for quantitation of the dose of dialysis therapy, where K is the hemodialyzer clearance, t is the duration of the dialysis session, and V is the volume of distribution of urea in the body. A Kt/V value of 1.25 for each hemodialysis session is currently considered to be the minimum dose. Because the V as a fraction of total body weight varies significantly among patients, Kt/V is tedious to determine precisely without a computer. The decrease in BUN during dialysis is often used as a simpler and alternative guide. A postdialysis-to-predialysis BUN ratio of 0.35 or a "urea reduction ratio"—calculated as (predialysis BUN − postdialysis BUN)/(predialysis BUN)—of 65% to 67% is roughly equivalent to a Kt/V of 1.20 to 1.25. The relationship between urea reduction ratio and Kt/V, however, varies depending on the ultrafiltration volume.

The results of a U.S. multicenter trial (the Hemodialysis or HEMO Study) on the clinical effects of higher urea Kt/V and high-flux membrane were published in 2003. In that study, comparisons were made between a urea Kt/V of 1.25, which is the level recommended by the practice guidelines in the United States, and a higher Kt/V of 1.65. Comparisons were also made between low-flux membranes (defined as β_2M clearance of less than 10 mL/minute) and high-flux membranes (defined as β_2M clearance of more than 20 mL/minute). There were no statistically significant differences in all-cause mortality between the two levels of Kt/V and between the two flux arms. However, secondary analysis showed that high-flux dialysis was associated with a decrease in cardiac death. Furthermore, higher urea Kt/V was associated with a decrease in all-cause mortality in women, but not in men. High-flux dialysis was associated with a decrease in all-cause mortality in patients who had been on dialysis for a long period of time (more than 3.7 years). This study did not specifically address different hemodialysis schedules, such as daily or nocturnal dialysis, nor did it address urea Kt/V level below 1.25. Yet, there is no doubt that a very low Kt/V level, such as 0.50, would be associated with poor clinical outcome in anuric patients. On the basis of these results and other epidemiologic studies, it is recommended that urea Kt/V should be maintained at a level above 1.25 for all patients. Consideration should be given to a higher Kt/V for women and the use of high-flux membranes in general. The potential benefits of high-flux membranes also lend support to toxic effects of uremic middle molecules and the removal of these molecules using β_2M as a marker. Further extrapolation of these data would suggest that intermittent hemodiafiltration is the preferred extracorporeal modality for ESRD; however, this notion requires further confirmatory studies.

The optimal amount of acute hemodialysis is even less clear. The dosage of dialysis for the treatment of toxins (e.g., salicylates and lithium) is often guided by the plasma levels of the toxin and the clinical status. Dosage of hemodialysis for acute renal failure has been guided by the plasma chemistries, including BUN, potassium, and bicarbonate, body fluid volume, and other clinical markers, with the objective of maintaining the BUN below about 80 mg/dL most of the time. For example, a patient with transient oliguric acute renal failure and severe hyperkalemia resulting from contrast-induced nephropathy should have the lowering of serum potassium as the primary goal. Whether acute hemodialysis should be quantified using urea Kt/V is unclear. Nonetheless, a randomized study showed that clinical outcome in acute renal failure was influenced by the level of hemofiltration using the ultrafiltered volume as a guide. Patients who were randomized to 35 mL/kg body weight/hour had a higher survival rate than those randomized to 20 mL/kg/hour. Since the removal of both small-sized solutes and middle molecules is increased with a higher ultrafiltration rate in hemofiltration, these results could not distinguish the relative importance of these solutes, but they do suggest that quantitation of extracorporeal therapy is also useful in acute renal failure. A larger multicenter trial comparing a lower dose of CRRT or thrice-weekly acute hemodialysis with a higher dose of CRRT or six times per week of hemodialysis is ongoing in the United States.

COMPLICATIONS OF HEMODIALYSIS

Although hemodialysis is a relatively safe procedure, several complications may still arise. Some are inherent side effects of the normal extracorporeal circuit; some result from technical errors, and yet others are due to abnormal reactions of patients to the procedure. Intradialytic hypotension is common and has been attributed variably to body volume depletion, shifting of fluid from extracellular to intracellular space as a result of a dialysis-induced decrease in serum osmolality, impaired sympathetic activity, vasodilatation in response to warm dialysate, sequestration of blood in the muscles, as well as splanchnic pooling of blood while eating during dialysis. Avoidance of large interdialytic fluid gain, administration of normal saline, hypertonic saline, hypertonic glucose, mannitol, or colloids, decreasing dialysate temperature to produce vasoconstriction, and avoidance of eating during dialysis are sometimes useful to reduce the frequency of hypotensive events. Other strategies that are used to minimize intravascular volume depletion include (1) varying ultrafiltration rates during the session ("ultrafiltration modeling"); (2) isolated ultrafiltration, which removes fluid in the absence of dialysate and therefore does not decrease plasma osmolality and cause intracellular fluid shifts; and (3) "sodium modeling," which tailors dialysate sodium concentrations (135 to 160 mEq/L) during the dialysis session.

Cardiac arrhythmias may occur as a result of rapid electrolyte changes, especially in patients on digitalis and dialyzed against very-low-potassium dialysate (0 to 1 mEq/L). The use of acetate dialysate also appears to induce arrhythmias, which can induce or aggravate hypotension and overt or silent myocardial ischemia. Avoiding rapid changes in electrolytes and fluid volumes by increasing the dialysis duration is perhaps the best strategy to prevent intradialytic arrhythmias.

Muscle cramps, nausea, and vomiting occur commonly during hemodialysis and are often a result of rapid fluid removal. Too rapid removal of urea and other small solutes may lead to the disequilibrium syndrome (see Chapter 67), manifested by headache with nausea and vomiting, altered mental status, seizure, coma, and even death. The pathophysiology of this syndrome is complex and may be related to the rapid decrease in plasma urea concentration and osmolality that causes fluid shifts into the brain and cerebral edema. Severe disequilibrium syndrome is now rare, because hemodialysis is usually initiated at an early stage when the BUN is not yet very high. Nonetheless, the practitioner should remain vigilant, and the efficiency of solute removal should be deliberately limited during the first hemodialysis session.

Dialyzers or dialysates that are contaminated with microorganisms or their toxins can cause fever and/or infection. Hepatitis B was prevalent in the United States in the 1970s, whereas hepatitis C infection is more common in hemodialysis units at present. The mode of transmission of hepatitis C in dialysis units has not been well established.

Anaphylactoid reactions during hemodialysis are rare. They are manifested by various combinations of hypertension or hypotension, pulmonary symptoms, chest and abdominal pain, vomiting, fever, chills, flushing, urticaria, and pruritus. Cardiopulmonary arrest and death rarely ensue. The etiologies are probably multifactorial and may involve activation of plasma complement by dialysis membranes, allergy to disinfectants, or the release of noxious substances that have contaminated the dialyzers during the manufacturing or disinfecting process. Another cause is the accumulation of vasoactive kinins as a result of enhanced activation of kininogen by dialysis membranes made of copolymers of acrylonitrile and methallyl sulfonate, and decreased kinin degradation as a result of the simultaneous administration of angiotensin-converting enzyme inhibitors, which are also kininase inhibitors. Measures to prevent anaphylactoid reactions include thorough rinsing of the dialyzer before use to remove residual ethylene oxide, and avoidance of the type of dialyzer, disinfectant, or medications to which a particular patient is hypersensitive.

Hypoxemia occurs commonly during hemodialysis using acetate, instead of bicarbonate, as the dialysate buffer. The primary mechanism appears to be the initial loss of bicarbonate and carbon dioxide by diffusion into the dialysate, which leads to hypoventilation. Dialysis membrane bioincompatibility may play a role by releasing mediators that impair gas exchange in some instances. A decrease in systemic partial oxygen pressure of 10 to 12 mm Hg is not uncommon, which could be deleterious for patients with underlying cardiopulmonary disease. Acetate dialysate also causes a transient intradialytic decrease in plasma pH. Dialysate containing bicarbonate is therefore preferable.

An array of technical errors associated with hemodialysis has been described, but fortunately they occur very rarely. Inadequate purification of the municipal water before use may result in high levels of contaminants in the dialysate and cause intoxication with metals, such as aluminum or calcium. Contamination of dialysate with chloramine (a disinfectant) and improper proportioning or overheating of dialysate by the dialysis machine lead to hemolysis. Rupture of the dialysis membrane by high transmembrane pressure causes blood loss into the dialysate and entry of microorganisms from the dialysate into the blood. Defective blood circuit and monitoring devices may result in air embolism. Difficult or improper puncture with the dialysis needle may cause a local hematoma around the vascular access or external bleeding, which can be aggravated by the intradialytic administration of heparin.

The most common posthemodialysis symptom is probably asthenia or a generalized "washed-out" sensation, which has been attributed to the relatively rapid changes in fluids and/or serum chemistry. Some patients appear to suffer from this symptom consistently, whereas others appear to be immune. It usually lasts for a few hours and disappears spontaneously.

DIALYZER REUSE

Hemodialyzers can be reused repeatedly on the same patient after thorough cleansing and disinfection. A variety of disinfectants have been used, including formaldehyde, glutaraldehyde, sodium hypochlorite (bleach), and the combination of hydrogen peroxide and peroxyacetic acid. The blood compartment must be thoroughly rinsed to remove all the disinfectants before the next use, because infusion of residual disinfectants into the body can be harmful. Inadequate disinfection, on the other hand, has been associated with infection by common or rare microorganisms. In general, reused dialyzers can clear small-sized solutes, such as urea, almost as effectively as new dialyzers unless a substantial portion of the hollow fibers has been occluded by clotted blood; in contrast, middle-molecule clearance is sometimes significantly impaired even when the clearance of small-sized solutes is maintained. The total volume of the hollow-fiber lumina is usually checked using an automated machine after each processing, and the dialyzer is discarded if the volume is below 80% of that of a new dialyzer. Other contraindications to reuse include a disrupted dialyzer casing and hepatitis B infection. Reports on the effect of reuse on long-term clinical outcome are conflicting. Because of the economic benefits and lack of definite harmful effects when practiced properly, dialyzer reuse is popular in the United States.

CHOICE OF HEMODIALYZERS

There are several considerations when choosing a hemodialyzer for clinical use. One of the most important considerations is the capacity (K_oA) of the membrane to clear urea, because urea removal seems to correlate with clinical outcome to a certain extent. Data presented earlier suggest that the removal of middle molecules is also beneficial; however, middle-molecule clearances are not quantified in clinical practice. Biocompatibility characteristics of dialysis membrane are taken into account by some, albeit not all nephrologists. Instead, many dialysis units and nephrologists simply use synthetic high-flux dialysis membranes. Purchase cost and reusability of the dialyzer are additional concerns.

DRUG USAGE IN HEMODIALYSIS

The removal of a drug by hemodialysis depends on the properties of the drug and dialysis membrane as well as the conditions of the dialysis procedure (see Chapter 41). Guidelines for dosing medications in kidney failure with or without dialysis have been published. It is imperative to refer to these publications if the physician is unfamiliar with the use of a particular drug in these settings. For example, different types of penicillins behave differently and the clearance of a drug by low-flux hemodialysis can be substantially different from that by hemofiltration or peritoneal dialysis. It is also important to note that these publications provide only rough guidelines. The information might be derived from conventional (low-efficiency and low-flux) hemodialysis and might not be applicable to high-efficiency, high-flux dialysis. Finally, the efficacy of the particular dialysis session must be taken into account. A short and difficult dialysis session plagued by vascular access problems would remove only a small amount of aminoglycosides, so that the postdialysis supplemental dose should be adjusted accordingly. Frequently, monitoring of drug levels is required.

CARE OF CHRONIC HEMODIALYSIS PATIENTS

The dialysis care of the ESRD patient in the United States is usually managed by the nephrologist, although in rare instances, dialysis treatments are supervised instead by other physicians. The nephrologist sees the patient during dialysis rounds, the frequency of which varies from thrice weekly to once monthly, depending on the stability of the patient, the proximity of the dialysis unit, and the standard of practice in the community. The attending nephrologist should evaluate a number of clinical and laboratory parameters that are particularly pertinent to the dialysis procedure or inherent to ESRD. These include: uremic symptoms; vascular access; nutritional status and serum potassium level; blood pressure; fluid status and estimated dry weight; anemia; iron stores and iron and erythropoietin dosage; serum calcium, phosphorus, and parathyroid hormone levels; and dosages of phosphate binders, vitamin D analogues, or cinacalcet. Whenever possible, these routine evaluations should be conducted in the outpatient dialysis unit and not during acute hospitalization, since the conditions in the two settings are often very different from each other. For example, the serum phosphorus level on a regulated hospital diet can be much lower than that obtained when the patient is living at home. Furthermore, communication lapses are common, and outpatient personnel may not even be made aware of the results of tests performed in the hospital. Since iron stores and parathyroid hormone levels, for instance, are monitored and treated on an ongoing basis in the outpatient setting, measuring these parameters in the hospital adds little to patient management and is not cost effective. In addition to seeing the patient during dialysis rounds, the physician should also see the patient in a more quiet and private environment of the clinic, at least annually, for more comprehensive evaluations.

The medical and psychosocial problems of the dialysis patient are often complex and are ideally dealt with using a team approach, involving the patient, family, nephrologist, dialysis nurse and/or technician, specialized dietitian, social worker, vascular surgeon, and sometimes a physician extender. The team should evaluate on a regular basis (e.g., monthly) various aspects of the patient, including medications, barriers to treatment compliance, and potential clinical depression that is frequently overlooked. The appropriateness of the current dialysis modality should also be assessed, and transfer to home hemodialysis or peritoneal dialysis or referral to the kidney transplant team should be made as necessary.

Some nephrologists are equipped to and prefer to manage the general medical problems of the chronic dialysis patients, whereas others prefer general practitioners to handle those problems. The responsibility for primary care, such as immunization and cancer screening, must be clearly delineated among these individual providers to ensure comprehensive patient care.

BIBLIOGRAPHY

Ambalavanan S, Rabetoy G, Cheung A: High efficiency and high flux hemodialysis. In Schrier RW (ed): Atlas of Diseases of the Kidney, vol 5. Philadelphia, Current Medicine, 1999, pp. 3.1–3.10.

Chelamcharla M, Leypoldt JK, Cheung AK: Dialyzer membranes as determinants of adequacy of dialysis. Semin Nephrol, 2005, in press.

Cheung AK, Leypoldt JK: Evaluation of hemodialyzer performance. Semin Dialysis 11:131–137, 1998.

Cheung AK, Agodoa LY, Daugirdas JT, et al: Effects of hemodialyzer reuse on clearances of urea and β2-microglobulin. The Hemodialysis (HEMO) Study Group. J Am Soc Nephrol 10: 117–127, 1999.

Cheung AK, Levin NW, Greene T, et al: Effects of high-flux hemodialysis on clinical outcomes: Results of the HEMO study. J Am Soc Nephrol 14:3251–3263, 2003.

Depner T, Daugirdas J, Greene T, et al: Hemodialysis Study Group: Dialysis dose and the effect of gender and body size on outcome in the HEMO Study. Kidney Int 65:1386–1394, 2004.

Eknoyan G, Beck GJ, Cheung AK, et al: Hemodialysis (HEMO) Study Group: Effect of dialysis dose and membrane flux in maintenance hemodialysis. N Engl J Med 347:2010–2019, 2002.

Gabutti L, Marone C, Colucci G, et al: Citrate anticoagulation in continuous venovenous hemodiafiltration: A metabolic challenge. Intensive Care Med 28:1419–1425, 2002.

Hakim RM, Held PJ, Stannard DC, et al: Effect of the dialysis membrane on mortality of chronic hemodialysis patients. Kidney Int 50:566–570, 1996.

Hakim RM, Wingard RL, Parker RA: Effect of the dialysis membrane in the treatment of patients with acute renal failure. N Engl J Med 331:1338–1342, 1994.

Held PJ, Port FK, Wolfe RA, et al: The dose of hemodialysis and patient mortality. Kidney Int 50:550–556, 1996.

Ing TS, Cheung AK, Golper TA, et al: National Kidney Foundation report on dialyzer reuse. Am J Kidney Dis 30:859–871, 1997.

Kaufman JS, O'Connor TZ, Zhang JH, et al; Veterans Affairs Cooperative Study Group on Hemodialysis Access Graft Thrombosis: Randomized controlled trial of clopidogrel plus aspirin to prevent hemodialysis access graft thrombosis. J Am Soc Nephrol 14:2313–2321, 2003.

Leypoldt JK, Cheung AK, Carroll CE, et al: Effect of dialysis membranes and middle molecule removal on chronic hemodialysis patient survival. Am J Kidney Dis 33:349–355, 1999.

National Kidney Foundation–Dialysis Outcomes Quality Initiative: NKF/DOQI clinical practice guidelines. Am J Kidney Dis 30(suppl 2 and 3), 1997.

Paulson WD, Ram SJ, Zibari GB: Vascular access: Anatomy, examination, management. Semin Nephrol 22:183–194, 2002.

Pereira BG, Cheung AK: Biocompatibility of hemodialysis

membrane. In Owen WF, Pereira BJG, Sayegh MH (eds): Dialysis and Transplantation: A Companion to Brenner & Rector's The Kidney. WB Saunders, Philadelphia, 2000, pp 32–56.

Ram SJ, Work J, Caldito GC, et al: A randomized controlled trial of blood flow and stenosis surveillance of hemodialysis grafts. Kidney Int 64:272–280, 2003.

Ronco C, Bellomo R, Homel P, et al: Effects of different doses in continuous veno-venous haemofiltration on outcomes of acute renal failure: A prospective randomised trial. Lancet 356:26–30, 2000.

Schwab SJ, Beathard G: The hemodialysis catheter conundrum: Hate living with them, but can't live without them. Kidney Int 56:1–17, 1999.

Vanholder RC, Ringoir SM: Adequacy of dialysis: A critical analysis. Kidney Int 42:540–558, 1992.

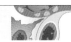

CHAPTER 61

Peritoneal Dialysis

Ram Gokal Alastair J. Hutchison

In the 1950s and 1960s, peritoneal dialysis (PD) was utilized predominantly to manage patients in acute renal failure. Patients with endstage renal disease (ESRD) were treated almost exclusively by hemodialysis (HD) and occasionally by intermittent PD (IPD). However, the introduction in 1976 of continuous ambulatory peritoneal dialysis (CAPD) transformed this situation. There has been a dramatic rise in the use of PD worldwide over the last 2 decades, especially in the developing world. However, this trend has not continued in the United States, where usage declined by nearly 5% between 1997 and 2001. Currently there are more than 140,000 patients on PD, comprising roughly 15% of the total world dialysis population. PD is still utilized for managing some cases of acute renal failure.

PRINCIPLES OF PERITONEAL DIALYSIS

The Peritoneal Membrane

The peritoneal membrane is used as the dialyzing surface in PD. The visceral peritoneal membrane covers the abdominal organs, whereas the parietal peritoneum lines the abdominal cavity. The peritoneal membrane consists of a single layer of mesothelial cells overlying an interstitium in which the blood and lymphatic vessels lie. The mesothelial cells are covered by microvilli that markedly increase the nominal 2 m^2 surface area of the peritoneum.

Solute Movement

Peritoneal dialysis represents solute and fluid exchange between the peritoneal capillary blood and dialysis solution in the peritoneal cavity across the peritoneal membrane. Solute movement occurs as a result of diffusion and convective transport, whereas fluid shifts relate to osmosis created by the addition of appropriate osmotic agents to the PD solutions. During PD, solutes such as urea, creatinine, and potassium move from the peritoneal capillaries across the peritoneal membrane to the peritoneal cavity, whereas other solutes such as lactate, bicarbonate, and calcium move in the opposite direction. Solute movement is mainly by diffusion and is thus based on the concentration gradient of the solute between dialysate and blood. Solutes also move across the peritoneal membrane by convection—the movement of solutes related to fluid removal.

Fluid Movement

Standard PD fluid contains a high concentration of glucose as the osmotic agent. Thus, dialysate is hyperosmolar in relation to serum, causing fluid removal (ultrafiltration) to occur. The volume of ultrafiltration depends on the concentration of glucose solution used for each exchange, the length of time the fluid dwells in the peritoneal cavity, and the individual patient's peritoneal membrane characteristics (see later). With increasing dwell time, transperitoneal glucose absorption diminishes the dialysate glucose concentration and the osmotic gradient. Ultrafiltration is therefore decreased with long dwell times, for example, with the overnight exchange on CAPD or the daytime exchange on automated PD (APD).

The crucial physiologic components of the PD system are, therefore, peritoneal blood flow and the peritoneal membrane (neither of which is amenable to any manipulation on a routine clinical basis), as well as the dialysate volume, dwell time, and number of exchanges/day (the only variables that can be manipulated to maximize solute and fluid removal). Various techniques and regimens have now emerged in the field of PD as a consequence of more recent understanding of the peritoneal membrane transport characteristics or permeability, and the amount of solute and fluid to be removed.

Measuring Solute and Fluid Transport to Determine Peritoneal Membrane Characteristics

Peritoneal dialysis effectively removes substances with low molecular weights, such as creatinine, urea, and potassium, which are not in the infused dialysis fluid. With increasing dwell time, solutes move across the peritoneal membrane toward equilibrium, and the ratio of dialysate to serum urea levels approaches one. Because the peritoneal membrane has a negative charge, negatively charged solutes such as phosphate will move across it more slowly than positively charged solutes such as potassium. Macromolecules such as albumin cross the peritoneum by mechanisms that are not completely understood but probably via lymphatics and through large pores in the capillary membranes. During a dwell, the osmotic gradient created by the dialysate within the abdominal cavity declines as the glucose is absorbed, resulting in fluid reabsorption into the systemic circulation. In addition, continuous lymphatic absorption diminishes net fluid removal.

The rate of movement of small solutes such as creatinine between dialysate and blood differs from one patient to another. Peritoneal function characteristics are monitored using the peritoneal equilibration test (PET; Fig. 61-1). In this standardized test, 2L of dialysate containing 2.5 g/dL glucose are infused, and the dialysate-to-plasma creatinine ratio (D/P) at the end of a 4-hour dwell is measured. Using this test, each patient's peritoneal membrane can be categorized as having high (D/P above 0.81), high average (0.65 to 0.81), low average (0.50 to 0.65), or low (less than 0.5) peritoneal transport capability. Using 2L of 4.25 g/dL glucose dialysate during the

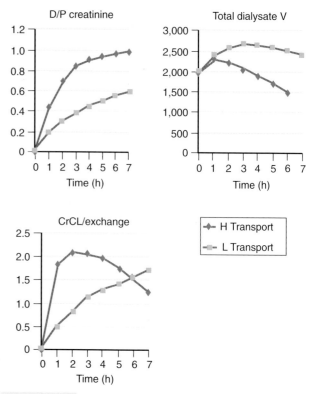

FIGURE 61-2 The intraperitoneal dialysate volume (V) profiles and solute transport of creatinine (creatinine clearance/exchange) in relationship to dwell time in hours, in high (H) and low (L) transporters. These profiles dictate the need for adjusting dwell times and setting the prescription. For long-dwell continuous ambulatory peritoneal dialysis, high transporters show both low fluid removal as well as creatinine clearance as compared with low transporters.

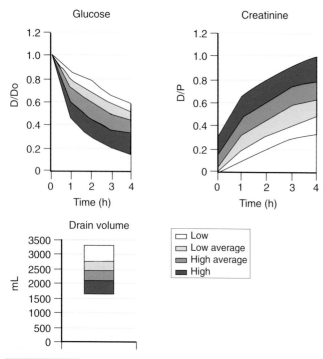

FIGURE 61-1 The peritoneal equilibration test (PET) measures the peritoneal transport characteristics of glucose movement from the peritoneal fluid and creatinine movement from plasma. The instillation volume for the PET is 2L. D/D_0 represents the ratio of dialysate glucose concentration (D) at various times to the dialysate glucose concentration at time 0 (D_0). D/P represents the ratio of dialysate (D) to plasma (P) concentrations. The rate of transport of these molecules will depend on the permeability of the membrane; the higher the permeability (high transporter), the more rapid the transport of glucose, with dissipation of the osmotic gradient and therefore less drain volume.

same dwell period as the PET permits the assessment of ultrafiltration failure for which an effluent volume of less than 2400 mL is diagnostic.

Removal of fluid and solutes is very dependent on the type of transporter status (Fig. 61-2). Patients with a high D/P creatinine ratio (high transporters) have rapid clearance of small molecules but poor ultrafiltration because of rapid glucose absorption and dissipation of the osmolar gradient between dialysate and blood. These patients will require short-dwell PD regimens to achieve adequate fluid removal. In addition, because the volume of fluid removed also dictates the solute clearance of equilibrated dialysate, high transporters will also have reduced solute clearance over long dwells because of low drain volumes. Patients with a low D/P creatinine ratio (low transporters) have low clearances for solutes and generally require increased numbers of dialysis exchanges and/or increased volume per exchange to avoid uremic symptoms once residual kidney function (RKF) is lost. Ultrafiltration in this category of patient is usually excellent. The majority of patients have high-average to low-average peritoneal transport and do well on either CAPD or APD.

TECHNIQUES OF PERITONEAL DIALYSIS

Continuous Ambulatory Peritoneal Dialysis

Continuous ambulatory PD utilizes the smallest volume of dialysate to prevent uremia; this usually means a daily volume of 8 to 10 L of dialysate to be equilibrated with body fluids. The CAPD technique usually entails three to five daily exchanges of 0.5 to 3.0 L each, with dialysis occurring continuously and occupying the entire 24-hour period. The prescription (volume, dwell time, number of exchanges) will depend on patient size, peritoneal permeability, and RKF.

Peritoneal dialysis fluid is initially instilled by gravity into the peritoneal cavity and drained out after a dwell period of several hours. The basic CAPD system, which to this day remains unchanged, consists of a plastic bag containing 0.5 to 3.0 L of PD fluid, a transfer set (tubing between the catheter and the plastic bag), and a permanent, indwelling, silastic catheter, which is implanted such that the tip of the intraperitoneal portion lies in the pelvis. The connection between the bag and the transfer set is broken three to five times a day (about 1500 exchanges/year), and the procedure must be performed using a strict, semisterile, nontouch technique, which the patient or helper performs at home. The most common connection device currently utilized is based on the "Y"-disconnect system. This entails drainage of the effluent after the connection has been made with the new bag, thereby permitting the "flushing out" of any touch contamination in the tubing before the infusion of new fluid into the peritoneal cavity (Fig. 61-3). This system reduces the incidence of infection and leaves the patient free from carrying the empty bag and transfer set, thus improving the psychologic aspects and quality of life of CAPD patients.

Automated Peritoneal Dialysis

Automated PD is a broad term that is used to refer to all forms of PD utilizing a mechanical device (called a cycler) to assist in the delivery and drainage of the dialysis fluid. APD variants range from IPD performed in patients with acute or chronic kidney failure three times a week in sessions of 24 hours, exchanging 20 to 60 L of dialysis fluid, to more sophisticated regimens. The latter include continuous cycling peritoneal dialysis (CCPD, three exchanges during the night and one during the day—a reversal of the CAPD regime), nightly intermittent peritoneal dialysis (NIPD, rapid exchanges during the night, with the abdomen kept dry during the "dry day"), nightly PD plus two exchanges during the day to allow for increased small-solute and fluid clearance (NIPD with "wet day"), and tidal peritoneal dialysis (TPD). During

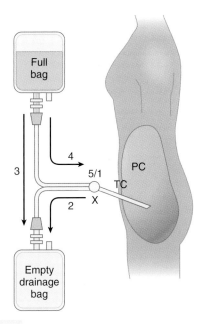

FIGURE 61-3 Diagrammatic representation of a CAPD exchange using a Y-set disconnect system. The Y-set consists of tubing with a full bag of dialysate at one end and an empty drainage bag at the other, placed on the floor. Fluid flow is by gravity, and the direction is controlled by clamps on the tubing. Between exchanges, the peritoneal cavity (PC) contains dialysate and only a short, capped extension tubing attached to the peritoneal Tenckhoff catheter (TC). The exchange procedure comprises five steps.

1. To begin the exchange, the patient connects the Y tubing to the short extension tubing at X.
2. Keeping the clamp on the full bag closed, the clamp on the peritoneal catheter extension tubing is opened to allow the fluid in the PC to drain into the drainage bag by gravity. Time: 10–15 min.
3. The patient closes the clamp on the peritoneal catheter extension tubing and opens the clamp on the full bag, allowing the fresh fluid to "flush" the tubing of air and any contamination into the drainage bag. Time: a few seconds (count of 5).
4. The patient closes the clamp on the drainage bag and opens the clamp on the peritoneal catheter extension tubing, allowing fresh dialysis fluid into the PC via the TC. Time: 10 min.
5. The final step is to close the clamp on the peritoneal catheter extension tubing, disconnect the Y tubing, and cap the short extension tubing.

TPD only 40% to 60% of the intraperitoneal fluid volume is replaced each exchange, so that continuous fluid-membrane contact improves the efficiency but requires 20 to 30 L of fluid per 24 hours. These regimens are illustrated in Table 61-1.

Automated PD regimes usually entail an increased number of short-dwell exchanges to enhance solute and fluid removal. The cycler delivers a set number of exchanges over 8 to 10 hours, the last fill constituting the long day dwell, which may be necessary to provide additional dialysis to achieve solute and fluid removal targets. The most obvious advantage of APD is that it eliminates

TABLE 61-1 Various Regimens Used in Peritoneal Dialysis

Type of Dialysis*	Number of Daytime Exchanges	Number of Night-time Exchanges	Volume of Exchanges (L)
CAPD	2–3	1–2[†]	1.0–3.0
CCPD	1	3–4	1.0–3.0
NIPD	0	3–5	2.0–3.0
NIPD "wet day"	1–2	3–5	2.0–3.0
TPD	0	20	1.0–1.5
IPD	5–10	5–10	1.0–2.0

CAPD, continuous ambulatory peritoneal dialysis; CCPD, continuous cycling peritoneal dialysis; IPD, intermittent peritoneal dialysis; NIPD, nocturnal intermittent peritoneal dialysis; TPD, tidal peritoneal dialysis.

*All regimens except CAPD utilize a cycler machine and are therefore variants of automated peritoneal dialysis.

[†]If an additional exchange is needed during CAPD to achieve adequate dialysis, a mechanical exchange device can be used to perform the exchange during the night while the patient is asleep.

the need for intensive manual involvement, with most of the dialysis occurring at night during sleep. In essence, APD entails only two procedures daily: an initial connection of catheter to the machine and a disconnection at the end of dialysis. There is increasing use of APD in the United States at the expense of CAPD. This trend may be due to the convenience of performing the dialysis connections and to the new cycler models, which are smaller and more attractive to patients.

Peritoneal Dialysis Solutions

Standard PD solutions (Table 61-2) contain varying concentrations of glucose as an osmotic agent and differing amounts of lactate, sodium, potassium, and calcium. Lactate was initially used as the buffer, because the low pH of such solutions prevented caramelization of the glucose during the autoclaving process. The biocompatibility of standard PD solutions has been intensively studied. There is no doubt that their unphysiologically

TABLE 61-2 Composition of Standard Peritoneal Dialysis Fluids Including the Osmotic Agents Used

Agent	Amount
Sodium	132 mEq/L
Chloride	96–102 mEq/L
Calcium	0, 1.20, 2.5, 3.5 mEq/L
Magnesium	0.5, 1.25 mEq/L
Lactate	35, 40 mEq/L
Glucose	1.5, 2.5, 4.25 g/dL*
Amino acids	1.1 g/dL
Icodextrin	7.5 g/dL

*Newer glucose-based solutions with low-glucose degradation products are now available in Europe.

low pH, high osmolality, and the presence of glucose degradation products (GDPs) generated during manufacture and autoclaving are harmful to peritoneal cells in vitro and, therefore, potentially harmful to the peritoneal membrane. Newer, more physiologic solutions have been developed that are low in GDPs, use bicarbonate as a buffer, and contain alternative osmotic agents.

Glucose is still the most common osmotic agent because of its low cost and ease of manufacture; however, larger molecules have interesting and attractive properties. Icodextrin is an isosmotic glucose polymer that produces ultrafiltration by colloid osmosis even with dwell periods of as long as 12 hours. Mixtures of amino acids can also generate osmosis and may have the additional benefit of acting as a protein supplement in malnourished patients. Both of these solutions are now available commercially.

Lactate is gradually being replaced by bicarbonate, a more physiologic buffer, which is separated from the other constituents of the fluid during the manufacturing process by means of a dual-chamber bag. This prevents caramelization during autoclaving, and the patient mixes the contents of the chambers immediately before infusion, producing a relatively pH-neutral solution. These newer solutions will be used increasingly to improve fluid balance and nutrition in PD, although it remains to be seen whether they will improve long-term outcome. Used in combination, they have the potential to preserve peritoneal membrane integrity and to reduce the metabolic side effects of glucose absorption.

Peritoneal Catheters

The access for PD is a catheter, which is inserted into the abdominal cavity, usually by either a surgeon or a nephrologist, and generally using local anesthetic with sedation. The catheter can be inserted surgically under direct vision, or percutaneously with or without peritoneoscopic guidance. Although there are numerous catheter designs such as the Swan-neck catheter (said to undergo less catheter tip migration and exit site infections), none offers a significant proven advantage over the original double-cuffed silastic Tenckhoff catheter. This original and simple design is still the most commonly used catheter. The intra-abdominal portion of the catheter has multiple perforations through which dialysate flows. With the deep cuff placed in a paramedian position in the rectus muscle, the extra-abdominal portion of the catheter is tunneled through the subcutaneous tissue to exit the skin, pointing laterally and caudally. The subcutaneous superficial cuff is located about 2 to 3 cm from the exit site of the catheter. PD can be initiated immediately after catheter placement if exchange volumes are small and the patient is kept recumbent. Ideally, PD should be deferred for at least 4 weeks until the insertion site is well healed, at which time the patient may be trained to perform CAPD or APD. HD can be used if necessary as a temporary measure until PD is initiated.

MANAGING PATIENTS ON PERITONEAL DIALYSIS

Peritoneal Dialysis Prescription

In arriving at a particular prescription for an individual patient, one needs to take into account the fixed components, including RKF, peritoneal membrane permeability, and size of the patient, as well as the variable components of dialysate volume, dwell times, concentration of glucose, and number of exchanges. A prescription will therefore entail modifications of the variable components to arrive at a regimen that provides for adequate solute and fluid removal to meet clinical needs and maintain reasonable quality of life. The setting of a PD prescription is outlined in Figure 61-4. Such a prescription takes into account the various factors (peritoneal permeability, RKF, size, dwell times, fill volume, number of exchanges) known to influence achievement of adequacy and nutritional targets. Dialysis "adequacy," fluid status, and clinical well-being are then monitored regularly (see later) and the prescription modified accordingly.

The overall clearance capacity of the peritoneum for small solutes is limited by the volume of dialysis fluid that can be provided daily. Many CAPD patients are prescribed four exchanges of 2-L volumes/day. Four 2-L CAPD exchanges/day with 2 L of ultrafiltration per day

represents a drain volume of 70 L/week, which is inadequate in the absence of significant RKF for most patients, especially large patients (greater than 80 kg). Initially, most patients have RKF, contributing to the total clearance. As kidney function is lost, patients require larger exchange volumes (2.5 or 3.0 L) and may also need five daily exchanges to avoid uremic symptoms and reach the target values of Kt/V and creatinine clearance (CrCl; see next section on Peritoneal Dialysis Adequacy). The fifth exchange may be provided by use of a device that will deliver a middle of the night exchange. Larger patients should be started on 2.5 or 3.0 L exchange volumes. APD can achieve higher clearance of small solutes, but it may necessitate 1 or 2 day dwells (wet day), in addition to three to four nocturnal exchange volumes of 2.5 to 3.0 L.

Peritoneal Dialysis Adequacy

Adequacy of PD is determined by clinical assessment, solute clearance measurements, and fluid removal. The well-dialyzed patient has a good appetite, no nausea, minimal fatigue, and feels well. In contrast, the uremic patient is anorectic with dysgeusia, nausea, and complaints of fatigue. In addition to these clinical parameters, the measures utilized to assess adequacy of solute removal include:

1. An index of peritoneal urea removal, expressed as Kt/V, which is urea clearance (K) per unit time (t) related to total body water (V). Kt is obtained by

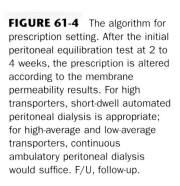

FIGURE 61-4 The algorithm for prescription setting. After the initial peritoneal equilibration test at 2 to 4 weeks, the prescription is altered according to the membrane permeability results. For high transporters, short-dwell automated peritoneal dialysis is appropriate; for high-average and low-average transporters, continuous ambulatory peritoneal dialysis would suffice. F/U, follow-up.

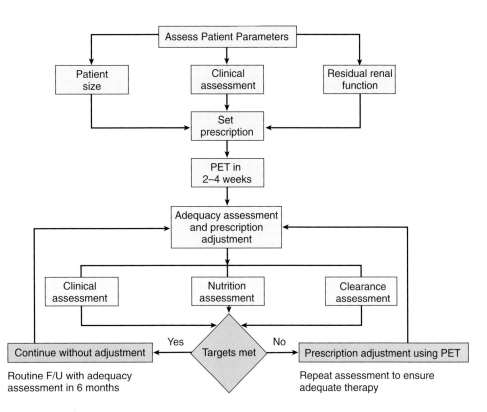

multiplying the effluent blood urea nitrogen concentration ratio (D/P$_{urea}$) by the 24-hour effluent drain volume. Renal urea nitrogen clearance is added to this. The daily value is multiplied by 7 to provide a weekly value. V can be estimated as 60% of weight in males and 55% of weight in females. A typical calculation is given in Table 61-3.

2. Creatinine clearance (both peritoneal and that due to RKF). Peritoneal CrCl is again obtained from the 24-hour collection of dialysate, but to this is added an estimate of the CrCl achieved by RKF. By tradition, residual renal clearance is arrived at by averaging creatinine and urea nitrogen clearance as an estimate of glomerular filtration rate. This is done to correct for tubular secretion of creatinine, which overestimates glomerular filtration rate at low levels of kidney function. An adjustment for body surface area is also usually applied.

Various national and international bodies have set minimum targets for these solute clearances, and most physicians would hope that their patients achieve both of them. However, this is not always possible, and doubt remains about the precise level at which these targets should be set. The National Kidney Foundation (NKF) in the United States has published the Dialysis Outcome Quality Initiative (DOQI) Practice Guidelines, which set a target minimum urea Kt/V of 2.0 and total weekly CrCl of 60 L, although the targets in other countries are lower. It is thought that failure to achieve these guidelines is likely to lead to uremic symptoms, decreased protein intake, and an increase in mortality, although this notion has recently been challenged. There have been two randomized controlled trials assessing outcomes with respect to amount of small-solute clearance. Both show no survival advantage of Kt/V of 1.7 compared with one of more than 2.0, or a weekly CrCl of 50 L compared with one of 60 L. Although this may indicate the minimum solute clearance targets required to achieve an acceptable long-term clinical outcome, some patients will need more dialysis to overcome uremic symptoms, and it must always be remembered that dialysis adequacy is not the same as overall "treatment" adequacy. Control of hypertension, serum lipids, and fluid balance, as well as management of other comorbidities will also hugely influence outcome in any dialysis patient. Despite these issues, anuric patients can be adequately managed on PD by appropriate prescription adjustments, including the use of APD regimes and icodextrin. It is now well recognized that RKF is extremely important in providing adequate solute clearance. Most studies show that RKF correlates with improved survival and less morbidity, and its preservation forms an important part of the management of a PD patient. To preserve RKF, nephrotoxic drugs such as aminoglycosides and nonsteroidal anti-inflammatory agents should be avoided whenever possible, and episodes of hypotension due to any cause should be corrected as rapidly as possible. RKF is better preserved in patients on PD than in those on HD, so that PD may be the better initial therapy option for endstage renal failure.

TABLE 61-3   An Example of Urea Kt/V Calculation*

Patient
70-kg female on CAPD (four exchanges/day)

Data to be obtained
24-hr dialysate volume (4 × 2 L infusion + 1 L net ultrafiltrate = 9 L)
D/P ratio for urea (0.9), determined by collecting the total dialysate for 24 hr
Residual kidney urea clearance, determined by dividing the 24-hr urine urea by blood urea (20 L/week, which corresponds to 2 mL/min)

Calculation

Peritoneal urea clearance/day (D/P × volume)	= 0.9 × 9 L = 8.1 L
Weekly peritoneal urea clearance	= 8.1 L/day × 7 days/week = 56.7 L/week
Residual renal urea clearance	= 20 L/week
Total urea clearance (Kt)	= 56.7 + 20 = 76.7 L/week
Volume (V) of urea distribution (0.55 × weight)†	= 38.5 L
Weekly Kt/V	= 76.7/38.5 = 2.0

CAPD, continuous ambulatory peritoneal dialysis; D/P ratio, dialysate-to-plasma creatinine ratio.

*It is more accurate to use the formula of Watson and Watson, which takes into account weight, height, gender, and age. For males, V(L) = 2.477 + (0.3362 × weight in kg) + (0.1074 × height in cm) − (0.09516 × age in years). For females, V(L) = −2.097 + (0.2466 × weight in kg) + (0.1069 × height in cm). The calculation of creatinine clearance (CrCl) is similar to that for Kt/V. However, the urinary component of CrCl is usually corrected for creatinine secretion by averaging it with the urinary urea clearance. The peritoneal CrCl is simply measured by dividing the creatinine content of the 24-hr dialysate by serum creatinine. The total CrCl (peritoneal + renal) is normalized to 1.73 m² body surface area.

†Volume can be estimated as 0.60 (male) or 0.55 (female) of body weight.

Fluid Removal on Peritoneal Dialysis

Peritoneal dialysis patients are generally regarded as being fluid overloaded, especially in the long term, when they lose their RKF and PD ultrafiltration capacity. It appears that fluid removal has a more direct impact on outcome than solute clearance. Ultrafiltration of at least 750 mL/day is associated with better survival in anuric patients, although the exact reason for this is unclear. Greater emphasis is now placed on optimizing fluid status, and algorithms are available that help in managing fluid overload in CAPD patients (Fig. 61-5). The use of icodextrin for the longest dwell achieves better fluid balance and results in improvement in left ventricular indices.

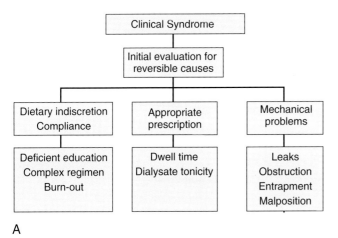

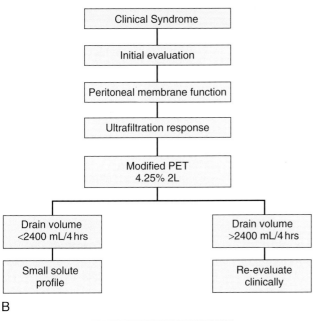

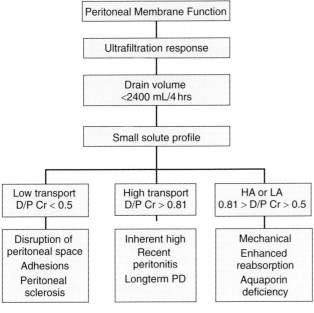

FIGURE 61-5 *A,* Evaluation of the clinical syndrome of fluid overload. This initially entails the evaluation and search for reversible causes. *B,* When reversible causes are excluded, then it is appropriate to evaluate peritoneal membrane function using the modified peritoneal equilibration test with 2 L of 4.25% glucose. *C,* Algorithm for further evaluation and treatment based on small-solute profile. For high-transport patients, the therapy is outlined. For low-transport patients peritoneal dialysis may not be possible and peritoneal sclerosis should be excluded, especially of the encapsulating variety (encapsulating peritoneal sclerosis). D/P, dialysate-to-plasma ratio; HA, high average; LA, low average.

Nutrition in the Peritoneal Dialysis Patient

As many as 40% of PD patients are thought to be protein malnourished according to anthropometric studies. This condition is in part due to losses of amino acids and protein in the dialysate, the latter generally being 8 to 12 g/day. Peritonitis markedly increases dialysate protein losses. The appetite of the patient may be suppressed by the absorbed dialysate glucose as well as from uremia resulting in lower protein and other nutrient intake. Both Kt/V and weekly CrCl correlate, albeit weakly, with dietary protein intake, suggesting that a certain minimum dose of dialysis is required for adequate protein intake. The serum albumin level is inversely related to both mortality and hospitalization in PD patients, although it must be remembered that serum albumin is greatly influenced by inflammation and is a poor marker of nutritional status when used alone. Although protein intake of at least 1.2 g/kg/day is recommended for PD patients, this is probably not necessary for most patients, many of whom ingest only 0.8 to 1.0 g/kg/day. The use of amino acid dialysate (in which amino acids replace the glucose) has been used on a limited basis as a means of correcting protein malnutrition, but proof of its long-term nutritional benefit is thus far lacking. Correction of malnutrition is especially difficult in PD patients when it is related to inflammation and comorbidity. This "type II" malnutrition may well be cytokine mediated, and its correction necessitates establishing an underlying cause for the "inflammation." Type I malnutrition is more readily amenable to protein and calorie supplementation.

The calories absorbed from dialysate glucose depend on the dextrose concentration used (1.50, 2.50, 4.25 g/dL) as well as on the membrane permeability of the patient. The development of obesity is therefore not unusual in PD patients, especially those who were already overweight at the start of dialysis. In addition, glucose absorption frequently results in hyperlipidemia, which may contribute to cardiovascular diseases.

COMPLICATIONS OF PERITONEAL DIALYSIS

Peritonitis

Peritonitis remains a major complication of PD, accounts for 15% to 35% of hospital admissions for these patients, and is the major cause of technique failure resulting in transfer to HD. Entry of bacteria into the catheter during an exchange procedure (touch contamination) is the most common source, but organisms can also track along the outside of the catheter or migrate into the peritoneum from another abdominal viscus. Diagnosis of peritonitis requires the presence of two of the following criteria in any combination:

- Organisms on Gram stain or subsequent culture
- Cloudy fluid (white cell count greater than 100/mm³; more than 50% neutrophils)
- Symptoms and signs of peritoneal inflammation

Cloudy dialysate effluent is almost invariably present, whereas abdominal pain is present in about 80% to 95% of cases. Gastrointestinal symptoms, chills, and fever are present in as many as 25% of the cases, whereas abdominal tenderness accompanies the symptoms in three quarters of the cases. Bacteremia is rare. Gram stain of the effluent is seldom helpful, except with fungal peritonitis, but cultures are generally positive. In many centers, 20% of peritonitis episodes result in a "no growth" culture result, predominantly as a result of inadequate culture techniques.

The etiologies of peritonitis are given in Table 61-4, together with the frequency of organisms. Peritonitis rates due to *Staphylococcus epidermidis* have decreased with the introduction of the Y-set and flush before fill, and *Staphylococcus aureus* and enteric organisms therefore account for a larger proportion of peritonitis episodes than in the past. Because patients with these organisms are more symptomatic than those with *S. epidermidis* peri-

tonitis, peritonitis has become a less frequent but more severe complication, often requiring hospital admission.

Peritonitis remains an important cause of hospitalization, catheter loss, and transfer to hemodialysis. Peritonitis rates, originally very high in the late 1970s and early 1980s, have decreased to less than an episode every 2 to 3 dialysis years, on account of improvements in the procedure for performing the dialysis tubing connections, which have decreased the risk of touch contamination (see Fig. 61-3). The catheter removal rate for peritonitis depends on the infecting microorganism. Peritonitis with *S. epidermidis* is less likely to result in catheter loss than peritonitis due to *S. aureus* or *Pseudomonas aeruginosa*. If these more virulent organisms are associated with a catheter tunnel or exit site infection, the catheter loss rate has been shown to be as high as 90%. Fungal peritonitis also almost invariably requires catheter removal, since a medical cure can only rarely be achieved. There is no apparent difference in rates of peritonitis between CAPD and APD.

The initial treatment of peritonitis is empiric and designed to cover both Gram-positive cocci and Gram-negative bacilli. A first-generation cephalosporin such as cefazolin or cephalothin may be used in conjunction with an aminoglycoside or a third-generation cephalosporin, with subsequent therapy tailored to the culture and sensitivity results. The latest International Society of Peritoneal Dialysis guidelines on peritonitis have advocated the use of a cephalosporin or vancomycin to provide Gram-positive coverage and ceftazidime or an aminoglycoside for Gram-negative coverage. There is the potential problem with the first-generation cephalosporins that they may not adequately cover methicillin-resistant organisms; in this situation, vancomycin should be used. Because of the concern about the emergence of vancomycin-resistant organisms, unnecessary use of vancomycin should be avoided, and aminoglycoside levels should be monitored to avoid accelerated loss of RKF or ototoxicity.

A listing of antibiotics and the dosing schedule is given in Table 61-5. Antibiotics are usually given intermittently once a day and administered intraperitoneally in the long-dwell exchange (overnight in CAPD and during the daytime long dwell in APD). They can also be given continuously in every exchange. The dosage may need adjustment if RKF is significant. Duration of therapy depends on the organisms and the severity of the peritonitis, which is usually 14 days for *S. epidermidis* infections and 3 weeks for most other infections.

It should be possible, in as many as 80% of cases, to achieve complete cure without having to resort to catheter removal. Persistent symptoms beyond 96 hours can occur in about 10% to 30% of episodes, and cure is then effected by removal of the catheter. Cure can be obtained if antibiotics are continued beyond 96 hours without catheter removal, but there is a high risk of damage to the peritoneum, and neither the short-term

TABLE 61-4 Microorganisms Causing Peritonitis

Microorganisms	Percent
Gram positive	
Staphylococcus epidermidis	30–40
Staphylococcus aureus	15–20
Streptococcus	10–15
Other Gram positive	2–5
Gram negative	
Pseudomonas	5–10
Enterobacter	5–20
Other Gram negative	5–7
Fungi	2–10
Other organisms	2–5
Culture negative	10–30

TABLE 61-5 Listing of Antibiotics and Dosing Schedules for Intraperitoneal Use Unless Otherwise Stated

Antibiotic	Initial Dose (mg/L)*	Subsequent Dose (mg/L each exchange)	Subsequent Doses (mg once daily)
Ampicillin	125	125	No data
Aztreonam	1000	250	1000 qd
Cefazolin	500	125	500 qd
Ceftazidime	500	125	1000 qd
Fluconazole	200 mg PO		200 mg PO qd
Aminoglycosides[†]	20 mg	4	20 mg
Metronidazole	500 mg PO/IV		500 mg PO/IV tid
Vancomycin	15–30 mg/kg	25	15–30 mg/kg q 5–7 days

*Once-daily antibiotics with the long dwell is preferred to antibiotic addition to each exchange; this has been shown to be efficacious for cefazolin, cephalothin, and ceftazidime. For ambulatory peritoneal dialysis (APD), patients may be changed to a continuous CAPD schedule. If patients stay on an APD schedule, the antibiotics are added to each exchange as shown in the second column.
[†]This group includes gentamicin, tobramycin, and netilmicin (same dose for all).

bacterial outcome nor the long-term peritoneal membrane effect is good. In a study in which antibiotics were continued for 10 days for "resistant" peritonitis without catheter removal, one third of patients died, another one third lost ultrafiltration, necessitating discontinuation of PD, and only one third were able to continue with PD.

Relapsing peritonitis is a feature in about 10% to 15% of episodes. Catheter removal is necessary in as many as 15% of these cases, and death is reported in about 1% to 3% of cases. Peritonitis results in a marked increase in acute peritoneal protein losses and a transient decrease in ultrafiltration; moreover, with long-term PD, the membrane may eventually become hyperpermeable, with an increase in solute transport and loss of ultrafiltration. Although peritoneal membrane changes are usually transient and related to acute peritonitis, peritoneal fibrosis, often referred to as sclerosing peritonitis, may result from severe episodes or as a cumulative effect of multiple episodes (see later).

Peritoneal Catheter Infection

Peritoneal catheter infections can involve the exit site (erythema or purulent drainage from the exit site) and the tunnel (edema, erythema, or tenderness over the subcutaneous pathway), and these can occur simultaneously. *Staphylococcus aureus* is the most common cause of exit site and tunnel infections, with *Pseudomonas* the next most frequent organism. *Staphylococcus aureus* exit site infections are difficult to treat, with frequent progression to tunnel infections and peritonitis, in which case catheter removal is required for resolution. *Staphylococcus aureus* nasal carriage is associated with an increased risk of *S. aureus* catheter infections. Treatment of nasal carriers with intranasal mupirocin twice a day for 5 days each month, mupirocin applied daily to the exit site, or oral rifampin 600 mg/day for 5 days every 12 weeks, are all effective in reducing *S. aureus* catheter infections. The

application of mupirocin at the exit site as part of routine exit site care has resulted in a dramatic reduction of exit site infections and peritonitis related to *S. aureus*. Bacteriologic monitoring of the PD population for *S. aureus* carriage is unnecessary when this approach is adopted, but there is concern that it may in the future encourage growth of resistant organisms. *Pseudomonas aeruginosa* catheter infections are also difficult to resolve and frequently relapse. Ciprofloxacin is used to treat such catheter infections, but if *P. aeruginosa* peritonitis develops, the catheter must be removed to resolve the infection.

Catheter Malfunction, Hernias, and Fluid Leaks

The most important noninfectious complications during PD are abdominal wall–related hernias, leakage of dialysis fluid, and inflow and outflow malfunction. Before PD treatment is started, all significant abdominal wall–related hernias should be corrected. With the presence of 2 to 3 L of dialysate in the abdominal cavity, there is an increased intra-abdominal pressure, and preexisting hernias will worsen during PD treatment. The most frequently occurring hernias after commencing PD are incisional, umbilical, and inguinal. Significant hernias should be repaired surgically, and intermittent PD may be continued postoperatively using low dwell volumes in a supine position.

Leakage of peritoneal fluid is related to catheter implantation technique, trauma, or patient-related anatomic abnormalities. It can occur early (less than 30 days) or late (greater than 30 days) after implantation and can have different clinical manifestation depending on whether the leak is external or subcutaneous. Early leakage is usually external, appearing as fluid through the wound or the exit site. Subcutaneous leakage may develop at the site of an incision and entry into the peritoneal cavity. The exact site of the leakage can be determined with computerized tomography after infusion of 2 L of dialysis fluid containing radiocontrast material. Scrotal or labial edema can be a sign of a fluid leak, usually through a patent processus vaginalis. Therapy usually entails a period off PD during which the patient, if needing dialysis, is maintained on HD or limited small-volume supine PD. For recurrent leaks, surgical repair is essential. Leakage of fluid into the subcutaneous tissue is sometimes occult and difficult to diagnose, and it may present as diminished drainage, which might be mistaken for ultrafiltration failure. Computerized tomography and abdominal scintigraphy may identify the leak.

Outflow/inflow obstruction is the most frequently observed early event within 2 weeks of the catheter implantation, although this complication can be seen later during other PD-related problems such as peritonitis. One-way outflow obstruction is the most frequent problem and is characterized by poor flow and failure to drain the peritoneal cavity. Common causes include both intraluminal factors (blood clot, fibrin) and extraluminal factors (constipation, occlusion of catheter holes by adjacent organs or omental wrapping, catheter tip dislocation out of the true pelvis, and incorrect catheter placement at implantation). A kidney, ureter, bladder (KUB) x-ray is useful in localizing the PD catheter tip and evaluating for malposition. Depending on the cause, appropriate therapy entails laxatives, heparinized saline flushes, urokinase instillation in the catheter, manipulation under fluoroscopy guidance (using a stiff wire or stylet manipulation combined with a "whiplash" technique), and revision or replacement of the catheter.

Peritoneal Membrane Changes and Loss of Ultrafiltration

The peritoneum undergoing PD reacts to changes in response to the new environment. There is thickening of the peritoneal interstitium and basement membrane reduplication, both in the mesothelium and in the capillaries. These changes occur in response to the nonphysiologic composition of standard dialysis solutions and also to the direct action of glucose and glucose degradation products, which causes advanced glycosylation end product formation and related changes in the peritoneal membrane. Changes of peritoneal microvessels and neovascularization occur, analogous to those seen in diabetic retinopathy, with deposition of type IV collagen. Other conditions that are important in the pathogenesis are acute peritonitis and chronic inflammatory reactions mediated by uremic or low-level bacterial activation of peritoneal macrophages, and intraperitoneal production of bioactive substances promoting inflammation and peritoneal fibrosis. A recent analysis from an international biopsy registry shows that thickening of the membrane usually occurs after 4 to 5 years of PD and is associated with increasing severity of vasculopathy, although these findings are variable with long duration of therapy. For patients who have been on PD for a long time (more than 5 years), it is prudent to be vigilant, because membrane changes can progress eventually to the rare encapsulating peritoneal sclerosis, which is characterized by dense fibrosis and thickening of the peritoneum with bowel adhesions and encapsulation.

Net ultrafiltration failure is the most important transport abnormality in long-term PD patients. On the basis of clinical symptoms, its prevalence has been reported to increase from 3% after 1 year on CAPD to about 30% after 6 years. Ultrafiltration failure is defined as net ultrafiltration of less than 400 mL after a 4-hour dwell using 2 L of 4.25% glucose containing dialysate. This condition is associated with a large vascular peritoneal surface area and impaired aquaporin channel-mediated water transport. These patients are best managed with frequent short dwells and elimination of long dwells, such as with nocturnal APD, combined with daytime icodextrin. Since icodextrin is a large molecule, its reabsorption is unaffected by membrane permeability and it is able to maintain gradual but sustained ultrafiltration for 12 hours or more. Improvement of peritoneal function can be brought about by minimizing glucose exposure, peritoneal rest (use of glucose-free dialysate), use of solutions low in GDPs, and use of icodextrin, which has been shown to extend therapy time on PD in patients with loss of ultrafiltration. Mortality in this group is higher than in other patients on PD, probably because of poor fluid control and increased protein losses in the dialysate.

Diabetic Patients on Peritoneal Dialysis

Diabetic glomerulosclerosis is the most common cause of kidney failure in PD patients. The vast majority of diabetic patients require insulin on PD, even if they did not require insulin before the initiation of dialysis. This condition is partly due to glucose absorption from the dialysate and the associated weight gain. Insulin can be given to PD patients via the intraperitoneal route (thought to be better because it is more physiologic, but evidence for this is lacking), the subcutaneous route, or a combination of both. If given intraperitoneally, the total daily dose of insulin required will increase as insulin adsorbs onto the polyvinylchloride bags. Patients on APD generally require long-acting subcutaneous insulin (with or without intraperitoneal regular insulin) for adequate glucose control. Injecting insulin regularly into dialysis fluid bags confers a theoretical risk of bacterial contamination and subsequent peritonitis, although no evidence of this occurring in practice exists. Nevertheless, it is not a widely used route of insulin administration for diabetic patients at present.

OUTCOMES IN PATIENTS ON PERITONEAL DIALYSIS

Survival of patients on PD is similar to those on HD. Underlying comorbidity very much dictates outcome, although several observational studies from Canada and Europe have shown that there is a survival advantage in commencing dialysis therapy with PD and then changing to HD when the therapy fails rather than starting on HD first. In this way, one can maximize the advantages that PD confers in the first few years of dialysis, in terms of preservation of RRF and better fluid control. If patient preference and medical conditions allow, PD may well be the preferred dialysis therapy when a patient reaches chronic kidney disease stage 5.

Patient and technique survival are improving. Various single-center and registry cohort long-term studies begun in the 1990s showed that the 5-year actuarial patient survival on PD ranged from 40% to 60%, whereas 5-year technique survival ranged from 55% to 70%. Risk factors for death on PD include increasing age, the presence of cardiovascular disease or diabetes mellitus, decreased serum albumin level, poor nutritional status, and inadequate dialysis. The leading causes of death are cardiovascular disease and infections.

Patients transfer from PD to HD for a multitude of reasons, including peritonitis or exit site infection, catheter malfunction, inability to perform the dialysis procedure, and inadequate clearance or ultrafiltration (particularly with loss of RKF) (see Fig. 61-5). In many cases, the patient who loses a catheter because of either peritonitis or a catheter infection may elect to switch to HD permanently. The increasing use of the Y-set and "flush before fill" systems is associated with improved technique survival on CAPD that is primarily due to lower peritonitis rates. It is hoped that long-term outcomes will improve with greater emphasis on adequacy, greater use of more physiologic PD solutions, and the use of PD in an integrated renal replacement treatment program, wherein PD is an equally important modality to HD and perhaps the first dialytic treatment for most ESRD patients.

Transplantation is the goal for most patients on dialysis. The allograft and patient survival of transplanted PD patients are similar to those of transplanted HD patients, but there is reduced delayed graft function in transplanted PD patients. Delayed graft function, in combination with rejection, is a strong predictor of graft survival. If the transplant does not initially function, PD can be continued as long as the peritoneal cavity was not entered during surgery. The peritoneal catheter is generally left in place for 2 to 3 months until the graft is functioning well.

Use of Peritoneal Dialysis in an Integrated Renal Replacement Therapy Program

The utilization of PD varies from 2% to 3% to over 80% of the dialysis population in different countries worldwide. Such discrepancies in utilization cannot be explained by medical variables alone. The major reasons reside in nonmedical factors, such as finance and reimbursement, plus physician biases and prejudices, which have a serious impact on therapy options conveyed to patients. There is a decline in the use of PD in many western countries, partly related to lack of patient choice and information.

PERITONEAL DIALYSIS FOR ACUTE RENAL FAILURE

Intermittent peritoneal dialysis can be successfully used to manage patients with acute renal failure. In this case, the peritoneal catheter is often inserted percutaneously using a stylet, without a subcutaneous tunnel and therefore with an increased risk of fluid leakage and peritonitis. Rapid exchanges are performed to maximize small-solute clearance, often one to two exchanges per hour using a cycler. The patient may be kept on a cycler for 48 hours or even longer, or IPD may be performed daily for 10 to 12 hours. Although extremely effective for volume control and better tolerated in the hemodynamically unstable patient than HD, clearance of small solutes may be inadequate in catabolic patients or patients on total parenteral nutrition receiving large protein loads. In addition, in the intensive care unit setting there is considerable risk of peritonitis. For these reasons, IPD has been largely replaced by HD and continuous hemodiafiltration for the management of acute renal failure.

BIBLIOGRAPHY

Abu-Alfa AK, Burkart J, Piraino B, et al: Approach to fluid management in peritoneal dialysis: A practical algorithm. Kidney Int 81(suppl):S8–S16, 2002.

Brown EA, Davies SJ, Rutherford P, et al: EAPOS Group. Survival of functionally anuric patients on automated peritoneal dialysis: The European APD Outcome Study. J Am Soc Nephrol 14:2948–2957, 2003.

Churchill DN, Thorpe KE, Nolph KD, et al: Increased peritoneal membrane transport is associated with decreased patient and technique survival for continuous peritoneal dialysis patients. J Am Soc Nephrol 9:1285–1293, 1998.

Coles G, Williams JD: What is the place of peritoneal dialysis in the integrated treatment of renal failure? Kidney Int 54:2234–2240, 1998.

Davies S, Phillips L, Griffiths A, et al: What really happens to people on long-term peritoneal dialysis? Kidney Int 54:2207–2217, 1998.

Davies SJ, Woodrow G, Donovan K, et al: Icodextrin improves the fluid status of peritoneal dialysis patients: Results of a double-blind randomized controlled trial. J Am Soc Nephrol 14:2338–2344, 2003.

Dinesh KC, Golper T, Gokal R: Adequacy, nutrition and cardiovascular outcome in peritoneal dialysis. Am J Kidney Dis 33: 617–632, 1999.

Fenton SSA, Schaulbel DE, Desmeules M, et al: Hemodialysis versus peritoneal dialysis: A comparison of adjusted mortality rates. Am J Kidney Dis 30:334–342, 1997.

Flanigan M, Gokal R: Peritoneal catheters and exit-site practices toward optimum peritoneal access—a review of current developments. Perit Dial Int 2005, in press.

Gokal R: New strategies for peritoneal dialysis solutions. Nephrol Dial Transplant 12(Suppl 1):74–77, 1997.

Gokal R: Peritoneal dialysis in the 21st century: An analysis of current problems and future developments. J Am Soc Nephrol 13(suppl 1):S104–S116, 2002.

Gokal R, Alexander SR, Ash S, et al: Peritoneal catheters and exit-site practices toward optimum peritoneal access: 1998 update. Perit Dial Int 18:11–33, 1998.

Hendriks PM, Ho-dac-Pannekeet MM, van Gulik TM, et al: Peritoneal sclerosis in chronic peritoneal dialysis patients: Analysis of clinical presentation, risk factors, and peritoneal transport kinetics. Perit Dial Int 17:136–143, 1997.

Lo WK, Ho YW, Li CS, et al: Effect of Kt/V on survival and clinical outcome in CAPD patients in a randomized prospective study. Kidney Int 64:649–656, 2003.

Mistry CD, Gokal R, Peers E, and the Midas Study Group: A randomised multicentre clinical trial comparing isosmolar dextrin 20 with hyperosmolar glucose solutions in Continuous Ambulatory Peritoneal Dialysis (CAPD): A 6 month study. Kidney Int 46:496–503, 1994.

Mujais S, Nolph K, Gokal R, et al: Evaluation and management of ultrafiltration problems in peritoneal dialysis. International Society for Peritoneal Dialysis Ad Hoc Committee on Ultrafiltration Management in Peritoneal Dialysis. Perit Dial Int 20(suppl 4):S5–S21, 2000.

Nakayama M, Kawaguchi Y, Yamada K, et al: Immunohistochemical detection of advanced glycosylation end-products in the peritoneum and its possible pathophysiological role in CAPD. Kidney Int 51:182–186, 1997.

National Kidney Foundation Dialysis Outcomes Quality Initiative (DOQI): Clinical practice guidelines: Peritoneal dialysis adequacy. Am J Kidney Dis 30(suppl 3):S67–S136, 1997.

Nissenson A, Prichard SS, Cheng IPS, et al: ESRD modality selection into the 21st century: The importance of non-medical factors. ASAIO J 43:143–150, 1997.

Paniagua R, Amato D, Vonesh E, et al: Effects of increased peritoneal clearances on mortality rates in peritoneal dialysis: ADEMEX, a prospective, randomized, controlled trial. J Am Soc Nephrol 13:1307–1320, 2002.

Piraino B, et al: ISPD Guidelines on management of peritonitis in peritoneal dialysis. Perit Dial Int 2005, in press.

Stenvinkel P, Chung SH, Heimburger O, Lindholm B: Malnutrition, inflammation, and atherosclerosis in peritoneal dialysis patients. Perit Dial Int. 21(suppl 3):S157–S162, 2001.

The Mupirocin Study Group: Nasal mupirocin prevents *Staphylococcus aureus* exit site infection during peritoneal dialysis. J Am Soc Nephrol 11:2403–2408, 1996.

Williams JD, Craig KJ, Topley N, et al: Peritoneal Biopsy Study Group. Morphologic changes in the peritoneal membrane of patients with renal disease. J Am Soc Nephrol 13:470–479, 2002.

CHAPTER **62**

Outcomes of Endstage Renal Disease Therapies

Akinlolu O. Ojo

In 2004, more than 450,000 endstage renal disease (ESRD) patients received renal replacement therapy (RRT) in the United States. The outcomes of ESRD therapy are largely determined by four variables: (1) the demographic characteristics of the patient; (2) the concomitant medical conditions or comorbidities at the initiation of ESRD therapy; (3) the modality of the RRT; and (4) new comorbid conditions that develop after the onset of ESRD. Among the three main RRT types, kidney transplantation is generally accepted to be associated with the best outcomes independent of all other factors, although there has never been a randomized trial to compare transplantation with dialytic therapies. It is more difficult to determine the superiority of one dialytic option over another because the decision to choose between hemodialysis and peritoneal dialysis are governed by numerous factors that are independent determinants of outcomes. Moreover, ESRD patients often change treatment modality, which further complicates the effort to isolate the independent survivorship effect of any one modality.

MORTALITY

In 2002, the adjusted annual mortality rate for all ESRD patients on treatment in the United States was 177 per 1000 patients, representing a death rate that was 20-fold higher than the corresponding rate of 9 per 1000 life-years in the overall U.S. general population. At age 45 years, the expected remaining life-years for the general U.S. population is 34.7 years, whereas an ESRD patient of the same age has a life expectancy of 6.2 years on dialysis and 19.5 years with a functioning kidney transplant. Given that mortality associated with ESRD is 100% without treatment, it is important that the comparison with the U.S. general population not obscure the huge survival benefits of ESRD therapy itself. Moreover, patients who begin ESRD treatment arrive with a proportionately higher burden of cardiovascular disease and other risk factors. Therefore, their underlying mortality risks would be significantly higher than the average for the overall U.S. population. Table 62-1 shows the mortality rates by ESRD diagnosis at two separate times: 1991

and 2002. There has been an encouraging trend in the overall ESRD mortality rate. In 2002, the overall, adjusted ESRD mortality rate was 11% lower than it was in 1991 (177 vs. 199 deaths per 1000 patient-years). This improvement can potentially be attributed to a number of factors, including the management of anemia, increased transplantation rates, improved dialysis delivery, and more attention to the management of cardiovascular risk factors.

CAUSES OF MORTALITY IN ENDSTAGE RENAL DISEASE PATIENTS

Cardiac diseases remain the predominant cause of death in ESRD patients, accounting for 39% of all deaths. Other leading causes of death are infection (15%), cerebrovascular disease (5%), and malignancy (4%; Fig. 62-1). The contrast in mortality due to cardiovascular disease in the general population and the ESRD population is striking (Fig. 62-2). The high rate of cardiac death reflects both the extraordinarily high burden of cardiac disease present at the onset of ESRD therapy and the accelerated progression of atherosclerosis that occurs during ESRD. Persistent volume overload, hemodynamic perturbations associated with the hemodialysis procedure, chronic inflammation due to uremia, and a host of nontraditional cardiovascular risk factors (hyperparathyroidism, hyperhomocysteinemia, anemia, and oxidative stress) have been identified as major contributors to cardiac death in ESRD patients. Among the individual cardiac causes of death, cardiac arrest or sudden death is listed as the most frequent cause of death (50%), followed by acute myocardial infarction (22%), arrhythmia (11%), cardiomyopathy (7%), and atherosclerotic heart disease (6%). Obviously, these cardiac diagnoses are not mutually exclusive; more than one cardiac diagnosis is often responsible for the proximate cause of death. These specific cardiac causes of death may not be absolutely accurate; errors associated with death certificates and data registries, such as the U.S. Renal Data System (USRDS), are of significant magnitude. Such inaccuracies notwithstanding, the majority of deaths in ESRD patients are due to cardiac disease regardless of the treatment modality being considered.

489

TABLE 62-1   Adjusted, Annual Mortality Rates per 1000 Patient-Years at Risk by Primary ESRD Diagnosis

Primary ESRD Diagnosis	1991	2002	Percent Change
All	199	177	−11.0
Diabetes mellitus	255	219	−14.1
Hypertension	181	168	−7.2
Glomerulonephritis	146	125	−14.4
Other	181	162	−10.5

ESRD, endstage renal disease.
Data from the U.S. Renal Data System: USRDS Annual Data Report: Atlas of End-Stage Renal Disease in the United States. Bethesda, MD, National Institutes of Health, National Institutes of Diabetes and Digestive and Kidney Diseases, 2004.

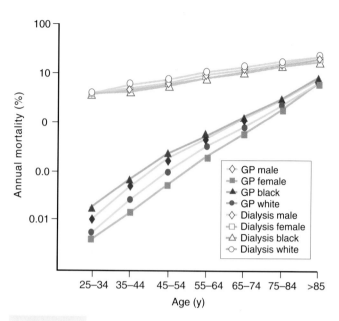

FIGURE 62-2   Cardiovascular disease mortality in the general population (GP) compared with that in the dialysis population. Data stratified by age, race, and gender. (From Foley RN, Parfrey PS, Sarnak MJ: Clinical epidemiology of cardiovascular disease in chronic renal disease. Am J Kidney Dis 32[suppl 3]:112–119, 1998.)

ESRD patients with cardiovascular, respiratory, or vascular access complications experience their highest mortality risk in the 6-month interval immediately following an event or medical procedure associated with the specific comorbid condition. For example, the risk for death following an acute myocardial infarction is greatest within the first 6 months and declines in the subsequent 18 months.

Pneumonia and blood-borne infection are the leading infectious causes of death in the ESRD population. The immunodeficient state of chronic uremia and frequent disruption of skin barrier by the vascular access penetration for hemodialysis and the transfer of pathogens during peritoneal dialysis bag exchanges are principal predisposing factors to infectious episodes in ESRD patients. Transplant recipients with good allograft function remain at increased risk for infectious deaths, particularly from opportunistic pathogens as a result of the chronic use of potent immunosuppressant drugs.

The most common malignancy in ESRD patients occurs in the urogenital system. The incidence of renal cell carcinoma is particularly high in ESRD patients with polycystic kidney disease. Renal cell carcinoma is sometimes diagnosed in other patients after the initiation of chronic dialysis. Most of these patients, however, die from cardiovascular disease before succumbing to the cancer.

FACTORS ASSOCIATED WITH MORTALITY

Demographics

Age, race, sex, and body mass index (BMI) are strong determinants of mortality in ESRD patients. Mortality increases substantially with increasing age. A small unexplained higher mortality rate is also noted in females compared with males (Fig. 62-3). Patients of Asian and African descent consistently have lower overall adjusted mortality rates compared with whites and Native Americans. The mortality advantage of African Americans is not evident when only patients with a functioning kidney transplant are considered. A notable paradoxical observation in both incident and prevalent dialysis patients is that, in contrast to the general population, higher BMI is associated with lower mortality except at the extremes of BMI distribution, in which the observations for general population also holds for dialysis patients. High BMI is associated with higher mortality risks in kidney transplant recipients.

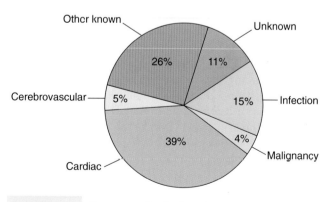

FIGURE 62-1   Percentage distribution of causes of death in ESRD patients receiving renal replacement therapy between 1991 and 2001. (Data from the U.S. Renal Data System: USRDS Annual Data Report: Atlas of End-Stage Renal Disease in the United States. Bethesda, MD, National Institutes of Health, National Institutes of Diabetes and Digestive and Kidney Diseases, 2003.)

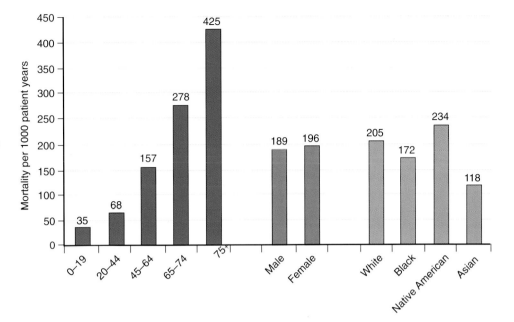

FIGURE 62-3 Death rates per 1000 patient-years at risk in ESRD patients by demographic characteristics. (Data from the U.S. Renal Data System: USRDS Annual Data Report: Atlas of End-Stage Renal Disease in the United States. Bethesda, MD, National Institutes of Health, National Institutes of Diabetes and Digestive and Kidney Diseases, 2004.)

Comorbidity

ESRD patients are plagued by a heavy burden of medical illnesses, which are principally related to preexisting cardiovascular risk factors, complications of dialytic therapy, and the underlying chronic uremia itself. The major coexisting medical conditions found in ESRD patients include diabetes mellitus, hypertension, coronary artery disease, congestive heart failure, peripheral vascular disease, anemia, uremic osteodystrophy, and vascular access or peritoneal catheter complications. Acute myocardial infarction (AMI) and decompensated congestive heart failures are two major problems in the ESRD population. The rate of acute myocardial infarction in

dialysis patients seems to be on the increase. In one registry report, the AMI rate in dialysis patients was 54 per 1000 patient-years in 1994 and 79 per 1000 patient-years in 2002. The average dialysis patient has two hospital admissions annually and the average kidney transplant recipient has one hospital admission annually (Fig. 62-4). In both dialysis and transplant groups, the annual hospitalization rate is 25% higher for patients with the primary ESRD diagnosis of diabetic nephropathy compared with the other diagnoses. The hospitalization rates translate into 14, 16, and 7 inpatient days per year for the average hemodialysis, peritoneal dialysis, and transplantation patient, respectively. Cardiac diagnoses and procedures account for 35% of all hospitalizations, with respiratory

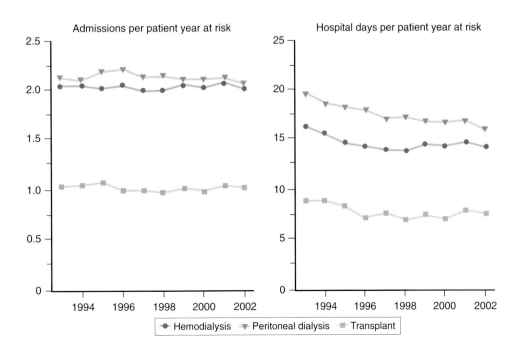

FIGURE 62-4 Adjusted hospital admissions and days in prevalent ESRD patients by modality. Rates adjusted for age, gender, race, and primary diagnosis. (Data from the U.S. Renal Data System: USRDS Annual Data Report: Atlas of End-Stage Renal Disease in the United States, Bethesda, MD, National Institutes of Health, National Institutes of Diabetes and Digestive and Kidney Diseases, 2004.)

disorders (mostly pneumonia) and infections accounting for 8% and 6% of hospital discharge diagnoses, respectively. According to the USRDS 2005 report, all-cause hospitalization rates for dialysis patients declined by 2% between 1993 and 2002. During the same period, admissions for vascular access declined by 26.4%, probably because of growth in outpatient interventional procedures. The rate of hospital admissions for cardiovascular disease and infection increased by 7% and 20%, respectively, during the same period.

Malnutrition contributes in large measure to the morbidity in ESRD patients. Serum albumin has been used as a traditional marker of nutritional status but it is now firmly established that serum albumin is also a marker of inflammation and nutritional status. Serum albumin concentration is a consistent reverse correlate of mortality in the ESRD population. Despite the improvement in the delivery of dialysis and correction of anemia witnessed in the past decade, the mean serum albumin level has changed little over time. According to the USRDS Nutrition Special Studies Report, 20% of prevalent dialysis patients have serum albumin levels below the lower limits of normal. In both incident and prevalent dialysis patients, a low serum albumin level is more prevalent in whites than in nonwhites.

Renal Replacement Modality

The choice of RRT modality is a strong predictor of outcome. However, this relationship is severely confounded, since the modality choice itself is governed by several independent predictors of mortality. Therefore, the true influence of the modality on clinical outcome is unclear. This is most glaringly illustrated by transplantation. ESRD patients achieve kidney transplant candidacy after a rigorous assessment of cardiovascular, nutritional, infectious, and psychosocial risks. Active status on the transplant waiting list implies that the candidate is well. Thus, the kidney transplant candidate is 45 years old on average, with either no clinically detectable or stable coronary artery disease and an annual morality risk of 6% to 8%, whereas the hemodialysis patient not on the transplant list has a mean age of 62 years, is hospitalized twice yearly for congestive heart failure, and has an annual mortality risk of 20% to 25%. Hence, fair comparison of the impact of hemodialysis versus kidney transplantation on patient outcome requires a comprehensive adjustment for the baseline differences in the characteristics between the patient groups receiving each type of RRT.

Of the prevalent ESRD population in the United States, 65% are on hemodialysis, 28% have a functioning kidney transplant, and 6% are on peritoneal dialysis. The latter are equally divided between continuous ambulatory peritoneal dialysis (CAPD) and automated peritoneal dialysis. Major differences in patient baseline characteristics notwithstanding, the survival curves are different among

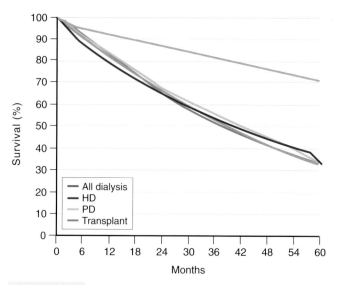

FIGURE 62-5 Adjusted survival by treatment modality: 1993–1997 incident patients. HD, hemodialysis; PD, peritoneal dialysis. (Data modified from the U.S. Renal Data System: USRDS Annual Data Report: Atlas of End-Stage Renal Disease in the United States. Bethesda, MD, National Institutes of Health, National Institutes of Diabetes and Digestive and Kidney Diseases, 2004.)

treatment modalities, as shown in Figure 62-5. Although controversies still exist, well-conducted analysis does not support a clear superiority of hemodialysis over peritoneal dialysis in patient survival. In the USRDS data of incident dialysis population, the adjusted 5-year survival rate was 34.3% and 33.0% for hemodialysis and peritoneal dialysis, respectively. Table 62-2 shows the adjusted annual death rates for hemodialysis, peritoneal dialysis, and transplant populations at 1, 2, and 3 years after the onset of ESRD. Aside from the consistently lower death rates in the transplant recipients, the relationship between modality and risks for death vary with time from the onset of ESRD, with no demonstrable superiority of hemodialysis over peritoneal dialysis. The impact of treatment modality on mortality is further confounded by the

TABLE 62-2 Adjusted Death Rates per 1000 Patient-Years at Risk by Modality among Incident Endstage Renal Disease Patients

	Adjusted Death Rate per 1000 Patient-Years		
Year Since Onset of ESRD	Hemodialysis	Peritoneal Dialysis	Renal Transplantation
First year	245.6	181.1	91.1
Second year	213.1	226.7	43.6
Third year	229.7	264.2	57.9

Data from the U.S. Renal System: USRDS Annual Data Report: Atlas of End-Stage Renal Disease in the United States. Bethesda, MD, National Institutes of Health, National Institutes of Diabetes and Digestive and Kidney Diseases, 2004.

cross-effect resulting from modality changes that occur in a significant proportion of patients.

Kidney transplantation offers the best survival outcomes in virtually all age categories of ESRD patients up to 74 years. Table 62-3 shows the expected additional life-years gained by deceased donor kidney transplantation when compared with dialysis patients who are also transplant candidates. On the average, kidney transplantation extends life by an additional 20 years. In absolute terms, younger patients gain more additional life-years from renal transplantation, but the proportional survival advantage of transplantation is equally large in older patients.

Treatment Parameters

The delivered dose of dialysis (as determined by urea Kt/V) and the membrane flux characteristics (which determine the sizes of the molecule removed) have been considered to be important determinants of mortality and morbidity (see Chapter 60). Observational studies support the notion that reduction in mortality can be achieved through the delivery of high urea Kt/V or the use of high-flux dialyzer membranes. These hypotheses were tested in a large randomized clinical trial of 1846 maintenance hemodialysis patients in the United States (the HEMO study). Neither high urea Kt/V nor high-flux membrane was associated with a decrease in the primary outcome of all-cause mortality. Because the HEMO study

was performed only in patients undergoing thrice weekly hemodialysis, a significant beneficial effect of daily hemodialysis treatment cannot be ruled out. A randomized trial on chronic peritoneal dialysis (the ADEMEX study) also failed to demonstrate a decrease in all-cause mortality by increasing the creatinine clearance of the dialysis.

Major treatment factors that influence the outcomes of kidney transplantation include donor source, immunosuppressive regimen, and follow-up care. In general, transplants from living donors have 20% to 25% longer graft half-life than kidneys from deceased donors. Independent of donor source, extremes of donor age are associated with diminished graft survival. The calcineurin inhibitors (cyclosporine and tacrolimus) are still the mainstay of maintenance immunosuppressive regimen for kidney transplantation, but the availability of target of rapamycin analogues (sirolimus and certican) has provided the impetus for the use of a calcineurin-free regimen. This, together with increasing use of steroid avoidance/minimization protocols, promises to reduce the immunosuppression-associated morbidity and mortality seen in transplant recipients. Lymphoproliferative disorders and malignant neoplasia of the genitourinary system, skin, and gastrointestinal tracts and opportunistic infections are major complications of prolonged immunosuppressive therapy used in kidney transplantation. The majority of kidney transplant recipients, however, die of cardiovascular disease with a functioning allograft.

TABLE 62-3   Life Expectancy among Recipients of First Cadaveric Renal Transplants (n = 23,275) Compared with Wait-Listed Dialysis Patients (n = 46,164), 1991–1997

Group	Relative Risk for Death 18 Months after Transplantation	Projected Years of Life (in Reference Group) without Transplantation	Projected Years of Life with Transplantation
All transplant recipients	0.32 (0.30–0.35)	10	20
Age (years)			
0–19	0.33 (0.12–0.87)	26	39
20–39	0.24 (0.20–0.29)	14	31
40–59	0.33 (0.29–0.37)	11	22
60–74	0.39 (0.33–0.47)	6	10
Sex			
Male	0.34 (0.30–0.38)	10	19
Female	0.30 (0.26–0.34)	11	23
Race			
Native American	0.50 (0.27–0.96)	9	14
Asian	0.43 (0.25–0.75)	15	23
Black	0.52 (0.44–0.62)	13	19
White	0.28 (0.25–0.30)	9	19
Cause of ESRD			
Diabetes	0.27 (0.24–0.30)	8	19
Glomerulonephritis	0.39 (0.31–0.48)	12	20
Other	0.38 (0.33–0.43)	12	20

ESRD, endstage renal disease.
Data from Wolfe RW, Ashby VB, Milford EL, et al: Comparison of mortality in all patients on dialysis, patients on dialysis awaiting transplantation, and recipients of a first cadaveric transplant. N Engl J Med 341:1725–1730, 1999.

QUALITY OF LIFE

Health-related quality of life (HRQOL) is an important measure in ESRD patients. Patients who perform poorly on HRQOL testing are more prone to suffer other untoward outcomes, including hospitalization and death. In the United States, blacks tend to have higher scores on all components of HRQOL, report better overall health, and have higher energy levels compared with whites. In the HEMO study, patients receiving high-dose dialysis tended to report better physical quality of life and less pain. Effective interventions to improve quality of life in ESRD patients are generally lacking, but aggressive treatment of anemia, musculoskeletal disorders, and minimization of hospital admissions have been shown to have positive impact of quality of life. Depression is prevalent in dialysis patients but is underrecognized and poorly treated.

REHABILITATION

In most situations, the onset of dialysis is associated with a progressive decline in socioeconomic status, and the ability to maintain gainful engagement in the labor force is often hampered by the physical and psychological limitations of ESRD itself and the tedious demand of dialysis therapy. Moreover, the median age of onset of ESRD (62 years) is close to the statutory retirement age in the United States.

Gainful employment is not the only component of successful rehabilitation. Ability to engage in volunteer and vocational activities, independent living, and exercise capacity are all essential features of successful rehabilitation, which bring benefits to the patient in terms of self-perception and to society at large. Kidney transplantation offers the best hope of rehabilitation, with a higher proportion of patients being able to participate in many normal activities. The annual national and international transplant games are a showcase of an impressive array of athletic ability and talents in ESRD patients who have received transplants. When judged by return to the labor force alone, however, the rate of successful rehabilitation in renal transplant recipients is only modestly higher than in dialysis patients. In the United States, it has been suggested that a large fraction of patients with a functioning transplant who are capable refrain from returning to gainful employment so that they may maintain Medicare disability benefits that include the insurance coverage of immunosuppressive drugs.

ECONOMIC COSTS

The ESRD population is growing rapidly and reached 450,000 patients in 2003. The number of incident patients reached 100,000 for the first time in 2003. Among Medicare dialysis patients, the per capita annual expenditure in 2002 was $63,000, including $53,000 from Medicare and $10,000 in deductibles and copayments. Among ESRD patients, dialysis cost is significantly higher than average in children, and total health-care costs are higher in patients over 65 years of age and in those with diabetes. Patients with a kidney transplant incur $100,000 in medical cost in the first year and $15,700 for each additional year of a functioning transplant. The expenditure of the major payer for the ESRD program, the Medicare system, has grown by 6.7% annually in the past decade, reaching $17.0 billion in 2002.

BIBLIOGRAPHY

Cheung AK, Levin NW, Greene T, et al: Effects of high-flux hemodialysis on clinical outcomes: Results of the HEMO study. Am Soc Nephrol 14:3251–3263, 2003.

Eknoyan G, Beck GJ, Cheung AK, et al, the Hemodialysis (HEMO) Study Group: Effect of dialysis dose and membrane flux in maintenance hemodialysis. N Engl J Med 347:2010–2019, 2002.

Hicks LS, Cleary PD, Epstein AM, Ayanian JZ: Differences in health-related quality of life and treatment preferences among black and white patients with endstage renal disease. Qual Life Res 13:1129–1137, 2004.

Mapes DL, Bragg-Gresham JL, Bommer J, et al: Health-related quality of life in the Dialysis Outcomes and Practice Patterns Study (DOPPS). Am J Kidney Dis 44(5 suppl 3):54–60, 2004.

Rocco MV, Dwyer JT, Larive B, et al, the HEMO Study Group: The effect of dialysis dose and membrane flux on nutritional parameters in hemodialysis patients: Results of the HEMO Study. Kidney Int 65:2321–2334, 2004.

U.S. Renal Data System: USRDS 2002 Annual Data Report: Atlas of End-Stage Renal Disease in the United States. Bethesda, MD, National Institutes of Health, National Institutes of Diabetes and Digestive and Kidney Diseases, 2004.

U.S. Renal Data System: USRDS 2003 Annual Data Report: Atlas of End-Stage Renal Disease in the United States. Bethesda, MD, National Institutes of Health, National Institutes of Diabetes and Digestive and Kidney Diseases, 2004.

van Doorn KJ, Heylen M, Mets T, Verbeelen D: Evaluation of functional and mental state and quality of life in chronic haemodialysis patients. Int Urol Nephrol 36:263–267, 2004.

Wolfe RA, Ashby VB, Milford EL, et al: Comparison of mortality in all patients on dialysis, patients on dialysis awaiting transplantation, and recipients of a cadaveric renal transplant. N Engl J Med 341:1725–1730, 1999.

CHAPTER 63

Nutrition and Kidney Disease

T. Alp Ikizler

During progression of chronic kidney disease (CKD), the requirements and utilization of different nutrients change significantly. These changes ultimately place kidney disease patients at higher risk for protein-calorie malnutrition. In addition, the presence of protein-calorie malnutrition is an important predictor of poor outcome in these patients. Understanding the applicable nutritional principles and the available methods for improving nutritional status of these patients is essential. National Kidney Foundation (NKF) Clinical Practice Guidelines for Chronic Kidney Disease and Nutrition in Chronic Kidney Disease provide in-depth information regarding these principles.

NUTRIENT METABOLISM IN KIDNEY DISEASE

Protein Metabolism and Requirements

Chronic Kidney Disease Patients

In general, the minimal daily protein requirement maintains a neutral nitrogen balance and prevents malnutrition; this minimum has been estimated to be a daily protein intake of approximately 0.6 g/kg in healthy individuals, with a safe level of protein intake equivalent to the minimal requirement plus 2 standard deviations, or approximately 0.75 g/kg/day. One of the most significant findings of advanced kidney disease is a decrease in appetite. Several studies have indicated that CKD patients spontaneously restrict their dietary protein intake, with levels less than 0.6 g/kg/day when glomerular filtration rate is less than 10 mL/minute (stage 5). Other markers of malnutrition, such as loss of weight, also correlate with decreasing kidney function and dietary protein intake as early as stage 3, suggesting that anorexia predisposes CKD patients to malnutrition. Accumulation of uremic toxins may not be the sole cause of decreased dietary nutrient intake. Table 63-1 depicts some of the factors that can cause decreased nutrient intake as well as other potential mechanisms that can cause protein-calorie malnutrition in kidney disease patients. Patients with kidney disease secondary to diabetes mellitus are more prone to malnu-

trition because of dietary restrictions and gastrointestinal symptoms such as gastroparesis, nausea, and vomiting, as well as bacterial overgrowth in the gut and pancreatic insufficiency. Depression, which is commonly seen in CKD patients, is also associated with anorexia. Diabetic CKD patients with poorly controlled blood sugar tend to have increased protein breakdown. In addition, CKD patients are usually prescribed a large number of medications, particularly sedatives, phosphate binders, and iron supplements, which are also associated with gastrointestinal complications. Finally, the socioeconomic status of the CKD patients, their lack of mobility, and their age are other predisposing characteristics for decreased dietary protein intake.

Protein Restriction in Chronic Kidney Disease Patients

Dietary protein restriction has been recommended as a therapeutic approach for retarding the progression of CKD. The results of several recent studies on this subject are conflicting. The results of the largest clinical trial, the Modification of Diet in Renal Disease (MDRD) study, did not demonstrate a benefit of dietary protein restriction on progression of kidney disease. On the other hand, three meta-analyses indicate that such diets may be beneficial in slowing the progression of disease, albeit only to a small extent. If such diets are to be used, it is important to assure that patients are not at risk for malnutrition. In the MDRD study, there were only minor changes in nutritional markers in the low-protein diet groups, suggesting that under close observation, protein-restricted diets provided with or without supplements of essential amino acids or their keto-analogues will maintain nutritional status. Indeed, patients with advanced CKD (stages 4 and 5) are shown to adjust their protein turnover rate appropriately in response to decreased protein intake, usually with no significant impact on net balance. However, the dedicated dietitian involvement with heavy emphasis on maintenance of caloric intake used in the MDRD study is not available to the majority of patients with CKD; thus, such dietary interventions should be tried only in highly motivated and closely supervised patients. Table 63-2 lists the recommended dietary prescriptions for protein intakes for patients at different stages of CKD.

TABLE 63-1 Variables Associated with Decreased Nutritional Status of Chronic Kidney Disease Patients

Increased protein and energy requirements
 Losses of nutrients (amino acids and/or proteins) during
  dialysis
 Increased resting energy expenditure

Decreased protein and calorie intake
 Anorexia
 Frequent hospitalizations
 Inadequate dialysis dose
 Comorbidities (diabetes mellitus, gastrointestinal diseases,
  ongoing inflammatory response)
 Multiple medications

Increased catabolism/decreased anabolism
 Dialysis-induced catabolism
  Bioincompatible hemodialysis membranes
  Amino acid losses
  Induction of inflammatory cascade
 Amino acid abnormalities
 Metabolic acidosis
 Hormonal derangements
  Hyperparathyroidism
  Insulin and growth hormone resistance

Chronic Dialysis Patients

Several treatment-related conditions predispose chronic dialysis patients to negative nitrogen balance (see Table 63-1). There are inevitable losses of amino acids during both hemodialysis (HD) and peritoneal dialysis (PD), ranging from 5 to 8 g of amino acids per HD session and 5 to 12 g/day of amino acids during PD. Losses may be higher with high-efficiency HD or when peritonitis is present. The absorption of glucose during PD may also predispose patients to anorexia due to the development of satiety. In addition, a feeling of fullness may be related to the fluid in the peritoneal cavity. One of the most important influences affecting the nutritional status of dialysis patients is the dose of dialysis. The amount of

dialysis should be adequate to prevent development of uremic malnutrition in both HD and PD patients.

Amino Acid Metabolism

Chronic kidney disease patients have well-defined abnormalities in their plasma and to a lesser extent in their muscle amino acid profiles. Commonly, essential amino acid concentrations are low and nonessential amino acid concentrations high. The etiology of this abnormal profile is multifactorial. An important influence is the progressive loss of kidney tissue, where metabolism of several amino acids takes place. Specifically, glycine and phenylalanine concentrations are elevated whereas serine, tyrosine, and histidine concentrations are decreased. Plasma and muscle concentrations of branched-chain amino acids (valine, leucine, and isoleucine) are reduced in chronic dialysis patients. Among these, valine displays the greatest reduction. In contrast, plasma citrulline, cystine, aspartate, methionine, and both 1- and 3-methylhistidine levels are increased. Although inadequate dietary intake possibly contributes to these abnormal essential amino acid profiles, certain abnormalities occur even in the presence of adequate dietary nutrient intake, indicating that the uremic milieu has an additional effect. Indeed, it has been suggested that the metabolic acidosis that is commonly seen in uremic patients plays an important role in increased oxidation of branched-chain amino acids.

Energy Metabolism

Patients with kidney failure have a less well-defined minimum energy requirement (see Table 63-2), which is dependent on the resting energy expenditure, the activity level of the patient, and other ongoing illnesses. Resting energy expenditure is elevated in chronic dialysis patients compared with normal controls matched for age,

TABLE 63-2 Recommended Intakes of Protein, Energy, and Minerals in Kidney Failure

	Protein	Energy	Phosphorus	Sodium
Chronic kidney disease				
Stages 1–3 (GFR >30 mL/min)	No restriction	No restriction	600–800 mg/day	<2 g/day*
Stages 4–5 (GFR <30 mL/min)	0.60–0.75 g/kg/day[†]	35 kcal/kg/day[‡]	600–800 mg/day[§]	<2 g/day
Endstage renal disease				
Hemodialysis	>1.2 g/kg/day	35 kcal/kg/day[‡]	600–800 mg/day[§]	<2 g/day
Peritoneal dialysis	>1.3 g/kg/day	35 kcal/kg/day[‡]	600–800 mg/day[§]	<2 g/day
Acute renal failure				
No dialysis	1.0–1.2 g/kg IBW/day	35 kcal/kg/day	600–800 mg/day[‖]	<2 g/day
Dialysis	1.0–1.2 g/kg IBW/day	35 kcal/kg/day	600–800 mg/day[‖]	<2 g/day

IBW, Ideal body weight.
*If hypertensive.
[†]With close supervision and frequent dietary counseling.
[‡]30 kcal/kg/day for individuals 60 years and older.
[§]Along with phosphate binders, as needed.
[‖]If phosphorus >5.5 mg/dL.

sex, and body mass index, and is further increased during the HD procedure when catabolism is at maximum due to amino acid losses. For stage 4 and 5 CKD patients, the recommended energy intake is 35 kcal/kg body weight/day for those who are younger than 60 years of age and 30 to 35 kcal/kg body weight/day for individuals 60 years and older.

Lipid Metabolism

Dyslipidemia is quite common in CKD patients, and abnormalities in lipid profiles can be detected in patients once kidney function begins to deteriorate, suggesting that uremia is associated with lipid disorders. The presence of nephrotic syndrome or other comorbidities such as diabetes mellitus and liver disease, as well as the use of medications altering lipid metabolism (e.g., thiazide diuretics, beta blockers), contribute additionally to the dyslipidemia seen in kidney disease.

In HD patients, the most common abnormalities are elevated serum triglycerides and very-low-density lipoproteins, and decreased low-density and high-density lipoproteins (LDLs, HDLs). The increased triglyceride component is thought to be related to increased levels of apolipoprotein CIII, an inhibitor of lipoprotein lipase. A substantial number of chronic HD patients also have elevated lipoprotein (a) (Lp[a]) levels. Patients on PD have higher concentrations of serum cholesterol, triglycerides, LDL cholesterol, and apolipoprotein B, even though the mechanisms that alter the lipid metabolism are similar to those seen in chronic HD patients. It is thought that this results from increased protein losses through the peritoneum, possibly by mechanisms that are operative in the nephrotic syndrome and the glucose load supplied by dialysate causing increased triglyceride synthesis and hyperinsulinemia. Patients on PD also have higher concentrations of Lp(a). It remains to be clarified whether these differences in dyslipidemia are clinically significant.

Dyslipidemia and Cardiovascular Risk in Dialysis Patients

Cardiovascular death is the leading cause of mortality in chronic dialysis patients. Hypercholesterolemia and other abnormalities in lipid profile have been associated with increased risk of atherosclerosis and cardiovascular events in the general population. However, it has not been well established whether this relationship applies to chronic dialysis patients. Indeed, large cross-sectional studies have identified that low rather than high cholesterol concentrations are associated with an increased risk of mortality in chronic dialysis patients. In contrast, a large multicenter study showed that, in a cohort of diabetic patients on HD, those who died from a cardiovascular event had higher median cholesterol, LDL cholesterol, LDL/HDL ratio, and apolipoprotein B concentrations at the time of initiation of dialysis. It is generally accepted that chronic dialysis patients with known risk factors for atherosclerosis and cardiovascular events should be treated with an appropriate regimen, including lipid-lowering agents when indicated. Given that chronic dialysis patients tend to have lower serum levels of cholesterol, a total cholesterol concentration higher than 200 mg/dL and/or LDL concentration higher than 100 mg/dL should be treated in these patients, preferably with 3-hydroxy-3-methylglutaryl coenzyme A reductase inhibitors. Whether this approach influences the overall outcome in these patients remains to be proved. The NKF Clinical Practice Guidelines for Managing Dyslipidemias in Chronic Kidney Disease provide in-depth review of this important subject.

Mineral, Vitamin, and Trace Element Requirements

Sodium intake should be restricted to less than 2 g/day in CKD patients with hypertension at any stage of disease. The restriction is similar in chronic dialysis patients, to control interdialytic fluid gain and reduce thirst. Potassium intake should be less than 2 g/day in patients with stage 4 and 5 CKD and in chronic dialysis patients, although PD patients may need a more liberal intake. In early kidney disease (stages 2 and 3), restriction of phosphorus intake to 600 to 800 mg/day is recommended. Because additional restriction of dietary phosphorus in clinical settings is impractical, once the creatinine clearance falls below 30 mL/minute (stages 4 and 5), phosphate binders are often necessary along with the dietary restriction. Use of calcium-containing binders will also provide the supplemental calcium needed in advanced kidney failure. Similar recommendations are appropriate for HD patients. A detailed review of calcium and phosphorus metabolism can be found in Chapter 64.

Vitamin A concentrations are usually elevated in chronic dialysis patients, and intake of even small amounts leads to excessive accumulation. There have been several reports on vitamin A toxicity in chronic dialysis patients, and therefore it should not be supplemented. Vitamin E levels in chronic dialysis patients are not well defined, and there have been reports of increased, decreased, or unchanged concentrations. Therefore, it is not clear whether vitamin E supplementation is required in chronic dialysis patients. The therapeutic use of pharmacologic doses of vitamin E as an antioxidant is under investigation. Vitamin K supplementation is usually not recommended in chronic dialysis patients unless they are at high risk for developing vitamin K deficiency, as with prolonged hospitalization, poor dietary intake, or antibiotic therapy. The derangements of vitamin D metabolism characteristic of CKD are discussed in detail in Chapter 64. The serum concentrations of the water-soluble vitamins are reported to be low in chronic dialysis patients, mainly because of decreased dietary intake and increased removal during HD. Multivitamin preparations designed specifically for patients with kidney failure are available and useful for correcting these low concentrations without inducing vitamin A toxicity. Nevertheless, it is important to recognize that the daily requirements of vitamin B_6, folic acid, and ascorbic acid are often increased in chronic dialysis patients. Monitoring levels may be appropriate for patients at risk of vitamin deficiency (e.g., patients not able take vitamin supplements, patients with moderate to severe malnutrition).

The concentrations of most of the trace elements are mainly dependent on the stage of CKD. Although there is an extensive list of trace elements that may have altered concentrations in body fluids in patients on chronic dialysis, only a few are thought to be important. Serum aluminum is the most important trace element in these patients, because elevated levels have been shown to be associated with dialysis dementia as well as bone disease. Aluminum intoxication can be caused either by use of inadequately purified water for HD (mostly eliminated with the use of reverse osmosis for water purification) or by use of phosphate binders that contain aluminum hydroxide. Because the prolonged ingestion of such binders is a risk factor for aluminum intoxication, patients consuming aluminum on a long-term basis should have repeated measurements of the element. A serum aluminum concentration well below 30 mg/L is the desired level in chronic HD patients. A detailed review of this subject can be found in Chapters 64 and 67.

METABOLIC AND HORMONAL DERANGEMENTS IN CHRONIC KIDNEY DISEASE PATIENTS

Metabolic acidosis, which commonly accompanies progressive kidney disease, also promotes malnutrition through increased protein catabolism. During metabolic acidosis, muscle proteolysis is stimulated by an adenosine triphosphate (ATP)-dependent pathway involving ubiquitin and proteasomes. Recent data suggest that correction of metabolic acidosis improves nutritional status in PD patients. The recommendation is to maintain the serum bicarbonate level within normal limits, supplementing with sodium bicarbonate as needed. Several hormonal derangements, including insulin resistance, increased glucagon concentrations, and secondary hyperparathyroidism, are also implicated in the development of malnutrition in CKD. Increased concentrations of parathyroid hormone have been shown to enhance amino acid release from muscle tissue. Resistance to anabolic actions of growth hormone and insulin-like growth factor-1 has been suggested as an important factor in the development of malnutrition in CKD patients. Although plasma concentrations of growth hormone actually increase during the progression of kidney failure, probably as a result of reduced renal clearance of the hormone, more recent evidence suggests that uremia per se is associated with the development of resistance to growth hormone action at cellular levels. This blunted response would be expected to attenuate the anabolic actions of these hormones, specifically protein synthesis.

INDICES OF NUTRITIONAL STATUS IN KIDNEY FAILURE PATIENTS

Although practical methods to assess nutritional status are imperative, the appropriate interpretation of nutritional markers in patients with kidney failure remains a challenge. Several markers utilized for nutritional purposes are influenced by many non-nutritional factors. In CKD patients, relatively simple biochemical measures reflecting the visceral protein stores, such as serum albumin, serum creatinine, and blood urea nitrogen (BUN), as well as less commonly used parameters such as prealbumin and insulin-like growth factor-1, have been proposed as nutritional markers. Serum albumin is probably the most extensively examined nutritional index in almost all patient populations, because of its readily available assay and strong association with outcome. However, serum albumin concentration may be affected by other coexisting problems in addition to malnutrition. Specifically, serum albumin is a negative acute-phase reactant; therefore, its serum concentration decreases sharply in response to inflammation and thus may not necessarily reflect the changes in nutritional status in acutely or chronically ill patients. Serum albumin concentration in CKD patients may also be affected by other non-nutritional factors, such as external losses (e.g., proteinuria), extravascular fluid volume, and liver disease.

Anthropometric studies can be used for body composition analysis in CKD patients. More reliable and accurate methods of body composition analysis such as prompt neutron activation analysis, which measures total body nitrogen content, and dual-energy x-ray absorptiometry require expensive equipment and are available only in specialized centers. A more recently proposed method to evaluate the nutritional status of CKD patients is subjective global assessment (SGA), a simple method that draws on the experience of a clinician to make an overall assessment of nutritional status in a standardized way. Its advantage is that it includes objective data (e.g., disease state and weight changes) and several manifestations of poor nutritional status. Its limitations are a heavy reliance on the clinical judgment and the inability to tailor a specific nutritional intervention. The usefulness of the SGA as a standard nutritional tool in kidney disease patients has yet to be determined.

Estimation of dietary protein intake can also be used as a marker of overall nutritional status in the CKD patient.

Although dietary recall is a direct and simple measure of dietary protein consumption, several studies have shown that this method lacks accuracy in estimating the actual intake. Therefore, other means of measuring dietary protein intake, such as 24-hour urine urea nitrogen excretion in CKD patients or urea nitrogen appearance (UNA) rate calculations derived from urea kinetic modeling in chronic dialysis patients, have been suggested as useful methods to estimate protein intake (equation 1). However, these indirect estimations of dietary protein intake are valid only in stable patients and may easily overestimate the actual intake in catabolic patients, in whom endogenous protein breakdown may lead to a high UNA.

Equation 1:

$$UNA\,(g/day) = urinary\ urea\ nitrogen\,(g/day)$$
$$+\ change\ in\ body\ urea\ nitrogen\,(g/day)$$

where

Change in body urea nitrogen
$$= (SUN_f - SUN_i[g/L/day]) \times BW_i(kg) \times (0.60\,L/kg)$$
$$+ (BW_f - BW_i[kg/d]) \times SUN_f(g/L) \times (1.0\,L/kg)$$

where SUN_i and SUN_f are the initial and final serum urea nitrogen values for the period of measurement (usually the entire interdialytic period), BW is body weight, $0.60\,L/kg$ is an estimate of the fraction of body weight that is water, and 1.0 is the volume of distribution of urea in the weight that is gained or lost.

In summary, there are many different methods available for assessing protein and energy nutritional status in CKD patients. Some are easy to perform, readily available, and inexpensive, whereas others are sophisticated, not available in many centers, and either expensive or have an unfavorable cost-to-benefit ratio. For example, a monthly nutritional screening can be easily performed at nearly any clinic or hospital by measuring serum albumin, serum prealbumin, serum transferrin, and bioimpedance values. However, if the goal is to follow changes in body composition precisely and longitudinally, then anthropometry, dual-energy x-ray absorptiometry, and even more sophisticated methods, if available, may be useful. For all indirect methods, repeated measures and technical standardization are extremely important to reduce variability of results.

EXTENT OF MALNUTRITION IN CHRONIC KIDNEY DISEASE PATIENTS

Virtually every study that has evaluated the nutritional status of advanced CKD patients (stages 3 through 5) has reported some degree of poor nutritional status. The prevalence of abnormalities has been estimated to range from approximately 20% to 60% in different studies using various nutritional parameters. In CKD patients not yet on chronic dialysis (stages 4 and 5), mild to severe malnutrition by subjective global assessment is reported in 44% of patients. Using the same method, the prevalence of moderate to severe malnutrition is reported at 30% in chronic HD patients and 40% in PD patients.

ASSOCIATION OF NUTRITION AND OUTCOME IN KIDNEY FAILURE

A number of studies have documented the increased mortality and morbidity in CKD patients suffering from poor nutritional status. In a comprehensive study of prevalent chronic dialysis patients, serum albumin concentration was identified as the most powerful indicator of mortality. Even serum albumin concentrations of 3.5 to 4.0 g/dL, which is considered a normal value by most laboratories, resulted in an increased relative risk of death as compared with 4.0 g/dL or higher. In addition, decreases in serum creatinine (an indicator of muscle mass) and percentage ideal body weight were also associated with increased risk of death in this patient population. Similar observations can be made for incident dialysis patients. Specifically, low serum creatinine and albumin concentrations at the time of initiation of maintenance dialysis are associated with increased risk of mortality and morbidity during the subsequent years on HD.

STRATEGIES FOR TREATMENT OF MALNUTRITION IN KIDNEY FAILURE PATIENTS

A list of general measures to prevent and/or to treat malnutrition in different stages of CKD is presented in Table 63-3. Considering the catabolic state associated with chronic uremia, it is clear that attempts to

---

TABLE 63-3 Interventions to Prevent and/or Treat Malnutrition in Advanced Kidney Failure

CKD patients
  Close supervision and nutritional counseling (especially for patients on protein-restricted diets)
  Initiation of dialysis or kidney transplant in advanced CKD patients with apparent uremic malnutrition despite vigorous attempts to rectify it

Maintenance dialysis patients
  Appropriate amount of dietary protein (>1.2 g/kg/day) and calorie (>35 kcal/kg/day) intake
  Optimal dose of dialysis (urea reduction ratio >70%)
  Use of biocompatible hemodialysis membranes
  Nutritional support in chronic dialysis patients who are unable to meet their dietary needs
    Oral supplements
    Tube feeds (if medically appropriate)
    Intradialytic parenteral nutritional supplements for hemodialysis patients
    Amino acid dialysate for peritoneal dialysis patients

CKD, chronic kidney disease.

encourage patients to maintain an adequate protein and calorie intake are essential. Most of these patients continue their predialysis diets while on chronic renal replacement therapy. It is important to ensure that the dietary protein and calorie intakes of these patients fulfill the increased requirements after initiation of dialysis. Repetitive comprehensive dietary counseling by an experienced dietitian is an important step to improve dietary intake; another is detection of early signs of malnutrition. Similar efforts should be spent not only in outpatient settings, but also during hospitalizations of these patients, since hospitalized patients have even lower dietary protein and calorie intake.

For cases in which dietary counseling to improve nutritional status is unsuccessful, other forms of supplementation such as enteral (including oral protein, amino acid, and energy supplementation; nasogastric feeding tubes; percutaneous endoscopic gastrostomy or jejunostomy tubes) and intradialytic parenteral nutrition (IDPN) may be considered. Only a limited number of studies evaluating the effects of enteral supplementation in malnourished chronic dialysis patients are available. Furthermore, most of these studies are uncontrolled and small in scope, and they demonstrate only a variable degree of success. It is usually a challenge to determine whether an enteral form of supplementation is effective and when to try more expensive and invasive measures such as IDPN.

Several reports have emphasized the effective use of IDPN as a potential therapeutic intervention in malnourished chronic dialysis patients. Recent studies suggest that IDPN acutely improves net protein synthesis and increases albumin fractional synthetic rate. In a retrospective analysis of more than 1500 chronic HD patients treated with IDPN, decreasing risk of death with the long-term use of IDPN was reported, particularly in patients with serum albumin concentrations below 3.5 g/dL and serum creatinine concentrations below 8 mg/dL. Studies using amino acid dialysate (AAD) in PD patients have provided conflicting results. In studies that suggested benefit from AAD, serum transferrin and total protein concentrations increased and plasma amino acid profiles tended toward normal with one or two exchanges of AAD per day. On the other hand, an increase in BUN concentration associated with exacerbations of uremic symptoms as well as metabolic acidosis are potential complications of AAD. Overall, the available evidence suggests that IDPN and AAD may offer alternative methods of nutritional intervention in a group of dialysis patients in whom oral or enteral intake cannot be maintained. Unfortunately, most studies evaluating IDPN and AAD are retrospective, uncontrolled, or short-term and subject to other design flaws. Until a controlled study comparing various forms of nutritional supplementation in similar patient groups is completed, one should be cautious in prescribing costly nutritional interventions.

NUTRITION IN ACUTE RENAL FAILURE

The nutritional hallmark of acute renal failure (ARF) is excessive catabolism. Numerous studies have shown that the protein catabolic rate in ARF patients requiring dialytic support is much higher than that seen in other patient populations; it can be massive (more than 2 g/kg ideal body weight/day). Several influences have been postulated as the underlying mechanism for the high rate of protein catabolism observed in ARF patients. Concurrent illnesses may initiate a sequence of catabolic events through several different processes. Specific cytokines including interleukins and tumor necrosis factor are stimulated during catabolic conditions such as sepsis and induce increased whole-body protein breakdown. In addition to increased catabolism, ARF patients may also encounter a diminished utilization and incorporation of available nutrients, presumably due to a combination of underlying diseases as well as metabolic abnormalities associated with acute uremia per se.

Proper nutritional indices should be used to identify ARF patients at risk for poor nutritional state, design appropriate nutritional support, and assess the response to nutritional supplementation. In ARF, the major process contributing to poor nutritional status is the metabolic response to ongoing morbidity or catabolism, whereas in other chronic states such as CKD, malnutrition is largely a response to chronic starvation. The nutritional markers that correlate best with efficacy of nutritional therapy and patient outcome may be considerably different in these two separate disease states and have not been well delineated in the ARF patient population. The determination of UNA and levels of biochemical markers such as serum albumin, prealbumin, and transferrin are influenced by many variables. Similarly, utilization of traditional measures of body composition such as anthropometry has limited application in ARF patients because of major shifts in body water.

The actual requirements for protein and energy supplementation in ARF patients are not well defined (see Table 63-2). Measurement of UNA, which reflects protein catabolism, may be cumbersome in clinical settings, because it requires urine collection on a daily basis. Measurement of energy expenditure by indirect calorimetry is also problematic. The fluid distribution and the fat-free mass may be considerably altered in ARF patients, especially during the oligoanuric phase. In the presence of diminished utilization due to altered metabolic state as well as diminished clearance due to decreased kidney function, excessive protein supplementation will result in increased accumulation of end products of protein and amino acid metabolism. This would be reflected as higher BUN concentrations. Provision of large quantities of nutrients may require more fluid administration and predispose patients to fluid overload. Aggressive nutrition may also cause hyperglycemia, hyperlipidemia, hypernatremia, hyponatremia, and abnormalities in amino acid profiles. Although most of these abnormalities can be managed by complementary dialytic support, the initiation and intensity, as well as the dose of dialysis treatment in ARF, are in themselves an area of controversy. In highly catabolic patients who are receiving excessive nutritional supplementation, even dialysis cannot fully prevent the undesirable accumulation of nitrogenous waste products.

BIBLIOGRAPHY

Chertow GM, Ling J, Lew NL, et al: The association of intradialytic parenteral nutrition with survival in hemodialysis patients. Am J Kidney Dis 24:912–920, 1994.

Ikizler TA, Greene J, Wingard RL, et al: Spontaneous dietary protein intake during progression of chronic renal failure. J Am Soc Nephrol 6:1386–1391, 1995.

Ikizler TA, Hakim RM: Nutrition in endstage renal disease. Kidney Int 50:343–357, 1996.

Ikizler TA, Himmelfarb J: Nutrition in acute renal failure. Adv Renal Replacement Ther 4(suppl 1):54–63, 1997.

K/DOQI clinical practice guidelines for nutrition in chronic renal failure. Am J Kidney Dis 6(suppl):S1–S140, 2000.

Klahr S, Levey AS, Beck GJ, et al: The effects of dietary protein restriction and blood-pressure control on the progression of chronic renal disease. N Engl J Med 330:877–884, 1994.

Kopple JD: The nutrition management of the patient with acute renal failure. JPEN. J Parenter Enteral Nutr 20:3–12, 1996.

Lowrie EG, Huang WH, Lew NL, Liu Y: The relative contribution of measured variables to death risk among hemodialysis patients. In Friedman EA (ed): Death on Hemodialysis. Amsterdam, Kluwer Academic Publishers, 1994, p 121.

Mitch WE, Goldberg AL: Mechanism of muscle wasting: The role of ubiquitin-proteasome pathway. N Engl J Med 335:1897–1905, 1997.

Owen WF, Jr, Lew NL, Liu Y, et al: The urea reduction ratio and serum albumin concentrations as predictors of mortality in patients undergoing hemodialysis. N Engl J Med 329:1001–1006, 1993.

Parker TF, III, Wingard RL, Husni L, et al: Effect of the membrane biocompatibility on nutritional parameters in chronic hemodialysis patients. Kidney Int 49:551–556, 1996.

Pupim LB, Flakoll PJ, Brouillette JR, et al: Intradialytic parenteral nutrition improves protein and energy homeostasis in chronic hemodialysis patients. J Clin Invest 110:483–492, 2002.

Qureshi AR, Alvestrand A, Danielsson A, et al: Factors predicting malnutrition in hemodialysis patients: A cross-sectional study. Kidney Int 53:773–782, 1998.

Stenvinkel P, Heimburger O, Paultre F, et al: Strong association between malnutrition, inflammation, and atherosclerosis in chronic renal failure. Kidney Int 55:1899–1911, 1999.

CHAPTER 64

Bone Disorders in Chronic Kidney Disease

Nadine DeLove Tanenbaum   L. Darryl Quarles

Chronic kidney disease (CKD) alters the regulation of calcium and phosphate homeostasis, leading to secondary hyperparathyroidism, metabolic bone disease, soft-tissue calcifications, and other metabolic derangements that have a significant impact on morbidity and mortality. Although bone disease and abnormalities of parathyroid function are historically the main clinical features of this disorder, cardiovascular diseases and extraskeletal calcifications are increasingly recognized as complications resulting from disordered mineral homeostasis or from treatment with calcium and vitamin D sterols. Earlier interventions and stringent management guidelines have been proposed for subjects with CKD by the National Kidney Foundation (NKF) Kidney Disease Outcomes Quality Initiative (K/DOQI), with the hope of more effectively and safely treating this disorder. In addition, new treatments with calcimimetic drugs based on a growing understanding of molecular targets that control parathyroid gland function are emerging.

PATHOGENESIS OF ABNORMAL MINERAL METABOLISM AND SECONDARY HYPERPARATHYROIDISM IN CHRONIC KIDNEY DISEASE

An increase in circulating parathyroid hormone (PTH) concentrations is the hallmark of secondary hyperparathyroidism. Diminished production of calcitriol $(1,25\text{-}(OH)_2$ vitamin $D_3)$, decreases in serum calcium, and increases in serum phosphorus are the major metabolic abnormalities leading to its increase. PTH is responsible for maintaining serum calcium concentrations in a narrow range through direct actions on the distal tubule of the kidney to increase calcium reabsorption and on bone to increase calcium and phosphate efflux (Fig. 64-1). PTH stimulates 1α-hydroxylase in the renal proximal tubule, thereby increasing calcitriol production. Vitamin D_3 is formed when 7-dehydrocholesterol in the skin absorbs solar radiation. Vitamin D_3 is also found in oily fish, such as salmon, and in fish liver oils. Vitamin D_3 undergoes hydroxylation in the liver to 25-hydroxyvitamin D (biologically inactive), in a conversion that is not tightly regulated. Then, 25-hydroxyvitamin D

undergoes 1α-hydroxylation in the renal proximal tubule to its active form. Calcitriol increases gastrointestinal absorption of calcium and phosphate and promotes osteoclast maturation.

The net effect of PTH is to create the positive calcium balance that is necessary to maintain calcium homeostasis. To prevent concomitant positive phosphate balance resulting from the skeletal effects of PTH and the gastrointestinal actions of calcitriol, PTH acts secondarily to increase renal phosphorus excretion mostly by decreasing activity of the sodium phosphate cotransporter in the proximal renal tubule. PTH is probably not the primary phosphaturic hormone, however. Instead, phosphaturic hormones, called phosphatonins, are probably the key regulators of phosphate homeostasis. The phosphatonin fibroblast growth factor 23 (FGF23) is increased in CKD and could potentially play a role in the adaptive response to loss of kidney function.

Parathyroid disease in CKD is a progressive disorder characterized by both increased PTH secretion and growth in the number of the PTH-secreting chief cells (hyperplasia). Elevations in serum PTH levels first become evident when the glomerular filtration rate (GFR) falls below $60\,\text{mL/minute/1.73}\,\text{m}^2$ (Fig. 64-2). This occurs before hyperphosphatemia, reductions in $1,25(OH)_2$ vitamin D_3 levels, and hypocalcemia are detectable by routine laboratory measurements (presumably as a result of the effects of increased PTH to restore homeostasis). PTH levels increase progressively as kidney function declines, such that all untreated subjects reaching stage 5 CKD (GFR less than $15\,\text{mL/minute/1.73}\,\text{m}^2$ or dialysis) would be expected to have elevated PTH levels.

Three molecular targets regulating parathyroid gland function have been identified. These targets include the G-protein-coupled calcium-sensing receptor (CaSR), the vitamin D receptor (VDR), and a putative extracellular phosphate sensor. Calcium acting through the CaSR is the major regulator of PTH transcription, secretion, and parathyroid gland hyperplasia. Calcitriol, which acts on the VDR in the parathyroid gland to suppress PTH transcription, but not PTH secretion, has overlapping functions with the CaSR. It appears, however, that the physiologic role of the VDR in regulating parathyroid

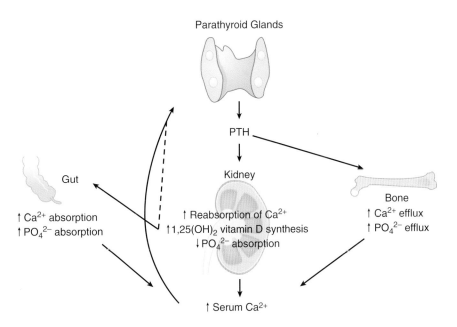

FIGURE 64-1 Regulation of systemic calcium homeostasis. Parathyroid hormone (PTH) is a calcemic hormone that targets the kidney to promote renal calcium conservation and bone to increase efflux of calcium and phosphorus. PTH-mediated $1,25(OH)_2$ vitamin D_3 production by the kidney increases gastrointestinal calcium and phosphate absorption. The phosphaturic actions of PTH on the kidney cause it to excrete the excess phosphate accompanying calcium absorption by the intestines and calcium efflux from bone. Changes in calcium, $1,25(OH)_2$ vitamin D_3, and phosphate levels exert feedback on the parathyroid glands (*dotted line*).

gland function may be subordinate to that of calcium. In this regard, secondary hyperparathyroidism and bone abnormalities in VDR-deficient mice can be corrected by normalizing serum calcium concentrations. Finally, extracellular phosphate has direct effects on parathyroid production, apparently through the regulation of PTH message stability. Hyperphosphatemia may also indirectly affect PTH production by lowering ionized calcium through chelation and by suppressing 1α-hydroxylase and hence calcitriol production by the kidney. Although animal studies have indicated that phosphate restriction alone is sufficient to prevent the development of secondary hyperparathyroidism in early CKD, these studies do not necessarily implicate hyperphosphatemia in a

primary role, since the increase in calcitriol production that accompanies dietary phosphate restriction can directly affect parathyroid gland function. Despite the relative importance of these molecular targets, the development of secondary hyperparathyroidism represents a compensatory response to reduced serum calcium and $1,25(OH)_2$ vitamin D_3 levels and to increased phosphorus.

Unless adequately treated, secondary hyperparathyroidism progresses inexorably, with the frequency of parathyroidectomy proportional to the number of years on dialysis. The difficulty in treating hyperparathyroidism is due in part to massive hyperplasia and possible adenomatous transformation of the parathyroid gland

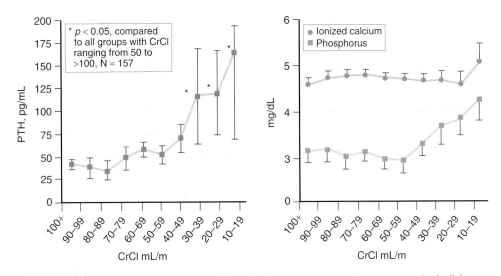

FIGURE 64-2 Secondary hyperparathyroidism develops as a compensatory response to declining kidney function and before detectable changes occur in serum calcium and phosphorus. Error bars reflect standard errors. (Data derived from Martinez I, Saracho R, Montenegro J, Llach F: The importance of dietary calcium and phosphorus in the secondary hyperparathyroidism of patients with early renal failure. Am J Kidney Dis 29:496–502, 1997.)

that occur as a result of the chronic stimulation of PTH production in CKD. Whereas enlarged hyperplastic parathyroid glands retain responsiveness to calcium-mediated PTH suppression (secondary hyperparathyroidism), hypercalcemia with an altered set point for PTH suppression, along with reductions in CaSR and VDR expression (tertiary hyperparathyroidism), can also develop. Some groups have sought to link parathyroid gland size by ultrasonography to the parathyroid gland's responsiveness to calcitriol and calcium-mediated suppression. Currently, however, there are no well-established methods for accurate parathyroid gland measurement.

HISTOLOGIC CLASSIFICATIONS OF BONE DISEASE ASSOCIATED WITH CHRONIC KIDNEY DISEASE

The specific types of histologic changes observed in CKD-associated bone disease depend on the age of the patient, duration of kidney failure, severity of serum PTH elevation, type of dialysis therapy used, and concurrent influences affecting bone. Both PTH and vitamin D receptors, as well as putative calcium sensing receptors, are present in osteoblasts. Osteoblast-mediated bone formation is coupled to osteoclast-mediated bone resorption through osteoblastic paracrine pathways. The circulating level of PTH is the primary determinant of bone turnover in CKD and a major determinant of the type of bone disease present. Acidosis, vitamin D status, accumulation of metals, and other conditions affecting mineralization of the extracellular matrix also contribute to the type of bone disease.

Bone disease associated with CKD (Fig. 64-3) has traditionally been classified histologically according to the degrees of abnormal bone turnover and impaired mineralization of the extracellular matrix. The current categories are: (1) secondary hyperparathyroidism/high-turnover bone disease or osteitis fibrosa, (2) mixed uremic bone disease (a mixture of high-turnover bone disease and osteomalacia), (3) osteomalacia (defective mineralization), and (4) adynamic bone disease (decreased rates of bone formation without a mineralization defect).

High-turnover bone disease caused by excess PTH is characterized by greater number and size of osteoclasts and an increase in number of resorption lacunae with scalloped trabeculae, as well as abnormally high numbers of osteoblasts. There is an increased amount of osteoid (unmineralized bone), which may have a woven appearance that reflects disordered collagen arrangement under conditions of rapid matrix deposition. The excess in osteoid surfaces that accompanies increased bone turnover has been described as mixed uremic bone disease but may reflect the normal response to increased turnover rather than superimposed defective mineralization. Peritrabecular fibrosis (and marrow fibrosis in severe cases), reflecting PTH stimulation of osteoblastic precursors, is observed in severe disease.

Osteomalacia is characterized by prolongation of the mineralization lag time as well as by increased thickness, surface area, and volume of osteoid. Osteomalacia was formerly linked to aluminum toxicity from both contamination of water in dialysis solutions and the use of aluminum-based phosphate binders. Other causes of osteomalacia that may be present in CKD patients include 25-hydroxyvitamin D deficiency (secondary to poor nutritional status and lack of exposure to sunlight from poor mobility and extended hospitalizations), metabolic acidosis (acidosis inhibits both osteoblasts and osteoclasts), and hypophosphatemia, such as seen in the Fanconi syndrome.

Adynamic bone disease is a low-turnover bone state that has received increased attention. In selected bone biopsy series, as many as 40% of hemodialysis patients and 50% of peritoneal dialysis patients have adynamic bone disease. In this disorder, the amount of osteoid thickness is normal or reduced, and there is no mineralization defect. The main findings are decreased numbers of osteoclasts and osteoblasts and very low rates of bone formation as measured by tetracycline labeling. High serum calcium levels sometimes seen in adynamic bone disease may be in part secondary to high oral calcium loads and suppression of PTH when calcium-based phosphate binders are used. There may also be a decreased ability of bone to buffer calcium loads in adynamic bone disease. The main risk factors for adynamic bone disease are peritoneal dialysis, older age, corticosteroid use, and diabetes. It is thought that adynamic bone disease represents a state of relative hypoparathyroidism in CKD.

Recently, this long-standing classification of CKD-associated bone disease has been questioned. One concern is that mixed uremic bone disease may not represent a distinct entity, since increased turnover is most often accompanied by variable degrees of reversible mineral deficit. Another problem is the uncertainty about the existence of adynamic bone disease, which in reality represents a low rate of bone formation that overlaps the normal range and is probably due to subnormal PTH secretion accompanying an excess of calcium and/or vitamin D treatment. Thus, so-called adynamic bone disease may not be a separate disease but a consequence of overtreatment of hyperparathyroidism with calcium and calcitriol.

CLINICAL MANIFESTATIONS OF BONE DISEASE ASSOCIATED WITH CHRONIC KIDNEY DISEASE

Most patients with CKD and mildly elevated circulating levels of PTH are asymptomatic. When present, clinical features of bone disease can be classified into musculoskeletal and extraskeletal manifestations.

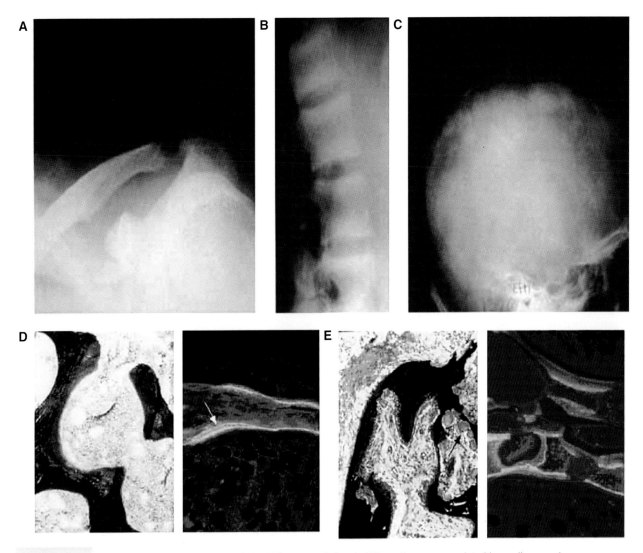

FIGURE 64-3 Radiographic (*A–C*) and histologic (*D, E*) features of chronic kidney disease–associated bone disease. *A*, Radiographic findings of severe erosion of the distal clavicle as a result of secondary hyperparathyroidism. *B*, An example of "rugger-jersey spine" resulting from sclerosis of the end plates. *C*, A "pepper-pot skull" with areas of erosion and patchy osteosclerosis. *D*, Histologic appearance of normal bone. Goldner Masson trichrome stain shows mineralized lamellar bone (*blue*) and adjacent nonmineralized osteoid surfaces (*red-brown, left*). Villanueva-stained section viewed under fluorescent light showing tetracycline labeling of freshly formed bone (double staining at arrow indicates amount of new bone laid down during the interval between periods of tetracycline administration) (*right*). *E*, Histologic appearance of osteitis fibrosa in a stage 5 CKD patient with elevated parathyroid hormone levels. Goldner Masson trichrome stain showing increased number of multinucleated osteoclasts at resorptive surfaces (*arrow*), and extensive bone marrow fibrosis, (as shown by light blue staining of marrow, *left*). Tetracyline labeling reveals marked increase in both the osteoid (*orange-red staining*) and sites of new bone formation as measured by the yellow-green bands below the osteoid surfaces (*right*). (*A–C*, From Martin KJ, González EA, Slatopolsky E: Renal osteodystrophy. In Brenner BM [ed]: Brenner and Rector's The Kidney, 7th ed. Philadelphia, Saunders, 2004, p 2280. With permission.)

Musculoskeletal Manifestations

Fractures, tendon rupture, and bone pain due to metabolic bone disease, muscle pain and weakness, and periarticular pain are the major musculoskeletal manifestations associated with CKD. The most clinically significant effect of metabolic bone disease in CKD is hip fracture, which is high among stage 5 CKD patients and is associated with an increased risk for death. Whereas there is a roughly 4.4-fold increase in hip fracture risk in dialysis patients compared to the general population,

studies attempting to link the type of histologic bone disease or a specific level of PTH to increased fracture risk have been inconclusive. The utility of bone mineral density (BMD) measurements as a measure of fracture risk have not been established in CKD.

Extraskeletal Manifestations

The most important evolution in the understanding of the clinical significance of disordered bone and mineral metabolism in CKD is the recognition that it a systemic disorder affecting soft tissues, particularly vessels, heart valves, and skin. Cardiovascular disease accounts for approximately half of all deaths of dialysis patients. Coronary artery and vascular calcifications occur frequently in stage 5 CKD and increase as a function of the number of years on dialysis. Gaining a better understanding of the etiology for this increased vascular calcification seen in patients with CKD and of how it may influence clinical cardiovascular events is of crucial importance.

Several patterns of vascular calcification have been described. The first occurs as focal calcification associated with lipid-laden foam cells seen in atherosclerotic plaques. These calcifications may increase both the fragility and risk for rupture of plaques. Some have questioned the negative role of calcification in the pathogenesis of the atherosclerotic vascular lesions, raising the possibility that it is an epiphenomenon with no pathologic consequences. The second pattern of vascular calcification is diffuse; it is not associated with atherosclerotic plaques and occurs in the media of vessels. This pattern is seen with aging, diabetes, and progressive kidney failure. This so-called "Mönckeberg's sclerosis" had been thought to be of little clinical significance for many years, but its effects of increasing blood vessel stiffness and reducing vascular compliance, resulting in a widened pulse pressure, increased afterload, and left ventricular hypertrophy, are potential mechanisms whereby vascular calcification could contribute to cardiovascular morbidity (Fig. 64-4). Coronary calcium load as detected by electron beam computed tomography (EBCT) has not been shown to correlate in dialysis patients with the degree of coronary vessel stenosis, however.

The exact mechanism of vascular calcification is not clear but probably reflects the combined effects of decreased mineralization inhibitors, such as matrix Gla protein (a calcification inhibitor known to be expressed by smooth muscle cells and macrophages in the artery wall), and increased mineralization inducers. Bone matrix proteins, such as osteopontin, osteocalcin, and the transcription factor osteoblast differentiation factor (Cbfa1) are found in calcified but not uncalcified vessels. Accumulating evidence suggests that vascular smooth muscle cells undergo a phenotypic transition to an osteoblast-like cell that may be important in driving the calcification process. An area of emerging study concerns how uremia may affect this process to accelerate calcification. Some studies suggest that calcitriol can modulate vascular smooth muscle growth and influence vascular calcification by up-regulation of its receptor and increased calcium uptake into smooth muscle cells. Vitamin D treatment enhances the extent of artery calcification in animal models given sufficient doses of warfarin to inhibit γ-carboxylation of matrix Gla protein. Phosphorus stimulates smooth muscle cells in culture to express bone-related proteins important in vascular calcification. An increased calcium × phosphate (Ca × P) product

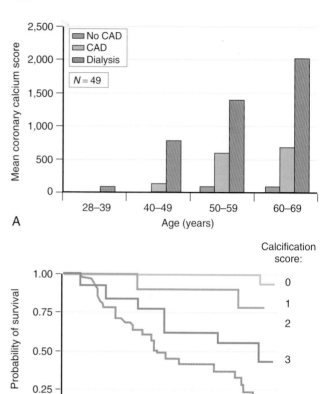

FIGURE 64-4 Increased risk of death and cardiovascular calcification in dialysis patients. *A,* Calcium score was determined by electron beam computed tomography. Mean coronary artery calcium score was significantly higher in hemodialysis patients than in nondialysis patients with documented cardiovascular disease. *B,* Risk of death in hemodialysis patients increases as a function of calcification score measured ultrasonographically. (p < 0.0001 for comparisons between all curres). (*A,* From Braun J, Oldendorf M, Moshage W, et al: Electron beam computed tomography in the evaluation of cardiac calcifications in chronic dialysis patients. Am J Kidney Dis 27:394–401, 1996. With permission from the National Kidney Foundation. *B,* From Blacher J, et al: Arterial calcification, arterial stiffness, and cardiovascular risk in end-stage renal disease. Hypertension 38:938, 2001. With permission.)

(obtained by by multiplying a patient's serum calcium, preferably corrected calcium, in mg/dL, by his or her serum phosphorus level in mg/dL) is associated with an increased risk of vascular and visceral calcification. Incremental elevations of serum phosphorus are an independent risk factor for increased mortality in patients on chronic maintenance hemodialysis.

Calciphylaxis, or calcemic uremic arteriolopathy, is another form of vascular calcification seen primarily, though not exclusively, in stage 5 kidney failure. The prevalence is not well established, but it may occur in between 1% and 4% of dialysis patients. Calciphylaxis presents with extensive calcifications of the skin, muscles, and subcutaneous tissues. Most often skin lesions occur on the breast, abdomen, and thighs. Unusual presentations, such as necrosis of the tongue and of the penis, as well as visceral involvement of the lungs, pancreas, and intestines, have been described. On examination there may be seen not only a violaceous rash, skin nodules, skin firmness, and eschars, but also livedo reticularis and painful hyperesthesia of the skin. Nonhealing ulcerations of the skin and gangrene resistant to medical therapy often lead to amputation, uncontrollable sepsis, and death. There is extensive medial calcification of small arteries, arterioles, capillaries, and venules, as well as intimal proliferation, endovascular fibrosis, and sometimes thrombosis. Whether the pathogenesis is similar to that of Mönckeberg's sclerosis is not clear. Cases reported to be associated with very high PTH levels improve following parathyroidectomy. However, there are reported cases in which the PTH levels are not markedly elevated. Anecdotal reports suggest that bisphosphonate therapy, thiosulfate, daily hemodialysis, hyperbaric oxygen treatment, and normalization of serum phosphate levels may improve outcomes. Other risk factors for calciphylaxis are obesity, advancing age, female gender, diabetes mellitus, warfarin use, recent trauma, hypotension, and calcium ingestion. Nanobacteria have recently been cultured from local calciphylaxis on the mitral valve, suggesting a role for infection and inflammation.

Musculoskeletal Abnormalities Not Related to Disordered Calcium and Phosphate Homeostasis: Amyloidosis

Patients who have been on dialysis for at least 7 to 10 years can develop osteoarticular amyloid depositions that consist of a protein called β_2-microglobulin (β_2M). This protein, which is found in the cell membrane and serves to stabilize the major histocompatibility complex (MHC) class I antigen on cell surfaces, is normally released into the plasma with cell turnover and cleared by the kidney. Severe forms of β_2M-deposition disease manifest as a destructive spondyloarthropathy, often in the cervical and lumbar spine, that can lead to spinal instability and neurologic compression. Magnetic resonance imaging (low signal intensity on both T1- and T2-weighted images) is important in distinguishing this entity from other destructive spinal processes. Carpal tunnel syndrome and arthritis are more frequent manifestations of β_2M amyloid deposition. β_2M deposits are found in periarticular areas, joints, and tendon sheaths. Bone cysts, especially in regions next to large joints where tendons insert, such as the hip, proximal humerus, and proximal tibia, can be seen in on radiography. There is no effective treatment except kidney transplantation to prevent ongoing bony damage from amyloidosis. A high-flux dialyzer that slightly lowers β_2M should be used.

DIAGNOSIS OF CHRONIC KIDNEY DISEASE–ASSOCIATED BONE DISEASE

Biochemical Parameters

Abnormal parathyroid gland function is assessed by measurement of random circulating PTH levels. Full-length PTH has a half-life of 2 to 4 minutes. PTH is cleaved into C-terminal (inactive), N-terminal (active), and midregional (inactive) PTH fragments in the peripheral tissues. These PTH fragments are excreted in the kidney and have a prolonged half-life in kidney failure. A two-site immunoreactive assay is currently used to measure circulating PTH concentrations. This "intact PTH" assay uses two antibodies: one detects an epitope near the N-terminal end, and the other detects the C-terminal end. The assay actually detects full-length bioactive PTH (amino acid residues 1 through 84; PTH[1–84]) as well as PTH fragments such as PTH(7–84). The PTH fragment, PTH(7–84), may lack biologic activity or potentially have distinct biologic effects. A new PTH assay ("whole PTH") has been developed that recognizes amino acid residues 1 through 4 of the N-terminal region of PTH and specifically detects full-length PTH(1–84). PTH levels using the whole PTH assay are approximately 50% lower than the "intact" PTH assay. The best way of using this assay has not been determined. The normal range of the intact PTH assay is 10 to 65 pg/mL in patients with normal kidney function. However, because of end-organ resistance to PTH that is more severe in later stages of CKD (possibly mediated by a decrease in PTH osteoblast receptors), the recommended PTH levels are about twofold to threefold above the upper value of the normal in dialysis patients. The recommended target ranges for serum intact PTH are 35 to 70 pg/mL, 70 to 110 pg/mL, and 150 to 300 pg/mL for CKD stages 3, 4, and 5, respectively (Table 64-1).

Parathyroid hormone levels are a direct measure of parathyroid gland function and an indirect measure of bone remodeling. PTH levels greater than 300 pg/mL correlate with the bony changes of secondary hyperparathyroidism and/or osteitis fibrosis. Patients with adynamic bone disease usually have intact PTH levels below 150 pg/mL, but these values also occur in subjects with normal bone.

Parathyroid hormone is only a crude, indirect measure of bone turnover, because factors other than PTH can affect bone. The predictive power of PTH levels as a measure of bone turnover can be increased by assessment of bone-specific alkaline phosphatase levels, which correlate with the degree of osteoblastic activity. Other biochemical markers of bone turnover are being developed that may provide a more accurate assessment of osteoblast and osteoclast activity in bone. For example, serum tartrate–resistant acid phosphatase 5b levels correlate well with histologic indices of osteoclasts and may serve as a specific marker for osteoclastic activity in CKD

TABLE 64-1   K/DOQI Clinical Practice Guidelines for Bone Metabolism and Disease in CKD

CKD Stage	GFR Range (mL/min/1.73 m²)	Recommended Serum Values			
		Phosphorus (mg/dL)	Calcium (corrected, mg/dL)	Ca × P (mg²/dL²)	Intact PTH (pg/mL)
3	30–59	2.7–4.6	8.4–10.2		35–70
4	15–29	2.7–4.6	8.4–10.2		70–110
5	<15, dialysis	3.5–5.5	8.4–9.5	<55	150–300

CKD, chronic kidney disease; Ca × P, calcium × phosphorus product; GFR, glomerular filtration rate; PTH, parathyroid hormone.
Modified from National Kidney Foundation. Kidney Disease Outcomes Quality Initiative. Clinical practice guidelines for bone metabolism and disease in chronic kidney disease. Am J Kidney Dis 43:S1–S201, 2004.

patients with bone disease. Efforts to correlate the different subtypes of bone disease with various markers of bone remodeling in both dialysis and predialysis patients is an area of ongoing research.

Bone Biopsy

Though no longer frequently performed, the gold standard for assessing and diagnosing the different types of bone disease in patients with CKD is an iliac crest bone biopsy with double tetracycline labeling. Bone histomorphometric analysis of the biopsy specimen includes assessment of bone and fibrosis volumes, amount of osteoid and mineralization, and numbers of osteoblasts and osteoclasts seen on bony surfaces. Bone biopsies should be considered in the setting of nontraumatic fracture with no other clear underlying etiology, suspected aluminum toxicity to confirm the diagnosis before chelation therapy or parathyroidectomy, and severe musculoskeletal symptoms and/or hypercalcemia with intermediate (100 to 500 pg/mL) intact PTH levels.

Imaging

In general, radiographic studies are not indicated in the diagnosis of the bone disorders seen in kidney failure. However, certain radiographic changes can be seen (see Fig. 64-3A to C). Increased osteoblast function, especially in the setting of severe elevations of PTH, can lead to increased trabecular bone volume and account for the sclerotic changes that manifest as a "rugger-jersey spine" on radiography. Osteoclast-mediated bone resorption of secondary hyperparathyroidism results in cortical thinning and the classical radiographic evidence of subperiosteal, intracortical, and endosteal bone resorption. Subperiosteal erosions are best seen at the distal ends of the phalanges and of the clavicles, and at the sacroiliac joints. Radiographically, expansile lytic lesions (brown tumors) can be seen in severe osteitis fibrosis. Pseudofractures, which show up as wide radiolucent bands perpendicular to the bone long axis, can be seen in osteomalacia.

There is currently no accurate correlation between BMD as measured by dual-energy x-ray absorptiometry (DEXA) and the type of CKD-associated bone disease present. Osteoporosis is defined as a BMD of 2.5 standard deviations or greater from the mean BMD of a young adult of the same gender and sex. Although patients with CKD generally have lower BMD than the general population, the interpretation of DEXA scans is further complicated in secondary hyperparathyroidism because of focal areas of osteosclerosis, the presence of extraskeletal calcifications, and variable presence of osteomalacia. Nevertheless, BMD should be assessed in patients who have had kidney transplantations or who have known risk factors or previous fractures and are candidates for osteoporosis therapy.

Deferoxamine Test

The deferoxamine (DFO) test is largely of historical interest, since the need to diagnosis aluminum toxicity has all but disappeared with the reduced exposure to aluminum in dialysate and phosphate binders. DFO chelates aluminum as well as iron, and its use increases the risk of serious mucormycosis and *Yersinia* infections because of the formation of ferrioxamine, which enhances the growth of these organisms. DFO is administered at 5 mg/kg at the end of dialysis after an initial serum aluminum level is drawn. Serum aluminum levels are measured again 2 days later. A test is positive if there is an increase in serum aluminum levels of 50 mg/L or more between the first and the second measurement.

TREATMENT OF DISORDERED BONE AND MINERAL METABOLISM IN CHRONIC KIDNEY DISEASE

The treatment of disordered mineral metabolism in CKD is directed toward normalizing serum calcium, phosphate, and PTH while minimizing the risk associated with the therapies. In the United States, the types of treatment chosen are currently influenced by the economic constraints of our current health care system, which reimburses for parenteral medications and limits the frequency of hemodialysis to three treatments per week. In addition, clinical practice guidelines for bone metabolism and disease in stages 3, 4, and 5 CKD have been developed by the NKF's K/DOQI. These are outlined in Table 64-1.

The K/DOQI recommendations are influenced by data linking an elevated serum phosphorus and Ca × P product to increased mortality and the growing recognition that excessive calcium exposure may increase the risk of cardiovascular calcification. However, there are no prospective studies that establish the efficacy and safety of the specific recommendations for biochemical target ranges included in these guidelines. The K/DOQI guidelines may be more conservative than would be supported by the existing data. For example, the risk of mortality associated with hyperphosphatemia increases at a serum phosphorus of greater than 6.2 mg/dL, whereas the recommended upper limit in K/DOQI in stage 5 CKD is 5.5 mg/dL. Also the recommendations set a new upper limit of corrected serum calcium at 9.5 mg/dL, which is below the upper limit of 10.2 mg/dL in normal individuals. (Note: corrected serum calcium = measured serum calcium + [0.8 × {4 − serum albumin in g/dL}].) In addition, achieving these targets with current treatment regimens may be difficult. For example, in a survey of 288 facilities that included 749 dialysis patients treated with vitamin D therapy, only 29% had average intact PTH levels within the defined target range. When serum phosphorus, Ca × P product, and serum calcium were included, the number of stage 5 CKD patients currently achieving K/DOQI guidelines was even lower. Nevertheless, these guidelines are a first step in standardizing the approach to manage this difficult disorder.

The various tools for treating secondary hyperparathyroidism and hyperphosphatemia include dietary phosphorus restriction, calcium- and noncalcium-based phosphate binders, calcitriol or other active vitamin D analogues, calcimimetics, and parathyroidectomy.

Controlling Serum Phosphorus

Dietary phosphorus restriction, though difficult to attain, should be initiated (800 to 1000 mg/day) for all subjects with stage 5 CKD. Dairy products, nuts, beer, and chocolate all have a high content of phosphorus. For patients who are on thrice-weekly dialysis and are receiving adequate nutrition, dietary phosphate restriction will be inadequate to correct the positive phosphate balance, especially in the presence of concurrent active vitamin D therapy. More frequent hemodialysis has been associated with better control of serum phosphorus levels, but with our current frequency and dose of dialysis, phosphate binders are almost invariably required.

The choice of phosphate binder used (i.e., calcium containing or nonaluminum, noncalcium containing) depends on many considerations, including efficacy of phosphate binding, side effects, and cost.

For many years calcium-based phosphate binders were the mainstay of therapy to control serum phosphate levels. Commonly used calcium-based phosphate binders include calcium carbonate and calcium acetate. Calcium carbonate contains 500 mg of elemental calcium in a 1250-mg tablet; calcium acetate contains 169 mg of elemental calcium in one 667-mg tablet. Calcium citrate should not be used as a phosphate binder, because citrate is reported to increase aluminum absorption from the gut. Calcium-based phosphate binders should be taken with meals so as to maximize binding of ingested phosphorus in the gut. When taken during fasting, more calcium is absorbed systemically and less phosphorus is bound. The concomitant use of active vitamin D sterols increases calcium absorption and the risk of hypercalcemia. While clinical studies are pending that will define the risk of calcium loading on mortality, the K/DOQI treatment recommendations in stage 5 CKD are to limit the total dose of calcium-based phosphate binders to 1500 mg elemental calcium per day and total intake of elemental calcium to 2000 mg/day. Calcium acetate has greater phosphorus-binding capacity than calcium carbonate, potentially allowing the use of lower doses of calcium binder. However, various small trials have not shown significant differences in the prevalence of hypercalcemia between these two compounds.

Vascular calcifications have been documented by EBCT to begin in the coronaries of childhood dialysis patients in their 20s. This, taken with growing concern about the possible clinical consequences of vascular calcifications, has lead to the greater use of noncalcium binders. Sevelamer is a noncalcium phosphate binder containing cross-linked poly-allylamine hydrochloride. It acts as an ion exchange polymer to bind phosphorus in the gut and is a less effective phosphate binder than calcium on a weight basis. However, in human trials, sevelamer, when titrated to meet serum phosphorus goals, appears equal in efficacy to the calcium-containing binders. Sevelamer has also been shown to decrease serum cholesterol and low-density lipoproteins and increase high-density lipoproteins in stage 5 CKD patients. Sevelamer has been associated with fewer arterial calcifications than calcium-based phosphate binders in dialysis patients. Whether this effect is due to less calcium loading, the lipid-lowering effect, or mild acidosis induced by sevelamer has not been established. Sevelamer is more costly than calcium binders and may be associated with gastrointestinal side effects at higher doses that can limit its use in some individuals. Nevertheless, regimens using vitamin D analogues to raise calcium and suppress PTH, along with sevelamer to lower phosphorus, are effective in controlling both the skeletal and extraskeletal complications of stage 5 CKD.

Although they are the most effective binders, aluminum-containing phosphate binders are not often used because of the potential of systemic absorption and subsequent neurologic, hematologic, and bone toxicity (see Chapter 67). Absorption of aluminum is increased by concomitant use of sodium citrate given for metabolic acidosis. Because of the potential for long-term toxicity, aluminum-containing antacids should be used only for a short period (less than 4 weeks) and for severe hyperphosphatemia that is refractory to other treatments.

A new noncalcium-based phosphate binder is lanthanum carbonate. Lanthanum, like aluminum, is a trivalent cation with an ability to chelate dietary phosphate, but it has low systemic absorption. In a phase III trial over a 1-year period, lanthanum carbonate controlled serum phosphorus levels in a comparable fashion to high-dose calcium carbonate. Mild gastrointestinal symptoms were the most common side effect in the lanthanum group. Because there is accumulation of small amounts of lanthanum in bone, it will be important to assess its long-term side effects. Polynuclear iron compounds that form insoluble complexes with phosphate are under early investigation.

Activating the Calcium-Sensing and Vitamin D Receptors to Suppress PTH Hyperfunction

Vitamin D Analogues

Treatment with 1,25-$(OH)_2$ vitamin D_3 (calcitriol) or an active vitamin D analogue (paricalcitol, doxercalciferol, alfacalcidol, or 22-oxacalcitrol) is also a means of controlling secondary hyperparathyroidism. By binding to the VDR on parathyroid tissue, the vitamin D analogue suppresses PTH production. There is not uniform agreement about the route, dose, and type of active vitamin D analogue that should be given. Some of the available vitamin D analogues apparently cause less hypercalcemia than calcitriol, although the mechanisms for this are still unclear. The "second-generation" analogue paricalcitol has generated interest, because studies suggest that it leads to less elevation of serum calcium and phosphorus as well as a greater PTH suppression than calcitriol. When compared to calcitriol in a large prospective nonrandomized 3-year trial, hemodialysis patients treated with paricalcitol had statistically significantly lower mortality rates. These results may imply toxicity of vitamin D and continue to raise questions about to what extent efforts to control secondary hyperparathyroidism with vitamin D analogues contribute to vascular disease.

Nevertheless, the current recommendations are to administer active vitamin D sterols to all hemodialysis or peritoneal dialysis patients with intact PTH values greater than 300 pg/mL, provided that their serum phosphorus is less than 5.5 mg/dL and their total serum calcium, corrected for serum albumin, is less than 9.5 mg/dL. Equipotent intravenous doses of calcitriol, paricalcitol, and doxercalciferol are 0.5, 2.5, and 5 µg, respectively, for PTH suppression. Whereas intermittent intravenous administration of active vitamin D analogues is common in the United States, in other countries daily oral therapy is more common. Whether intravenous administration of calcitriol is more effective than daily oral calcitriol in lowering serum PTH and reducing toxicity remains to be established. Typical doses of calcitriol are 0.5 to 8 µg intravenously after each hemodialysis session. Calcitriol can also be given intraperitoneally. Typical oral doses are 0.25 to 1 µg/day.

Stage 5 CKD patients whose PTH levels drop below 150 pg/mL during treatment for secondary hyperparathyroidism require a reduction in their phosphate binders and/or active vitamin D analogue. In patients suspected of having low-turnover bone disease, the risk for aluminum toxicity should be assessed. In patients with presumed adynamic bone disease, the intact PTH level should be allowed to drift up to levels within target range for the particular degree of kidney failure by decreasing vitamin D analogues and/or phosphate binders. Individuals who develop hypercalcemia on vitamin D analogues can be switched to a lower calcium dialysate bath and their vitamin D dose decreased or stopped. The treatment of stage 5 CKD patients who also have low 25-hydroxyvitamin D levels with 25-hydroxyvitamin D is not recommended, because these patients would not be expected to be able to convert this intermediary to calcitriol.

Calcimimetics

An emerging class of drugs called calcimimetics offers novel approaches to treating secondary hyperparathyroidism without raising serum calcium or using active vitamin D analogues. Calcimimetics are calcium receptor–sensing agonists that act on the parathyroid gland's CaSR by allosterically increasing the sensitivity of the receptor to calcium. Cinacalcet, the first available of this group, was approved by the Food and Drug Administration (FDA) in 2004 to treat secondary hyperparathyroidism in stage 5 CKD. Treatment with cinacalcet caused significant decreases in PTH without elevating serum calcium or phosphorus. In fact, there was a reduction in serum calcium and a tendency to reduce serum phosphorus in protocols using calcimimetics in conjunction with standard therapy. The use of cinacalcet resulted in approximately 41% of patients attaining PTH and Ca × P values recommended by the K/DOQI guidelines, compared with less than 10% achieving optimal control in the group treated with phosphate binders and vitamin D analogues alone. Given the importance of the CaSR in regulating parathyroid function and the current suspected toxicity of combined therapy with calcium and high-dose vitamin D, calcimimetics offer the promise of more effective and safe treatment of secondary hyperparathyroidism in stage 5 CKD. Additional studies are needed to evaluate the effect of cinacalcet to alter the

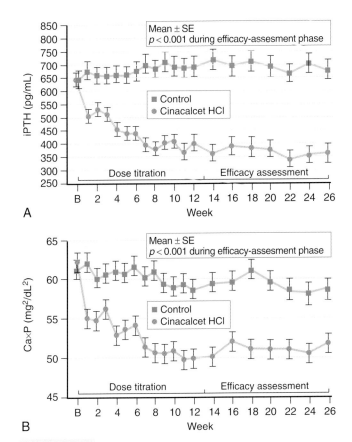

FIGURE 64-5 Effects of cinacalcet to suppress PTH without elevation of the calcium × phosphorus product in hemodialysis patients with secondary hyperparathyroidism not adequately controlled by treatment with phosphate binders and vitamin D analogues. (From Block GA, Martin KJ, de Francisco AL, et al: Cinacalcet for secondary hyperparathyroidism in patients receiving hemodialysis. N Engl J Med 350:1516–1525, 2004. With permission.)

natural history of parathyroid gland hyperplasia and the impact of lowering the Ca × P product with this drug on subsequent vascular calcifications (Fig. 64-5).

Parathyroidectomy

An option remaining for patients with uncontrolled hyperparathyroidism, parathyroidectomy should be considered for persistently elevated intact PTH levels (greater than 800 pg/mL) associated with hypercalcemia and/or hyperphosphatemia despite medical management, and for calciphylaxis or severe bone pain and fractures in the presence of elevated intact PTH levels. Either a subtotal parathyroidectomy or a total parathyroidectomy with forearm gland implantation can be performed. There is a 15% to 30% recurrence rate of hyperparathyroidism. Forearm implantation is done to avoid the need for repeated invasive neck surgery if hyperparathyroidism recurs. Both subtotal and total parathyroidectomy with implantation are effective methods, and there are no studies comparing these approaches. Percutaneous ethanol injection into the gland for hyperparathyroidism

refractory to medical management is performed in some centers. "Hungry bone" syndrome is a frequent complication of parathyroidectomy, especially when markedly elevated PTH values are acutely reduced. This syndrome is characterized by hypocalcemia, hypophosphatemia, and hypomagnesemia secondary to increased bone uptake of these three ions. For unclear reasons, hyperkalemia is occasionally seen. When severe and/or symptomatic hypocalcemia develops, treatment with a continuous calcium infusion is necessary. Concomitant treatment with oral calcitriol before and after parathyroidectomy may minimize the duration of treatment and the severity of hungry bone syndrome.

Patients with Stage 3 and Stage 4 Chronic Kidney Disease

Treatment of subjects with stage 3 and 4 CKD who are not yet on dialysis has not been well studied; however, the early development of parathyroid gland hyperplasia due to chronic stimulation and frequent progression to tertiary hyperparathyroidism suggests that treatment should focus on prevention of parathyroid gland hyperplasia early in CKD. Phosphate restriction, phosphate binders, and calcium supplementation are the mainstays of treatment in stages 3 and 4 CKD. Chronic metabolic acidosis should be corrected with sodium bicarbonate supplementation. The need for and timing of starting therapy with active vitamin D analogues in stages 3 and 4 CKD have not been firmly established, but this intervention should probably be restricted to the latter stages and used only for persistently elevated intact PTH levels after administration of phosphate binders and calcium supplementation. CKD patients are at increased risk for low 25-hydroxyvitamin D levels for several potential reasons, including lack of sunlight if chronically ill and/or bedridden, poor oral intake of foods with vitamin D, lower vitamin D skin production in individuals with reduced GFR, and the presence of nephrotic syndrome causing loss of 25-hydroxyvitamin D and vitamin D–binding protein in the urine. Although the level of 25-hydroxyvitamin D in CKD that is diagnostic of hypovitaminosis D has not been firmly established, levels less than 30 ng/mL are associated with rising PTH levels. Stage 3 and 4 CKD patients with vitamin D deficiency can be supplemented with ergocalciferol (vitamin D_2) or cholecalciferol (vitamin D_3), although the risks and benefits of correcting vitamin D deficiency have not been evaluated in a clinical trial. In patients without CKD, correcting vitamin D deficiency increases BMD and decreases fracture rate. Cinacalcet has not been tested in patients with CKD 3 and 4 and to date is not FDA-approved for these patients.

Kidney Transplantation

The bony changes of secondary hyperparathyroidism improve following transplantation; however, in patients with severe pretransplant hyperparathyroidism, elevated levels of PTH can persist for as long as 10 years after transplantation. The incidence of parathyroidectomy remains high following kidney transplantation, probably reflecting the irreversible hyperplasia of parathyroid glands that occurs in CKD. It is not uncommon for patients to develop hypophosphatemia following kidney transplantation. This reduction in serum phosphorus may be mediated by persistent PTH elevations as well as by other variables unrelated to PTH that reduce renal phosphate reabsorption. Typically, phosphate supplementation is reserved for severe hypophosphatemia (less than 1.5 mg/dL). More aggressive use of phosphate supplementation may exacerbate secondary hyperparathyroidism. Transplantation also prevents but does not reverse bone damage from amyloidosis caused by β_2M deposition. Symptoms of amyloidosis frequently abate after transplantation, perhaps because of concomitant steroid therapy.

Although kidney transplantation corrects many of the conditions that lead to disordered mineral metabolism associated with kidney failure, the immunosuppressive therapy (i.e., prednisone) used to prevent rejection in patients leads to increased bone fragility, osteoporosis, and increased fracture rates. DEXA scans are indicated in kidney transplant patients at the time of the surgery and at least yearly for the first several years thereafter to evaluate for osteoporosis. There are currently no trials that evaluate whether the use of bisphosphonates reduces fracture risk in this population. Calcium and vitamin D supplementation may be effective in counteracting the effects of glucocorticoids to reduce gastrointestinal calcium absorption. Intravenous bisphosphonate given at the time of transplant and every 3 months during the first year or at 1 month after transplant appears to decrease the rate of bone loss, but there are currently no consensus recommendations.

Avascular necrosis is another frequent complication of kidney transplantation. It most typically occurs in the femoral heads or other weight-bearing joints and is characterized by collapse of surface bone and cartilage. The pathogenesis of this disorder is not clear, but it is related to prednisone therapy. Magnetic resonance imaging is the most sensitive technique for evaluating patients with hip pain after transplant for the presence of avascular necrosis. Surgical therapies include core decompression and hip replacement.

BIBLIOGRAPHY

Block GA: Association of serum phosphorus and calcium × phosphate product with mortality risk in chronic hemodialysis patients: A national study. Am J Kidney Dis 31:607–617, 1998.

Block GA, Martin KJ, de Francisco AL, et al: Cinacalcet for secondary hyperparathyroidism in patients receiving hemodialysis. N Engl J Med 350:1516–1525, 2004.

Bricker NS, Fine LG: Uremia: Formulations and expectations. The trade-off hypothesis: Current status. Kidney Int 8:S5–S8, 1978.

Brown EM, Gamba G, Riccardi D, et al: Cloning and characterization of an extracellular Ca^{2+}-sensing receptor from bovine parathyroid. Nature 366:575–580, 1993.

Chertow GM, Burke SK, Raggi P, et al: Sevelamer attenuates the progression of coronary and aortic calcification in hemodialysis patients. Kidney Int 62:245–252, 2002.

Davies MR, Hruska KA: Pathophysiological mechanisms of vascular calcification in end-stage renal disease. Kidney Int 60:472–479, 2001.

D'Haese PC, Spasovski GB: A multicenter study on the effects of lanthanum carbonate (Fosrenol) and calcium carbonate on renal bone disease in dialysis patients. Kidney Int 85:S73–S78, 2003.

Drueke TB: β_2-Microglobulin and amyloidosis. Nephrol Dial Transplant 15:17–24, 2000.

Goodman WG, Coburn JW, Slatopolsky E, et al: Renal osteodystrophy in adults and children. In Favus MJ (ed); Primer on the Metabolic Bone Diseases and Disorders of Mineral Metabolism, 5th ed. Washington, DC, American Society for Bone and Mineral Research, 2003, pp 430–447.

Goodman WG, Goldin J, Kuizon BD, et al: Coronary-artery calcification in young adults with end-stage renal disease who are undergoing dialysis. N Engl J Med 342:1478–1483, 2000.

Indridason OS, Heath H, III, Khosla S, et al: Non-suppressible parathyroid hormone secretion is related to gland size in uremic secondary hyperparathyroidism. Kidney Int 50:1664–1671, 1996.

Parfitt AM: Renal bone disease: A new conceptual framework for the interpretation of bone histomorphometry. Curr Opin Nephrol Hypertens 12:387–403, 2003.

Price PA, Faus SA, Williamson MK: Warfarin-induced artery calcification is accelerated by growth and vitamin D. Arterioscler Thromb Vasc Biol 20:317–327, 2000.

Qi Q, Monier-Faugere MC, Geng Z, et al: Predictive value of serum parathyroid hormone levels for bone turnover in patients on chronic maintenance dialysis. Am J Kidney Dis 26:622–631, 1995.

Quarles LD, Lobaugh B, Murphy G: Intact parathyroid hormone overestimates the presence and severity of parathyroid-mediated osseous abnormalities in uremia. J Clin Endocrinol Metab 75:145–150, 1992.

Quarles LD, Sherrard DJ, Adler S, et al: The calcimimetic AMG 073 as a potential treatment for secondary hyperparathyroidism of end-stage renal disease. J Am Soc Nephrol 14575–14583, 2003.

Reichel H, Esser A, Roth HJ, et al: Influence of PTH assay methodology on differential diagnosis of renal bone disease. Nephrol Dial Transplant 18:759–768, 2003.

Sprague SM, Llach F, Amdahl M, et al: Paricalcitol versus calcitriol in the treatment of secondary hyperparathyroidism. Kidney Int 63:1483–1490, 2003.

Stehman-Breen CO, Sherrard DJ, Alem AM, et al: Risk fractures for hip fracture among patients with end-stage renal disease. Kidney Int 58:2200–2205, 2000.

Sugarman JR, Frederick PR, Frankenfield DL, et al: Developing clinical performance measures based on the Dialysis Outcomes Quality Initiative Clinical Practice Guidelines: Process, outcomes and implications. Am J Kidney Dis 42:806–812, 2003.

Teng M, Wolf M, Lowrie E, et al: Survival of patients undergoing hemodialysis with paricalcitol or calcitriol therapy. N Engl J Med 349:446–456, 2003.

CHAPTER 65

Cardiac Function and Cardiac Disease in Endstage Renal Disease

Robert N. Foley

Since the 1960s, cardiac disease has been shown repeatedly to be the major cause of death in endstage renal disease (ESRD). This is still the case, with older and sicker patients being accepted for renal replacement therapy. The excessive cardiac mortality of ESRD crosses the divides of nationality, race, gender, and cause of ESRD. Cardiac disease also accounts for a substantial degree of comorbidity. Most studies in industrialized nations show that between one third and one half of new dialysis patients have symptomatic ischemic heart disease and cardiac failure before the initiation of ESRD therapy. The probability that a dialysis patient will develop ischemic heart disease or cardiac failure is about 20% per year, orders of magnitude higher than in otherwise comparable members of the general population. Several recent studies, performed in a community setting, suggest that earlier stages of chronic kidney disease (CKD) act as a risk multiplier, in those with and without established cardiovascular disease, and after accounting for traditional cardiovascular risk factors.

EPIDEMIOLOGY

Prevalence

Echocardiographic left ventricular hypertrophy (LVH), coronary artery disease, and cardiac failure are conservatively estimated to be between two and five times more prevalent in ERSD patients than in an age-matched general population.

Abnormalities of left ventricular (LV) structure and function are very common in patients starting renal replacement therapy. Concentric LVH (where wall thickening occurs in response to pressure overload) and LV dilation (increase in cavity size in response to volume overload, often associated with systolic dysfunction) are approximately similarly represented. Systolic dysfunction (inadequate contractility, often defined on echocardiography as a fractional shortening less than 25%) is also common in uremic patients. Several studies of patients with CKD suggest that these abnormalities develop early in CKD and progress rapidly as kidney function declines. In one patient population with progressive renal impairment, 27% of patients with creatinine clearance greater than 50 mL/minute had LVH; this figure rose to 31% for clearances between 25 and 50 mL/minute and 45% for clearances less than 25 mL/minute.

Nearly one half of all hemodialysis patients in the United States have clinically evident ischemic heart disease. Silent coronary artery disease is also common in dialysis patients, especially in those with diabetes mellitus. The situation is confounded by the observation that more than one quarter of dialysis patients with typical angina have normal coronary arteriograms. Cardiac failure is also very common in dialysis patients; data from the U.S. Renal Data System (USRDS) registry suggest that almost one half of all patients have a history of clinically evident cardiac failure.

Valvular dysfunction is common in dialysis patients. Some studies have noted mitral or aortic valvular abnormalities in one half of all patients with CKD. Mild to moderate mitral regurgitation, usually secondary to LV dilatation and calcification of the mitral valve, are the most commonly reported abnormalities. The prevalence of hemodynamically important valvular dysfunction is not well described in the literature. In one study, approximately 10% of dialysis patients had hemodynamically important abnormalities of the mitral or aortic valves.

Stiffness of large arteries, though difficult to measure accurately in clinical practice, is also strongly prognostic in CKD populations and may prove useful as a surrogate in clinical trials. Increased pulse pressure (defined as systolic blood pressure minus diastolic blood pressure), a useful clinical manifestation of arterial stiffening, is highly prevalent in dialysis patients.

Coronary artery calcification is an accurate indicator of the total burden of coronary atherosclerosis in the general population. Atherosclerosis is a disease of the arterial intima. In contrast to extracoronary arteries, where medial calcification can occur without atherosclerosis, the degree of calcification in coronary arteries parallels closely the extent of atherosclerosis. Coronary calcification is very common in CKD and seems to be responsive to interventions such as lowering lipid and phosphorus levels, suggesting a phenomenon that is not inevitable, even in dialysis populations. Coronary calcification scores can be measured accurately with techniques such as electron beam computed tomography (EBCT) and multiple-gated spiral CT.

New instances of ischemic heart disease, congestive heart failure, stroke, and peripheral vascular disease are also very common after the inception of maintenance dialysis therapy. In one study from the USRDS, the incidence of new-onset acute coronary syndrome, congestive heart failure, stroke, and peripheral vascular disease over 2.2 years were 10.2%, 13.6%, 2.2%, and 14%, respectively. CKD patients not yet on renal replacement therapy also show much higher rates of cardiovascular disease than otherwise expected. Most studies until now have suggested that cardiovascular risk increases monotonically with declining glomerular filtration rate (GFR); thus, even GFR levels between 60 and $89\,mL/minute/1.73\,m^2$ have been associated with higher cardiovascular risk than normal GFR levels.

Risk Factors

Many of the traditional, Framingham-type risk factors apply also to cardiac disease in chronic uremia. Older age and diabetes mellitus have been consistently associated with cardiovascular mortality in ESRD patients. Paradoxically, low serum cholesterol and low BP have been associated with mortality in large-scale epidemiologic studies of dialysis patients. It is probable that low serum cholesterol levels, acting as a negative acute-phase reactant, reflect inflammation and malnutrition, both of which are major predictors of mortality in ESRD populations. Recently, C-reactive protein levels have been shown to modulate the association between cholesterol and mortality in dialysis patients. Thus, the association of total cholesterol level with mortality in dialysis patients may be due to the cholesterol-lowering effect of systemic inflammation and malnutrition, rather than a protective effect of high cholesterol concentrations. In one study, even moderate degrees of hypertension were associated with progressive cardiac enlargement and subsequent cardiac failure in dialysis patients; two thirds of all deaths were preceded by a hospital admission for cardiac failure. Hypertension was also associated with the development of new symptomatic ischemic heart disease. After the development of cardiac failure, low BP was the single greatest predictor of subsequent mortality. These data suggest that the association between low BP and mortality reflects the very high frequency of advanced cardiomyopathy in dialysis patients. They also suggest that aggressive management of hypertension is needed in patients without clinically apparent cardiac disease. Although the actual BP target that minimizes cardiac risk in chronic uremia has not been conclusively defined, recent guidelines recommend levels below $130/80\,mm\,Hg$ (predialysis in dialysis patients). Although it is often suggested that achieving normal BP is not feasible in dialysis populations, it remains true that average BP levels come close to recommended levels immediately after a conven-

tional hemodialysis session, and using quotidian therapies. Thus, normalizing time-averaged BP in dialysis patients seems to be a difficult, but feasible, goal for many patients. Emerging data suggest that arterial stiffness is a dominant feature of advanced CKD; arterial pulse pressure may be a more discriminating measurement than either systolic or diastolic BP alone, in terms of mortality associations in epidemiologic studies. Several recent studies show direct relationships between pulse pressure and mortality in dialysis populations. Recent studies confirm the long-held belief that normalization of extracellular fluid volume (ECFV) is a critical hurdle for achieving BP goals.

Several studies suggest that smoking is an independent risk factor for cardiovascular disease and death in ESRD. Smoking and diabetes seem to constitute a particularly adverse combination of risk factors.

Recent epidemiologic data suggest that many conditions related to the uremic state may be associated with cardiac disease. For example, anemia is clearly associated with LVH, congestive heart failure, hospitalization, and mortality. Other variables amenable to correction include dialysis dose and abnormalities of calcium-phosphorus metabolism; however, the lack of controlled evidence means that suggested current treatment targets and recommendations are largely based on associations seen in observational studies. Chronically uremic patients also have an increased prevalence of hyperhomocystinemia, inflammation, oxidative stress, and endothelial dysfunction, compared with patients who have normal kidney function. Two small randomized trials, one using vitamin E, another using acetylcysteine, suggest that antioxidant therapy improves cardiovascular outcome in dialysis patients. As yet, there is no evidence showing that treating hyperhomocystinemia reduces cardiovascular disease in uremic patients. However, high-dose folic acid has been shown to lower levels of homocysteine in patients with advanced CKD. Elevated levels of serum lipoprotein (a) (Lp[a]) are also seen in patients with declining kidney function and are associated with an increased incidence of cardiovascular disease. The kidney has a probable role in the catabolism of Lp(a), and, therefore, kidney dysfunction may lead directly to a high serum Lp(a) concentration.

The effects of uremia on thrombogenesis and platelet function are complex. Elevated fibrinogen levels are associated with cardiovascular disease in patients with normal kidney function. The epidemiologic impact of fibrinogen levels in uremia, as well as altered antithrombin III, protein C, and protein S activity have yet to be determined. In addition, other effects such as platelet dysfunction occur in uremia, and, therefore, although uremia clearly affects thrombogenesis in many different ways, it cannot be thought of as simply a prothrombotic or antithrombotic state.

Finally, the uremic microenvironment has a profound impact on cardiovascular health in animal models, suggesting that strategies that slow progression of kidney disease and strategies that ensure adequate clearance of uremic toxins may improve cardiovascular prognosis.

Prognosis

Systolic dysfunction, concentric LVH, and LV dilatation are antecedents of cardiovascular events in dialysis patients. It is probable that these associations partly reflect a direct causal relationship; it is also plausible that shared risk factors (leading to both LV abnormalities and cardiovascular events) may account for this association, without a direct causal relationship. Coronary artery disease predicts mortality independently of age and diabetes. Clinically defined cardiac failure is a rapidly lethal condition in ESRD patients, much the same as it is in the general population. Figure 65-1 shows survival of ESRD patients with the major clinical and structural manifestations of cardiac disease.

DIAGNOSIS

Cardiomyopathy

Chest x-rays and electrocardiograms (ECGs) are not sufficiently sensitive to detect cardiac enlargement. Echocardiography is noninvasive and relatively easy to perform. It provides information about cardiac dimensions; about valve, systolic, and diastolic function; and about abnormal wall motion, which indicates regional ischemia. Cardiac magnetic resonance imaging shows great promise as a tool to measure cardiac dimensions, exceeding echocardiography in overall accuracy, but it is not yet routinely available. Thus, echocardiography remains the most commonly used test of global cardiac function. Cardiomyopathy often progresses rapidly in chronic uremia, and many of the causes of this rapid progression are treatable. It is not clear how often echocardiography should be performed in patients with ESRD. Annual echocardiography is performed in many centers, partly as a tool to assess continued suitability for transplantation. There are, however, no comparative studies available to demonstrate the optimum use of echocardiography in chronic uremic patients, although it is clearly indicated when symptomatic cardiac dysfunction develops. It is important that echocardiography be carried out after ultrafiltration to as close to dry weight as possible, preferably within 1 kg.

Although dialysis patients with normal hearts can develop pulmonary edema with the rapid accumulation of large amounts of salt and water, it is safer to assume cardiac dysfunction as opposed to simple ECFV expansion in patients who develop pulmonary edema. Therefore, patients with pulmonary edema should undergo further cardiac workup, initially by echocardiography. Brain natriuretic peptide (BNP) is a useful serologic

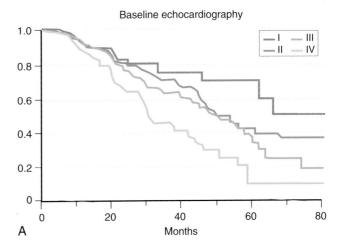

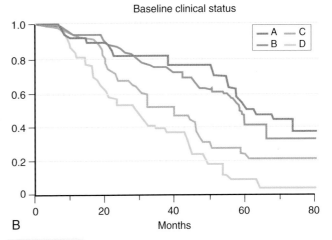

FIGURE 65-1 *A*, Survival according to baseline echocardiography in patients starting endstage renal disease (ESRD) therapy. (I) Normal left ventricle (LV); (II) concentric LV hypertrophy; (III) LV dilatation; (IV) systolic dysfunction. *B*, Survival according to presence or absence of ischemic heart disease and cardiac failure in patients starting ESRD therapy. (A) No ischemic heart disease, no cardiac failure; (B) ischemic heart disease, no cardiac failure; (C) cardiac failure, no ischemic heart disease; (D) both ischemic heart disease and cardiac failure. (*A*, Data from Foley RN, et al: J Am Soc Nephrol 5:2024–2031, 1995; Parfrey PS, et al: Nephrol Dial Transplant 11:1277–1285, 1996. *B*, Data from Harnett JD, et al: Kidney Int 47:884–890, 1995; Parfrey PS, et al: Kidney Int 49:1428–1434, 1996. With permission.)

marker of congestive heart failure in the general population. GFR and BNP levels are negatively correlated, which means that diagnostic BNP cutoff points indicative of cardiac failure are higher, especially as GFR falls below $60\,mL/minute/1.73\,m^2$. In practice, distinguishing cardiac failure from simple fluid overload remains a difficult clinical problem.

Ischemic Heart Disease

Diagnostic techniques in cardiovascular medicine are in a state of rapid flux, and a detailed review is beyond the scope of this chapter. There is a broad consensus, however, that CKD patients with symptoms of ischemic heart disease, diabetic patients, and older patients undergoing pretransplant assessment should undergo coronary angiography. The role of noninvasive testing is still unclear. Exercise-based stress tests are often not informative in ESRD patients, because most are unable to achieve an adequate level of exercise intensity. Of the other noninvasive screening tests available, adenosine thallium-201, dipyridamole thallium-201, and dobutamine stress echocardiography appear useful. All these techniques are highly operator dependent, and the choice of technique depends on the clinical center. Coronary calcification scores on EBCT are very useful for prognostic discrimination, but they do not detect individual stenotic lesions when revascularization is being considered.

TREATMENT

Risk Factor Management

The cardiac morbidity and mortality of uremic patients without coronary disease or cardiomyopathy probably exceeds that of survivors of myocardial infarction in the general population. For all CKD patients, the following targets may be appropriate to minimize the risk of new cardiac disease and the progression of existing cardiac disease: attainment of ideal body mass index, nonsmoking, regular exercise, euglycemia, BP less than 130 systolic and 80 diastolic, total low-density lipoprotein cholesterol less than 100 mg/dL, hemoglobin 11 to 12 g/dL, calcium × phosphorus product less than 55 mg^2/dL^2, intact parathyroid hormone less than 300 ng/L, and GFR not allowed to fall below 15 mL/minute/1.73 m^2 without adding renal replacement therapy. For hemodialysis patients, Kt/V$_{urea}$ (urea clearance, K, per unit time, t, related to total body water, V) should be greater than 1.2, and for peritoneal dialysis patients, Kt/V$_{urea}$ should be at least 2.0 per week with a total creatinine clearance of at least 60 L/week/1.73 m^2 for high and high-average transporters, and 50 L/week/1.73 m^2 in low and low-average transporters.

In CKD patients, there is considerable evidence that angiotensin-converting enzyme (ACE) inhibitors or angiotensin receptor blockers (ARBs) are the antihypertensive agents of choice because of their ability to retard the progression to ESRD. Beta blockers have been shown to reduce mortality in one small trial of ESRD patients with systolic dysfunction, and they appear useful as second-line antihypertensive agents. Concurrent cardiovascular diseases are common in CKD, and the nature and severity of these diseases are important considerations in the decision to use specific classes of agents. Malnutrition is a major problem in dialysis patients, most of whom are already on restricted diets; therefore, the threshold for using pharmacologic treatment for hyperlipidemia should be low. Statins are well tolerated and generally safe for patients with CKD. Statins undergo hepatic metabolism; with the exception of pravastatin, all are metabolized by the hepatic cytochrome P450 system. Thus, the potential for drug interactions must be considered when statins are being chosen. For kidney transplant patients receiving calcineurin inhibitors, for example, it is recommended that cyclosporine or tacrolimus levels be monitored closely as statins are introduced or discontinued, and that creatine kinase values be followed to exclude rhabdomyolysis. Erythropoietin and darbepoetin are agents of choice to treat renal anemia, and intravenous iron is often needed, especially in hemodialysis patients. Erythropoietin and darbepoetin, mostly via hemoglobin increments but also via direct pressor mechanisms, will lead to an increase in BP in as many as one third of patients. For most patients, this increase in BP is readily reversible with standard antihypertensive treatment. For most patients the benefits of partial correction of renal anemia outweigh the potential risks. The risks and benefits of normalizing hematocrit in hemodialysis patients with cardiac disease have been evaluated in randomized trials. The enhanced quality of life with normal hemoglobin targets appears to be offset by increased thrombotic risk, which is most apparent for dialysis vascular access. Thus, a recommendation to normalize hemoglobin cannot be advocated in all dialysis patients, and levels of 11 to 12 g/dL appear to be a reasonable compromise.

Management of Coronary Artery Disease

As in the general population, antiplatelet therapy should be used unless otherwise contraindicated. Beta blockers, calcium channel blockers, and nitrates are the cornerstones of symptomatic therapy. Risk factor management should be aggressive in this group. ESRD patients with symptoms of ischemic heart disease should have coronary arteriography to identify target lesions suitable for angioplasty or surgical bypass. Dialysis patients fulfilling the anatomic and functional criteria used in the general population are likely to benefit from coronary revascularization. The perioperative morbidity and mortality rates associated with coronary artery bypass surgery are higher in dialysis patients than in the general population. Most recent studies suggest that these rates are acceptable and justifiable on the basis of good subsequent survival rates. Observational evidence suggests that in the dialysis population, coronary artery bypass surgery is marginally better than angioplasty in terms of overall survival, cardiac death, and myocardial infarction, although prospective trials comparing revascularization procedures have not been undertaken.

Management of Cardiomyopathy

Of prevalent dialysis patients, 80% or more have cardiomyopathy, which can progress rapidly. All patients who develop cardiac failure should have echocardiography to rationalize therapeutic management. BP reduction is the primary therapeutic target in concentric LVH. In practice, the use of multiple antihypertensives is often necessary to achieve BP control. Data from the nonuremic population indicate that ACE inhibitors and beta blockers are used as initial therapy in patients with LV dilatation, systolic dysfunction, and symptomatic cardiac failure. Digoxin may benefit patients with cardiac failure in the presence of systolic dysfunction and atrial fibrillation, but it is best avoided in patients with diastolic dysfunction. Nitrates are useful for symptomatic relief in frank cardiac failure, whether due to systolic or diastolic dysfunction. Although aldosterone inhibitors are valuable in patients with systolic dysfunction who have preserved kidney function, they have not been assessed in patients with advanced CKD. In particular, their propensity to cause serious hyperkalemia, when added to ACE inhibitors or ARBs, has yet to be defined.

PERICARDITIS IN UREMIC PATIENTS

Clinically important pericarditis is now an infrequent occurrence, although small pericardial effusions are not uncommon on echocardiography in dialysis patients. Uremic pericarditis is most commonly seen in patients with ESRD who have never received dialysis therapy. Pericarditis may also occur in individuals already on dialysis. The uremic milieu is responsible for the former condition, although the specific culprits are unknown; the latter condition often has a viral etiology. About one half of all patients who develop pericarditis while on dialysis therapy improve after intensified dialysis therapy, suggesting that uremia is not causative in all these cases.

The major clinical findings are due to inflammation (precordial pain, dyspnea, fever, generalized systolic changes on ECG) and fluid in the pericardial sac leading to a restriction to ventricular filling (fluid overload and intolerance of ultrafiltration). With large effusions, frank cardiac tamponade and cardiogenic shock may occur. It is more likely that a given volume of pericardial fluid will lead to cardiac tamponade when it accumulates quickly. Uremic pericardial effusions are usually exudates in their initial phase. It is thought that refilling of pericardial effusions is more common with fluid overload. Thus, later-phase pericardial effusions can be a mixture of exudate and transudate. Echocardiography should be performed to estimate the volume of fluid within the pericardium. Daily hemodialysis is usually recommended in the presence of moderate-sized effusions, to increase clearance of the uremic solutes that may have initiated pericarditis, and to gradually eliminate ECFV expansion. Heparin avoidance and analgesia are integral parts of management. The use of nonsteroidal anti-inflammatory agents remains controversial, because they can sometimes exacerbate bleeding tendencies. Surgical drainage is needed for large, nonresponsive effusions or where cardiac tamponade is imminent.

BIBLIOGRAPHY

Besarab A, Bolton WK, Browne JK et al: The effects of normal as compared with low hematocrit values in patients with cardiac disease who are receiving hemodialysis and epoetin. N Engl J Med 339:584–590, 1998.

Blacher J, Guerin AP, Pannier B, et al: Arterial calcifications, arterial stiffness, and cardiovascular risk in endstage renal disease. Hypertension 38:938–942, 2001.

Boaz M, Smetana S, Weinstein T, et al: Secondary prevention with antioxidants of cardiovascular disease in endstage renal disease (SPACE): Randomised placebo-controlled trial. Lancet 356:1213–1218, 2000.

Chertow GM, Burke SK, Raggi P: Treat to Goal Working Group. Sevelamer attenuates the progression of coronary and aortic calcification in hemodialysis patients. Kidney Int 62:245–252, 2002.

Cice G, Ferrara L, D'Andrea A, et al: Carvedilol increases two-year survival in dialysis patients with dilated cardiomyopathy: A prospective, placebo-controlled trial. J Am Coll Cardiol 41:1438–1444, 2003.

Eknoyan G, Beck GJ, Cheung AK, et al, Hemodialysis (HEMO) Study Group: Effect of dialysis dose and membrane flux in maintenance hemodialysis. N Engl J Med 347:2010–2019, 2002.

Eknoyan G, Levin A, Levin NW: Bone metabolism and disease in chronic kidney disease. Am J Kidney Dis 42(4 suppl 3):1–201, 2003.

Foley RN, Parfrey PS, Harnett JD, et al: Clinical and echocardiographic disease in endstage renal disease: Prevalence, associations and prognosis. Kidney Int 47:186–192, 1995.

Foley RN, Parfrey PS, Morgan J, et al: Effect of hemoglobin levels in hemodialysis patients with asymptomatic cardiomyopathy. Kidney Int 58:1325–1335, 2000.

Herzog CA, Ma JZ, Collins AJ: Long-term outcome of dialysis patients in the United States with coronary revascularisation procedures. Kidney Int 56:324–332, 1999.

Holdaas H, Fellstrom B, Jardine AG, et al; Assessment of LEscol in Renal Transplantation (ALERT) Study Investigators: Effect of fluvastatin on cardiac outcomes in renal transplant recipients: A multicentre, randomised, placebo-controlled trial. Lancet 361:2024–2031, 2003.

Levin A, Singer J, Thompson CR, et al: Prevalent left ventricular hypertrophy in the predialysis population: Identifying opportunities for intervention. Am J Kidney Dis 27:347–354, 1996.

Liu Y, Coresh J, Eustace JA, et al: Association between cholesterol level and mortality in dialysis patients: Role of inflammation and malnutrition. JAMA 291:451–459, 2004.

Murphy SW, Parfrey PS: Screening for cardiovascular disease in dialysis patients. Curr Opin Nephrol Hypertens 5:532–540, 1996.

Oparil S: Treating multiple-risk hypertensive patients. Am J Hypertens 12:1215–1295, 1999.

Paniagua R, Amato D, Vonesh E, et al; Mexican Nephrology Collaborative Study Group: Effects of increased peritoneal clearances on mortality rates in peritoneal dialysis: ADEMEX, a prospective, randomized, controlled trial. J Am Soc Nephrol 13:1307–1320, 2002.

Tonelli M, Moye L, Sacks FM, et al; Cholesterol and Recurrent Events (CARE) Trial Investigators: Pravastatin for secondary prevention of cardiovascular events in persons with mild chronic renal insufficiency. Ann Intern Med 138:98–104, 2003.

CHAPTER **66**

Hematologic Manifestations of Chronic Kidney Disease

Jonathan Himmelfarb

ANEMIA

Pathogenesis

The pathogenesis of anemia of chronic kidney disease (CKD) is multifactorial. Erythropoietin (EPO) deficiency, shortened erythrocyte (RBC) survival, the presence of uremic inhibitors of erythropoiesis, hemolysis, bleeding, blood loss in hemodialysis circuits, and iron deficiency are all contributors. In normal subjects, circulating plasma EPO levels are minute, but they increase exponentially in response to anemia. In contrast, in anemic patients with progressive kidney disease, the normal relationship between the degree of anemia and plasma EPO is lost (Fig. 66-1). Therefore, it is clear that the major cause of anemia in CKD is deficient EPO production.

Normal erythropoiesis is primarily regulated by circulating EPO. When EPO binds to specific receptors on bone marrow erythroid progenitor cells, their proliferation, differentiation, and development into mature RBCs is enhanced. The kidney produces as much as 90% of circulating EPO, accounting for its pivotal role in erythropoiesis. In situ hybridization techniques have shown that the major site of EPO production is the renal peritubular interstitial fibroblasts. Most extrarenal EPO is produced in the liver by centrilobular hepatocytes. However, extrarenal EPO production is rarely able to provide for significant erythropoiesis in the anephric state, suggesting that the liver is less sensitive than the kidney to hypoxic stimuli. The precise mechanisms by which hypoxia stimulates renal EPO secretion remain incompletely understood.

Support for the hypothesis that uremic toxins retained in the plasma inhibit bone marrow erythroid production rests on in vitro experiments demonstrating that uremic human serum blunts the growth of erythroid colony-forming units (CFU-E). This erythroid inhibition has been thought to be due to plasma polyamines such as spermine or putrescine as well as "middle molecules" that are as yet unidentified. However, studies using human autologous cultured bone marrow cells have not demonstrated inhibition of erythroid progenitor cell growth by uremic serum. Furthermore, in vivo studies involving the infusion of recombinant EPO into normal subjects and

hemodialysis patients demonstrate that erythropoiesis, as quantitated by ferrokinetics and the reticulocyte response, are not blunted in dialysis subjects. Almost all patients with CKD, if iron replete and free of inflammation or infection, will have an appropriate erythropoietic response to EPO. Thus, current evidence suggests that uremic inhibitors of erythropoiesis play a minimal role, if any, in the pathogenesis of the anemia of CKD.

A decrease in RBC survival has also been postulated to contribute to the anemia of CKD. Decreased RBC survival in uremic patients may be related to reduced resistance to both complement-mediated RBC lysis and oxidant stress. RBC survival is 60 to 90 days in uremic patients as compared with 120 days in normal individuals, and it generally does not improve with dialysis therapy. The use of EPO may also extend RBC survival by preventing neocytolysis, a physiologic process by which the youngest RBCs in the circulation undergo hemolysis.

Laboratory and Clinical Manifestations of Anemia of Chronic Kidney Disease

The anemia of CKD is morphologically a normocytic, normochromic anemia. Corrected reticulocyte count and serum EPO levels are inappropriately low when compared with values seen in patients with similar degrees of anemia without kidney disease. Iron parameters should be normal. The bone marrow examination is usually normal and is not usually necessary for the hematologic evaluation.

Patients with CKD who develop anemia should undergo screening for causes of anemia other than EPO deficiency. This evaluation should include measurement of RBC indices, reticulocyte count, iron parameters, and a test for stool occult blood. An abnormal platelet count or white blood cell count may reflect a more generalized disturbance of bone marrow function. RBC indices, reticulocyte counts, and iron parameters are helpful in detecting many anemias that are not due to EPO deficiency. Microcytosis can reflect iron deficiency, aluminum intoxication, and certain hemoglobinopathies. Macrocytosis may be associated with vitamin B_{12} or folate deficiency.

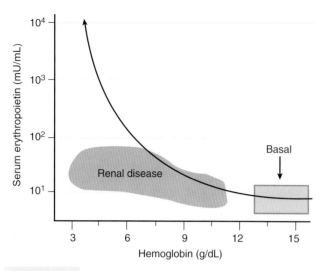

FIGURE 66-1 Erythropoietin (EPO) levels in kidney disease. The box entitled "Basal" refers to serum EPO levels in normal individuals. The upward arrow reflects the typical rise in serum EPO levels in patients with anemia not due to chronic kidney disease. (Adapted from Hillman RS, Ault KA: Hematology in Clinical Practice. New York, McGraw-Hill, 1995, with permission from the McGraw-Hill Companies.)

As kidney disease progresses, there is an increased likelihood of developing anemia, because diseased kidneys are unable to produce sufficient quantities of EPO. Figure 66-2 depicts the relationship between the change in hematocrit and the serum creatinine in more than 900 patients. Whereas the mean hematocrit drops below 30% at a serum creatinine of approximately 6 mg/dL, there are considerable interpatient variations. There is even less

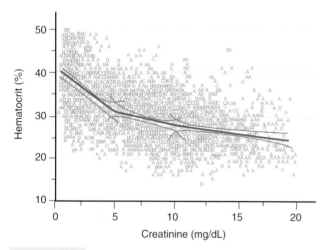

FIGURE 66-2 The change of hematocrit with creatinine in chronic kidney disease. This figure represents approximately 4000 data points obtained from 911 patients followed without treatment with erythropoietin on dialysis. The 95% confidence limit of the slope is shown around each line. Each letter represents the number of data points at that value (e.g., A = 1 data point, B = 2 data points). (Adapted from Hakim RM, Lazarus JM: Biochemical parameters in chronic kidney disease. Am J Kidney Dis 11:238–247, 1988.)

correlation between the blood urea nitrogen (BUN) and hematocrit.

In patients whose kidney disease is the result of polycystic kidney disease, the hemoglobin level and hematocrit may be higher than in patients with a comparable level of kidney dysfunction due to other causes. On the other hand, patients who have undergone bilateral nephrectomies generally have more severe anemia than other patients on dialysis therapy. Even when kidneys are devoid of excretory function, they usually retain some capability for EPO biosynthesis.

Patients with severe anemia, regardless of its etiology, display signs and symptoms attributable to tissue hypoxia. However, many of the symptoms usually attributable to anemia may be clinically difficult to distinguish from symptoms related to uremia. For most patients, symptoms develop when the hematocrit decreases to 30% or less. Therapy is indicated at a higher level of hematocrit if angina pectoris or other significant symptoms develop. Younger patients often will adjust better to anemia. When anemia develops gradually, an intraerythrocytic increase in 2,3-diphosphoglycerate (2,3-DPG) occurs, which shifts the oxygen dissociation curve to the right and allows oxygen to be unloaded at the tissue level more readily. Thus, many patients may not be as severely symptomatic as might be expected from the degree of anemia. Additional cardiovascular compensatory mechanisms may also develop over time, thereby limiting symptoms directly attributed to anemia.

The symptoms of anemia include weakness, fatigue, and dyspnea, particularly with exertion. Decreased exercise tolerance is common, and many patients experience difficulty with concentration, attention span, and memory. Sexual dysfunction, cold intolerance, and anorexia may also be side effects related to anemia.

Treatment of Anemia

The therapeutic modalities available today for treatment of the anemia of kidney disease include administration of recombinant erythropoietic agents, institution of renal replacement therapy including dialysis and kidney transplantation, and packed RBC transfusions. With the introduction of recombinant EPO to treat the anemia of CKD, it became evident that the contribution of anemia to the morbidity of CKD was greater than originally assumed. The clinical benefits of improved tissue oxygenation include improvements in exercise capacity, central nervous system function, endocrine and cardiac function, as well as a reduction in hospital admissions. The most important benefit in treating the anemia of CKD may be in the reduction of cardiovascular morbidity and mortality.

Chronic anemia and consequent tissue hypoxia result in a compensatory increase in cardiac contractility, which contributes to the development of left ventricular hypertrophy. The development of left ventricular hypertrophy with consequent diastolic dysfunction and myocardial ischemia is a risk factor for mortality in patients on dialysis therapy. Correction of the anemia of CKD generally results in improvement but not resolution of left ventricular hypertrophy. Anemia correction also lowers the rate of hospitalization for myocardial infarction and cardiac disease in general and markedly improves exercise capacity. See Chapter 65 for further details.

The use of EPO to improve anemia in hemodialysis patients is also associated with improvement in cognitive function. This improvement has been documented by normalization of electroencephalograms as well as improvement on neuropsychiatric testing. Normalization of cerebral blood flow has also been demonstrated with improvement in anemia. These improvements in cognition have translated into a lessening of depression and improvements in indicators of quality of life. Endocrine changes also occur in response to EPO therapy in CKD. Sexual function improves in some men after increase in hematocrit. Some (but not all) studies have demonstrated an increase in serum testosterone levels. Serum prolactin levels have decreased in some (but not all) male hemodialysis patients. Anemia may also play a role in growth retardation in pediatric patients. See Chapter 67 for further details on endocrine effects of EPO.

Recombinant Erythropoietin

The first clinical trials of recombinant human EPO in hemodialysis patients began in 1984 and demonstrated a clear-cut relationship between the dose of EPO and the rate of rise in hematocrit (Fig. 66-3). EPO responsiveness is dependent on dose, route, and frequency of parenteral administration. Absorption following subcutaneous administration of EPO is incomplete. Subcutaneous EPO administration results in a slower increase in serum EPO levels, with maintenance of a stable serum level for hours. Although EPO administered intravenously has 100% bioavailability, most of the administered intravenous dose is probably biologically ineffective once the relatively few EPO receptors on erythroid progenitor cells are saturated. As a result, subcutaneous dosing is more efficient than intravenous dosing because of more sustained serum EPO levels. Several studies have demonstrated that 20% to 40% less EPO is required to maintain a target level of hematocrit with subcutaneous as opposed to intravenous dosing, a finding confirmed by meta-analysis. EPO can also be administered intraperitoneally, a method that may be preferable for children treated with peritoneal dialysis.

It is currently recommended that the initial administration of EPO for treatment of anemia in predialysis, peritoneal dialysis, and hemodialysis patients should be subcutaneous at a dose of 80 to 120 units/kg/week in two to three divided doses to achieve the target hematocrit (see Fig. 66-3). Children under 5 years of age frequently require higher doses than adults (300 units/kg/week).

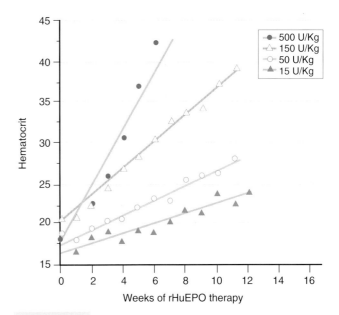

FIGURE 66-3 The response in hematocrit to recombinant human erythropoietin (rHuEPO) therapy. Each line represents the response to the given dose of rHuEPO administered intravenously three times a week to hemodialysis patients. (Adapted from Eschbach JW, Egrie JC, Downing MR, et al: Correction of the anemia of endstage renal disease with recombinant human erythropoietin. N Engl J Med 316:73–78, 1987. Reprinted with permission. Copyright © 1987 Massachusetts Medical Society. All rights reserved.)

The site of EPO injection should be rotated with each administration.

The appropriate target hemoglobin and hematocrit for patients with CKD on EPO therapy, whether or not receiving dialysis, remains incompletely defined. The original target hematocrit recommended by the U.S. Food and Drug Administration (FDA) in 1989 was 30% to 33%, but this was subsequently widened to a target hematocrit range of 30% to 36% in June 1994. Extensive evaluation by the National Kidney Foundation (NKF) led to a recommended hematocrit of 33% to 36% with a corresponding hemoglobin target of 11 to 12 g/dL. This is the current generally accepted target. Several investigators have suggested that using EPO to normalize hematocrit (target hematocrit 42%) may have additional benefits in improving cardiac function, cognition, and quality of life. Several randomized trials have examined the consequences of normalizing hemoglobin in hemodialysis patients. In the largest prospective randomized trial, more than 1200 long-term dialysis patients who had signs or symptoms of congestive heart failure or ischemic heart disease were randomized to receive EPO to a target hematocrit of either 30% ± 3% or 42% ± 3% (Fig. 66-4). In an unexpected finding, the incidence of death and nonfatal myocardial infarction was higher in the normal as compared with the low-hematocrit group (relative risk 1.3, 95% confidence interval, 0.9 to 1.9). Other studies examining patients with less severe documented heart

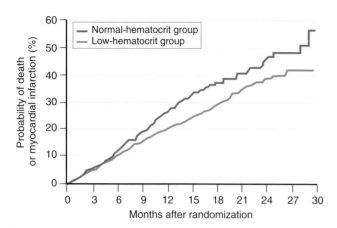

Number at risk

Normal
hematocrit   618 540 476 415 353 259 186 124 69 26

Low
hematocrit   615 537 485 434 391 292 216 131 80 20

FIGURE 66-4 Kaplan-Meier estimates of the probability of death or a first nonfatal myocardial infarction in patients randomized to the normal-hematocrit and low-hematocrit groups. (Adapted from Besarab A, Bolton WY, Browne JK, et al: The effects of normal as compared with low hematocrit values in patients with cardiac disease who are receiving hemodialysis and epoietin. N Engl J Med 339:584–590, 1998. Copyright © 1998 Massachusetts Medical Society. All rights reserved.)

disease have demonstrated improved quality of life and decreased hospitalization with no apparent excess mortality with hemoglobin normalization. Observational studies have demonstrated that higher hemoglobin levels are associated with lower hospitalization rates and no excess mortality compared with a target hemoglobin of 11 to 12 g/dL. On balance, the NKF's Kidney Disease Outcomes Quality Initiative (K/DOQI) target guidelines for hemoglobin concentration seem prudent, especially for the U.S. hemodialysis population, where there is a high prevalence of cardiovascular comorbidity. Additional studies are required examining a target hemoglobin of 12 to 13 g/dL. Selected patients at low risk for cardiovascular events may achieve additional quality-of-life benefits with normalized hemoglobin levels. Whether higher hemoglobin targets would be beneficial for CKD patients not receiving hemodialysis is currently being investigated.

Darbepoietin Alfa

Darbepoietin alfa is a novel RBC-stimulating protein that has been developed for the treatment of anemia. Though similar to EPO, darbepoietin alfa is a glycoprotein with a threefold longer terminal half-life than EPO in hemodialysis patients, thus allowing it to be administered less frequently. In controlled clinical trials, an equivalent number of patients receiving darbepoietin alfa and recombinant EPO achieved a target hemoglobin increase.

The frequencies of adverse events, withdrawals, and deaths reported in clinical trials do not differ between patients receiving darbepoietin alfa and recombinant EPO. The longer half-life of darbepoietin compared with EPO may be particularly beneficial in the treatment of anemia in patients with CKD, who have less frequent health care encounters than dialysis patients. For these patients, darbepoietin alfa is usually initiated as a single weekly injection.

Iron Therapy

A crucial aspect of EPO therapy is the maintenance of adequate iron stores for the production of new RBCs. Normally, three quarters of body iron is present in circulating RBCs, and one quarter exists as storage iron primarily in the liver and bone marrow. Because the demands for iron by the erythroid marrow frequently exceed iron stores once EPO therapy has been initiated, iron supplementation is essential to assure adequate response. In the era before EPO therapy, advanced kidney disease and its associated hypoproliferative anemia were frequently accompanied by excess storage iron due to frequent RBC transfusions. Since the widespread use of EPO therapy, iron overload is now uncommon, whereas iron deficiency has become more common.

Iron status in patients receiving EPO is monitored by measuring both the serum ferritin and the percentage transferrin saturation. Serum ferritin and percentage transferrin saturation are complementary tests, because they measure different pools of body iron. The serum ferritin is proportional to storage iron, and a low serum ferritin is highly specific for EPO resistance. However, the serum ferritin is also an acute-phase reactant that may be increased in the presence of acute or chronic inflammation. Thus, a low serum ferritin is a specific but not a sensitive marker for absolute iron deficiency.

In contrast, the percentage transferrin saturation (measured as the serum iron divided by the total iron-binding capacity multiplied by 100), reflects iron that is readily available for erythropoiesis or functional iron. The transferrin molecule contains two receptors for molecular iron transported from storage iron sites to erythroid progenitor cells. The percentage transferrin saturation is decreased not only with absolute iron deficiency, but also with functional iron deficiency. The latter exists when, despite having a serum ferritin level above 100 ng/mL, a patient demonstrates an augmented erythropoietic response to additional supplementation with iron. Thus, transferrin saturation appears to be a better predictor of iron responsiveness than the serum ferritin level. The reticulocyte hemoglobin content is a test of iron status that may have a higher sensitivity and specificity for utilizable iron stores in hemodialysis than monitoring based on serum ferritin and transferrin saturation. Other tests of iron status such as RBC ferritin or zinc protoporphyrin do not appear to increase diagnostic sensitivity or specificity and are less widely available. The gold standard test for iron status, bone marrow stainable iron, is invasive and expensive and need not be used on a routine basis. For optimal responsiveness to EPO, current recommendations are that the serum ferritin should be maintained between 100 and 800 ng/mL, and the percentage transferrin saturation should be maintained between 20% and 50%.

Iron can be administered either orally as iron salts or intravenously. Oral iron should be given as 200 mg of elemental iron per day in two to three divided doses. For optimal absorption, oral iron should be given more than 1 hour before meals or more than 2 hour after meals or ingestion of phosphate binders. In the majority of dialysis patients receiving EPO, oral iron is insufficient to maintain adequate iron status, and intravenous iron is required. Iron dextran, iron sucrose, and iron gluconate complex are all forms of intravenous iron currently approved by the U.S. FDA. Until recently, the only FDA-approved source of parenteral iron in the United States had been iron dextran. Dextran binds relatively tightly to iron, thereby allowing for less dissociation, with less potential for adverse effects from the release of free iron into the circulation. However, iron dextran administration has been associated with anaphylactoid reactions in some patients who produce antidextran antibodies. Life-threatening anaphylactoid reactions to iron dextran have been reported to occur in as many as 0.7% of hemodialysis patients treated with this agent, and at least 30 deaths in the United States have been attributed to its use. The two newer forms of parenteral iron for use in the United States, iron sucrose and iron gluconate complex, are associated with substantially lower rates of adverse drug events than iron dextran. Both iron sucrose and iron gluconate complex have come into widespread use in the dialysis patient population.

Recently, questions have been raised about the safety of routine intravenous iron administration with the view that iron administration may result in an increased risk of infection and cardiovascular complications. Iron is an important growth factor for bacteria, and organisms such as staphylococci have developed mechanisms to acquire iron during infection. Iron-overloaded hemodialysis patients may have defective phagocytic cell function and host defense. However, a recent large, multicenter, prospective study of risk factors for bacteremia in chronic hemodialysis patients did not identify iron overload (as measured by a high serum ferritin) as a risk factor for infection. It has also been suggested that the administration of high doses of intravenous iron would overwhelm plasma iron-binding capacity, leading to the presence of free ferrous iron in the plasma, which could increase oxidative stress. However, serum transferrin and other host defense mechanisms can handle a great deal of excess plasma iron without allowing free ferrous iron in the plasma. Thus, at the present time, the idea that intravenous iron administration contributes to septicemia or cardiovascular toxicity in chronic hemodialysis patients remains speculative. It may be prudent, however, to withhold intravenous iron therapy in dialysis patients with evidence of acute-phase inflammation or active infections, because of theoretical risks of exacerbating infection risk and oxidant stress-induced tissue injury.

Erythropoietin Resistance

True resistance to EPO therapy for the treatment of CKD is rare (Table 66-1). In the largest clinical trial, more than 96% of iron-replete dialysis patients responded when EPO was given at approximately 50 units/kg intravenously three times a week. The median dose of EPO needed to maintain the target hematocrit was 75 units/kg intravenously three times a week. The most common cause of a poor response to EPO is either an inadequate EPO dose or the presence of iron deficiency. Other causes of EPO resistance include the presence of inflammation or infection. Inflammation results in a deficient iron supply by blocking the release of iron from the reticuloendothelial system despite the presence of normal to increased iron stores and by decreasing oral iron absorption. Bone marrow fibrosis from osteitis fibrosa cystica as a consequence of hyperparathyroidism can cause true EPO resistance. The definitive diagnosis of osteitis fibrosa cystica requires a bone biopsy, since hyperparathyroidism without osteitis fibrosa cystica does not blunt the effect of EPO. Aluminum intoxication, now a rarity in maintenance dialysis patients, contributes to anemia by decreasing bone marrow hemoglobin synthesis. It can be suspected in the iron-replete patient who has a low RBC mean corpuscular volume, and it can be confirmed by measuring an increased serum aluminum level after deferoxamine administration or by positive staining for aluminum in a bone biopsy. Rarely, folate or vitamin B_{12} deficiency can be a cause of EPO resistance. Resistance to EPO therapy has also been documented due to anti-N_{form} hemolysis in patients with chronic formaldehyde exposure related to sterilization of reused dialyzers. Occult bleeding also needs to be considered in EPO-resistant patients.

TABLE 66-1   Causes of Apparent Erythropoietin Resistance

Inadequate EPO dose
Inflammation and infection
Osteitis fibrosa cystica
Aluminum intoxication
Folate deficiency
Severe malnutrition
Hemolysis or blood loss
Primary hematologic diseases
Anti-EPO antibodies (PRCA)

EPO, erythropoietin; PRCA, pure red cell aplasia.

Anti-Erythropoietin Antibodies and Pure Red Cell Aplasia

Immunization of rabbits with human EPO can cause them to develop EPO resistance and progressive anemia. From the 1980s through 1998, reports of anti-EPO antibodies causing pure red cell aplasia (PRCA) and progressive anemia in patients receiving recombinant human EPO were extremely rare. However, since 1998, the number of reported cases of PRCA has increased dramatically. The vast majority of these cases have been associated with the administration of epoietin alfa outside the United States. Most reported cases involved subcutaneous administration of EPO. A temporal coincidence has been noted with a change in the formulation of epoietin alfa (removal of serum albumin from the formulation and replacement with Tween 80). It has been postulated that this change in formulation may have changed the stability or otherwise changed the immunogenicity of EPO.

Patients developing PRCA due to anti-EPO antibodies typically have been on therapy for 6 to 18 months when a decline in hemoglobin concentration is noted despite continued therapy. Reticulocyte counts declined to very low levels (generally fewer than 20,000 cells/mm³). Corollary laboratory findings are a frequent minor drop in platelet count within the normal range and a marked increase in transferrin saturation and ferritin levels. Definitive diagnosis requires a bone marrow examination and the demonstration of serum anti-EPO antibodies (Table 66-2). Both types of investigations should be performed when the diagnosis is suspected. Once the diagnosis of PRCA is suspected, EPO therapy should be discontinued. To achieve remission, immunosuppressive therapy may be required in addition to stopping EPO administration. To date, no relapse of PRCA has been reported after stopping immunosuppressive therapy. Kidney transplantation has been reported to result in rapid recovery from PRCA.

Side Effects of Erythropoietin Therapy

Early experiences suggested that accelerated hypertension, the development of seizures, and hyperkalemia frequently accompanied correction of anemia with EPO therapy. However, extensive clinical experience has now demonstrated that the adverse effects of EPO therapy are infrequent and generally manageable. The most frequent adverse effect is aggravation of hypertension in 20% to 30% of patients. An increase in blood pressure usually occurs in association with a rapid increase in hematocrit or at higher doses of EPO. The development or worsening of hypertension is thought to be related to an increase in vascular wall reactivity as well as hemodynamic changes that occur as a consequence of increasing red cell mass. Worsening hypertension associated with EPO therapy can be treated by initiating or increasing antihypertensive therapy, by intensifying ultrafiltration in dialysis patients with evidence of volume expansion, or by reducing EPO dose.

The initial multicenter study with EPO in the United States noted a higher incidence of seizures during the first 3 months of the study compared with historical controls. These findings have not been subsequently confirmed. With the exception of patients with hypertensive encephalopathy, there does not appear to be evidence of increased seizures in patients in whom appropriate close monitoring and titration recommendations are followed. A history of seizures is not considered a contraindication to the use of EPO. Although serious hyperkalemia was observed during the early clinical experiences, recent studies have not demonstrated a higher incidence of hyperkalemia in EPO-treated patients.

It remains a matter of controversy whether increasing the hematocrit with EPO increases the likelihood of developing vascular-access thrombosis in hemodialysis patients. Most studies have not demonstrated an increase in the rate of either native fistulae or prosthetic graft thrombosis when the hematocrit is kept at or below a target of 36%. An exception is the Canadian multicenter trial that suggested that EPO increased the rate of thrombosis in synthetic grafts. Vascular-access thrombosis clearly increases when hematocrits are normalized with EPO therapy.

OTHER HEMATOLOGIC MANIFESTATIONS OF KIDNEY DISEASE

Erythrocytosis in Uremic Patients

Erythrocytosis is occasionally seen in previously anemic uremic patients who develop a renal cell carcinoma or large renal cyst and is occasionally seen in patients with polycystic kidney disease. Erythrocytosis has also been reported to occur in as many as 17% of kidney transplant recipients. The pathogenesis of post-transplant erythrocytosis is poorly understood and is not usually related to higher circulating EPO levels. Angiotensin-converting enzyme inhibitors and angiotensin receptor blockers can often correct kidney transplant erythrocytosis by a mechanism that is as yet undefined and can contribute to post-transplant anemia. Phosphodiesterase inhibitors such as

---

TABLE 66-2   Clinical and Diagnostic Features of Erythropoietin-Induced Pure Red Cell Aplasia

Weekly hemoglobin decline of approximately 1 g/dL or weekly transfusion requirement
Reticulocyte count <20,000/mm³
No major decline in platelet and leukocyte counts
Presence of serum anti-erythropoietin antibodies
Bone marrow aspirate with normal cellularity and <4% erythroblasts

theophylline can also correct post-transplant erythrocytosis. Because erythrocytosis of any etiology enhances the risks of thromboembolic disease, therapy for post-transplant erythrocytosis is recommended. Standard therapy includes discontinuation of cigarette smoking or diuretic use. Although serial phlebotomy has been the recognized standard of care, most transplant centers now use low-dose angiotensin-converting enzyme inhibitor therapy to manage post-transplant erythrocytosis successfully. Angiotensin receptor blockers have been used for the same purpose in patients intolerant of angiotensin-converting enzyme inhibitors.

Platelet Dysfunction in Uremia

Clinical bleeding in patients with uremia is due to an acquired qualitative platelet defect and has best been correlated with a prolonged bleeding time. At present, however, there is no single unifying pathogenetic mechanism to explain the acquired platelet dysfunction seen in patients with uremia. No single intrinsic defect in platelet function can be consistently linked to the bleeding tendency; uremic platelet dysfunction is thus multifactorial. Defects in platelet aggregation in vitro, diminished thromboxane A2 production, abnormal intracellular calcium mobilization, and increased intracellular cyclic adenosine monophosphate (cAMP) have all been described in uremic platelets. Several studies have emphasized a defect in platelet adhesion to vascular subendothelium in uremic patients. Platelet adhesiveness to subendothelium depends on the cooperative interactions of platelet glycoproteins with von Willebrand factor in the vascular wall. Platelet glycoprotein function is abnormal in hemodialysis patients. Fibrinogen fragments that interfere with platelet adhesion and aggregation may also accumulate in uremia. There are conflicting data as to whether patients with uremia have decreased von Willebrand factor activity. Uremia may also be associated with increased release of endothelial prostacyclin and nitric oxide, both of which inhibit adhesion of platelets.

The mainstay of treatment of the bleeding diathesis of uremia has been dialysis, although it is not consistently effective. In addition to dialysis, a number of therapeutic approaches are available to correct the bleeding diathesis in patients who are experiencing serious bleeding complications (Table 66-3). The synthetic vasopressin derivative desmopressin (DDAVP) has been shown to shorten the bleeding time rapidly and improve clinical bleeding in uremia. The mechanism of action of DDAVP is thought to be related to release of multimeric von Willebrand factor from endothelial cells and platelets, although this has not been conclusively demonstrated. A limitation to DDAVP therapy is the development of tachyphylaxis after two to three doses. Other therapeutic approaches have included the administration of cryoprecipitate or conjugated estrogens. Similar to DDAVP, the mechanism of action of these agents is thought to be related either to release of von Willebrand factor multimers or to endothelial functional changes. Unfortunately, all of these agents have variable clinical efficacy in uremia.

Increasing the hematocrit to above 30%, either via packed RBC transfusions or the by use of EPO, has been demonstrated to improve the bleeding time in most anemic patients. Although the primary pathogenetic mechanism of increasing the hematocrit in improving the bleeding time may be rheologic, additional evidence suggests that increasing hemoglobin concentration may inactivate the platelet-inhibiting effects of nitric oxide.

Leukocyte Dysfunction in Uremia

Infection remains a major cause of morbidity and mortality in the dialysis patient. Vascular access infections, particularly with *Staphylococcus* species, remain the leading source of serious infection. Most infections in chronic hemodialysis patients are due to common catalase-producing bacteria rather than to opportunistic organisms. The pattern of infectious organisms in chronic dialysis patients is similar to patients with chronic granulomatous disease whose phagocytic cells cannot produce reactive oxygen species.

The number and morphology of granulocytes in patients with uremia are normal except for a tendency toward hypersegmentation in some patients. Numerous studies have documented alterations in granulocyte function in patients with uremia or on chronic dialysis,

TABLE 66-3 Treatment of Uremic Platelet Dysfunction

Therapy	Dose or Goal	Onset	Duration	Comment
Increase hematocrit (EPO, RBC transfusion)	>30	Immediate	Prolonged	Highly effective
DDAVP	0.3 µg/kg intravenous	Immediate	4–8 hr	Rapid tachyphylaxis, use just before needed
Cryoprecipitate	10 units	1–4 hr	24 hr	Hepatitis, HIV risk
Conjugated estrogens	0.6 mg/kg/day × 5 days	6 hr	14 days	Hot flashes, HTN, abnormal LFTs

DDAVP, desmopressin; EPO, erythropoietin; HTN, hypertension; LFT, liver function test; RBC, red blood cell.

including chemotaxis, granulocyte adherence, phagocytic capability, and reactive oxygen species production. Iron overload may contribute to phagocytic dysfunction.

In addition to changes in granulocyte function associated with uremia, it is now well documented that hemodialysis with cellulosic membranes results in complement-mediated granulocyte activation and subsequent dysfunction. Changes in granulocyte function as a consequence of dialysis with cellulosic membranes include modulation of chemotactic receptors, changes in granulocyte reactive oxygen species production, alterations in granulocyte adherence, and alterations in granulocyte expression of cell adhesion molecules. A cohort study using the U.S. Renal Data System (USRDS) database demonstrated a correlation between the use of unmodified cellulosic dialysis membranes and the risk of mortality due to infection in chronic hemodialysis patients. In current clinical practice, the use of unmodified cellulosic membranes has virtually disappeared.

Changes in monocyte function as well as a reduction in number and function of lymphocytes in patients with uremia lead to altered immunity in this patient population. Evidence of altered immunity includes alterations in T-cell-dependent humoral responses such as reduced responsiveness to vaccinations, diminished delayed hypersensitivity responses, and a dramatic attenuation of autoimmune disease activity with uremia. The chronic use of cellulosic dialysis membranes may also exacerbate the underlying defect in immunity in patients with uremia.

BIBLIOGRAPHY

Besarab A, Bolton WK, Browne JK, et al: The effects of normal as compared with low hematocrit values in patients with cardiac disease who are receiving hemodialysis and erythropoietin. N Engl J Med 339:584–590, 1998.

Besarab A, Kaiser JW, Frinak S: A study of parenteral iron regimens in hemodialysis patients. Am J Kidney Dis 34:21–28, 1999.

Besarab A, Reyes CM, Hornberger J: Meta-analysis of subcutaneous versus intravenous epoetin in maintenance treatment of anemia in hemodialysis patients. Am J Kidney Dis 40:439–446, 2002.

Beusterein KM, Nissenson AR, Port FK, et al: The effects of recombinant human erythropoietin on functional health and well-being in chronic dialysis patients. J Am Soc Nephrol 7:763–773, 1996.

Casadevall N, Nataf J, Viron B, et al: Pure red-cell aplasia and antierythropoietin antibodies in patients treated with recombinant erythropoietin. N Engl J Med 346:469–475, 2002.

Chandler G, Harchowal J, Macdougall IC: Intravenous iron sucrose: Establishing a safe dose. Am J Kidney Dis 38:988–991, 2001.

Churchill DN, Muirhead N, Goldstein M, et al: Effect of recombinant human erythropoietin on hospitalization of hemodialysis patients, Clin Nephrol 43:184–188, 1995.

Collins AJ, Li S, St Peter W, et al: Death, hospitalization, and economic associations among incident hemodialysis patients with hematocrit values of 36 to 39%. J Am Soc Nephrol 12:2465–2473, 2001.

Eschbach JW, Egrie JC, Downing MR, et al: Correction of anemia of endstage renal disease with recombinant human erythropoietin: Results of a combined phase I and II clinical trial. N Engl J Med 316:73–78, 1987.

Eschbach JW, Kelly MR, Haley NR, et al: Treatment of the anemia of progressive kidney disease with recombinant human erythropoietin. N Engl J Med 321:158–163, 1989.

Eschbach JW, Haley NR, Egrie JC, Adamson JW: A comparison of the responses to recombinant human erythropoietin in normal and uremic subjects. Kidney Int 42:407–416, 1992.

Feldman HI, Santanna J, Guo W, et al: Iron administration and clinical outcomes in hemodialysis patients. J Am Soc Nephrol 13:734–744, 2002.

Fishbane S, Frei GL, Maesaka J: Reduction in recombinant human erythropoietin doses by the use of chronic intravenous iron supplementation. Am J Kidney Dis 26:41–46, 1995.

Fishbane S, Shapiro W, Dutka P, et al: A randomized trial of iron deficiency testing strategies in hemodialysis patients. Kidney Int 60:2406–2411, 2001.

Foley RN, Parfrey PS, Harnett JD, et al: The impact of anemia on cardiomyopathy, morbidity and mortality in endstage renal disease. Am J Kidney Dis 28:53–61, 1996.

Foley RN, Parfrey PS, Morgan J, et al: Effect of hemoglobin levels in hemodialysis patients with asymptomatic cardiomyopathy. Kidney Int 58:1325–1335, 2000.

Goldblum SE, Reed WP: Host defenses and immunologic alterations associated with chronic hemodialysis. Ann Intern Med 93:597–613, 1980.

Hakim RM, Lazarus JM: Biochemical parameters in chronic kidney disease. Am J Kidney Dis 11:238–247, 1988.

Ibbotson T, Goa KL: Darbepoetin alfa [Review]. Drugs 61:2097–2104, 2001.

Kaufman JS, Reda DJ, Fye CL, et al: Subcutaneous compared with intravenous epoetin in patients receiving hemodialysis. N Engl J Med 339:578–583, 1998.

Lewis SL, Van Epps DE: Neutrophil and monocyte alterations in chronic dialysis patients. Am J Kidney Dis 9:381–395, 1987.

Locatelli F, Olivares J, Walker R, et al: Novel erythropoesis stimulating protein for treatment of anemia in chronic renal insufficiency. Kidney Int 60:741–747, 2001.

Macdougall IC, Gray SJ, Elston O, et al: Pharmacokinetics of novel erythropoiesis stimulating protein compared with epoetin alfa in dialysis patients. J Am Soc Nephrol 10:2392–2395, 1999.

Michael B, Coyne DW, Fishbane S, et al: Sodium ferric gluconate complex in hemodialysis patients: Adverse reactions compared to placebo and iron dextran. Kidney Int 61:1830–1839, 2002.

Moreno F, Sanz-Guajardo D, Lopez-Gomez JM, et al: Increasing the hematocrit has a beneficial effect on quality of life and is safe in selected hemodialysis patients. Spanish Cooperative Renal Patients Quality of Life Study Group of the Spanish Society of Nephrology. J Am Soc Nephrol 11:335–342, 2000.

Owen WF: Optimizing the use of parenteral iron in endstage renal disease patients: Focus on issues of infection and cardiovascular disease. Introduction. Am J Kidney Dis 34(4 suppl 2):S1–S2, 1999.

Powe NR, Griffiths RI, Watson AJ, et al: Effect of recombinant erythropoietin on hospital admissions, readmissions, length of stay, and costs of dialysis patients. J Am Soc Nephrol 4:1455–1465, 1994.

Ratcliff PJ: Molecular biology of erythropoietin. Kidney Int 44:887–904, 1993.

Rice L, Alfrey CP, Driscoll T, et al: Neocytolysis contributes to the anemia of renal disease. Am J Kidney Dis 33:59–62, 1999.

Rossert J, Casadevall N, Eckardt K: Anti-erythropoietin antibodies and pure red cell aplasia. J Am Soc Nephrol 15:398–406, 2004.

Steiner RW, Coggins C, Carvalho ACA: Bleeding time in uremia: A useful test to assess clinical bleeding. Am J Hematol 7:107–117, 1979.

CHAPTER 67

Endocrine and Neurologic Manifestations of Kidney Failure

Eugene C. Kovalik

ENDOCRINE MANIFESTATIONS

Chronic kidney disease (CKD), endstage renal disease (ESRD), and kidney transplantation all affect the endocrine system. Alterations in signal-feedback mechanisms and in production, transport, metabolism, elimination, and protein binding of hormones occur, as do a variety of drug interactions (Tables 67-1 and 67-2). As a result, the levels of some hormones, including growth hormone, prolactin, and catecholamines, are genuinely elevated in CKD. In addition, hormonal assays may give aberrant results in patients with kidney disease. This can occur if the assay cross-reacts with inactive metabolites that are excreted by the normal kidney but accumulate with a falling glomerular filtration rate (GFR). Glucagons and calcitonin are two examples of the latter.

Hypothalamic-Hypophyseal Axes

Thyroid

Thyroid abnormalities have been well documented in CKD and ESRD patients. As many as 58% of uremic patients have evidence of a goiter by palpation, thought to be caused by an uncharacterized circulating goitrogen that accumulates as GFR falls. Total thyroxine (T_4) is either normal or decreased, and triiodothyronine (T_3) levels are depressed. Free T_4 levels may be low without clinical hypothyroidism. The use of reverse T_3 (rT_3) to differentiate between hypothyroid states and the "euthyroid sick" state is not helpful in patients with CKD, since levels are often normal. Although binding globulin levels are normal, circulating inhibitors bring about decreased globulin binding and interfere with the older resin uptake–based tests of thyroid function. These abnormalities tend to worsen with the progression of CKD. Thyroid-stimulating hormone (TSH) concentrations tend to be normal despite the abnormalities in thyroid hormone levels and therefore are the best indicator of thyroid function for the diagnosis of hypothyroidism or hyperthyroidism, especially with the availability of ultrasensitive TSH assays. The basal metabolic rate is also normal in CKD.

Although TSH levels are normal in patients with CKD, subtle abnormalities exist in the hypothalamic-hypophyseal axis. Exogenous thyrotropin-releasing hormone (TRH) stimulation brings about a blunted TSH response. The usual nocturnal TSH surge is absent. TSH administration results in an increase in T_3 levels but not in the expected rise in T_4. It has been postulated that two different problems occur in patients with CKD. First, there is an inappropriate response to decreased thyroid hormone levels due to a reset in the normal feedback loop to a lower level of TSH secretion for a given level of thyroid hormone. Second, thyroid gland resistance to TSH also occurs. For unknown reasons, the use of recombinant erythropoietin normalizes the TSH response to TRH but not the thyroid response to TSH. The mildly impaired thyroid axis may play a role in protecting the body by maintaining a positive nitrogen balance despite the uremic state. After kidney transplantation, thyroid function tests normalize, although some patients may still have an abnormal TSH response to TRH due to glucocorticoid suppression of TSH secretion.

Growth Hormone

Although plasma growth hormone (GH) levels are elevated in patients with CKD and ESRD, because of both increased secretion and impaired clearance of the hormone, this change has no apparent clinical significance in adults, in whom the role of GH for general health is controversial. Insulin-like growth factor (IGF) levels are normal. Dynamic testing of the GH axis demonstrates several abnormalities. Oral glucose loading does not suppress GH levels, whereas intravenous glucose, glucagon, or TRH paradoxically increases GH levels. GH-releasing hormone (GHRH) and L-dopa infusions also cause prolonged and exaggerated responses in GH secretion. On the other hand, insulin-induced hypoglycemia does not stimulate GH secretion. Correction of anemia with erythropoietin corrects the paradoxic response of GH secretion to TRH and insulin-induced hypoglycemia, although the prolonged GHRH response remains.

In children, uremia results in growth retardation despite normal or elevated GH and IGF levels.

527

TABLE 67-1 Pathogenetic Mechanisms of Endocrine Dysfunction in CKD

Increased circulating hormone levels
  Impaired renal or extrarenal clearance (e.g., insulin, glucagon, PTH, calcitonin, prolactin)
  Increased secretion (e.g., PTH, aldosterone?)
  Accumulation of immunoassayable hormone fractions that may lack bioactivity (e.g., glucagon, PTH, calcitonin, prolactin)

Decreased circulating hormone levels
  Decreased secretion by diseased kidney (e.g., EPO, renin, 1,25(OH)$_2$ vitamin D$_3$)
  Decreased secretion by other endocrine glands (e.g., testosterone, estrogen, progesterone)

Decreased sensitivity to hormones
  Altered target tissue response (e.g., insulin, glucagon, 1,25(OH)$_2$ vitamin D$_3$, EPO, PTH)

CKD, chronic kidney disease; EPO, erythropoietin; PTH, parathyroid hormone.
From Mooradian AD: In Becker KL (ed): Principles and Practice of Endocrinology and Metabolism. Philadelphia, Lippincott, 1995, p 1759.

Contributing variables include protein malnutrition, chronic acidosis, recurrent infections, hyperparathyroidism, and decreased bioactive IGF. The assurance of adequate nutrition and dialysis as well as correction of acidosis and hyperparathyroidism improve but do not normalize growth. Kidney transplantation does not by itself reverse the abnormal growth patterns observed in children, probably because of the effects of exogenous

TABLE 67-2 Directional Changes of Hormones in CKD

Hypothalamopituitary axis
  GH ↑ prolactin ↑

Thyroid
  TT$_4$ N or ↓, FT$_4$ N or ↓
  TT$_3$ ↓, FT$_3$ ↓, rT$_3$ N, TSH N

Gonads
  Testosterone ↓, spermatogenesis ↓
  Estrogen N or ↓, progesterone ↓
  LH N or ↑, FSH N

Pancreas
  Insulin ↑, glucagon ↑

Adrenal glands
  Aldosterone N or ↓, cortisol N or ↑
  ACTH N or ↑
  Catecholamines N or ↑

Kidney
  EPO ↓, renin ↓, 1,25(OH)$_2$ vitamin D$_3$ ↓

ACTH, adrenocorticotropic hormone; CKD, chronic kidney disease; EPO, erythropoietin; FSH, follicle-stimulating hormone; FT$_3$, free triiodothyronine; FT$_4$, free thyroxine; GH, growth hormone; LH, luteinizing hormone; N, no change; rT$_3$, reverse triiodothyronine; TT$_3$, total triiodothyronine; TT$_4$, total thyroxine; TSH, thyroid-stimulating hormone.
From Lim VS: In Greenberg A (ed): Primer on Kidney Diseases. San Diego, Academic Press, 1994, p 315.

glucocorticoids used for immunosuppression. The availability and use of recombinant human growth hormone (rHGH) has greatly improved the well-being of children with CKD, restoring growth velocity and increasing muscle mass without adversely affecting epiphyseal closure. rHGH does not affect glucose tolerance in children but does tend to aggravate preexisting hyperinsulinemia. The use of rHGH after kidney transplantation in children also significantly improves growth without increasing adverse events.

Prolactin

Prolactin secretion is normally under inhibition via prolactin inhibitory factor (PIF), which is in turn controlled by dopaminergic neurons. Basal levels of prolactin are elevated up to six times normal in patients with CKD because of a decrease in dopaminergic activity. Many medications that have antidopaminergic effects also contribute to the increased prolactin levels by decreasing the tonic inhibitory effects of dopamine. The major effects of increased prolactin levels are reflected in the reproductive abnormalities observed in CKD and ESRD patients: gynecomastia, impotence, and amenorrhea. Bromocriptine can reduce prolactin levels, but its effectiveness in relieving symptoms has not been well established. Side effects such as nausea and gastrointestinal upset lead to discontinuation of therapy in one third of patients. Again, erythropoietin therapy can normalize prolactin levels and improve sexual dysfunction in men and menstrual regularity in women, although the mechanism of the effect is not well established.

Any medications that can increase prolactin levels should be minimized or avoided if possible (i.e., α-methyldopa, phenothiazines, neuroleptics, metoclopramide, and H$_2$ blockers, especially cimetidine), particularly if gynecomastia becomes painful or cosmetically displeasing for male patients. As also observed in pubertal males, gynecomastia in men with CKD may be related in part to the increased estrogen-to-androgen ratio that commonly occurs in this setting. Mammography should be performed in patients with true gynecomastia (firm subareolar tissue as opposed to fat deposition), since breast cancer does occur, though rarely, in men. Alternative therapies for gynecomastia in men include subcutaneous mastectomies or breast bud irradiation.

Glucocorticoids

Patients with CKD exhibit normal to elevated levels of adrenocorticotropic hormone (ACTH) without clinical significance. The ACTH response to corticotropin-releasing hormone (CRH) can be blunted or normal. Correction of anemia with erythropoietin can lead to an exaggerated ACTH response to CRH. The standard ACTH stimulation test for diagnosing hypocortisolism is not affected by the uremic state.

Basal cortisol levels in CKD patients are normal. Circadian rhythm of cortisol secretion remains intact. The usual oral low-dose 1-mg overnight or 2-day dexamethasone suppression tests used to evaluate hypercortisolism do not suppress cortisol levels in patients with CKD, partly because of decreased oral absorption of the hormone and an altered set point of the axis. The 1-mg intravenous or 8-mg oral high-dose overnight dexamethasone test will suppress cortisol levels in CKD patients. Although insulin-induced hypoglycemia fails to raise serum cortisol levels, the response to major stress such as surgery is preserved.

Gonadotropins

Males

Loss of libido, impotence, testicular atrophy, gynecomastia, and infertility may occur in males with CKD or ESRD. Testosterone is decreased, and testosterone-binding globulin levels are normal. Levels of luteinizing hormone (LH), which controls testosterone production, are increased. Follicle-stimulating hormone (FSH) levels are elevated, indicating that spermatogenesis feedback is abnormal, and testicular biopsy confirms abnormal sperm maturation. Prolonged stimulation with human chorionic gonadotropin (HCG) can result in increased testosterone levels, suggesting some preservation of testicular reserve. The response to administration of LH-releasing hormone (LHRH) is unpredictable; blunted and normal as well as exaggerated, prolonged responses have all been observed. Thus it appears that both a central hypothalamic insensitivity and peripheral testicular failure exist in men with CKD or ESRD. Hyperprolactinemia and elevated parathyroid hormone (PTH) levels may contribute to the combined central and peripheral problem. Treatment with erythropoietin can improve symptoms of fatigue and lack of energy without actually affecting testosterone levels by increasing a patient's sense of well-being and decreasing prolactin and PTH levels. Zinc deficiency has also been thought to contribute to the hypogonadism, although replacement therapy has yielded varying results. A trial of zinc supplementation can be attempted for those with documented zinc deficiency. Although kidney transplantation reverses many of the symptoms, the hypogonadism may worsen as a consequence of glucocorticoid administration.

Impotence may also be caused by neuropathies or vasculopathies. Drugs that can contribute to impotence (i.e., beta blockers) should be discontinued or reduced in dose. Sildenafil and its newer analogue have significantly improved the ability to treat impotence and should be used as first-line agents. Due to their vasoconstrictor effects, cavernous injections should be used with caution in severely hypertensive patients. Unfortunately, many patients fail to respond to these measures and require vacuum erector devices or penile implants. Figure 67-1 outlines an approach to sexual dysfunction in the male patient.

Females

Women with CKD and ESRD may have diminished libido or an inability to achieve orgasms. Approximately half of postpubertal women on dialysis become amenorrheic, and those who still have menses find their menstrual cycles progressively irregular and anovulatory as kidney function declines. Fewer than 10% of women on dialysis have regular menses. Estradiol, estrone, progesterone, and testosterone levels are normal to low. FSH levels are normal with mildly elevated LH, resulting in an increased LH/FSH ratio that is similar to prepubertal patterns, and in a defect in the positive hypothalamic feedback mechanism in response to estrogen. Without positive feedback, the midcycle LH and FSH surge fails to occur; anovulation results. Nonetheless, women who have some residual renal function and who are well dialyzed may rarely become pregnant and carry to term, although the fetus tends to be premature and small for gestational age (see Chapter 56). Unlike premenopausal women, postmenopausal women with CKD or ESRD have the expected increases in both LH and FSH. Hyperprolactinemia may also be present. Hormone replacement therapy in postmenopausal women should follow the recommendations for women with normal kidney function. The use of estrogen replacement to prevent bone loss in premenopausal CKD and ESRD women has not been investigated.

Transplantation rapidly restores fertility to premenopausal women. Ovulation can start within a month of transplantation. Appropriate counseling should be undertaken to stress the need for contraception. Current guidelines call for women who wish to become pregnant to wait 2 years with stable graft function (creatinine under 1.8 mg/dL), with minimal immunosuppression and normal or readily controlled blood pressure. Good data on the use of oral contraceptives in the transplant patient group are lacking. Referral to a gynecologist should be made if this mode of contraception is considered because of the possible increased risk of thromboembolic disease. Figure 67-2 outlines an approach to sexual dysfunction in uremic women. The evaluation focuses on menstrual irregularities and libido, the latter of which is more difficult to treat. Besides hormonal evaluation including thyroid, prolactin, estrogen, and androgen profiles, mechanical issues such as dyspareunia should be addressed. Again, referral to a gynecologist or endocrinologist is useful.

Carbohydrate Metabolism

Patients with CKD can develop what has been termed "pseudodiabetes." The condition results from a combination of peripheral resistance to insulin, circulating inhibitors of insulin action, and decreased islet cell

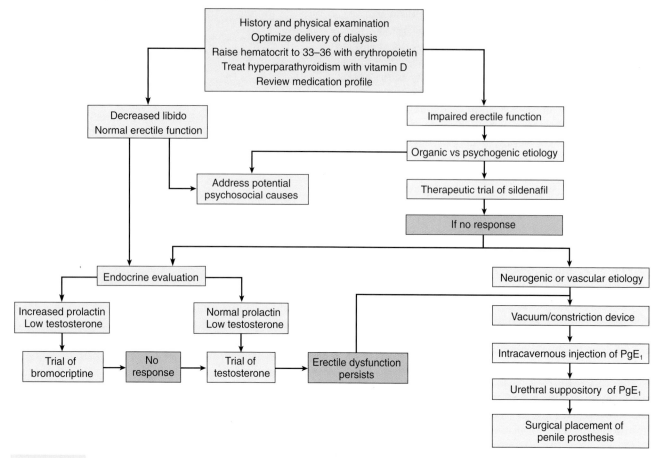

FIGURE 67-1 An approach to sexual dysfunction in the male patient. (From Palmer BF: Sexual dysfunction in uremia. J Am Soc Nephrol 10:1384, 1999.)

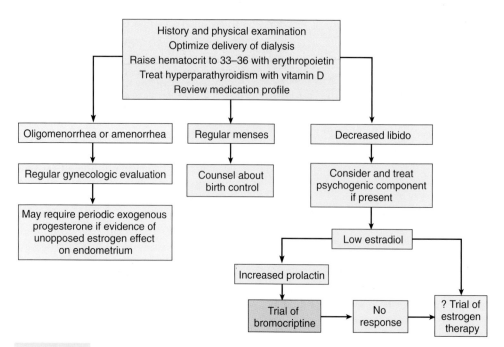

FIGURE 67-2 An approach to sexual dysfunction in uremic women. (From Palmer BF: Sexual dysfunction in uremia. J Am Soc Nephrol 10:1386, 1999.)

insulin release. Blood glucose levels are generally less than 140 mg/dL. Dialysis corrects these defects. In contrast, diabetics with CKD and ESRD often find that their need for oral hypoglycemic agents or insulin decreases as a result of reduced insulin clearance by the kidney. In the case of patients with type 2, non-insulin-dependent diabetes mellitus (NIDDM), a condition mostly due to peripheral insulin resistance, endogenous insulin half-life is prolonged, resulting in a decreased or eliminated need for medication. In addition, the decreased clearance of oral hypoglycemic agents (primarily first-generation sulfonylureas) can lead to prolonged hypoglycemia. Agents that are primarily hepatically metabolized (second-generation sulfonylureas) or insulin should be used to treat type 2 patients. Metformin is contraindicated in patients with CKD because of the increased risk of lactic acidosis, but newer agents that decrease peripheral insulin resistance (i.e., thiazolidinediones) appear safe. Type 1 insulin-dependent diabetes mellitus (IDDM) patients may need their insulin dose reduced, but never discontinued, since their underlying problem is a lack of endogenous insulin production. Glycemic control can worsen in peritoneal dialysis patients as a result of the glucose load absorbed from the peritoneal dialysis fluid. Intraperitoneal insulin administration, based on a sliding scale, may facilitate management. New peritoneal dialysis fluids containing icodextrins instead of dextrose can cause spurious hyperglycemia, since some of the absorbed metabolites interfere with the reagents used in some glucometers. Patients may need to use special glucometers.

Although many patients have glucose intolerance, fasting hyperglycemia with a glucose value over 140 mg/dL suggests that frank diabetes mellitus is present. Glycosylated hemoglobin values may underestimate the degree of hyperglycemia because of the shortened erythrocyte life span seen in uremia.

Transplantation often reveals an underlying abnormality of glucose metabolism in patients due to the high doses of steroids used for immunosuppression. Patients not previously thought to be diabetic can develop diabetes mellitus and require oral hypoglycemic or insulin therapy. Those already known to be diabetic may require conversion from an oral hypoglycemic agent to insulin or a significant increase in their insulin dosage because of steroid-induced peripheral resistance to insulin action. Calcineurin inhibitors can be diabetogenic. This effect seems more common with tacrolimus than cyclosporine, although most studies show no statistical difference in the rate of development of posttransplant diabetes mellitus in patients using tacrolimus- versus cyclosporine-based immunosuppression over long-term follow-up.

Spontaneous and fasting hypoglycemia can occur in CKD and ESRD patients because of malnutrition, impaired glycogenolysis, and carnitine deficiency. Besides nutritional evaluation and supplementation, carnitine levels should be measured and a trial of supplementation attempted if levels are decreased and hypoglycemia persists despite efforts to improve inadequate nutrition.

Mineralocorticoids

As a result of the progressive loss of renal tissue with CKD as well as suppression due to volume expansion, renin production is generally decreased but aldosterone levels can be low, normal, or even elevated. The renin-angiotensin-aldosterone response to volume contraction or hypotension is blunted. Measurements of renin levels are not particularly useful in evaluating hypertension in CKD patients. With renin levels low, hyperkalemia becomes the most important stimulus for aldosterone secretion. Aldosterone in turn stimulates colonic loss of potassium, an often-overlooked means of potassium removal in CKD patients. The elevated serum levels of aldosterone may play a role in the progression of kidney disease on account of their enhancement of high blood pressure and direct effects on mesangial and vascular collagen synthesis. Urinary aldosterone secretion is a strong predictor of urinary albumin secretion.

In general, it is difficult to diagnose hyperaldosteronism in CKD patients as kidney disease progresses. Elevated 24-hour urine aldosterone levels in the setting of new-onset hypertension should prompt renal artery or adrenal imaging studies.

Adrenal Medulla

Basal levels of catecholamines in CKD and dialysis patients are elevated because of several influences, including both decreased degradation and decreased neuronal reuptake of catecholamines. Hemodialysis treatments remove catecholamines but not in sufficient amounts to cause intradialytic hypotension. The diagnosis of pheochromocytoma is difficult in patients with CKD. Suppression testing has not been validated in this setting. The observation of high levels of catecholamines should be combined with appropriate radiologic studies to make the diagnosis.

Lipids and Atherogenesis

Patients with CKD and ESRD only infrequently have hypercholesterolemia or elevated levels of low-density lipoprotein (LDL), but hypertriglyceridemia is observed in half. Conversely, levels of intermediate-density lipoprotein (IDL) and small, dense LDL are increased as a result of poor hepatic clearance. Low levels of high-density lipoprotein (HDL) are also common. Nephrotic patients are an exception: they have elevated levels of all these lipid fractions that improve as the underlying kidney disease is treated. When disease is active, these abnormalities are often resistant to treatment with statins.

Heparin administration during hemodialysis causes release of both hepatic and endothelial lipoprotein lipase, resulting in a depletion of these enzymes and an impairment of the metabolism of triglycerides (TGs), particularly of highly atherogenic, triglyceride-rich remnant IDL particles.

Elevated lipoprotein (a) (Lp[a]) and homocysteine levels are considered to be independent risk factors for atherosclerosis in the general population. Studies of Lp(a) demonstrate increased levels in CKD and ESRD patients, but the isoform distribution is similar to that of patients without renal failure. Homocysteine levels are elevated in 75% to 90% of peritoneal dialysis and hemodialysis patients. Isotope studies suggest that in hemodialysis patients, hyperhomocysteinemia is due to a decrease in homocysteine remethylation to methionine rather than defects in the transsulfuration pathway. The hyperhomocysteinemia seen in hemodialysis patients has been associated with a 4% increased risk of vascular access thrombosis for every $1\mu M$ increase in serum homocysteine level.

Until additional data are available, treatment of lipid disorders in CKD and dialysis patients should follow general guidelines used in patients with normal kidney function. Patients with elevated LDL levels should be started on therapeutic life-style modifications and then advanced to pharmacologic therapy. Bile acid resin binders, such as cholestyramine and colestipol, should be avoided, since they may worsen hypertriglyceridemia. Fibric acid derivatives such as gemfibrozil and clofibrate should be used with careful monitoring in CKD and ESRD patients, since they are cleared primarily by the kidney, and their accumulation increases the risk of rhabdomyolysis. The safest agents are statins. High statin doses may increase the risk of myalgias and rhabdomyolysis and require close patient follow-up. Because of its many side effects, such as insulin resistance and gastric irritation, nicotinic acid is not a good lipid-lowering agent in the CKD population. Experience with its use is limited, but it can be used with close follow-up.

Although initial studies demonstrated the possible protective effects of vitamin E on cardiovascular mortality in the general population, later randomized trials found no benefit of vitamin E in preventing cardiovascular events in the general population and no evidence-based role in CKD patients. Reducing homocysteine levels by supplementing with folic acid is safe in the CKD population as a means to reduce cardiac risk and, theoretically, slow the progression of cardiac disease. Unfortunately, at least one randomized trial of folic acid for the prevention of cardiovascular events in dialysis patients showed no improvement in outcomes with doses up to 15 mg of folic acid per day. In fact, evidence suggests that homocysteine levels may be inversely related to hospitalization and mortality rates, probably as a reflection of nutritional status. Further trials are ongoing, and until further data are available, folate supplementation is a reasonable practice in those with elevated homocysteine

levels. Vitamin C also acts as an antioxidant. Unfortunately, it is relatively contraindicated in CKD and ESRD patients, since its metabolic by-product (oxalate) is excreted by the kidney, and its use can result in elevated serum oxalate levels or hyperoxaluria and stone formation in CKD and ESRD patients.

As in dialysis patients, cardiovascular disease is the major cause of death in the transplant population, and every effort should be made to reduce risk factors. However, kidney transplant patients should be considered separately from other CRF patients when it comes to lipid abnormalities. Total cholesterol, TG, LDL, oxidized LDL, Lp(a), and homocysteine levels are elevated, whereas HDL levels are variable. In addition to the increased cardiac risk of posttransplant lipid abnormalities, some evidence suggests that dyslipidemia may also contribute to chronic graft rejection. Treatment of lipid abnormalities in transplant patients is similar to that of CRF patients. Bile resin binders should be avoided because they interfere with cyclosporine absorption from the gastrointestinal tract. Fibrates have an increased risk of causing rhabdomyolysis with decreased GFR, particularly in combination with cyclosporine. Statins have been safely used in studies on transplant patients without major side effects. At least one study has shown a reduction in acute rejection episodes using pravastatin. The use of vitamin E, vitamin C, or folic acid has not been investigated, although a multicenter trial of the latter is currently underway.

NEUROLOGIC MANIFESTATIONS

Nervous system dysfunction commonly occurs in patients with kidney disease. The spectrum of abnormalities includes mild to severe alterations in the sensorium, cognitive dysfunction, generalized weakness, and peripheral neuropathies. These problems can occur before the initiation of dialytic therapy and can progress despite ostensibly adequate renal replacement therapy.

Uremic Encephalopathy

The term uremic encephalopathy refers to the central nervous system (CNS) signs and symptoms that result from a decline in kidney function. The threshold for development of uremic encephalopathy is a fall in GFR to a level below 10% of normal. Symptoms are more severe and abrupt in onset when associated with an acute rather than a chronic loss of kidney function. Psychomotor behavior, cognition, memory, speech, perception, and emotion can all be affected. In this respect, uremic encephalopathy resembles and can be difficult to distinguish from organic brain syndromes due to other etiologies.

Uremic encephalopathy should be suspected in patients with kidney failure if there are clinical signs and symptoms consistent with CNS deterioration. However, overlap with symptoms resulting from other intercurrent illnesses or drug toxicities complicates diagnosis. In patients with both advanced liver and kidney disease, particularly those with hepatorenal syndrome, it is often difficult to determine whether the encephalopathy is due to hepatic or renal causes or both. In such patients, the blood urea nitrogen (BUN) and serum creatinine do not always reflect the degree of kidney functional impairment. Mildly elevated BUN and creatinine levels may underestimate the magnitude of the loss of kidney function due to malnutrition and/or a diminished capacity to generate urea and creatinine. The diagnosis may be made by exclusion if other causes such as hypercalcemia, hypernatremia, hyponatremia, hyperglycemia, hypoglycemia, hypoxia, and hypercapnia are excluded, or in retrospect after improvement is observed in response to dialysis or other specific therapy such as treatment of hepatic encephalopathy or discontinuation of narcotics, benzodiazepines, or other medications that can affect the sensorium.

The initial neurologic presentation of patients with acute renal failure may include signs of psychosis, lassitude, and lethargy, with disorientation and confusion occurring later. Physical findings may include cranial nerve signs, nystagmus, dysarthria, abnormal gait, and motor signs manifested by weakness (both symmetric and asymmetric), fasciculations, and asymmetric variation in deep tendon reflexes. These findings may progress to asterixis and hyperreflexia with unsustained clonus at the ankle. Spontaneous myoclonus may be present and has the same significance as asterixis. If uremia is left untreated and allowed to progress, seizures and coma often supervene.

Electroencephalograms (EEGs) in patients with acute renal failure are generally grossly abnormal when the diagnosis of severe acute renal failure is first made and are not usually improved by dialysis during the first few weeks of treatment. The EEG may remain abnormal for as long as 6 months after initial presentation with severe acute renal failure, despite adequate renal replacement therapy. Completely normal tracings may not be reached until the patient receives a kidney transplant or recovers kidney function. Despite the presence of these EEG abnormalities, it is not a tool used in diagnosing uremic encephalopathy, since similar findings can be seen in other toxic and metabolic encephalopathies.

Pathogenesis

Although many influences may contribute to uremic encephalopathy, no precise correlation exists between the degree of encephalopathy and any of the commonly measured blood chemistries associated with renal dysfunction (BUN, creatinine, bicarbonate, or pH). There are numerous potential or putative uremic toxins, including PTH and other nitrogenous wastes (see Chapter 58). Unfortunately levels of these agents do not reliably correlate with the severity of symptoms.

Peripheral Neuropathies

Neuropathy of some degree is probably present in about 65% of patients with CKD and ESRD. The findings may be subtle, and abnormal nerve conduction may be present in the absence of symptoms or physical findings. Specific questions about paresthesias, diminished sensation, sexual dysfunction, or presyncope may elicit a history of sensory/autonomic neuropathy that can be confirmed by careful physical examination. Uremic neuropathy is a distal, symmetric, mixed polyneuropathy and is also associated with a secondary demyelinating process in the posterior columns of the spinal cord and the CNS. Motor and sensory modalities are both generally affected, and the lower extremities are more severely involved than are the upper extremities. Dysfunction is usually maximal distally and is characterized by mixed motor and sensory abnormalities, resulting in weakness and wasting in the arms and legs with sensory changes in a "glove and stocking" distribution. Isolated or multiple isolated lesions of the peripheral nerves are designated as mononeuropathies. Like uremic encephalopathy, the pathophysiology of uremic neuropathy has not been well established. Although many uremic toxins have been implicated, no single one can explain all the observed abnormalities of peripheral nerve function. Uremic neuropathy may, in part, also be related to anatomic nerve damage of unknown etiology and to the cumulative effects of multiple toxic agents over months to years.

Symptoms and Signs

The restless-leg syndrome is a common early manifestation of kidney failure in CKD. Clinically, patients experience sensations such as crawling, prickling, and pruritus in their lower extremities. The sensations are generally worse distally and are usually more prominent in the evening. Patients are awakened because they cannot find a comfortable sleeping position. The burning-foot syndrome, which is present in fewer than 10% of patients with kidney failure, actually represents swelling and tenderness of the distal lower extremities. The physical signs of peripheral nerve dysfunction often begin with loss of deep tendon reflexes, particularly in the ankle and knee. Sensory modalities that are lost include pain, light touch, vibration, and pressure. Clinically, uremic neuropathy cannot easily be distinguished from the neuropathies associated with diabetes mellitus, chronic alcoholism, and other nutritional deficiency states. The occurrence of uremic neuropathy bears no relationship to the type of underlying kidney disease. However, some disorders, including amyloidosis, multiple myeloma, systemic lupus erythematosus, polyarteritis nodosa, diabetes mellitus, and hepatic failure, can cause both peripheral neuropathy and kidney disease.

Diagnosis and Treatment

Motor nerve conduction velocity has very limited utility in detecting moderately impaired peripheral nerve function in CKD and ESRD patients because of a daily test variability of as much as 20%. Sensory nerve conduction velocity testing is more sensitive, but its performance can be painful.

No one treatment appears to be uniformly effective, probably because of the multifactorial etiologies of the neuropathies. Analgesics (nonsteroidal agents, cyclo-oxygenase 2 inhibitors, opiates, quinine, and muscle relaxants), anticonvulsants (e.g., gabapentin and carbamazepine), antidepressants (e.g., tricyclics), anxiolytics (e.g., benzodiazepines), and antiarrythmics have all been utilized with varying results. Dopaminergic agents and L-dopa may have specific benefit for restless-leg syndrome. Often a trial-and-error method is the only way to find the best therapy for an individual. There is no reliable evidence to suggest that increasing the intensity of dialysis in ESRD patients ameliorates symptoms.

Autonomic and Cranial Nerve Dysfunction

Autonomic dysfunction is quite common in CRF and is usually associated with postural hypotension, impaired sweating, impotence, and gastrointestinal motility disturbances. Hemodialysis-associated hypotension is often associated with autonomic insufficiency, especially in patients with diabetes or amyloidosis. Hand-grip dynamometer, heart rate response to the Valsalva maneuver, beat-to-beat heart rate respiratory variability, and vascular response to norepinephrine infusion can all be used to evaluate autonomic dysfunction.

Cranial nerve involvement in uremia often manifests as transient nystagmus, miosis, heterophoria, and facial asymmetry. Eighth-nerve involvement including both auditory and vestibular function can occur and must be distinguished from deafness due to hereditary nephritis and drug ototoxicity such as that caused by aminoglycosides or high-dose furosemide.

Intellectual Dysfunction

Intellectual dysfunction is not well characterized and is without distinctive anatomic lesions. On the basis of psychologic testing, progressive loss of kidney function in CKD is associated with organic-like loss of intellectual function. Since patients are often older, they are also susceptible to other conditions that can cause a decline in intellectual function such as Alzheimer's, multi-infarct dementia, and chronic alcoholism. It is often quite difficult to establish a clear etiology for the declining function.

Complications of Dialysis Therapy

Dialysis Disequilibrium Syndrome

Several CNS disorders may occur as a consequence of dialytic therapy. One such disorder is dialysis disequilibrium syndrome (DDS), which can occur acutely in patients who have recently initiated hemodialysis, usually during or after the first several treatments. The symptom complex is quite variable and may include muscle cramps, anorexia, restlessness, dizziness, headache, nausea, emesis, blurred vision, muscular twitching, disorientation, hypertension, tremors, seizures, and obtundation. It occurs most often in the elderly and in children. The syndrome is generally associated with intense initiation of hemodialysis but is rarely seen today because of a more gradual and earlier initiation of hemodialysis. DDS has not been described in peritoneal dialysis patients.

It is thought that DDS results from overly rapid correction of plasma osmolality, causing cerebral edema. As kidney function declines, the brain increases intracellular osmolality to protect itself from the associated extracellular hyperosmolality. If brain osmolality did not increase, the brain would lose water and shrink. Such a reduction in brain volume is undesirable, because it can lead to intracranial hemorrhage. The brain increases intracellular osmolality by generating intracellular organic acids, amino acids, methylamines, and polyols, the "idiogenic osmoles." A similar process occurs with hyperglycemia and hypernatremia. Thus, any treatment, such as hemodialysis, that acutely lowers plasma osmolality without allowing adequate time for the internal removal of neuronal intracellular idiogenic osmoles runs the risk of establishing a substantial brain-to-plasma osmolar gradient, which can result in brain water uptake and cerebral edema. To avoid DDS, nephrologists typically select an initial dialysis prescription that is deliberately inefficient (low blood flow, shortened treatment times, and small–surface area dialyzer) so as to permit a gradual lowering of the plasma-to-CNS osmolar gradient and allow the brain to dissipate the "idiogenic osmoles." During subsequent treatments, both the duration of dialysis and the blood flow rate and surface area of the dialyzer are increased. Other measures to prevent DDS include ultrafiltration followed by dialysis, use of bicarbonate instead of acetate as the dialysate base, and the addition of mannitol, glycerol, or glucose osmoles to the dialysate solution or as intravenous bolus injections.

Dialysis Dementia

Dialysis dementia is a progressive, frequently fatal neurologic disease that is seen almost exclusively in patients who are being treated with chronic hemodialysis. Dialysis dementia can occur in isolation or in association with osteomalacia, proximal myopathy, and anemia, and it occurs in three settings: an epidemic form, a sporadic form, and with childhood kidney disease. Initial symptoms of this disorder include dysarthria, apraxia, and slurring of speech with stuttering and hesitancy. Later in the course of the disease, symptoms progress to personality changes, psychosis, myoclonus, seizures, and eventually dementia and death within 6 months after the onset of symptoms. The diagnosis of dialysis dementia depends on the presence of the typical clinical picture, the characteristic EEG findings (multifocal bursts of high-amplitude delta activity with spikes and sharp waves), and, most importantly, exclusion of other causes of CNS dysfunction.

The epidemic form, which occurred mainly in the 1970s, has now been clearly linked to aluminum (see later). It occurred in dialysis units that did not use water purification techniques such as reverse osmosis or deionization that would remove aluminum from source water. Dialysate aluminum concentrations were thus high, and patients were exposed to aluminum during hemodialysis. Numerous patients in these units developed dialysis dementia along with painful fracturing osteomalacia. This disorder disappeared once its relationship to aluminum exposure had been established and water purification standards were upgraded. The sporadic form occurred in patients who had been on chronic hemodialysis for more than 2 years and was also thought to be due to long-term aluminum exposure in aluminum-based phosphate binders and drinking water.

Dialysis dementia has been reported in children with kidney failure. Many received high doses of oral aluminum-containing phosphate binders, but some were neither on dialysis nor exposed to aluminum. Therefore, encephalopathy in such children cannot be ascribed to aluminum alone and may represent developmental neurologic defects resulting from exposure of the growing brain to the uremic milieu.

Role of Aluminum in Dialysis Dementia

Aluminum content in the brain is more than threefold greater in patients with dialysis dementia than in those on chronic hemodialysis without dementia. Increased aluminum levels in CKD and ESRD are due to both an increase in gastrointestinal absorption and a decrease in renal elimination. Normally, only a minimal amount of orally administered aluminum is absorbed and later excreted by the kidneys. For unknown reasons, absorption appears to be increased in patients with kidney failure, a condition that, when coupled with the decrease in excretion, leads to toxicity. Aluminum sources include drinking water, cooking pots, and medications such as aluminum-containing antacids. Citrate and sucralfate preparations increase aluminum absorption from the gastrointestinal tract. Before deionization of the water used in hemodialysis became routine, most of the aluminum in dialysis patients came from dialysate water. Aluminum is clearly responsible for the development of the epidemic form of dialysis dementia. However, whether aluminum plays an important role in the other types of dialysis dementia (sporadic and childhood) is still unresolved. Deionization of dialysate water removes not only aluminum but also cadmium, mercury, lead, manganese, copper, nickel, thallium, boron, and tin. Thus, not only aluminum, but several other trace elements and minerals may be involved in the pathogenesis of dialysis dementia. Fortunately, with improved water treatment and the elimination of routine use of aluminum-containing antacids, the incidence of epidemic and sporadic dialysis dementia has fallen markedly.

Treatment

Although diazepam and clonazepam appear to be useful in controlling initial seizure activity associated with dialysis dementia, the drugs usually become ineffective and do not appear to alter the usually fatal outcome. Improvement in symptoms has been reported in several patients treated with deferoxamine, which, when given intravenously, chelates aluminum and promotes its removal during hemodialysis.

BIBLIOGRAPHY

Endocrine

Bostom AG, Gohh RY, Tsai MY, et al: Excess prevalence of fasting and postmethionine-loading hyperhomocysteinemia in stable renal transplant recipients. Atherosclerosis Thrombosis Vasc Biol 17:1894–1900, 1997.

Deck KA, Fischer B, Hillen H: Studies on cortisol metabolism during hemodialysis. Eur J Clin Invest 9:203–207, 1979.

Grundy SM: Management of hyperlipidemia of kidney disease. Kidney Int 37:847–853, 1990.

Haffner D, Nissel R, Wuhl E, et al: Metabolic effects of long-term growth hormone treatment in pubertal children with chronic renal failure and after kidney transplantation. Pediatr Res 43:209–215, 1998.

Holdsworth S, Atkins RC, Kretser DM: The pituitary-testicular axis in men with chronic renal failure. N Engl J Med 296:1245–1249, 1977.

Hostetter T, Ibrahim H: Aldosterone in chronic kidney and cardiac disease. Kidney Int 14:2395–2401, 2003.

Kalantar-Zadeh K, Block G, Humphreys MH, et al: Reverse epidemiology of cardiovascular risk factors in maintenance dialysis patients. Kidney Int 63:793–808, 2003.

Katznelson S, Wilkinson AH, Kobashigawa JA, et al: The effect of pravastatin on acute rejection after kidney transplantation—a pilot study. Transplantation 61:1469–1474, 1996.

Kokot F, Wiecek A, Grzeszczak W, et al: Influence of erythropoietin treatment on function of the pituitary-adrenal axis and somatotropin secretion in hemodialyzed patients. Clin Nephrol 33:241–246, 1990.

Lim VS: Reproductive function in patients with renal insufficiency. Am J Kidney Dis 9:363–367, 1987.

Lim VS, Flanigan MJ, Zavala DC, et al: Protective adaptation of low serum triiodothyronine in patients with chronic renal failure. Kidney Int 28:541–549, 1985.

Massey ZA, Kasiske BL: Post-transplant hyperlipidemia: Mechanisms and management. J Am Soc Nephrol 7:971–977, 1996.

Mooradian AD: Endocrine dysfunction due to renal disease. In Becker KL (ed): Principles and Practice of Endocrinology and Metabolism. Philadelphia, Lippincott, 1995, pp 1759–1762.

Moustapha A, Gupta A, Robinson K, et al: Prevalence and determinants of hyperhomocysteinemia in hemodialysis and peritoneal dialysis. Kidney Int 55:1470–1475, 1999.

N'Gankam V, Uehlinger U, Dick B, et al: Increased cortisol metabolites and reduced activity of 11 β-hydroxysteroid dehydrogenase in patients on hemodialysis. Kidney Int 61:1859–1866, 2002.

Palmer BF: Sexual dysfunction in uremia. J Am Soc Nephrol 10:1381–1388, 1999.

Ramirez G: Abnormalities in the hypothalamic-hypophyseal axes in patients with chronic renal failure. Semin Dial 7:138–146, 1994.

Ramirez G, Butcher DE, Newton JL, et al: Bromocriptine and the hypothalamic hypophyseal function in patients with chronic renal failure on chronic hemodialysis. Am J Kidney Dis 6:111–118, 1985.

Schaefer RM, Kokot F, Geiger H, et al: Improved sexual function in hemodialysis patients on recombinant erythropoietin: A possible role for prolactin. Clin Nephrol 31:1–5, 1989.

Sechi LA, Zingaro L, Catena C, et al: Lipoprotein (a) and apolipoprotein (a) isoforms and proteinuria in patients with moderate renal failure. Kidney Int 56:1049–1057, 1999.

Shemin D, Lapane KL, Bausserman L, et al: Plasma homocysteine and hemodialysis access thrombosis: A prospective study. J Am Soc Nephrol 10:1095–1099, 1999.

Van Guldener C, Kulik W, Berger R, et al: Homocysteine and methionine metabolism in ESRD: A stable isotope study. Kidney Int 56:1064–1071, 1999.

Wrone EM, Hornberger JM, Zehnder JL, et al: Randomized trial of folic acid for prevention of cardiovascular events in endstage renal disease. J Am Soc Nephrol 15:420–426, 2004.

Neurology

Andreoti SP, Bergstein JM, Sherrard DJ: Aluminum intoxication from aluminum containing phosphate binders in children with azotemia not undergoing dialysis. N Engl J Med 310:1079–1084, 1984.

Arieff AI: Dialysis disequilibrium syndrome: Current concepts on pathogenesis and prevention. Kidney Int 45:629–635, 1994.

Arnaud CD: Hyperparathyroidism and renal failure. Kidney Int 4:89–95, 1973.

Fraser CL, Arieff AI: Nervous system complications in uremia. Ann Intern Med 109:143–153, 1988.

Fraser CL, Arieff AI: Nervous system manifestations of renal failure. In Schrier RW, Gottschalk CW (eds): Diseases of the Kidney, 5th ed. Boston, Little, Brown, 1997, pp 2625–2646.

Slatopolsky E, Martin K, Hruska K: Parathyroid hormone metabolism and its potential as a uremic toxin. Am J Physiol 238:F1–F12, 1980.

CHAPTER 68

Evaluation of Patients for Kidney Transplantation

Bertram L. Kasiske

Studies of patients who have received a kidney transplant indicate that their survival is generally better than survival on dialysis. This is true irrespective of the sex, race/ethnicity, cause of kidney disease, or the age of the recipient. Therefore, transplantation is probably the treatment of choice for most patients with endstage renal disease (ESRD). Nevertheless, not all patients are suitable for transplantation, and a patient's nephrologist usually performs the initial evaluation to decide if and when to refer a patient to a transplant center.

WHO IS A CANDIDATE FOR KIDNEY TRANSPLANTATION?

There are few absolute contraindications for kidney transplantation. There is no absolute age that precludes transplantation, and patients over age 50 are the most rapidly growing segment of the deceased-donor transplant waiting list (Fig. 68-1). However, physiologic age and overall health status should be carefully considered, especially in individuals who are over age 60. Probably the most common reason not to refer a patient is that the patient's overall condition is so poor that the patient is not expected to survive, even if transplanted, for more than 2 years. This may include patients who are severely debilitated, patients with incurable cancer, and patients with severe cardiovascular disease that is not amenable to treatment. In questionable cases, it is best to refer the patient to the transplant center but to make it clear to the center and the patient that the purpose of the referral is to consider whether transplantation is suitable, and that the referral will not necessarily result in the patient's being approved for transplantation.

EARLY REFERRAL

Outcomes are better for patients who undergo transplantation before they begin chronic maintenance dialysis (i.e., preemptive transplantation) than they are for patients who are transplanted after they initiate dialysis. Therefore, early referral to a transplant center is important. On the other hand, it is equally important to be sure that the transplant candidate has ESRD. A small percentage of patients presenting with presumed ESRD (e.g., patients with renal vascular disease or interstitial nephritis) may regain function. Knowing the cause of kidney disease (e.g., type 1 diabetes typically progresses inexorably) and the rate of decline in estimated kidney function (plots of the reciprocal of serum creatinine concentration versus time) can help in the determination of when a patient should be referred to a transplantation center.

In general, patients with stage 3 or 4 chronic kidney disease (CKD) should be referred to a nephrologist, and patients with stage 4 CKD should be referred by their nephrologist to a transplant center, unless they are clearly not transplant candidates. Stage 3 refers to patients with measured or estimated (by any of several formulas) glomerular filtration rate (GFR) of 30 to 59 mL/minute/1.73 m^2. Stage 4 refers to patients with measured or estimated GFR of 15 to 29 mL/minute/1.73 m^2. In the United States, patients can begin accumulating waiting time on the United Network for Organ Sharing (UNOS) waiting list for a deceased-donor transplant when the measured or estimated GFR is 20 mL/minute or lower. In general, it is better to refer too early than too late.

WHO IS A CANDIDATE FOR PANCREAS TRANSPLANTATION?

Patients whose quality of life is poor because they have diabetes that is difficult to control may want to consider pancreas transplantation. Pancreas transplantation undertaken before kidney transplantation may be appropriate for some, but it runs the risk of accelerating the decline in native kidney function from the use of immunosuppressive agents such as calcineurin inhibitors. Simultaneous deceased-donor kidney and pancreas transplantation usually requires that the patient spend time waiting for an available kidney. Because the waiting time for a deceased-donor pancreas is currently much shorter than the waiting time for a kidney, many

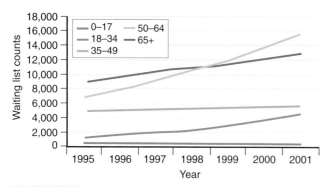

FIGURE 68-1 Growth in the deceased-donor United Network for Organ Sharing kidney transplantation waiting list 1995–2001, by recipient age in years. (Data from the United States Renal Data System 2003 Annual Data Report.)

patients opt to have a living-donor kidney followed by a deceased-donor pancreas transplantation. Usually, the pancreas transplantation can occur within 3 to 6 months after the kidney transplantation.

Although pancreas transplantation may prevent recurrence of diabetic nephropathy, recurrent diabetic nephropathy is rarely the cause of kidney graft failure. Therefore patients should understand that the reason for pancreas transplantation is to improve the quality of life, not to prevent chronic complications. Indeed, it has never been shown that the additional risk of pancreas transplantation outweighs any benefits with regard to long-term complications; diabetes control and some long-term complications may be reduced by kidney transplantation alone.

RISK OF RECURRENT KIDNEY DISEASE

Many kidney diseases other than diabetes recur after transplantation, but rarely does the risk of recurrence prohibit transplantation. The most common cause of recurrence that results in graft failure is idiopathic focal segmental glomerulosclerosis (FSGS). The risk of recurrence in the first kidney transplant is probably about 25% to 30%. However, patients who have lost a transplanted kidney because of recurrent FSGS have at least a 50% chance of losing the second transplant to FSGS, and these odds probably increase with each subsequent transplant. Therapy with plasma exchange may reduce proteinuria from recurrent FSGS and may prolong the life of the graft. Plasma exchange is thought to work by removing a glomerular permeability factor that causes proteinuria in some patients with idiopathic FSGS.

Patients with nondiarrheal hemolytic-uremic syndrome or thrombotic thrombocytopenic purpura may have recurrence of the disease after transplantation. However, the true rate of recurrence is difficult to ascer-

tain, because the syndrome can also be caused by the immunosuppressive agents cyclosporine, tacrolimus, and probably sirolimus.

Type 1 membranoproliferative glomerulonephritis (MPGN) recurs in 20% to 30% of transplant recipients, whereas type 2 MPGN (dense-deposit disease) recurs in 90% to 100%. However, even with type 2 MPGN, recurrence may be slow enough for many, if not most, patients to benefit from transplantation. Membranous glomerulonephritis recurs in approximately 25% of transplant recipients.

Immunoglobulin A (IgA) nephropathy and Henoch-Schönlein purpura frequently cause IgA deposition in the transplanted kidney, but they only infrequently cause graft failure. The estimated recurrence rate of clinically apparent IgA nephropathy (associated with elevated serum creatinine and/or proteinuria) is approximately 30%.

Antineutrophil cytoplasmic antibody (ANCA)–associated vasculitis may recur in as many as 20% of transplant recipients. Unfortunately, the presence or absence of ANCA at the time of transplantation does not appear to predict recurrence. Antiglomerular basement membrane (anti-GBM) disease recurs in 10% to 25% of cases, but there is no effective way to predict when this will happen. Ironically, about 10% of patients with Alport's syndrome may develop de novo anti-GBM disease after transplantation, because of the production of antibodies against GBM antigens that their immune systems encounter for the first time after transplantation. Systemic lupus erythematosus recurs infrequently, and recurrence rarely results in graft failure.

Primary oxalosis is rare, but without treatment oxalate deposition quickly recurs in the transplanted kidney. Fortunately, intensive treatment with orthophosphate and pyridoxine, with or without liver transplantation to provide a source of the deficient enzyme, is often successful.

Secondary amyloidosis (with the deposition of amyloid AA fibrils) frequently recurs in the allograft if the underlying cause of the disease is still present. In addition, patients with secondary amyloidosis often have severe, progressive cardiovascular disease from amyloid deposition. Nevertheless, the course of secondary amyloidosis may be slow enough to allow transplantation, and some patients may survive for years with a successful kidney transplant. Patients with primary amyloidosis (amyloid AL) should generally have any underlying plasma cell dyscrasias treated and controlled before transplantation. However, treatment may include bone marrow or stem cell transplantation that may actually reduce the requirement for long-term immunosuppression.

Patients with sickle cell nephropathy can be successfully transplanted if their overall condition does not preclude surgery. Graft survival has generally been reported to be about 75% at 1 year.

CANCER

Immunosuppression may favor the growth of malignant tumors, and an active malignancy is usually an absolute contraindication to transplantation. Exceptions are locally invasive basal or squamous cell skin carcinomas. Some have argued that applying guidelines for cancer screening (that have been designed for use in the general population) to transplant candidates may not be warranted, given the shorter life expectancy of patients with ESRD compared with the general population. However, the risk of cancers that can be detected with screening seems to be higher in transplant patients, and the cost effectiveness of screening may actually be enhanced by the investment of resources (including the donated kidney) necessitated by transplantation. Therefore, most recommend that all patients undergo routine screening with a physical examination, chest x-ray, and stool sample for occult blood. Individuals over age 50 years should also have flexible sigmoidoscopy or colonoscopy or other appropriate imaging of the colon. Women should have mammography, pelvic examination, and Pap test following the guidelines established for the general population.

Immunosuppression probably increases the risk of cancer recurrence. Data from registries, though imperfect, provide some guidance on the chances of recurrence of different malignant tumors. The overall recurrence rate for malignancies treated before transplantation is 20% to 25%. Since more than half of these recurrences are in patients treated within 2 years before transplantation, many centers recommend a 2-year disease-free interval before kidney transplantation. However, a waiting period of as long as 5 years may be prudent for lymphomas; for breast, prostate, and colon cancer; as well as for symptomatic renal cell carcinomas (especially if they are greater than 5 cm in diameter). It is probably not necessary to delay transplantation for incidentally discovered renal cell carcinomas and adequately treated in situ carcinomas of the skin or uterine cervix.

INFECTIONS

Immunosuppression greatly increases the risk for life-threatening infections. Immunizations for influenza (yearly), pneumococcus, and hepatitis B are mandatory. In general, the effectiveness of these vaccinations is not well documented in ESRD, but their potential benefits outweigh their negligible risks. Patients should also be screened for infections that may become problematic with immunosuppression. Sites of occult infection include the lung, urinary tract, and dialysis catheters. Dialysis-related peritonitis within 3 to 4 weeks is a relative contraindication to transplantation.

Patients should be screened for human immunodeficiency virus (HIV). Before the era of highly active antiretroviral therapy, HIV was considered an absolute contraindication to kidney transplantation. However, some centers are reporting encouraging preliminary results among patients who were HIV positive but without active disease at the time of transplantation. Interactions between antiretroviral drugs and immunosuppressive agents make it mandatory that HIV-positive transplant patients be managed in centers with appropriate expertise.

Tuberculosis is common in the ESRD population. Screening should include a high index of suspicion, a chest x-ray, and a purified protein derivative skin test, unless there is already a history of a positive skin test. High-risk individuals are those (1) with a past history of active disease, (2) from a high-risk population (e.g., from endemic areas or immunocompromised), and (3) with an abnormal chest x-ray consistent with active or inactive tuberculosis. High-risk individuals should receive prophylactic therapy. Most authors recommend prophylaxis for 6 to 12 months, but it probably is not necessary to delay transplantation once therapy has begun.

Although cytomegalovirus (CMV) infection is common and is often transmitted with the transplanted organ, the presence of CMV antibodies in donors and recipients should not preclude transplantation. Most centers routinely use prophylactic therapy (e.g., ganciclovir or valganciclovir) for CMV-seronegative recipients of kidneys from CMV-seropositive donors. Some centers also use prophylaxis for CMV-seropositive recipients of kidneys from CMV-seropositive donors, and for CMV-seropositive recipients of kidneys from CMV-seronegative donors. However, few use prophylaxis if both donor and recipient are seronegative. Potential recipients who are seronegative for the varicella zoster virus are at risk for disseminated infection and should be identified before transplantation. Patients from tropical regions should be screened for *Strongyloides stercoralis*, and transplantation should occur only if response to treatment is satisfactory.

Particularly difficult to evaluate are patients who are being evaluated for another transplant and who have had a viral infection that may have caused the graft to fail. However, second transplants have been successful in patients who have had Epstein-Barr virus–associated B-cell lymphomas. Similarly, patients who have lost a kidney transplant due to BK virus nephropathy have had successful kidney transplants, with or without removal of the failed allograft.

LIVER DISEASE

Liver failure is a major cause of morbidity and mortality after kidney transplantation, and kidney transplant candidates should be carefully screened for liver disease. The hepatitis A and E viruses do not cause chronic liver disease, whereas hepatitis B virus (HBV) and hepatitis C virus (HCV) can cause chronic active hepatitis after transplant. Transplant recipients who are hepatitis B surface antigen (HBsAg) positive are at increased risk of dying from liver disease in the posttransplant period; however, HBsAg per se is not a contraindication to transplantation. Patients who are HBsAg positive and have serologic evidence of viral replication (by polymerase chain reaction assay or the presence of HBeAg) should probably forgo transplantation. Likewise, HBsAg-positive patients who also have hepatitis D (fortunately rare) often develop severe liver disease and therefore should not receive a transplant. Otherwise, HBsAg-positive patients with elevated liver enzymes should undergo biopsy, and those with chronic active hepatitis may be candidates for antiviral therapy (e.g., lamivudine). The decision as to whether such patients should undergo transplantation or remain on dialysis is often difficult. Patients with liver disease that is severe may be candidates for simultaneous liver and kidney transplantation. Fortunately, the incidence of HBV is declining in the ESRD population, largely because of effective vaccination and isolation procedures.

Although the natural history of HCV is less well defined, patients who test positive for HCV antibodies should probably undergo liver biopsy if enzymes are elevated, and possibly even if enzymes are not elevated, since disease may occur without enzyme elevation in ESRD. Patients with HCV and evidence of viral replication (by polymerase chain reaction) and/or chronic active hepatitis on biopsy are probably at increased risk for progressive liver disease after transplantation. Antiviral therapy (e.g., interferon-α and/or ribavirin) has been used to induce remission of HCV disease before transplantation; however, the long-term results of antiviral therapy in patients with ESRD are unclear.

ISCHEMIC HEART DISEASE

Ischemic heart disease (IHD) is a major cause of death after kidney transplantation. Patients with CKD should be considered to be in the highest risk category (i.e., equivalent to someone with diabetes or IHD) for risk factor management. Risk factors should be optimized both before and after transplantation. Low-density lipoprotein cholesterol should be less than 100 mg/dL, blood pressure should ideally be less than 130/90 mm Hg, and patients should be strongly encouraged to abstain from cigarette smoking. Perioperative beta blockade should also be used unless contraindicated, and aspirin prophylaxis should be considered.

With the increased risk of perioperative IHD events, most centers screen for asymptomatic IHD, although firm evidence for the cost effectiveness of this approach is lacking. Nevertheless, most centers select high-risk patients (e.g., patients with known cardiovascular disease, diabetes, age older than 45 to 50 years, or multiple risk factors) for a noninvasive cardiac stress test. Unfortunately, noninvasive stress tests are often less sensitive in patients with ESRD than in the general popula-

tion. Nevertheless, patients whose stress test is positive for reversible ischemia usually undergo coronary angiography with angioplasty or bypass surgery if there are serious lesions. Long waiting times for a deceased-donor kidney transplant mean that high-risk patients should be rescreened periodically.

CEREBROVASCULAR DISEASE

There is also an increased risk of atherosclerotic cerebrovascular disease complications after kidney transplantation. Patients with a history of transient ischemic attacks or other cerebral vascular disease events should be evaluated for possible treatment and should be free of symptoms for at least 6 months before transplant surgery. Whether asymptomatic patients should undergo screening with a carotid ultrasound examination is unclear. In the general population, controlled clinical trials have shown that the success of prophylactic carotid endarterectomy is dependent on the center and on the selection of patients. However, all patients should be managed with appropriate risk factor intervention.

OBESITY

Obesity, an increasingly important problem in patients with ESRD, carries an increased risk of postoperative complications, particularly wound infections and type 2 diabetes. Obesity is also associated with an increased risk of graft failure. Although there are few studies examining the safety and efficacy of a weight reduction diet in ESRD, obese patients who have a body mass index of 30 to 39 kg/m^2 should be encouraged to lose weight. A 10% reduction in body weight is generally achievable by diet. Patients with body mass indices of 40 kg/m^2 or higher may need bariatric surgery to lose weight before transplantation.

PSYCHOSOCIAL EVALUATION

Transplant candidates should be screened for cognitive or psychologic impairments that may interfere with their ability to give informed consent. Failure to adhere to immunosuppressive therapy is a major cause of kidney allograft failure, and the psychologic assessment should also attempt to identify patients who are at risk. However, reliably identifying patients who will not adhere to therapy is difficult at best, and care should be exercised to avoid unjustifiably refusing transplantation. Most centers require that patients with a history of chemical dependency undergo treatment and demonstrate a period of abstinence, generally 6 months, before transplantation. Major psychiatric disorders are usually apparent during the routine pretransplantation evaluation, and appropriate psychiatric care can be sought.

UROLOGIC EVALUATION

In the absence of a history of chronic infection and/or bladder dysfunction, urologic evaluation and a voiding cystourethrogram are probably not necessary. High-risk patients (e.g., diabetics) can be screened by obtaining a postvoid residual urine volume. If the postvoid urine volume is greater than 100 mL, a voiding cystourethrogram and urologic evaluation should be obtained. In patients with a dysfunctional bladder, every effort should be made to avoid urinary diversion. A few patients may need to use intermittent self-catheterization for optimal bladder drainage.

Pretransplant native kidney nephrectomies may be indicated in some patients. Indications for pretransplant nephrectomy include: reflux associated with chronic infection, polycystic kidneys that are symptomatic and/or too large to allow placement of the allograft, severe nephrotic syndrome, nephrolithiasis associated with infection, renal carcinoma, and difficult-to-control hypertension.

GASTROINTESTINAL EVALUATION

Patients with symptomatic, recurrent cholecystitis should undergo cholecystectomy, because cholecystitis in an immunocompromised transplant recipient may be more severe and more difficult to diagnose and treat. However, most centers no longer routinely screen patients with ultrasonography, and most no longer perform cholecystectomy for asymptomatic cholelithiasis. Similarly, patients with symptomatic diverticulitis may be considered for partial colectomy, but most centers do not conduct screening and surgery for asymptomatic diverticular disease. Peptic ulcer disease is common in the posttransplantation period. However, it can usually be managed medically, and most centers do not routinely perform endoscopy as part of the pretransplantation evaluation.

PULMONARY EVALUATION

Patients with chronic obstructive lung disease are at increased risk for surgical complications and postoperative pneumonia. Patients with a history of cigarette smoking and dyspnea on exertion should undergo pulmonary function testing to allow better assessment of this surgical risk. Patients should be offered nicotine replacement therapy and, if possible, a formal smoking cessation program. It is reasonable to refuse transplantation until patients demonstrate abstinence from smoking for a period of time.

BLOOD AND TISSUE TYPING

Three major immunologic barriers to transplantation need to be addressed: (1) Transplants should generally be ABO blood group compatible; (2) the degree of matching at the major histocompatibility complex (MHC) loci A, B, and DR correlate with long-term graft survival and is used in the UNOS system for allocating deceased-donor kidneys; and (3) the presence of preformed antibodies, and how broadly they react to a random panel of antigens from the general population, correlates directly with the likelihood of a positive cross-match when an organ becomes available and is also used in the UNOS kidney allocation scheme.

Blood and MHC tissue type is determined when it is apparent that the patient will be a suitable transplant candidate. Serum is collected at the initial evaluation and at least quarterly to measure preformed antibodies. An estimate of the number of preformed antibodies is made by reacting the potential recipient's blood against a panel of lymphocytes from a random sample of the general population. The percentage of cells that react is called the percent panel-reactive antibody (PRA). A high PRA indicates that it will be more difficult to find a donor with a negative cross-match for that recipient. A high PRA is also associated with decreased graft survival, even if the final cross-match is negative. Patients have a high PRA due to prior blood transfusion, transplantation, or pregnancy. A recipient's PRA may fall over time, especially if blood transfusions are avoided.

As a final screen, the recipient's most recent serum is tested against donor antigens, since a positive cross-match indicates the presence of preformed antibodies that can cause hyperacute rejection (see Chapter 69). Not all reacting antibodies cause hyperacute rejection, so other laboratory tests are also performed to determine whether the recipient's reacting antibody should preclude transplantation. Usually, the serum with the highest previous PRA is also tested at the time of final cross-matching. Recipients with a negative cross-match but a positive "historical" cross-match may be transplanted, but some studies indicate that the risk of graft failure is increased.

Some centers use plasmapheresis and the infusion of large doses of polyclonal intravenous immunoglobulin (IVIG) to overcome ABO blood group incompatibility and positive cross-matches. Pheresis removes preformed antibodies, and IVIG suppresses subsequent antibody production. These procedures (sometimes combined with splenectomy and rituximab therapy) have allowed a number of patients to receive kidney transplants from blood group–incompatible donors, or from donors with a positive cross-match. However, the risk of antibody-mediated rejection and graft failure are nevertheless increased. As an alternative, some centers are exploring innovative organ exchange programs, whereby kidneys from donors that are immunologically incompatible with the desired recipients are exchanged for kidneys from comparable donors that are compatible.

ALLOCATION OF DECEASED-DONOR KIDNEYS IN THE UNITED STATES

A patient ready for transplantation can be placed on the UNOS waiting list to receive a deceased-donor kidney. Kidneys are allocated by UNOS (under contract from the U.S. government) according to a priority system that is designed to balance equity with efficiency. Equity demands that all patients be given the same access to kidneys, regardless of race, ethnicity, gender, or socioeconomic status. Efficiency dictates that kidneys are given to the patients who are likely to benefit the most, usually patients in whom the longest graft survival can be expected. Unfortunately, the goals of equity and efficiency often conflict. Although the UNOS point system is designed to allocate organs, the final decision to accept a particular organ once it is offered rests in the hands of the patient's physician.

Mandatory Sharing of Zero-MHC Antigen Mismatched Kidneys

Except for kidneys procured for simultaneous kidney and nonkidney organ transplantation, kidneys are first offered to any blood group–compatible recipient who has zero-MHC antigen mismatches. These kidneys are allocated locally first, then regionally, and then nationally.

Blood Group Priority

If there are no zero-MHC antigen–mismatched candidates, then blood type O kidneys must be transplanted into blood type O patients, and blood type B kidneys must be transplanted into blood type B patients. In addition, all patients who have an ABO blood type that is compatible with that of the donor and who are listed as active on the UNOS waiting list will be assigned points and priority according to waiting time, MHC DR mismatches, PRA, pediatric status, and prior organ donation history.

Waiting Time

For candidates under 18 years old, waiting time begins at listing; for candidates 18 years of age or older, waiting time begins when measured or calculated creatinine clearance or GFR is 20 mL/minute or less, or the patient has been initiated on dialysis. Patients can be listed if they have GFR higher than 20 mL/minute, but generally such patients will only receive a deceased-donor kidney that is perfectly matched (through the zero-MHC antigen mismatch program). Otherwise, kidneys are preferentially allocated to those with the longest waiting time. One point is assigned to the patient waiting for the longest period, with fractions of points being assigned proportionately to all other patients, according to their relative time of waiting. For each full year of waiting, an additional point is assigned. The calculation of points is conducted separately for each geographic (local, regional, and national) level of kidney allocation.

DR Mismatches

Two points are assigned if there are no DR mismatches, and 1 point if there is one DR mismatch.

Panel-Reactive Antibody

A patient is assigned 4 points for PRA of 80% or more on the basis of historical or current serum samples, and there is a negative preliminary cross-match between the donor and that patient.

Pediatric Kidney Transplant Candidates

Kidney transplant candidates under 11 years old receive 4 additional points; candidates older than 11 years but under 18 years old receive 3 additional points. These points are assigned when the candidate is registered on the list and retained until the candidate reaches 18 years of age.

Donation Status

A patient receives 4 points if he or she has donated for transplantation in the United States a vital organ or a segment of a vital organ (e.g., kidney, liver segment, lung segment, partial pancreas, small bowel segment).

Recently, the UNOS established a policy whereby patients agreeing to accept a high-risk, "expanded-criteria donor" kidney would be offered such a kidney before it would be offered to those accepting only "standard" kidneys. The UNOS defines expanded-criteria donor kidneys as those from deceased donors 60 years of age and older, or those from deceased donors 50 to 59 years of age and having either: (1) cerebral vascular accident as cause of death and a history of hypertension, or (2) cerebral vascular accident as cause of death and serum creatinine greater than 1.5 mg/dL, or (3) hypertension and creatinine greater than 1.5 mg/dL. Patients agreeing to accept an expanded-criteria donor kidney are also offered standard kidneys according to the usual allocation scheme. In either case, the same allocation rules as those already described apply.

LIVING DONORS

The number of new transplantations has not kept pace with the growth in the number of patients developing ESRD (Fig. 68-2), and there has been a growing shortage of deceased-donor kidneys. With this shortage, a greater

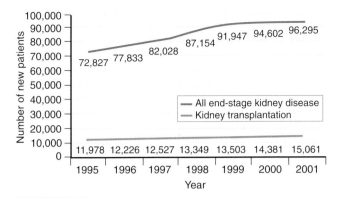

FIGURE 68-2 The number of new endstage kidney disease patients (including kidney transplant patients) and the number of new kidney transplantations in the United States, 1995–2001. (Data from the United States Renal Data System 2003 Annual Data Report.)

emphasis has been placed on living donations (Fig. 68-3). Kidneys from living donors generally survive longer than deceased-donor kidneys. The duration of graft survival based on the source of the donor kidney is, on average, identical twin, longer than two-haplotype-matched sibling, longer than one-haplotype-matched sibling or parent, equal to zero-haplotype-matched sibling, equal to distantly related or unrelated (emotionally related) living donor, greater than deceased-donor kidney. Living-donor kidneys have the added advantages of more easily allowing preemptive transplantation and sparing more kidneys for individuals who do not have suitable living donors.

Potential living (blood-related and emotionally related) donors should be counseled about both the short- and long-term risks of donation. Mortality from donation is approximately 0.03%, whereas major morbidity is about 0.23%. The recent introduction of laparoscopic nephrectomy has substantially reduced the morbidity of kidney donation, without compromising long-term outcomes for the recipient. With regard to long-term risk for the donor, a meta-analysis of 48 studies

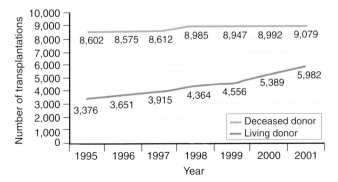

FIGURE 68-3 The number of deceased-donor and living-donor transplantations in the United States, 1995–2001. (Data from the United States Renal Data System 2003 Annual Data Report.)

including 3124 patients and 1703 controls found little evidence of progressive kidney dysfunction among normal individuals with only one kidney. Although there was a small increase in blood pressure, this increase was not enough to raise the prevalence of hypertension in patients who had a single kidney. There was also a statistically significant increase in proteinuria, but the increase was probably too small to be of clinical relevance.

In general, proteinuria greater than 150 mg/24 hours should be considered a contraindication to donation. Microhematuria and pyuria should be investigated to rule out underlying kidney disease that would preclude donation. Kidney function should generally be normal, after adjusting for gender, age, and possible dietary influences on GFR.

Blood typing and cross-matching are often the first steps in evaluating a living donor. If a potential donor and recipient are blood group compatible and cross-match negative, further evaluation can then be carried out. This should include a psychologic evaluation to ensure that the donation is truly voluntary and that the donor can give informed consent. A complete medical evaluation should also be carried out to uncover conditions that would increase the risk of surgery. Potential donors should be screened for conditions such as hypertension that may be made worse by having only one kidney. A controversial issue involves the extent to which possible incipient diabetes in donors with a positive family history or other risk factors for diabetes should be tested. This is because the effect of having one kidney on the rate of progression of diabetic nephropathy (if diabetes occurred) is uncertain. It is reasonable to screen with a fasting and 2-hour postprandial blood glucose. Consideration should be given to the risk of inherited kidney diseases such as autosomal dominant polycystic kidney disease and hereditary nephritis. Finally, the medical evaluation should ensure that the donor is free of diseases that could be transmitted with the kidney, including malignancies, HIV, viral hepatitis, and tuberculosis.

If there is more than one potential living donor, selection should be based on both medical and nonmedical criteria, and good matching need not be the only determinant of donor choice. Although the best donor is usually a member of the recipient's immediate family, most centers would consider an emotionally related donor. Once a potential donor has been selected and evaluated, the final step is usually arteriography or an equivalent imaging technique to define the renal vasculature and to look for potential anatomic abnormalities.

THE TRANSPLANTATION PROCEDURE

The kidney is usually placed retroperitoneally in the iliac fossa. The renal artery is usually anastomosed (end-to-end) with the internal iliac artery. Different techniques are available for dealing with multiple renal arteries and atherosclerosis in the recipient's iliac artery. The renal vein is usually anastomosed (end-to-end) with the external iliac vein. The ureter is implanted via a long submucosal tunnel into the bladder. In general, this surgical approach has made the transplant procedure relatively routine, although immunosuppression delays wound healing and increases the risk of postoperative infection.

BIBLIOGRAPHY

Andresdottir MB, Assmann KJ, Hoitsma AJ: Recurrence of type I membranoproliferative glomerulonephritis after renal transplantation. Transplantation 63:1628–1633, 1997.

Artero M, Biava C, Amend W, et al: Recurrent focal glomerulosclerosis: Natural history and response to therapy. Am J Med 92:375–383, 1992.

Birkeland SA, Hamilton-Dutoit S, Bendtzen K: Long-term follow-up of kidney transplant patients with posttransplant lymphoproliferative disorder: Duration of posttransplant lymphoproliferative disorder–induced operational graft tolerance, interleukin-18 course, and results of retransplantation. Transplantation 76:153–158, 2003.

Bumgardner GL, Amend WC, Ascher NL, Vincenti FG: Single-center long-term results of renal transplantation for IgA nephropathy. Transplantation 65:1053–1060, 1998.

Conlon PJ, Brennan DC, Pfaf WW, et al: Renal transplantation in adults with thrombotic thrombocytopenic purpura/hemolytic-uraemic syndrome. Nephrol Dial Transplant 11:1810–1814, 1996.

Couchoud C, Pouteil-Noble C, Colon S, Touraine JL: Recurrence of membranous nephropathy after renal transplantation. Transplantation 59:1275–1279, 1995.

Droz D, Nabarra B, Noel LH, et al: Recurrence of dense deposits in transplant kidneys. Kidney Int 15: 386–395, 1979.

Frohnert PP, Donadio JV Jr, Velosa JA, et al: The fate of renal transplants in patients with IgA nephropathy. Clin Transplant 11:127–133, 1997.

Ginevri F, Pastorino N, de Santis R, et al: Retransplantation after kidney graft loss due to polyoma BK virus nephropathy: Successful outcome without original allograft nephrectomy. Am J Kidney Dis 42:821–825, 2003.

Kasiske BL, Cangro CB, Hariharan S, et al: The evaluation of renal transplant candidates: Clinical practice guidelines. Am J Transplant 2:5–95, 2002.

Kasiske BL, Ma JZ, Louis TA, Swan SK: Long-term effects of reduced renal mass in humans. Kidney Int 48: 814–819, 1995.

Kasiske BL, Ravenscraft M, Ramos EL, et al: The evaluation of living renal transplant donors: Clinical practice guidelines. J Am Soc Nephrol 7:2288–2313, 1996.

Kasiske BL, Snyder JJ, Matas AJ, et al: Preemptive kidney transplantation: The advantage and the advantaged. J Am Soc Nephrol 13:1358–1364, 2002.

Penn I: Evaluation of transplant candidates with pre-existing malignancies. Ann Transplant 2:14–17, 1997.

Roland ME, Stock PG: Review of solid-organ transplantation in HIV-infected patients. Transplantation 75:425–429, 2003.

United States Renal Data System: USRDS 2003 Annual Data Report: Atlas of End-Stage Renal Disease in the United States. Bethesda, MD, National Institutes of Health, National Institute of Diabetes and Digestive Kidney Diseases, 2003.

CHAPTER 69

Kidney Transplantation: Management and Outcome

Richard N. Formica, Jr.   Fadi G. Lakkis

Kidney transplantation has become a mainstay treatment for patients with endstage renal disease. Advances in the management of transplant recipients over the past two decades have resulted in improved short-term and long-term allograft survival. This success has translated into enhanced patient survival, thus permitting the inclusion of more elderly and complex patients in the transplant recipient pool. In this chapter, post-transplant management of the kidney allograft recipient is described, and long-term graft and patient outcomes following kidney transplantation are summarized.

INPATIENT MANAGEMENT: RECOVERY ROOM THROUGH HOSPITAL DISCHARGE

The week after kidney transplantation is characterized by dramatic changes in the recipient's health and kidney function. When the allograft functions immediately, rapid improvement in the metabolic derangement of uremia and the recipient's overall sense of well-being occurs. When graft function is delayed, a balance must be struck between managing the medical issues that arise and protecting the allograft. Management during the first week after kidney transplantation, therefore, consists of monitoring the patient for life- and allograft-threatening surgical complications, initiating the immunosuppressive regimen, monitoring for rejection and other medical issues that ensue, and educating the patient about caring for the allograft.

Initial Evaluation

The initial evaluation of the patient after kidney transplantation occurs in the postoperative recovery room, where an assessment of the patient's respiratory and hemodynamic condition is made. Large volumes of crystalloid are used during surgery, and if delayed graft function occurs, the patient is at risk for pulmonary edema. The transplanted kidney is very sensitive to blood flow postoperatively, and, therefore, hypotension, or a decrease in blood pressure relative to the patient's baseline, is corrected with normal saline infusions. In some

centers, postoperative renal Doppler ultrasonography is performed to verify that there is adequate blood flow to the kidney. This study can diagnose potential surgical problems in the renal vasculature, and the patient can be returned to the operating room for surgical re-exploration. The immediate surgical emergencies that could arise include bleeding and renal artery or renal vein thrombosis. Renal artery thrombosis is usually correctable, whereas venous thrombosis necessitates removal of the allograft.

Delayed Graft Function

For the recipient of a living-donor kidney, excellent initial function is expected unless complications arise during the transplantation procedure. For the recipient of a deceased-donor kidney, the postoperative course is dependent on several variables, including the graft ischemic time, quality of the organ, and the manner in which the donor died. Prolonged warm ischemia time (longer than 20 minutes), prolonged cold ischemia time (longer than 24 hours), donor age over 50 years, presence of comorbidities in the donor that affect kidney function such as hypertension, and traumatic brain injury as cause of donor death predispose the recipient to delayed graft function. Delayed graft function is defined as need for dialysis within the first week after transplantation and can manifest either as primary nonfunction of the allograft or initial function followed by rapid decline. On histopathologic examination, delayed graft function has the same features as acute tubular necrosis. Knowledge of the factors that predispose the recipient to delayed graft function, therefore, allows the transplant nephrologist to anticipate the need for dialysis after transplantation.

Monitoring the Urine Output

Under most circumstances, urine output serves as a poor marker of kidney function, because significant urine output can occur despite minimal solute clearance. In kidney transplantation, urine output does not assess solute clearance but rather serves as a noninvasive measure of renal blood flow and patency of the urinary tract. Additionally, if the patient produced urine before the transplant (residual urine production), then the total urine output may not reflect the condition of the transplanted kidney. A decrease in urine output in a patient with primary allograft function prompts the following initial maneuvers: The urinary catheter is flushed with normal saline to remove any obstructing blood clots, and a central venous pressure is obtained. If volume depletion is present, the deficit is corrected. If no improvement in urine output occurs, prompt ultrasonographic examination of the allograft is obtained to evaluate for urinary obstruction, vascular complications, and perinephric fluid collections. Perinephric collections in the early postoperative period include hematomas, urinomas due to a leak at the ureterocystic anastomosis, and occasionally lymphoceles (lymphatic fluid accumulations). Compromised arterial blood flow or fluid collections causing compression of the allograft or the ureter require immediate surgical evaluation.

Rejection

An acute rise in serum creatinine always raises the suspicion of allograft rejection irrespective of the time interval since transplantation. Several categories of rejection have been characterized (Table 69-1). However, only the acute forms of rejection can occur within the first 7 days after transplantation.

Hyperacute Rejection

Hyperacute rejection occurs within minutes to hours after reperfusion of the transplanted kidney. Preformed antibodies to human leukocyte antigens (HLAs) or blood group antigens (ABO) cause this type of rejection. These antibodies bind to endothelial cells, where they activate the complement system and initiate the coagulation cascade, resulting in diffuse thrombosis of the allograft. Hyperacute rejection leads to loss of the allograft, but it rarely occurs in modern transplantation because of strict ABO matching and careful HLA cross-matching before transplantation to exclude presensitized patients. Hyperacute rejection is diagnosed clinically when the kidney is observed to thrombose in the operating room.

Accelerated Acute Rejection

Accelerated acute rejection usually occurs within the first 5 days after transplantation. It also occurs in presensitized recipients but results from the activation of memory T and/or B lymphocytes rather than from preformed antibodies. Causes of presensitization in transplant recipients are previous blood transfusion, prior transplantation, and pregnancy. Presensitization that causes accelerated acute rejection is not detected during the cross-match, because memory cells specific to donor antigens occur at a low frequency and are not yet activated. However, after transplantation they proliferate rapidly in response to the allograft and bring about an accelerated form of rejection. Accelerated acute rejection has histologic features of both antibody-mediated (hyperacute) and cell-mediated (acute) rejection involving tubules and blood vessels. Staining for C4d, a component of the complement cascade and a marker of humoral rejection, can be observed in the peritubular capillaries. The diagnosis depends on the clinical circumstances, rapid rejection within the first 5 days after transplantation, and an allograft biopsy containing the features just described.

TABLE 69-1   Types of Kidney Allograft Rejection

	Hyperacute Rejection	Accelerated Acute Rejection	Acute Rejection	Chronic Rejection
Onset after transplantation	Minutes to hours (sensitized recipient)	Days (sensitized recipient)	Days to months	Months to years
Proposed mechanisms	Preformed anti-HLA or anti-ABO antibodies bind to the vascular endothelium and activate the complement and coagulation cascades	Memory cellular and humoral immune response to donor antigens, including HLA	Acute cellular and occasionally humoral immune response to donor antigens including HLA	Insidious cellular and humoral immune response to foreign HLA Nonimmunologic influences such as hypertension and reduced renal mass
Pathology	Intravascular thrombi Neutrophilic infiltrates Interstitial edema Cortical infarcts	Mononuclear and neutrophilic cell infiltrate causing tubulitis and often vasculitis	Mononuclear cell infiltrate causing tubulitis and less often vasculitis	Vasculopathy Glomerulopathy Glomerulosclerosis Interstitial fibrosis Mononuclear infiltrate
Progression to graft failure	Minutes to hours Irreversible	Days Potentially reversible	Days to weeks Reversible	Months to years Irreversible

HLA, human leukocyte antigen.

Acute Rejection

Acute cellular rejection usually occurs 5 days or later after transplantation. It is most common during the first 3 months following transplantation, declines in frequency over the next 3 months, and is a rare event thereafter. Most episodes are cell mediated and do not have a humoral component. Acute rejection is graded histopathologically according to the structures involved. Mild rejections are characterized by tubulitis, whereas severe forms are characterized by both tubulitis and vasculitis. The classical constitutional symptoms of rejection, which include fevers, chills, arthralgias, myalgias, and pain over the allograft, rarely occur because of the enhanced efficacy of current immunosuppressive regimens. Therefore, acute rejection has become primarily a laboratory diagnosis confirmed by a biopsy. A subacute rise in serum creatinine that occurs over 1 to 2 weeks and cannot readily be attributed to another etiology should also prompt an allograft biopsy to exclude acute rejection.

Immunosuppressive Drugs

Modern immunosuppressive medications have reduced the incidence of acute allograft rejection to less than 15% and improved both 1-year and long-term allograft survival. An advantage of modern immunosuppression is the ability to target different phases of the immune response simultaneously with currently available agents. This allows for additive and often synergistic immunosuppression with fewer side effects.

Antibodies

Polyclonal and monoclonal antibody preparations that target T-lymphocyte surface antigens are used in organ transplantation to deplete or inactivate peripheral T lymphocytes. This prevents the initiation of the immune response to the allograft. Two polyclonal antibody preparations are available for general use: horse antithymocyte globulin (Atgam) and rabbit antithymocyte globulin (Thymoglobulin), both of which are produced by immunizing animals with human leukocytes, then collecting the serum and purifying the antibody. Since these are animal proteins, the major side effect is serum sickness in the recipient. Because they are polyclonal and given at dosages that overwhelm the immune system, antibodies in the recipient against these preparations rarely diminish their clinical effectiveness.

OKT3 (Muromonab) is the only monoclonal antibody in common use. It is a mouse antibody against one of the proteins forming the CD3 complex on human T lymphocytes. Binding of this antibody to CD3 causes its removal from the cell surface and renders the T-cell receptor for antigen incapable of transmitting an activating signal to the cell. The significant side effect of OKT3 is initial release of T-lymphocyte-derived cytokines into the circulation. This cytokine release syndrome occurs with the first few doses and causes fever, capillary leak, and neurologic symptoms such as headache and aseptic meningitis. Because the epitope-recognizing region of OKT3 is of mouse origin and directed against only one target, antibodies can form against it and render it ineffectual, because they block binding to the cell surface CD3 molecule. Therefore, before a second course of therapy the recipient's serum is tested for the presence of anti-OKT3 antibodies.

The monoclonal anti-CD25α antibodies, basiliximab (Simulect) and daclizumab (Zenapax), are humanized (genetically engineered to resemble human immunoglobulin) monoclonal antibodies directed against the α-subunit of the high-affinity interleukin 2 (IL-2) receptor expressed exclusively on activated T lymphocytes. IL-2 is an important T-lymphocyte mitogen. It is suspected that anti-IL-2 antibodies do not deplete T cells from the circulation but rather prevent them from responding to IL-2. They are associated with few if any side effects, because they are humanized and generate little human antimouse response. In addition, they have a very long half-life in the serum that results in a prolonged period of protective immunosuppression.

Calcineurin Inhibitors

The calcineurin inhibitors cyclosporine and tacrolimus, though chemically distinct and acting through different intracellular proteins, ultimately exert their immunosuppressive action by binding to the intracellular phosphatase calcineurin. Calcineurin cleaves phosphates from regulatory cytosolic proteins and allows them to translocate to the nucleus and facilitate the expression of cytokine genes. By inhibiting this function of calcineurin, cyclosporine A and tacrolimus disrupt the signal from the T-cell receptor to the nucleus and prevent T-lymphocyte activation. Their actions, unfortunately, are not limited to T lymphocytes and are therefore associated with various side effects. These include nephrotoxicity, neurotoxicity (seizures, tremor, and rarely leukoencephalopathy), diabetes, hypertension, hirsutism (cyclosporine), and alopecia (tacrolimus).

Target of Rapamycin Inhibitors

The target of rapamycin (TOR) inhibitors sirolimus and everolimus are chemically similar to the macrolide antibiotics. They exert their immunosuppressive effects on T lymphocytes and to a lesser extent on B lymphocytes by binding to the intracellular protein mammalian TOR. This protein is a regulatory kinase in the pathway downstream of the IL-2 receptor, as well as other mitogenic receptors, that causes activated cells to enter the cell cycle. TOR inhibitors block progression from G_1 to S phase, thus allowing cells to become activated but preventing them from proliferating. Side effects of this class of immunosuppressive medications include delayed wound healing due to impaired fibroblast proliferation, lymphoceles, hyperlipidemia, and hematologic abnormalities, particularly thrombocytopenia. Additive nephrotoxicity can occur when TOR inhibitors are combined with full-dose calcineurin inhibitors.

Mycophenolate Mofetil

Mycophenolate mofetil (MMF) has replaced azathioprine as the antiproliferative agent of choice in kidney transplantation. The active metabolite of MMF, mycophenolate, works by inhibiting the enzyme inosine monophosphate dehydrogenase (IMPDH), which is a critical rate-limiting enzyme in the de novo synthesis of guanine nucleotides. Because T lymphocytes lack the ability to scavenge guanine nucleotides, they must produce their own. MMF inhibits this ability and blocks T-lymphocyte proliferation by preventing DNA synthesis. The most common side effects of MMF are hematologic, primarily leukopenia, and gastrointestinal, primarily diarrhea.

Corticosteroids

Corticosteroids have widespread effects, because most mammalian cells have glucocorticoid receptors in their cytosol. The immunosuppressive actions of corticosteroids result from the direct effect they exert on antigen-presenting cells (e.g., dendritic cells and macrophages) and T lymphocytes, in which they inhibit cytokine production. Corticosteroids also exert more general anti-inflammatory effects that are the result of their ability to block the production of chemokines that signal immune cells to migrate to an area of inflammation and to directly block the migration of these cells.

Choice of Immunosuppressive Drugs

The choices for initial immunosuppression have broadened substantially over the past 10 years, and it is no longer a one-size-fits-all approach. Many centers employ "induction" therapy consisting of either a monoclonal or polyclonal antibody regimen given in the perioperative period. Anti-CD25α monoclonal antibodies are commonly used, because they are well tolerated and result in a significant reduction in acute rejection rates. The use of T-lymphocyte-depleting antibodies such as Thymoglobulin and Atgam is generally reserved for patients at high risk for acute rejection. Patients at high risk are those with a high panel-reactive antibody (PRA), previous kidney transplant, history of losing a prior allograft to rejection within the first year after transplantation, and recipients of a simultaneous kidney and pancreas transplant. Additionally, the use of these polyclonal antibodies for patients with delayed graft function allows kidney function to recover before starting a calcineurin inhibitor.

Whether or not "induction" therapy leads to improved long-term survival remains a matter of debate.

The term "base immunosuppression" refers to the primary maintenance immunosuppressive medications around which the therapeutic regimen is constructed. Currently there are two widely used options. Most commonly used is calcineurin inhibitor–based immunosuppression consisting of either tacrolimus or cyclosporine. These medications are used at conventional dosing and monitored by measuring 12-hour trough drug levels. They are combined with MMF and prednisone. This regimen yields an acute rejection rate between 15% and 20% during the first year following transplantation. A second option is TOR inhibitor–based immunosuppression. In this regimen, sirolimus or everolimus is administered in combination with reduced-dose calcineurin inhibitors and prednisone. Reducing the dose of calcineurin inhibitors is hypothesized to lessen the risk of nephrotoxicity without increasing the risk of acute rejection because of the potent immunosuppressive properties of TOR inhibitors. Available data suggest that TOR inhibitor–based immunosuppression achieves protection from acute rejection comparable to calcineurin inhibitor–based strategies. TOR inhibitor–based immunosuppressive regimens are currently being studied to explore the possibility of eliminating either calcineurin inhibitors or steroids in selected patients at low risk for acute rejection.

The choice of which base immunosuppressive regimen to prescribe is tailored to the individual patient and how the side effect profiles of a specific agent may affect them. For example, patients at risk for delayed wound healing may benefit from a regimen that excludes TOR inhibitors, whereas patients at high risk for type 2 diabetes mellitus are perhaps best prescribed a regimen that does not employ standard-dose tacrolimus. Hirsutism caused by cyclosporine is unacceptable to most women, and, therefore, a tacrolimus-based regimen may be a better option.

Kidney transplant recipients with rare exception require lifelong immunosuppression to preserve their allograft. The dosages are kept high immediately after transplantation to protect the kidney from rejection. During the first year, the initial regimen is tapered to a maintenance regimen based on center-specific practices. Patients are instructed never to taper or stop their immunosuppression unless directed to do so by the transplant team.

Treatment of Acute Rejection

Only acute rejection is readily responsive to treatment. More than 95% of acute rejection episodes can be reversed with currently available immunosuppressive agents. Milder forms of acute rejection are treated with a 3-day intravenous pulse of methylprednisolone. More severe forms of acute rejection, or those episodes that do not respond to methylprednisolone, require therapy with either OKT3 or one of the polyclonal antibody preparations. Accelerated acute rejection is less responsive to therapy. Strategies currently employed to salvage the allograft involve the simultaneous use of plasmapheresis (to remove donor-specific antibodies), with or without intravenous immunoglobulin, and high-dose immunosuppression employed for the treatment of acute rejection. Hyperacute rejection is irreversible and requires allograft nephrectomy to prevent systemic complications that could result from the necrotic graft.

Initiation of Prophylaxis Against Infection

Bacterial Prophylaxis

Patients who are not allergic to sulfa-containing drugs receive antimicrobial prophylaxis with a single-strength trimethoprim-sulfamethoxazole tablet daily. This provides protection from *Pneumocystis carinii* pneumonia (PCP) infection as well as urinary tract and sinus infections. Practice varies, with some transplant programs stopping therapy at 6 months to 1 year and others continuing indefinitely. For a patient with sulfa allergy, PCP prophylaxis is achieved with dapsone or monthly inhaled pentamidine given for 1 year.

Fungal Prophylaxis

Nystatin swish-and-swallow solution is started immediately after transplantation or at the first signs of oral thrush to prevent or treat oral and esophageal candidiasis. This treatment is continued until the prednisone dosage has been lowered to 10 mg/day or less; this level is usually attained by 2 months after transplantation.

Viral Prophylaxis

The choice of viral prophylaxis depends on the recipient's viral exposure history. Cytomegalovirus (CMV) antibody–negative recipients who receive a kidney from a CMV antibody–positive donor are at highest risk of acquisition of CMV disease. If either the recipient or donor has antibodies to CMV, valganciclovir is prescribed to prevent CMV disease. Valganciclovir dosing is adjusted according to renal clearance and is continued for 3 months after transplantation. If both the recipient and donor are negative for antibodies to CMV, acyclovir is prescribed to prevent herpes simplex virus (HSV) infection. Patients receiving valganciclovir do not require acyclovir as well because the former is active against HSV. Because of the high cost of antiviral drugs, some centers use surveillance strategies. Patients are monitored at regular intervals for CMV blood antigenemia, and therapy is reserved for patients who turn positive.

OUTPATIENT MANAGEMENT: 1 WEEK TO 6 MONTHS

Outpatient management during the first 6 months after transplantation is focused on monitoring the recipient for acute rejection, delayed surgical complications, infection, and treating medical conditions associated with kidney transplantation and immunosuppression.

Frequency of Follow-up

The frequency of outpatient visits following kidney transplantation is largely determined by the clinical course of the individual recipient. At the minimum, patients are seen either by a physician or a combination of physician visit and laboratory check, two times per week for the first 2 weeks, then once a week for the next 6 weeks, then every 2 weeks until 6 months after transplantation. This schedule ensures that an elevated creatinine, which serves as a marker for acute allograft rejection or acute renal failure, does not go undetected for an extended period of time. Additionally, frequent patient visits allow for managing other medical issues such as hypertension, hyperlipidemia, hematologic abnormalities, bone disease, and electrolyte and mineral disorders.

Acute Rise in Serum Creatinine

A rise in serum creatinine during this period has a broad differential diagnosis. The evaluation of the patient is directed at quickly eliminating reversible causes such as volume depletion, calcineurin inhibitor nephrotoxicity, and urinary tract obstruction. If none of these conditions is present, a kidney allograft biopsy is indicated to exclude rejection (discussed in the previous section). The clinic evaluation therefore includes a thorough history, with special attention to the possibility of noncompliance, and a thorough physical exam. In addition to routine laboratory tests, cyclosporine or tacrolimus levels are checked to exclude calcineurin inhibitor toxicity. Cyclosporine and tacrolimus occasionally cause rhabdomyolysis, especially when combined with lipid-lowering agents; therefore, it is also important to measure the serum creatine kinase. Finally, an ultrasonogram of the allograft is obtained to determine if urinary tract obstruction or a fluid collection compressing the kidney is present.

Volume Depletion

The transplanted kidney is defective at volume regulation not only because of calcineurin inhibitor effects on the afferent arteriole but also because it is denervated. Transplant recipients are advised to consume at least 2 L of fluids per day. Gastrointestinal disease causing significant fluid loss through diarrhea or inability to take oral liquids due to nausea and vomiting warrants intravenous fluid replacement.

Calcineurin Inhibitor Toxicity

Calcineurin inhibitors cause vasoconstriction of the afferent arteriole of the glomerulus. This induces a prerenal state and can result in a significant rise in serum creatinine. A serum level of calcineurin inhibitor that is clearly in the toxic range or elevated compared with the patient's normal levels can cause an elevation in serum creatinine. Additionally, in a patient with volume depletion, calcineurin inhibitors, even dosed in an appropriate fashion, can bring about a dramatic rise in serum creatinine. Another laboratory feature of calcineurin inhibitor toxicity is hyperkalemia. Fortunately, the rise in both serum creatinine and potassium levels is reversible once appropriate drug levels have been restored.

Rarely, calcineurin inhibitors can cause a renal microangiopathy similar to that observed in the hemolytic uremic syndrome, leading to an acute rise in serum creatinine and thrombocytopenia. This condition does not correlate with high calcineurin inhibitor levels and could occur in patients in whom drug levels are within the therapeutic range. Moreover, it does not appear that the microangiopathy occurs more often with one agent (cyclosporine or tacrolimus) than the other. If this condition is suspected, a kidney allograft biopsy is indicated to make the diagnosis and to exclude acute humoral rejection, which can also cause microangiopathic lesions in the glomeruli. In this situation, microangiopathy on biopsy will classically show thrombosis in the capillary loops of the glomeruli, whereas humoral rejection will show margination of leukocytes in the peritubular capillaries. The accepted management of calcineurin inhibitor–induced microangiopathy is to discontinue the calcineurin inhibitor and initiate plasmapheresis.

Urinary Tract Obstruction and Perinephric Fluid Collections

Obstruction to bladder outflow caused by an enlarged prostate or by bladder dysfunction due to prolonged disuse can lead to a rise in serum creatinine. Because this is readily correctable, it must be diagnosed rapidly. Perinephric fluid collections can result from bleeding, urinary leak (urinoma), or lymphoceles. Urinomas usually result from leakage of urine at the ureterocystic junction, whereas lymphoceles are due to disruption of the lymphatic channels surrounding the iliac vessels and accumulation of lymph in the retroperitoneal space around the allograft. A diagnostic aspiration of the fluid collection is indicated to differentiate between urinoma and lymphoceles, because the two conditions have similar ultrasonographic and radiographic characteristics. A fluid creatinine level comparable to a concurrent serum creatinine indicates the presence of a lymphocele,

whereas a fluid creatinine level significantly greater than serum creatinine indicates a urinoma. Prompt fluid drainage is required, because extrinsic compression of the allograft or its ureter by these collections can cause an acute rise in serum creatinine, and a urine leak leads to reabsorption of urea, creatinine, and other excreted solutes. A urinary leak is also managed with placement of a urinary catheter or ureteral stent, or surgical revision of the ureterocystic anastomosis. Definitive treatment of large lymphoceles involves surgical marsupialization to the peritoneal cavity. Occasionally, compression of the iliac vein leads to venostasis and deep venous thrombosis in the ipsilateral lower extremity.

Rhabdomyolysis

Kidney transplant patients receiving statins are at higher risk for rhabdomyolysis than the nontransplant patient, because higher dosages are required to control hypercholesterolemia and an interaction with calcineurin inhibitors results in higher serum levels of the statin. In comparison with healthy individuals, kidney transplant patients are more susceptible to rhabdomyolysis. The reason for this is not known; however, it could be due to synergistic nephrotoxicity of myoglobinuria and calcineurin inhibitors.

Nonsteroidal Anti-Inflammatory Drugs

Kidney transplant recipients are instructed not to use any over-the-counter pain medication other than acetaminophen unless instructed to do so by the transplant team. Nonsteroidal anti-inflammatory drugs (NSAIDs) cause acute renal failure, since they block prostaglandin production and further enhance afferent arteriolar vasoconstriction caused by calcineurin inhibitors. NSAIDs and trimethoprim-sulfamethoxazole occasionally cause acute interstitial nephritis in the kidney transplant recipient.

Infection

Kidney transplant recipients are predisposed to a variety of infections that afflict the immunocompromised host. The type of infection that arises is generally determined by the intensity of immunosuppression and the time elapsed since transplantation. Infections related to the surgical procedure (wound infection) and hospital-acquired infections (pneumonia, urinary tract infections, and *Clostridium difficile*–associated diarrhea) occur in the immediate post-transplant period. Viral and fungal infections tend to peak between the second and sixth post-transplant months. The most common viral etiologies are the herpes family of viruses, specifically CMV and Epstein-Barr virus. Recurrence of hepatitis B or C or de novo infection with these viruses at the time of transplantation can also manifest within 6 months to 1 year. *Candida* is the most common fungal etiology and usually presents as oral or esophageal candidiasis, whereas aspergillosis and histoplasmosis are less common and often depend on either historical or current exposure. For example, aspergillosis outbreaks have been reported in association with hospital renovation, with diabetics being at higher risk than other patients. Other infections that could occur in the first year after transplantation include PCP, toxoplasmosis, tuberculosis, and crypto-coccal or listerial meningitis. *Pneumocystis* and *Toxoplasma* infections, however, have become exceeding rare because of prophylaxis with trimethoprim-sulfamethoxazole. Although the risk of infection declines after the first year following transplantation, allograft recipients remain at higher risk than the general population, especially if immunosuppression is increased to treat acute rejection.

Management of Hypertension

Most kidney transplant recipients have hypertension. Hypertension in this patient population can be attributed to their underlying endstage renal disease and the effects of calcineurin inhibitors on sodium handling by the nephron (increased sodium avidity) and vasomotor tone (increased tone). Treating hypertension in kidney transplant recipients is essential not only for reducing cardiovascular and cerebrovascular events, which are the leading cause of mortality among these patients, but also for prolonging the survival of the allograft. There is reasonable evidence that controlling systolic blood pressure to 140 mm Hg (or below?) improves long-term allograft survival. In addition, a stepwise increase in allograft loss has been observed for a rise in systolic blood pressure above 140 mm Hg.

The same medication guidelines used for treating essential hypertension in the general population apply to kidney transplant recipients. However, a few caveats apply. Unless used intentionally to decrease the dosage of cyclosporine or tacrolimus needed to obtain a therapeutic serum level, nondihydropyridine calcium channel blockers such as diltiazem and verapamil should be avoided, because they increase levels of calcineurin inhibitors. In contrast, the dihydropyridine class of calcium channel blockers, including amlodipine, felodipine, and isradipine, are both safe and effective. There is a growing body of evidence and clinical experience demonstrating safety and efficacy of either angiotensin-converting enzyme inhibitors or angiotensin II receptor blockers in kidney transplant recipients.

Management of Hyperlipidemia

Hyperlipidemia is a common problem following kidney transplantation. An elevation in low-density lipoprotein (LDL) is the most common abnormality, followed by an elevation in total cholesterol. This is attributed to the use of immunosuppressive agents, mainly TOR inhibitors (sirolimus and everolimus) and corticosteroids. Patients on sirolimus have a disproportionate rise in serum triglyceride levels. In addition, calcineurin inhibitors can contribute to hypercholesterolemia. This medication side effect is superimposed on the predisposition to dyslipidemia already present in this patient population. Since kidney transplant recipients have multiple cardiovascular risk factors, lowering serum cholesterol to the target set by the National Cholesterol Education Program for patients with coronary artery disease or risk equivalents is appropriate (LDL cholesterol less than 100 mg/dL). Statins are recommended. If target cholesterol is not achieved, niacin or bile acid sequestrants such as cole-sevelam hydrochloride can be added. Fibric acid analogues, with the exception of gemfibrozil, should be avoided because of the risk of myositis and rhabdomyolysis. Combination therapy with gemfibrozil and a statin, however, should be used cautiously, since the risk of myositis and rhabdomyolysis is greatly increased for patients taking calcineurin inhibitors.

Hematologic Abnormalities

Leukopenia is a common disorder encountered after kidney transplantation. The differential diagnosis includes medications, both immunosuppressive (MMF, azathioprine, sirolimus, and everolimus) and antiviral (valganciclovir) agents, and viral infections, specifically CMV. Leukopenia usually responds to decreasing the dose of immunosuppressive or antiviral medication. Valganciclovir, if not properly dosed according to the level of kidney function, is a common cause of leukopenia. Absolute neutropenia is treated with granulocyte colony-stimulating factor to avoid the risk of sepsis.

Anemia occurs in the kidney transplant recipient most often as the allograft fails. However, many patients have a hematocrit lower than would be expected for their serum creatinine. Evaluation consists of measurement of iron stores, since iron deficiency could result from surgical blood loss or increased iron utilization due to erythropoietin production by the allograft. If the patient has adequate iron stores, other causes of anemia such as viral infection with parvovirus B19, which causes suppression of red blood cell progenitor cells and results in pure red cell aplasia, and use of angiotensin-converting enzyme inhibitors or angiotensin II receptor blockers should be considered.

Post-transplant erythrocytosis affects 10% to 20% of kidney transplant patients. The etiology is unclear and does not appear to be due to increased erythropoietin production. If the hematocrit exceeds 50%, increased blood viscosity may lead to cerebrovascular accidents, and immediate phlebotomy is required. Fortunately, post-transplant erythrocytosis responds predictably to angiotensin II–converting enzyme inhibitors or angiotensin II receptor blockers. Chronically, these agents can be used to maintain the hematocrit within normal range. Just as the etiology of post-transplant erythrocytosis is unclear, so is the mechanism of response to these medications.

Calcium and Phosphorus Disorders

Most patients presenting for kidney transplantation already have secondary hyperparathyroidism. Elevated parathyroid hormone levels act on the transplanted kidney to cause phosphate wasting and increased calcium reabsorption. Therefore, hypophosphatemia is common following transplantation, and efforts should be made to keep the serum phosphate concentration above 2 mg/dL by increasing the intake of dairy products or dark-colored soda, and phosphorus supplementation if required. Hypercalcemia in patients after kidney transplantation is usually mild, and secondary hyperparathyroidism resolves spontaneously in most patients. However, periodic monitoring of parathyroid hormone is recommended to diagnose the occasional patient who has persistent hypercalcemia due to a parathyroid adenoma.

Gout

Gout occurs in approximately 10% of kidney allograft recipients and may manifest at any time after transplantation. The prevalence of hyperuricemia is even greater because of decreased uric acid clearance by the transplanted kidney, which is thought to be due to the effect of calcineurin inhibitors on proximal tubule secretion of uric acid. Additionally, many patients are on diuretics, and the resultant volume depletion enhances proximal tubule uric acid reabsorption. Although immunosuppression may slightly alter the threshold at which symptoms are perceived, the clinical presentation of gout in the kidney transplant patient is similar to that in the general population. As with the general population, every effort should be made to establish the definitive diagnosis by arthrocentesis. Acute gout attacks are treated by increasing the dose of corticosteroids or with colchicine. Short-term colchicine therapy is effective and safe when adjustment for kidney function is made to avoid bone marrow suppression. Long-term colchicine use in the transplant recipient who is also receiving cyclosporine is associated with increased risk of myopathy. NSAIDs should be avoided because of their nephrotoxicity. Chronic or tophaceous gout is treated with allopurinol given in dosages appropriate for the degree of kidney function. Allopurinol should be avoided in patients who are taking azathioprine, because allopurinol inhibits the metabolism of azathioprine, leading to bone marrow suppression or hepatotoxicity. In contrast, the concomitant use of allopurinol and MMF is safe. Uricosuric agents

in general have no place in the therapy of gout in the kidney transplant population, because the glomerular filtration rate is rarely sufficient to allow significant clearance of uric acid and because of the risk of developing uric acid stones.

LONG-TERM MANAGEMENT

Frequency of Follow-up

Patients are usually seen monthly until the end of the first year following transplantation, after which the frequency decreases to once every 3 months unless the clinical situation dictates more intensive follow-up. Acute allograft rejection is very rare after the first year and occurs primarily in the setting of noncompliance with immunosuppressive medications. The main causes of allograft loss after the first year are death of the patient with a functioning graft, chronic rejection, and recurrence of primary kidney disease. Therefore, long-term management is concerned with the same medical issues addressed during the first 6 months, including the monitoring for chronic allograft dysfunction and recurrent kidney disease, as well as long-term complications of immunosuppression such as bone disease and cancer.

Chronic Allograft Nephropathy

Chronic allograft nephropathy, also known as chronic rejection, is the leading cause of chronic allograft dysfunction and is second only to death of the recipient as the most common cause of kidney allograft loss. Clinically, chronic allograft nephropathy presents as a slow decline in kidney function, often accompanied by proteinuria. The histologic changes are interstitial fibrosis, tubular dropout, glomerulosclerosis, and a vasculopathy characterized by concentric intimal thickening that causes narrowing of arterial lumina. Dispersed mononuclear cell infiltrates are often present in the parenchyma but without evidence of tubulitis or vasculitis typical of acute rejection. Some patients also develop a transplant glomerulopathy, the main feature of which is glomerular capillary wall thickening with a double-contour appearance. Immunologic risk factors for chronic allograft nephropathy are histocompatibility mismatch, acute rejection, and suboptimal immunosuppression. An important differential diagnosis of chronic allograft nephropathy is calcineurin inhibitor toxicity. If the classic finding of calcineurin inhibitor toxicity, striped fibrosis, is present, the patient may benefit from switching to an immunosuppressive regimen that minimizes or eliminates the calcineurin inhibitor. There is no specific treatment for chronic rejection. However, strict blood pressure and lipid control may be beneficial.

BK Virus Nephropathy

BK virus, a member of the polyomavirus family, is an important cause of late allograft loss. Unlike the other polyomavirus that causes disease in humans, JC virus, BK virus pathology is limited to the genitourinary tract. In the kidney transplant recipient BK virus nephropathy and ureteral stenosis are most common, whereas urothelial carcinomas and vasculopathy are reported in individual cases. BK virus nephropathy is caused by both primary infection and reactivation of latent disease. It is rare in the first months after transplantation and increases in frequency up to 1 year after transplantation. The prevalence of BK virus nephropathy is increasing over time, with current studies reporting a prevalence of as much as 10%. The increase in prevalence is attributed to more potent immunosuppressive regimens, increased awareness of this agent, and improved diagnostic tools.

The accurate and timely diagnosis of BK virus nephropathy remains a challenge. A patient with BK virus nephropathy has a rising creatinine that is clinically indistinguishable from rejection. The biopsy findings are patchy interstitial infiltrates consistent with acute rejection, a distinction important to make since treatment for acute rejection worsens the outcome of BK virus nephropathy. If BK virus nephropathy is present, urine cytology is positive for decoy cells, which are tubular epithelial cells that appear malignantly transformed but on close inspection have viral inclusions. Many asymptomatic patients shed virus in the urine, but viremia, as demonstrated with polymerase chain reaction analysis of the blood, is highly sensitive and specific for BK virus nephropathy. Immunohistochemistry of kidney biopsy specimens, using an antibody to simian virus 40 that cross-reacts with BK virus, is still experimental. The mainstay of treatment is the reduction of immunosuppression. Successful treatment depends on early diagnosis. Early reports suggest that leflunomide or perhaps cidofovir may prove to be useful antiviral agents.

Recurrent Kidney Disease

As long-term allograft survival has improved, recurrent kidney disease has become a greater clinical concern and is in fact the third most common cause of allograft loss after the first post-transplant year. It is important to note that the rate of recurrence and the rate of allograft loss due to recurrence are different. For example, diabetic changes develop commonly in allografts transplanted into diabetic patients, but graft loss due to diabetic nephropathy is rare. In contrast, certain glomeru-

TABLE 69-2 Biopsy-Proven Recurrent Glomerulonephritis in Kidney Allograft Recipients

Disease	Histological Recurrence Rate	Allograft Loss Due to Recurrent Disease
Mesangiocapillary glomerulonephritis	10.2	14.4
Focal segmental glomerulosclerosis*	7.2	12.7
Membranous nephropathy	6.2	12.5
IgA nephropathy	2.8	9.7
Pauci-immune crescentic glomerulonephritis	2.0	7.7
Other types of glomerulonephritis	1.0	3.1

*Includes all forms of focal segmental glomerulosclerosis.
Adapted from Briganti EM, Russ GR, McNeil JJ, et al: Risk of renal allograft loss from recurrent glomerulonephritis. N Engl J Med 347:103–109, 2002.

lonephritides such as familial focal segmental glomerulosclerosis recur in 30% to 40% of allografts, and up to 60% of the grafts in which it recurs are lost. The glomerulonephritides that tend to recur in the transplanted kidney, according to biopsy data both before and after transplantation, and cause allograft loss are summarized in Table 69-2.

Cancer

Neoplasia is an important complication of immunosuppression. Kidney transplant recipients are at approximately 100-fold increased risk of developing skin cancer compared with the general population. The majority of these cancers, however, are of the squamous cell variety. Kidney transplant recipients are also at a 3.5-fold increased risk of developing nonskin malignancies compared to age-matched controls. Of these, malignant lymphoma, usually of the non-Hodgkin's type, is the most common (7- to 10-fold increased risk). Epstein-Barr virus–driven B-cell proliferation occurs in approximately 1% of kidney transplant recipients and is referred to as post-transplant proliferative disease (PTLPD). Only 15% of PTLPD patients have monoclonal B-cell proliferation leading to the malignant non-Hodgkin's lymphoma just described. The remainder either has polyclonal benign proliferation or early malignant transformation that usually responds to reduction in immunosuppression.

Non-Hodgkin's lymphoma in transplant recipients differs from that in the general population. It involves extranodal sites more commonly (including the allograft itself), is more aggressive, and responds poorly to therapy.

Other cancers that arise more frequently in transplanted patients include Kaposi's sarcoma (due to human herpesvirus 8), genitourinary malignancies, esophageal cancer, thyroid carcinoma, and hematologic malignancies other than lymphoma. The risk for developing cancer after transplantation does not appear to be due to a specific immunosuppressive agent but rather is proportional to the total dose of immunosuppression given to the patient.

Bone Health

Bone loss is a major health concern for both male and female kidney transplant recipients. This problem is caused by immunosuppression (predominantly corticosteroids) compounded by the fact that endstage renal disease patients arrive at transplantation with established bone disease. Bone disease in transplanted patients can be caused by either high (osteoporosis) or low bone turnover, with the latter being more common than in dialysis patients. Kidney transplant recipients should be screened periodically, starting as early as 3 months after transplantation, with bone mineral density measurements. Patients with low bone mass and evidence for high-turnover disease (as measured by elevated urinary cross-links, deoxypyridinoline and pyridinoline, which are markers of bone matrix degradation) benefit from therapy with antiresorptive agents (bisphosphonates). Unless hypercalcemia is present, it is recommended that all kidney transplant recipients receive oral calcium and adequate amounts of vitamin D through either diet or supplementation.

LONG-TERM OUTCOMES

The results of kidney transplantation continue to improve as more effective and less toxic immunosuppressive regimens are introduced. When censored for death of the patient, deceased-donor kidneys have a projected half-life of approximately 15 years and living-donor kidneys of 20 years or more. Predictors of poor long-term outcomes are rejection events in the first year and elevated serum creatinine (above 1.6 mg/dL) at 1 year. The latter is not only dependent on prior rejection episodes but is also influenced by the status of the donor kidney at the time of transplantation. For example, kidneys from older or hypertensive donors and kidneys that develop delayed graft function tend to fare more poorly. Importantly, HLA-mismatched, living-unrelated kidneys fare better than HLA-matched, deceased-donor kidneys. This further underscores the importance of the status of the kidney at the time of transplantation in determining long-term allograft outcome.

Despite the success of kidney transplantation over the past 20 years, several challenges still lie ahead. These include increasing the availability of suitable organs for transplantation, developing therapies for chronic rejection, and minimizing immunosuppressive side effects to protect recipients from death due to cardiovascular disease and infections.

BIBLIOGRAPHY

Briganti EM, Russ GR, McNeil JJ, et al: Risk of renal allograft loss from recurrent glomerulonephritis. N Engl J Med 347:103–109, 2002.

Clinical Practice Guidelines of the American Society of Transplantation. J Am Soc Nephrol 11(suppl 1):S1–S86, 2000.

Danovitch GM: Handbook of Kidney Transplantation. Philadelphia, Lippincott Williams & Wilkins, 2001.

Gaber AO, First MR, Tesi RJ, et al: Results of the double-blind, randomized, multicenter, phase III clinical trial of Thymoglobulin versus Atgam in the treatment of acute graft rejection episodes after renal transplantation. Transplantation 66:29–37, 1998.

Ginns LC, Cosimi AB, Morris PJ: Transplantation. Los Angeles, Blackwell Science, 1999.

Hariharan S, Johnson CP, Bresnahan BA, et al: Improved graft survival after renal transplantation in the United States, 1988 to 1996. N Engl J Med 342:605–612, 2000.

Kasiske BL, Vazquez MA, Harmon WE, et al: Recommendations for the outpatient surveillance of renal transplant recipients. American Society of Transplantation. J Am Soc Nephrol 11(suppl 15):S1–S86, 2000.

MacDonald AS: A worldwide, phase III, randomized, controlled, safety and efficacy study of a sirolimus/cyclosporine regimen for prevention of acute rejection in recipients of primary mismatched renal allografts. Transplantation 71:271–280, 2001.

Nashan B, Moore R, Amlot P, et al: Randomised trial of basiliximab versus placebo for control of acute cellular rejection in renal allograft recipients. CHIB 201 International Study Group. Lancet 350:1193–1198, 1997.

Pirsch JD, Miller J, Deierhoi MH, et al: A comparison of tacrolimus (FK506) and cyclosporine for immunosuppression after cadaveric renal transplantation. FK506 Kidney Transplant Study Group. Transplantation 63:977–983, 1997.

A randomized clinical trial of cyclosporine in cadaveric renal transplantation. N Engl J Med 309:809–815, 1983.

Solez K, Axelsen RA, Benediktsson H, et al: International standardization of criteria for the histologic diagnosis of renal allograft rejection: The Banff working classification of kidney transplant pathology. Kidney Int 44:411–422, 1993.

Sollinger HW: Mycophenolate mofetil for the prevention of acute rejection in primary cadaveric renal allograft recipients. U.S. Renal Transplant Mycophenolate Mofetil Study Group. Transplantation 60:225–232, 1995.

Wolfe RA, Ashby VB, Milford EL, et al: Comparison of mortality in all patients on dialysis, patients on dialysis awaiting transplantation, and recipients of a first cadaveric transplant. N Engl J Med 341:1725–1730, 1999.

Hypertension

CHAPTER 70

Pathogenesis of Hypertension

Christopher S. Wilcox

Hypertension implies an increase in either cardiac output (CO) or total peripheral resistance (TPR). Essential hypertension developing in young adults is often initiated by an increase in CO, associated with signs of overactivity of the sympathetic nervous system; the blood pressure (BP) is labile and the heart rate is increased. Later, the BP increases further because of a rise in TPR with the restoration of a normal CO. Therefore, most patients encountered in clinical practice with sustained hypertension have an elevated TPR. This is accompanied by vasoconstriction of resistance vessels, but, over time, vascular remodeling contributes a structural component to increased vascular resistance.

Left ventricular systole creates a shock wave that is reflected back from the peripheral resistance vessels. During early diastole, this wave reaches the ascending aorta, where it is visible as the dicrotic notch in tracings of aortic pressure. With aging and loss of elasticity, the pressure wave is transmitted more rapidly to and fro within the arterial tree. Eventually, this shock wave in the aorta coincides with the upstroke of the aortic systolic pressure wave, leading to an abrupt increase in the height of the systolic blood pressure (SBP). This accounts for the frequent finding of isolated, or predominant, systolic hypertension in the elderly. In contrast, systolic hypertension in the young usually reflects an enhanced cardiac contractility and output.

PATHOPHYSIOLOGY OF HYPERTENSION

When a normal person arises, there is an abrupt fall in venous return. An ensuing drop of 30% to 50% in CO elicits a baroreflex response, as resistance vessels contract to buffer the immediate fall in BP and as capacitance vessels contract to restore venous return. The outcome is only a small drop in the SBP, with a modest rise in diastolic blood pressure (DBP) and heart rate. During prolonged standing, increased renal sympathetic nerve activity enhances the reabsorption of sodium chloride (NaCl) and fluid by the renal tubules, as well as the release of renin from the juxtaglomerular apparatus, with the subsequent generation of angiotensin II (Ang II) and aldosterone, which maintain the BP and the volume of the circulation. In contrast, the BP of patients with autonomic insufficiency declines progressively on standing,

often to the point of syncope. These patients illustrate vividly the crucial importance of a stable BP for efficient function of the brain, heart, and kidneys. Thus, it is no surprise that evolution has provided multiple, coordinated BP-regulatory processes. The understanding of the cause for a sustained change in BP, such as hypertension, requires knowledge of a number of interrelated pathophysiologic processes. The most important and well understood of these are discussed in this chapter.

Renal Mechanisms and Salt Balance

The kidney has a unique role in BP regulation. Renal salt and water retention sufficient to increase the extracellular fluid (ECF) and blood volumes enhances venous return, CO, and BP. In fact, the kidney is so effective in excreting excess NaCl and fluid during periods of surfeit, or retaining them during periods of deficit, that the ECF and blood volumes normally vary less than 15% with changes in salt intake. Consequently, the role of body fluids in hypertension is subtle. For example, a 10-fold increase in daily NaCl intake in normal subjects leads to an increase in ECF volume (ECFV) of less than 1 L (about 7%) and normally does not increase BP. Conversely, a diet with no salt content leads to the loss of approximately 1 L of body fluid over 3 to 5 days and only a trivial fall in BP. Quite different effects are seen in patients with chronic kidney disease (CKD), whose BP increases quite predictably with the level of salt intake. This "salt-sensitive" component to BP increases progressively with loss of kidney function in patients with vascular or glomerular kidney diseases. Among normotensive subjects, a salt-sensitive component to BP is apparent in about 30% and appears to be genetically determined. Salt sensitivity is almost twice as frequent in patients with hypertension and is particularly common among African Americans, the elderly, and those who develop CKD. It is generally associated with a lower level of plasma renin activity (PRA).

What underlies salt sensitivity? The normal kidneys are exquisitely sensitive to BP. A rise in mean arterial pressure (MAP) of a little as 1 to 3 mm Hg elicits a subtle increase in renal NaCl and fluid elimination. This "pressure natriuresis" also conserves NaCl and fluid during decreases in BP. It is rapid, quantitative, and fundamental for normal homeostasis. It is due primarily to changes in tubular NaCl reabsorption rather than total renal blood flow or glomerular filtration rate (GFR). Renal hemodynamics are indeed accurately autoregulated in healthy kidneys across a wide range of BPs. Two primary mechanisms of pressure natriuresis have been identified. First, a rise in renal perfusion pressure increases blood flow selectively through the medulla, which is not autoregulated. This increase in pressure and flow enhances renal interstitial hydraulic pressure throughout the kidney and impairs fluid uptake into the bloodstream. Therefore, net NaCl and fluid reabsorption is diminished. Second, the degree of stretch of the afferent arteriole regulates the secretion of renin into the bloodstream, and hence the generation of Ang II. Therefore, an increase in BP that is transmitted to this site reduces renin secretion. Ang II coordinates the body's salt and fluid retention mechanisms by stimulating thirst and enhancing NaCl and fluid reabsorption in the proximal, loop, and distal nephron segments. By stimulating secretion of aldosterone and arginine vasopressin and inhibiting atrial natriuretic peptic (ANP), Ang II further enhances reabsorption in the distal nephron. Thus, during normal homeostasis, an increase in BP is matched by a decrease in PRA. It follows that a normal or elevated value for PRA in hypertension is effectively "inappropriate" for the level of BP and is thereby contributing to the maintenance of hypertension.

The relationships between long-term changes in salt and the renin-angiotensin-aldosterone system (RAAS) and BP are shown diagrammatically in Figure 70-1. Normal human subjects regulate the RAAS closely with changes in salt intake. A challenge in the form of an increase in salt intake brings about only a modest and transient rise in MAP, because the RAAS is suppressed and the highly effective pressure natriuresis mechanism rapidly increases renal NaCl and fluid elimination sufficiently to restore a normal blood volume and BP. Expressed quantitatively in Figure 70-1, the slope of the increase in NaCl excretion with BP is almost vertical. The steepness of this slope, or the gain of the pressure natriuresis, reflects reciprocal changes in the RAAS with BP that dictate appropriate changes in salt handling by the kidney. Thus, when the RAAS is artificially fixed, the slope of the pressure natriuresis relationship flattens, leading to salt sensitivity. The set point is displaced, leading to a change in ambient BP. For example, an infusion of Ang II into a normal subject raises the BP. Since Ang II is being infused, the kidney cannot reduce Ang II levels appropriately by reducing renin secretion. Therefore, the pressure natriuresis mechanism is prevented, and the BP elevation is sustained without an effective and complete renal compensation. In contrast, normal subjects treated with an angiotensin-converting enzyme (ACE) inhibitor to block Ang II generation or an angiotensin receptor blocker (ARB) to block AT$_1$ receptors have a fall in BP. Again, the kidney cannot dictate an appropriate rise or effect in Ang II and aldosterone that would be required to retain sufficient NaCl and fluid to buffer the fall in BP. Thus, when the RAAS is fixed the BP changes as a function of salt intake and becomes highly "salt sensitive" (see Fig. 70-1). These studies demonstrate the unique role of the RAAS in long-term BP regulation and its importance in isolating BP from NaCl intake.

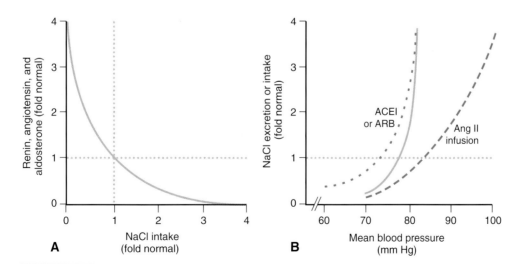

FIGURE 70-1 Diagrammatic representation of the steady-state relationships between (*A*) plasma renin, angiotensin II (Ang II), and aldosterone concentrations and dietary salt intake, and (*B*) between sodium excretion, relative to intake, and mean arterial pressure in normal subjects (*solid line*) and those given an angiotensin-converting enzyme inhibitor (ACEI) or an angiotensin receptor blocker (ARB) (*short dashes*) or an infusion of Ang II (*long dashes*) to prevent adaptive changes in Ang II levels. See text for explanation. (After Guyton AC et al: In Laragh JH, Brenner BM [eds]: Hypertension, Pathophysiology, Diagnosis and Management. New York, Raven, 1995, pp 1311–1326.)

Three compelling lines of evidence implicate the kidney and RAAS in long-term BP regulation. First, transplantation studies between genetically hypertensive and normotensive rat strains show that normotensive animals receiving a kidney from a hypertensive animal become hypertensive, and vice versa. Similarly, human kidney transplant recipients frequently become hypertensive if they receive a kidney from a hypertensive donor. Apparently, the kidney in hypertension is programmed to retain salt and water inappropriately for a normal level of BP, thereby resetting the pressure natriuresis to a higher level of BP and dictating the appearance of hypertension in the recipient even if the neurohumoral environment is that of normotension. A second observation is that an ACE inhibitor, an ARB, or an aldosterone receptor antagonist normally reduces BP by 5% to 20%. The fall in BP is greatest in those with elevated PRA values and is enhanced by dietary salt restriction (see Fig. 70-1). Third, nearly 90% of patients approaching end-stage renal disease (ESRD) have hypertension.

Total-Body Autoregulation

An increase in CO necessarily increases peripheral blood flow. However, each organ has intrinsic mechanisms that adapt blood flow to its metabolic needs. Therefore, over time, an increase in CO is translated into an increase in TPR. Organ blood flow is maintained, but hypertension becomes sustained. This "total-body autoregulation" is demonstrated in human subjects given salt-retaining mineralocorticosteroid hormones. An initial rise in CO is translated in most into sustained hypertension and a raised TPR over 5 to 15 days.

Structural Components to Hypertension

Hypertension causes not only hypertrophic remodeling in the distributing and resistance vessels and the heart, but also fibrotic and sclerotic changes in the kidney glomeruli and interstitium. Hypertrophy of resistance vessels limits the lumen wall diameter and dictates a fixed component to TPR. This is evident as a higher TPR of hypertensive subjects during maximal vasodilatation. Moreover, thickened and hypertrophied resistance vessels have greater reductions in vessel diameter during agonist stimulation, which is apparent as an increase in vascular reactivity to pressor agents. Sclerotic and fibrotic changes in renal glomeruli and interstitium, combined with hypertrophy of the afferent arterioles, limit the sensing of BP in the juxtaglomerular apparatus and interstitium of the kidney. This blunts renin release and pressure natriuresis, thereby contributing to salt sensitivity and sustained hypertension. Rats receiving intermittent weak electrical stimulation of the hypothalamus to raise their BP respond initially with an abrupt increase in BP and an abrupt reduction after the cessation of the stimulus. However, after about 6 weeks, the baseline BP increases in parallel with the appearance of hypertrophy of their resistance vessels. These structural components may explain why it often takes some weeks or months to achieve maximal antihypertensive action from a drug, a reduction in salt intake, or correction of a renal artery stenosis. Vascular and left ventricular hypertrophy is largely, but not completely, reversible during treatment of hypertension, whereas fibrotic and sclerotic changes unfortunately are not.

Sympathetic Nervous System, Brain, and Baroreflexes

A rise in BP elicits a baroreflex-induced reduction in tone of the sympathetic nervous system and an increase in tone of the parasympathetic nervous system. Paradoxically, human hypertension is often associated with an increase in heart rate, maintained or increased plasma catecholamine levels, and an increase in directly measured sympathetic nerve discharge despite the stimulus to the baroreceptors. What is the cause of this inappropriate activation of the sympathetic nervous system in hypertension? First, studies in animals show that the baroreflex "resets" to the ambient level of BP after 2 to 5 days. It no longer continues to "fight" the elevated BP but defends it at the new elevated level. This adaptation occurs within the baroreceptors themselves. Second, animal models of hypertension have identified central mechanisms that alter the gain of the baroreflex process, and therefore the sympathetic tone, in hypertension. The importance of central mechanisms in human hypertension is apparent from the effectiveness of drugs, such as clonidine, that act within the brain to decrease the sympathetic tone. Third, with aging and atherosclerosis, the walls of the carotid sinus and other baroreflex sensing sites become less distensible. Therefore, the BP is less effective in stretching the afferent nerve endings, and the sensitivity of the baroreflex is diminished. This may explain the enhanced sympathetic nerve activity and plasma catecholamines that are characteristic of elderly hypertensive subjects.

Endothelium and Oxidative Stress

Calcium-mobilizing agonists, such as bradykinin or acetylcholine, or shear forces produced by the flow of blood, release endothelium-dependent relaxing factors, predominantly nitric oxide (NO). NO has a half-life of only a few seconds because of inactivation by oxyhemoglobin or reactive oxygen species (ROS) such as oxygen radicals (O_2^{-}). Animal models and humans with essential hypertension have defects in endothelium-dependent relaxing factor responses of peripheral vessels, and diminished NO generation. One underlying mechanism is oxidative stress. Excessive O_2^- formation inactivates NO, leading to a functional NO deficiency. Another mechanism is the appearance of circulating inhibitors of nitric oxide synthase (NOS) that include asymmetric dimethyl arginine (ADMA). Finally, atherosclerosis, prolonged hypertension, or the development of malignant hypertension causes structural changes of the endothelium that limit NO generation further. In the kidney, NO inhibits renal NaCl reabsorption. Therefore, NO deficiency could not only induce vasoconstriction but also diminish renal pressure natriuresis. Functional NO deficiency in large blood vessels also contributes to vascular inflammation and atherosclerosis.

Genetic Contributions

The heritability of human hypertension can be assessed from differences in the concordance of hypertension between identical twins, who share all genes, and a similar environment with nonidentical twins, who share only a similar environment. These studies suggest that genetics contributes less than half to the development of hypertension in modern humans. Studies in mice with targeted disruption of individual genes, or insertions of extra copies of genes, provide direct evidence for critical regulatory roles for certain gene products in hypertension. Deletions of the gene for endothelial NOS or ANP lead to salt-dependent hypertension in mice. The BP of mice with deletion or insertion of the gene encoding ACE increases with the number of copies of the gene. These are compelling examples of circumstances where a single gene can sustain hypertension. However, studies with genetically altered mice can produce results that are not in keeping with expectations, sometimes reflecting novel effects of a gene on development. Moreover, there is increasing recognition of the complexity and importance of gene-gene interaction and the crucial effects expressed by the genetic background on the changes in BP that accompany insertion or deletion of a gene. Presently, compelling evidence for individual gene defects in human essential hypertension is lacking. However, certain rare forms of hereditary hypertension are due to single-gene defects. For example, dexamethasone-suppressible hyperaldosteronism is due to a chimeric rearrangement of the gene encoding aldosterone synthase that renders the enzyme responsive to adrenocorticotropic hormone. Liddle's syndrome is due to a mutation in the gene encoding one component of the endothelial sodium channel that is expressed in the distal convoluted tubule. The mutated form has lost its normal regulation, leading to a permanent "open state" of the sodium channel that dictates inappropriate renal NaCl retention and salt-sensitive, low-renin hypertension (see Chapters 9, 43, and 72).

AGENTS IMPLICATED IN HYPERTENSION

Alterations in the synthesis, secretion, degradation, or action of numerous substances are implicated in certain categories of hypertension. The most important of these are described in the following paragraphs.

Renin, Angiotensin II, and Aldosterone

The PRA is not appropriately suppressed in the majority of patients with essential hypertension and is increased above normal values in approximately 15%. Subjects with normal or high PRAs have a greater antihypertensive response to single-agent therapy with an ACE inhibitor, an ARB, or a beta blocker than patients with low-renin hypertension, who respond especially to salt restriction and diuretic therapy. The RAAS is particularly important in the maintenance of BP in patients with renovascular hypertension, although its importance wanes during the chronic phase when structural alterations in blood vessels or damage in the kidney dictate a RAAS-independent component to the hypertension.

Sympathetic Nervous System and Catecholamines

Pheochromocytoma is a catecholamine-secreting tumor, often in the adrenal medulla, that increases plasma catecholamines 10- to 1000-fold. However, even such extraordinary increases in pressor amines are rarely fatal, because an intact renal pressure natriuresis mechanism reduces the blood volume, thereby limiting the rise in BP. Indeed, such patients can have orthostatic hypotension between episodes of catecholamine secretion (see Chapter 72).

An increased sympathetic nerve tone to resistance vessels in human essential hypertension causes α_1-receptor-mediated vasoconstriction to blood vessels and β_1-receptor-mediated increases in contractility and output of the heart that are only modestly offset by β_2-receptor-mediated vasorelaxation of peripheral blood vessels. Increased sympathetic nerve discharge to the kidney leads to α_1-mediated enhancement of NaCl reabsorption and β_1-mediated renin release.

Dopamine

Dopamine is synthesized in the brain and renal tubular epithelial cells independent of sympathetic nerves. Dopamine synthesis in the kidney is enhanced during volume expansion and contributes to decreased reabsorption of NaCl, especially in the proximal tubule. Defects in tubular dopamine responsiveness are apparent in genetic models of hypertension, but its role in human essential hypertension is unclear. Dopamine, acting on type I dopaminergic receptors, lowers BP and increases renal blood flow and NaCl excretion in normal human subjects.

Arachidonate Metabolites

Arachidonate is esterified as a phospholipid in cell membranes. It is released by phospholipases that are activated by agents such as Ang II. Arachidonate is metabolized principally by three enzymes. Cyclo-oxygenase (COX) generates unstable intermediates whose subsequent metabolism by specific enzymes yields prostaglandins that are either vasodilator (e.g., PGI_2), vasoconstrictor (e.g., thromboxane), or of mixed effect (e.g., prostaglandin E_2, PGE_2). COX-1 is expressed in many tissues, including platelets, resistance vessels, glomeruli, and cortical collecting ducts. COX-2 is induced by inflammatory mediators. However, the normal kidney is unusual in expressing substantial COX-2, which is located in macula densa cells, tubules, renal medullary interstitial cells, and arterioles. The net effect of blocking COX-1 is to cause fluid and NaCl retention, leading to a modest salt-sensitive increase in BP. COX-2 is implicated in renin secretion and renovascular hypertension. Blockade of COX-2 has little effect on normal BP but can increase BP in those with essential hypertension. Nonsteroidal anti-inflammatory agents exacerbate hypertension, blunt the antihypertensive actions of most commonly used agents, predispose to acute renal failure during volume depletion or hypotension, and blunt the natriuretic action of loop diuretics. Metabolism of arachidonate by cytochrome P450 monooxygenase yields 19,20-hydroxyeicosatetraenoic acid (HETE), which is a vasoconstrictor of blood vessels but inhibits tubular NaCl reabsorption. Metabolism by epoxygenase leads to epoxyeicosatrienoic acids (EETs), which are powerful vasodilators. Arachidonate metabolites act primarily as modulating agents in normal physiology; however, their role in human essential hypertension remains elusive.

L-Arginine–Nitric Oxide Pathway

Nitric oxide is generated by three isoforms of NOS that are widely expressed in the body. NO interacts with many iron-centered enzymes. Activation of guanylyl cyclase generates cyclic guanosine monophosphate, which is a powerful vasorelaxant and inhibits NaCl reabsorption in the kidney. Defects in NO generation in the endothelium of blood vessels in human essential hypertension may contribute to increased peripheral resistance, vascular remodeling, and atherosclerosis, whereas defects in renal NO generation may contribute to inappropriate renal NaCl retention and salt sensitivity. Recent studies have shown a profound reduction in conversion of arginine to NO in hypertensive human subjects and those with CKD.

Reactive Oxygen Species

The incomplete reduction of molecular oxygen, either by the respiratory chain during cellular respiration, or by oxidases such as nicotamine adenine dinucleotide phosphate dehydrogenase (NADPH) oxidase or NOS yields ROS including $O_2^{.-}$ and generates peroxynitrite ($ONOO^-$), which has long-lasting effects through oxidizing and nitrosylating reactions. Reaction of ROS with lipids yields oxidized low-density lipoprotein (LDL) that promotes atherosclerosis and isoprostanes that cause vasoconstriction, salt retention, and platelet aggregation. ROS are difficult to quantitate, but indirect evidence suggests that hypertension, and especially CKD, are states of oxidative stress. Drugs that effectively reduce $O_2^{.-}$ reduce BP in animal models of hypertension, but are largely unexamined in human hypertension.

Endothelins

Endothelins are produced especially in cells of the vascular endothelium and tubules. Discrete receptors mediate either increased vascular resistance (type A) or the release of NO (type B). Endothelin type A receptors potentiate the vasoconstriction accompanying Ang II infusion or blockade of NOS. Endothelin is released by hypoxia, specific agonists such as Ang II, salt loading, and cytokines. Nonspecific blockade of endothelin receptors lowers BP in models of volume-expanded hypertension. The role of endothelin in human essential hypertension is unclear.

Atrial Natriuretic Peptide

Atrial natriuretic peptide is released from the heart during atrial stretch. It acts on receptors that increase GFR, decrease NaCl reabsorption in the distal nephron, and inhibit renin secretion. ANP is released during volume expansion and contributes to the natriuretic response. Its role in essential hypertension is unclear. Endopeptidase inhibitors that block ANP degradation are natriuretic and antihypertensive but unfortunately also inhibit the metabolism of kinins. Although an increase in kinins may contribute to the fall in BP with endopeptidase or ACE inhibitors, kinins can cause an irritant cough or a more serious anaphylactoid reaction.

PATHOGENESIS OF HYPERTENSION IN CHRONIC KIDNEY DISEASE

As CKD progresses, the prevalence of salt-sensitive hypertension increases in proportion to the fall in GFR. Hypertension is almost universal in patients with CKD due to primary glomerular or vascular disease, whereas those with primary tubulointerstitial disease are often normotensive or, occasionally, salt losing.

With declining nephron number, CKD limits the ability to adjust NaCl excretion rapidly and quantitatively during changes in intake. The role of ECFV expansion is apparent from the ability of hemodialysis to lower BP, often to normotensive levels, in patients with ESRD.

Additional mechanisms besides primary renal fluid retention contribute to the increased TPR and hypertension in patients with CKD. The RAAS is often inappropriately stimulated. The ESRD kidney generates abnormal renal afferent nerve impulses that entrain an increased sympathetic nerve discharge that is reversed by bilateral nephrectomy. Plasma levels of endothelin increase with kidney failure. CKD induces oxidative stress, which contributes to vascular disease and impaired endothelium-dependent relaxing factor responses. Additionally, a decreased generation of NO from L-arginine relates to the accumulation of ADMA, which inhibits NOS. ADMA is removed by hemodialysis. The thromboxane prostanoid receptor is activated and contributes to vasoconstriction and structural damage.

Clearly, hypertension in CKD is multifactorial, but volume expansion and salt sensitivity are predominant. Pressor mechanisms mediated by Ang II, catecholamines, endothelin, or thromboxane prostanoid receptors become more potent during volume expansion. This may underlie the importance of these systems in the ESRD patients. Finally, many of the pathways that contribute to hypertension in ESRD, such as impaired NO generation and excessive production of endothelin, ROS, and ADMA, also contribute to atherosclerosis, cardiac hypertrophy, and progressive renal fibrosis and sclerosis. Indeed, in poorly treated hypertension, kidney damage leads to additional hypertension, which itself engenders further kidney damage, generating a vicious spiral culminating in accelerated hypertension, progressively diminishing kidney function, and the requirement for renal replacement therapy. Therefore, rational management of hypertension in CKD first entails vigorous salt-depleting therapy with a salt-restricted diet and diuretic therapy. Patients frequently require additional therapy to combat the enhanced vasoconstriction and to attempt to slow the rate of progression.

BIBLIOGRAPHY

Brady HR, Wilcox CS (eds): Therapy in Nephrology and Hypertension, 2nd ed. Philadelphia, WB Saunders, 2003.

Folkow B: The "structural factor" in hypertension with special emphasis on the hypertrophic adaptations of the systemic resistance vessels. In Laragh JH, Brenner BM (eds): Hypertension, Pathophysiology, Diagnosis and Management. New York, Raven, 1990, pp 565–582.

Guyton AC, Hall JE, Coleman TG, Manning RD: The dominant role of the kidneys in the long-term regulation of arterial pressure in normal and hypertensive states. In Laragh JH, Brenner BM (eds): Hypertension, Pathophysiology, Diagnosis and Management. New York, Raven, 1990, pp 1029–1052.

JNC VII: The seventh report of the Joint National Committee on Detection, Evaluation and Treatment of High Blood Pressure. Hypertension 43:1–3, 2004.

Wilcox CS, Schrier RW (eds): Atlas of Diseases of the Kidney: Hypertension and the Kidney. Philadelphia, Current Medicine, 1998.

CHAPTER 71

Evaluation and Management of Hypertension

Arshad Asghar George L. Bakris

Hypertension is the most common disease-specific reason for Americans to visit a physician. High blood pressure (BP), especially systolic elevation, is a powerful risk factor that increases the likelihood of developing a stroke, myocardial infarction (MI), or heart failure, which are the most common causes of death in people with kidney disease. Despite progress in identifying the risks associated with elevated BP and the development of many ways to lower BP and improve long-term survival, BP control remains suboptimal.

The Joint National Committee (JNC) is an advisory panel on prevention, evaluation, and treatment of high BP. The National High Blood Pressure Education Program of the National Heart, Lung, and Blood Institute impanels the JNC. Developed using a consensus process, the JNC 7 report is based on the latest scientific research and reflects the state-of-the-art approach to hypertension. The JNC 7 has redefined the approach to high BP by making the diagnostic criteria simple and easy to relate to risk and treatment. The updated categorization and treatment model is presented in Table 71-1. Whereas normal BP is less than 120/80 mm Hg, a new category called "prehypertension" is introduced and encompasses the BP range between 120 to 139/80 to 89 mm Hg. The reason for this designation is that risk for cardiovascular events is higher in this range than it is in persons with normal blood pressure (Fig. 71-1).

EVALUATION OF THE HYPERTENSIVE PATIENT

Six key issues must be addressed during the initial office evaluation of a person with an elevated BP reading.
1. Documenting an accurate diagnosis of hypertension. This will require two separate readings with the patient's feet on the floor and arm relaxed at the level of the heart.
2. Defining the presence or absence of target organ damage related to hypertension.
3. Screening for other cardiovascular risk factors that often accompany hypertension.
4. Stratifying risk for cardiovascular disease.
5. Assessing whether the person is likely to have an identifiable cause of hypertension (i.e., secondary causes).
6. Integrating clinical and laboratory data that may be helpful in the initial or subsequent choice of therapy.

ROUTINE EVALUATION IN ALL HYPERTENSIVE PATIENTS

The approach in assessing for the presence or absence of target organ damage includes a thorough history, physical examination, and laboratory analysis including blood urea nitrogen (BUN), creatinine, electrolytes, urinalysis, and electrocardiogram (ECG). In individuals with diabetes or kidney disease, spot urine for albumin-to-creatinine ratio should be part of every annual checkup.

The physical examination should be focused on clues to identify secondary causes of hypertension such as an abdominal or flank bruit, which could be a sign of renal arterial disease, or an abdominal or flank mass consistent with polycystic kidney disease. Another important aspect of the physical examination is visualization of the optic fundi. The optic fundus is the only site in the entire body where blood vessels can be examined directly. The impact of controlling hypertension on ophthalmic end points, such as visual loss, retinal hemorrhages, and laser photocoagulation procedures, is clinically relevant, particularly among diabetic hypertensive patients.

Cardiac Evaluation

One of the most important features of the physical examination of hypertensive patients is the cardiac examination. An atrial (S_4) gallop is a very common finding and may suggest hypertensive heart disease, although it is not a very sensitive or specific indicator. The ECG is currently recommended as a part of the initial evaluation of all persons with hypertension. Not only is the ECG useful in documenting previously undetected MI, myocardial ischemia, and/or cardiac rhythm disturbance, it is the least expensive and possibly most cost-effective way to diagnose and/or exclude left ventricular hypertrophy (LVH). Both in the Framingham Heart Study and in dialysis patients, ECG evidence of LVH was associated with more than a threefold increase in the incidence of cardiovascular events. LVH can be associated with intimal hyperplasia of the epicardial coronary arteries, increased

TABLE 71-1 Staging and Recommended Treatment of Hypertension to Prevent Cardiovascular Events

BP Classification	SBP* (mmHg)	DBP* (mmHg)	Life-style Modification	Initial Drug Therapy	
				Without Compelling Indications	With Compelling Indications
Normal	<120	and <80	Encourage		
Prehypertension	120–139	or 80–89	Yes	No antihypertensive drug indicated	Drug(s) for compelling indications[‡]
Stage 1 hypertension	140–159	or 90–99	Yes	Thiazide-type diuretics for most. May consider ACEI, ARB, BB, CCB, or combination	Drug(s) for the compelling indications[‡]
Stage 2 hypertension	≥160	or ≥100	Yes	Two-drug combination for most[†] (usually thiazide-type diuretic and ACEI or ARB or BB or CCB)	Other antihypertensive drugs (diuretics, ACEI, ARB, BB, CCB) as needed

ACEI, angiotensin-converting enzyme inhibitor; ARB, angiotensin receptor blocker; BB, beta blocker; CCB, calcium channel blocker; DBP, diastolic blood pressure; SBP, systolic blood pressure.
*Treatment determined by highest BP category.
[†]Initial combined therapy should be used cautiously in those at risk for orthostatic hypotension.
[‡]Treat patients with chronic kidney disease or diabetes to BP goal of <130/80 mmHg.
Reprinted with permission from Chobanian AV, Bakris GL, Black HR, et al: Seventh Report of the Joint National Committee on Prevention, Detection, Evaluation, and Treatment of High Blood Pressure. Hypertension 42:1206–1252, 2003.

coronary vascular resistance, and reduced diastolic relaxation, in some cases resulting in symptoms of heart failure with preserved systolic function.

Kidney Evaluation

Current recommendations for the evaluation of kidney function in the general population include measurement of serum BUN and creatinine as well as a dipstick for proteinuria. Figure 59-3 shows the recommendations for evaluation of albuminuria in individuals with suspected

kidney disease made by a recent National Institutes of Health (NIH) and National Kidney Foundation (NKF) consensus panel. In patients with diabetes or kidney disease at any stage, a spot urine albumin-to-creatinine ratio is recommended by the NKF, JNC 7, and the American Diabetes Association. Microalbuminuria (MA), which is defined as a urine albumin concentration between 30 and 300 mg/g creatinine, is a powerful and independent risk factor for cardiovascular events in those patients with and without diabetes.

The prevalence of MA in type 2 diabetics is 20%, with a range of 12% to 36%, and it is more common (about

FIGURE 71-1 Impact of high-normal blood pressure (BP) on cardiovascular disease risk. Optimal BP: <120/80 mmHg; normal BP: 120–129/80–84 mm Hg; high-normal BP: 130–139/ 85–89 mmHg. Please note that the JNC 6 definitions were used in this analysis. JNC 7 definitions would define the optimal group as normal and the other two groups as prehypertensive. (Reprinted with permission from Vasan RS, Larson MG, Leip EP, et al: Impact of high-normal blood pressure on the risk of cardiovascular disease. N Engl J Med 345:1291–1297, 2001.)

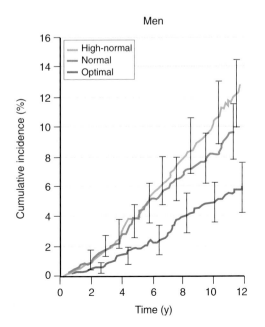

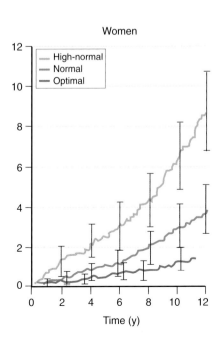

30%) in those older than 55 years. The prevalence of MA ranges from 5% to 40% in nondiabetic hypertensives.

In addition to measurement of albuminuria, an estimated glomerular filtration rate (GFR) should be used to define kidney function. The GFR can be calculated using the methods described in Chapters 3 and 59.

Evaluation of Identifiable Causes of Hypertension

There are many identifiable causes of hypertension (secondary hypertension; Table 71-2). In patients with some of these causes, the elevation of BP can be ameliorated or eliminated with specific treatment such as angioplasty, surgery, or avoidance of the ingested agent that caused the hypertension. Other etiologies, such as specific enzyme deficiencies, coarctation of the aorta, and Ask-Upmark kidney, are distinctly rare. Secondary causes of hypertension are discussed in detail in Chapter 72.

TREATMENT OF HYPERTENSION

Once the diagnosis of hypertension has been recognized and established in a patient, it can be best managed through an integrated approach, starting with life-style modifications and choosing a treatment regimen depending on the stage of hypertension and comorbid conditions such as chronic kidney disease (CKD) and

TABLE 71-2   Identifiable Causes of Hypertension

Obesity
Chronic kidney disease
Coarctation of the aorta
Cushing's syndrome and other glucocorticoid excess states including chronic steroid therapy
Drug-induced or drug-related
  Nonsteroidal anti-inflammatory drugs; cyclooxygenase-2 inhibitors
  Cocaine, amphetamines, other illicit drugs
  Sympathomimetics (decongestants, anorectics)
  Oral contraceptive hormones
  Adrenal steroid hormones
  Cyclosporine and tacrolimus
  Erythropoietin
  Licorice (including some chewing tobacco)
  Selected over-the-counter dietary supplements and medicines (e.g., ephedra, ma haung, bitter orange)
Obstructive uropathy
Pheochromocytoma
Primary aldosteronism and other mineralocorticoid excess states
Renovascular hypertension
Sleep apnea
Thyroid or parathyroid disease

Adapted from Chobanian AV, Bakris GL, Black HR, et al: Seventh Report of the Joint National Committee on Prevention, Detection, Evaluation, and Treatment of High Blood Pressure. Hypertension 42:1206–1252, 2003.

cardiovascular disease. Age and ethnic background also play an important role in the selection of hypertensive drugs. The JNC 7 provides guidelines for initiation of hypertensive agents that are primarily based on outcome trials, the largest of which, to date, is the "Antihypertensive and Lipid-Lowering Treatment to Prevent Heart Attack Trial" (ALLHAT).

The ALLHAT was a randomized prospective study of a little more than 43,000 patients with hypertension and one additional risk factor for coronary heart disease such as LVH or type 2 diabetes. This trial was designed to evaluate whether the incidence of adverse coronary and cardiovascular outcomes differed among those randomly assigned to chlorthalidone (a thiazide-like diuretic) compared to one of three other antihypertensive drugs: amlodipine (a dihydropyridine calcium channel blocker), lisinopril (an angiotensin-converting enzyme [ACE] inhibitor), or doxazosin (an α-adrenergic blocker). The primary outcomes were fatal coronary heart disease and nonfatal MI, whereas the secondary outcomes were all-cause mortality, stroke, and combined cardiovascular disease events. Because diuretics were the reference group against which the other agents were compared, and because it was a "superiority" rather than an "equivalence" trial, the principal findings indicated that diuretics were superior to the other classes tested, since the other classes did not have fewer coronary heart disease deaths or nonfatal MIs. It must be kept in mind that these results apply to people with demographic characteristics similar to the individuals enrolled in the trial (i.e., age over 55 years with high cardiovascular risk).

Life-Style Modification

The JNC 7 report builds on a recent advisory from the National High Blood Pressure Education Program to recommend weight loss for obese hypertensive patients, modification of dietary sodium intake to 100 mmol/day or less, and modification of alcohol intake to no more than two drinks per day. All recommendations for life-style modifications include smoking cessation. Because tobacco avoidance protects cardiovascular health and because smoking induces a rise in BP, the recommendation not to smoke is clearly appropriate. In general, patients should be encouraged to lose weight; restrict sodium intake; eat generous amounts of potassium, magnesium, calcium, and fish; exercise regularly; moderate their alcohol consumption; stop smoking; and reduce stress.

For those with stage 1 hypertension and no compelling indications for antihypertensive medicines, life-style modification should be tried for 6 months before pharmacologic treatment for hypertension is initiated. For those with stage 2 hypertension, pharmacologic treatment should be initiated along with life-style modification (see Table 71-1).

Pharmacologic Therapy

Antihypertensive medications should be initiated if on two separate occasions at least 2 months apart the systolic pressure is persistently 140 mm Hg or higher and/or the diastolic pressure is 90 mm Hg or higher in the office despite attempted life-style modification. Table 71-3 lists all the approved antihypertensive drugs available in the United States.

Initial Drug Therapy

The JNC 7 recommends that a thiazide diuretic be the initial choice for most patients. The word "most" refers to the category of patients in whom diuretics have reduced cardiovascular events in trials (i.e., generally individuals aged 55 and older). Thus, diuretics are not recommended for initial therapy for everyone. Moreover, if compelling indications are present (i.e., diabetes or kidney disease), all guidelines (JNC 7, American Diabetes Association, and NKF) recommend that an ACE inhibitor or an angiotensin receptor blocker (ARB) be used as initial therapy, with a diuretic as an "add-on" drug if needed to achieve the BP goal. If the BP goal is not achieved within 2 to 3 months with monotherapy, appropriately up-titrated to doses used in trials, then a second agent should be added.

Sequence of Additional Drugs

It is obvious from many trials, including ALLHAT, that only about 25% of people with hypertension will achieve target BP with monotherapy. Moreover, in individuals with stage 2 hypertension, initiation of combination therapy is recommended, since virtually all such patients will require two or more drugs to get to their BP goal. In these circumstances, if a thiazide diuretic was the initial agent, then an ACE inhibitor, ARB, beta blocker, or calcium channel blocker can be used as the second agent to attain the BP goal, depending on the concomitant conditions.

Achievement of Blood Pressure Goal

The BP goal should be achieved within 6 to 9 months of initiating therapy. This is important, because in all clinical trials, events start to separate the groups at 6 months, and almost always this separation is due to differences in BP.

One of the perceived limitations to achieving the goal of under 130/80 mm Hg in individuals with kidney disease or diabetes is the fear that lowering BP excessively might be harmful. Clinical trial evidence does not substantiate this perception. Specifically, the Systolic Hypertension in the Elderly Patients (SHEP) trial demonstrated that lowering the diastolic BP to as low as 67 mm Hg is well tolerated and prevents MI and strokes better than in patients with an average of 71 mm Hg. This was also noted in the Systolic Hypertension in Europe (Syst-Eur)

trial. Thus, a low diastolic pressure should not be a deterrent from achieving a low systolic pressure in older people, since in everyone over the age of 50 years, systolic pressure is a much stronger predictor of cardiovascular events than is diastolic pressure.

Factors to Consider in Building an Antihypertensive Drug Regimen

Several issues should always be considered when antihypertensive drug therapy is chosen.

Comorbidities and Other Risk Factors

JNC 7 recognizes two other possible influences that may alter the choice of initial treatment in an individual hypertensive patient: (1) comorbid conditions such as osteoporosis where thiazide diuretics are useful, and angina pectoris where beta blockers and now verapamil are useful; (2) compelling conditions, defined as the presence of other medical conditions that are commonly associated with hypertension.

Specific Risk Factors

Dyslipidemia

With the exception of beta blockers and diuretics, all other classes of antihypertensive agents are considered lipid neutral. It should be noted that these agents have been repeatedly shown to reduce adverse cardiovascular outcomes, and thus the potential to raise lipid levels does not translate into a major clinical issue, at least over 5 years duration, as noted in trials. Moreover, cholesterol-lowering agents are used in many patients who require these antihypertensive agents and thus do not result in a management problem.

New-Onset Diabetes Mellitus

Some antihypertensive drugs may affect glucose metabolism and worsen or improve insulin sensitivity. Peripheral alpha blockers, ACE inhibitors, and ARBs generally improve insulin sensitivity. Calcium antagonists are neutral on insulin sensitivity but improve it more effectively than does either diuretics or beta blockers, a factor that translates into changes in cardiovascular morbidity. Both moderate- to high-dose thiazide and beta blockers worsen insulin sensitivity and can precipitate glucose intolerance and frank diabetes.

Left Ventricular Hypertrophy

Left ventricular hypertrophy is a robust independent risk factor for cardiovascular and premature mortality, probably because it reflects the degree of BP control over the long term. LVH is especially common in the elderly, particularly women, and often is associated with diastolic dysfunction. Virtually all patients studied with endstage

TABLE 71-3   Oral Antihypertensive Drugs*

Class	Drug (Trade Name)	Usual Dose Range (mg/day)	Usual Daily Frequency*
Thiazide diuretics			
	Chlorothiazide (Diuril)	125–500	1–2
	Chlorthalidone (generic)	12.5–25	1
	Hydrochlorothiazide (Microzide, HydroDIURIL†)	12.5–50	1
	Polythiazide (Renese)	2–4	1
	Indapamide (Lozol†)	1.25–2.5	1
	Metolazone (Mykrox)	0.5–1.0	1
	Metolazone (Zaroxolyn)	2.5–5	1
Loop diuretics			
	Bumetanide (Bumex†)	0.5–2	2
	Furosemide (Lasix†)	20–80	2
	Torsemide (Demadex†)	2.5–10	1
Potassium-sparing diuretics			
	Amiloride (Midamor†)	5–10	1–2
	Triamterene (Dyrenium)	50–100	1–2
Aldosterone receptor blockers			
	Eplerenone (Inspra)	50–100	1
	Spironolactone (Aldactone†)	25–50	1
Beta blockers			
	Atenolol (Tenormin†)	25–100	1
	Betaxolol (Kerlone†)	5–20	1
	Bisoprolol (Zebeta†)	2.5–10	1
	Metoprolol (Lopressor†)	50–100	1–2
	Metoprolol extended release (Toprol XL)	50–100	1
	Nadolol (Corgard†)	40–120	1
	Propranolol (Inderal†)	40–160	2
	Propranolol long-acting (Inderal LA†)	60–180	1
	Timolol maleate (Blocadren†)	20–40	2
Beta blockers with intrinsic sympathomimetic activity			
	Acebutolol (Sectral†)	200–800	2
	Penbutolol (Levatol)	10–40	1
	Pindolol (generic)	10–40	2
Combined alpha and beta blockers			
	Carvedilol (Coreg)	12.5–50	2
	Labetalol (Normodyne, Trandate†)	200–800	2
Angiotensin-converting enzyme inhibitors			
	Benazepril (Lotensin†)	10–40	1
	Captopril (Capoten†)	25–100	2
	Enalapril (Vasotec†)	5–40	1–2
	Fosinopril (Monopril)	10–40	1
	Lisinopril (Prinivil, Zestril†)	10–40	1
	Moexipril (Univasc)	7.5–30	1
	Perindopril (Aceon)	4–8	1
	Quinapril (Accupril)	10–80	1
	Ramipril (Altace)	2.5–20	1
	Trandolapril (Mavik)	1–4	1
Angiotensin II antagonists			
	Candesartan (Atacand)	8–32	1
	Eprosartan (Teveten)	400–800	1–2
	Irbesartan (Avapro)	150–300	1
	Losartan (Cozaar)	25–100	1–2
	Olmesartan (Benicar)	20–40	1
	Telmisartan (Micardis)	20–80	1
	Valsartan (Diovan)	80–320	1–2
Calcium channel blockers— non-Dihydropyridines			
	Diltiazem extended release (Cardizem CD, Dilacor XR, Tiazac†)	180–420	1
	Diltiazem extended release (Cardizem LA)	120–540	1
	Verapamil immediate release (Calan, Isoptin†)	80–320	2
	Verapamil long-acting (Calan SR, Isoptin SR†)	120–480	1–2
	Verapamil (Coer, Covera HS, Verelan PM)	120–360	1

TABLE 71-3 Oral Antihypertensive Drugs*—*Continued*

Class	Drug (Trade Name)	Usual Dose Range (mg/day)	Usual Daily Frequency*
Calcium channel blockers—Dihydropyridines			
	Amlodipine (Norvasc)	2.5–10	1
	Felodipine (Plendil)	2.5–20	1
	Isradipine (Dynacirc CR)	2.5–10	2
	Nicardipine sustained release (Cardene SR)	60–120	2
	Nifedipine long-acting (Adalat CC, Procardia XL)	30–60	1
	Nisoldipine (Sular)	10–40	1
Alpha-1 blockers			
	Doxazosin (Cardura)	1–16	1
	Prazosin (Minipress[†])	2–20	2–3
	Terazosin (Hytrin)	1–20	1–2
Central alpha-2 agonists and other centrally acting drugs			
	Clonidine (Catapres[†])	0.1–0.8	2
	Clonidine patch (Catapres-TTS)	0.1–0.3	1 wkly
	Methyldopa (Aldomet[†])	250–1000	2
	Reserpine (generic)	0.1–0.25	1
	Guanfacine (Tenex[†])	0.5–2	1
Direct vasodilators			
	Hydralazine (Apresoline[†])	25–100	2
	Minoxidil (Loniten[†])	2.5–80	1–2

*In some patients treated once daily, the antihypertensive effect may diminish toward the end of the dosing interval (trough effect). BP should be measured just before dosing to determine if satisfactory BP control is obtained. Accordingly, an increase in dosage or frequency may need to be considered. These dosages may vary from those recommended in the package inserts.
[†]Available now or soon to become available in generic preparations.
Chobanian AV, Bakris GL, Black HR, et al: Seventh Report of the Joint National Committee on Prevention, Detection, Evaluation, and Treatment of High Blood Pressure. Hypertension 42:1206–1252, 2003.

renal disease (ESRD) have LVH, as do many patients with stage 3 or higher CKD. All antihypertensive agents except direct vasodilators reduce LV mass.

Heart Failure

Hypertension is a major risk factor for the subsequent development of heart failure, typically many years later. For many hypertensives, LVH is an important intermediate step, resulting in hypertensive heart disease with impaired LV filling and increased ventricular stiffness. This is commonly referred to as heart failure with preserved systolic function. The more common type of systolic dysfunction associated with a reduced LV ejection fraction is most often due to previous myocardial ischemia. Distinguishing between the two subtypes of heart failure is most easily done by estimating the LV ejection fraction; moreover, the results dictate therapy. Patients with a low ejection fraction (systolic heart failure) improve both their BP and long-term prognosis with ACE inhibitors and diuretics, to which can be added beta blockers, aldosterone receptor antagonists, and/or other drugs as needed. Treatment of hypertension in patients with preserved systolic function and heart failure has not been well studied, but most authorities recommend using drugs that reduce heart rate, increase diastolic filling time, and allow the heart muscle to relax more fully: beta blockers or nondihydropyridine calcium

channel blockers. Although these suggestions make physiologic sense, there are no clinical trial data to support them.

Microalbuminuria and Proteinuria

The normal rate of albumin excretion is less than 20 mg/day. Persistent values between 30 and 299 mg/day define the range for microalbuminuria. A number of studies in different patient populations support the concept that microalbuminuria is an important risk factor for cardiovascular disease and associated early cardiovascular mortality in patients with and without diabetes, irrespective of the presence of hypertension. The risk of an adverse cardiovascular event grows progressively as absolute levels of microalbuminuria increase. Unfortunately, there is no conclusive evidence from outcome trials to establish that reducing microalbuminuria results in less cardiovascular risk. Both ACE inhibitors and ARBs have the most consistent data showing reduction in microalbuminuria and delaying its progression to macroalbuminuria (proteinuria). These agents reduce albuminuria by reducing intraglomerular pressure and altering membrane permeability at the level of the podocyte.

Conversely, retrospective analyses of clinical trials in advanced CKD demonstrate that reducing proteinuria by 30% to 35% below baseline is associated with marked slowing in progression to ESRD. In two specific trials, the African-American Study of Kidney Disease, a nondiabetic cohort, and the Irbesartan Diabetic Nephropathy Trial, the randomized groups in whom proteinuria was not reduced did not experience the same magnitude of slowing of progression of CKD as those groups in whom proteinuria declined, despite similar BP control. Figure 71-2 integrates the recommendations of the JNC7, the American Diabetes Association, and the NKF to provide an approach to achieving the BP goal and reducing the risk of kidney disease progression. It is also relevant to note that achievement of the goal BP is particularly important, especially in people with greater than 1 g/day of proteinuria (Fig. 71-3).

Coronary Artery Disease

Because hypertension is a major risk factor for coronary artery disease (CAD), it is not surprising that a large number of patients have both conditions. The presence of CAD in a patient with hypertension should influence both the choice of drugs used to treat the patients and the BP goal to be achieved. Both beta blockers and nondihydropyridine calcium channel blockers (e.g., verapamil) are effective antihypertensive agents with major antianginal efficacy. In the ALLHAT trial, amlodipine was equal in its protection against heart attack to chlorthalidone and lisinopril.

After Stroke

In the immediate setting of acute stroke (within 72 hours), most neurologists avoid antihypertensive drugs unless BP is very high (e.g., BP higher than 185/110 mm Hg). If treatment is necessary at this time, an intravenously administered, short-acting drug is preferred, because it can be discontinued quickly if the patient's neurologic condition deteriorates acutely. After this period, the use of a combination of an ACE inhibitor with a thiazide diuretic reduces recurrent events.

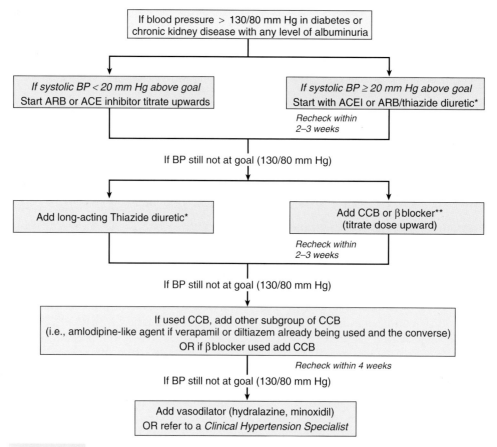

FIGURE 71-2 Integrated approach to achieving blood pressure goal in patients with kidney disease or diabetes. *Doses of 12.5 or 25 mg/day should be used. Doses of 50 mg/day and higher have not demonstrated cardiovascular risk reduction. Thiazides are not useful in individuals with serum creatinine values above 2 mg/dL. Loop diuretics should be substituted. **Beta blockers should be preferred if coronary disease is present or the patient has recently suffered a myocardial infarction. Once-daily beta blockers are preferred. Note that verapamil can be substituted for a beta blocker in those with coronary disease, since it is as efficacious as the beta blockers for reducing mortality in large outcome trials. ACEI, angiotensin-converting enzyme inhibitor; ARB, angiotensin receptor blocker; BB, beta blocker; CCB, calcium channel blocker.

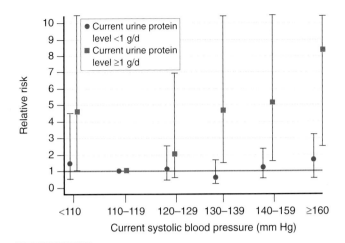

FIGURE 71-3 The relationship between relative risk of kidney disease progression, blood pressure, and level of proteinuria. The reference group for each level of proteinuria is the systolic blood pressure interval 110 to 119 mm Hg. Note that with proteinuria of less than 1 g/day, blood pressure recommendations of lower than 130 mm Hg for those with nondiabetic kidney disease is appropriate. If proteinuria is greater than 1 g/day, then systolic blood pressure should be lower than 120 mm Hg if possible for this subgroup. Please refer to the National Kidney Foundation K/DOQI Clinical Practice Guidelines (see Bibliography). (Reprinted with permission from Jafar TH, Stark PC, Schmid CH, et al: Progression of chronic kidney disease: The role of blood pressure control, proteinuria, and angiotensin-converting enzyme inhibition: A patient-level meta-analysis. Ann Intern Med 139:244–252, 2003.)

Safety: Adverse Reactions and Side Effects

The two primary types of adverse reactions and the side effects that occur with antihypertensive drugs are clinical and biochemical. The clinical side effects are more evident to the patients and are perceived by the patients or the clinician to be related to the drug. The appearance of these adverse reactions requires that the drug be stopped, the dose reduced, or the patient be willing to remain on therapy until he or she becomes able to tolerate the side effect or until it disappears. Weight gain, erectile dysfunction, depression, bronchospasm, and bradycardia are common with beta blockers. Calcium channel blockers may cause constipation, headache, dizziness, or lightheadedness, flushing, and peripheral edema. ACE inhibitors are commonly associated with cough and angioedema. ACE inhibitor cough may develop in about 15% to 20% of patients. Cough is class specific and usually occurs within 1 to 2 weeks of the initiation of the treatment, but its onset may occur after as long as 6 months. It is also more common in women and resolves within a week of discontinuing the offending agent. When cough is the main presenting symptom, switching to an ARB commonly alleviates the problem. When patients develop angioedema on an ACE inhibitor, however, changing to an ARB is advised with great caution. The mechanism for the associated cough and

angioedema with ACE inhibitors is not known, although it may be related to inhibition of bradykinin degradation.

The biochemical side effects consist of alterations in electrolyte balance and lipid profiles, which may or may not be perceived by the patient or the provider. These abnormalities are usually detected by laboratory analysis or other diagnostic tests such as ECG. The widespread use of thiazide diuretics is not free of risk; although lower doses in the range of 12.5 to 25 mg/day may be associated with fewer side effects, individual variation in clinical practice is not uncommon. A higher dose of thiazide diuretics (more than 25 mg/day) can lead to hyperuricemia and may result in gouty arthritis. The other electrolyte abnormalities seen with thiazide diuretics are hypokalemia, hyponatremia, hypercalcemia, and hypomagnesemia. Long-term use of thiazide diuretics also predisposes to hyperglycemia and diabetes. In two very large trials, about 11% of people taking thiazide diuretics who had body mass indexes higher than 30 and were over age 55 developed new-onset diabetes. This was significantly higher than those taking ACE inhibitors or calcium channel blockers. Lipid abnormalities are also seen with certain antihypertensive agents. High doses of thiazide diuretics (more than 25 mg/day) produces an elevation of total and low-density lipoprotein cholesterol. Beta blockers have little effect on cholesterol level, but their use leads to increases in triglycerides and an associated drop in cardioprotective high-density lipoprotein cholesterol. Carvedilol, a relatively new beta blocker, is a combined nonselective beta and alpha-1 blocker that prevents lipid peroxidation and is not associated with lipid abnormalities. Hyperkalemia is also a common abnormality in patients treated with agents such as spironolactone, ACE inhibitors, and ARBs. The overall incidence of hyperkalemia (defined as a plasma potassium concentration above 5.5 mEq/L) is approximately 5% with ACE inhibitors. More prominent hyperkalemia may be seen in patients with impaired kidney function. Among those with stage 3 or higher CKD (GFR 30 mL/minute or less), limited evidence suggests that increases in serum potassium may be less pronounced with an ARB than with an ACE inhibitor.

Special Circumstances

Hypertension is present in about 10% of pregnancies and is a major cause of perinatal morbidity and mortality in most developing countries (see Chapter 56).

Hypertensive Emergencies and Urgencies

Hypertensive emergency is defined as a spectrum of clinical manifestations associated with an acute and life-threatening elevation of BP (systolic higher than 180 mm Hg), which untreated may result in target organ damage. There are two major clinical syndromes induced by severe hypertension. Malignant hypertension is manifested by marked hypertension with retinal hemorrhage, exudates, or papilledema. Hypertensive encephalopathy refers to the presence of signs of cerebral edema resulting from a sudden rise in BP. Patients with hypertensive emergencies should be diagnosed quickly and started promptly on effective parenteral therapy in an intensive care unit. BP should be reduced gradually and by about 25% over 2 to 3 hours. Oral antihypertensive therapy should be instituted after 6 to 12 hours of parenteral therapy; evaluation of secondary causes of hypertension may be considered after transfer from the intensive care unit. A general approach to the treatment of patients with hypertensive emergencies is summarized in Table 71-4.

Many physicians still prefer nitroprusside or another intravenous vasodilator to lower blood pressure quickly, because it can be discontinued quickly if BP goes too low. Patients who present with hypertensive emergency involving cardiac ischemia/infarction or pulmonary edema can be managed with either nitroglycerin or nitroprusside. Efforts to preserve the myocardium and the opening of the obstructed coronary artery by thrombolysis, angioplasty, or surgery are also indicated. Patients with aortic dissection are managed somewhat differently. Once the diagnosis has been confirmed, reduction of the systolic BP to 100 to 120 mm Hg, or the lowest level that is tolerated, is indicated. Moreover, initial treatment consists of an intravenous beta blocker to reduce heart rate below 60 beats/minute. Beta blockers are the agents of choice, since they both reduce pressure and lower heart rate, resulting in reduced shear stress in the aorta and a lower risk of further dissection. Nitroprusside can be used after adequate beta blockade has been achieved, provided kidney function is preserved. Nitroprusside should not be used without beta blockers, since vasodilatation induces reflex activation of the sympathetic nervous system, leading to enhanced ventricular contraction and increased aortic shear stress. Hydralazine should not be used in this setting, because it tends to cause reflex tachycardia and the BP-lowering effect of hydralazine is not always predictable.

Hypertensive emergency may also result in malignant nephrosclerosis, which leads to acute renal failure, hematuria, and proteinuria. Within the kidney, fibrinoid necrosis in arterioles and capillaries is observed. The renal vascular disease in this circumstance results in glomerular ischemia and activation of the renin-angiotensin system, which leads to further deterioration of BP. Lowering BP is the most important aspect of the management of this condition and should be the main objective, even in the presence of worsening kidney function. Some physicians prefer the dopamine-1 selective agent, fenoldopam, to nicardipine or nitroprusside in this setting because of its lack of toxic metabolites and specific renal vasodilating effects. Depending on the height of the initial systolic pressure, the goal is to get the systolic BP to around 140 mm Hg within 2 to 3 hours, because that will reduce

TABLE 71-4 Types of Hypertensive Crises, with Suggested Drug Therapy and BP Targets

Type of Crisis	Drug of Choice	Blood Pressure Target
Neurologic		
Hypertensive encephalopathy	Nitroprusside*	25% reduction in MAP over 2 to 3 hr
Intracranial hemorrhage or acute stroke in evolution	Nitroprusside* (controversial)	0% to 25% reduction in MAP over 6 to 12 hr (controversial)
Acute head injury/trauma	Nitroprusside*	0% to 25% reduction in MAP over 2 to 3 hr (controversial)
Subarachnoid hemorrhage	Nimodipine	Up to 25% reduction in MAP in previously hypertensive patients
Cardiac		
Ischemia/infarction	Nitroglycerin or nicardipine	Reduction in ischemia
Heart failure	Nitroprusside* or nitroglycerin	Improvement in failure (typically 10% to 15% decrease in BP)
Aortic dissection	Beta blocker + nitroprusside*	120 mm Hg systolic in 30 min (if possible)
Renal		
Hematuria or acute renal failure	Fenoldopam	0% to 25% reduction in MAP over 1 to 12 hr
Catecholamine excess states		
Pheochromocytoma	Phentolamine	To control paroxysms
Abrupt drug withdrawal	Withdrawn drug	Typically only one dose necessary
Pregnancy-related		
Eclampsia	Methyldopa, hydralazine, MgSO$_4$	Typically <90 mm Hg diastolic, but often lower

BP, blood pressure; MAP, mean arterial pressure.
*Some physicians prefer an intravenous infusion of either fenoldopam or nicardipine, neither of which has potentially toxic metabolites, over nitroprusside. Recent studies have also shown improvements in kidney function during therapy with the former, as compared to nitroprusside.
Adapted from Elliott WJ: Hypertensive emergencies. Crit Care Clin 17:435–451, 2001.

the risk of stroke. Once at this level, additional lowering should be pursued with agents that block the renin-angiotensin system.

Hypertensive emergencies resulting from catecholamine-excess states (e.g., pheochromocytoma, monoamine oxidase inhibitor crises, cocaine intoxication) are best managed with long-acting alpha blockade, such as phenoxybenzamine. In patients with pheochromocytoma, acute bouts of hypertension may occur before or during surgical intervention, and under these circumstances should be treated with phentolamine, administered intravenously. Phentolamine is a short-acting, nonselective, α-adrenergic blocker. Effective α-adrenergic blockade permits expansion of blood volume, which is usually severely decreased because of excessive adrenergic vasoconstriction. A β-adrenergic blocker may then be added to overcome tachycardia, but it should never begin the regimen because blockade of vasodilatory peripheral β-adrenergic receptors with unopposed β-adrenergic receptor stimulation can lead to an additional elevation in BP.

Hypertensive urgency is defined the as presence of severe hypertension (systolic higher than 180 mm Hg) in an asymptomatic patient. Hypertensive urgencies are situations in which acute target organ damage is not present; they require somewhat less aggressive management and nearly always can be handled with oral antihypertensive agents without admission to the hospital. Clonidine, captopril, labetolol, and several other short-acting antihypertensive drugs have been used for this problem. Short-acting nifedipine has been reported to cause precipitous hypotension, stroke, MI, and death. Thus, sublingual nifedipine is contraindicated in such patients, because it has been associated with a high mortality in this situation.

Drug Interactions

The most commonly used antihypertensive agents do not have any serious interactions with anticoagulants, platelet inhibitors, or antibiotics. Nondihydropyridine calcium channel blockers, beta blockers, and telmisartan (an ARB) must be used with care if prescribed with digoxin. The nodal blocking effect of the nondihydropyridine calcium channel blockers and the beta blockers can be additive with that of digoxin. In addition, these calcium channel blockers and telmisartan reduce digoxin elimination, potentially leading to digoxin toxicity. Nonsteroidal anti-inflammatory agents may raise BP and

interfere with the activity of all antihypertensive agents. The newer cyclooxygenase-2 inhibitors also increase BP, but the magnitude of the rise is less marked with some agents, such as celecoxib, because of their shorter half-life (see Chapter 40). Use of multiple antihypertensive agents may be problematic under certain circumstances. Beta blockers in concert with nondihydropyridine calcium antagonists are warranted if a hyperdynamic circulation is present, such as a young person with elevated BP and tachycardia. In contrast, in older people such a combination should be used with caution and an ECG checked before such use. In the presence of second-degree heart block, this combination is contraindicated. Moreover, it is contraindicated to use beta blockers or verapamil with clonidine in the presence of any type of heart block, because this combination may precipitate complete heart block and prompt the need for a pacemaker. The combination of ACE inhibitors or ARBs with spironolactone or epleronone may precipitate hyperkalemia, particularly if CKD is present. In the EPHESUS trial (Eplerenone Post-AMI Heart Failure Efficacy and Survival Study), this combination resulted in a 13% further risk reduction of cardiovascular death among those with systolic heart failure who were already receiving either an ACE inhibitor or ARB and a beta blocker. This benefit existed until the serum potassium reached 6 mEq/L. Thus, it is safe and beneficial to use such combinations, although patients should be warned about use of nonsteriodal anti-inflammatory agents, cyclooxygenase-2 inhibitors, or foods high in potassium (e.g., fruits and potatoes). Potassium levels should be checked with the use of these combinations within 2 to 4 weeks of their institution.

CONCLUSIONS

Even though treating hypertension can be costly and at times seems unrewarding, the benefits to individual patients and to society make the effort worthwhile. Physicians must be careful not to become apathetic about hypertension. This important public health problem has not been solved and will not be solved until all hypertensive patients are able to avail themselves of what has been among the most successful examples of preventive medicine.

For prevention of hypertension-related kidney disease and in individuals with diabetes, it is essential to reduce systolic BP at least to 130 mm Hg, if possible, with agents that inhibit the renin-angiotensin-aldosterone system.

BIBLIOGRAPHY

Bakris GL, Weir MR: Angiotensin-converting enzyme inhibitor–associated elevations in serum creatinine: Is this a cause for concern? Arch Intern Med 160:685–693, 2000.

Bakris GL, Weir MR, Secic M, et al: Differential effects of calcium antagonist subclasses on markers of nephropathy progression. Kidney Int 65:1991–2002, 2004.

Bakris GL, Weir MR, Shanifar S, et al: Effects of blood pressure level on progression of diabetic nephropathy: Results from the RENAAL study. Arch Intern Med 163:1555–1565, 2003.

Black HR, Bakris GL, Elliott WJ: Hypertension: Epidemiology, pathophysiology, diagnosis and treatment. In Fuster V,

Alexander W, O'Rourke R et al (eds): Hurst's: The Heart. New York, McGraw-Hill, 2001, pp 1553–1604.

Chobanian AV, Bakris GL, Black HR, et al: Seventh Report of the Joint National Committee on Prevention, Detection, Evaluation, and Treatment of High Blood Pressure. Hypertension 42:1206–1252, 2003.

Eknoyan G, Hostetter T, Bakris GL, et al: Proteinuria and other markers of chronic kidney disease: A position statement of the National Kidney Foundation (NKF) and the National Institute of Diabetes and Digestive and Kidney Diseases (NIDDK). Am J Kidney Dis 42:617–622, 2003.

Elliott WJ: Hypertensive emergencies. Crit Care Clin 17:435–451, 2001.

2003 European Society of Hypertension–European Society of Cardiology guidelines for the management of arterial hypertension. J Hypertens 21:1011–1053, 2003.

Garg JP, Bakris GL: Microalbuminuria: Marker of vascular dysfunction, risk factor for cardiovascular disease. Vasc Med 7:35–43, 2002.

Gashti CN, Bakris GL: The role of calcium antagonists in chronic kidney disease. Curr Opin Nephrol Hypertens 13:155–161, 2004.

Jacobsen P, Andersen S, Jensen BR, Parving HH: Additive effect of ACE inhibition and angiotensin II receptor blockade in type I diabetic patients with diabetic nephropathy. J Am Soc Nephrol 14:992–999, 2003.

Jafar TH, Stark PC, Schmid CH, et al: Progression of chronic kidney disease: The role of blood pressure control, proteinuria, and angiotensin-converting enzyme inhibition: A patient-level meta-analysis. Ann Intern Med 139:244–252, 2003.

Jones CA, Francis ME, Eberhardt MS, et al: Microalbuminuria in the US population: Third National Health and Nutrition Examination Survey. Am J Kidney Dis 39:445–459, 2002.

Levy D, Larson MG, Vasan RS, et al: The progression from hypertension to congestive heart failure. JAMA 275:1557–1562, 1996.

Nakao N, Yoshimura A, Morita H, et al: Combination treatment of angiotensin-II receptor blocker and angiotensin-converting-enzyme inhibitor in non-diabetic renal disease (COOPERATE): A randomised controlled trial. Lancet 361:117–124, 2003.

National Kidney Foundation. K/DOQI Clinical Practice Guidelines on Hypertension and Antihypertensive Agents in Chronic Kidney Disease. Am J Kidney Dis 43(5 suppl 2):1–290, 2004.

Pepine CJ, Handberg EM, Cooper-DeHoff RM, et al: A calcium antagonist vs a non-calcium antagonist hypertension treatment strategy for patients with coronary artery disease. The International Verapamil-Trandolapril Study (INVEST): A randomized controlled trial. JAMA 290:2805–2816, 2003.

Summary of Revisions for the 2004 Clinical Practice Recommendations. Diabetes Care 27:S1–S146, 2004.

Vasan RS, Larson MG, Leip EP, et al: Impact of high-normal blood pressure on the risk of cardiovascular disease. N Engl J Med 345:1291–1297, 2001.

Voyaki SM, Staessen JA, Thijs L, et al: Follow-up of renal function in treated and untreated older patients with isolated systolic hypertension. Systolic Hypertension in Europe (Syst-Eur) Trial Investigators. J Hypertens 19:511–519, 2001.

CHAPTER 72

Secondary Hypertension

Colin Mason   Peter Conlon

Hypertension is the second most common cause of consultation to primary care physicians in the developed world, accounting for many millions of visits every year. Although the vast majority of these cases constitute essential or idiopathic hypertension, about 10% reflect an underlying pathophysiology and thus constitute secondary hypertension. It is important that physicians can identify those patients for whom screening for secondary hypertension is appropriate so as to minimize overinvestigation of essential hypertension while not failing to diagnose the potential readily treatable underlying conditions that may be present. Many of the causes of secondary hypertension are reversible, and specific treatment may allow significant improvement in or normalization of the blood pressure.

Table 72-1 lists some clinical clues that may suggest the presence of secondary hypertension. Categorized in Table 72-2 are the many causes of secondary hypertension. This chapter will provide a concise overview of these conditions and suggest a practical clinical approach to the diagnosis and treatment of the patient with suspected secondary hypertension.

RENAL CAUSES OF SECONDARY HYPERTENSION

Renovascular Hypertension

Renovascular disease is the most frequent correctable cause of secondary hypertension. Its prevalence varies according to the clinical circumstances, being relatively uncommon in patients with mild hypertension but quite common (incidence 10% to 45%) in patients with severe or refractory hypertension. Although it was previously thought to be much less common in the African-American population, some studies now suggest that the prevalence is similar to that among whites, particularly when clinical situations similar to those in Table 72-3 are present.

Renal artery stenosis consists of narrowing of the renal artery of greater than 50% and may be unilateral or bilateral. Associated clinical syndromes include renovascular hypertension, ischemic renal function impairment, and otherwise unexplained recurrent episodes of acute pulmonary edema. Renovascular hypertension is medi-

ated by activation of the renin-angiotensin-aldosterone system (RAAS) as a result of renal underperfusion resultant from unilateral or bilateral renal artery stenosis. Patients with renal artery stenosis can be classified into those with fibromuscular dysplasia (FMD) and those with atherosclerotic renal artery stenosis (ARAS). Rarely, renal artery stenosis may be caused by extrinsic renal artery compression, neurofibromatosis type I, or Williams syndrome.

Fibromuscular dysplasia is a nonatherosclerotic, noninflammatory vascular disease that causes stenosis in medium and small arteries, most commonly the renal and carotid arteries. Renovascular hypertension is the most common manifestation, usually presenting in 30- to 50-year-old women. The progression of stenosis is slow, and renal function is usually well preserved. The most frequent subtype of the disease causes medial dysplasia of the affected artery with multiple contiguous stenoses causing a "string of beads" appearance on imaging. It has an estimated prevalence in hypertensive patients of less than 1%, but this may well be an underestimation because of the probable high rate of undetected cases. It can be a familial disease. Diagnosis of renal artery FMD should prompt screening of the carotid arteries for associated lesions.

Atherosclerotic renal artery stenosis is generally found in patients over 50 years old who are cigarette smokers and who often have other associated cardiovascular risk factors. It constitutes more than 85% of all renovascular disease. Lesions tend to progress, and there is often coexistent renal function impairment. The treatment of these patients is much less well defined and is discussed in detail later.

Diagnosis

The several well-recognized clinical situations that suggest the presence of renovascular disease are summarized in Table 72-3. Clinical examination may reveal evidence of systemic atherosclerotic disease, such as carotid or femoral bruits or absent pedal pulses. The presence or absence of abdominal bruits is not particularly useful. The urine sediment is usually bland, with mild to moderate proteinuria.

The gold standard diagnostic investigation for renal artery stenosis is conventional arteriography (Fig. 72-1). Most centers do not proceed directly to arteriography

TABLE 72-1   Clues to the Presence of Secondary Hypertension

Young age of onset
Sudden onset of hypertension
Uncontrolled/refractory hypertension
Malignant hypertension
Features of a recognized underlying cause

TABLE 72-3   Clinical Clues to the Presence of Renovascular Disease

Abrupt onset of or accelerated hypertension at any age
Episodes of flash pulmonary edema with normal ventricular function
Acute unexplained rise in serum creatinine after an angiotensin-converting enzyme inhibitor or angiotensin receptor blocker
Elevated serum creatinine in patients with severe or refractory hypertension
Asymmetric renal size
Moderate to severe hypertension in a patient with diffuse atherosclerotic disease

because of the risk of contrast nephrotoxicity, cholesterol embolization, and damage to the renal or femoral arteries. Whereas captopril renography was formerly utilized extensively, the most popular screening tests at present are magnetic resonance angiography (MRA), duplex ultrasonography, or computed tomography (CT) spiral angiography with contrast.

Magnetic resonance angiography is the screening investigation of choice for renal artery stenosis in most centers (Fig. 72-2). Advantages are that it is noninvasive, avoids ionizing radiation, and uses a non-nephrotoxic contrast agent (gadolinium). Meta-analyses comparing MRA, with or without gadolinium, to conventional angiography show that gadolinium-enhanced MRA is 97% sensitive and 93% specific for renal artery stenosis and is considerably better at depicting accessory renal arteries than nongadolinium scans.

Duplex ultrasonography of the renal arteries also reliably detects renal artery stenosis. With an experienced ultrasonographer, the sensitivity and specificity has been

TABLE 72-2   Causes of Secondary Hypertension

Renal
Renovascular hypertension
Renal parenchymal hypertension

Endocrine
Primary hyperaldosteronism
Cushing's syndrome
Pheochromocytoma
Hyperreninism
Hypothyroidism
Hyperparathyroidism

Cardiovascular/cardiopulmonary
Coarctation of the aorta
Obstructive sleep apnea

Drugs
Glucocorticoids
Nonsteroidal anti-inflammatory drugs
Combined oral contraceptive pill
Calcineurin inhibitors
Phenylephrine, caffeine
Licorice

Inherited
Glucocorticoid–remediable aldosteronism
Syndrome of apparent mineralocorticoid excess (SAME)
Gordon's syndrome (type 2 pseudohypoaldosteronism)
Liddle's syndrome
Congenital adrenal hyperplasia

as high as 97% to 99% in one trial in patients who later undergo conventional angiography. This method is time consuming, however, but is the preferred screening test at a number of institutions, where the considerable expertise required is available. Sensitivity and specificity of Doppler ultrasonography is estimated at best at about 80% to 85% in most published trials.

Spiral CT with CT angiography is also highly sensitive and specific compared with conventional angiography. Accuracy is reduced in patients with serum creatinine levels above 2 mg/dL, probably because of reduced renal blood flow. The need for a significant contrast load in patients with coexistent impairment of kidney function is a limitation.

Isotope renogram (DTPA scan) after an angiotensin-converting enzyme (ACE) inhibitor is no longer popular. Although the sensitivity and specificity of this method in high-risk populations may be greater than 90% for high-grade lesions, its sensitivity and specificity is much reduced in low-risk patients and in patients with bilateral

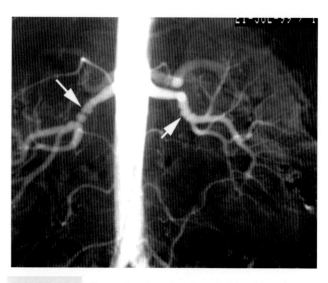

FIGURE 72-1   Conventional renal angiography demonstrating the classic "beadlike" appearance of fibromuscular dysplasia in both renal arteries. (Courtesy of Professor Mick Lee, Beaumont Hospital, Dublin, Ireland.)

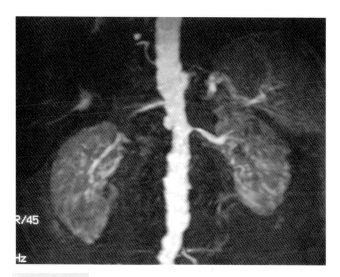

FIGURE 72-2 Magnetic resonance angiography of the aorta and renal arteries showing diffuse atherosclerotic disease of the aorta and right renal artery and a tight ostial stenosis of the left renal artery. (Courtesy of Professor Mick Lee, Beaumont Hospital, Dublin, Ireland.)

disease of equal severity. It is also more cumbersome to perform than the other available screening tests.

Plasma renin activity is often elevated with significant renal artery stenosis, but this is by no means universal. Plasma renin activity is also elevated in other important causes of secondary hypertension, as well as by many antihypertensive drugs, and therefore measurement is not sufficiently specific to have a major role in diagnosis of renal artery stenosis.

Intravenous pyelography has no role in the modern diagnosis of renal artery stenosis.

Treatment

All patients with renal artery stenosis should be on appropriate antihypertensive, lipid-lowering, and antiplatelet therapy.

Hypertensive patients with FMD should initially be treated with an ACE inhibitor or angiotensin receptor blocker (ARB). If they remain hypertensive, the treatment of choice is revascularization with percutaneous angioplasty (PTRA). PTRA in FMD is almost always technically successful, with a low restenosis rate, minimal risk, and usually an improvement or complete cure of the associated hypertension (see Fig. 72-1). There is very little literature addressing the use of stenting in this disease, presumably because of the high rate of prolonged success with angioplasty alone. Stenting is an option in cases of restenosis, although, in view of the young age of many of these patients, surgical revascularization is usually the best long-term option.

Management of ARAS is not so straightforward. Nonselective correction of stenotic lesions has led to disappointing results. It is clear that not all lesions are functionally significant. It is helpful to decide before recommending revascularization procedures whether the indication for intervention is for treatment of renovascular hypertension, preservation of kidney function, or both.

Renovascular Hypertension

Renovascular hypertension typically presents as an abrupt onset of severe hypertension or a marked deterioration from a previously stable baseline. Chronic stable hypertension present for many years is unlikely to be due to progressive renal artery stenosis and, therefore, unlikely to respond to intervention. Some useful criteria can help to predict whether a patient suspected to have renovascular hypertension will or will not respond to revascularization. First, most recent data suggest that angioplasty, with or without stenting, will not improve blood pressure in patients who have already lost more than 60% of kidney function. Second, evaluation of the renal resistance index with Doppler ultrasonography or captopril scintigraphy, in centers with appropriate expertise, has emerged as an excellent method to classify patients as responders or nonresponders. A renal resistance index value of 80 or more reliably predicts patients in whom revascularization will not improve kidney function, blood pressure, or kidney survival. Evaluation of the renal resistance index has not been part of the routine assessment for patients with FMD. A recent large metaanalysis of studies comparing balloon angioplasty to medical management of patients with uncontrolled hypertension and renal artery stenosis suggested that angioplasty has at least a significant but modest effect on blood pressure but that complete cure of hypertension is rare.

Preservation of Kidney Function

The issue of revascularization for preservation of kidney function, particularly in patients with well-controlled or normal blood pressure, is much more controversial. The same meta-analysis mentioned previously suggested no benefit of PTRA over medical therapy for preservation or improvement of kidney function. It is well established that ARAS tends to progress in a large percentage of patients usually within only a few years of diagnosis and that this progression has been associated with a progressive decline in kidney function. The problem seems to be that patients, particularly those with serum creatinine levels of 2.5 mg/dL or above, already have significant irreversible renal parenchymal disease and that this is unlikely to be affected by revascularization unless a coincident improvement in associated renovascular hypertension, if present, is beneficial. There must also be signs of salvageability of the kidney or of kidneys being revascularized. Signs of poor salvageability are size less than 9 cm, reduced function on a renal flow scan, a renal resistive index greater than 80 on Doppler ultrasonography,

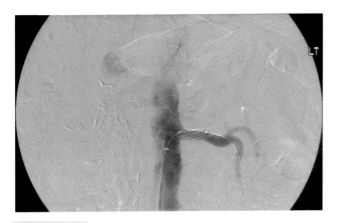

FIGURE 72-3 A stent in the ostium of the left renal artery. (Courtesy of Professor Mick Lee, Beaumont Hospital, Dublin, Ireland.)

serum creatinine greater than 2.5 mg/dL, significant proteinuria or evidence of an alternative renal diagnosis, or findings of marked chronicity on kidney biopsy.

A good policy seems to be to follow serial kidney function over a period of time and identify those patients with known renal artery stenosis greater than 60% who are progressively losing function but who still have evidence of salvageability. There is some evidence that this group responds better to intervention than those with chronic stable kidney function impairment.

Once the decision has been made to intervene, most centers then proceed to PTRA rather than surgical repair. Because of the high rate of initial failure or early restenosis, current evidence suggests that angioplasty with stenting is the treatment of choice for ostial renal artery stenosis, giving better technical success rate and better long-term patency than angioplasty alone. The role of primary stenting in nonostial lesions is as yet unclear. Stenting has previously been used when the results of angioplasty have been suboptimal and in restenotic lesions. Surgery is reserved for patients with restenotic or technically difficult lesions, although in centers with dedicated renovascular surgeons, referral may be earlier and even may be the primary recommendation, particularly in young fit patients with ostial lesions.

Contrast nephrotoxicity, atheroembolism to the kidneys and distal vasculature (see Chapter 37), and local damage to the femoral artery are complications of PTRA and occur in as many as 20% of patients. Figure 72-3 shows a stent in the left renal artery after percutaneous intervention.

Renal Parenchymal Hypertension

Hypertension is a common feature of much of acute and chronic kidney disease (CKD), particularly with glomerular and vascular disorders. Hypertension results from a combination of a positive salt balance, increased activity of the RAAS, and hyperstimulation of the sympathetic system. Treatment of hypertension in CKD thus consists of dietary salt restriction and promotion of salt excretion with diuretics, inhibition of the RAAS system with ACE inhibition and ARBs, and/or inhibition of the sympathetic nervous system. Clues to the presence of renal parenchymal disease in hypertensive patients are elevated serum creatinine and/or abnormal urinalysis. A kidney ultrasonogram is a useful noninvasive screening test to assess kidney size and asymmetry and to rule out major renal structural abnormalities or obstructive lesions. The variety of disorders and the treatments available are wide, and a discussion of each is beyond the scope of this chapter.

ENDOCRINE CAUSES OF SECONDARY HYPERTENSION

Hypertension is a feature of several endocrine conditions (see Table 72-2). However, the most well-characterized associations are those with primary hyperaldosteronism, Cushing's syndrome, and pheochromocytoma.

Primary Hyperaldosteronism

Primary hyperaldosteronism is the most common cause of hypertension due to an endocrinopathy. The prevalence is much debated in the literature, with recent studies suggesting that it may be a cause of hypertension in as many as 15% of hypertensive patients in some ethnic groups. Most groups, however, would report a rate of primary hyperaldosteronism in about 1% to 2% of their hypertensive populations.

Primary hyperaldosteronism may be due to an aldosterone-secreting adrenal adenoma (70% to 80% of cases), bilateral adrenal hyperplasia (idiopathic hyperaldosteronism), or, rarely, a secretory adrenal carcinoma or inherited endocrinopathies (see later). Patients with adrenal adenomas tend to be younger and have a more severe clinical picture than those with adrenal hyperplasia. Adenomas are more common in females.

Clinical Syndrome

Conn first described the clinical syndrome in 1955. Patients may complain of symptoms related to hypertension and hypokalemia. In particular, spontaneous hypokalemia, moderate to severe hypokalemia induced by diuretic therapy, and persistent hypokalemia refractory to replacement therapy with or without ACE inhibitor therapy should arouse suspicions as to the presence of primary hyperaldosteronism.

Diagnosis

There is much debate about the optimum screening method. It is not recommended for all hypertensive patients. Those who benefit most are young patients,

patients with difficult to control or refractory hypertension, and patients with spontaneous or diuretic-induced hypokalemia. Screening tests used include serum potassium measurement, plasma aldosterone-to-renin ratio (ARR), 24-hour urinary potassium excretion, and abdominal imaging with either CT or magnetic resonance imaging (MRI).

Serum Potassium

Serum potassium is normal in at least 20% of patients and is not reliable in excluding hyperaldosteronism. Hypokalemia, when present, however, is an important clue to the diagnosis.

Plasma Aldosterone-to-Renin Ratio

Measurement of the ARR is recommended when there is a strong clinical suspicion for primary hyperaldosteronism but not for all hypertensive patients. It is widely accepted as the screening test of choice for primary hyperaldosteronism. Plasma aldosterone concentration should be markedly elevated in primary hyperaldosteronism, but levels can be extremely variable, even within the same individual. At the same time, renin activity is suppressed and usually very low (less than 1 ng/mL/hour), distinguishing it from secondary hyperaldosteronism, renin-secreting tumors, and renovascular hypertension. In normal individuals, the ARR is 4 to 10. In primary hyperaldosteronism, the ratio is often between 30 and 50.

A morning ambulatory blood sample is the best vehicle for ARR testing. Intercurrent antihypertensive drug therapy, in particular spironolactone, ACE inhibitors, amiloride, and triamterene, may interfere with testing and should be stopped at least 2 to 3 weeks in advance if possible. Beta blockers reduce serum renin levels, whereas the acute use of calcium channel blockers increases them. Alpha blockers and calcium channel blockers used chronically do not affect testing. The ratio is strongly denominator dependent, varying markedly with the level of renin detected by the individual hospital laboratory. There is variation in the literature as to the appropriate cutoff for a positive ARR, but most consider a ratio greater than 20 with a simultaneous plasma aldosterone concentration of greater than 15 ng/dL to be a positive screening test.

24-Hour Urinary Potassium Excretion

A 24-hour urine collection demonstrating a potassium excretion greater than 30 mEq/day in a patient with hypokalemia supports the presence of hyperaldosteronism and is a useful screening test. Patients should be well hydrated and have a normal serum bicarbonate to ensure accurate interpretation. The test is not useful when the serum potassium is normal or when patients are taking kaliuretic diuretics.

Dynamic Tests

The purpose of dynamic testing is to confirm autonomous adrenal production of aldosterone. One such test is the aldosterone suppression test. An oral sodium chloride load over 3 days or an intravenous saline load (2 L over 4 hours) is administered, and lack of suppression of aldosterone levels is demonstrated. Measurement of 24-hour aldosterone levels, in the presence of normokalemia, after 3 days of oral salt loading can also be a sensitive and specific test to confirm primary hyperaldosteronism. Another such test is the fludrocortisone suppression test, where lack of suppression of aldosterone is again demonstrated.

Such dynamic tests require hospitalization and are not without risk, especially in older patients with cardiac disease. They are generally cumbersome and time consuming. Most centers would now directly proceed to imaging after a positive biochemical screening test (e.g., ARR).

Radiology

The adrenal glands are imaged with a CT or MRI scan to determine the etiology of the primary hyperaldosteronism. Adenomas of 10 mm in diameter and sometimes even smaller can be detected.

The relative merits of CT and MRI are not entirely clear, however. One study showed MRI to be much more sensitive than CT for adrenal adenoma detection but to have a higher rate of false-positive scans. It is estimated that with CT alone, as many as 40% of adenomas could be missed. Radionuclide scintigraphy with [131I]iodocholesterol has been reported to be sensitive for adenomas; however, it is not widely available, and there are several case reports of missed lesions.

A major problem is the high incidence of radiologically detected nonfunctioning adenomas, particularly after the age of 40. Before the age of 40, if an adenoma larger than 1 cm is found and the contralateral adrenal gland appears normal on scanning, it is thought to be reasonable to proceed to adrenalectomy. In older people, adrenal vein sampling should be performed where possible if an adenoma is detected. If the adrenal glands are normal on scanning, patients should also proceed directly to adrenal vein sampling (AVS).

Adrenal vein sampling is highly predictive of a successful result of unilateral adrenalectomy. It must be performed by an experienced radiologist and is more accurate when performed after adrenocorticopic hormone (ACTH) stimulation. Position in the adrenal vein is confirmed by measuring simultaneous adrenal vein and peripheral vein cortisol levels. A greater than fivefold increase in plasma aldosterone concentration (PAC) compared with the contralateral side should be demonstrated on the side of an adenoma. In adrenal hyperplasia, there should be little difference between the two adrenals. Occasionally the adenoma may be extra-adrenal, and adrenal vein sampling is normal. If imaging and adrenal vein sampling are negative, the rare diagnosis of glucocorticoid-remediable aldosteronism (see later) should be considered.

Treatment

Adenomas should be referred surgically for unilateral laparoscopic adrenalectomy. Removal of well-localized unilateral lesions is very successful. Selective hypoaldosteronism may occur for some months after surgery, so potassium supplementation should be cautious in this period. The drugs of choice for medical management of adrenal hyperplasia and preoperative management of adenomas in the past have been spironolactone, amiloride, and ACE inhibitors. Eplerenone, a new selective aldosterone receptor antagonist, is now popular, because it causes much less gynecomastia than spironolactone. There are some case reports of embolization of adenomas with ethanol in patients medically unfit for surgery.

Hyperreninism

Renin-secreting tumors are very rare. Patients will be hypertensive and hypokalemic, with high plasma renin activity along with elevated aldosterone levels and urinary potassium excretion. These tumors usually originate from the juxtaglomerular apparatus in the kidney, but renin production has been reported with other malignancies in the literature including teratomas and ovarian tumors.

Cushing's Syndrome

Cushing's syndrome is a clinical condition resulting from excess effects of either exogenous or endogenous glucocorticoids. Patients develop a characteristic clinical appearance, with the classic Cushingoid "moon facies" related to facial fat deposition, along with truncal obesity, abdominal striae, hirsutism, and kyphoscoliosis. There is varying multiorgan involvement with diabetes mellitus, cataracts, neuropsychiatric disorders, cataracts, proximal myopathy, avascular necrosis of humeral and femoral heads, osteoporosis, and secondary hypertension among the more prominent of its manifold possible complications. The original syndrome described by Cushing related to a patient with pituitary ACTH excess driving excess cortisol production. As a consequence, pituitary-dependent disease is known as Cushing's disease. Hypertension, resulting from the mineralocorticoid effect of the glucocorticoids, is a common feature. Causes of Cushing's syndrome are listed in Table 72-4. The most common cause of endogenous excess is a pituitary adenoma.

TABLE 72-4 Causes of Cushing's Syndrome

Exogenous glucocorticoid administration

Endogenous glucocorticoid excess
ACTH
  Ectopic production
  Pituitary secretory adenoma (Cushing's disease)
Cortisol
  Adrenal cortical adenoma or carcinoma

Diagnosis

The presence of cortisol excess must first be confirmed biochemically. This can be achieved with the "low-dose" dexamethasone suppression test, measurement of 24-hour urinary free-cortisol levels, or assessment of circadian pattern of cortisol secretion.

Overnight/"Low-Dose" Dexamethasone Suppression Test

A 2-mg dose of dexamethasone is taken at 11 PM, and then a plasma cortisol sample is drawn at 9 AM the next morning. Suppression is defined as a cortisol level of less than 5 mg/dL.

Circadian Testing of Cortisol Secretion

Cortisol levels are measured at 9 AM and 11 PM. They are usually high in the morning and lowest at night.

Other causes of abnormally high cortisol secretion should be considered, such as stress, endogenous depression, and chronic excess alcohol consumption. A normal response to an insulin suppression test is suggestive of endogenous depression.

When cortisol excess is confirmed, further testing to elucidate a pituitary, adrenal, or ectopic source should follow. Extremely high plasma or urinary cortisol levels are suggestive of adrenal carcinoma or ectopic ACTH secretion. An adrenal carcinoma often causes marked virilization and a severe hypokalemic metabolic alkalosis.

Plasma Adrenocorticotropic Hormone

If there is an adrenal source of glucocorticoids, then ACTH levels should be suppressed below the normal range. A normal or moderately raised level is suggestive of pituitary disease. High levels suggest ectopic disease.

"High-Dose" Dexamethasone Suppression Test

Dexamethasone, 2 mg every 6 hours, is given for 2 days. Cortisol levels are taken at 9 AM on day 1 and day 3. Suppression of cortisol to less than 50% of the day 1 level is defined as suppression. Pituitary-dependent Cushing's disease should respond in this way, whereas ectopic ACTH production should not.

Imaging

Either CT or MRI of the adrenals or the pituitary, depending on the clinical suspicion, should be performed. If ectopic ACTH is diagnosed, a bronchial neoplasm should be aggressively ruled out.

Treatment

If the cause is exogenous steroid use, efforts should be made to withdraw the medication dose carefully and slowly if the patient can do so or if the clinical condition being treated allows. Steroid-sparing agents may help.

Endogenous Cushing's syndrome is best treated by surgical excision. If imaging does not reliably demonstrate a pituitary lesion, then radiation may be used. If there is adrenal overactivity and tumor localization is not possible, or if there is symptomatic ectopic ACTH activity, symptoms may be relieved by suppressing the adrenal gland with medications such as metyrapone, aminoglutethimide, or mitotane.

Pheochromocytoma

Pheochromocytoma is a secretory tumor of neurochromaffin cells in the adrenal medulla. It is a rare condition that causes less than 0.2% of all hypertension. Symptoms are due to catecholamine hypersecretion.

Patients classically present with the triad of episodic headache, sweating, and tachycardia; most will have at least two of these. Pallor, paroxysmal hypotension, orthostatic hypotension, visual blurring, papilledema, high erythrocyte sedimentation rate, weight loss, polyuria, polydipsia, psychiatric disorders, hyperglycemia, dilated cardiomyopathy, and, rarely, secondary erythrocytosis are other less common clinical features. About half of patients have paroxysms of hypertension, whereas most of the rest have apparently essential hypertension. Many have no symptoms and are detected by serendipity with abdominal radiology, at surgery, or at postmortem examination.

When referring to these tumors, the "10% rule" is often cited and is still clinically useful, with approximately 10% of cases extra-adrenal, 10% malignant, 10% bilateral, and 10% associated with familial syndromes, the rest being sporadic.

There are two main familial syndromes associated with pheochromocytoma.

1. Von Hippel-Lindau syndrome—pheochromocytoma in 10% to 20%.
2. Multiple endocrine neoplasia syndrome type II—associated with medullary thyroid carcinoma and hyperparathyroidism. Pheochromocytoma occurs in 20% to 50% of affected individuals.

More rarely, pheochromocytoma is found in neurofibromatosis type I (less than 5%). Genetic screening is recommended if the patient is under 21 years old, has extra-adrenal/bilateral disease, or has multiple paragangliomas.

Diagnosis

A classic history of the typical triad of symptoms and/or a family history if present may suggest the diagnosis. The screening tests used are measurements of urinary and plasma catecholamines or their metabolites.

Urinary and Plasma Catecholamine Levels

Assays of urinary and plasma catecholamines are equally effective and are up to 95% sensitive in symptomatic patients. Nearly all of these have increased urinary catecholamine metabolites (metanephrines and vanillylmandelic acid) and free catecholamines. Urinary metanephrines are the best indicator, because they are the most sensitive and their production is unaffected by food ingestion. However, one should be careful, because false-positive urinary metanephrine results can occur with some drugs, particularly labetalol.

Plasma catecholamine levels should be drawn from an indwelling intravenous catheter at least 30 minutes after insertion. Norepinephrine and epinephrine levels greater than 2000 pg/mL are diagnostic; levels greater than 950 pg/mL are highly suggestive. If levels are suggestive but not diagnostic, a clonidine suppression test may be performed. Plasma metanephrine tests had in the past been recommended as sensitive and specific, but there has been concern more recently about an unacceptably high false-positive rate (as high as 15%).

Clonidine Suppression Test

Clonidine is given after all antihypertensives have been held for at least 12 hours; plasma catecholamines 3 hours later should fall to less than 500 pg/mL in patients without a pheochromocytoma. The clonidine suppression test is more than 90% sensitive for a pheochromocytoma.

Radiology

Radiology should be performed after biochemical confirmation of the diagnosis using the assays already described and not before. Ninety-five percent of pheochromocytomas are intra-abdominal, with 90% being in the adrenal glands themselves. CT or MRI is the initial modality of choice (Fig. 72-4); both are up to 98% sensitive but are only about 70% specific because of the high prevalence of nonfunctional adrenal adenomas, particularly with increasing age.

If CT or MRI is negative despite positive screening assays, the diagnosis should be reconsidered. If there is still a strong suspicion, an MIBG ([123I]metaiodobenzylguanidine) radioisotope scan or total-body MRI should be considered. MIBG is an analogue of norepinephrine.

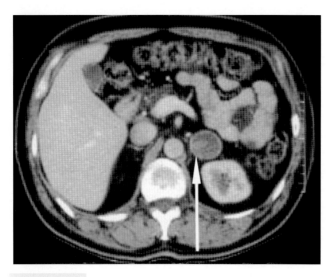

FIGURE 72-4   A computed tomography (CT) scan showing a pheochromocytoma arising from the left adrenal gland. (Courtesy of Professor Mick Lee, Beaumont Hospital, Dublin, Ireland.)

MIBG scans are used to detect pheochromocytomas in cases where CT or MRI is negative, or to detect extra-adrenal or metastatic disease. Positron emission tomographic scanning may have a future role in detecting metastatic disease.

Treatment

The definitive treatment for a pheochromocytoma is surgical excision, but medical treatment to control the effects of the catecholamine excess is crucial preoperatively. There are several accepted approaches. The most widely used is to give the alpha blocker phenoxybenzamine, starting at a dose of 10 mg once daily and increasing the dose every few days until blood pressure and symptoms are controlled. A beta blocker may then be added to control tachycardia. A beta blocker should never be given first, because the subsequent unopposed alpha-agonist vasoconstrictive action can precipitate markedly worse hypertension. Indeed, a hypertensive crisis precipitated by a beta blocker may be a clue to the presence of a pheochromocytoma in a patient with hypertension. Using this approach, a patient should be ready for surgery in 10 to 14 days.

Surgery for pheochromocytoma has a perioperative mortality of 2.4% and a morbidity of 24%. If there are metastases, they should be resected if possible. Skeletal lesions may be irradiated. Chemotherapy may be used in selected patients.

Prognosis

Long-term follow-up is indicated in all patients, because there is a high incidence of recurrent hypertension even with complete tumor removal, especially in older patients with a family history of hypertension.

Tumor recurs in about 10% of patients, and usually when it does it is associated with familial cases. A significant proportion of recurrences are malignant.

CARDIOVASCULAR/ CARDIOPULMONARY CAUSES OF SECONDARY HYPERTENSION

Coarctation of the Aorta

Coarctation is a congenital narrowing of the aortic lumen, occurring most commonly just distal to the origin of the left subclavian artery. Clinically, the patient will have hypertension when measured in the upper limbs, with reduced or unmeasurable blood pressure in the legs. If the coarctation is proximal to the origin of the left subclavian artery, the blood pressure and brachial pulsation in the left upper limb may both be reduced. The femoral pulses may be delayed or diminished when compared with the radial or brachial pulses, and there may be an audible bruit over the patient's back. Diagnosis is confirmed with aortic imaging, and treatment is surgical.

Sleep Apnea Syndrome

The association of obesity, obstructive sleep apnea, and hypertension has long been recognized. Although the pathophysiology is not entirely clear, the apneic syndrome itself seems to contribute directly to the hypertension, along with other comorbid conditions such as obesity. Many cases of obstructive sleep apnea go undiagnosed unless a high index of suspicion is maintained. In most studies of assessment of hypertension before and after treatment of sleep apnea, daytime and nighttime levels of blood pressure were improved significantly.

INHERITED CAUSES OF SECONDARY HYPERTENSION

There are several mendelian disorders associated with hypertension. Although all are probably significantly underdiagnosed, they are rare. Most are associated with defects in sodium-reabsorptive processes in the distal nephron. There are at least two genetic disorders associated with features of hyperaldosteronism, namely glucocorticoid-remediable aldosteronism (GRA) and the syndrome of apparent mineralocorticoid excess (AME). In Liddle's syndrome (pseudohyperaldosteronism), hypertension is associated with reduced plasma aldosterone levels. Gordon's syndrome (type 2 pseudohypoaldosteronism) is a volume-dependent form of inherited hypertension associated with hypertension and a variable phenotype including hyperkalemia. Although all of these conditions are rare, they are important because the associated hypertension may be refractory to conventional therapy but may respond well to specific therapy.

Glucocorticoid-Remediable Aldosteronism

Glucocorticoid-remediable aldosteronism is a rare subtype of primary hyperaldosteronism in which the hyperaldosteronism can be reversed with steroid administration. GRA is inherited and should be suspected in patients with an early onset of hypertension and a positive family history of early hypertension or intracerebral hemorrhage. Individuals are otherwise usually phenotypically normal.

Glucocorticoid-remediable aldosteronism is inherited as an autosomal-dominant (AD) trait. It may be suspected from a positive family history and an early onset of hypertension before the age of 21. Plasma potassium may be low but is often normal. Severe hypokalemia after administration of a thiazide diuretic (due to increased sodium delivery to the aldosterone-sensitive potassium-secretory site in the cortical collecting tubule) can be a clue. As many as 18% of patients suffer a cerebrovascular complication, mainly hemorrhage from ruptured berry aneurysms. The rate of aneurysm occurrence is similar to that in patients with adult polycystic kidney disease. Surveillance MRA has been recommended, but the benefit of this approach is not yet proven. Mean age of onset of cerebral hemorrhage if an aneurysm is present is 32 years.

Pathogenesis

In the adrenal cortex, aldosterone is normally synthesized in the zona glomerulosa, whereas glucocorticoids are predominantly synthesized in the adjacent zona fasciculosa. Two isozymes of the enzyme, 11β-hydroxylase, encoded by chromosome 8, are responsible for the synthesis of aldosterone and cortisol. The isozyme in the zona glomerulosa (CYP 11 B2) encodes aldosterone production under the influence of potassium and angiotensin II, whereas that in the zona fasciculata (CYP 11 B1) encodes cortisol production under the influence of ACTH. In GRA, the promoter region for CYP 11 B1 fuses with the coding sequences of the aldosterone synthase enzyme, CYP 11 B2, resulting in ACTH-dependent aldosterone synthesis in the zona fasciculata.

Diagnosis

Diagnosis may be achieved by dexamethasone suppression testing demonstrating the production of 18-carbon oxidation products of cortisol. However, a genetic test demonstrating the pathologic chimeric gene is now recommended, because there is a significant false-positive rate in patients with primary hyperaldosteronism when tested with dexamethasone. This test can be obtained from the International Registry for Glucocorticoid-Remediable Aldosteronism at http://www.bwh.partners.org/gra.

Treatment

Corticosteroids suppress ACTH and lower the blood pressure to normal. Target dose should be enough to suppress aldosterone levels sufficiently without causing debilitating side effects.

Syndrome of Apparent Mineralocorticoid Excess

In aldosterone-selective tissues, cortisol is usually metabolized enzymatically to steroids with little or no activity for the mineralocorticoid receptor. In AME, this enzyme (11β-hydroxysteroid dehydrogenase) is deficient, and cortisol acts on the mineralocorticoid receptor, causing a syndrome of apparent aldosteronism despite suppressed aldosterone levels.

These patients usually present at very young ages, usually less than 12 years old, with hypertension and a hypokalemic alkalosis. The oldest reported case in the literature was in a 21-year-old. Plasma renin and aldosterone levels are low. The hypertension is often severe and causes hypertension-related fatalities in a significant number of patients. Although the genetic defect at present remains uncharacterized, there is often a history of a similar syndrome in a sibling and consanguinity in the parents.

Differential diagnosis includes the other common causes of pediatric hypertension (especially renal structural abnormalities). Among other mendelian forms of hypertension, GRA is distinguished by the elevated aldosterone, the elevated 18-oxocortisol level, and the positive genetic test. Liddle's syndrome (see later) can present similarly but with AD inheritance and normal cortisol-to-cortisone ratios, whereas 11β-hydroxylase deficiency shows autosomal-recessive (AR) inheritance, and patients are abnormally virilized and have elevated deoxycortisone and deoxycortisol levels.

Because cortisol is the endogenous mineralocorticoid in AME, suppression with dexamethasone is used and is effective in correcting blood pressure and potassium. Adjunctive spironolactone is also used along with other antihypertensives if necessary to normalize blood pressure.

A mild acquired variant may be encountered in patients with excessive licorice intake. In addition to an inherent weak mineralocorticoid effect, the principal metabolite of licorice (glycyrrhizic acid) inhibits the same enzyme that is deficient in AME. An old treatment for peptic ulcers, carbenoxolone, was associated with hypertension for similar reasons.

Gordon's Syndrome (Type 2 Pseudohypoaldosteronism)

Gordon and colleagues first described this syndrome of hypertension and hyperkalemia in 1970. It has now been characterized as an AD disorder caused by mutations in two members of the WNK family of serine-threonine kinases, a group of enzymes involved in regulating the activity of the thiazide-sensitive Na-Cl cotransporter (NCCT) molecule in the distal convoluted tubule.

WNK4 inhibits surface expression of the NCCT. Missense mutations in the WNK4 gene (chromosome 17) produce mutant proteins that allow increased NCCT expression. WNK1 is predominantly a cytoplasmic protein that inhibits WNK4 function. Large deletions in the WNK1 gene (chromosome 12) increase WNK1 production, leading to excess WNK4 inhibition and thus, also, to increased NCCT expression. Both WNK kinase mutations, therefore, cause overactivity of the NCCT with resultant excess salt reabsorption. This results in volume-dependent hypertension and suppression of the RAAS. In addition, augmented absorption at this site reduces collecting duct sodium delivery, which leads to potassium and acid retention and hyperkalemic metabolic acidosis. Aldosterone levels are variable and may be increased by hyperkalemia, but not enough to correct it. This was formerly a rare diagnosis, but with the advent of the ARR (see earlier) as a screening test in patients with suspected secondary hypertension, it may be increasingly detected as a false-positive ARR. In severe cases, there may be associated short stature, intellectual impairment, and muscle weakness.

Treatment typically involves a combination of dietary salt restriction and low-dose thiazide or loop diuretics and is usually very effective. WNK kinases and their targets may offer novel targets for future antihypertensive agents.

Liddle's Syndrome

Liddle's syndrome is a rare congenital defect due to enhanced activity of the luminal membrane sodium channel (ENaC; see Chapter 9) in the principal cells of the cortical collecting tubule, causing them to behave as if constantly stimulated by aldosterone. The resultant increase in sodium absorption results in hypertension and is usually, but not always, associated with hypokalemia and a metabolic alkalosis. Inheritance is AD. Presentation is usually at a young age, although it is sometimes not detected until adulthood due to varying phenotypic expression. The consistent diagnostic finding, apart from the suggestive history and family history, is decreased urinary excretion of aldosterone. Patients are treated with drugs that directly close the hyperactive sodium channels, and these include amiloride or triamterene, but not spironolactone because the increased sodium reabsorption in this disorder is independent of aldosterone.

Congenital Adrenal Hyperplasia

Congenital adrenal hyperplasia is an AR inherited inability to synthesize cortisol. In this condition, defects in the final steps of steroid biosynthesis result in excess mineralocorticoid and androgen effects with coincident signs of glucocorticoid deficiency. The most common forms, 17α-hydroxylase deficiency and 11β-hydroxylase deficiency, may cause hypertension due to overproduction of excess cortisol precursors that are, or are metabolized to, mineralocorticoid agonists.

CONCLUSIONS

Secondary hypertension constitutes as much as 10% to 15% of all hypertension encountered in clinical practice. Causes can be endocrine, drug-related, cardiovascular, or genetic, but the most common underlying diagnosis is renal parenchymal or vascular disease. Knowledge of this is important, because there is now good evidence that percutaneous intervention can significantly improve blood pressure and reduce the need for medication in selected patients with renovascular disease. Endocrine diseases are relatively uncommon, although the incidence of primary hyperaldosteronism as a cause for hypertension has probably been markedly underestimated. Other endocrine causes include Cushing's syndrome and pheochromocytoma, both of which may reflect underlying malignant disease. Coarctation is rare but can readily be detected clinically and radiologically if the diagnosis is suspected. Inherited mendelian disorders causing hypertension are rare but may be suspected in young patients with a strong family history of hypertension, intracerebral hemorrhage, or potassium abnormalities.

BIBLIOGRAPHY

Conlon PJ, O'Riordan E, Kalra PA: New insights into the epidemiologic and clinical manifestations of atherosclerotic renovascular disease. Am J Kidney Dis 35:573–587, 2000.

Conn JW: Primary hyperaldosteronism, a new clinical syndrome. J Lab Clin Med 45:3–17, 1955.

Nadar S, Lip GY, Beevers DG: Primary hyperaldosteronism. Ann Clin Biochem 40(Pt 5):439–452, 2003.

Nordmann AJ, Woo K, Parkes R, et al: Balloon angioplasty or medical therapy for hypertensive patients with atherosclerotic renal artery disease? A meta-analysis of randomized-controlled trials. Am J Med 114:44–50, 2003.

Pohl MA: Renal artery stenosis, renal vascular hypertension and ischemic nephropathy. In Schrier RW, Gottschalk CW (eds): Diseases of the Kidney, 6th ed. Boston, Little, Brown, 1997, pp 1367–1425.

Radermacher J, Chavan A, Bleck J, et al: Use of Doppler ultra-sonography to predict the outcome of therapy for renal artery stenosis. N Engl J Med 344:410–417, 2001.

Radermacher J, Weinkove R, Haller H: Techniques for predicting a favourable response to renal angioplasty in patients with renovascular disease. Curr Opin Nephrol Hypertens 10: 799–805, 2001.

Ramos F, Kotliar C, Alvarez D, et al: Renal function and outcome of PTRA and stenting for atherosclerotic renal artery stenosis. Kidney Int 63:276–282, 2003.

Rossi GP, Chiesura-Corona M, Tregnaghi A, et al: Imaging of aldosterone-secreting adenoma: A prospective comparison of computed tomography and magnetic resonance imaging in 27 patients with suspected primary hyperaldosteronism. J Hum Hypertens 7:357–363, 1993.

Safian RD: Atherosclerotic renal artery stenosis. Curr Treat Options Cardiovasc Med 5:91–101, 2003.

Slovut DP, Olin JW: Fibromuscular dysplasia. N Engl J Med 350:1862–1871, 2004.

Tan KT, van Beek EJ, Brown PW, et al: Magnetic resonance angiography for the diagnosis of renal artery stenosis: A meta-analysis. Clin Radiol 58:257, 2003.

Wilson FH, Disse-Nicodeme S, Choate KA, et al: Human hypertension caused by mutations in WNK kinases. Science 293:1030, 2001.

Appendix

Following are DOQI and K/DOQI guidelines, listed in chronologic order. Current versions are also available on line at www.kdoqi.org along with a GFR calculator, Clinical Action Plans, and other interpretive material. An additional source for information about kidney disease and its management is the National Kidney Foundation website: www.kidney.org

NKF-DOQI clinical practice guidelines for hemodialysis adequacy. Am J Kidney Dis 30(suppl 2):S15–S66, 1997.

NKF-DOQI clinical practice guidelines for peritoneal dialysis adequacy. Am J Kidney Dis 30(suppl 2): S67–S136, 1997.

NKF-DOQI clinical practice guidelines for vascular access. Am J Kidney Dis 30(suppl 3):S150–S191, 1997.

NKF-DOQI clinical practice guidelines for the treatment of anemia of chronic renal failure. Am J Kidney Dis 30(suppl 3):S192–S240, 1997.

K/DOQI clinical practice guidelines for nutrition in chronic renal failure. Am J Kidney Dis 35(suppl 2): S1–S140, 2000.

NKF-K/DOQI clinical practice guidelines for hemodialysis adequacy, peritoneal dialysis adequacy, vascular access, anemia of chronic kidney disease: update 2000. Am J Kidney Dis 37(suppl 1):S1–S238, 2001.

K/DOQI clinical practice guidelines for chronic kidney disease: evaluation, classification and stratification. Am J Kidney Dis 39(suppl 1):S1–S266, 2002.

K/DOQI clinical practice guidelines for managing dyslipidemias in chronic kidney disease. Am J Kidney Dis 41(suppl 3):S1–S92, 2003.

K/DOQI clinical practice guidelines for bone metabolism and disease in chronic kidney disease. Am J Kidney Dis 42(suppl 3):S1–S202, 2003.

K/DOQI clinical practice guidelines on hypertension and antihypertensive agents in chronic kidney disease. Am J Kidney Dis 43(suppl 1):S1–S290, 2004.

Index

Note: Page numbers followed by f refer to figures; page numbers followed by t refer to tables.